THE ESSENTIAL *life*

A Simple Guide to Living the Wellness Lifestyle

Thank you to the many contributors for their collective Genius in bringing this work together and sharing a vision of how plants and natural remedies bring new levels of wellness to powerfully impact our lives.

6th EDITION

The information contained in this book has not been evaluated or approved by the U.S. Food and Drug Administration or any other regulatory agency. The information is not intended to diagnose, treat, cure, prevent or otherwise reduce the effects of any disease or ailment. The information is not, and nothing contained herein is claimed to be, written, edited, endorsed or researched by a licensed health care provider or medical professional or borne out by any specific medical science. In fact, it is not. The information referenced herein is intended for educational purposes only and is not meant to and should not otherwise be implied to substitute for seeking qualified medical care from a licensed medical doctor or to seek a prescribed treatment in lieu of a treatment prescribed by any licensed medical professional for a specific health condition. Consult a licensed and qualified health care provider for diagnosis, medical care and treatment.

The information contained in this book does not in any way seek to promote or endorse any specific brand of essential oils, nutritional products or other products offered or provided by any specific company. Any mention in this book of a specific brand name is not an endorsement or recommendation of any specific product or company.

The authors of this book have expressed their good faith opinions, which are not established by conventional medical professionals. Total Wellness Publishing, LLC and any contributor to this book expressly disclaim any liability arising from the use of the information contained in this book or for any adverse outcome resulting from the use of the information contained herein for any reason, including but not limited to any misdiagnosis of any condition or any misunderstanding, misapplication or misinterpretation of the information set forth herein. In no event shall the authors of this book or Total Wellness Publishing, LLC be liable for any direct, indirect, consequential, special, exemplary, or other damages related to the use of the information contained in this book.

DISCLAIMER: Total Wellness Publishing, LLC is a third-party company that does not benefit financially from the sales of essential oils. Total Wellness Publishing, LLC is not affiliated with, sponsored by, or endorsed by any essential oil company. The trademarked and copyrighted names in this publication are owned by doTERRA Holdings, LLC. Total Wellness Publishing is not affiliated with, sponsored by, or endorsed by doTERRA Holdings, LLC. The material in this publication is a third-party presentation of and commentary on the essential oils, blends, supplements, and other products produced by doTERRA, Inc.

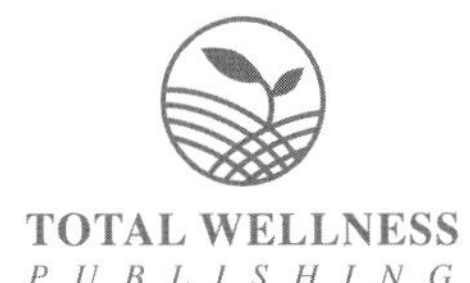

TOTAL WELLNESS
PUBLISHING

ISBN 9 781532 384103

TABLE OF CONTENTS

SECTION 1 introduction

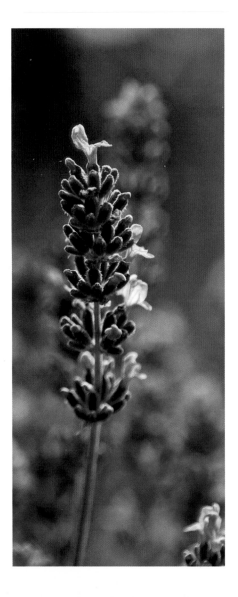

SECTION 2 quick reference

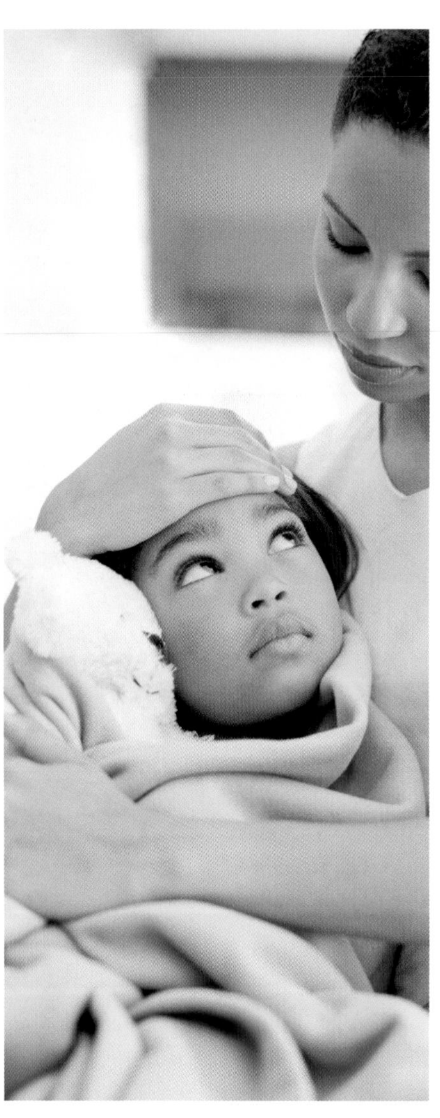

SECTION 3 natural solutions

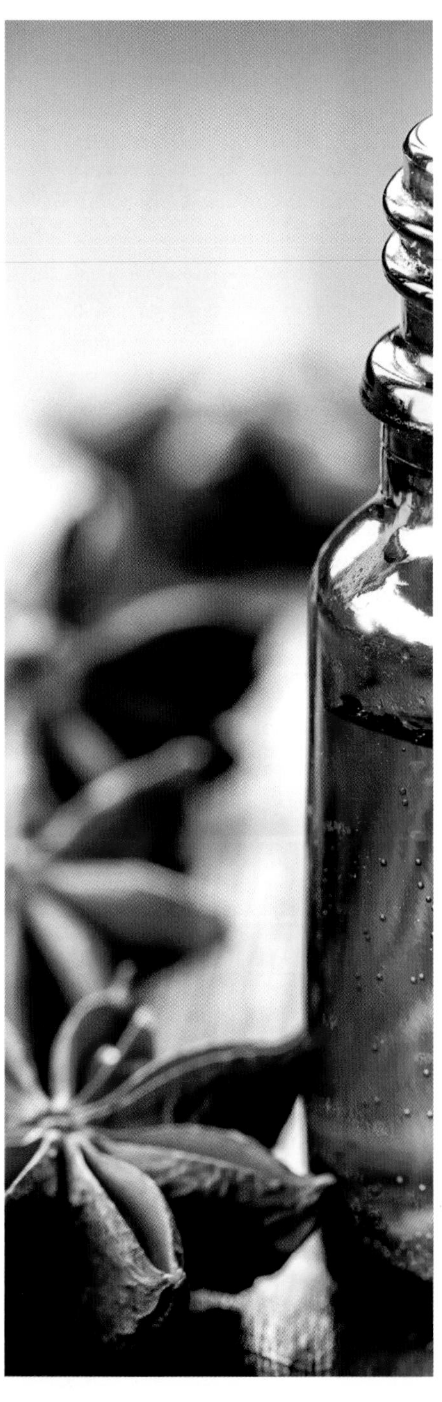

SECTION 4

body systems & focus areas

SECTION 5

essential lifestyle

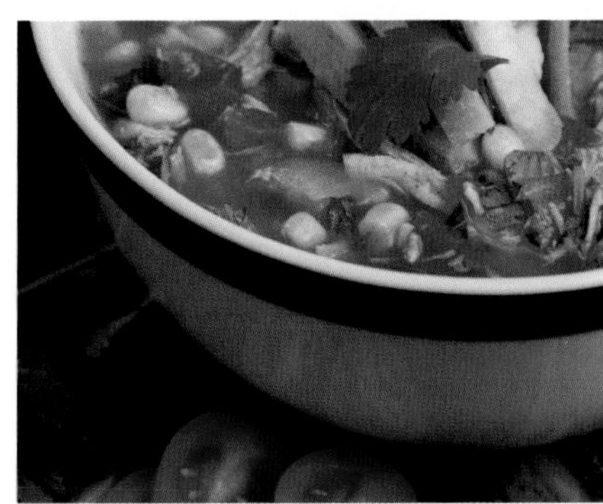

SECTION 6

supplemental

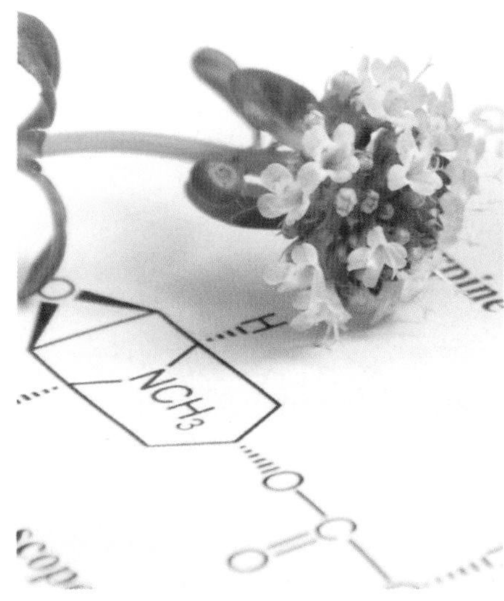

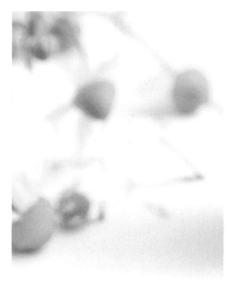

SECTION 1

INTRODUCTION

For both the new and the experienced essential oil user, THE ESSENTIAL LIFE is a composition of everything needed to create positive and profound results. Providing both simple quick-reference information and expert-level knowledge, this book brings together the best research and proven solutions to provide you, the user, a trusted, credible, and comprehensive guide.

Reach for your oils and refer to this book often. Enjoy THE ESSENTIAL LIFE!

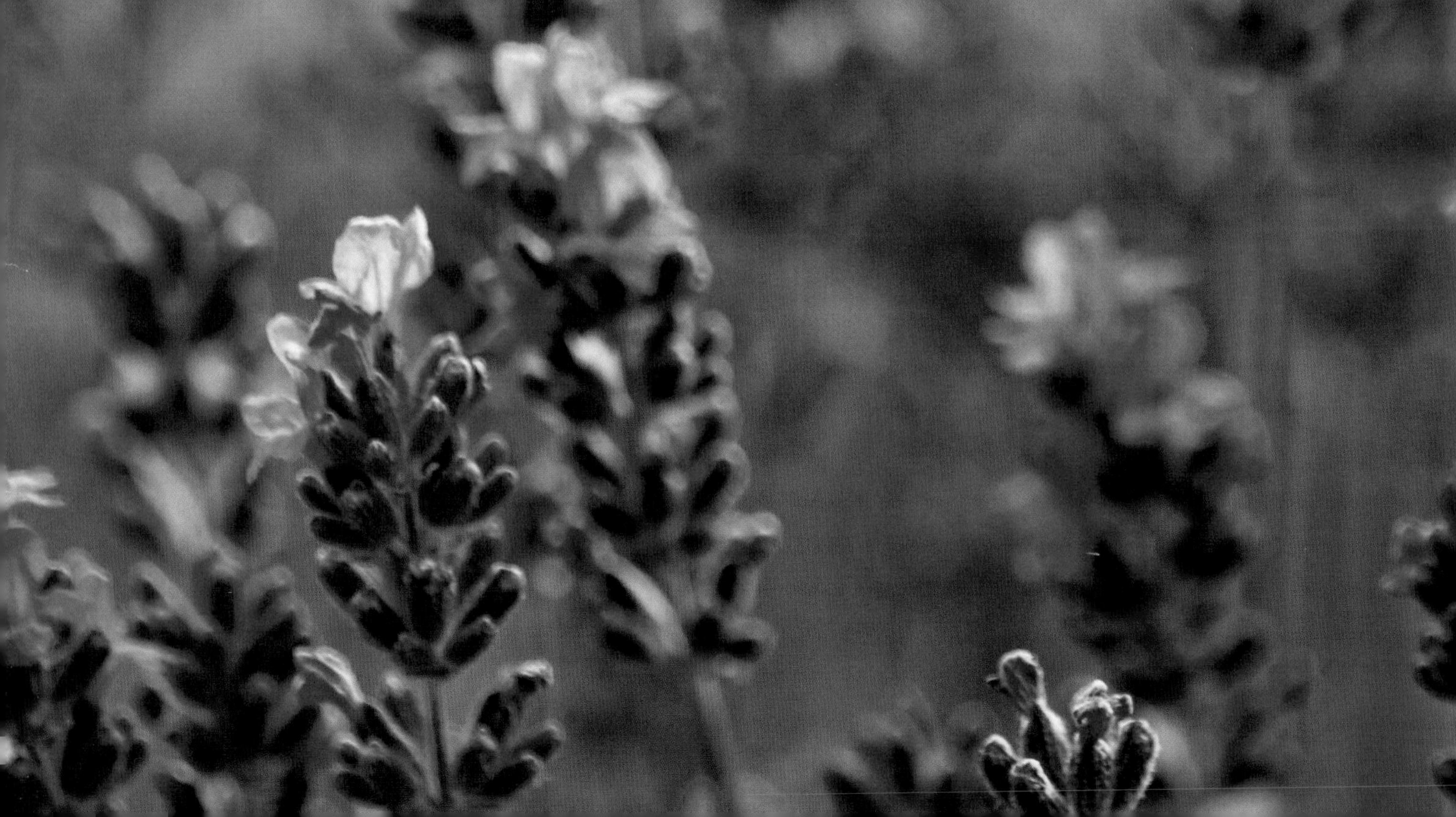

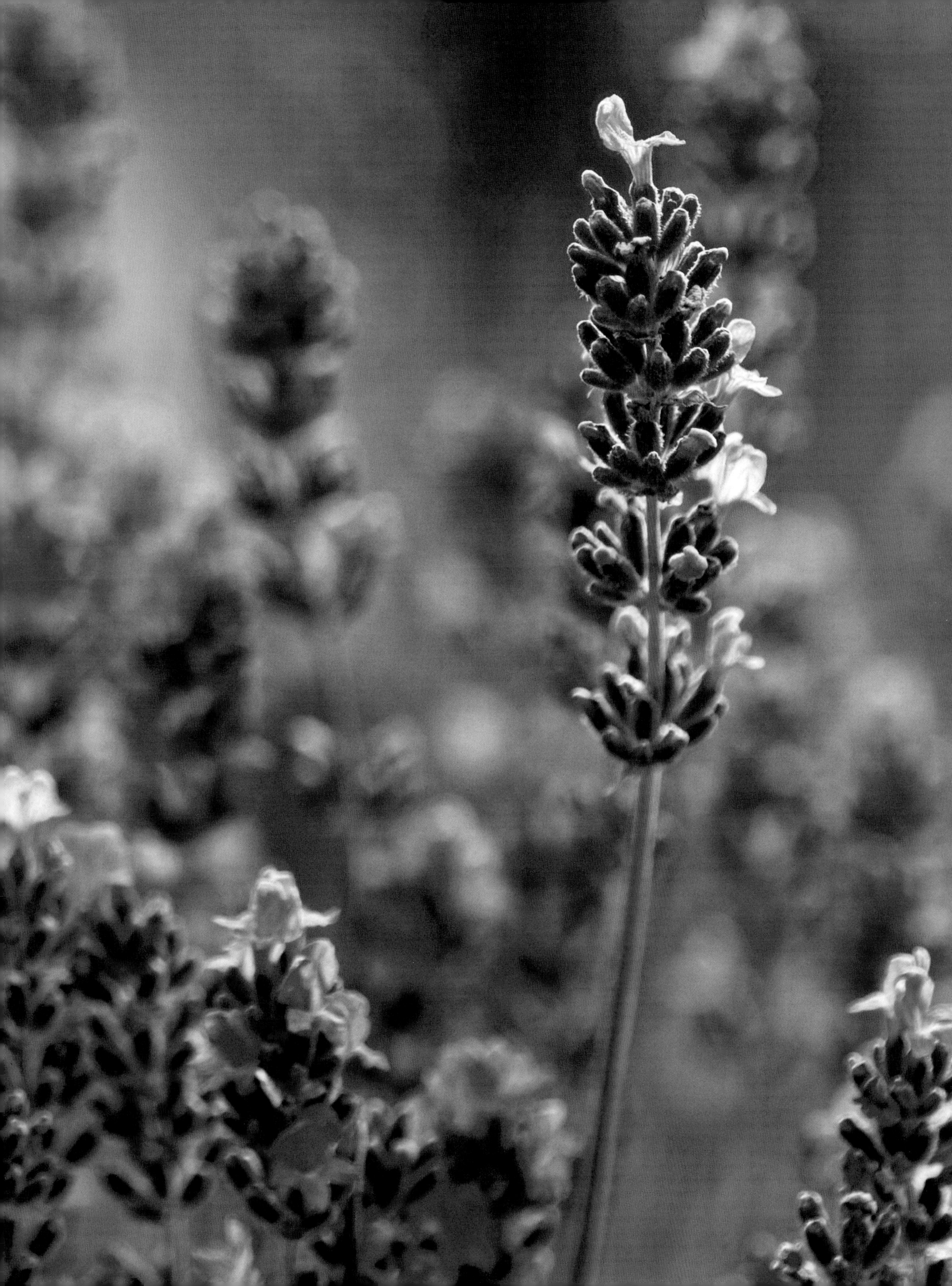

How to Use this Guide

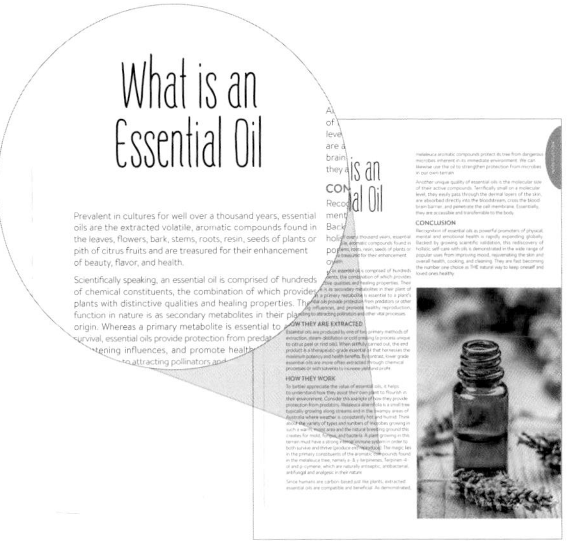

introduction

Establish a foundation of simple knowledge for using essential oils. Learn what oils are, where they come from, and how to use them safely and effectively.

quick reference

Quickly look up any ailment and link it to the top recommended used essential oils with this A-Z index of ailments. Learn basic application methods and find cross references for more in-depth understanding and other (recommended remedies).

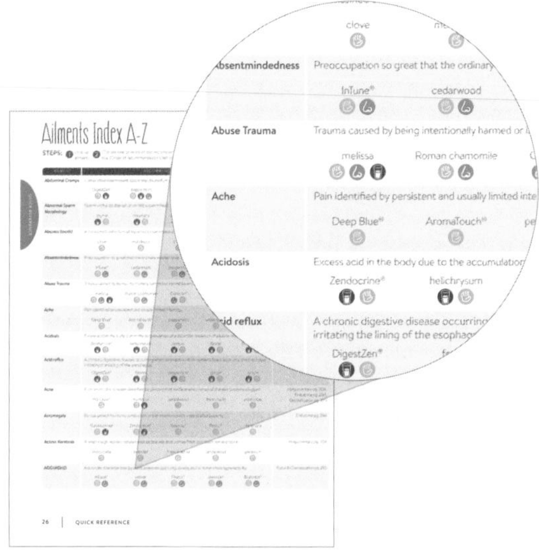

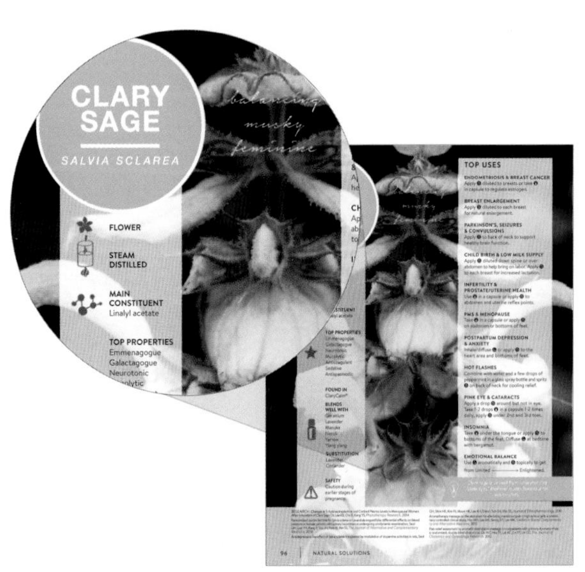

natural solutions

Become familiar with individual essential oils, essential oil blends, and supplementary products. Discover how each oil is derived, common uses, basic emotional benefits, and insights.

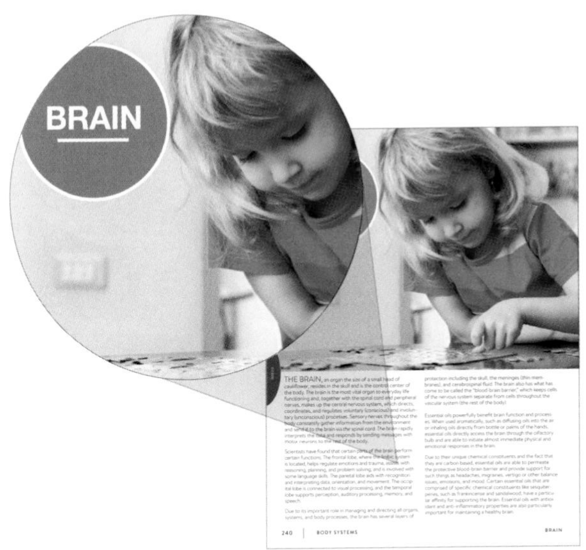

body systems & focus areas

Reference this section to experience expanded levels of knowledge and learn to address wellness in a more holistic way. Explore both disease symptoms and body symptoms to better identify root causes and corresponding healing remedies and resources.

essential lifestyle

Explore and enjoy the benefits of using essential oils for cleaning, cooking, gardening, fitness, intimacy, weight loss, children, pets, on-the-go, and more. Integrate the power of essential oils into every part of your life!

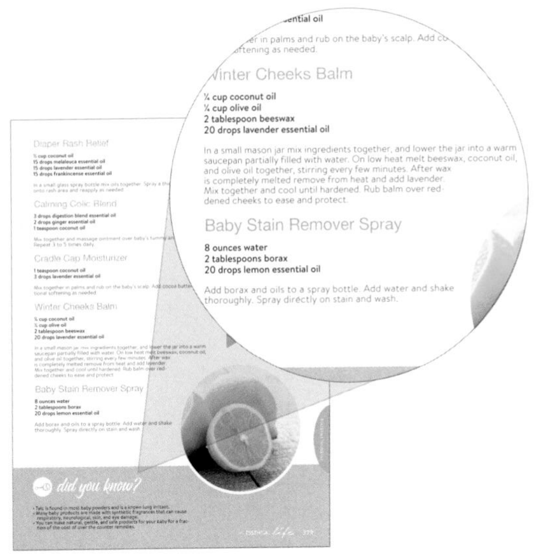

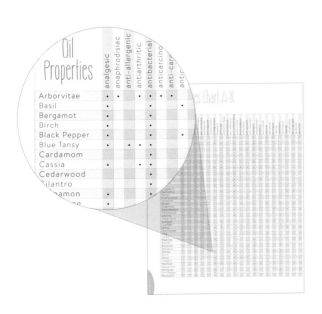

supplemental

Explore in-depth essential oil insights through informative charts, indexes, and other resources.

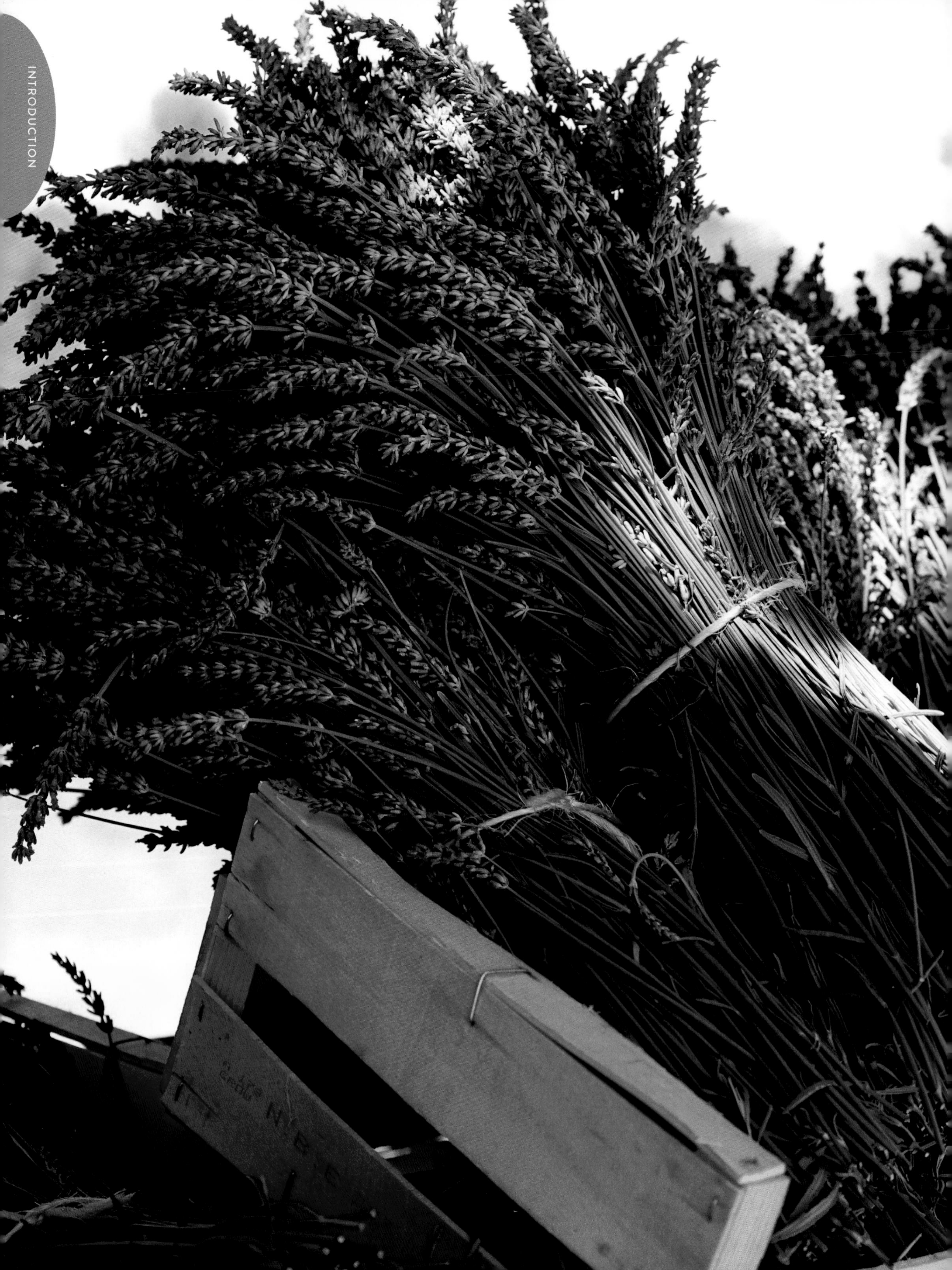

What is an Essential Oil

Prevalent in cultures for well over a thousand years, essential oils are the extracted volatile, aromatic compounds found in the leaves, flowers, bark, stems, roots, resin, seeds of plants or pith of citrus fruits and are treasured for their enhancement of beauty, flavor, and health.

Scientifically speaking, an essential oil is comprised of hundreds of chemical constituents, the combination of which provides plants with distinctive qualities and healing properties. Their function in nature is as secondary metabolites in their plant of origin. Whereas a primary metabolite is essential to a plant's survival, essential oils provide protection from predators or other threatening influences, and promote healthy reproduction, contributing to attracting pollinators and other vital processes.

HOW THEY ARE EXTRACTED

Essential oils are produced by one of two primary methods of extraction, steam-distillation or cold pressing (a process unique to citrus peel or rind oils). When skillfully carried out, the end product is a therapeutic-grade essential oil that harnesses the maximum potency and health benefits. By contrast, lower grade essential oils are more often extracted through chemical processes or with solvents to increase yield and profit.

HOW THEY WORK

To better appreciate the value of essential oils, it helps to understand how they assist their own plant to flourish in their environment. Consider this example of how they provide protection from predators. Melaleuca alternifolia is a small tree typically growing along streams and in the swampy areas of Australia where weather is consistently hot and humid. Think about the variety of types and numbers of microbes growing in such a warm, moist area and the natural breeding ground this creates for mold, fungus, and bacteria. A plant growing in this terrain must have a strong internal immune system in order to both survive and thrive (produce and reproduce). The magic lies in the primary constituents of the aromatic compounds found in the melaleuca tree, namely a- & y-terpinenes, Terpinen-4-ol and p-cymene, which are naturally antiseptic, antibacterial, antifungal and analgesic in their nature.

Since humans are carbon-based just like plants, extracted essential oils are compatible and beneficial. As demonstrated, melaleuca aromatic compounds protect its tree from dangerous microbes inherent in its immediate environment. We can likewise use the oil to strengthen protection from microbes in our own terrain.

Another unique quality of essential oils is the molecular size of their active compounds. Terrifically small on a molecular level, they easily pass through the dermal layers of the skin, are absorbed directly into the bloodstream, cross the blood-brain barrier, and penetrate the cell membrane. Essentially, they are accessible and transferrable to the body.

CONCLUSION

Recognition of essential oils as powerful promoters of physical, mental and emotional health is rapidly expanding globally. Backed by growing scientific validation, this rediscovery of holistic self-care with oils is demonstrated in the wide range of popular uses from improving mood, rejuvenating the skin and overall health, cooking, and cleaning. They are fast becoming the number one choice as THE natural way to keep oneself and loved ones healthy.

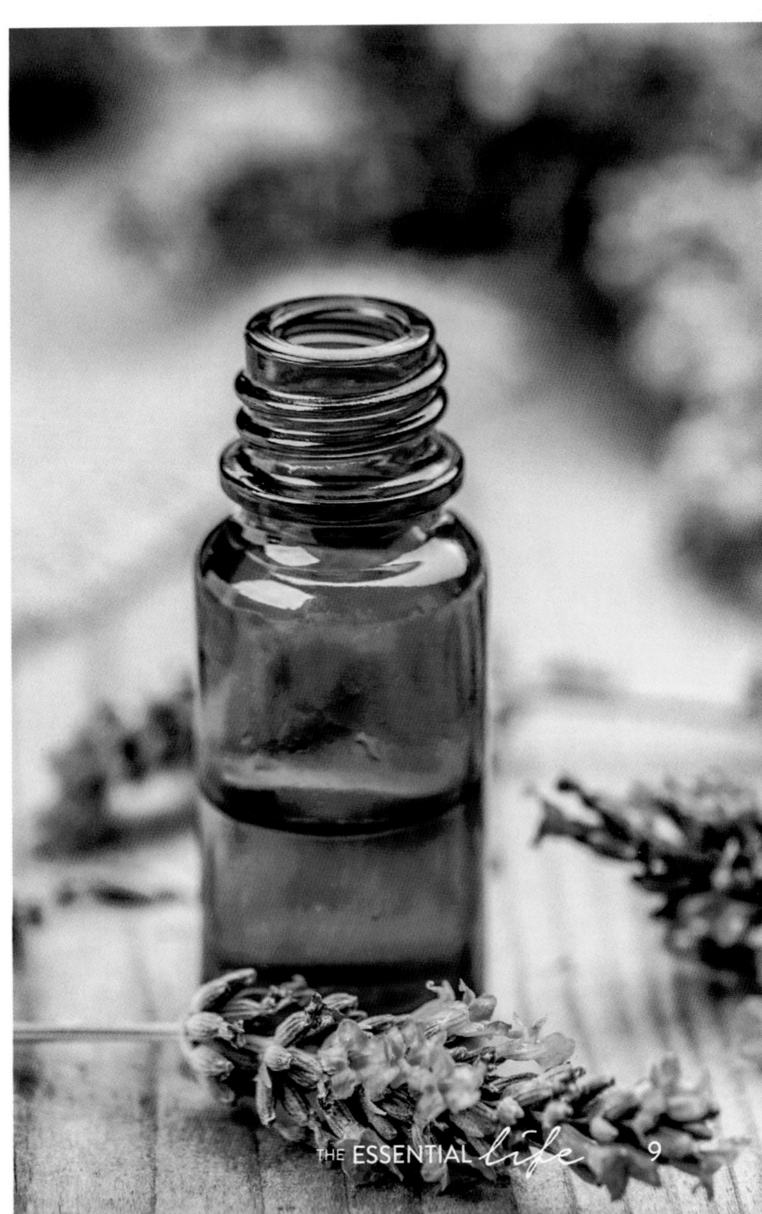

Essential Oil Classifications

Understanding plant classifications helps you come to know essential oils categorically. This gives you a broader knowledge of the general attributes and characteristics, improving your ability to identify oils that best serve in specific circumstances. Keep in mind that while oils within a classification have common characteristics, each individual oil has far more specific and even unique properties. See **Oil Properties** (pg. 478) to learn more.

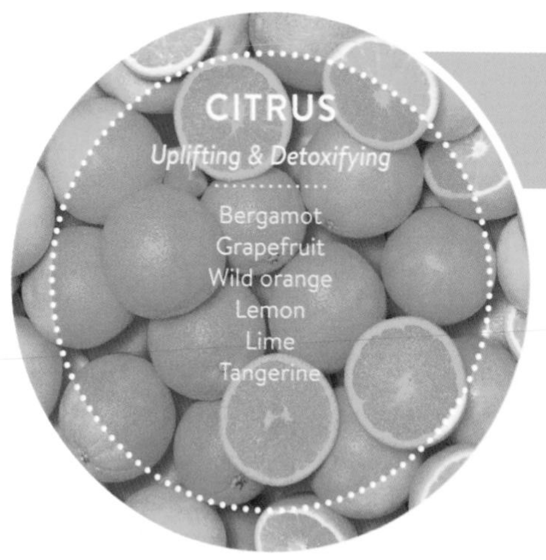

Citrus trees grow juicy fruit with a pulpy rind in warm climates. Oils are cold-pressed or steam distilled from the rind.

Top Properties:
- Stimulating
- Uplifting
- Antiseptic
- Calming
- Antimicrobial
- Energizing
- Antioxidant

Positive energy and emotions heightened by citrus oils:
- Invigorated, joy, energized, validated, feeling worthy, enlivened, restored, productive, mindful

Negative energy and emotions addressed by citrus oils:
- Discouraged, gloomy, distressed, depleted, drained, oppressed, faint, mindless

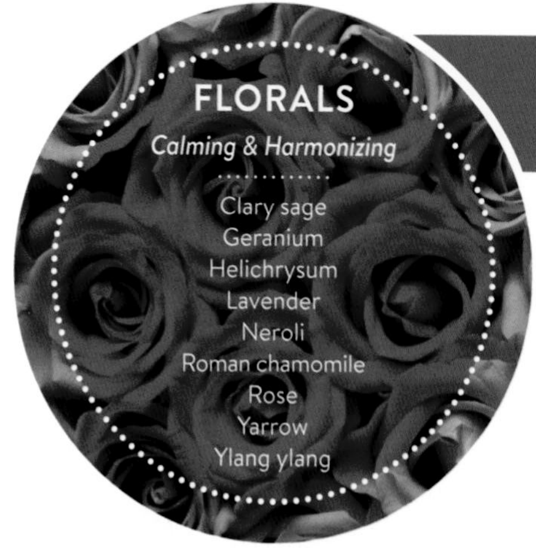
FLORALS
Calming & Harmonizing
Clary sage
Geranium
Helichrysum
Lavender
Neroli
Roman chamomile
Rose
Yarrow
Ylang ylang

Florals are flowers. Oils are distilled from the petals or aerial parts of plants.

Top Properties:
- Antiinflammatory
- Antispasmodic
- Relaxant
- Antihistamine
- Analgesic
- Regenerative
- Antiviral

Positive energy and emotions heightened by floral oils:
- Better able to express oneself, reassured, mended, purposeful, light-filled, loved, exuberant, expressive

Negative energy and emotions addressed by floral oils:
- Fearful, worried, hurt, unheard, wounded, neglected, frustrated, depressed, isolated, burdened

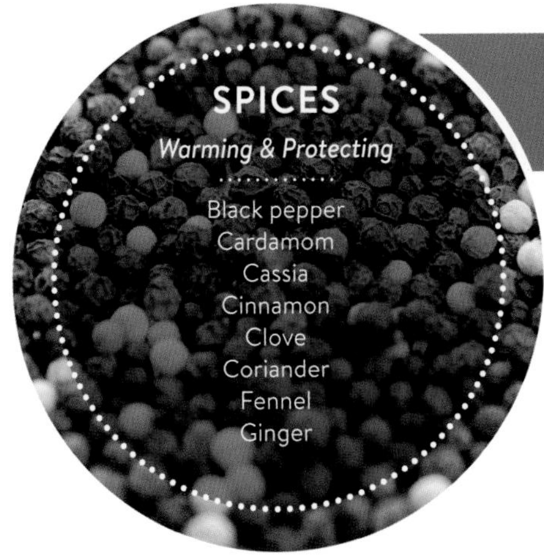
SPICES
Warming & Protecting
Black pepper
Cardamom
Cassia
Cinnamon
Clove
Coriander
Fennel
Ginger

Spices are aromatic, flavorful plants. Oil is distilled from the bark, roots, seeds, and buds of the plant.

Top Properties:
- Warming
- Digestive stimulant
- Immunostimulant
- Aphrodisiac
- Antiemetic
- Anti-infectious
- Anti-parasitic

Positive energy and emotions heightened by spice oils:
- Honest, charitable, bold, receptive, supported, participating, activated, empowered

Negative energy and emotions addressed by spice oils:
- Repressed, self-centered, uncertain, denied, dominated, apprehensive, apathetic, somber, disinterested, bored

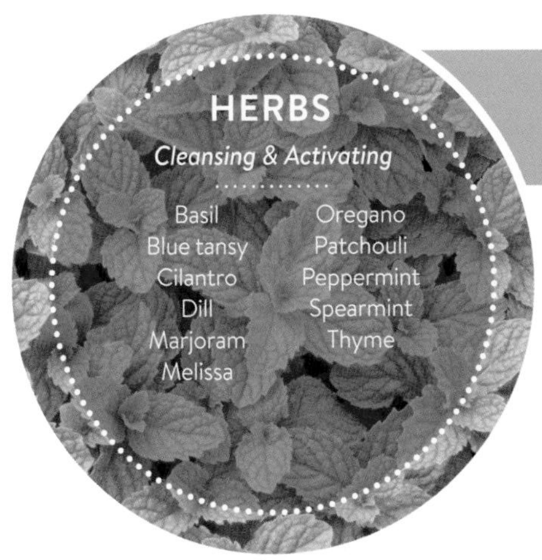

Herbs are seed-bearing, flowering plants that do not have woody tissue in the stem. Oils are distilled from the green leafy part of these low-growing plants.

Top Properties:
- Immunostimulant
- Detoxifier
- Antiviral
- Antifungal
- Carminative
- Antibacterial
- Anti-parasitic

Positive energy and emotions heightened by herb oils:
- Accepting, yielding, open-minded, invigorated, enhanced, unattached, trusting, progressing, enlightened, relieved

Negative energy and emotions addressed by herb oils:
- Stubborn, angry, unyielding, confused, hindered, degraded, obstinate, doubtful, stalled, limited, inundated

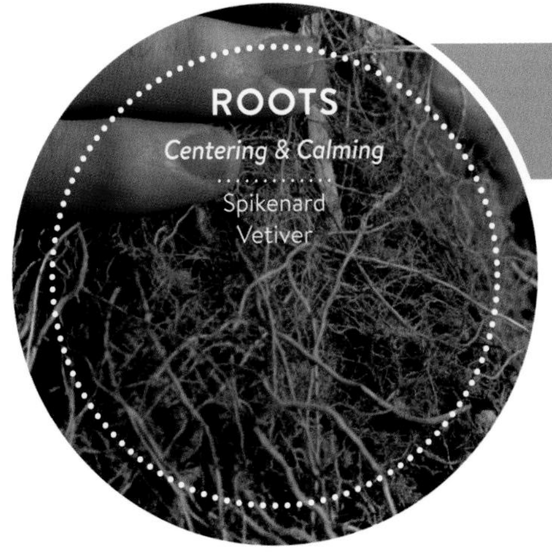
ROOTS
Centering & Calming
Spikenard
Vetiver

Roots are the plant fibers that attach it to the ground and receive water and nourishment for the plant. Oils are distilled from roots.

Top Properties:
- Calming
- Nervine
- Grounding
- Neurotonic
- Sedative
- Restorative
- Neuroprotective

Positive energy and emotions heightened by root oils:
- Rooted, flowing, centered, elevated, aware, peaceful, meditative, prioritized

Negative energy and emotions addressed by root oils:
- Ungrounded, obstructed, discontented, erratic, unattentive, agitative, scattered

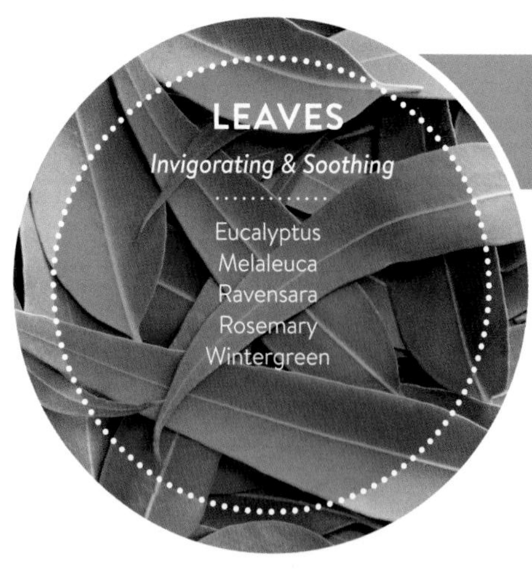
LEAVES
Invigorating & Soothing
Eucalyptus
Melaleuca
Ravensara
Rosemary
Wintergreen

Leaves are an outgrowth of the plant stem that manufacture plant nutrients by photosynthesis. Oils are steam distilled from the leaves.

Top Properties:
- Antiseptic
- Invigorating
- Anti-inflammatory
- Insecticide
- Analgesic
- Antibacterial
- Antimicrobial

Positive energy and emotions heightened by leaf oils:
- Accepting, yielding, receiving, invigorated, enhanced, unattached, trusting, progressing, enlightened, relieved

Negative energy and emotions addressed by leaf oils:
- Stubborn, refusing, unyielding, confused, hindered, degraded, obstinate, doubtful, stalled, limited, inundated

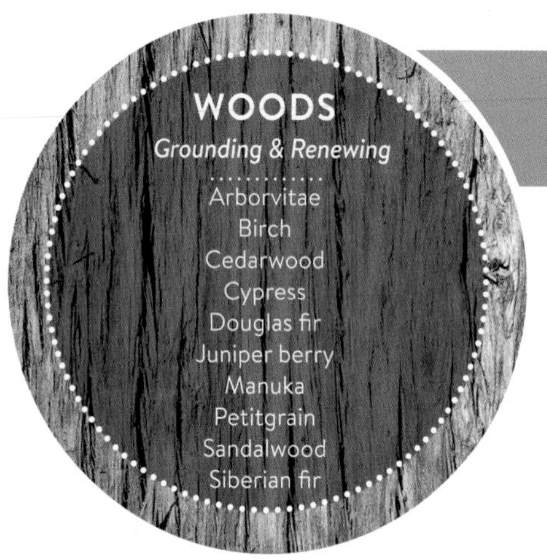
WOODS
Grounding & Renewing
Arborvitae
Birch
Cedarwood
Cypress
Douglas fir
Juniper berry
Manuka
Petitgrain
Sandalwood
Siberian fir

Woods typically grow high off the ground and are characterized by a single trunk. Oils are distilled from the leaves, twigs, branches, needles, berries, bark, and wood.

Properties:
- Anticatarrhal
- Regenerative
- Relaxant
- Grounding
- Steroidal
- Analgesic
- Astringent

Positive energy and emotions heightened by wood oils:
- Receiving, devoted, collected, stimulated, progressing, alone, courageous, composed

Negative energy and emotions addressed by wood oils:
- Blocked, uninspired, unsure, congested, stalled, connected, cowardly, overzealous, grieving, sad, ashamed

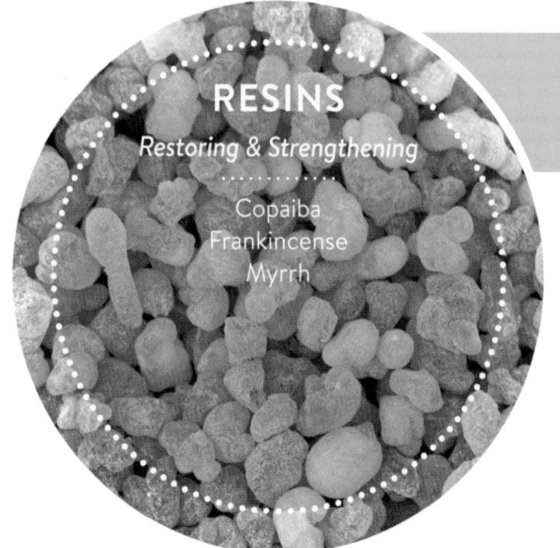
RESINS
Restoring & Strengthening
Copaiba
Frankincense
Myrrh

Resins are a natural sticky substance that come from certain trees and are insoluble in water. Oils are distilled from hardened resins.

Properties
- Anti-inflammatory
- Cytophylactic
- Analgesic
- Restorative
- Antidepressant
- Immunostimulant
- Antimutagenic

Positive energy and emotions heightened by resin oils:
- Unified, connected, grounded, nurtured, enlightened, inoculated, bonded, awakened

Negative energy and emotions addressed by resin oils:
- Separated, disconnected, stressed, malnourished, unprotected, abandoned, darkened, weak

Why Quality Matters

SOURCING

When it comes to sourcing essential oils, the terrain and soil of origin matter. If a field is sprayed with toxic chemicals, or these chemicals are added to the soil, it affects the chemistry of the plants. The distillation process, temperature, and the use of toxic solvents and chemicals for extraction also affect the purity and potency of the essential oil.

Variations in the natural chemistry of oils is permitted, as this is a legitimate expression of nature. As one truly studies the art of growing, harvesting, and distilling essential oils, one discovers the grower's craft and the beauty of this expert human art. Today we experience the best of tradition in growers' expertise and wisdom handed down through the generations, combined with advancements in science, farming, and distillation practices.

SUPPLIER

When it comes to healing, choosing a supplier of essential oils who is well known for quality and efficacy is, well, "essential." Every oil has specific constituents, which provide varying levels of therapeutic effects. Therefore, it is necessary to sort through dozens of species of a single plant source, from a myriad of geographical locations, to find the right combination of therapeutic compounds.

This is one of the supplier's greatest tasks: to responsibly search the world for the highest quality compounds that produce the best possible essential oils nature can provide. One of the best ways this is accomplished is by creating trusted alliances with honest growers and distillers.

AUTHENTICITY

Regulation of therapeutic grade essential oils is limited and standards are minimal. This leaves suppliers to self-regulate quality. The term "therapeutic grade" is simply insufficient to identify a level of quality. There exists, therefore, two very distinctly different views. In one, compromised sourcing is permissible and synthetic additives are acceptable components. In the other, true holistic healing requires unprocessed oils that are sourced directly from nature with nothing added. These strict standards allow the oils to remain rich and complex as nature created them. One should expect to pay a higher price for these genuine, authentic, pure, and potent superior-grade essential oils.

QUALITY

To be truly therapeutic and superior grade, an essential oil needs to be tested and certified as pure, potent, genuine, and authentic. Each of these terms is important and meaningful in reference to measurements of quality. It is vital to note that although chemists have successfully recreated multiple constituents of plants, they have never replicated a complete essential oil. Why? They simply have not discovered or identified every compound nature produces.

PROCESS

To protect and maintain the highest quality essential oils, plants must be patiently harvested by those who are knowledgeable, honest, and committed to gathering only the "one" specie, and who allow the plant proper maturation time.

After harvesting, the plant material is ready for distillation. In order to carefully extract the precious constituents, this process must be conducted gently, slowly, and skillfully. Quality distillation requires reduced pressure and temperature, protecting these essences from being oxidized or destroyed by excessive heat.

Once distillation is complete, the essential oils are moved to distribution companies or to middlemen, known as brokers. As a general rule, the farther down the supply chain you go, the less likely you are to get pure product. Most companies that sell essential oils have no ability (or in many cases no desire) to verify the quality of the oils they receive from their supplier before they pass it on to their customers. Look for companies that work directly with growers, sourced from all over the world.

There is a growing number of products falsely claiming to be an essential oil or to contain essential oils. Too often, these products use fragrant synthetic chemical substitutes to dilute or replace more expensive essential oil extracts. These claims deceive many consumers who believe they are using natural products.

Essential oils are comprised of only three elements: carbon, hydrogen, and oxygen. The molecules in essential oils are primarily monoterpenes, sesquiterpenes, and their oxygenated derivatives. Essential oils are volatile organic liquids. There are no vitamins, minerals, essential fatty acids, or hormones in essential oils. Any claim of such ingredients simply reveals the impurity of a product.

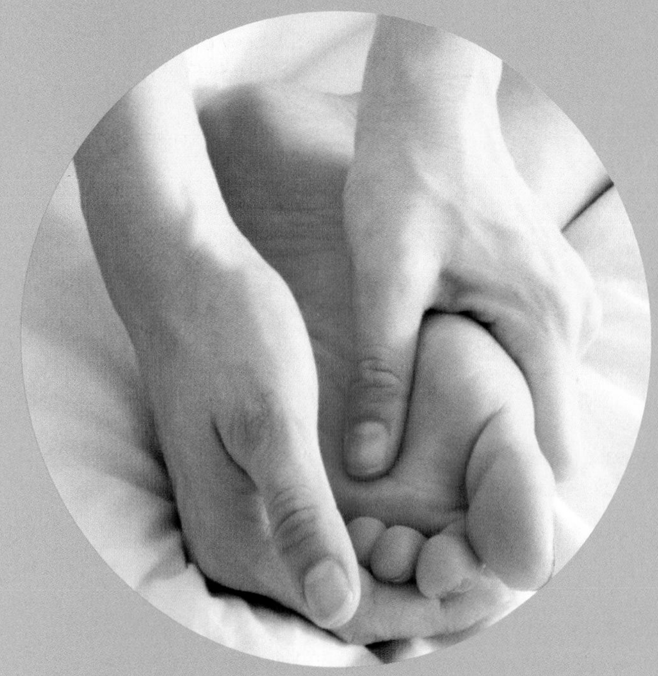

- The oil is not the product of a mixture of plants or weeds growing alongside the species.
- The oil is comprised of and distilled from only the plant parts clearly identified.
- In total, the oil is characterized precisely so as to clearly identify its healing qualities through consistently occurring compounds.

Genuine

The term "Genuine" is equivalent to the term "Unadulterated," meaning:

- **The essential oil is 100 percent natural** and contains no addition of any other substances – even other natural substances. It contains NO synthetics, agents, diluents, or additives.
- **The essential oil is 100 percent pure** and contains NO similar essential oil or hybrid, added to extend supply.
- **The essential oil is 100 percent complete** and has been fully distilled. Almost all essential oils are distilled in a single process. Ylang ylang is an exception, as it passes through more than one distillation to be complete. Distillation processes that are disrupted can produce I, II, III, and "extra" essential oil classes.

Pure

Purity alone does not necessarily mean an oil is good quality. A pure oil can be distilled incorrectly or may be obtained from a particular variety of inferior plant species. Additionally, oils may contain contaminants, pesticides, herbicides, solvents, inferior and/or unlabeled plant sources, other unlabeled species, and synthetic compounds. The distillation process may magnify the concentration of these undesirable elements.

Potent

Essential oils are the most potent form of plant material. The chemical constituents found in the plant material will either increase or decrease the potency of the essential oil. The climate and soil composition affect the potency of plant matter. This is why sourcing an oil from its native habitat is essential.

Aroma

One of the most telling ways to detect pure, high-quality oils is by the aroma. Superb aroma is earned and is the result of quality plant sourcing, quality distillation processes, and the absence of chemical solvents. Generally, the more pure and "sweet" an aroma, the greater the purity and the better the sourcing.

SUPPLIER RESPONSIBILITY

It is the distributing company's responsibility to provide the consumer with carefully extracted, pure (no fillers or artificial ingredients) essential oils. Rigorous quality testing, above and beyond the minimum required, helps ensure oils are free of contaminants. Look for companies that verify the quality and purity multiple times prior to making the product available to the consumer. Additionally, the distributor is responsible for labeling products according to FDA GRAS (Generally Regarded As Safe) standards.

MEASURING QUALITY

Measurements of quality fall under specific categories of genuine, authentic, pure, and potent.

Authentic

In the world of essential oils, the term "Authenticity" means:

- The composition of an oil is equal to the plant specified on the label.
- The oil is not a mixture of plant species, rather the plant specified.

PERSONAL RESPONSIBILITY

When it comes to obtaining quality essential oils, the consumer must do his own research, use common sense, exercise prudence, and do what is best for himself and his family. Education is key to becoming a skilled user of these potent plant extracts.

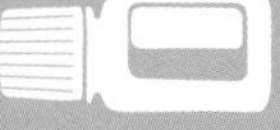

How To Know Which Oils To Use

The greater the number of oils you have at your disposal, the more choices you make and results you can create. Deciding which oil to use in certain circumstance can at times be overwhelming, especially with so many options for use and overlapping qualities and properties. Good news! You can't go wrong!

The skill to develop here is learning to make better choices to create even better results. Remember this: oils, to the best of their ability, move you to the more balanced state of homeostasis. Necessarily then, ask yourself, "What might I experience on my way to greater balance and wholeness (e.g. temporary discomfort or symptoms due to detoxification from an unhealthy terrain)? Am I providing proper support for my body's needs (e.g. adequate nutrition & rest, proper diet) to help get me where I want to be in the most successful way?"

Following are a number of highly beneficial ways to make oil selections. Enjoy the process of getting to know each oil as if it were a friend you've learned to count on in times of need or want. The most important factors in your decision-making are you and your experiences. Interactions with the oils vary from person to person. Even with the same condition, people are drawn to and benefited by different solutions. Keep a log or journal, or simple notations right here in the pages of this book, about what you've learned. Become your own best advocate, knowing greater health and wellness, modeling it for generations to come, and inviting those around you to do the same.

SELECTION TOOLS

On-Hand – In a moment of need, your go-to choices are what you have on hand. Put each of your oils to work for you by looking them up in this book and learning what they do best. As your interest grows in making essential oils your first line of response, identify health issues (and desired changes and results), research them here in the book, and then increase your personal collection accordingly. It's what you do every day that matters most.

Intuition – Nothing could be more powerful in essential oil use than simply paying attention to what you are attracted to. Trust that feedback and act on it. Again, make notations so you can repeat what you've done before and, with experience, better your results.

Look Things Up in the Book

A-Z Quick Reference (pg. 26) Find the health condition you want to resolve. Pay attention to the five oils listed and considered to be among the top choices for that particular ailment. This immediately narrows your focus to just a few options.

Oil Properties (pg. 478) The last section of this book is designated for the more experienced and committed Power User. Utilize the resources provided. The **Oil Properties** chart is a superb advanced way to learn about how oils work. Notice as well that on the second page of every **Body Systems** section you will find oils listed by "Related Properties." In other words, certain essential oil properties excel in their capacity to address unique aspects of each body system.

Body Systems – Look up your condition(s) in **Body Systems & Focus Areas** (pg. 226). First go to the body system that relates to your concern (e.g. **Respiratory** for a cough; **Cardiovascular** for a heart or circulation issue), and then look for specific conditions or symptoms you want to relieve. Note both oil suggestions and remedies are provided.

Online – If you need more detailed knowledge about what to address, first look up your condition online so you better understand it. For example, learn about the different facets of whatever ails you and discover what body parts are involved. With these specific areas of focus identified, now utilize the book as described above to pursue your essential oil solutions.

Smell – Like intuition, the value of smelling an oil to discover what you love or are drawn to cannot be overemphasized. This is one of the most wonderful aspects of essential oil use. After all, it is called **aromatherapy**! Don't limit your thinking to what is taught. Deliberately choose to make selections by aroma. It is both scientific (every oil has very precise chemistry hence a unique aroma) and traditional to do so. There is a reason why smelling oils prior to selection is so commonplace and the natural inclination. Even animals and small children quickly identify their favorites and what their body most needs.

Emotions (pg. 378) – Perhaps the idea of matching an oil to an emotional state is new to you. However, it is the number one way to narrow selections. Here's why. Consider two people have arthritis. One is impatient and the other is resigned. In each case, a different emotional profile is found as well as different needs to be met. Learn more about the connection between essential oils and emotions by first reading **Emotional Well-Being** (pg. 378). The science and chemistry behind this correlation make it well worth your understanding and application. Then at the end of that section, use the charts in the **Emotions Index** to introduce the connection of what oil for what emotion. Also, see **Mood & Behavior** (pg. 319). Consider acquiring additional resources on this topic.

Oil Personalities – Learn your oils by their 'personalities' and get a sense for which oils and blends work best for you. Where and how they grow, plant parts used, and chemistry contained, are all significant aspects of the oils, revealing much about the 'energy' profile they provide. Here is an example. Cinnamon, considered a spice oil (see *Emotions Index* (pg. 384) to learn more), has warming properties (see pg. 477-481 for more information). This heat both wards off unwanted predators and warms up a cold heart or body, serving as both an Immunostimulant and Aphrodisiac (two more properties). Upon use, the user has a sense of feeling more protected, safe, and warm, and is thus more willing to be intimate and sexually/emotionally vulnerable.

Individual Test – Utilize a personal digital scan or applied kinesiology (also known as muscle response testing) to quickly identify what resonates as beneficial to your body at the time of evaluation.

How to Use Essential Oils

Application Methods

AROMATIC 

The very term **Aromatherapy** was derived from the fact that essential oils are, by nature, aromatic. Their aromas can elicit powerful physiologic, mental, and emotional responses. Essential oils are also volatile, meaning they evaporate quickly and are rapidly absorbed into the body. The process of conveying aromas to the brain is called olfaction, or simply, smelling. It happens courtesy of the olfactory system.

As a person inhales an essential oil, the molecules of oil go up into the back of each nostril to the postage-sized epithelium patch. There the molecules attach to receptors on the cilia hairs, which convert to nerves on the other side of the mucous patch. These nerves send the odor information to the olfactory bulb in the brain. This means the essential oil itself is not sent to the brain, but instead a neural translation or "message" of the complex chemistry it contains is delivered. The millions of nerves enter the olfactory bulb, which communicates directly with the amygdala, hippocampus, and other brain structures.

The amygdala, a center for emotions in the limbic system, links our sense of smell to our ability to learn emotionally. Here, aromatic information is connected to the emotions of the situation. This capacity to pair the two, information and emotions, is inextricably connected to our survival ability, making essential oils a powerful partner in creating and maintaining emotional health. Inhalation of essential oils is also received through the alveoli of the lungs and, from there, into the bloodstream.

The easiest way to aromatically use essential oils is to open a bottle and simply breathe in the aroma through the nose. This technique is known as **direct inhalation**. To enhance this method, place a drop of an oil or blend in the hands, rub them together, and then cup around the nose and mouth (not necessary to make contact with the face) and breathe in. Additionally, oil drops can be placed on a piece of cloth or tissue, held close to the face, and inhaled.

Diffusing essential oils aromatically is beneficial for affecting mood, killing airborne pathogens, and changing the aroma of a space such as a room, office, or car. Other uses include a targeted approach for relaxing or stimulating the mind.

Additionally, one of the most effective ways to impact a respiratory condition is to use a diffuser as an inhalation device, whether being in a room where diffusing is occurring or purposely breathing in the vapor. **Diffusers** are devices that can be used to evaporate an essential oil into a surrounding environment. There are four main types of diffusers: atomizing, vaporizing or humidification, fan, and heat. The best diffusers are atomizing and employ a cold air pump to force the essential oil through an atomizer, separating the oil into tiny particles that create a micro-fine vapor in the air. The essential oil bottle is, in some manner, directly connected to the diffuser, and no water is involved. Atomizing diffusers are normally more expensive and usually create a little bit of noise due to the mechanisms in action. Vaporizing or humidification diffusers employ water with the essential oil and use ultrasonic waves to emit the oil and water particles into the air. Fan and heat diffusers are usually low cost and mainly used for small areas such as cars. The amount of oil used varies with each diffuser type.

Different diffusers provide different capacities for covering the square footage of a room. Other features may include timers, some allowing both constant and intermittent distribution options. Essential oils can be added to water or alcohol (such as vodka) in a **spray bottle** (preferably glass). The mixture can then be sprayed in the air (e.g. air freshener), on surfaces (e.g. countertop), or on the body (e.g. for cooling and soothing benefits).

The best **dosage** for aromatic use of essential oils is smaller doses implemented multiple times throughout the day. It is best to avoid having infants and young children inhale oils at a close distance, as it is harder to determine dosage.

TOPICAL 

Essential oils are fat-soluble. Because of their chemical compounds, they are readily absorbed and enter the bloodstream when they are **applied directly**. This is one reason why quality of oils is important. Many quality oils are safe to use NEAT (i.e., applied topically to the skin with no carrier oil). One location that is most universally accepted as best for NEAT application is the bottoms of the feet.

The other primary method of distributing essential oils topically is to combine them with a carrier oil (i.e., a different kind of oil used for dilution such as fractionated coconut oil) for both dilution and prevention of evaporation. Using a carrier oil PRIOR to applying an oil slows down the absorption process (does not prohibit), therefore slowing the therapeutic onset. Applying a carrier oil AFTER essential oil application enhances therapeutic onset. Either way, the carrier oil prevents potential rapid evaporation.

By taking the time to massage an essential oil thoroughly into the skin, absorption is enhanced by increasing the blood flow to the area thus allowing the skin to more efficiently absorb valued compounds. Applying essential oils with a carrier oil and then **massaging** the skin or applying warm heat such as a rice bag or **moist cloth compress** helps drive the oil deeper into the tissues. This is especially helpful for muscle pain, body aches, and injured tissue. Carrier oils also protect the skin from irritation. Children, the elderly, and those with sensitive skin or compromised systems are advised to always use a carrier oil.

Some of the more popular **carrier oils** are fractionated coconut oil, virgin coconut oil, jojoba oil, grapeseed oil, almond oil, avocado oil, and extra virgin olive oil. Competing aroma is one consideration when selecting the carrier oil of choice. Fractionated coconut oil is a favorite and is created by removing the fatty acids from regular coconut oil, which is solid at 76 degrees. Fractionating, or removing the fatty acids, keeps the oil in a liquid state, making it easier for use in application (e.g., while giving a massage) and to combine with essential oils in containers such as spray and roll-on bottles. The fractionating process also increases shelf life and makes it odorless and colorless. It's great on the skin and doesn't clog the pores.

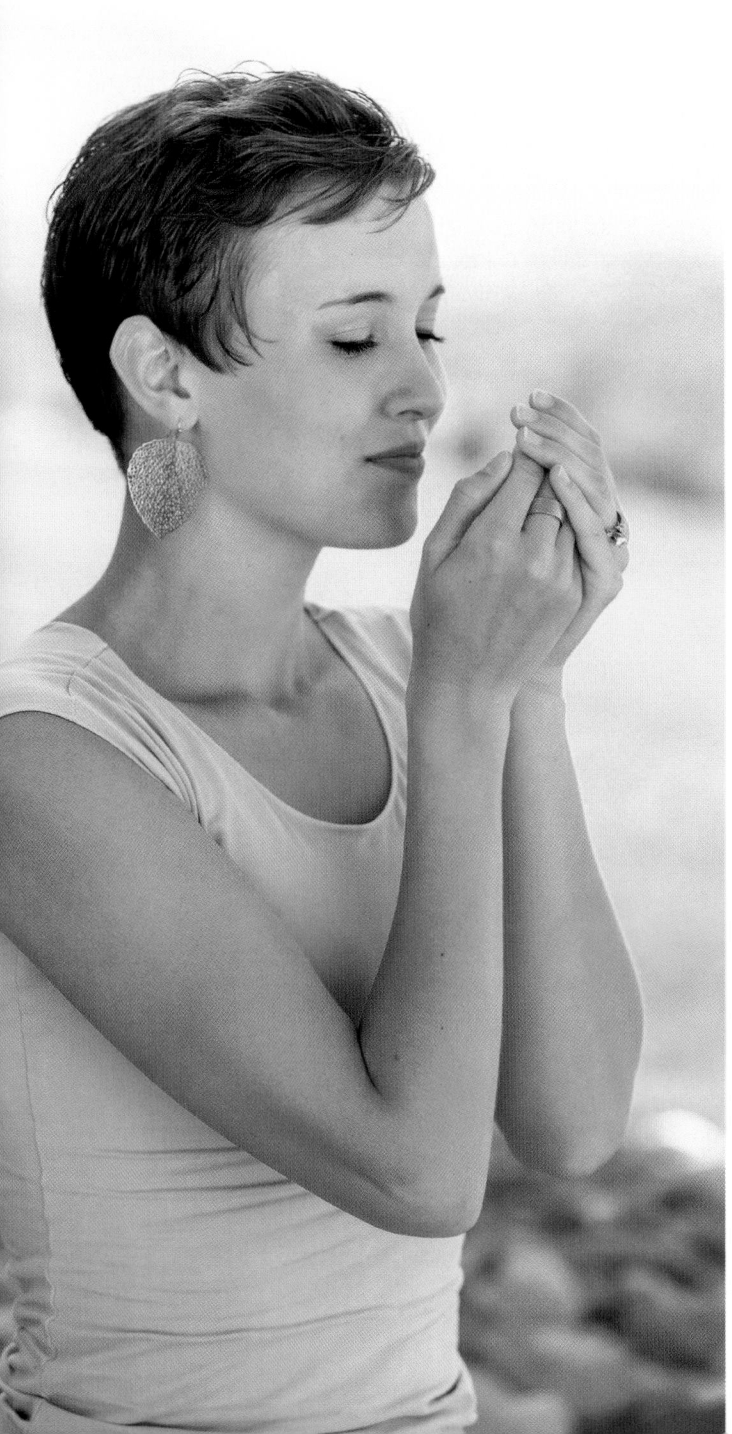

Topical application methods can vary considerably. Most frequently, oils are simply placed either on the skin of any area of concern or on the bottoms of the feet. Additional methods of distribution can include combining oils in an unscented lotion, or with a carrier oil or water in a spray, balm, or roller bottle. Limiting the number of drops used and diluting is the best way to safely use essential oils topically. It's generally unnecessary to use exaggerated amounts to achieve a therapeutic effect. Every drop of essential oil contains a vast bouquet of potent chemical constituents made by nature to deliver powerful effects in sometimes as little as one or a few drops.

The appropriate **dosage** for topical use of essential oils is different for each individual and should be tailored to their personal circumstances. The age and size of an individual are the biggest considerations as is the individual's overall health status. It is best to use smaller amounts more often rather than greater amounts less often. Start with the lowest amount that makes sense, and then increase the dose as needed to achieve the desired outcome. A topical dose of essential oils can be repeated every twenty minutes in an acute situation or every two to six hours as needed otherwise. A recommended ratio for dilution follows:

Babies	0.3 % dilution	(1 drop to 1 tablespoon)
Children	1.0 % dilution	(1 drop to 1 teaspoon)
Adults	2.0-4.0% dilution	(3-6 drops to 1 teaspoon)

When applying essential oils topically, avoid sensitive skin areas such as eyes, inner ears, genitals, and broken, damaged, or injured skin. After applying essential oils, the residue can be enjoyed and massaged into the palms for therapeutic benefit. However, if immediate contact with sensitive areas, such as the eyes, is predicted be sure to thoroughly wash hands.

A favorite use for essential oils is in a **bath**, which functions both as a topical and aromatic method. Using an emulsifier such as shampoo, bath gel, milk, or honey with an essential oil before placing in the bath water disperses the oil throughout the water rather than it floating on top. Or add 3 to 10 drops of essential oils to **bath salts** (use amount per product instructions) or 1 cup Epsom salts, and then dissolve in bath.

Essential oils can be applied to **reflex points** or nerve endings in the feet or hands. Oils can also be applied to various points on the rim and parts of the ears, referred to as **auricular therapy**, which are similar to the reflex points on the hands or feet. Refer to "Reflexology" later in this section.

Layering is the process of applying more than one oil to a desired location to intensify the effect of an oil or to address multiple concerns at once. For example, frankincense is often used as the first oil applied to an area on the skin to magnify the effects of subsequent oils layered on top. If an individual is sensitive to or dislikes the smell of an oil(s), they may resist its use. Applying an oil to the bottoms of one's feet (perhaps the least preferred aroma is applied first) and then layering a second and even third oil on top to "deodorize" and create a different aroma can be effective. Putting on socks after application can "contain" the aroma to a degree as an additional option. For example, apply vetiver then layer lavender on top. If satisfactory, then the process is complete. If not, add a third oil such as wild orange or Citrus Bliss®. The last oil applied will be the strongest aroma initially. After time, a more base note oil lingers longer than a top note oil.

INTERNAL 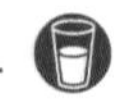

Just as plants are eaten fresh, dried for herbs, used in hot water infusions (tea), taken internally for therapeutic benefits, and used for improved flavor of foods, essential oils can be taken internally for these same uses. We consume essential oils when we eat food. Fresh aromatic plants normally contain 1 to 2 percent by weight of volatile compounds or essential oils. When plants are distilled for the extraction of their essential oils, the properties are concentrated. Essential oils are more potent than whole plant material. Small amounts should be used when taking oils internally.

Essential oils are fat-soluble, so they are readily delivered to all organs of the body, including the brain. They are then metabolized by the liver and other organs. Internal use of essential oils is the most potent method of use, and proper dosing for internal use should be followed according to labeling recommendations and other professional guidelines to avoid unnecessary overuse or toxicity. All ingested food can be toxic if taken in too high of doses. Some traditional essential oil users profess that internal use of essential oils is not safe. However, modern research as well as internal use by hundreds of thousands of users over many years indicates that internal use following appropriate and safe dosing guidelines is perfectly and appropriately safe. Dosage guidelines for internal use vary depending on the age and size of the person as well as an individual's health status.

Essentials oils can be **ingested** internally under the tongue (1 to 2 drops sublingually), in a gelatin cap (often referred to as a "gel cap"), in a vegetable capsule (often referred to as a "veggie cap"), in a tea, in food, or in water. Some essential oils, such as cinnamon and oregano, are best used internally. Heat affects the compounds in an oil. Therefore, it is best to add oils to hot liquids after the heating process has occurred.

Another method of internal essential oil use is **vaginal insertion**. Oils can be diluted in a carrier oil, inserted using a vaginal syringe, and held in place using a tampon. Oils can also be diluted in a carrier oil and then absorbed into a tampon. The tampon is inserted and kept in usually overnight. Essential oils can also be diluted in water and used to irrigate the vaginal area with a vaginal syringe.

Rectal insertion is an appropriate and safe way to apply essential oils, especially for internal conditions. Oils can be deposited into the rectum using a rectal syringe, or oils can be placed in a capsule and the capsule then inserted and retained in the rectum overnight. Consult an aromatherapy professional for using essential oils in **suppositories**.

Keep in mind that a single drop of essential oil is obtained from a large amount of plant material. One drop of essential oil can contain hundreds of compound constituents and is very potent. These two facts should be considered in determining the amount of oil to ingest. For example, it takes one lemon to make about five drops of lemon essential oil. A common internal dose for an adult is 1 to 5 drops of essential oil every one or two to six hours (depending on the oils selected), but preferably no more than 25 drops of essential oils divided into doses in a 24-hour period. This methodology allows the body, especially the liver, time to process each dosage. This dosage should be adjusted for a person's age, size, and health status. For extended internal use a lower daily dose is advised. If a higher dose is desired, consult a healthcare professional.

Some oils are not considered safe to ingest. Those include oils from the needles of trees such as pine essential oil and some bark oils such as cypress and some varieties of eucalyptus. Verifying a "Safe for Supplemental Use" or "Supplement Facts" label on an essential oil bottle serves as guide for oils that are appropriate to be taken internally. Other oils such as wintergreen and birch are required by law to have childproof lids on them, because the benefit of thinning blood could be hazardous to a young child or baby if ingested.

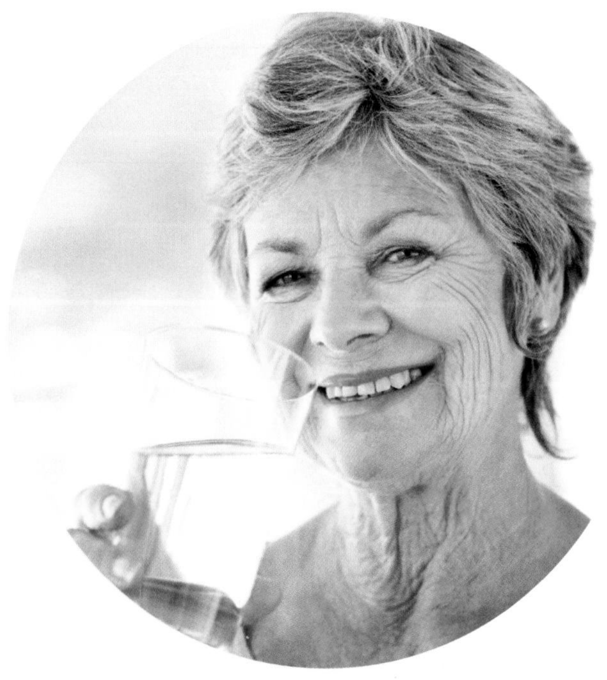

Oil Touch Technique

Essential oils have a powerful effect on well being. These effects are specific and unique to each oil that nature has provided. When we understand these healing properties and how our bodies naturally respond to them, we can use essential oils to promote a superior state of being. The Oil Touch technique provides a way to use these gifts to maximizes emotional and physical healing.

The Oil Touch technique is comprised of four stages. Each stage utilizes two oils or oil blends. Do not substitute other essential oils. Because these essential oils are applied full strength (NEAT) to the skin, it is very important that you use only the highest quality essential oil. Oils need to be both pure and potent. The method of distillation, growing and harvesting standards, plant species, even the region of the world from which it comes, greatly affect the content of the essential oil. Much like the raw materials entering a factory completely determine the end product, an Oil Touch is effective if the essential oil used has consistent and whole chemistry.

WHAT IS THE OIL TOUCH TECHNIQUE

Oil Touch is an interaction between nature's chemistry and neurology (brain and healing communication system). It supports the body to move toward a healing state. Health is created as the body achieves and maintains balance. This balance can be interrupted by heightened stress, environmental toxins, or traumas. Oil Touch promotes balance so healing can continue and is recommended as an integral part of preventive care even for healthy people.

Oil Touch is not a treatment for any specific disease or condition. The body's natural healing abilities are miraculous. Awakening these abilities in others is a simple and precious gift.

HOW DOES IT WORK

Balance in your body looks something like a series of connected teeter-totters. To illustrate, consider the process of standing up. In order for you to stand and walk, your body is maintaining a delicate balance between falling forward and falling backwards. Just like leaning too much to either side will make you fall over, your body inside is maintaining similar delicate balances. For example, your nervous system is either in a stressed state or a rested state. Like a teeter-totter, both sides can't be high at the same time. Your immune system is the same and will mirror the nervous system's actions. It is either moving infection out of your body or it is pushing it in deeper for you to deal with later. Your body works this way with regard to your senses too. When injured your body sends pain; we call this nociception. When it is not in pain, it sends good sensations we call proprioception. When all of these are in balance with each other you become more healthy and heal much better. Oil Touch can help restore this balance. It can be compared to re-booting a computer for optimal functioning. This condition is called homeostasis.

The Oil Touch Technique

Oil Touch technique is divided into four stages. Each stage supports a shift in how your body heals and adapts to stress and injury.

Step 1 shifts the nervous system from stress to rest. Step 2 encourages the body to move from the secondary immune system to the primary immune system. Step 3 reduces pain and inflammation. During the entire process, good feeling (proprioception) is stimulated. As the technique progresses, the effects compound, and a dramatic shift occurs in all three factors.

Once your recipient is in this state, they are ready for step 4. In this step, you nudge them back the other direction. The body takes over and finds its balance. This is why it is like re-booting a computer. You turn it off and then back on. The body knows where to stay to get the healing job done right.

In order to do this, you will need to learn a few easy skills and perform them in the right order.

Setting up for an Oil Touch:

You should find a quiet, comfortable place. Using a massage table is best. A headpiece that angles up and down can be helpful for comfort. You may wish to bolster the recipient's ankles with a rolled towel or blanket. Your goal is to make your recipient as comfortable as possible. Your recipient will need a blanket for warmth and modesty as they will need to remove their clothing from the waist up and lie face down on the table. They will have their arms at their sides with their shoes and socks off. They will remain in this position for the duration of the technique. Encourage the recipient to completely relax and receive.

Applying Oil

When applying oil, hold the bottle at a 45-degree angle over the recipient and let a drop fall onto the back. You will typically apply 3 to 4 drops along the spine. It is preferable to start at the low back and move up to the neck. In stage 4 you will apply a couple of drops to each foot.

Distributing the Oil

When distributing along the spine spread the oil from the base of the low back to the top of the head. This is done by gently using the pads of the finger tips. This is a very light touch and is complete when you have spread the oil along the spine with three passes.

Palm Circles through the Heart Area:

Making a triangle with the thumbs and first fingers, place your hands on the center of the back at the level of the heart. Slide the hands in a clockwise fashion over the skin, creating a circle about eight inches wide. Complete three circles and hold for a moment. After pausing, separate the hands, sliding them along the spine. One hand stops on back of the head while the other hand stops and rests just below the waistline. Pause, leaving your hands in this position. Connect with your recipient, and feel their breathing. Focus on being present with them to find a rhythm that is theirs and not yours.

The Alternating Palm Slide:

This movement is a rhythm created by sliding the hands along the surface of the skin. Stand to the side of the recipient, and place your hand on the low back with your fingers pointing away from you at the level just below their waistline. Place your palm against the far side of the spine. Slide your hand away from you with very mild pressure. That is the basic movement. Begin this motion with your fingertips at the spine and lower your palm to their skin as you slide your hand away from you. The slide ends when your hand starts to turn down the recipient's side. Follow your first slide with a second using your other hand and, while alternating hands, move up the body toward the head with each horizontal slide. Keep your touch very light and keep it rhythmic. It is kind of like mowing a lawn, one stroke overlapping the other as it moves up the back toward the head. This movement continues up the back, the shoulders, the neck, and finally up on the head until you reach the level just above the ears.

Repeat this three times, beginning each time at the waistline. Move to the recipient's other side, and complete three passes on the opposite side.

5 Zone Activation:

Imagine broad vertical pinstripes running from the waistline to the shoulders five to the left of the spine and five to the right running parallel with the spine. The two-inch area directly on either side of the spine is Zone 1. The spaces on both sides directly adjacent to Zone 1 are Zone 2 and so forth. Zone 5 is the farthest out, located on both sides at the angle of the ribs where they start to turn down to the recipient's sides. Standing at the head of the table, place both hands on either side of the spine at the waistline as close together as you can. Drag your palms with light pressure up the spine, allowing your fingers to trail behind like the train of a wedding dress. Continue this motion through the neck and head, allowing your hands to gently continue the motion lightly to the crown of the head. That completes Zone 1. Now move to Zone 2. Place your hands at the waistline again, but separate them about two inches (this is Zone 2). Pull your palms up toward the shoulders in a straight line as you did for Zone 1. However, once your hands reach the shoulders, turn the fingertips in, drag your palms out along the shoulder blade, rotate the

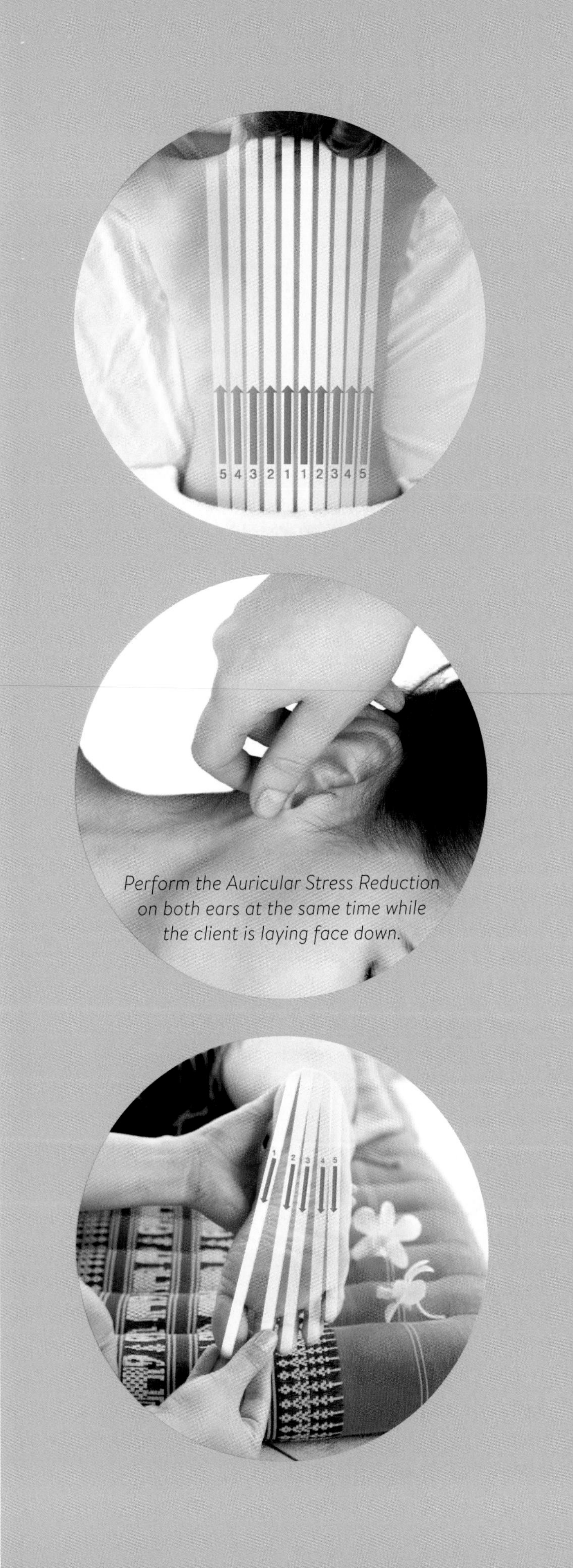

Perform the Auricular Stress Reduction on both ears at the same time while the client is laying face down.

fingers out, and slide them under the front of the shoulders as you drag your palms lightly back to toward the spine, continue up the neck and head as you did for Zone 1. Repeat for Zones 3, 4, and 5 as you did for zone 2, starting with your hands on the zone just outside the previous one. Complete just one pass per zone.

Auricular Stress Reduction:

Stand at the head of the table. Using your thumbs and forefingers, take hold of both earlobes. Massage them in a circular motion, much like you might rub a penny. Massage along the edge of the ears from the lobe to the top. Drag your fingers back down to the earlobe and repeat three times.

Thumb Walk Tissue Pull:

Stand at your recipient's side near the hips. Place your hands on the back at the waistline with your thumbs on the muscles running directly on either side of the spine. In a circular motion with your thumbs, massage the muscle on either side as you walk up the spine in an alternating fashion until you reach the back of the head. Repeat three times.

Autonomic Balance on the Feet:

There are three steps for the feet. Apply the oils (wild orange and peppermint) together, and spread on the bottom of the foot. You may wish to apply some fractionated coconut oil here as well.

Grip the foot with your hands and, using a circular motion with your thumbs similar to the thumb tissue pull, wipe the oil into the skin. Start at the side of the heel and move across it horizontally, then move down one half inch and work your way across the other direction almost like you are tilling a garden. Repeat this pattern until you reach the end of the forefoot. You will have just pushed the oil quickly into the skin.

Divide the foot into five zones, just like on the back. The strip running from the heal to the big toe is Zone 1, the strip including the second toe is Zone 2, and so forth. To trigger the reflexes in the foot, place one thumb near the other thumb, starting at the heel on the inside (Zone 1), walk down the foot, pushing into the bottom of the foot with the thumbs using medium pressure. Let one thumb trail the other thumb, so each spot is triggered twice. Complete one pass for each of the five zones, continuing to the tips of the toes.

Gripping the foot, swipe down each zone with your thumb as you slightly compress the foot with your hand. Similar to lightly milking a cow, alternating your hands, swipe Zone 1 three times and then continue through all five zones. Make one pass.

Complete these steps again on the second foot.

The Lymphatic Pump:

If your recipient falls asleep let them sleep, or perform the Lymphatic Pump. This will help them get moving again and be less disoriented when they arise. Do this by taking both feet in the hands, saddling your thumbs just in front of the heel at the arch. Push toward the head crisply one time, giving them a forward shake. Their body will rebound back toward you. Repeat the motion, matching the rebound. Create a pulse going back and forth. Do this for about ten seconds and repeat a couple of times.

STEP 1 Balance®
- Apply & distribute oil
- Heart Area Circles

Lavender
- Apply & distribute oil
- Alternating Palm Slide
- 5-Zone Activation
- Auricular Stress Reduction

STEP 2 Melaleuca
- Apply & distribute oil
- Alternating Palm Slides
- 5-Zone Activation

On Guard®
- Apply & distribute oil
- Alternating Palm Slides
- 5-Zone Activation
- Thumb Walk Tissue Pull

STEP 3 AromaTouch®
- Apply & distribute oil
- Alternating Palm Slides
- 5-Zone Activation

Deep Blue®
- Apply & distribute oil
- Alternating Palm Slides
- 5-Zone Activation
- Thumb Walk Tissue Pull

STEP 4 Wild orange & Peppermint
- Apply oil to feet
- Autonomic Balance on feet
- Apply & distribute oil to spine
- Heart Area Circles
- Lymphatic Pump

tips

- If for some reason a particular essential oil cannot be used, do not substitute it with another oil. Just remove it from the technique and use fractionated coconut oil on that stage.
- The Oil Touch technique is designed to be performed on a massage table. If you do not have access to one, adapt, and do the best you can.
- Once you establish contact with your recipient, stay in contact with at least one hand on the body at all times.
- You can use fractionated coconut oil at any time during this process, but if you are using it to lubricate the skin you are pressing too hard. You should be able to perform this on dry skin. Complete the following steps in order, referencing the descriptions above.

What To Do When an Oil Doesn't Seem To Be Working

Although temporarily frustrating or bewildering, occasionally essential oil choices seem insignificant. Oils have undeniably potent chemistry and are capable of impacting the body in significant and meaningful ways, yet an oil chosen may still not work due to a number of circumstances. Consider the following ideas to assist you in identifying ways to enhance results from your essential oil use.

APPLICATION METHOD – There are three basic ways to use essential oils: aromatic, topical, and internal. Each method impacts the body and its numerous layers and parts in different ways. For example, to eliminate a respiratory infection, both topical and internal use may be needed to address the multiple facets of that temporary issue. As the condition progresses, a change in application methods may be called for. Pay attention to body cues and adjust as needed. Take a moment to consider the variety of aspects of any situation and how you can address them by using more than one oil in more than one way. For further and detailed knowledge on how to use essential oils, refer to *Application Methods* (pg. 16). Also consider learning a special method, *The Oil Touch Technique,* taught on pg. 19.

FREQUENCY OF USE – A best rule of essential oil use is: use less more often. With the powerful chemistry packed in every drop, a little goes a long way. For example, 1-2 drops of an oil every 20-30 minutes (e.g. stomach flu or food poisoning, sprained ankle) or every 1-2 hours (e.g. cold & flu, exhaustion) until desired relief is achieved, is likely to far more effective and fast-acting then 10 drops used one time per day. The body can only chemically process so much at any given time. Therefore, repeated usage such as every 15-30 minutes for an acute condition and 2-4 times daily for a more chronic or long-lasting condition, is far more likely to drive the results you are looking for. Wondering where to start with your oil use for a particular health goal? Consider: a couple drops, a couple times per day, in, on or around you.

OIL SELECTION – One of the most beautiful things about essential oils is if a legitimate reference or expert says, "This oil does that," it is likely true more than 80% of the time. For the occasional time that it doesn't work, it's often found that a user simply doesn't know the true nature of their issue and therefore made a less effective choice. Perhaps a stomach issue was suspected so a favorite digestion blend was used yet no effect. Really the gall bladder was the issue and grapefruit and geranium oils would have been the better selection. Additionally, as individual's body chemistry, composition, and level of health differ, effects of oils differ as well. See the section in this book titled *How to Know Which Oils to Use* on page15, to familiarize yourself with methods of selection. You will discover there are many ways to approach oil choices throughout the book. Dive in and become your own expert user!

QUALITY – The quality of essential oils offered in the marketplace radically differ. Many are adulterated and deceptively labeled. For example, it's common practice for a broker to dilute pure oils with synthetic counterparts or add a less expensive oil (e.g. add cypress to frankincense or lemongrass to melissa) to extend oil yield. Though the dealer may have found momentary profit, their choice drastically reduces the effects for the end user. Because chemical profiles have some similarities, common methods of testing for quality are inferior and won't identify the adulterations, allowing for the deception to prevail. Choosing a reliable source is imperative to safe and successfully use. Be sure to read *Why Quality Matters* on pg. 13.

BODY HEALTH – What many people don't realize is that essential oils work chemically with and within the body. Acting as messenger molecules, or what is known as exogenous ligands, they enter the body like a hired outside management consulting firm, rapidly identifying what's needed and immediately sending instructions to whatever department need be involved. Imagine if no one were in the office, nothing would get done. If the body is void of necessary nutrition, then the oils have no way for their powerful instructions to be carried out. One of the most crucial habits for successful results from essential use is to make a healthy diet and use of high-quality dietary supplements vital daily wellness habits.

LIFESTYLE – Assessing lifestyle and self-care patterns may be necessary to find the culprits of compromise. Lack of sleep or proper consumption of water, poor quality drinking water, lack of regular exercise or movement, consumption of acid-producing beverages (e.g. carbonated or caffeinated drinks), high levels of stress, etc. may be overriding the benefits of essential oils as the demands on the body are simply too high. It is possible the ratio of offense (e.g. a bad habit) is higher than the ratio of solutions (e.g. good habits like essential oil use) and frequency of oil use may need to be adjusted along with overall changes in personal choices. Oils can make up for a 'myriad of sins', but lifestyle has a significant impact on the results you experience.

Safety and Storage

Essential oils are concentrated, potent plant extracts and should be used with reasonable care. Essential oils are very effective and safe when used appropriately. It takes a small amount to induce a powerful therapeutic benefit.

Never apply oils directly to the eyes or ear canals. After applying essential oils, avoid eye contact or the touching of sensitive areas. If essential oils enter the eyes, place a drop of carrier oil, such as fractionated coconut oil or olive oil, in the eye and blink until the oils clear. Never use water, as oils and water don't mix or help with dilution.

Some oils are "warm," creating a heat-like sensation on the skin, and should be diluted with a carrier oil when used topically. These oils can include birch, cassia, cinnamon, clove, eucalyptus, ginger, lemongrass, oregano, peppermint, thyme, and wintergreen. With babies, children, and those with sensitive skin or compromised health, it is particularly important to exercise caution or avoidance with these same oils, as they can be a temporary irritant or overly potent to delicate skin. When using these oils internally, it is best to consume in a gelatin or vegetable capsule.

Some oils contain furocoumarins, a constituent that can cause skin to be photosensitive. Photosensitive oils react to sources of UV rays. The higher the concentration of furanoids, the greater the sensitivity. Oils with concentrated amounts of furanoids include any cold pressed citrus oil such as bergamot, grapefruit, lemon, and lime, with lesser amounts in wild orange. Internal use of these oils is typically not a problem. It is best to wait a minimum of twelve hours after topical application of photosensitive oils before being exposed to UV rays.

Most essential oils applied topically and used reasonably are safe to be used during pregnancy and nursing. Some individuals prefer to avoid internal use during pregnancy and some use essential oils only aromatically during the first trimester. Several oils may be helpful during and after delivery. Internal use of peppermint essential oil should be avoided while nursing as it may reduce milk supply.

Persons with critical health conditions should consult a healthcare professional or qualified aromatherapist before using essential oils and may want to research individual oils prior to using them. In general, those with low seizure thresholds should be cautious in using or avoid altogether fennel, basil, rosemary, birch, and any digestive blend that contains fennel. Those with high blood pressure should be cautious with or avoid thyme and rosemary essential oils.

On occasion a person may experience a cleansing reaction, which takes place when the body is trying to rid itself of toxins faster than it is able. When this happens, increase water intake and decrease application of essential oils, or change the area of application.

safety tips

- Avoid eyes, ears, and nose
- Avoid exposing area of application to sunlight for 12 hours after using citrus oils topically
- Dilute oils for children and sensitive skin with fractionated coconut oil
- Refer to the Natural Solutions section for specific oil safety and usage

The compounds in essential oils are best preserved when stored and kept from light, heat, air, and moisture. Long exposure to oxygen begins to break down and change the chemical makeup of an essential oil. This process is called oxidation and an oil is said to have "oxidative breakdown." This process is slow but can, over time, promote skin sensitivity with some oils. Citrus oils and blue tinted oils are especially prone to this breakdown.

For optimum storage of these types of oils for longer than a year, refrigeration is best. A carrier oil can also be added to slow the oxidation process. Keep air space in essential oil bottles to a minimum for those that are opened and kept for a long period of time. Consider combining partially used bottles. Some oils with compounds such as sesquiterpenes (e.g. myrrh and sandalwood) can actually get better with age. Essential oils can be flammable and should be kept clear of open flame, spark, or fire hazards.

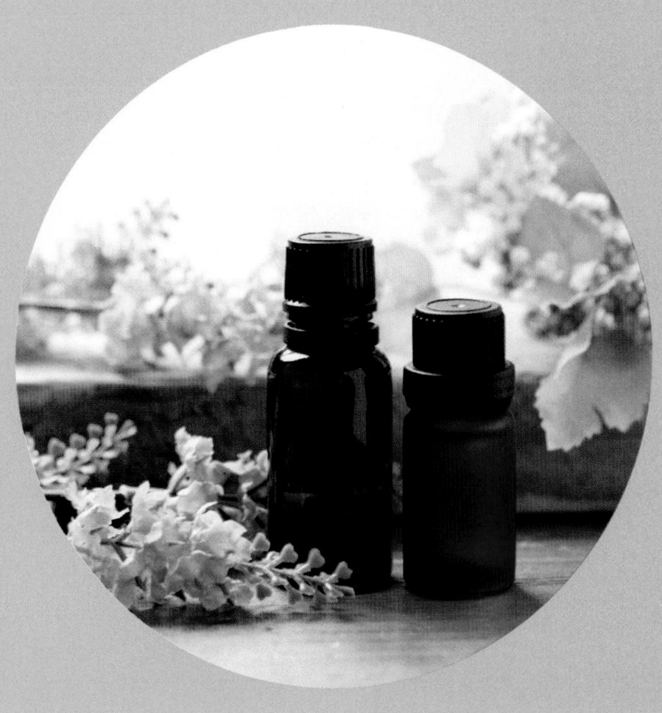

QUICK REFERENCE

How to Use This Section

Ailments are listed alphabetically. Start by searching for the ailment in question, then note the recommended essential oils for each ailment. Oils are listed in order of most common use. Application methods are also recommended for each oil. Here are key applications for you to choose from:

= Aromatic:

Diffuse with a diffuser.
Inhale from cupped hands (your personal diffuser).
Inhale directly from oil bottle.
Wear an oil pendant.

= Topical:

Apply to area of pain or concern (dilute as needed).
Apply under nose, to back of neck, forehead, or wrists.
To affect entire body, apply to bottoms of feet, spine, or navel.
To affect specific organs or body systems, apply to reflex points on the ears, hands, or feet (See *Reflexology* pg. 474).
*Add warm compress or massage to drive oils deeper into body tissues.

= Internal:

Put a drop or two of oil under tongue, hold a few seconds, and then swallow.
Drink a few drops in a glass of water.
Put a few drops of oil in an empty capsule and swallow.
Put a drop of oil on the back of your hand and lick.

For more specific instruction, see *Application Methods* on page 16. For more in-depth information, see *Be a Power User* on page 462.

Frequency:
For acute conditions use every fifteen to twenty minutes until symptoms subside, then apply every two to six hours as needed. For chronic or ongoing conditions, repeat one to two times per day, typically a.m. and p.m.

For more information on a particular ailment, see the corresponding *Body Systems* page.

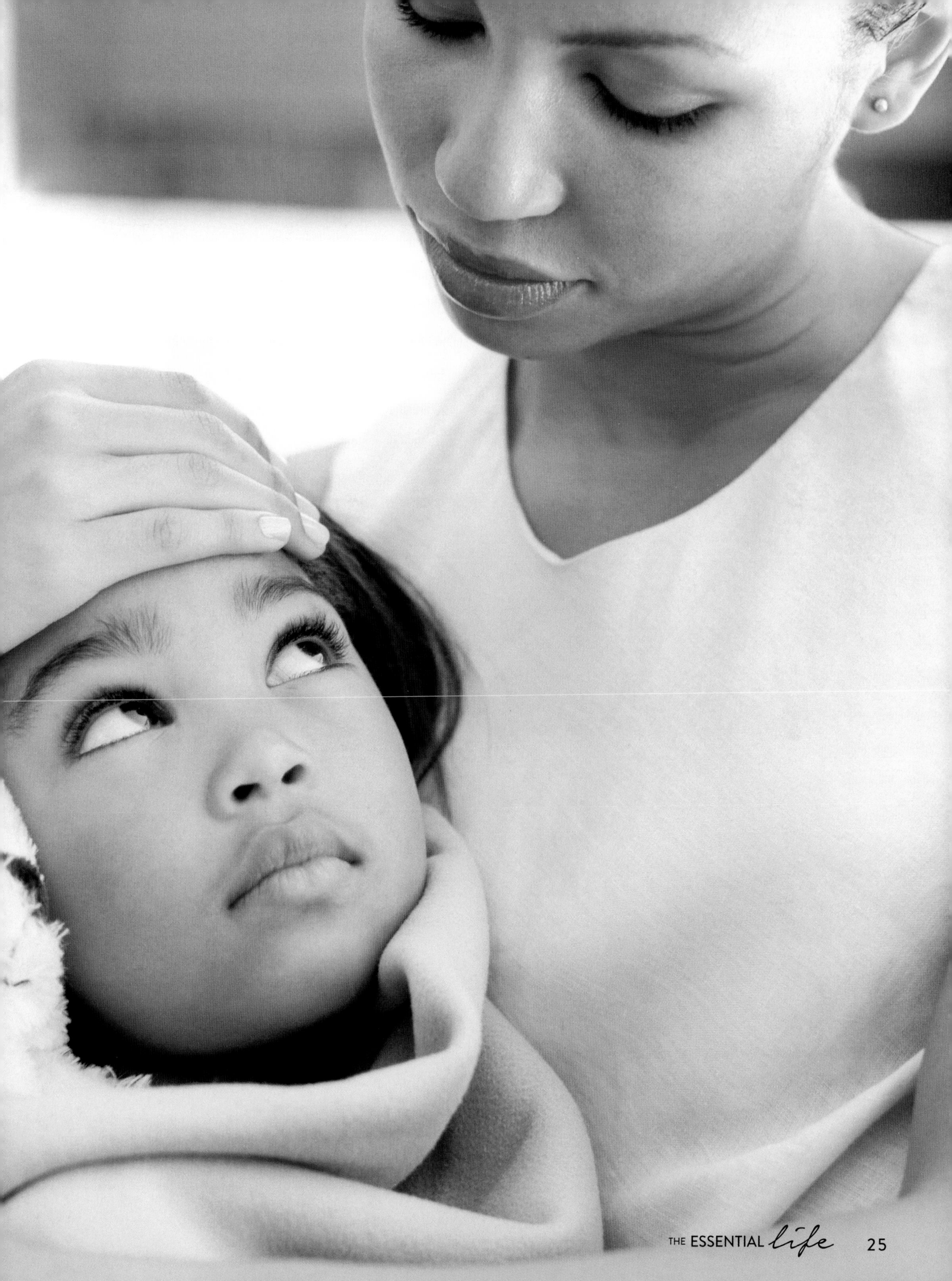

Ailments Index A-Z

STEPS: **1** Look up ailment. **2** Choose one or more of the recommended oils. (Order of recommendation is left to right.) **3** Use oil(s) as indicated. **4** Learn more in corresponding body system/focus area. **5** Find more solutions at essentiallife.com

QUICK REFERENCE

AILMENT	RECOMMENDED OILS AND USAGE	BODY SYSTEM/FOCUS AREA
Abdominal Cramps	Constrictive intermittent abdominal discomfort resulting from the spasm of an internal organ. DigestZen® · peppermint · petitgrain · ginger · ClaryCalm®	Digestive & Intestinal pg. 275; Women's Health pg. 374; Pain & Inflammation pg. 334
Abnormal Sperm Morphology	Sperm with a double tail or no tail; a sperm head that is crooked, has double heads, or is too large. thyme · rosemary · clary sage · DDR Prime® · Zendocrine®	Men's Health pg. 316
Abscess (tooth)	A contained collection of liquefied tissue known as pus reacting as a defense to foreign material. clove · melaleuca · thyme · frankincense · Purify	Oral Health pg. 331
Absentmindedness	Preoccupation so great that the ordinary insistence on attention is avoided. InTune® · cedarwood · peppermint · patchouli · vetiver	Brain pg. 248; Focus & Concentration pg. 295
Abuse Trauma	Trauma caused by being intentionally harmed or injured by another person. melissa · Roman chamomile · Console® · frankincense · Elevation™	Mood & Behavior pg. 319; Limbic pg. 313
Ache	Pain identified by persistent and usually limited intensity. Deep Blue® · AromaTouch® · peppermint · wintergreen · cypress	Muscular pg. 323; Skeletal pg. 355; Pain & Inflammation pg. 334; Immune & Lymphatic pg. 299
Acidosis	Excess acid in the body due to the accumulation of acid or the depletion of alkaline reserves. Zendocrine® · helichrysum · lemon · fennel · DDR Prime®	Detoxification pg. 270
Acid reflux	A chronic digestive disease occurring when stomach acid or content flows back into the food pipe irritating the lining of the esophagus. DigestZen® · fennel · peppermint · ginger · lemon	Digestive & Intestinal pg. 275
Acne	A common skin disease identified by pimples that surface when pores of the skin become clogged. HD Clear® · melaleuca · sandalwood · Immortelle · arborvitae	Integumentary pg. 304; Endocrine pg. 284; Detoxification pg. 270
Acromegaly	Excess growth hormone production in the anterior pituitary gland after puberty. frankincense · Zendocrine® · Balance® · Peace® · rosemary	Endocrine pg. 284
Actinic Keratosis	A small rough reddish colored spot on the skin that comes from too much sun exposure. Immortelle · lavender · frankincense · sandalwood · geranium	Integumentary pg. 304
ADD/ADHD	A disorder characterized by short attention span, impulsivity, and in some cases hyperactivity. InTune® · vetiver · Peace® · lavender · Motivate®	Focus & Concentration pg. 295

Aromatic: Inhale from cupped hands or diffuse into the air.

Topical: Apply directly to affected area(s) or bottom of feet.

Internal: Take in a capsule, glass of water, or on/under tongue.

TIP For adults use 2-3 drops; for children use 1-2 drops.

AILMENT	RECOMMENDED OILS AND USAGE	BODY SYSTEM/FOCUS AREA
Addictions	The repeated involvement with a substance or activity, despite the potential substantial harm it may cause, because that involvement was (and may continue to be) pleasurable and/or valuable. copabia · helichrysum · black pepper · bergamot · cinnamon	Endocrine pg. 284; Autoimmune pg. 240
Addison's Disease	A long-term endocrine disorder in which the adrenal glands do not produce enough steroid hormones. clove · basil · cinnamon · Zendocrine® · rosemary	Endocrine pg. 284; Autoimmune pg. 240
Adrenal Fatigue	A decrease in the adrenal glands' ability produce a diversity of hormones essential to life, commonly caused by chronic stress. rosemary · basil · geranium · Zendocrine® · ylang ylang	Endocrine pg. 284; Energy & Vitality pg. 288
Age Spots	Flat tan, brown, or black spots that vary in size that usually appear on the face, hands, shoulders, and arms. Immortelle · frankincense · sandalwood · spikenard · petitgrain	Integumentary pg. 304
Agitation	A feeling of restlessness associated with increased motor activity. Serenity® · Deep Blue® · Peace® · Balance® · lavender	Mood & Behavior pg. 319; Focus & Concentration pg. 295
AIDS or HIV	A disease in which there is a severe loss of the body's cellular immunity, greatly lowering the resistance to infection and malignancy. cinnamon · On Guard® · melissa · melaleuca · DDR Prime®	Immune & Lymphatic pg. 299
Alcohol Addiction	The frequent intake of large amounts of alcohol, commonly noted by the impairment of regular functioning. helichrysum · Forgive® · cinnamon · Zendocrine® · Slim & Sassy®	Addictions pg. 230; Limbic pg. 313
Alertness	A measure of being mentally keen, active, and rapidly aware of one's environment. peppermint · rosemary · Motivate® · Breathe® · InTune®	Brain pg. 248; Focus & Concentration pg. 295; Energy & Vitality pg. 288
Alkalosis	Uncommonly high alkalinity of blood and body fluids. geranium · Balance® · On Guard® · Citrus Bliss® · rosemary	Detoxification pg. 270
Allergies (insect)	A hypersensitive reaction to an insect allergen. lavender · Purify · Roman chamomile · arborvitae · blue tansy	First Aid pg. 291; Integumentary pg. 304; Allergies pg. 234
Allergies (pet dander)	An overreaction of the immune system to ordinarily harmless pet dander resulting in skin rash, sneezing or wheezing. lavender · Roman chamomile · Zendocrine® · Breathe® · Purify	Allergies pg. 234
Allergies (respiratory)	Uncommon reactions of the respiratory system that arise in response to otherwise inoffensive substances. lavender · lemon · peppermint · Roman chamomile · Breathe®	Respiratory pg. 349; Allergies pg. 234; First Aid pg. 291; Digestive & Intestinal pg. 275
Alzheimer's Disease	A progressive neurological disease that destroys memory and other important mental functions. DDR Prime® · frankincense or black spruce · thyme · clove or tumeric · cilantro	Brain pg. 248

STEPS: 1 Look up ailment. 2 Choose one or more of the recommended oils. (Order of recommendation is left to right.) 3 Use oil(s) as indicated. 4 Learn more in corresponding body system/focus area. 5 Find more solutions at essentiallife.com

QUICK REFERENCE

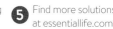

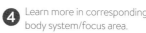

AILMENT	RECOMMENDED OILS AND USAGE	BODY SYSTEM/FOCUS AREA
Amenorrhea	Women who have missed at least three menstrual periods in a row, as do girls who haven't begun menstruation by age 15. ClaryCalm® · basil · rosemary · DDR Prime® · clary sage	Women's Health pg. 374
Amnesia	A partial or total loss of memory. peppermint · InTune® · Forgive® · Peace® · frankincense	Brain pg. 248
Amyotrophic Lateral Sclerosis (ALS) / Lou Gehrig's Disease	Also known as Lou Gehrig's disease, ALS is a neurological disease that attacks the nerve cells that control voluntary muscles. cypress · DDR Prime® · melissa · patchouli · frankincense	Autoimmune pg. 240; Nervous pg. 327; Muscular pg. 323
Anemia	A condition in which there is an unusually low number of red blood cells in the bloodstream. Zendocrine® · cinnamon · helichrysum · geranium · DDR Prime®	Cardiovascular pg. 256
Aneurysm	Excessive localized enlargement or ballooning of an artery caused by a weakening of the artery wall. helichrysum · cypress · DDR Prime® · frankincense · marjoram	Cardiovascular pg. 256
Anger	A strong feeling of annoyance, displeasure, or hostility. Forgive® · Balance® · helichrysum · Peace® · Serenity®	Mood & Behavior pg. 319; Children pg. 265; Focus & Concentration pg. 295;
Angina	A condition marked by severe pain in the chest caused by an inadequate blood supply to the heart. Douglas fir · thyme · basil · cinnamon · rosemary	Cardiovascular pg. 256
Ankylosing Spondylitis	An inflammatory arthritis affecting the spine and large joints. wintergreen · AromaTouch® · birch · Balance® · Deep Blue®	Skeletal pg. 355; Pain & Inflammation pg. 334
Anorexia	An emotional disorder characterized by an obsessive desire to lose weight by refusing to eat. grapefruit · patchouli · Slim & Sassy® · bergamot · Peace®	Eating Disorders pg. 280; Addictions pg. 230; Weight pg. 369
Anosmia	Loss of the sense of smell, usually caused by a nasal condition or brain injury. peppermint · basil · lemongrass · helichrysum · arborvitae	Respiratory pg. 349
Anthrax	A rare but serious bacterial illness typically affecting livestock but can be spread to humans affecting the intestines, skin, or lungs. oregano · melissa · thyme · clove · frankincense	Immune & Lymphatic pg. 299
Anxiety	A mental health disorder characterized by feelings of worry, nervousness, or fear that are strong enough to interfere with one's daily activities. Serenity® · Adaptiv® · lavender + wild orange · Peace® · Balance®	Mood & Behavior pg. 319; Stress pg. 363; Focus & Concentration pg. 295
Apathy	A lack of, absence, indifference, or suppression of emotion. ginger · Motivate® · Passion® · ylang ylang · Citrus Bliss®	Mood & Behavior pg. 319

Aromatic: Inhale from cupped hands or diffuse into the air.
Topical: Apply directly to affected area(s) or bottom of feet.
Internal: Take in a capsule, glass of water, or on/under tongue.
TIP For adults use 2-3 drops; for children use 1-2 drops.

AILMENT	RECOMMENDED OILS AND USAGE	BODY SYSTEM/FOCUS AREA
Appetite (loss of)	Absence of the desire to eat. Peace®, Slim & Sassy®, Console®, wild orange, cardamom	Digestive & Intestinal pg. 275; Stress pg. 363; Eating Disorders pg. 280; Weight pg. 369
Appetite (overactive)	Excessive feelings of hunger. Slim & Sassy®, grapefruit, ginger, cinnamon, peppermint	Weight pg. 369; Eating Disorders pg. 280; Addictions pg. 230
ARDS	Acute Respiratory Distress Syndrome is a condition in which fluid collects in the lungs' air sacs, depriving organs of oxygen. rosemary, melissa, eucalyptus, Breathe®, cardamom	Respiratory pg. 349
Arrhythmia	An irregularity in the strength or rhythm of the heartbeat. lavender, ylang ylang, basil, rosemary, melissa	Cardiovascular pg. 256
Arteriosclerosis	A chronic disease involving the thickening and hardening of the walls of the arteries, occurring typically in old age. black pepper, lemongrass, cinnamon, juniper berry, On Guard®	Cardiovascular pg. 256
Arthritic Pain	Inflammation and stiffness of the joints followed by pain, and swelling that can worsen with age. Deep Blue®, copaiba, turmeric, frankincense, black pepper	Skeletal pg. 355; Pain & Inflammation pg. 334
Arthritis (reactive)	A chronic form of arthritic joint pain and swelling triggered by an infection. Deep Blue®, lemongrass, On Guard®, AromaTouch®, wintergreen	Immune & Lymphatic pg. 299; Pain & Inflammation pg. 334; Autoimmune pg. 240; Skeletal pg. 355
Asthma	A respiratory condition characterized by spasms in the bronchi of the lungs, causing difficulty in breathing. Typically results from an allergic reaction or other forms of hypersensitivity. Breathe®, eucalyptus, rosemary, peppermint, cardamom	Respiratory pg. 349; Allergies pg. 234; Digestive & Intestinal pg. 275
Ataxia	Loss of the full control to coordinate bodily muscular movement. frankincense, sandalwood, helichrysum, marjoram, DDR Prime®	Brain pg. 248; Muscular pg. 323
Atherosclerosis	The increase of a waxy plaque on the inside of blood vessels. marjoram, lemongrass, Slim & Sassy®, cinnamon, On Guard®	Cardiovascular pg. 256
Athlete's Foot	A fungus infection that typically begins between the toes in which the skin starts cracking and peeling away, becoming itchy and sore. melaleuca, cinnamon, oregano, HD Clear®, arborvitae	Athletes pg. 237; Candida pg. 252; Integumentary pg. 304
Auditory Processing Disorder	A disorder affecting the ability to understand speech in noisy environments, follow directions, and distinguish between similar sounds. helichrysum, basil, Peace®, Douglas fir, DDR Prime®	Brain pg. 248; Nervous pg. 327
Autism / Asperger's	A serious developmental disorder, present from early childhood, that impairs the ability to communicate, interact, and regulate behavior. clary sage, Serenity®, Balance®, Zendocrine®, frankincense	Brain pg. 248; Mood & Behavior pg. 319; Nervous pg. 327

STEPS: **1** Look up ailment. **2** Choose one or more of the recommended oils. (Order of recommendation is left to right.) **3** Use oil(s) as indicated. **4** Learn more in corresponding body system/focus area. **5** Find more solutions at essentiallife.com

QUICK REFERENCE

AILMENT	RECOMMENDED OILS AND USAGE	BODY SYSTEM/FOCUS AREA
Autoimmune Disorder	A disease in which the body's immune system attacks healthy cells. DDR Prime®, turmeric, lemongrass, Zendocrine®, thyme	Autoimmune pg. 240
Autointoxication	Poisoning by toxins or metabolic waste formed within the body itself. Zendocrine®, cilantro, clove, geranium, thyme	Detoxification pg. 270; Weight pg. 369
Avoidant Restrictive Food Intake Disorder	A type of eating disorder where the consumption of certain foods is limited based on the food's appearance, smell, taste, texture, or a past negative experience with the food. Previously known as selective eating disorder (SED). Slim & Sassy®, patchouli, Passion®, Forgive®, bergamot	Eating Disorders pg. 280
Back Muscle Fatigue	A state of fatigue or loss of strength and/or muscle endurance following arduous activity associated with the accumulation of lactic acid in muscles. AromaTouch®, Deep Blue®, ginger, wintergreen, marjoram	Muscular pg. 323
Back Pain	A pain in the lumbar regions of the back varying in sharpness and intensity. Deep Blue®, copaiba, wintergreen, Siberian fir, frankincense	Pain & Inflammation pg. 334; Skeletal pg. 355; Muscular pg. 323
Back Stiffness	Persistent throbbing or stiffness anywhere along the spine, from the base of the neck to the tail bone. AromaTouch®, peppermint, Deep Blue®, Siberian fir, PastTense®	Pain & Inflammation pg. 334; Muscular pg. 323; Skeletal pg. 355
Bacteria	Single-celled microorganisms that can exist either as independent (free-living) organisms or as parasites (dependent on another organism for life) that thrive in diverse environments. melaleuca, oregano, cinnamon, Purify, cilantro	Immune & Lymphatic pg. 299
Bags Under the Eyes	The appearance of mild swelling or puffiness in the tissues under the eyes caused by fluid buildup. lime, Immortelle, juniper berry, cedarwood, Roman chamomile	Integumentary pg. 304; Sleep pg. 359
Balance Problems	Symptoms include light-headedness to dizziness and may be caused by viral or bacterial infections in the ear, a head injury, or blood circulation disorders that affect the inner ear or brain. rosemary, cedarwood, frankincense, ylang ylang, Douglas fir	Brain pg. 248; Cardiovascular pg. 256; Immune & Lymphatic pg. 299
Baldness	Having little or no hair on the scalp. DDR Prime®, ylang ylang, rosemary, thyme, clary sage	Integumentary pg. 304; Men's Health pg. 316
Basal Cell Carcinoma	A slow-growing form of skin cancer with a low metastatic risk. It is the most common skin cancer. DDR Prime®, frankincense, sandalwood, Zendocrine®, melissa	Cellular Health pg. 261; Integumentary pg. 304
Bed Bugs	Small, oval, brownish parasitic insects that live on the blood of animals or humans. TerraShield®, arborvitae, eucalyptus, Siberian fir, peppermint	On the Go pg. 450
Bed Sores	A painful reddened area of ulcerated skin caused by pressure and lack of movement. lavender, myrrh, geranium, frankincense, cypress	Integumentary pg. 304
Bed-wetting	Involuntary urination while asleep after the age at which bladder control typically happens. cypress, juniper berry, cinnamon, copaiba, Peace®	Children pg. 265; Urinary pg. 366; Mood & Behavior pg. 319

Aromatic: Inhale from cupped hands or diffuse into the air.
Topical: Apply directly to affected area(s) or bottom of feet.
Internal: Take in a capsule, glass of water, or on/under tongue.
TIP For adults use 2-3 drops; for children use 1-2 drops.

AILMENT	RECOMMENDED OILS AND USAGE	BODY SYSTEM/FOCUS AREA
Bee Sting	An injury caused by the venom of bees, usually followed by swelling and pain. Purify, lavender, Roman chamomile, clove, basil	First Aid pg. 291
Bell's Palsy	A weakness or paralysis of the muscles on one side of the face causing that side of the face to droop. Usually the result of a virus, respiratory, cranial, nerve or blood sugar issue. frankincense, basil, thyme, On Guard®, helichrysum	Nervous pg. 327; Immune & Lymphatic pg. 299; Muscular pg. 323
Benign Prostatic Hyperplasia	A noncancerous case of the prostate that causes overgrowth of the prostate tissue and obstructing urination. clary sage, thyme, DDR Prime®, juniper berry, sandalwood	Cellular Health pg. 261; Men's Health pg. 316
Binge Eating Disorder (BED)	A serious eating disorder characterized by recurrent episodes of compulsively consuming unusually large amounts of food quickly and feeling unable to stop. A person with BED will not use compensatory behaviors, such as self-induced vomiting or over-exercising after binge eating. Slim & Sassy®, cinnamon, Elevation™, Console®, Adaptiv® or cedarwood	Eating Disorders pg. 280; Digestive & Intestinal pg. 275; Weight pg. 369
Bipolar Disorder	A mood disorder characterized by extreme episodes of mania and depression. Individuals with severe episodes may experience psychotic symptoms. Also known as manic-depressive illness. melissa, Elevation™, Peace®, Serenity®, bergamot	Limbic pg. 313
Bladder Control	Urinary incontinence is unexpected loss of urine that is sufficient enough in regularity and amount to cause physical and/or emotional concern in the person experiencing it. Forgive®, thyme, rosemary, coriander, spearmint	Urinary pg. 366; Mood & Behavior pg. 319
Bladder Infection (Cystitis)	Inflammation of the urinary bladder, typically due to a bacterial infection of the bladder. lemongrass, wintergreen, oregano, thyme, lemon	Urinary pg. 366; Candida pg. 252
Bleeding	The discharge of blood from the vascular system as a result of harm to a blood vessel. helichrysum, yarrow, geranium, lavender, frankincense	Cardiovascular pg. 256; First Aid pg. 291
Blisters from Sun	A local swelling of the skin that contains watery fluid, caused by overexposure to the sun. lavender, myrrh, Immortelle, helichrysum, sandalwood	Integumentary pg. 304
Blisters on Feet	A local swelling of the skin that contains watery fluid, caused by moisture or friction. myrrh, frankincense, patchouli, lavender, eucalyptus	Integumentary pg. 304
Bloating	Any abnormal general swelling of the abdominal area with symptoms including feeling full, tight, or in pain. peppermint, ginger, DigestZen® or Tamer™, fennel, Slim & Sassy®	Digestive & Intestinal pg. 275; Holiday pg. 446
Blood Clot	A thickened lump in the blood formed to stop bleeding, such as at the site of a cut. coriander, DDR Prime®, fennel, helichrysum, AromaTouch®	Cardiovascular pg. 256
Blood Pressure (high)/ Hypertension	A condition in which the force of the blood against the artery walls is too strong. Commonly known as hypertension. marjoram, ylang ylang, celery seed, petitgrain, clove	Cardiovascular pg. 256; Urinary pg. 366

QUICK REFERENCE

STEPS: **1** Look up ailment. **2** Choose one or more of the recommended oils. (Order of recommendation is left to right.) **3** Use oil(s) as indicated. **4** Learn more in corresponding body system/focus area. **5** Find more solutions at essentiallife.com

QUICK REFERENCE

AILMENT	RECOMMENDED OILS AND USAGE	BODY SYSTEM/FOCUS AREA
Blood Pressure (low)/Hypotension	A condition in which a person's blood pressure is not satisfactory for tissue oxygenation. Commonly known as hypotension. thyme, DDR Prime®, basil, rosemary, lime	Cardiovascular pg. 256; Endocrine pg. 284
Blood Sugar (low) Hypoglycemia	An uncommonly low concentration of glucose in the circulating blood. cassia, lavender, Zendocrine®, cypress, juniper berry	Blood Sugar pg. 245; Endocrine pg. 284
Blood Sugar (high) Hyperglycemia	A condition in which the body does not handle glucose effectively. Blood glucose levels may fluctuate outside of the body's optimal blood glucose range. coriander, cinnamon, cassia, Slim & Sassy®, fennel	Blood Sugar pg. 245; Endocrine pg. 284;
Blood Toxicity	Occurs when bacteria causing infection in another part of the body enters the bloodstream. geranium, Zendocrine®, celery seed or turmeric, DDR Prime®, frankincense	Blood Sugar pg. 245; Endocrine pg. 284;
Body Dysmorphic Disorder	A type of chronic mental illness in which one cannot stop thinking about a minor or imagined flaw in appearance. Appearance seems so shameful that the individual does not want to be seen by anyone. clove, frankincense, arborvitae, DDR Prime®, rosemary	Brain pg. 248; Limbic pg. 313; Mood & Behavior pg. 319
Body Myositis	Inflammation of a muscle, especially a voluntary muscle, characterized by pain, tenderness, and sometimes spasm in the affected area. marjoram, lemongrass, AromaTouch®, cypress, wintergreen	Muscular pg. 323; Pain & Inflammation pg. 334
Body Odor	An unpleasant smell produced by bacteria on the skin that breaks down the acids in perspiration. petitgrain, cilantro, Purify, Zendocrine®, arborvitae	Detoxification pg. 270; Personal Care pg. 454
Boils	Painful, pus-filled bumps under the skin caused by infected, inflamed hair follicles. myrrh, Immortelle, melaleuca, Purify, lavender	Integumentary pg. 304
Bone Pain	Any pain that is associated with an unusual condition within a bone, such as osteomyelitis. Deep Blue®, helichrysum, wintergreen, Siberian fir, birch	Skeletal pg. 355; Pain & Inflammation pg. 334
Bone Spurs	Bony projections that develop along the edges of bones. Also referred to as osteophytes. cypress, eucalyptus, basil, lemongrass, wintergreen	Skeletal pg. 355
Brain Fog	A condition defined by decreased clarity of thought, confusion, and forgetfulness which may lead to minor depression. peppermint, Motivate®, rosemary, lemon, Douglas fir	Brain pg. 248; Focus & Concentration pg. 295;
Brain Injury	A comprehensive term for any injury occurring in the brain that is typically traumatic. frankincense, Balance®, DDR Prime®, Forgive®, bergamot	Brain pg. 248
Breastfeeding (milk supply)	Giving a baby milk from the breast, suckling or nursing. clary sage, ClaryCalm®, basil, fennel, geranium	Pregnancy, Labor & Nursing pg. 341

Aromatic: Inhale from cupped hands or diffuse into the air.
Topical: Apply directly to affected area(s) or bottom of feet.
Internal: Take in a capsule, glass of water, or on/under tongue.
TIP For adults use 2-3 drops; for children use 1-2 drops.

AILMENT	RECOMMENDED OILS AND USAGE	BODY SYSTEM/FOCUS AREA
Breathing Problems	A condition in which respiratory function is insufficient to meet the needs of the body when physical activity increases. Breathe® (Topical); eucalyptus (Topical); Douglas fir (Topical); cardamom (Topical, Internal); peppermint (Topical, Internal)	Respiratory pg. 349
Brittle Nails	Brittleness with breakage of finger or toenails. myrrh (Topical); lemon (Topical); frankincense (Topical); grapefruit (Topical); eucalyptus (Topical)	Integumentary pg. 304
Broken Bone	A break in continuity of bone. Siberian fir (Topical); birch (Topical); helichrysum (Topical, Internal); Deep Blue® (Topical); wintergreen (Topical)	Skeletal pg. 355
Broken Capillaries	Break in the tiniest blood vessels with the smallest diameter. cypress (Topical); geranium (Internal, Topical); helichrysum (Internal, Topical); yarrow (Internal, Topical); lavender (Internal, Topical)	Cardiovascular pg. 256
Broken Heart Syndrome	A severe but short-term condition in which extreme stress can lead to heart muscle failure, feeling similar to the sensation of a heart attack. Console® (Aromatic, Topical); ylang ylang (Aromatic, Topical, Internal); geranium (Aromatic, Topical, Internal); lime (Aromatic, Topical, Internal); clary sage (Aromatic, Topical, Internal)	Cardiovascular pg. 256; Mood & Behavior pg. 319; Emotional pg. 378
Bronchitis	Inflammation of the lining of bronchial tubes, which carry air to and from the lungs, resulting in hoarseness and a vigorous cough. Breathe® (Topical); eucalyptus (Topical); cardamom (Internal, Topical); thyme (Internal, Topical); On Guard® (Internal, Topical)	Respiratory pg. 349; Immune & Lymphatic pg. 299
Bruise	An injury appearing as an area of discolored skin on the body, caused by a blow or impact rupturing underlying blood vessels. Siberian fir (Topical); Roman chamomile (Topical); geranium (Topical); helichrysum (Topical); Deep Blue® (Topical)	Cardiovascular pg. 256; Integumentary pg. 304; First Aid pg. 291
Bruised Muscles	A deep bruise on a muscle can occur when the underlying fibers and connective tissue of the muscle are crushed without breaking through the skin. Also known as a contusion. Deep Blue® (Topical); helichrysum (Topical); birch (Topical); AromaTouch® (Topical); Siberian fir (Topical)	Muscular pg. 323
Buerger's Disease	A blood vessel disease with swelling and blockage from blood clots. Typically caused by smoking. clary sage (Aromatic, Topical, Internal); arborvitae (Aromatic, Topical); cypress (Aromatic, Topical); lemongrass (Aromatic, Topical, Internal); cinnamon (Aromatic, Topical, Internal)	Cardiovascular pg. 256
Bulimia	A chronic eating disorder involving repeated episodes of uncontrolled eating followed by self-induced purging. melissa (Internal, Topical); cinnamon (Internal, Topical, Aromatic); grapefruit (Topical, Internal, Aromatic); Forgive® (Topical, Aromatic); patchouli (Topical, Internal, Aromatic)	Eating Disorders pg. 280; Addictions pg. 230
Bunions	A bony bump that forms on the joint at the base of the big toe. eucalyptus (Topical); cypress (Topical); ginger (Topical); wintergreen (Topical); basil (Topical)	Skeletal pg. 355
Burns	Injuries to tissues caused by electricity, radiation, heat, friction, or chemicals. lavender (Topical); peppermint (Topical); Immortelle (Topical); myrrh (Topical); helichrysum (Topical)	Integumentary pg. 304; First Aid pg. 291
Bursitis	Inflammation of the fluid-filled pads that act as cushions to the joints. Deep Blue® (Topical); birch (Topical); wintergreen (Topical); Siberian fir (Topical); cypress (Topical)	Skeletal pg. 355

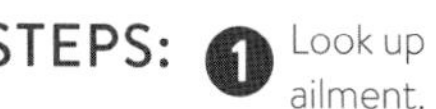

STEPS: 1 Look up ailment. 2 Choose one or more of the recommended oils. (Order of recommendation is left to right.) 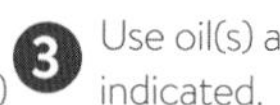 3 Use oil(s) as indicated. 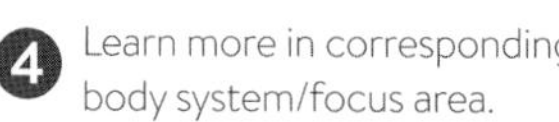 4 Learn more in corresponding body system/focus area. 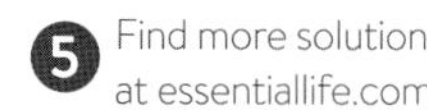 5 Find more solutions at essentiallife.com

AILMENT	RECOMMENDED OILS AND USAGE	BODY SYSTEM/FOCUS AREA
Calcified Spine	A spine that is hardened by calcium deposits. birch · DDR Prime® · lemongrass · Deep Blue® · wintergreen	Skeletal pg. 355
Calluses	A thickened and hardened part of the skin or soft tissue, especially in an area that has been subjected to friction. Roman chamomile · cypress · HD Clear® · Siberian fir · oregano	Integumentary pg. 304
Cancer (bladder)	A growth of abnormal cells forming masses called tumors in the bladder. frankincense · DDR Prime® · lemongrass · rosemary · cinnamon	Cellular Health pg. 261
Cancer (blood)	A cancer of blood-forming tissues, hindering the body's ability to fight infection. Also known as Leukemia. frankincense · DDR Prime® · turmeric · helichrysum · Siberian fir	Cellular Health pg. 261
Cancer (bone)	A skeletal malignancy typified by a mass of unusual cells growing in a bone. frankincense · DDR Prime® · helichrysum · lemongrass & turmeric · Siberian fir	Cellular Health pg. 261
Cancer (brain)	A mass or growth of abnormal cells in the brain or central spinal canal. arborvitae · DDR Prime® · clove · frankincense · thyme	Cellular Health pg. 261
Cancer (breast)	The development of uncontrolled breast cells causing a malignant tumor. Usually only occurs in women but sometimes is present in men. frankincense · thyme · grapefruit · DDR Prime® · eucalyptus	Cellular Health pg. 261
Cancer (cervical)	A malignant tumor of the cervix, the lowermost part of the uterus. frankincense · DDR Prime® · Siberian fir · tangerine · sandalwood	Cellular Health pg. 261
Cancer (colon)	A cancer of the colon or rectum, located at the digestive tract's lower end. geranium · Zendocrine® · rosemary · turmeric · DDR Prime®	Cellular Health pg. 261
Cancer (follicular thyroid)	Occurs when cells in the thyroid undergo genetic changes (mutations). The mutations allow the cells to multiply and grow rapidly. Characterized by capsular invasion and vascular invasion by tumor cells. rosemary · clary sage · frankincense · tangerine · sandalwood	Cellular Health pg. 261
Cancer (hurthle cell thyroid)	An unusual form of cancer that affects the thyroid gland. melissa · frankincense · DDR Prime® · clary sage · thyme	Cellular Health pg. 261
Cancer (liver)	A rare form of cancer that is either initiated in the liver or spread from another part of the body. Zendocrine® · turmeric · tangerine · DDR Prime® · clove	Cellular Health pg. 261
Cancer (lung)	Malignant growths of the lung believed to be caused by inhaled carcinogens. frankincense · Breathe® · DDR Prime® · rosemary · thyme	Cellular Health pg. 261

Aromatic: Inhale from cupped hands or diffuse into the air.
Topical: Apply directly to affected area(s) or bottom of feet.
Internal: Take in a capsule, glass of water, or on/under tongue.
TIP For adults use 2-3 drops; for children use 1-2 drops.

AILMENT	RECOMMENDED OILS AND USAGE	BODY SYSTEM/FOCUS AREA
Cancer (lymph)	A cancer characterized by the formation of solid tumors in the immune system which impact white blood cells. Also known as lymphoma. lemongrass, frankincense, DDR Prime®, tangerine, turmeric	Cellular Health pg. 261
Cancer (mouth)	Cancer that develops in any part of the mouth typically induced by tobacco use, heavy alcohol use, and HPV. Also known as oral cavity cancer. myrrh, turmeric, DDR Prime®, frankincense, black pepper	Cellular Health pg. 261
Cancer (ovarian)	A cancer that begins in the female organs that produce eggs (ovaries). frankincense, tangerine, Zendocrine®, grapefruit, DDR Prime®	Cellular Health pg. 261
Cancer (pancreatic)	An uncontrolled multiplication of cells in the pancreas (the organ lying behind the lower part of the stomach) that impacts endocrine and exocrine functions. turmeric, DDR Prime®, cinnamon, Zendocrine®, frankincense	Cellular Health pg. 261
Cancer (prostate)	A disease in which cells in the prostate gland become atypical and start to grow uncontrollably, forming tumors. thyme, Zendocrine®, oregano, turmeric, DDR Prime®	Cellular Health pg. 261
Cancer (skin)	The abnormal growth of skin cells caused by genetics, chemical carcinogens, fumes, or overexposure to the sun or other sources of ultraviolet light. Immortelle, sandalwood, turmeric, tangerine, frankincense	Cellular Health pg. 261
Cancer (throat)	A group of cancers of the mouth, sinuses, nose, tonsils or throat. frankincense, DDR Prime®, thyme, lavender, cinnamon	Cellular Health pg. 261
Cancer (thyroid)	A disease in which malignant cells are found in the tissues of the thyroid gland. DDR Prime®, turmeric, thyme, lemongrass, frankincense	Cellular Health pg. 261
Cancer (tongue)	A form of cancer that begins in the cells of the tongue. geranium, DDR Prime®, turmeric, frankincense, Zendocrine®	Cellular Health pg. 261
Cancer (uterine)	Cancer of the womb (uterus) is a common cancer that affects the female reproductive system. It's also called uterine cancer and endometrial cancer. clary sage, DDR Prime®, tumeric, frankincense, geranium	Cellular Health pg. 261
Candida	A variety of yeast like fungi that are generally part of the normal flora of the mouth, skin, intestinal tract, and vagina, but can cause an array of infections. thyme, oregano, DDR Prime®, pink pepper & melaleuca, arborvitae	Candida pg. 252
Canker Sores	Small white or yellow colored sores or ulcers that grow inside the mouth. They are painful to the touch, self-healing, and can reappear. On Guard®, myrrh, black pepper, melaleuca, birch	Oral Health pg. 331

STEPS: 1 Look up ailment. 2 Choose one or more of the recommended oils. (Order of recommendation is left to right.) 3 Use oil(s) as indicated. 4 Learn more in corresponding body system/focus area. 5 Find more solutions at essentiallife.com

AILMENT	RECOMMENDED OILS AND USAGE	BODY SYSTEM/FOCUS AREA
Cardiovascular Disease	Heart conditions that include diseased vessels, structural problems, and blood clots. AromaTouch® · black pepper · basil · cypress · PastTense®	Cardiovascular pg. 256
Carpal Tunnel Syndrome	A numbness, tingling, and weakness in the hand and arm caused by a pinched nerve in the wrist. Deep Blue® · lemongrass · cypress · ginger · copaiba	Nervous pg. 327
Cartilage Injury	An injury to the fibrous, flexible, and connective tissue found in adults resulting in joint pain and stiffness. Deep Blue® · lemongrass · helichrysum · birch · wintergreen	Skeletal pg. 355; Athletes pg. 237
Cataracts	A medical condition in which the lens of the eye becomes progressively opaque, resulting in blurred vision and may lead to blindness. lemongrass · clary sage · cardamom · Immortelle · black pepper	Nervous pg. 327
Cavities	The decayed part of a tooth that has developed into a hole. clove · On Guard® · birch · wintergreen · helichrysum	Oral Health pg. 331
Celiac Disease	A genetic disease defined by malabsorption of nutrients from food and an immune response to eating gluten (a protein found in wheat, barley, and rye). lemongrass · DigestZen® · cardamom · Slim & Sassy® · Zendocrine®	Autoimmune pg. 240; Digestive & Intestinal pg. 275
Cellulite	A fatty deposit causing an uneven or dimpled appearance, commonly found around the thighs. eucalyptus · grapefruit · Slim & Sassy® · spikenard · lemongrass	Detoxification pg. 270; Weight pg. 369
Chapped Skin	Skin that is rough, cracked, or reddened by exposure to cold or excessive moisture. Roman chamomile · petitgrain · sandalwood · Immortelle · myrrh	Integumentary pg. 304; Baby pg. 388
Chemical Imbalance	A disequilibrium of one or more neurotransmitters. Chemical imbalances show a strong association with mental illnesses. Zendocrine® · Elevation™ · cilantro · DDR Prime® · melissa	Brain pg. 248; Mood & Behavior pg. 319
Chemical Sensitivity Reaction	An allergic condition attributed to extreme sensitivity to various environmental chemicals, such as water, food, air, building materials, or fabrics. Zendocrine® · cilantro · Purify · coriander · arborvitae	Allergies pg. 234
Chest Infection	An infection in the airways or lungs, commonly resulting in coughing up yellow or green phlegm (thick mucus). Zendocrine® · On Guard® · Breathe® · eucalyptus · melaleuca	Immune & Lymphatic pg. 299
Chest Pain	A sharp, burning, or crushing sensation in the chest. marjoram · Douglas fir · AromaTouch® · basil · On Guard®	Cardiovascular pg. 256; Stress pg. 363; Respiratory pg. 349; Pain & Inflammation pg. 334
Chicken Pox	A highly contagious viral infection causing an itchy, blister-like rash on the skin and fever. Most cases occur in children under the age of 16. melaleuca · patchouli · blue tansy · On Guard® · thyme	Immune & Lymphatic pg. 299

Aromatic: Inhale from cupped hands or diffuse into the air.
Topical: Apply directly to affected area(s) or bottom of feet.
Internal: Take in a capsule, glass of water, or on/under tongue.
TIP For adults use 2-3 drops; for children use 1-2 drops.

AILMENT	RECOMMENDED OILS AND USAGE	BODY SYSTEM/FOCUS AREA
Chiggers	Red bugs similar to a tick from the Trombiculidae family; however, chiggers do not burrow into the skin but have feeding structures that insert into the skin. lemongrass (Topical); Purify (Aromatic, Topical); TerraShield® (Topical); lavender (Topical); clove (Topical, Internal)	Parasites pg. 338; First Aid pg. 291
Cholera	A bacterial disease causing severe diarrhea and dehydration, usually spread in water. cinnamon (Internal, Topical, Aromatic); rosemary (Internal, Topical, Aromatic); Zendocrine® (Internal, Topical, Aromatic); Breathe® (Topical, Aromatic); melissa (Topical, Internal, Aromatic)	Immune & Lymphatic pg. 299
Cholesterol (high)	Abnormally high levels of cholesterol (a waxy substance found in the fats in the blood) that can lead to an increased risk of heart disease. Slim & Sassy® (Internal, Topical); lemongrass (Internal, Topical); coriander (Internal, Topical); cinnamon (Internal, Topical); lemon (Internal, Topical)	Cardiovascular pg. 256
Chondromalacia Patella	Damage to the cartilage under the kneecap, also known as "runner's knee." AromaTouch® (Topical); helichrysum (Topical, Internal); birch (Topical); Siberian fir (Topical); sandalwood (Topical)	Skeletal pg. 355
Chronic Fatigue	A disease characterized by profound fatigue, sleep abnormalities, pain, and other symptoms that are made worse by exertion. rosemary (Internal, Topical, Aromatic); Passion® (Topical, Aromatic); geranium (Internal, Topical); black pepper (Internal, Topical); basil (Internal, Topical, Aromatic)	Energy & Vitality pg. 288; Limbic pg. 313; Endocrine pg. 284
Chronic Pain	Persistent pain that lasts weeks to years from a disease or unknown cause. Deep Blue® (Topical); helichrysum (Topical, Internal); copaiba (Topical, Internal); wintergreen (Topical); peppermint (Topical, Internal)	Pain & Inflammation pg. 334; Muscular pg. 323; Skeletal pg. 355; Sleep pg. 359
Circulation (Poor)	A poor circulation of blood and lymph through the body, consisting of the heart, blood vessels, blood, lymph, and the lymphatic vessels and glands. cypress (Topical); AromaTouch® (Topical); geranium (Topical, Internal); cassia (Internal, Topical); peppermint (Topical, Internal)	Cardiovascular pg. 256
Cirrhosis	A continual degenerative disease in which normal liver cells are impaired and then replaced by scar tissue. Zendocrine® (Internal, Topical); geranium (Internal, Topical, Aromatic); myrrh (Internal, Topical); helichrysum (Internal, Topical); marjoram (Internal, Topical)	Digestive & Intestinal pg. 275
Clogged Pores	A plug of sebum and keratin within a hair follicle. HD Clear® (Topical); cedarwood (Topical); juniper berry (Topical, Internal); DDR Prime® (Topical, Internal); petitgrain (Topical, Internal)	Integumentary pg. 304
Club Foot	A condition in which one or both feet are twisted into an unusual position before birth. basil (Topical); AromaTouch® (Topical); wintergreen (Topical); marjoram (Topical, Internal); helichrysum (Topical, Internal)	Skeletal pg. 355; Muscular pg. 323
Cold Body Temperature	A body temperature below 97.6 degrees Fahrenheit (36.4 degrees Celsius). "Normal" body temperature is 98.6 degrees Fahrenheit (37 degrees Celsius). Passion® (Topical); cypress (Topical); AromaTouch® (Topical); wintergreen (Topical); eucalyptus (Topical)	Cardiovascular pg. 256
Cold (common)	A viral infection of the upper respiratory system including the throat, nose, and sinuses. Sneezing, coughing, and temperature are common symptoms. On Guard® (Topical, Internal, Aromatic); black pepper (Topical, Internal); Breathe® (Topical, Aromatic); thyme (Topical, Internal, Aromatic); yarrow (Topical, Internal, Aromatic)	Immune & Lymphatic pg. 299
Cold Hands/Feet/Nose	Relative to problems with poor blood circulation, small blood vessels, and the body attempting to maintain its natural core temperature. AromaTouch® (Topical); Motivate® (Topical, Aromatic); cassia (Topical, Internal); DDR Prime® (Topical, Internal); Passion® (Topical, Aromatic)	Cardiovascular pg. 256

STEPS: **1** Look up ailment. **2** Choose one or more of the recommended oils. (Order of recommendation is left to right.) **3** Use oil(s) as indicated. **4** Learn more in corresponding body system/focus area. **5** Find more solutions at essentiallife.com

AILMENT	RECOMMENDED OILS AND USAGE	BODY SYSTEM/FOCUS AREA
Cold Sores/Fever Blisters	Infection with the herpes simplex virus around the border of the lips. melaleuca, melissa, arborvitae, On Guard®, bergamot	Oral Health pg. 331; Immune & Lymphatic pg. 299
Colic	Persistent, unexplained crying in a healthy baby between two weeks and five months of age. DigestZen® or Tamer™, fennel, Roman chamomile, Serenity® or Adaptiv®, ylang ylang	Children pg. 265; Digestive & Intestinal pg. 275; Baby pg. 388
Colitis	An inflammatory reaction in the colon or large bowel, often resulting in ulcers. cardamom, DigestZen®, peppermint, copaiba, ginger	Digestive & Intestinal pg. 275
Coma	A state of severe unresponsiveness, in which an individual shows no voluntary movement or behavior. frankincense, spikenard, vetiver, ginger, cedarwood	Brain pg. 248; Blood Sugar pg. 245
Concentration (poor)	The inability to focus the mind or concentrate. InTune®, vetiver & lavender, Peace®, cedarwood, Motivate®	Focus & Concentration pg. 295; Brain pg. 248
Concussion	A trauma-induced change in mental status with or without a brief loss of consciousness. frankincense, sandalwood, cedarwood, clove, petitgrain	Athletes pg. 237; Brain pg. 248
Confidence (lack of)	The low belief that you have in yourself and your abilities. Self-esteem affects how you think and act, how you feel about others, and how successful you are in life. bergamot, Motivate®, patchouli, jasmine, Passion®	Mood & Behavior pg. 319
Confusion	Impaired orientation in terms of time, place, or person; a disturbed mental state or lack of clarity or discernment. peppermint, frankincense, rosemary, Douglas fir, Motivate®	Mood & Behavior pg. 319; Focus & Concentration pg. 295;
Congenital Heart Disease	An abnormality in the heart's structure that develops before birth. geranium, ylang ylang, helichrysum, basil, Passion®	Cardiovascular pg. 256
Congestion	The existence of an unusual amount of fluid in a vessel or organ causing obstruction. lemon, peppermint, DigestZen®, Breathe®, eucalyptus	Respiratory pg. 349; Allergies pg. 234; Digestive & Intestinal pg. 275
Conjunctivitis (Pink Eye)	Inflammation or infection of the outer membrane of the eyeball and the inner eyelid. lavender, melaleuca, Douglas fir, rosemary, melissa	Immune & Lymphatic pg. 299; Children pg. 265
Connective Tissue Injury	Injury to tissue that binds and supports other connecting ligaments and tendons. lemongrass, helichrysum, wintergreen, Siberian fir, clove	Skeletal pg. 355; Muscular pg. 323
Constipation	A condition in which bowel movements occur less often than normal or consist of hard, dry stools that are painful and difficult to pass. DigestZen® or Tamer™, marjoram, Zendocrine®, ginger, peppermint	Digestive & Intestinal pg. 275; Children pg. 265
Convalescence	Recuperation time spent recovering from an illness or medical treatment. petitgrain, frankincense, spikenard, Console®, myrrh	Brain pg. 248

Aromatic: Inhale from cupped hands or diffuse into the air.

Topical: Apply directly to affected area(s) or bottom of feet.

Internal: Take in a capsule, glass of water, or on/under tongue.

TIP For adults use 2-3 drops; for children use 1-2 drops.

AILMENT	RECOMMENDED OILS AND USAGE	BODY SYSTEM/FOCUS AREA
Convulsions	A sudden violent contraction of a group of muscles. Also referred to a seizures. petitgrain, sandalwood, spikenard, frankincense, clary sage	Brain pg. 248
Corns	Thick and hardened layers of skin caused by friction and pressure, usually found on a toe. arborvitae, lemon, DDR Prime®, clove, ylang ylang	Integumentary pg. 304
Cortisol Imbalance	An imbalance in the naturally produced cortisol hormone generated from the adrenal glands that helps the body use sugar and fat for energy, and to manage stress. geranium, Adaptiv®, ylang ylang, black spuce, petitgrain	Endocrine pg. 284
Cough	A strong release of air from the lungs that can be heard. Coughing protects the respiratory system by clearing it of secretion and irritants. Breathe®, rosemary, DigestZen®, cardamom, lemon	Respiratory pg. 349;
Cough (whooping)	A highly contagious respiratory tract infection causing spasms of uncontrollable coughing. clary sage, Roman chamomile, Breathe®, blue tansy, cardamom	Respiratory pg. 349
Cradle Cap	White or yellow scaly patches on an infant's scalp. lavender, melaleuca, sandalwood, frankincense, Immortelle	Baby pg. 388
Cramps (intestinal)	An uncontrolled, spasmodic muscular contraction in the lower abdomen causing severe pain. DigestZen® or Tamer™, marjoram, ginger, turmeric, cardamom	Digestive & Intestinal pg. 275
Creutzfeldt-Jakob Disease	A degenerative neurological disorder that leads to dementia and is incurable. Also called a human form of mad cow disease. spikenard, frankincense, DDR Prime®, clove, Zendocrine®	Brain pg. 248; Immune & Lymphatic pg. 299
Crohn's Disease	A type of inflammatory bowel disease (IBD), followed by swelling and dysfunction of the intestinal tract. DigestZen® or Tamer™, copaiba, frankincense, peppermint, pink pepper	Autoimmune pg. 240 Digestive & Intestinal pg. 275
Croup	An upper airway infection that blocks breathing and has a distinctive barking cough, typical to children. thyme, lemon, eucalyptus, marjoram, Breathe®	Children pg. 265 Respiratory pg. 349
Crying Baby	A sudden, loud automatic or voluntary vocalization in response to fear, pain, or a startle reflex. Serenity®, Roman chamomile, Peace® or Tamer™, lavender, Console®	Children pg. 265
Cushing's Syndrome	A condition that occurs from exposure to inappropriately high cortisol levels over a long period of time. clove, black pepper, DDR Prime®, geranium, Citrus Bliss®	Endocrine pg. 284
Cuts	The separation of skin or other tissue created by a sharp edge. melaleuca, frankincense, geranium, lavender, helichrysum	First Aid pg. 291 Integumentary pg. 304

QUICK REFERENCE

STEPS: 1 Look up ailment. 2 Choose one or more of the recommended oils. (Order of recommendation is left to right.) 3 Use oil(s) as indicated. 4 Learn more in corresponding body system/focus area. 5 Find more solutions at essentiallife.com

AILMENT	RECOMMENDED OILS AND USAGE	BODY SYSTEM/FOCUS AREA
Cyst	An abnormal membranous sac or cavity in the body containing semisolid material or liquid. Douglas fir, On Guard®, lemon, thyme, cardamom	Integumentary pg. 304
Cystic Fibrosis	An inherited life-threatening disorder that damages the lungs and digestive system. eucalyptus, lemon, Douglas fir, Breathe®, frankincense	Respiratory pg. 349
Dandruff	A common scalp condition in which small pieces of dry skin flake off of the scalp. melaleuca, wintergreen, patchouli, rosemary, petitgrain	Integumentary pg. 304
Deep Vein Thrombosis	A blood clot in a deep vein, usually in the legs. frankincense, cypress, wintergreen, DDR Prime®, Zendocrine®	Cardiovascular pg. 256
Dehydration	A condition that occurs when the loss of body fluids, mostly water, exceeds the amount that is taken in. wild orange, lemon, Slim & Sassy®, Zendocrine®, juniper berry	First Aid pg. 291 Athletes pg. 237 Urinary pg. 366
Dementia	A chronic disorder of the mental processes caused by brain disease or injury and marked by memory disorders, personality changes, and impaired reasoning. DDR Prime®, frankincense, thyme, sandalwood, clove	Brain pg. 248
Dengue Fever	A mosquito-borne viral disease occurring in tropical and subtropical areas. Symptoms include fever, headache, muscle and joint pain, and a measle-like rash. eucalyptus, melissa, On Guard®, thyme, melaleuca	Immune & Lymphatic pg. 299
Dental Infection	An infection of the jaw, face mouth, or throat that begins as a tooth cavity or infection. clove, On Guard®, myrrh, melaleuca, cinnamon	Oral Health pg. 331
Depression	A mental state of altered mood associated by feelings of despair, sadness, and discouragement. melissa, Elevation™, Cheer®, frankincense, neroli	Mood & Behavior pg. 319 Limbic pg. 313 Pregnancy, Labor & Nursing pg. 341
Deteriorating Spine	A deterioration of the series of vertebrae that provide support and form a flexible bony case for the spinal cord. wintergreen, birch, DDR Prime®, helichrysum, Siberian fir	Skeletal pg. 355
Detoxification	The process of removing toxic substances or qualities from the body which is mainly carried out by the liver. Zendocrine®, grapefruit, Slim & Sassy®, clove, lemon	Detoxification pg. 270
Diabetes	A disease identified by an inability to process sugars in the diet, due to a decrease in or total absence of insulin production. cinnamon, coriander, Slim & Sassy®, juniper berry, cassia	Blood Sugar pg. 245
Diabetes (gestational)	A condition in which women without previously diagnosed diabetes show high blood glucose levels during pregnancy, especially after the third trimester. cinnamon, Zendocrine®, coriander, cassia, juniper berry	Pregnancy, Labor & Nursing pg. 341 Blood Sugar pg. 245

Aromatic: Inhale from cupped hands or diffuse into the air.
Topical: Apply directly to affected area(s) or bottom of feet.
Internal: Take in a capsule, glass of water, or on/under tongue.
TIP For adults use 2-3 drops; for children use 1-2 drops.

AILMENT	RECOMMENDED OILS AND USAGE	BODY SYSTEM/FOCUS AREA
Diabetic Sores	Open wounds or sores that normally occur on the bottom of the feet over weight-bearing areas. myrrh, lavender, patchouli, sandalwood, geranium	Integumentary pg. 304; Blood Sugar pg. 245
Diaper Rash	Irritation of the genitals, buttocks, lower abdomen, or thigh folds of an infant or toddler. Balance®, Roman chamomile, lavender, myrrh, patchouli	Baby pg. 388 Children pg. 265
Diarrhea	The fast movement of fecal matter through the intestines resulting in poor absorption of nutritive elements and persistent watery stools. DigestZen® or Tamer™, cardamom, black pepper, melaleuca, ginger	Digestive & Intestinal pg. 275
Digestive Discomfort	Symptoms may include bloating, diarrhea, gas, stomach pain, and stomach cramps. DigestZen® or Tamer™, cardamom, peppermint, ginger, fennel	Digestive & Intestinal pg. 275
Diphtheria	A contagious disease that commonly involves the throat, nose, and air passages. eucalyptus, Breathe®, On Guard®, DigestZen®, thyme	Respiratory pg. 349 Immune & Lymphatic pg. 299
Diverticulitis	An inflammation or infection in one or more small pouches in the digestive tract. DigestZen®, Slim & Sassy®, basil, DDR Prime®, AromaTouch®	Digestive & Intestinal pg. 275
Dizziness	A disturbed sense of relationship to space involving light-headedness and a sensation of unsteadiness. rosemary, peppermint, cedarwood, arborvitae, Zendocrine®	Cardiovascular pg. 256
Do Quervain's Tenosynovitis	Inflammation of the tendons on the side of the wrist at the base of the thumb. Commonly causes pain when grasping anything, turning the wrist, or making a fist. lemongrass, cypress, AromaTouch®, Deep Blue®, birch	Muscular pg. 323; Skeletal pg. 355
Down Syndrome	A genetic chromosome 21 disorder causing developmental and intellectual delays. Balance®, frankincense, melissa, DDR Prime®, cedarwood	Brain pg. 248
Drug Addiction	An overwhelming desire to continue taking a drug because of a particular effect, typically an alteration of mental status. Zendocrine®, Serenity®, peppermint, Motivate®, Purify	Addictions pg. 230
Dry Skin	Epidermis that lacks sebum or moisture, often identified by a pattern of fine lines, scaling, and itching. myrrh, petitgrain, patchouli, sandalwood, Immortelle	Integumentary pg. 304
Dumping Syndrome	A condition which occurs when food, especially sugar, moves from the stomach into the small bowel too quickly. Can develop after bypass stomach surgery. fennel, ginger, frankincense, helichrysum, DigestZen®	Digestive & Intestinal pg. 275
Dysentery	An infection of the intestines resulting in severe diarrhea with potential mucus and flood in feces. peppermint, ginger, On Guard®, myrrh, spearmint	Digestive & Intestinal pg. 275
Dysmenorrhea	The existence of painful cramps during menstruation. ClaryCalm®, clary sage, AromaTouch®, marjoram, thyme	Women's Health pg. 374

STEPS: 1 Look up ailment. 2 Choose one or more of the recommended oils. (Order of recommendation is left to right.) 3 Use oil(s) as indicated. 4 Learn more in corresponding body system/focus area. 5 Find more solutions at essentiallife.com

AILMENT	RECOMMENDED OILS AND USAGE					BODY SYSTEM/FOCUS AREA
Dysphagia	Difficulty swallowing foods or liquids arising from the throat or esophagus.					Digestive & Intestinal pg. 275; Oral Health pg. 331
	peppermint	arborvitae	black pepper	Serenity®	lavender	
Earache	A pain in the ear, sensed as dull, sharp, intermittent, burning or constant.					Respiratory pg. 349
	melaleuca	helichrysum	basil	lavender	rosemary	
Ear Infection	The existence and growth of bacteria or viruses in the ear.					Respiratory pg. 349
	On Guard®	thyme	basil	melaleuca	helichrysum	
Ear Mites	The existence of tiny parasites that feed on the wax and oils in the ear canal.					Parasites pg. 338; Respiratory pg. 349
	Purify	cedarwood	thyme	clove	melaleuca	
E. Coli	Bacteria found in the environment, foods, and intestines of warm-blooded organisms. Most E. Coli are harmless but some can cause serious infection.					Immune & Lymphatic pg. 299
	cinnamon	On Guard®	cassia	oregano	clove	
Eczema	Chronic or acute noncontagious inflammation of patches of the skin. Defined mainly by itchy red lesions that may become scaly and encrusted.					Integumentary pg. 304; Candida pg. 252
	cedarwood	neroli	HD Clear®	yarrow	black spruce	
Edema	A condition of unusually large fluid volume in the circulatory system or in tissues between the body's cells.					Cardiovascular pg. 256; Pregnancy, Labor & Nursing pg. 341
	cypress	lemon	lemongrass	celery seed or juniper berry	grapefruit	
Ehrlichiosis	A bacterial illness transmitted by ticks that causes flu-like symptoms ranging from mild body aches to severe fever.					Immune & Lymphatic pg. 299
	oregano	On Guard®	thyme	Zendocrine®	rosemary	
Electrical Hypersensitivity Syndrome	A group of symptoms caused by exposure to electromagnetic fields resulting in effects similar to allergic reactions.					Limbic pg. 313
	vetiver	frankincense	Zendocrine®	Balance®	Purify	
Emotional Trauma	An extremely disturbing, overwhelming, and stressful event that exceeds one's ability to cope that can lead to emotional impairment.					Mood & Behavior pg. 319; Limbic pg. 313
	frankincense	melissa	helichrysum	Forgive®	Peace®	
Emphysema	A progressive disease of the lungs that primarily causes shortness of breath due to over-inflation of the air sacs in the lung.					Respiratory pg. 349
	Douglas fir	Breathe®	eucalyptus	black pepper	frankincense	
Endometriosis	A condition in which part of the tissue similar to the lining of the uterus grows in other parts of the body.					Women's Health pg. 374
	clary sage	thyme	geranium	DDR Prime®	rosemary	
Endurance (poor)	A weak ability to continue an activity over an extended period of time.					Energy & Vitality pg. 288; Fitness pg. 440
	peppermint	basil	Slim & Sassy®	Breathe®	Motivate®	

Aromatic: Inhale from cupped hands or diffuse into the air.
Topical: Apply directly to affected area(s) or bottom of feet.
Internal: Take in a capsule, glass of water, or on/under tongue.
TIP For adults use 2-3 drops; for children use 1-2 drops.

AILMENT	RECOMMENDED OILS AND USAGE	BODY SYSTEM/FOCUS AREA
Energy (lack of)	The strength and vitality required for sustained physical or mental activity. peppermint, pink pepper, Citrus Bliss®, Motivate®, Passion®	Energy & Vitality pg. 288; Fitness pg. 440
Engorgement	A condition where the breasts become painfully firm and swollen from being overfull with milk. peppermint, AromaTouch®, Deep Blue®, PastTense®, ginger	Pregnancy, Labor & Nursing pg. 341;
Epilepsy	A neurological disorder defined by recurrent seizures with or without a loss of consciousness. spikenard, frankincense, clary sage, cedarwood, DDR Prime®	Brain pg. 248
Epstein-Barr (EBV)	The most common viral infection in humans and the best known cause of mononucleosis. Zendocrine®, rosemary, basil, ylang ylang, Passion®	Immune & Lymphatic pg. 299; Energy & Vitality pg. 288
Erectile Dysfunction	The inability to achieve or sustain an erection for satisfactory sexual activity; also known as impotence. cypress, Zendocrine®, sandalwood, ylang ylang, Passion®	Men's Health pg. 316; Intimacy pg. 448
Esophagitis	Inflammation that damages the tube running from the throat to the stomach (esophagus). peppermint, DigestZen®, frankincense, fennel, coriander	Digestive & Intestinal pg. 275
Estrogen Imbalance	A condition where a woman can have deficient or excessive levels of estrogen, but has little or no progesterone to balance its effects in the body. grapefruit, thyme, ClaryCalm®, Zendocrine®, basil	Women's Health pg. 374; Detoxification pg. 270
Exhaustion	A state of extreme loss of mental or physical abilities caused by illness or fatigue. Motivate®, Passion®, basil, Citrus Bliss®, wild orange	Energy & Vitality pg. 288; Endocrine pg. 284; Athletes pg. 237
Eyes (dry)	Dryness of the cornea caused by a deficiency of tear secretion resulting in a gritty sensation and irritation. sandalwood, frankincense, lavender, wild orange, Zendocrine®	Respiratory pg. 349
Eyes (swollen)	Uncommon enlargement of the eyes not due to an underlying disease. Immortelle, cypress, lemon, frankincense, Zendocrine®	Nervous pg. 327
Fainting	Loss of consciousness caused by a brief lack of oxygen to the brain. peppermint, rosemary, Citrus Bliss®, sandalwood, frankincense	Cardiovascular pg. 256; First Aid pg. 291
Fatigue	Physical and/or mental exhaustion that can be triggered by stress, overwork, medication, or physical and mental illness or disease. Motivate®, Passion®, basil, Citrus Bliss®, wild orange	Energy & Vitality pg. 288
Fear	A feeling of dread and agitation caused by the presence or imminence of danger or perceived threat. Peace® or Adaptiv®, Motivate®, Console®, bergamot, Passion®	Mood & Behavior pg. 319
Fear of Flying	A fear of being on an airplane or other flying vehicle, such as a helicopter, while in flight. It is also referred to as flying phobia. Causes great anxiety or panic attacks. Peace®, Balance®, Serenity®, cassia, On Guard®	Mood & Behavior pg. 319

STEPS: ❶ Look up ailment. ❷ Choose one or more of the recommended oils. (Order of recommendation is left to right.) 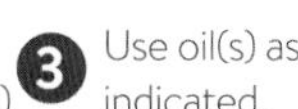 ❸ Use oil(s) as indicated. ❹ Learn more in corresponding body system/focus area. ❺ Find more solutions at essentiallife.com

AILMENT	RECOMMENDED OILS AND USAGE	BODY SYSTEM/FOCUS AREA
Fever	Any body temperature elevation above 100° F (37.8° C). peppermint · spearmint · eucalyptus · pink pepper · yarrow	Immune & Lymphatic pg. 299
Fibrillation	Fast, uncoordinated contractions of the lower or upper chambers of the heart. ylang ylang · black pepper · lime · marjoram · AromaTouch®	Cardiovascular pg. 256
Fibrocystic Breasts	Noncancerous changes that give a breast a lumpy or rope-like texture. frankincense · thyme · grapefruit · sandalwood · geranium	Endocrine pg. 284; Women's Health pg. 374
Fibroids (uterine)	Growths in the uterus which are non-cancerous (benign). sandalwood · frankincense · thyme · lemongrass · DDR Prime®	Immune & Lymphatic pg. 299; Women's Health pg. 374;
Fibromyalgia	A chronic neurosensory disorder defined by widespread joint stiffness, muscle pain, and fatigue with pain moving throughout the body. DDR Prime® · AromaTouch® · ginger · Deep Blue® · oregano	Muscular pg. 323
Fifth's Disease (Human Parvovirus B19)	A common and highly contagious childhood ailment causing a distinctive face rash. Sometimes referred to as "slapped-cheek disease." On Guard® · DDR Prime® · black pepper · oregano · Purify	Children pg. 265 Immune & Lymphatic pg. 299
Fleas	Small flightless external parasites of warm-blooded animals, living by hematophagy off the blood of mammals. lemon eucalyptus or eucalyptus · arborvitae · cedarwood · TerraShield® · lavender	Parasites pg. 338 First Aid pg. 291 Pets pg. 456
Floaters	Spots in vision that look like black or gray specks or strings that drift across the eye. Immortelle · sandalwood · frankincense · lavender · DDR Prime®	Nervous pg. 327
Flu (influenza)	A common viral infection of the nose and throat with common symptoms including chills, fever, runny nose, sore throat, muscle pain, and fatigue. On Guard® · thyme · melissa · yarrow · oregano	Immune & Lymphatic pg. 299 Children pg. 265
Focal Brain Dysfunction (brain injury)	Injuries confined to one specific area of the brain, often the result of a severe head trauma. helichrysum · frankincense · DDR Prime® · sandalwood · Balance®	Brain pg. 248 Limbic pg. 313
Focus	The ability to concentrate or direct one's attention or efforts. InTune® · frankincense & wild orange · vetiver & lavender · cedarwood · peppermint	Focus & Concentration pg. 295;
Food Addiction	A compulsive behavior of uncontrolled eating, often consuming food past the point of being comfortably full, followed by feelings of guilt and depression. grapefruit · Slim & Sassy® · peppermint · ginger · basil	Addictions pg. 230; Weight pg. 369
Food Poisoning	Illness caused by food contaminated with bacteria marked by diarrhea, cramps, nausea, vomiting, and fever. DigestZen® · Zendocrine® · melaleuca · clove · lemon	Digestive & Intestinal pg. 275; Parasites pg. 338; Immune & Lymphatic pg. 299

Aromatic: Inhale from cupped hands or diffuse into the air.
Topical: Apply directly to affected area(s) or bottom of feet.
Internal: Take in a capsule, glass of water, or on/under tongue.
TIP For adults use 2-3 drops; for children use 1-2 drops.

AILMENT	RECOMMENDED OILS AND USAGE	BODY SYSTEM/FOCUS AREA
Fragile Hair	Damaged or dry hair that is prone to breaking because of weakness. rosemary (Topical); DDR Prime® (Topical, Internal); thyme (Topical); cedarwood (Topical); geranium (Topical)	Integumentary pg. 304
Frozen Shoulder	A condition characterized by stiffness and pain in the shoulder joint. Also known as adhesive capsulitis. Deep Blue® (Topical); wintergreen (Topical); Siberian fir (Topical); lemongrass (Topical); birch (Topical)	Skeletal pg. 355; Muscular pg. 323
Fungal Skin Infection	Any inflammatory skin condition caused by a fungus, including athlete's foot, ringworm, jock itch, and yeast infections. melaleuca (Topical, Internal); HD Clear® (Topical); DDR Prime® (Topical, Internal); turmeric (Topical); myrrh (Topical, Internal)	Integumentary pg. 304; Candida pg. 252
Fungus	A condition in which primitive organisms duplicates by spores. oregano (Topical, Internal, Aromatic); DDR Prime® (Topical, Internal, Aromatic); cinnamon (Topical, Internal, Aromatic); melaleuca (Topical, Internal, Aromatic); arborvitae (Topical, Aromatic)	Immune & Lymphatic pg. 299; Candida pg. 252; Integumentary pg. 304
Gallbladder Issues	Disruptions that affect normal function of the gallbladder. geranium (Topical, Internal); grapefruit (Internal, Topical); Zendocrine® (Topical, Internal); Slim & Sassy® (Internal, Topical); turmeric (Internal, Topical)	Digestive & Intestinal pg. 275; Detoxification pg. 270
Gallbladder Infection	Generally categorized as inflammation of the gallbladder which can be caused by gallstones, excessive alcohol consumption, infections, or tumors causing bile buildup. Zendocrine® (Topical, Internal); Slim & Sassy® (Topical, Internal); On Guard® (Topical, Internal); cinnamon (Topical, Internal); rosemary (Topical, Internal)	Digestive & Intestinal pg. 275
Gallstones	Small stone-like masses in the gallbladder that are formed by excessive bile or calcium salt buildup. geranium (Internal, Topical); celery seed + juniper berry (Internal, Topical); lemon & grapefruit (Internal, Topical); Zendocrine® (Internal, Topical); wintergreen (Topical)	Digestive & Intestinal pg. 275
Ganglion Cyst	Round or oval lumps that most frequently develop in the wrist and are filled with a jelly-like fluid. DDR Prime® (Topical, Internal); frankincense (Topical, Internal); lemongrass (Topical, Internal); lemon (Topical, Internal); basil (Topical, Internal)	Skeletal pg. 355; Cellular Health pg. 261
Gangrene	The death or decay of a tissue or an organ caused by a lack of blood supply. cypress (Topical); AromaTouch® (Topical, Aromatic); Slim & Sassy® (Topical, Internal); cinnamon (Topical, Internal); myrrh (Topical)	Cardiovascular pg. 256; Immune & Lymphatic pg. 299; Blood Sugar pg. 245
Gas (flatulence)	An overabundance of gas in the digestive tract. ginger (Internal, Topical); DigestZen® or Tamer™ (Internal, Topical); black pepper (Internal, Topical); coriander (Internal, Topical); peppermint (Internal, Topical)	Digestive & Intestinal pg. 275
Gastritis	Inflammation of the lining of the stomach. Symptoms include abdominal discomfort or burning. peppermint (Internal, Topical); DigestZen® (Internal, Topical); coriander (Internal, Topical); petitgrain (Internal, Topical); fennel (Internal, Topical)	Digestive & Intestinal pg. 275
Gastroenteritis/ stomach flu	An intestinal infection marked by diarrhea, cramps, nausea, vomiting, and fever. cardamom (Internal, Topical); peppermint (Internal, Topical); ginger (Internal, Topical); DigestZen® (Internal, Topical); thyme (Internal, Topical)	Digestive & Intestinal pg. 275; Children pg. 265
Gastroesophageal Reflux Disease (GERD)	A digestive disease in which stomach acid or bile irritates the food pipe lining. Zendocrine® (Internal, Topical); lemon (Internal, Topical); DigestZen® (Internal, Topical); ginger (Internal, Topical); coriander (Internal, Topical)	Digestive & Intestinal pg. 275
Genital Warts	Growths in the genital area generated by a sexually transmitted papillomavirus. frankincense (Topical, Internal); arborvitae (Topical); thyme (Topical, Internal); melissa (Topical, Internal); geranium (Topical, Internal)	Immune & Lymphatic pg. 299; Women's Health pg. 374; Men's Health pg. 316; Integumentary pg. 304

STEPS: 1 Look up ailment. 2 Choose one or more of the recommended oils. (Order of recommendation is left to right.) 3 Use oil(s) as indicated. 4 Learn more in corresponding body system/focus area. 5 Find more solutions at essentiallife.com

AILMENT	RECOMMENDED OILS AND USAGE	BODY SYSTEM/FOCUS AREA
Giardia	An intestinal infection caused by a microscopic parasite that causes diarrheal illness. thyme, oregano, rosemary, cardamom, On Guard®	Parasites pg. 338 Digestive & Intestinal pg. 275
Gingivitis	Inflammation of the gums, identified by redness and swelling. myrrh, clove, On Guard®, frankincense, black pepper	Oral Health pg. 331
Glaucoma	A condition that is linked to a buildup of pressure inside the eye that can lead to loss of vision and even blindness. lemongrass, DDR Prime®, frankincense, black pepper, Immortelle	Nervous pg. 327
Goiter	A swelling of the thyroid gland, sometimes leading to a swelling of the larynx (voice box) or neck. myrrh, lemongrass, DDR Prime®, frankincense, patchouli	Autoimmune pg. 240; Endocrine pg. 284
Gout	A form of intense arthritis that causes severe swelling, tenderness, and pain in the joints. copaiba, lemongrass, turmeric, wintergreen, Deep Blue®	Skeletal pg. 355; Pain & Inflammation pg. 334
Grave's Disease	A thyroid dysfunction characterized by generalized overactivity of the entire gland. myrrh, frankincense, lemongrass, rosemary, Zendocrine®	Endocrine pg. 284
Grief	The commonly emotional response to an external and consciously recognized loss. Console®, Elevation™, Peace®, Serenity®, magnolia	Mood & Behavior pg. 319
Growing Pains	Pains in the joints and limbs of children or adolescents frequently appearing at night and often attributed to rapid growth. cypress, AromaTouch®, Siberian fir, marjoram, Deep Blue®	Children pg. 265; Muscular pg. 323
Gulf War Syndrome	A prominent condition affecting Gulf War Veterans with symptoms including fatigue, headaches, joint pain, indigestion, insomnia, dizziness, respiratory problems, and memory issues. frankincense, clove, thyme, patchouli, Passion®	Limbic pg. 313; Nervous pg. 327; Pain & Inflammation pg. 334; Digestive & Intestinal pg. 275
Gum Disease	Often appears in the form of gingivitis and bone loss to toxins produced by bacteria in plaque collecting along the gum line. On Guard®, myrrh, clove, melaleuca, cinnamon	Oral Health pg. 331
Gums (bleeding)	Gums that bleed during and after tooth brushing. myrrh, helichrysum, frankincense, clove, melaleuca	Oral Health pg. 331
H. Pylori	Spiral-shaped bacteria that grow in the digestive tract and have a tendency to attack the stomach lining. Responsible for the majority of stomach and intestine ulcers. cassia or cinnamon, black pepper, oregano, ginger, thyme	Immune & Lymphatic pg. 299; Digestive & Intestinal pg. 275
Hair (dry)	Occurs when the scalp does not produce enough oil to moisturize the hair or the hair does not absorb moisture. sandalwood, patchouli, geranium, copaiba, rosemary	Integumentary pg. 304

QUICK REFERENCE

Aromatic: Inhale from cupped hands or diffuse into the air.

Topical: Apply directly to affected area(s) or bottom of feet.

Internal: Take in a capsule, glass of water, or on/under tongue.

TIP For adults use 2-3 drops; for children use 1-2 drops.

AILMENT	RECOMMENDED OILS AND USAGE	BODY SYSTEM/FOCUS AREA
Hair Loss	The lack of all or a significant part of the hair on the head or other parts of the body. clary sage (topical, internal); DDR Prime® (topical); thyme (topical, internal); rosemary (topical); arborvitae (topical)	Integumentary pg. 304
Hair (oily)	Excessive sebum production caused by heredity, unhealthy eating habits, medications or improper hygiene. petitgrain (topical, internal); lemon (topical, internal); arborvitae (topical); rosemary (topical, internal); citronella (topical)	Integumentary pg. 304
Halitosis	The condition of having revolting-smelling breath. peppermint (internal); spearmint (internal); Slim & Sassy® (internal); On Guard® (internal); cardamom (internal)	Oral Health pg. 331
Hallucinations	Seeing, hearing, or experiencing sensations that appear to be real but are actually created within the mind. Balance® (aromatic, topical); frankincense (topical, aromatic, internal); cedarwood (topical, aromatic); Peace® (aromatic, topical); Serenity® (topical, aromatic)	Limbic pg. 313
Hand, Foot & Mouth Disease	A mild, contagious viral infection common in young children that is defined by sores in the mouth and a rash on the feet and hands. thyme (internal, topical); cinnamon (internal, topical); melaleuca (internal, topical); melissa (internal, topical); wintergreen (topical)	Immune & Lymphatic pg. 299
Hangover	A group of disagreeable physical effects, including thirst, nausea, headache, fatigue, and irritability, resulting from the heavy consumption of alcohol and/or certain drugs. Zendocrine® (internal, topical); Slim & Sassy® (internal); lemon (internal); geranium (internal); PastTense® (topical)	Addictions pg. 230; Detoxification pg. 270
Hardening of Arteries	A chronic condition defined by hardening and thickening of the arteries and the build-up of plaque on the arterial walls. black pepper (internal, topical); lemongrass (internal, topical); cinnamon (internal, topical); grapefruit (internal, topical); lemon (internal, topical)	Cardiovascular pg. 256
Hashimoto's Disease	An autoimmune disease of the thyroid gland in which immune cells mistakenly attack healthy thyroid tissue, causing inflammation. DDR Prime® (internal, topical); myrrh (topical, internal); Zendocrine® (topical, internal); lemongrass (topical, internal); peppermint (topical, internal, aromatic)	Endocrine pg. 284; Autoimmune pg. 240
Hay Fever	An allergic reaction caused by an abnormal sensitivity to airborne pollen, typically defined by nasal discharge and itchy/watery eyes. lavender (internal, topical, aromatic); lemon (internal, topical, aromatic); Breathe® (aromatic, topical); Purify (topical, aromatic); cilantro (internal, topical, aromatic)	Allergies pg. 234; Respiratory pg. 349
Head Lice	A wingless parasite that spends their entire lives on the human scalp and feeding exclusively on human blood. Transmitted in crowded conditions. cinnamon (topical); arborvitae (topical); eucalyptus (topical); rosemary (topical); thyme (topical, internal)	Parasites pg. 338; Integumentary pg. 304; First Aid pg. 291
Headache	A painful sensation in any part of the head, ranging from sharp to dull. PastTense® (topical); peppermint (topical, aromatic); Siberian fir (internal, topical); copaiba (topical, internal); frankincense (topical, aromatic)	Pain & Inflammation pg. 334; Nervous pg. 327; Muscular pg. 323; Women's Health pg. 374
Headaches (blood sugar)	Pain in the head caused by blood sugar levels being either too high or too low. cassia (internal); Zendocrine® (topical, internal); Slim & Sassy® (internal); On Guard® (internal); coriander (topical, aromatic, internal)	Blood Sugar pg. 245
Headache (sinus)	The buildup of pressure in the sinuses resulting in sensitive pressure which may worsen when bending over. basil (topical, aromatic, internal); cedarwood (topical, aromatic); rosemary (topical, internal, aromatic); peppermint (topical, aromatic, internal); eucalyptus (topical, aromatic)	Pain & Inflammation pg. 334; Respiratory pg. 349

STEPS: 1 Look up ailment. 2 Choose one or more of the recommended oils. (Order of recommendation is left to right.) 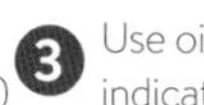 3 Use oil(s) as indicated. 4 Learn more in corresponding body system/focus area. 5 Find more solutions at essentiallife.com

AILMENT	RECOMMENDED OILS AND USAGE	BODY SYSTEM/FOCUS AREA
Headache (tension)	A common form of headache that is defined by severe muscle contractions triggered by overexertion or stress. PastTense® · peppermint · Deep Blue® · AromaTouch® · frankincense	Muscular pg. 323; Pain & Inflammation pg. 334
Hearing in a Tunnel	The ability to hear only one thing at a time with the accompanying sensation of hearing noise as if standing in a tunnel. helichrysum · lemon · clary sage · cardamom · Purify	Respiratory pg. 349
Hearing Problems	An impairment of any degree of the ability to apprehend sound. helichrysum · basil · lemon · frankincense · patchouli	Respiratory pg. 349
Heartburn	A burning pain or discomfort in the upper chest. DigestZen® · peppermint · cardamom · black pepper · Zendocrine®	Digestive & Intestinal pg. 275; Pregnancy, Labor & Nursing pg. 341
Heart Failure	Sudden interruption or inadequate supply of blood to the heart, commonly resulting from occlusion or obstruction of a coronary artery and often defined by severe chest pain. lemongrass · marjoram · ylang ylang · thyme · rosemary	Cardiovascular pg. 256
Heart Issues	Generally refers to conditions that involve narrowed or blocked blood vessels that can lead to a heart attack, chest pain or stroke. ylang ylang · cypress · marjoram · geranium · AromaTouch®	Cardiovascular pg. 256
Heat Exhaustion	A condition deriving from exposure to intense heat. Defined by dizziness, abdominal cramp, and prostration. Also called heat prostration. peppermint · lime · lemon · petitgrain · eucalyptus	First Aid pg. 291; Athletes pg. 237; Outdoors pg. 452
Heatstroke	A serious condition caused by the body overheating, usually as a result of prolonged exposure to or physical exertion in high temperatures. peppermint · petitgrain + lemon · black pepper · Zendocrine® · spearmint	First Aid pg. 291; Athletes pg. 237; Outdoors pg. 452
Heavy Metal Toxicity	The toxic buildup of heavy metals in the soft tissues of the body, most commonly associated with lead, mercury, arsenic and cadmium. cilantro · Zendocrine® · arborvitae · thyme · black pepper	Detoxification pg. 270
Hematoma	A localized swelling filled with blood emerging from a break in a blood vessel. cypress · helichrysum · geranium · AromaTouch® · lemongrass	Cardiovascular pg. 256
Hemochromatosis	An inherited blood disorder that causes the body to retain more than normal amounts of iron, leading often to cirrhosis of the liver. Zendocrine® · DDR Prime® · arborvitae · geranium · helichrysum	Digestive & Intestinal pg. 275
Hemophilia	One of a group of inherited bleeding disorders that cause abnormal or exaggerated bleeding and poor blood clotting. geranium · helichrysum · lavender · Roman chamomile · vetiver	Cardiovascular pg. 256

Aromatic: Inhale from cupped hands or diffuse into the air.

Topical: Apply directly to affected area(s) or bottom of feet.

Internal: Take in a capsule, glass of water, or on/under tongue.

TIP For adults use 2-3 drops; for children use 1-2 drops.

AILMENT	RECOMMENDED OILS AND USAGE	BODY SYSTEM/FOCUS AREA
Hemorrhage	An emergency condition in which a ruptured blood vessel causes bleeding that is difficult to control. helichrysum, yarrow, geranium, wild orange, lavender	Cardiovascular pg. 256
Hemorrhoids	Swollen and inflamed veins in the rectum and anus that cause discomfort and bleeding. cypress, helichrysum, yarrow, myrrh, Balance®	Cardiovascular pg. 256; Digestive & Intestinal pg. 275; Integumentary pg. 304; Pregnancy, Labor & Nursing pg. 341
Hepatitis	An inflammation of the liver, with accompanying liver cell damage or cell death. Created frequently by viral infection, but also by certain poisons, drugs, or chemicals. Zendocrine®, melaleuca, myrrh, helichrysum, geranium	Digestive & Intestinal pg. 275; Immune & Lymphatic pg. 299
Hernia, Hiatal	Occurs when part of the stomach pushes upward through the diaphragm. basil, arborvitae, helichrysum, ginger, juniper berry	Digestive & Intestinal pg. 275
Hernia, Incisional	A type of hernia caused by an incompletely-healed surgical wound. helichrysum, geranium, basil, arborvitae, cypress	Integumentary pg. 304
Herniated Disc	A condition which refers to a swelling or fragmented disk between the spinal bones. birch, wintergreen, Siberian fir, eucalyptus, AromaTouch®	Skeletal pg. 355; Pain & Inflammation pg. 334
Herpes Simplex	A virus causing contagious sores, most often around the mouth or on the genitals. melissa, melaleuca, peppermint, On Guard®, basil	Immune & Lymphatic pg. 299; Autoimmune pg. 240
Hiccups	The outcome of an involuntary, spasmodic contraction of the diaphragm followed by the closing of the throat. Zendocrine®, peppermint, Serenity®, arborvitae, basil	Respiratory pg. 349; Children pg. 265
Hives	An allergic skin reaction resulting in localized redness, swelling, and itching. Roman chamomile, rosemary, frankincense, peppermint, lavender	Allergies pg. 234; Children pg. 265
Hoarse Voice	An inflammation of the voice box from overuse, irritation, or infection. lemon or lime, ginger, frankincense or myrrh, peppermint, cinnamon	Oral Health pg. 331
Hodgkin's Disease	A malignant form of lymphoma defined by painless enlargement of the lymph nodes, liver, and spleen. cardamom, DDR Prime®, lemongrass, myrrh, frankincense	Cellular Health pg. 261
Hormonal Imbalance (female)	Subtle changes in the endocrine system with an estrogen decline causing a change in the ratio of estrogen to testosterone in the body. ClaryCalm®, geranium, clary sage, Whisper®, ylang ylang	Women's Health pg. 374; Detoxification pg. 270
Hormone Imbalance (male)	A testosterone decline with advancing age which causes a change in the ratio of estrogen to testosterone in the body. sandalwood, juniper berry, rosemary, Balance®, ylang ylang	Men's Health pg. 316; Detoxification pg. 270

STEPS: 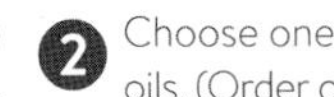 Look up ailment. 2 Choose one or more of the recommended oils. (Order of recommendation is left to right.) 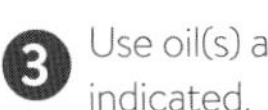 Use oil(s) as indicated. 4 Learn more in corresponding body system/focus area. 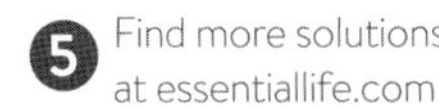 Find more solutions at essentiallife.com

AILMENT	RECOMMENDED OILS AND USAGE	BODY SYSTEM/FOCUS AREA
Hot Flashes	Troublesome warmth beginning in the upper chest, neck, and face followed by chills and sweating. ClaryCalm® · peppermint · eucalyptus · clary sage · PastTense®	Women's Health pg. 374
Huntington's Disease	A rare hereditary condition that causes mental deterioration and progressive jerky muscle movements that ends in dementia. DDR Prime® · frankincense · clove · thyme · rosemary	Brain pg. 248; Nervous pg. 327; Autoimmune pg. 240
Hydrocephalus	An unusual expansion of cavities (ventricles) within the brain that is caused by the accumulation of cerebrospinal fluid. spikenard · frankincense · basil · juniper berry · sandalwood	Brain pg. 248
Hyperactivity	Excessive or abnormally increased muscular activity or function. vetiver · lavender · InTune® · petitgrain · Peace®	Focus & Concentration pg. 295; Children pg. 265; Energy & Vitality pg. 288
Hyperpnea	Fast and deep respiration that appears normally after exercise or abnormally when associated with fevers or other disorders. peppermint · cardamom · patchouli · Breathe® · ylang ylang	Respiratory pg. 349
Hypersomnia	Excessive daytime sleepiness. People who have hypersomnia can fall asleep at any time, even while driving. Zendocrine® · peppermint · lemon · Douglas fir · eucalyptus	Sleep pg. 359; Focus & Concentration pg. 295; Energy & Vitality pg. 288
Hyperthyroidism	A medical condition that results from an excess of thyroid hormone in the blood. DDR Prime® · rosemary · myrrh · ginger · juniper berry	Endocrine pg. 284
Hypoglycemia	Occurs when blood glucose or blood sugar concentrations fall below a level necessary to support the body's need for energy stability at the cellular level. cassia · lavender · Zendocrine® · cypress · juniper berry	Blood Sugar pg. 245
Hypothermia	A condition in which core temperature drops below the needed temperature for normal metabolism and body functions which is defined as 35.0° C (95.0° F). cinnamon · clove · ginger · wintergreen · AromaTouch®	First Aid pg. 291
Hypothyroidism	A condition in which the thyroid gland doesn't produce enough thyroid hormone. clove · peppermint · blue tansy · lemongrass · myrrh	Endocrine pg. 284
Hysteria	A psychiatric disorder characterized by violent emotional outbreaks, disturbances of sensory and motor functions. Roman chamomile · melissa · neroli · Balance® · petitgrain	Mood & Behavior pg. 319; Women's Health pg. 374
Ichthyosis Vulgaris	An inherited skin condition that occurs when the skin does not shed its dead cells. Also known as "fish scale disease" because of the similar appearance. frankincense · geranium · sandalwood · patchouli · cedarwood	Integumentary pg. 304

Aromatic: Inhale from cupped hands or diffuse into the air.

Topical: Apply directly to affected area(s) or bottom of feet.

Internal: Take in a capsule, glass of water, or on/under tongue.

TIP For adults use 2-3 drops; for children use 1-2 drops.

AILMENT	RECOMMENDED OILS AND USAGE	BODY SYSTEM/FOCUS AREA
Impetigo	A highly contagious skin infection that causes red sores on the face. geranium, oregano, vetiver, Purify, lavender	Integumentary pg. 304
Impotence	The inability to maintain or achieve an erection long enough to engage in sexual intercourse. cypress, Passion®, ylang ylang, ginger, AromaTouch®	Men's Health pg. 316; Intimacy pg. 448
Incontinence	Loss of bladder control, varying from a slight loss of urine after sneezing, coughing, or laughing to complete inability to control urination. cypress, basil, thyme, AromaTouch®, lemongrass	Urinary pg. 366; Men's Health pg. 316; Women's Health pg. 374
Indigestion	A broad term covering a group of universal symptoms in the digestive tract including bloating, heartburn, nausea, or gas discomfort. DigestZen® or Tamer™, peppermint, black pepper, Slim & Sassy®, cardamom	Digestive & Intestinal pg. 275; Weight pg. 369; Detoxification pg. 270
Infant Reflux	A condition where the contents of the stomach are spit out shortly after feeding. Also known as infant acid reflux. fennel, DigestZen® or Tamer™, peppermint, lavender, Roman chamomile	Children pg. 265
Infected Wounds	Infiltration of microorganisms in body tissues. melaleuca, Purify, frankincense, copaiba, On Guard®	Integumentary pg. 304; First Aid pg. 291
Infection	Multiplication of microorganisms in body tissues, mainly causing cellular injury due to competitive toxins. oregano, On Guard®, cinnamon, thyme, melissa	Immune & Lymphatic pg. 299
Infertility	The inability to conceive a pregnancy after trying for at least one full year. thyme, clary sage, spikenard, ylang ylang, grapefruit & Zendocrine®	Men's Health pg. 316; Women's Health pg. 374
Inflammation	A protective tissue response process by which the body's white blood cells and substances they produce protect from infection. frankincense, peppermint, massage & Deep Blue®, DDR Prime®, turmeric	Pain & Inflammation pg. 334
Inflammatory Bowel Disease	A chronic disorder of the gastrointestinal tract defined by inflammation of the intestine and resulting in persistent diarrhea and abdominal cramping. DigestZen®, ginger, marjoram, copaiba, basil	Digestive & Intestinal pg. 275; Autoimmune pg. 240
Inflammatory Myopathies	A disease featuring weakness and inflammation of muscles. Another term for chronic muscle tissue inflammation is myositis. lemongrass, AromaTouch®, Deep Blue®, Siberian fir, wintergreen	Muscular pg. 323; Autoimmune pg. 240
Ingrown Toenail	Abnormal growth of a toenail with one edge growing deeply into the nail groove and surrounding tissues. arborvitae, DDR Prime® or lemongrass, eucalyptus, myrrh, melaleuca	Integumentary pg. 304

STEPS: 1 Look up ailment. 2 Choose one or more of the recommended oils. (Order of recommendation is left to right.) 3 Use oil(s) as indicated. 4 Learn more in corresponding body system/focus area. 5 Find more solutions at essentiallife.com

AILMENT	RECOMMENDED OILS AND USAGE	BODY SYSTEM/FOCUS AREA
Injury (muscle, bone, connective tissue, bruising (skin))	Harm or damage caused to the body, specifically to the muscles, bones, or other connective tissue. helichrysum · Deep Blue® · lemongrass · wintergreen · copaiba	First Aid pg. 291; Muscular pg. 323; Skeletal pg. 355
Insect Bites	An adverse response to a bite or sting of an insect such as bees, wasps, hornets, ticks, mosquitoes, or ants. lavender · Purify · Roman chamomile · blue tansy · basil	First Aid pg. 291; Allergies pg. 234
Insect Repellent	A substance applied to clothing or skin which discourages insects from landing or climbing on that surface. TerraShield® · citronella · cedarwood · lemon eucalyptus eucalyptus · arborvitae	First Aid pg. 291; Outdoors pg. 452
Insomnia	The inability to access a satisfactory amount or quality of sleep. Serenity® · lavender · petitgrain · Roman chamomile · vetiver	Sleep pg. 359
Insulin Imbalances	Irregular levels of insulin produced by the pancreas to help the body use glucose for storing energy. coriander · cinnamon · Slim & Sassy® · cassia · geranium	Blood Sugar pg. 245
Insulin Resistance	A physiological condition in which cells fail to respond to the normal actions of the hormone insulin. lavender · Slim & Sassy® · tumeric or ginger · Zendocrine® · oregano	Blood Sugar pg. 245
Iris Inflammation	Inflammation of the iris caused by eye trauma. (Do not put oil directly in eye.) juniper berry · helichrysum · patchouli · frankincense · arborvitae	Nervous pg. 327
Irritable Bowel Syndrome	An intestinal disorder causing pain in the belly, gas, diarrhea, and constipation. DigestZen® or Tamer™ · ginger · peppermint · cardamom · Zendocrine®	Digestive & Intestinal pg. 275
Itching	An acute disturbing irritation or tickling sensation that may be felt all over the skin's surface or confined to just one area. Roman chamomile · Zendocrine® · blue tansy · lavender · myrrh	Integumentary pg. 304; Allergies pg. 234
Jaundice	A yellowish tinge to the skin, whites of the eyes, and mucous membranes caused by elevated levels of the bile pigment bilirubin. (See dilution recommendation for infants). frankincense · lemon · geranium · Zendocrine® · juniper berry	Digestive & Intestinal pg. 275
Jet Lag	A condition marked by insomnia, fatigue, and irritability that is caused by air travel through changing time zones, probably as the result of disrupting circadian rhythms in the body. peppermint · Serenity® · rosemary · Citrus Bliss® · Slim & Sassy®	Sleep pg. 359; Energy & Vitality pg. 288; On the Go pg. 450
Jock Itch	A fungal infection that causes an itchy, red rash to the skin of the groin area, inner thighs and buttocks. melaleuca · myrrh · cedarwood · thyme · patchouli	Men's Health pg. 316; Candida pg. 252
Joint Pain	Discomfort, pain, and/or inflammation originating from any part of the joint. turmeric & copaiba · Deep Blue® · Siberian fir · pink & black pepper · wintergreen	Skeletal pg. 355; Pain & Inflammation pg. 334

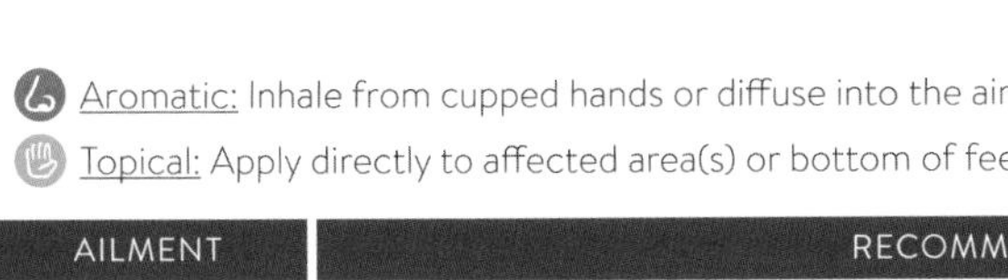

Aromatic: Inhale from cupped hands or diffuse into the air.
Topical: Apply directly to affected area(s) or bottom of feet.

Internal: Take in a capsule, glass of water, or on/under tongue.

TIP For adults use 2-3 drops; for children use 1-2 drops.

AILMENT	RECOMMENDED OILS AND USAGE	BODY SYSTEM/FOCUS AREA
Kidney Infection	The condition that occurs when microbes from the bladder or blood (bacteria, fungi or viruses) invade the tissues of the kidney(s) and reproduce. lemongrass · juniper berry · thyme · cinnamon · cardamom	Urinary pg. 366
Kidney Stones	Small, hard mineral deposits that form inside the kidneys. lemon · eucalyptus · wintergreen · lemongrass · celery seed	Urinary pg. 366
Kidneys	A bean-shaped organ that regulates fluid and excretes waste products through urine. juniper berry · lemon · DDR Prime® · rosemary · eucalyptus	Urinary pg. 366
Knee Cartilage Injury	When damage occurs to the cartilage (tough, flexible connective tissue) in the knee, resulting in pain, stiffness and inflammation. lemongrass · wintergreen or birch · helichrysum · copaiba · Siberian fir	Skeletal pg. 355
Labor	The process during which the uterus contracts and the cervix opens to allow the transition of a baby into the vagina. ylang ylang · ClaryCalm® · Serenity® · clary sage · frankincense	Pregnancy, Labor & Nursing pg. 341;
Lactation Problems	Conditions which prevent or discourage breastfeeding, including engorged breasts, sore nipples, mastitis (infection), thrush, and low milk supply that new nursing mothers may experience. fennel · basil · clary sage · ylang ylang · Deep Blue®	Pregnancy, Labor & Nursing pg. 341;
Lactose Intolerance	Failure of the body to digest lactose, a compound found in dairy products, due to lack of the enzyme lactase in the small intestine. cardamom · DigestZen® · ginger · Slim & Sassy® · coriander	Digestive & Intestinal pg. 275; Allergies pg. 234
Laryngitis	Inflammation of the larynx followed by hoarseness of the voice and a painful cough. lemon · On Guard® · myrrh · sandalwood · frankincense	Respiratory pg. 349; Oral Health pg. 331
Lead Poisoning	A potentially fatal buildup of lead in the body, usually over months or years. cilantro · Zendocrine® · helichrysum · rosemary · frankincense	Detoxification pg. 270
Leaky Gut Syndrome	A type of gastrointestinal tract dysfunction that allows bacteria, fungi, toxins and parasites to permeate the intestinal wall and leak into the bloodstream. myrrh · lemongrass · cardamom · dill · DigestZen®	Digestive & Intestinal pg. 275
Learning Difficulties	An impairment or significantly reduced ability to learn, understand, organize, retain and/or use new information. vetiver & lavender · Balance® · InTune® · peppermint · cedarwood	Focus & Concentration pg. 295; Brain pg. 248
Leg Cramps	An abrupt, involuntary, spasmodic muscular contraction causing severe pain, often existing in the leg or shoulder as the result of chill or strain. AromaTouch® · marjoram · basil · Deep Blue® · Douglas fir	Muscular pg. 323; Pregnancy, Labor & Nursing pg. 341

STEPS: 1 Look up ailment. 2 Choose one or more of the recommended oils. (Order of recommendation is left to right.) 3 Use oil(s) as indicated. 4 Learn more in corresponding body system/focus area. 5 Find more solutions at essentiallife.com

AILMENT	RECOMMENDED OILS AND USAGE	BODY SYSTEM/FOCUS AREA
Legg-Calve-Perthes Disease	Occurs when too little blood is supplied to the ball part of the hip joint. Without ample blood flow, the bone stops growing, begins to die and breaks more easily. AromaTouch® · lemongrass · peppermint · cypress · cassia	Children pg. 265; Skeletal pg. 355
Legionnaires' Disease	A severe form of pneumonia (lung inflammation caused by infection) which is typically caused by inhaling a bacteria called legionella. melaleuca · black pepper · thyme · eucalyptus · birch	Respiratory pg. 349; Immune & Lymphatic pg. 299
Leukemia	A progressive, malignant cancer of blood-forming tissues, hindering the body's ability to fight infection. frankincense · DDR Prime® · lemongrass · Zendocrine® · geranium	Cellular Health pg. 261
Libido (low) for Men	The inhibition of a man's sex drive or natural desire for sexual activity. ylang ylang · patchouli · Passion® · cinnamon · neroli	Intimacy pg. 448; Men's Health pg. 316
Libido (low) for Women	The inhibition of a woman's sex drive or natural desire for sexual activity. ylang ylang · Whisper® · jasmine · Passion® · neroli	Intimacy pg. 448; Women's Health pg. 374
Lichen Nitidus	A chronic inflammatory skin condition defined by small, glistening, skin-colored bumps on the surface of the skin. Purify · patchouli · DDR Prime® · Zendocrine® · geranium	Integumentary pg. 304
Lipoma	A benign, rubbery, encapsulated tumor of fatty tissue that is not tender and feels doughy to the touch. DDR Prime® · clove · arborvitae · frankincense · eucalyptus	Cellular Health pg. 261
Lips (dry)	Skin on the lips that has lost moisture, often due to dehydration, too much sun or wind, or constant licking or picking. myrrh · geranium · sandalwood · lavender · frankincense	Integumentary pg. 304
Listeria Infection	A food-borne bacterial illness that is often contracted by eating improperly processed deli meats and unpasteurized dairy products. cinnamon · oregano · On Guard® · melaleuca · Purify	Immune & Lymphatic pg. 299
Liver Disease	Any condition or damage that lowers or stops the functioning of the liver. Zendocrine® · geranium · copaiba · turmeric · lemon & grapefruit	Digestive & Intestinal pg. 275
Lockjaw (Tetanus)	An early symptom of tetanus that affects the central nervous system by causing painful muscular contractions that result in difficulty opening the jaw. Deep Blue® · cypress · rosemary · clove · eucalyptus	Immune & Lymphatic pg. 299; Nervous pg. 327; Muscular pg. 323
Long QT Syndrome	A heart rhythm disorder that can cause fast, chaotic heartbeats, which may trigger a seizure, sudden fainting spell, or death. ylang ylang · melissa · rosemary · On Guard® · Zendocrine®	Cardiovascular pg. 256
Lou Gehrig's Disease (ALS)	A rapidly progressive neurodegenerative disease that attacks and kills the nerve cells responsible for controlling voluntary muscles. melissa · DDR Prime® · frankincense · copaiba · cypress	Nervous pg. 327; Autoimmune pg. 240; Muscular pg. 323

Aromatic: Inhale from cupped hands or diffuse into the air.
Topical: Apply directly to affected area(s) or bottom of feet.
Internal: Take in a capsule, glass of water, or on/under tongue.
TIP For adults use 2-3 drops; for children use 1-2 drops.

AILMENT	RECOMMENDED OILS AND USAGE	BODY SYSTEM/FOCUS AREA
Lumbago	An old term used to describe pain in the muscles and joints of the lower back. Deep Blue® (Topical); AromaTouch® (Topical); frankincense (Topical); Siberian fir (Topical); cardamom (Topical)	Muscular pg. 323; Skeletal pg. 355
Lupus	A chronic inflammatory disease caused when the immune system attacks its own tissues. DDR Prime® (Internal, Topical); Zendocrine® (Internal, Topical); clove (Internal, Topical); copaiba (Internal, Topical); AromaTouch® (Topical)	Autoimmune pg. 240
Lyme Disease	An inflammatory disease caused by bacteria carried by ticks. oregano (Internal); thyme (Topical, Internal); clove (Topical, Internal); cassia (Internal, Topical); frankincense (Internal, Topical, Aromatic)	Immune & Lymphatic pg. 299
Lymphoma	A type of blood cancer that starts in the lymphatic tissues of the body, causing white blood cells to behave abnormally. DDR Prime® (Internal, Topical); frankincense (Internal, Topical); thyme (Internal, Topical); clove (Internal, Topical); wild orange (Internal, Topical, Aromatic)	Cellular Health pg. 261
Macular Degeneration	A progressive deterioration of a critical region of the retina called the macula which can cause severe vision impairment. Immortelle (Topical); helichrysum (Topical, Internal); coriander (Topical, Internal); juniper berry (Internal, Topical); frankincense (Topical, Internal)	Nervous pg. 327
Malabsorption Syndrome	A condition that prevents absorption of nutrients through the small intestine. sandalwood (Topical, Internal); fennel (Topical, Internal); Citrus Bliss® (Topical); DigestZen® (Topical, Internal); ginger (Topical, Internal)	Digestive & Intestinal pg. 275
Malaria	A life-threatening blood disease transmitted by the bite of infected mosquitoes. thyme (Internal, Topical); cinnamon (Internal, Topical); Zendocrine® (Topical, Internal); lemon eucalyptus or eucalyptus (Topical, Aromatic); TerraShield® (to avoid) (Topical, Aromatic)	Immune & Lymphatic pg. 299; Parasites pg. 338
Marfan Syndrome (Connective Tissue Disorder)	A genetic disorder that affects connective tissue and causes excessive bone elongation, joint flexibility, and abnormalities of the cardiovascular system. lemongrass (Topical, Internal); helichrysum (Topical, Internal); AromaTouch® (Topical); Siberian fir (Topical); basil (Topical, Internal)	Cardiovascular pg. 256; Skeletal pg. 355; Muscular pg. 323
Mastitis	A bacterial infection in the mammary glands of the breast which typically only occurs in women who are breastfeeding. lavender (Topical); DDR Prime® (Internal, Topical); thyme (Internal); peppermint (Topical, Internal); oregano (Internal)	Pregnancy, Labor & Nursing pg. 341
Measles	A highly contagious viral infection which causes full-body rash and other symptoms, mostly in children. On Guard® (Internal, Topical, Aromatic); yarrow (Topical, Internal); melaleuca (Topical, Internal, Aromatic); coriander (Topical, Internal); blue tansy (Topical)	Immune & Lymphatic pg. 299
Melanoma	The least common but most deadly form of skin cancer which typically develops in pigment-containing cells. frankincense (Topical, Internal); sandalwood (Topical, Internal); DDR Prime® (Internal, Topical); Immortelle (Topical); lemongrass (Topical, Internal)	Cellular Health pg. 261
Melatonin Imbalances/ Insufficiencies	Melatonin is a hormone produced at the onset of darkness to aid in sleep. Imbalances or insufficiencies may lead to sleep deprivation or sleeping disorders. vetiver (Internal, Topical, Aromatic); lavender (Internal, Topical, Aromatic); Serenity® (Topical, Aromatic); petitgrain (Internal, Topical, Aromatic); Roman chamomile (Internal, Topical, Aromatic)	Endocrine pg. 284; Sleep pg. 359
Memory (poor)	The weak mental capacity of retaining facts or recalling previous experiences. peppermint (Topical, Aromatic); rosemary (Internal, Topical, Aromatic); frankincense (Topical, Internal, Aromatic); thyme (Aromatic, Topical, Internal); sandalwood (Aromatic, Topical, Internal)	Focus & Concentration pg. 295; Brain pg. 248

STEPS: 1 Look up ailment. 2 Choose one or more of the recommended oils. (Order of recommendation is left to right.) 3 Use oil(s) as indicated. 4 Learn more in corresponding body system/focus area. 5 Find more solutions at essentiallife.com

AILMENT	RECOMMENDED OILS AND USAGE	BODY SYSTEM/FOCUS AREA
Meningitis	Inflammation of brain and spinal cord membranes, typically caused by a viral or bacterial infection, characterized by serious symptoms. melaleuca · On Guard® · clove · DDR Prime® · basil	Immune & Lymphatic pg. 299
Meniere's Disease	Inner disorder with symptoms including vertigo, tinnitus, hearing loss and a sensation of pressure. helichrysum · frankincense · juniper berry · ginger · basil	Women's Health pg. 374
Menopause	The period of permanent cessation of menstruation, typically occurring between the ages of 45 and 55 ClaryCalm® · Zendocrine® · Passion® · thyme · clary sage	Women's Health pg. 374
Menorrhagia (excessive menstrual bleeding)	Extremely heavy menstrual flow with cycles of normal length or prolonged uterine bleeding lasting longer than seven days. ClaryCalm® · helichrysum · Zendocrine® · geranium · DDR Prime®	Women's Health pg. 374
Menstrual Cycle (irregular or scanty)	Uncommonly slight or infrequent menstrual flow. ClaryCalm® · geranium · rosemary · yarrow · Zendocrine®	Women's Health pg. 374
Menstrual Pain/ Cramps	Also referred to as dysmenorrhea, a female condition of painful, debilitating menstrual cycles that ranges from dull to severe. ClaryCalm® · clary sage · marjoram · PastTense® · copaiba	Women's Health pg. 374
Mental Fatigue	A cognitive or emotional state associated with decreased ability to function, typically caused by prolonged mental exertion or emotional duress. rosemary · basil · peppermint · Motivate® · Citrus Bliss®	Brain pg. 248
Mesenteric Lymphadentis	Painful inflammation of the lymph nodes that attach the intestine to the abdominal wall, typically a temporary condition in children. Purify · DDR Prime® · basil · cardamom · Zendocrine®	Immune & Lymphatic pg. 299
Mesothelioma	A cancerous tumor of the epithelium lining the lungs, heart, or abdomen often associated with exposure to asbestos dust. Zendocrine® · basil · black pepper · DDR Prime® · HD Clear®	Cellular Health pg. 261
Metabolic Muscle Disorders	A condition that interferes with the body's ability to draw and utilize energy from food, resulting in muscle weakness or pain. basil · cypress · ginger · peppermint · cassia	Muscular pg. 323
Metabolism (Low)	A low basal metabolic rate normally leads to low energy expenditure. As a result, the number of calories a person normally expends is likely less than the number of calories consumed. grapefruit · Slim & Sassy® · cinnamon · DDR Prime® · clove	Weight pg. 369
Migraine	A severe recurring headache over the course of 3 hours to 4 days associated with sharp pain, nausea and sensitivity to light. peppermint · copaiba · frankincense · lavender · PastTense®	Pain & Inflammation pg. 334; Muscular pg. 323

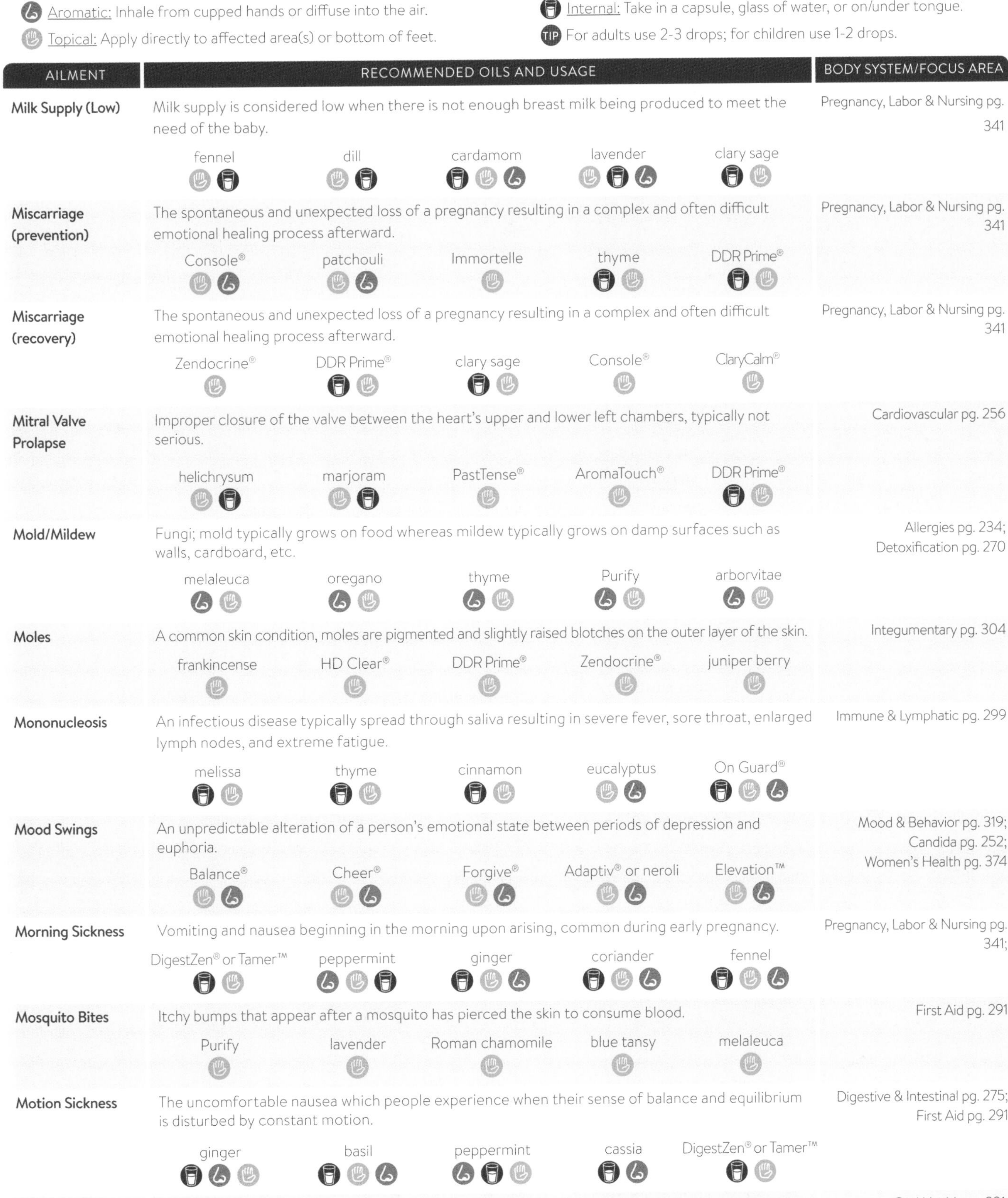

Aromatic: Inhale from cupped hands or diffuse into the air.

Topical: Apply directly to affected area(s) or bottom of feet.

Internal: Take in a capsule, glass of water, or on/under tongue.

TIP For adults use 2-3 drops; for children use 1-2 drops.

AILMENT	RECOMMENDED OILS AND USAGE	BODY SYSTEM/FOCUS AREA
Milk Supply (Low)	Milk supply is considered low when there is not enough breast milk being produced to meet the need of the baby. fennel (Topical, Internal); dill (Topical, Internal); cardamom (Internal, Topical, Aromatic); lavender (Topical, Internal, Aromatic); clary sage (Internal, Topical)	Pregnancy, Labor & Nursing pg. 341
Miscarriage (prevention)	The spontaneous and unexpected loss of a pregnancy resulting in a complex and often difficult emotional healing process afterward. Console® (Topical, Aromatic); patchouli (Topical, Aromatic); Immortelle (Topical); thyme (Internal, Topical); DDR Prime® (Internal, Topical)	Pregnancy, Labor & Nursing pg. 341
Miscarriage (recovery)	The spontaneous and unexpected loss of a pregnancy resulting in a complex and often difficult emotional healing process afterward. Zendocrine® (Topical); DDR Prime® (Internal, Topical); clary sage (Internal, Topical); Console® (Topical); ClaryCalm® (Topical)	Pregnancy, Labor & Nursing pg. 341
Mitral Valve Prolapse	Improper closure of the valve between the heart's upper and lower left chambers, typically not serious. helichrysum (Topical, Internal); marjoram (Topical, Internal); PastTense® (Topical); AromaTouch® (Topical); DDR Prime® (Internal, Topical)	Cardiovascular pg. 256
Mold/Mildew	Fungi; mold typically grows on food whereas mildew typically grows on damp surfaces such as walls, cardboard, etc. melaleuca (Aromatic, Topical); oregano (Aromatic, Topical); thyme (Aromatic, Topical); Purify (Aromatic, Topical); arborvitae (Aromatic, Topical)	Allergies pg. 234; Detoxification pg. 270
Moles	A common skin condition, moles are pigmented and slightly raised blotches on the outer layer of the skin. frankincense (Topical); HD Clear® (Topical); DDR Prime® (Topical); Zendocrine® (Topical); juniper berry (Topical)	Integumentary pg. 304
Mononucleosis	An infectious disease typically spread through saliva resulting in severe fever, sore throat, enlarged lymph nodes, and extreme fatigue. melissa (Internal, Topical); thyme (Internal, Topical); cinnamon (Internal, Topical); eucalyptus (Topical, Aromatic); On Guard® (Internal, Topical, Aromatic)	Immune & Lymphatic pg. 299
Mood Swings	An unpredictable alteration of a person's emotional state between periods of depression and euphoria. Balance® (Topical, Aromatic); Cheer® (Topical, Aromatic); Forgive® (Topical, Aromatic); Adaptiv® or neroli (Topical, Aromatic); Elevation™ (Topical, Aromatic)	Mood & Behavior pg. 319; Candida pg. 252; Women's Health pg. 374
Morning Sickness	Vomiting and nausea beginning in the morning upon arising, common during early pregnancy. DigestZen® or Tamer™ (Internal, Topical); peppermint (Aromatic, Topical, Internal); ginger (Internal, Topical, Aromatic); coriander (Internal, Topical, Aromatic); fennel (Internal, Topical, Aromatic)	Pregnancy, Labor & Nursing pg. 341;
Mosquito Bites	Itchy bumps that appear after a mosquito has pierced the skin to consume blood. Purify (Topical); lavender (Topical); Roman chamomile (Topical); blue tansy (Topical); melaleuca (Topical)	First Aid pg. 291
Motion Sickness	The uncomfortable nausea which people experience when their sense of balance and equilibrium is disturbed by constant motion. ginger (Internal, Aromatic, Topical); basil (Internal, Topical, Aromatic); peppermint (Aromatic, Internal, Topical); cassia (Internal, Aromatic); DigestZen® or Tamer™ (Internal, Topical)	Digestive & Intestinal pg. 275; First Aid pg. 291
Mouth Ulcers	Ulcers of the oral mucosa commonly caused by a secondary bacterial infection of less severe mucosal lesions. clove (Topical, Internal); On Guard® (Topical, Internal); cinnamon (Topical, Internal); melaleuca (Topical, Internal); myrrh (Topical, Internal)	Oral Health pg. 331; Autoimmune pg. 240

QUICK REFERENCE

STEPS: 1 Look up ailment. 2 Choose one or more of the recommended oils. (Order of recommendation is left to right.) 3 Use oil(s) as indicated. 4 Learn more in corresponding body system/focus area. 5 Find more solutions at essentiallife.com

AILMENT	RECOMMENDED OILS AND USAGE	BODY SYSTEM/FOCUS AREA
MRSA	An infection caused by a type of staph bacteria that has become resistant to many of the antibiotics used to treat ordinary staph infections. cinnamon, oregano, thyme, On Guard®, clove	Immune & Lymphatic pg. 299
Mucus	A thick, gel-like, viscous material that functions to protect and moisten inner body surfaces. lemon, DigestZen®, fennel, eucalyptus, cardamom	Respiratory pg. 349; Digestive & Intestinal pg. 275; Allergies pg. 234
Multiple Chemical Sensitivity Reaction	A medical condition identified by symptoms to low-level chemical exposure. Substances include pesticides, smoke, plastics, petroleum products, scents, and paints. cilantro, Zendocrine®, Douglas fir, geranium, coriander	Allergies pg. 234
Multiple Sclerosis	A potentially disabling disease of the brain and spinal cord in which the immune system eats away at the protective covering of nerves. Zendocrine®, frankincense, sandalwood, DDR Prime®, cypress	Nervous pg. 327; Autoimmune pg. 240
Mumps	A mild short-term viral infection of the salivary glands that commonly occurs during childhood. On Guard®, DDR Prime®, Zendocrine®, yarrow, lavender	Immune & Lymphatic pg. 299
Muscular Cramps / Charley Horse	An immediate, uncontrolled, spasmodic muscular contraction causing severe pain, often occurring in the leg or shoulder as the result of a strain or chill. marjoram, AromaTouch®, Deep Blue®, PastTense®, Siberian fir	Athletes pg. 237; Muscular pg. 323
Muscle Pulls, Strains	Partial or total breach of muscle fibers due to sudden applied force or overuse. copaiba, lemongrass, Deep Blue®, marjoram, AromaTouch®	Muscular pg. 323; Athletes pg. 237; Pain & Inflammation pg. 334
Muscle Pain	Pain in a muscle or group of muscles that is typically shared by a feeling of unease. AromaTouch®, Deep Blue®, Siberian fir, marjoram, peppermint	Muscular pg. 323; Athletes pg. 237; Pain & Inflammation pg. 334; Fitness pg. 440
Muscle Spasms	A quick, involuntary contraction of a muscle or group of muscles. AromaTouch®, marjoram, copaiba, Roman chamomile, basil	Muscular pg. 323; Athletes pg. 237; Sleep pg. 359
Muscle Stiffness	The rigidity of muscles due to inadequate use and movement. PastTense®, AromaTouch®, Siberian fir, ginger, marjoram	Muscular pg. 323; Athletes pg. 237
Muscle Weakness / Lack of Growth	Muscle development from exercise and exertion. When a muscle is pushed to its limits, it will repair and rebuild itself for future exertion. wintergreen or birch, helichrysum, ginger, lemongrass, Siberian fir	Muscular pg. 323; Athletes pg. 237
Muscular Dystrophy	A group of inherited disorders in which muscle bulk and strength gradually drop. lemongrass, frankincense, PastTense®, DDR Prime®, marjoram	Muscular pg. 323
Myasthenia Gravis	A weakness and rapid fatigue of muscles under voluntary control. helichrysum, ginger, lemongrass, cypress, DDR Prime®	Muscular pg. 323; Autoimmune pg. 240
Myelofibrosis	A severe bone marrow disorder that disrupts the body's normal production of blood cells. helichrysum, Zendocrine®, ginger, frankincense, Siberian fir	Skeletal pg. 355

Aromatic: Inhale from cupped hands or diffuse into the air.

Topical: Apply directly to affected area(s) or bottom of feet.

Internal: Take in a capsule, glass of water, or on/under tongue.

TIP For adults use 2-3 drops; for children use 1-2 drops.

AILMENT	RECOMMENDED OILS AND USAGE	BODY SYSTEM/FOCUS AREA
Myotonic Dystrophy	A genetic disorder that causes progressive muscle weakness. Douglas fir [Topical]; DDR Prime® [Internal, Topical]; helichrysum [Internal, Topical]; Siberian fir [Topical]; lemongrass [Internal, Topical]	Muscular pg. 323
Nails	The hard, cutaneous plate on the dorsal surface of the end of a finger or toe. sandalwood [Topical]; lemon [Topical]; wild orange [Topical]; arborvitae [Topical]; ClaryCalm® [Topical]	Integumentary pg. 304
Narcolepsy	A disorder distincted by extreme daytime sleepiness, cataplexy and uncontrollable sleep attacks. sandalwood [Internal, Topical, Aromatic]; Console® [Topical, Aromatic]; Motivate® [Topical, Aromatic]; wild orange [Aromatic, Internal, Topical]; InTune® [Topical, Aromatic]	Sleep pg. 359; Brain pg. 248
Nasal Polyp	A rounded, stretched piece of pulpy, dependent mucosa that projects into the nasal cavity. rosemary [Topical, Aromatic]; melissa [Topical]; Breathe® [Topical, Aromatic]; On Guard® [Topical, Aromatic]; sandalwood [Topical, Aromatic]	Respiratory pg. 349; Cellular Health pg. 261
Nausea	An undesirable queasy sensation including an urge to vomit. DigestZen® or Tamer™ [Internal, Topical, Aromatic]; ginger [Internal, Topical, Aromatic]; peppermint [Internal, Topical, Aromatic]; pink pepper [Internal, Topical, Aromatic]; Zendocrine® [Internal, Topical, Aromatic]	Digestive & Intestinal pg. 275
Neck Pain	Pain in response to injury or another stimulus that resolves when the injury stimulus is removed or healed. Deep Blue® [Topical]; PastTense® [Topical]; copaiba [Topical]; AromaTouch® [Topical]; wintergreen [Topical]	Muscular pg. 323
Nerves, Weakened / Damaged	A dysfunction or breakdown of the nervous system. vetiver [Topical]; helichrysum [Topical, Internal]; petitgrain [Topical, Internal]; copaiba [Topical, Internal]; patchouli [Topical]	Nervous pg. 327
Nervous Fatigue	A form of fatigue associated with changes in the synaptic concentration of neurotransmitters within the central nervous system. peppermint [Topical, Aromatic, Internal]; Citrus Bliss® [Topical, Aromatic]; basil [Topical, Aromatic, Internal]; yarrow [Topical, Internal]; Zendocrine® [Topical, Aromatic]	Energy & Vitality pg. 288; Stress pg. 363
Nervousness	A state of concern, with great physical and mental unrest. Peace® [Topical, Aromatic]; Balance® [Topical, Aromatic]; Serenity® [Topical, Aromatic]; Motivate® [Topical, Aromatic]; petitgrain [Internal, Topical, Aromatic]	Mood & Behavior pg. 319; Stress pg. 363
Neuralgia	Characterized as an extreme stabbing or burning pain caused by irritation of or damage to a nerve. helichrysum [Topical, Internal, Aromatic]; PastTense® [Topical]; wintergreen [Topical]; clove or neroli [Topical, Internal]; Douglas fir [Topical]	Nervous pg. 327; Muscular pg. 323; Pain & Inflammation pg. 334
Neuritis	The inflammation of a nerve or group of nerves that is defined by loss of reflexes, pain and atrophy of the affected muscles. cardamom [Topical, Internal]; patchouli [Topical, Internal]; helichrysum [Topical, Internal]; ginger [Topical, Internal]; Deep Blue® [Topical]	Nervous pg. 327
Neuromuscular Disorders	A broad term that encompasses many different diseases that affect the function of the skeletal muscles that move the limbs and trunk. marjoram [Topical]; arborvitae [Topical]; ginger [Topical]; basil [Topical]; AromaTouch® [Topical]	Muscular pg. 323
Neuropathy	A condition affecting the nerves supplying the legs and arms. cypress [Topical]; AromaTouch® [Topical]; Deep Blue® [Topical]; basil [Topical]; wintergreen [Topical]	Nervous pg. 327
Night Eating Syndrome (NES)	An eating disorder characterized by abnormal food intake patterns during the night, not to be confused with binge eating disorder. cinnamon [Internal, Aromatic]; Slim & Sassy® [Internal, Aromatic]; grapefruit [Internal, Aromatic, Topical]; ginger [Internal, Aromatic, Topical]; peppermint [Internal, Aromatic, Topical]	Eating Disorders pg. 280; Weight pg. 369

STEPS:  Look up ailment. 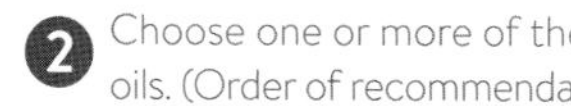 Choose one or more of the recommended oils. (Order of recommendation is left to right.) 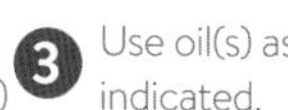 Use oil(s) as indicated. 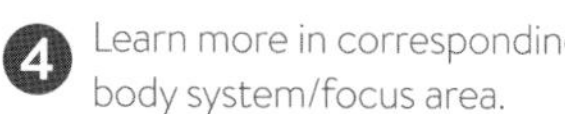 Learn more in corresponding body system/focus area. 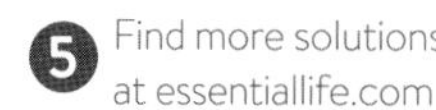 Find more solutions at essentiallife.com

AILMENT	RECOMMENDED OILS AND USAGE	BODY SYSTEM/FOCUS AREA
Night Sweats	Profuse episodes of sweating at night that soak nightclothes or bedding. peppermint, DDR Prime®, ClaryCalm®, Whisper®, spearmint	Women's Health pg. 374
Nighttime Urination	Nocturia, or nocturnal polyuria, is the medical term for excessive urination during the night. rosemary, cypress, juniper berry, Slim & Sassy®, thyme	Children pg. 265
Nipples, Sore	Increased sensitivity due to breastfeeding, friction, running, or hormonal imbalances. myrrh, melaleuca, sandalwood, frankincense, geranium	Pregnancy, Labor & Nursing pg. 341
Nose (dry)	Irritation caused from insufficient mucus in the nasal cavity. myrrh, wild orange, geranium, sandalwood, lavender	Respiratory pg. 349
Nosebleed	Bleeding from the nose, either spontaneous or induced by nose picking or trauma. helichrysum, geranium, myrrh, On Guard®, lavender	Respiratory pg. 349
Numbness	Loss of sensation or feeling. peppermint, cypress, PastTense®, ginger, basil	Nervous pg. 327; Cardiovascular pg. 256
Obesity	Obesity is an uncommon quantity of body fat, usually 20% or more over an individual's ideal body weight. Slim & Sassy®, cinnamon, grapefruit, ginger, bergamot	Weight pg. 369; Endocrine pg. 284; Stress pg. 363; Blood Sugar pg. 245
Obsessive-Compulsive Disorder (OCD)	A type of anxiety disorder marked by distressing excessive thoughts (obsessions) that lead to repetitive ritualized behaviors (compulsions) that interfere with daily life. Adaptiv® or cedarwood, Serenity®, Forgive®, InTune®, ylang ylang	Mood & Behavior pg. 319; Limbic pg. 313
Ocular Rosacea	A common inflammatory condition affecting the eyes. Often develops in individuals who have rosacea, a chronic condition that affects the face and chest. myrrh, frankincense, Zendocrine®, Immortelle, sandalwood	Nervous pg. 327; Integumentary pg. 304; Respiratory pg. 349
Olfactory Loss	The inability to perceive odor or loss of the sense of smell. Also known as anosmia. lavender or helichrysum, peppermint, Adaptiv® or basil, DDR Prime®, arborvitae	Respiratory pg. 349; Allergies pg. 234
Oppositional Defiant Disorder	A disorder in a child marked by defiant and disobedient behavior to authority figures. Peace®, PastTense®, Forgive®, cardamom, Cheer®	Mood & Behavior pg. 319
Oral Health	The state of health of the mouth, throat, tooth and other capacities to allow for biting, chewing, smiling, and speaking. Topical use can indicate brushing with or rubbing oil(s) on affected area. myrrh, clove, peppermint, On Guard®, turmeric	Oral Health pg. 331; Personal Care pg. 454
Osgood-Schlatter Disease	A childhood repetitive-use injury that causes a painful lump below the kneecap. cypress, ginger, lemongrass, AromaTouch®, birch	Skeletal pg. 355

Aromatic: Inhale from cupped hands or diffuse into the air.
Topical: Apply directly to affected area(s) or bottom of feet.
Internal: Take in a capsule, glass of water, or on/under tongue.
TIP For adults use 2-3 drops; for children use 1-2 drops.

AILMENT	RECOMMENDED OILS AND USAGE	BODY SYSTEM/FOCUS AREA
Osteoarthritis	A form of arthritis, occurring commonly in older persons, that is defined by chronic degeneration of the cartilage of the joints. black pepper (Topical, Internal); frankincense (Topical, Internal); Siberian fir (Topical); Deep Blue® (Topical); wintergreen (Topical)	Skeletal pg. 355; Pain & Inflammation pg. 334
Osteomyelitis	Inflammation of bone caused by infection, generally in the legs, arm, or spine. thyme (Topical); melissa (Topical); lemongrass (Topical); wintergreen (Topical); clove (Topical)	Immune & Lymphatic pg. 299; Skeletal pg. 355
Osteoporosis	A disease defined by loss in bone mass and density, occurring commonly in postmenopausal women, resulting in a predisposition to fractures and bone deformities such as vertebral collapse. Siberian fir (Topical); clove (Internal, Topical); wintergreen (Topical); geranium (Topical, Internal); lemongrass (Topical, Internal)	Skeletal pg. 355
Ovarian Cyst	A solid or fluid-filled sac or pocket within or on the surface of an ovary. Commonly benign. Zendocrine® (Internal, Topical); DDR Prime® (Internal, Topical); clary sage (Internal, Topical); basil (Internal, Topical, Aromatic); rosemary (Topical, Internal)	Women's Health pg. 374; Cellular Health pg. 261
Overactive Bladder (OAB)	The leakage of urine in large amounts at unexpected times, including during sleep. cypress (Topical); thyme (Internal, Topical); juniper berry (Topical, Internal); ginger (Topical, Internal); Zendocrine® (Topical, Internal)	Urinary pg. 366
Overeating	Uncontrolled ingestion of sizable quantities of food in a discrete interval, usually with a lack of control over the activity. Slim & Sassy® (Topical, Internal); coriander (Topical, Internal, Aromatic); grapefruit (Topical, Internal, Aromatic); cinnamon (Topical, Internal, Aromatic); ginger (Topical, Internal)	Weight pg. 369; Stress pg. 363; Eating Disorders pg. 280
Over-Exercised	Overuse of muscle and connective tissue that may cause injury or exhaustion. peppermint (Topical); Deep Blue® (Topical); AromaTouch® (Topical); marjoram (Topical); eucalyptus (Topical)	Muscular pg. 323; Athletes pg. 237
Overheated	An elevated body temperature due to failed thermoregulation. peppermint (Topical, Internal); eucalyptus (Topical); PastTense® (Topical); petitgrain (Topical, Internal); spearmint (Topical)	First Aid pg. 291; Athletes pg. 237
Overwhelmed	To feel overcome completely in mind or body, usually by large amounts of stress. Peace® (Aromatic, Topical); InTune® (Aromatic, Topical); rosemary (Aromatic, Topical); Adaptiv® or Serenity® (Aromatic, Topical); lemon (Aromatic, Topical)	Mood & Behavior pg. 319
Ovulation (lack of)	The failure of an egg to rupture from the ovary at mid-cycle. The cause is a lack of progesterone. basil (Topical, Internal); ClaryCalm® (Topical, Aromatic); thyme (Topical, Internal); ylang ylang (Topical, Aromatic); clary sage (Topical)	Women's Health pg. 374; Blood Sugar pg. 245
Paget's Disease	A disease that disrupts the replacement of old bone tissue with new bone tissue. DDR Prime® (Internal, Topical); myrrh (Topical); wintergreen (Topical); clove (Topical, Internal); ClaryCalm® (Topical)	Skeletal pg. 355; Cellular Health pg. 261
Pain	An undesirable sensation occurring in varying degrees of severity as a consequence of disease, injury, or emotional disorder. turmeric or copaiba (Topical, Internal); peppermint (Topical, Internal); Deep Blue® (Topical); helichrysum (Topical, Internal); wintergreen or birch (Topical)	Pain & Inflammation pg. 334
Palpitations	A sensitivity in which a person is aware of an intermittent, hard, or rapid heartbeat. ylang ylang (Topical, Internal, Aromatic); petitgrain (Internal, Topical); lavender (Aromatic, Topical, Internal); neroli (Topical); rosemary (Aromatic, Topical, Internal)	Cardiovascular pg. 256
Pancreatitis	An inflammation of the pancreas, an organ that is essential in digestion. coriander (Internal, Topical); rosemary (Internal, Topical); geranium (Internal, Topical); cinnamon (Internal, Topical); Zendocrine® (Internal, Topical)	Endocrine pg. 284

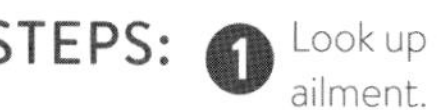 Look up ailment. ❷ Choose one or more of the recommended oils. (Order of recommendation is left to right.) 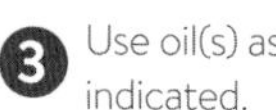 Use oil(s) as indicated. ❹ Learn more in corresponding body system/focus area. ❺ Find more solutions at essentiallife.com

AILMENT	RECOMMENDED OILS AND USAGE	BODY SYSTEM/FOCUS AREA
Panic Attacks	Periods of intense apprehension or fear typically characterized by hyperventilation that occur suddenly and of variable duration from minutes to hours. petitgrain · Adaptiv® or Serenity® · neroli · magnolia · Balance®	Mood & Behavior pg. 319
Paralysis	Complete or partial loss of strength or muscle function. frankincense · cypress · melissa · ginger · DDR Prime®	Nervous pg. 327; Muscular pg. 323; Cardiovascular pg. 256; Immune & Lymphatic pg. 299; Autoimmune pg. 240
Parasites	An organism that feeds, grows, and is sheltered on or in a different organism while contributing nothing to the survival of its host. clove · oregano · thyme · turmeric · lemongrass	Parasites pg. 338; Detoxification pg. 270; Digestive & Intestinal pg. 275; Integumentary pg. 304
Parathyroid Disorder	Overactivity of one or more of the parathyroid lobes, which make too much parathyroid hormone, causing a potentially serious calcium imbalance. ClaryCalm® · Zendocrine® · melissa · ginger · Citrus Bliss®	Endocrine pg. 284
Parkinson's Disease	A gradual nervous disease appearing most often after the age of 50, associated with the ruin of brain cells that produce dopamine. copaiba + frankincense · Zendocrine® · marjoram · bergamot or melissa · DDR Prime®	Brain pg. 248; Nervous pg. 327; Muscular pg. 323; Addictions pg. 230
Pelvic Pain Syndrome	Pain in the pelvis that arises in endometritis, appendicitis, and oophoritis. ginger · geranium · thyme · copaiba · rosemary	Women's Health pg. 374; Digestive & Intestinal pg. 275
Perforated Ear Drum	Occurs when there is a rupture or hole in the eardrum (the thin membrane that separates the outer ear canal from the middle ear. Do not drop oil(s) directly in ear. basil · ylang ylang · On Guard® · arborvitae · patchouli	Respiratory pg. 349
Pericardial Disease	Occurs when there is too much fluid buildup around the heart. rosemary · juniper berry · marjoram · lemongrass · Zendocrine®	Cardiovascular pg. 256
Perimenopause	The three to five year period before menopause during which progesterone and estrogen levels decline and symptoms of hormone deprivation begin. Zendocrine® · Whisper® · DDR Prime® · clary sage · rosemary	Women's Health pg. 374
Perineal Tearing, Lack of Elasticity	An unintended laceration of women's skin and other soft tissue structures which separate the vagina from the anus. geranium · frankincense · sandalwood · Roman chamomile · lavender	Pregnancy, Labor & Nursing pg. 341;
Periodic Limb Movement Disorder	Repetitive cramping or jerking of the legs during sleep. AromaTouch® · PastTense® · marjoram · basil · lavender	Sleep pg. 359
Pernicious Anemia	A severe anemia associated with poor intake or absorption of vitamin B12, defined by defective production of red blood cells. helichrysum · geranium · Zendocrine® · cinnamon · lemon	Autoimmune pg. 240; Cardiovascular pg. 256

QUICK REFERENCE

Aromatic: Inhale from cupped hands or diffuse into the air.

Topical: Apply directly to affected area(s) or bottom of feet.

Internal: Take in a capsule, glass of water, or on/under tongue.

TIP For adults use 2-3 drops; for children use 1-2 drops.

AILMENT	RECOMMENDED OILS AND USAGE	BODY SYSTEM/FOCUS AREA
Perspiration (excessive)	An inherited disorder of the eccrine sweat glands in which emotional stimuli cause abnormal amounts of sweating. coriander, geranium, petitgrain, Zendocrine®, Douglas fir	Endocrine pg. 284; Athletes pg. 237; Urinary pg. 366; Detoxification pg. 270
Phantom Pains	Pain, itching, tingling, or numbness in the place where amputated parts used to be. helichrysum, basil, frankincense, Deep Blue®, AromaTouch®	Pain & Inflammation pg. 334; Nervous pg. 327
Phlebitis	Inflammation of a vein. cypress, helichrysum, Zendocrine®, basil, lemongrass	Cardiovascular pg. 256
Pica	Craving and chewing substances that have no nutritional value, such as ice, clay, soil, or paper. multivitamin supplements, patchouli, cilantro, cinnamon, peppermint	Eating Disorders pg. 280; Children pg. 265
Pinkeye	Inflammation or infection of the outer membrane of the eyeball and the inner eyelid, causing the eye to become pink in color. frankincense, melaleuca, spikenard, lavender, clary sage	Immune & Lymphatic pg. 299; Children pg. 265
Pinworms	A parasitic nematode worm infecting the rectum, colon, and anus of humans. clove, oregano, thyme, lemongrass, On Guard®	Parasites pg. 338
Plantar Fasciitis	An inflammation of a thick band of tissue that connects the heel bone to the toes. copaiba, lemongrass, AromaTouch®, wintergreen, Siberian fir	Skeletal pg. 355; Muscular pg. 323
Plantar Warts	An unpleasant verrucous lesion on the sole of the foot. cinnamon, melissa, Purify, oregano, frankincense	Integumentary pg. 304
Plaque	An semi-hardened accumulation of substances from fluids that surround an area. Examples include dental plaque and cholesterol plaque. On Guard®, clove, thyme, myrrh, lemon	Oral Health pg. 331; Cardiovascular pg. 256
Pleurisy	An infection of the membrane that surrounds and protects the lungs. cinnamon, Breathe®, rosemary, eucalyptus, melissa	Respiratory pg. 349
Pneumonia	Infection that inflames air sacs in one or both lungs which many fill with fluid. Breathe®, arborvitae, copaiba, Roman chamomile, eucalyptus	Respiratory pg. 349
Poison Ivy	A poisonous North American vine or shrub that is well known for causing itching, irritation, and rash on skin that has come in contact with its leaves. geranium, Purify, Roman chamomile, lavender, frankincense	First Aid pg. 291; Integumentary pg. 304; Outdoors pg. 452
Polio	A highly infectious viral disease that may attack the central nervous system and can cause paralysis. melissa, lemongrass, patchouli, spikenard, frankincense	Immune & Lymphatic pg. 299; Nervous pg. 327
Polycystic Ovary Syndrome (PCOS)	A hormonal disorder causing enlarged ovaries with small cysts on the outer edges. Hormonal symptoms include acne and facial hair. thyme, basil, geranium, Zendocrine®, DDR Prime®	Women's Health pg. 374; Blood Sugar pg. 245; Cellular Health pg. 261

STEPS: 1 Look up ailment. 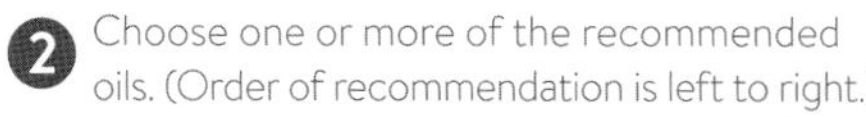 2 Choose one or more of the recommended oils. (Order of recommendation is left to right.) 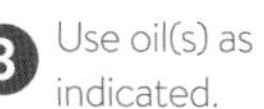 3 Use oil(s) as indicated. 4 Learn more in corresponding body system/focus area. 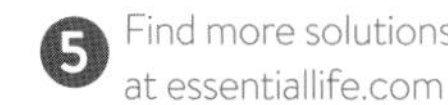 5 Find more solutions at essentiallife.com

AILMENT	RECOMMENDED OILS AND USAGE	BODY SYSTEM/FOCUS AREA
Polymyositis	A disease featuring inflammation of the muscle fibers. ginger, black pepper, Balance®, Deep Blue®, DDR Prime®	Muscular pg. 323; Pain & Inflammation pg. 334
Polyps	A tumor with a small flap that attaches itself to the wall of different vascular organs such as the rectum, uterus and nose. rosemary, ginger, peppermint, clove, lemongrass	Digestive & Intestinal pg. 275; Cellular Health pg. 261; Women's Health pg. 374; Respiratory pg. 349
Porphyria	Disorders resulting from buildup of certain chemicals related to red blood cell proteins. Zendocrine®, frankincense, lemongrass, geranium, DDR Prime®	Nervous pg. 327; Integumentary pg. 304; Detoxification pg. 270
Postpartum Depression	An emotional disorder that starts after childbirth and typically lasts beyond six weeks. Cheer®, frankincense, clary sage, Zendocrine®, Elevation™	Pregnancy, Labor & Nursing pg. 341
Post-Traumatic Stress Disorder (PTSD)	A disorder characterized by failure to recover after experiencing or witnessing a terrifying event. Individuals who are triggered can relive the event as if it was happening again in the present. melissa, Roman chamomile, helichrysum & vetiver, Adaptiv® or Balance®, neroli	Limbic pg. 313; Mood & Behavior pg. 319
Precocious Puberty	A condition in which a child's body begins changing into that of an adult too soon. Zendocrine®, frankincense, Whisper®, ClaryCalm®, DDR Prime®	Endocrine pg. 284; Women's Health pg. 374; Men's Health pg. 316
Preeclampsia	A condition during pregnancy that results in high blood pressure, large amounts of protein in the urine and swelling that doesn't go away. Also called toxemia. marjoram, frankincense, Zendocrine®, AromaTouch®, cypress	Pregnancy, Labor & Nursing pg. 341
Pregnancy	The time from conception until birth, typically lasting 9 months or 40 weeks, with three stages or trimesters. DigestZen®, lavender, geranium, ylang ylang, Slim & Sassy®	Pregnancy, Labor & Nursing pg. 341; Women's Health pg. 374
Pregnancy (post-term)	Delivery on or after 41 weeks plus three days of gestation, or 10 days over the estimated date of delivery. myrrh, clary sage, Zendocrine®, basil, Whisper®	Pregnancy, Labor & Nursing pg. 341
Premenstrual Syndrome	A group of symptoms including irritability, bloating, and fatigue that occur in women, typically between ovulation and a period. ClaryCalm®, geranium, DDR Prime®, clary sage, Whisper®	Women's Health pg. 374; Mood & Behavior pg. 319
Preterm Labor	Labor before the thirty-seventh week of pregnancy. marjoram, ylang ylang + wild orange, lavender & neroli, Balance®, Serenity®	Pregnancy, Labor & Nursing pg. 341
Pre-Workout Muscle Prep	To help insure a good workout and decrease chance of injury, preparation or stretching should be implemented before a workout. Deep Blue®, peppermint, marjoram, wild orange, Slim & Sassy®	Athletes pg. 237
Prostatitis	Enlargement or inflammation of the prostate gland which is relatively typical in adult males. rosemary, Balance®, juniper berry, DDR Prime®, cypress	Men's Health pg. 316; Cardiovascular pg. 256

Aromatic: Inhale from cupped hands or diffuse into the air.
Topical: Apply directly to affected area(s) or bottom of feet.
Internal: Take in a capsule, glass of water, or on/under tongue.
TIP For adults use 2-3 drops; for children use 1-2 drops.

AILMENT	RECOMMENDED OILS AND USAGE	BODY SYSTEM/FOCUS AREA
Psoriasis	A continual, non-contagious skin disease defined by inflamed lesions covered with silvery-white scabs of dead skin. Zendocrine® (internal); Roman chamomile (topical, internal); turmeric (topical, internal); copaiba (internal, topical); geranium (topical, internal)	Integumentary pg. 304; Digestive & Intestinal pg. 275; Candida pg. 252; Parasites pg. 338
Purging Disorder	An eating disorder characterized by recurrent self-induced vomiting, misuse of laxatives, diuretics, or enemas to control weight or shape in the absence of binge eating episodes. melissa (internal, topical); cinnamon (internal, topical, aromatic); Balance® (aromatic, topical); patchouli (aromatic, internal, topical); Slim & Sassy® (internal, topical)	Eating Disorders pg. 280
Pyorrhea	A serious gum infection that damages gums and can destroy the jawbone. clove (topical); myrrh (topical, internal); cedarwood (topical); frankincense (topical, internal); On Guard® (topical, aromatic)	Oral Health pg. 331
Q Fever	A sickness caused by a type of Coxiella burnetii bacteria and resulting in a rash and fever. oregano (internal, topical); On Guard® (topical, internal); thyme (internal, topical); eucalyptus (topical); arborvitae (topical)	Immune & Lymphatic pg. 299
Radiation Damage	Radiation can damage the DNA inside a cell's nucleus, and if the DNA becomes sufficiently damaged, the cell can become cancerous. peppermint (internal, topical); Zendocrine® (internal, topical); patchouli (topical); cilantro (internal, topical); geranium (internal, topical)	Cellular Health pg. 261; Detoxification pg. 270
Rashes	A spotted, pink, or red skin outbreak that may be followed by itching. cedarwood (topical); Zendocrine® (internal); neroli (topical); lavender (topical); Immortelle (topical)	Integumentary pg. 304; Allergies pg. 234; Autoimmune pg. 240; Parasites pg. 338
Raynaud's Disease	A disorder in which the toes or fingers suddenly experience reduced blood circulation. black pepper (internal, topical); cypress (topical); AromaTouch® (topical); lemongrass (internal, topical); Console® (topical)	Cardiovascular pg. 256; Endocrine pg. 284
Reactive Attachment Disorder (RAD)	A rare but severe condition in which an infant or young child does not establish healthy attachments with parents or caregivers, resulting in markedly disturbed and developmentally inappropriate ways of relating socially. frankincense (topical, aromatic); Balance® (topical, aromatic); Forgive® (topical, aromatic); Console® (topical, aromatic); Peace® (topical, aromatic)	Limbic pg. 313; Mood & Behavior pg. 319; Stress pg. 363
Reiter's Arthritis	Joint pain and swelling triggered by an infection in another part of the body. basil (topical, internal); thyme (topical, internal); Deep Blue® (topical); AromaTouch® (topical); Forgive® (topical)	Immune & Lymphatic pg. 299; Digestive & Intestinal pg. 275; Skeletal pg. 355
Renal Artery Stenosis	The narrowing of one of the renal arteries that can impede blood flow to the target kidney, resulting in a secondary type of high blood pressure. Zendocrine® (internal, topical); ylang ylang (internal, topical); lemon (internal, topical); Citrus Bliss® (topical); lemongrass (internal, topical)	Cardiovascular pg. 256; Urinary pg. 366
Respiratory Issues	Respiratory problems can be as minor as the common cold or as serious as pneumonia. They may affect the upper respiratory system (nose, mouth, sinuses, and throat) or the lower bronchial tubes and lungs. Breathe® (aromatic, topical); cardamom (topical, internal, aromatic); rosemary (aromatic, topical, internal); arborvitae (aromatic, topical); eucalyptus (topical, aromatic)	Respiratory pg. 349
Restless Leg Syndrome	A condition characterized by a nearly irresistible urge to move the legs, typically in the evenings. AromaTouch® (topical); Deep Blue® (topical); PastTense® (topical); cypress (topical); Serenity® (topical)	Cardiovascular pg. 256; Sleep pg. 359
Restlessness	A failure to achieve relaxation; perpetually agitated or in motion; unquiet or uneasy. Balance® (topical, aromatic); lavender (topical, aromatic); Peace® (topical, aromatic); patchouli (topical, aromatic); Adaptiv® or Serenity® (topical, aromatic)	Sleep pg. 359; Energy & Vitality pg. 288; Mood & Behavior pg. 319

QUICK REFERENCE

STEPS: 1 Look up ailment. 2 Choose one or more of the recommended oils. (Order of recommendation is left to right.) 3 Use oil(s) as indicated. 4 Learn more in corresponding body system/focus area. 5 Find more solutions at essentiallife.com

AILMENT	RECOMMENDED OILS AND USAGE	BODY SYSTEM/FOCUS AREA
Retinitis Pigmentosa	An eye disease in which the back wall of the eye (retina) is damaged. patchouli, helichrysum, juniper berry, DDR Prime®, cardamom	Nervous pg. 327
Rheumatic Fever	A sickness which emerges as a complication of untreated or inadequately treated strep throat. oregano, ginger, wintergreen, eucalyptus, thyme	Immune & Lymphatic pg. 299; Pain & Inflammation pg. 334
Rheumatism	Any disease marked by inflammation and pain in the joints, muscles, or fibrous tissue (especially rheumatoid arthritis). turmeric, Deep Blue®, celery seed, lemongrass, Siberian fir	Muscular pg. 323; Skeletal pg. 355
Rheumatoid Arthritis	A chronic disease of the musculoskeletal system defined by swelling and inflammation of the joints (hands, wrists, knees, and feet). Deep Blue®, frankincense, AromaTouch®, Siberian fir, marjoram	Skeletal pg. 355; Pain & Inflammation pg. 334; Autoimmune pg. 240
Rhinitis	An infection of the mucous lining of the nose. Breathe®, On Guard®, peppermint, eucalyptus, oregano	Respiratory pg. 349
Ringworm	A highly contagious fungal infection of the skin or scalp. petitgrain, HD Clear®, melaleuca, Purify, myrrh	Integumentary pg. 304; Immune & Lymphatic pg. 299
Rosacea	A condition that causes redness and often small, red, pus-filled bumps on the face. Roman chamomile, sandalwood, helichrysum, myrrh, DDR Prime®	Integumentary pg. 304; Nervous pg. 327; Parasites pg. 338
Roseola	A common viral infection in young children that may cause high fever and a rash. melissa, melaleuca, On Guard®, copaiba, myrrh	Children pg. 265; Immune & Lymphatic pg. 299
RSV (Respiratory Syncytial Virus)	A virus that causes infections of the lungs and respiratory tract. The virus is so common that most children have been infected by age two. rosemary, eucalyptus, melissa, Siberian fir, Breathe®	Children pg. 265; Respiratory pg. 349
Rubella	An extremely contagious viral disease, spread through contact with discharges from the throat and nose of an infected person. On Guard®, melaleuca, lime, thyme, clove	Immune & Lymphatic pg. 299
Rumination Disorder	An eating disorder in which a person (usually an infant or young child) brings back up and re-chews partially digested food that has already been swallowed. DigestZen®, Zendocrine®, grapefruit, Balance®, peppermint	Eating Disorders pg. 280
Scabies	A somewhat contagious infection caused by a tiny burrowing mite. Purify, peppermint, thyme, arborvitae, On Guard®	Parasites pg. 338; Integumentary pg. 304
Scarlet Fever	An acute contagious bacterial illness that develops in some individuals who have strep throat. Produces a bright red rash that covers most of the body. oregano, On Guard®, melaleuca, sandalwood, thyme	Children pg. 265; Immune & Lymphatic pg. 299

Aromatic: Inhale from cupped hands or diffuse into the air.

Topical: Apply directly to affected area(s) or bottom of feet.

Internal: Take in a capsule, glass of water, or on/under tongue.

TIP For adults use 2-3 drops; for children use 1-2 drops.

AILMENT	RECOMMENDED OILS AND USAGE	BODY SYSTEM/FOCUS AREA
Scarring	The fibrous tissue that replaces normal tissue ruined by disease or injury. frankincense, helichrysum, lavender, sandalwood & neroli, Immortelle	Integumentary pg. 304
Schizophrenia	A long-term mental disorder characterized by extremely impaired emotions, thinking, hallucinations, and behaviors. frankincense, Roman chamomile, juniper berry, spikenard, patchouli	Brain pg. 248; Limbic pg. 313; Mood & Behavior pg. 319
Schmidt's Syndrome	A combination of Addison's disease with autoimmune hypothyroidism and/or type 1 diabetes. Zendocrine®, spikenard, Motivate®, cardamom, On Guard®	Autoimmune pg. 240; Endocrine pg. 284; Nervous pg. 327
Sciatica	An inflammation of the sciatic nerve, commonly defined by pain and tenderness along the course of the nerve through the leg and thigh. Deep Blue®, Douglas fir, frankincense, Siberian fir, basil	Nervous pg. 327; Pain & Inflammation pg. 334; Athletes pg. 237
Scleroderma	A gradual hardening and contraction of the skin and connective tissue, either locally or throughout the body. sandalwood, helichrysum, Douglas fir, ginger, coriander	Autoimmune pg. 240; Integumentary pg. 304; Skeletal pg. 355; Muscular pg. 323
Scoliosis	An abnormal side-to-side curve of the spine. Deep Blue®, lemongrass, helichrysum, AromaTouch®, wintergreen	Skeletal pg. 355
Scurvy	Disease caused by a deficiency of vitamin C. cypress, Zendocrine®, lemon, helichrysum, ginger	Immune & Lymphatic pg. 299; Energy & Vitality pg. 288
Seasonal Affective Disorder (SAD)	A type of depression that tends to occur as the days grow shorter in the fall and winter. Cheer®, bergamot, Motivate®, Elevation™, Passion®	Mood & Behavior pg. 319; Limbic pg. 313
Sebaceous Cyst	Noncancerous small bumps beneath the skin that can appear anywhere on the skin, but are most common on the face, neck and trunk. fennel, cedarwood, basil, black pepper, coriander	Integumentary pg. 304
Seizures	A convulsion or attack, commonly from a stroke or epileptic fit. spikenard, frankincense, petitgrain, cedarwood, sandalwood	Brain pg. 248; Children pg. 265
Sepsis	A bacterial infection in the body tissues or bloodstream. This is a very broad term covering the presence of many types of microscopic disease-causing organisms. oregano, marjoram, thyme, copaiba, On Guard®	Immune & Lymphatic pg. 299
Sex Drive (excessive)/ Hypersexuality	An obsession with sexual thoughts, urges, or behaviors that may cause distress and negatively affect one's health, job, relationships, or other parts of life. marjoram, arborvitae, Zendocrine®, neroli, Console®	Intimacy pg. 448
Sex Drive (low)	The inhibition of the sex drive or natural desire for sexual activity. Passion®, jasmine, cinnamon, ylang ylang, Whisper®	Intimacy pg. 448; Men's Health pg. 316; Women's Health pg. 374

STEPS: 1 Look up ailment. 2 Choose one or more of the recommended oils. (Order of recommendation is left to right.) 3 Use oil(s) as indicated. 4 Learn more in corresponding body system/focus area. 5 Find more solutions at essentiallife.com

AILMENT	RECOMMENDED OILS AND USAGE					BODY SYSTEM/FOCUS AREA
Shigella Infection	An intestinal disease caused by a family of bacteria known as shigella. The main sign of shigella infection is bloody diarrhea.					Immune & Lymphatic pg. 299; Digestive & Intestinal pg. 275
	eucalyptus	clove	black pepper	thyme	On Guard®	
Shingles	A viral infection that causes a painful rash, most often as a stripe of blisters that wraps around the torso.					Immune & Lymphatic pg. 299; Nervous pg. 327
	patchouli	melissa	yarrow	melaleuca	black pepper	
Shin Splints	Acute pain in the shin and lower leg caused by moderate to heavy physical activity. Commonly occurs in athletes who have recently intensified or changed their training routines.					Skeletal pg. 355; Athletes pg. 237
	AromaTouch®	Deep Blue®	lemongrass	wintergreen	basil	
Shock	Critical condition brought on by a sudden drop in blood flow through the body often accompanying severe injury or illness.					First Aid pg. 291; Nervous pg. 327; Stress pg. 363
	peppermint	Peace® or Adaptiv®	lavender	Roman chamomile	Balance®	
Sickle Cell Anemia	Disorder of the blood characterized by distorted red blood cells which are fragile and prone to rupture. The decrease in number of red blood cells results in anemia.					Cardiovascular pg. 256; Detoxification pg. 270
	Zendocrine®	frankincense	lemongrass	geranium	cassia	
Silent Thyroiditis	Inflammation of the thyroid gland, commonly occurring in the middle-aged women.					Autoimmune pg. 240; Endocrine pg. 284
	Zendocrine®	basil	DDR Prime®	AromaTouch®	Console®	
Sinus Congestion	Blockage of the nasal passage, also known as a stuffy nose.					Respiratory pg. 349; Digestive & Intestinal pg. 275
	Breathe®	eucalyptus	rosemary	On Guard®	helichrysum	
Sinusitis	Inflammation of the nasal sinus.					Respiratory pg. 349
	peppermint	Breathe®	cedarwood	Passion®	thyme	
Sjogren's Syndrome	A chronic, autoimmune disease characterized by dryness of the mouth and eyes.					Autoimmune pg. 240
	cinnamon	black pepper	Zendocrine®	Roman chamomile	DDR Prime®	
Skin (dry)	Chapped or flaky skin caused from dehydration, lack of omega 3s, or sun or wind damage.					Integumentary pg. 304
	sandalwood	cedarwood	copaiba	Immortelle	myrrh	
Skin (oily)	Excessively oily skin caused by excessive discharge of sebum from the sebaceous glands.					Integumentary pg. 304
	HD Clear®	petitgrain	lemon	wild orange	ylang ylang	
Skin Issues	A variety of issues that occur on the skin, causing irritation, outbreaks, or a breach in the surface.					Integumentary pg. 304
	lavender	Immortelle	geranium	sandalwood	frankincense	
Skin Ulcers	A lesion of a mucous membrane or the skin.					Integumentary pg. 304
	frankincense	helichrysum	lavender	geranium	myrrh	
Sleep Apnea	Disorder characterized by one or more pauses in breathing or shallow breaths while asleep.					Sleep pg. 359; Respiratory pg. 349
	Breathe®	thyme	rosemary	peppermint	lemongrass	

Aromatic: Inhale from cupped hands or diffuse into the air.

Topical: Apply directly to affected area(s) or bottom of feet.

Internal: Take in a capsule, glass of water, or on/under tongue.

TIP For adults use 2-3 drops; for children use 1-2 drops.

AILMENT	RECOMMENDED OILS AND USAGE	BODY SYSTEM/FOCUS AREA
Sleepwalking	Purposeful moving or walking while in a deep stage of sleep. vetiver · Serenity® · lavender · Peace® · Balance®	Sleep pg. 359
Smell (loss of)	Inability to perceive odor. sandalwood · peppermint · lavender or Adaptiv® · arborvitae or basil · helichrysum	Immune & Lymphatic pg. 299; Respiratory pg. 349
Smoking Addiction	A physical addiction or strong craving for nicotine, a chemical found in tobacco products. black pepper · clove · On Guard® · cilantro · Zendocrine®	Addictions pg. 230; Mood & Behavior pg. 319
Snake Bites	A bite from a snake which may be nonpoisonous or poisonous. basil · Purify · On Guard® · myrrh · Zendocrine®	First Aid pg. 291
Snoring	A sound achieved during sleep by vibration of loose tissue in the upper airway. To breathe during sleep with harsh, snorting noises caused by pulsing of the soft palate. Breathe® · peppermint · rosemary · eucalyptus · Douglas fir	Respiratory pg. 349; Sleep pg. 359
Social Anxiety Disorder	Excessive and unreasonable fear of social situations, arising from a fear of being closely watched, judged, and criticized by others. Peace® · bergamot & patchouli · Douglas fir · Adaptiv® or Serenity® · Console®	Brain pg. 248; Mood & Behavior pg. 319
Sore Feet	Pain or discomfort in the foot. AromaTouch® · Deep Blue® · ginger · copaiba · wintergreen	Athletes pg. 237; Muscular pg. 323; Skeletal pg. 355
Sore Muscles	Pain and stiffness felt in muscles several hours to days after unaccustomed or strenuous exercise. AromaTouch® · Deep Blue® · peppermint · PastTense® · marjoram	Muscular pg. 323; Pain & Inflammation pg. 334; Athletes pg. 237
Sore Throat	Any of various inflammations of the pharynx, tonsils, or larynx defined by pain in swallowing. On Guard® · melaleuca · myrrh · lime · thyme	Oral Health pg. 331; Immune & Lymphatic pg. 299; Respiratory pg. 349
Spina Bifida	Birth defect of the spine in which part of the spinal cord is exposed through a gap in the backbone. Siberian fir · clove · DDR Prime® · wintergreen · Deep Blue®	Skeletal pg. 355; Nervous pg. 327
Sprains	An injury to a ligament when the joint is carried through a range of motion larger than its normal range without dislocation or fracture. Deep Blue® · lemongrass · marjoram · copaiba · wintergreen	Muscular pg. 323; Pain & Inflammation pg. 334; First Aid pg. 291
Staph Infection	Infections caused by staphylococcus bacteria. On Guard® · Purify · geranium · oregano · myrrh	Immune & Lymphatic pg. 299
Stevens-Johnson Syndrome	Disorder of the skin and mucous membranes in which cell death causes the epidermis to separate from the dermis. Zendocrine® · melaleuca · frankincense · myrrh · arborvitae	Integumentary pg. 304

STEPS: **1** Look up ailment. **2** Choose one or more of the recommended oils. (Order of recommendation is left to right.) **3** Use oil(s) as indicated. **4** Learn more in corresponding body system/focus area. **5** Find more solutions at essentiallife.com

AILMENT	RECOMMENDED OILS AND USAGE	BODY SYSTEM/FOCUS AREA
Stomach Ache	Pain in the abdomen or stomach area. DigestZen® or Tamer™, peppermint, ginger, wild orange, black pepper	Digestive & Intestinal pg. 275
Strep Throat	A sore throat with fever caused by streptococcal infection. oregano, On Guard®, melaleuca, lemon, cinnamon	Immune & Lymphatic pg. 299
Stress	An organism's total response to environmental pressures or demands. Adaptiv® or Peace®, Balance®, lavender, Serenity®, neroli	Stress pg. 363
Stress Fractures	A fracture of bone caused by replicated application of a heavy load, such as the constant pounding on a surface by runners, dancers, and gymnasts. birch, helichrysum, Siberian fir, wintergreen, Deep Blue®	Skeletal pg. 355
Stretch Marks	Streaks or stripes on the skin, especially the abdomen, caused by prolonged stretching of the skin. Immortelle, geranium, sandalwood, lavender, frankincense	Integumentary pg. 304; Pregnancy, Labor & Nursing pg. 341; Weight pg. 369
Stroke	The sudden death of brain cells in a localized area due to insufficient blood flow. cassia, helichrysum, cypress, basil, fennel	Brain pg. 248
Stye	Infection of the sebaceous gland of an eyelash. Do not drop oil directly in eye. melaleuca, DDR Prime®, patchouli, frankincense, myrrh	Respiratory pg. 349
Sunburn	Overexposure to the sun that causes redness and inflammation. lavender, peppermint, Immortelle, frankincense, helichrysum	Integumentary pg. 304; First Aid pg. 291; Outdoors pg. 452
Swimmer's Ear	Infection of the outer ear canal that runs from the eardrum to the outside of the head. Often caused by water remaining in the ear after swimming. (Do not drop oil directly in ear canal) rosemary, clove, On Guard®, lavender, oregano	Respiratory pg. 349; Fitness pg. 440
Swimmer's Itch	Rash usually caused by an allergic reaction to parasites that burrow into the skin while swimming or wading in warm water. Purify, lemongrass, Zendocrine®, frankincense, Roman chamomile	Parasites pg. 338; Integumentary pg. 304
Tachycardia	A fast heart rate which is above 100 beats per minute in an adult. Balance®, ylang ylang, lavender, rosemary, melissa	Cardiovascular pg. 256
Taste, Loss	Loss of taste functions of the tongue. Also refers to alterations in taste (such as metallic taste, etc.). peppermint, lime, Zendocrine®, melissa, helichrysum	Respiratory pg. 349; Nervous pg. 327
Tear Duct (blocked)	A blocked nasolacrimal duct which typically moves tears from the eyes to the nose. myrrh, lavender, clary sage, eucalyptus, melaleuca	Respiratory pg. 349

Aromatic: Inhale from cupped hands or diffuse into the air.
Topical: Apply directly to affected area(s) or bottom of feet.
Internal: Take in a capsule, glass of water, or on/under tongue.
TIP For adults use 2-3 drops; for children use 1-2 drops.

AILMENT	RECOMMENDED OILS AND USAGE	BODY SYSTEM/FOCUS AREA
Teeth, Discolored	Occurs when the outer layer of the tooth is stained by smoking, coffee, wine, cola or other drinks or foods. wintergreen [topical] · lemon [topical] · peppermint [topical] · lime [topical] · Zendocrine® [topical]	Oral Health pg. 331; Personal Care pg. 454
Teeth Grinding	The habit of grinding and clenching one's teeth at night during sleep. Roman chamomile [topical, internal, aromatic] · lavender [aromatic, topical, internal] · marjoram [topical, aromatic] · Serenity® [topical, aromatic] · geranium [topical, aromatic]	Oral Health pg. 331
Teething Pain	Pain experienced when an infant's first teeth emerge through the gums. clove [topical] · Roman chamomile [topical] · myrrh [topical] · On Guard® [topical] · helichrysum [topical]	Oral Health pg. 331; Children pg. 265; Baby pg. 388
Tendonitis	The inflammation of a tendon, a hard rope-like tissue that connects muscle to bone. Deep Blue® [topical] · AromaTouch® [topical] · copaiba & marjoram [topical] · lemongrass [topical] · Siberian fir [topical]	Muscular pg. 323; Athletes pg. 237
Tennis Elbow	Inflammation of the tendons of the elbow caused by overuse of the muscles of the forearm. AromaTouch® [topical] · Deep Blue® [topical] · basil [topical] · ginger [topical] · lemongrass [topical]	Skeletal pg. 355; Muscular pg. 323
Tension (muscle)	Condition in which muscles of the body remain semi-contracted for an extended period. PastTense® [topical] · AromaTouch® [topical] · peppermint [topical] · marjoram [topical] · ginger [topical]	Muscular pg. 323; Fitness pg. 440
Testosterone (low)	Abnormally low levels of testosterone, a hormone required for male development and sexual function. sandalwood [topical, internal] · rosemary [topical, internal] · Passion® [topical, aromatic] · rose or ylang ylang [topical, internal, aromatic] · black spruce [topical, aromatic]	Men's Health pg. 316
Thrush	A contagious disease caused by a Candida albicans, fungus that appears most often in children and infants, defined by small whitish outbreaks on the mouth, throat, and tongue. spikenard [topical, internal] · arborvitae [topical] · clary sage [topical, internal] · melaleuca [topical, internal] · myrrh [internal, topical]	Candida pg. 252; Children pg. 265; Pregnancy, Labor & Nursing pg. 341; Women's Health pg. 374
Tick Bites	Bites from any of numerous small bloodsucking parasitic arachnids of the group Ixodidae and Argasidae, many of which spread febrile diseases. Purify [topical] · HD Clear® [topical] · melaleuca [topical] · lemon eucalyptus or eucalyptus [topical] · peppermint [topical]	Parasites pg. 338; First Aid pg. 291
Tinnitis	Hearing buzzing, ringing, or other sounds without an external cause. helichrysum [topical] · basil [topical] · cypress [topical] · Zendocrine® [topical] · juniper berry [topical]	Respiratory pg. 349
TMJ (TempoRo-mandibular Joint Dysfunction)	Pain in the jaw joint and in the muscles that control jaw movement. AromaTouch® [topical] · marjoram [topical] · PastTense® [topical] · Siberian fir [topical] · Deep Blue® [topical]	Muscular pg. 323; Oral Health pg. 331
Toe Fungus	A nail fungus causing thickened, brittle, crumbly, or ragged nails. melaleuca [topical, internal] · cinnamon [topical, internal] · copaiba [topical, internal] · HD Clear® [topical] · arborvitae [topical]	Athletes pg. 237; Candida pg. 252; Integumentary pg. 304
Tonsillitis	A swelling and infection of the tonsils, which are oval-shaped masses of lymph gland tissue located on both sides of the back of the throat. On Guard® [internal, topical] · myrrh [internal, topical] · lemon [internal, topical] · melaleuca [topical] · eucalyptus [topical]	Immune & Lymphatic pg. 299; Oral Health pg. 331
Toothache	A soreness or pain around or within a tooth, indicating inflammation and possible infection. clove [topical] · birch [topical] · helichrysum [topical] · On Guard® [topical] · melaleuca [topical]	Oral Health pg. 331

STEPS: 1 Look up ailment. 2 Choose one or more of the recommended oils. (Order of recommendation is left to right.) 3 Use oil(s) as indicated. 4 Learn more in corresponding body system/focus area. 5 Find more solutions at essentiallife.com

AILMENT	RECOMMENDED OILS AND USAGE	BODY SYSTEM/FOCUS AREA
Tourette Syndrome	Disorder of the nervous system characterized by involuntary tics and vocalizations. spikenard, DDR Prime®, patchouli, frankincense, vetiver	Nervous pg. 327; Brain pg. 248; Mood & Behavior pg. 319
Toxemia	Blood poisoning by toxins from a local bacterial infection. Frequently used to refer to preeclampsia, a condition in pregnancy characterized by high blood pressure. Zendocrine®, Slim & Sassy®, patchouli, cypress, frankincense	Pregnancy, Labor & Nursing pg. 341
Toxicity	The degree to which a substance can damage an organism. Zendocrine®, lemongrass, lemon or celery seed, DDR Prime®, petitgrain	Detoxification pg. 270; Fitness pg. 440; On the Go pg. 450; Personal Care pg. 454
Transverse Myelitis	Inflammation across both sides of one level, or segment, of the spinal cord. patchouli, clove, spikenard, wintergreen, Roman chamomile	Nervous pg. 327
Trigeminal Neuralgia	A disorder of the trigeminal nerve that causes episodes of stabbing, sharp pain in the lips, cheek, gums, or chin on one side of the face. wintergreen, juniper berry, helichrysum, spikenard, Roman chamomile	Nervous pg. 327
Tuberculosis	Infectious bacterial disease characterized by the growth of nodules in the tissues, especially the lungs. thyme, black pepper, rosemary, eucalyptus, Breathe®	Respiratory pg. 349; Immune & Lymphatic pg. 299
Tularemia	Rare infectious disease that typically attacks the skin, eyes, lymph nodes and lungs, characterized by ulcers, fever, and loss of weight. oregano, melaleuca, Zendocrine®, rosemary, thyme	Immune & Lymphatic pg. 299
Tumor	An uncommon growth of tissue resulting from uncontrolled, continuous multiplication of cells. DDR Prime®, frankincense, thyme, copaiba, sandalwood	Cellular Health pg. 261
Turner Syndrome	Chromosomal disorder affecting only females characterized by the absence of part or all of a second sex chromosome in some or all cells. thyme, clary sage, myrrh, ylang ylang, frankincense	Endocrine pg. 284
Typhoid	An infectious bacterial fever with an eruption of red spots on the chest and abdomen and severe intestinal irritation. clove, oregano, eucalyptus, cinnamon, peppermint	Immune & Lymphatic pg. 299
Ulcers (Duodenal)	An ulcer that occurs in the duodenum, the beginning of the small intestine. frankincense, myrrh, wintergreen, DigestZen®, fennel	Digestive & Intestinal pg. 275
Ulcers (Gastric)	An ulcer of the inner wall of the stomach. DigestZen®, peppermint, bergamot, yarrow, geranium	Digestive & Intestinal pg. 275
Ulcers (Leg)	An ulcer in the leg. geranium, frankincense, AromaTouch®, yarrow, helichrysum	Integumentary pg. 304; Cardiovascular pg. 256

Aromatic: Inhale from cupped hands or diffuse into the air.

Topical: Apply directly to affected area(s) or bottom of feet.

Internal: Take in a capsule, glass of water, or on/under tongue.

TIP For adults use 2-3 drops; for children use 1-2 drops.

AILMENT	RECOMMENDED OILS AND USAGE	BODY SYSTEM/FOCUS AREA
Ulcers (Peptic)	Ulcers in the upper duodenum and stomach (first portion of the small intestine) caused by a bacterium and stomach acid called Helicobacter pylori. cinnamon, fennel, peppermint, DigestZen®, juniper berry	Digestive & Intestinal pg. 275
Ulcers (Varicose)	Loss of skin surface in the drainage area of a varicose vein, typically in the leg, emerging from stasis and infection. PastTense®, helichrysum, cypress, geranium, coriander	Cardiovascular pg. 256; Integumentary pg. 304
Ureter Infection	Infection in the tube that transfers urine from the kidney to the bladder. coriander, On Guard®, lemongrass, DDR Prime®, cinnamon	Urinary pg. 366; Immune & Lymphatic pg. 299
Urinary Tract Infection (UTI)	An infection in any part of the urinary system, ureters, kidneys, bladder and urethra. lemon, geranium, lemongrass, juniper berry, cypress	Urinary pg. 366; Immune & Lymphatic pg. 299
Urination (Painful/Frequent)	Discomfort or burning with urination, usually felt in the urethra or perineum. cinnamon, melaleuca, lemongrass, Zendocrine®, On Guard®	Urinary pg. 366
Urine Flow (poor)	Abnormally slight or infrequent urination. Zendocrine®, Slim & Sassy®, juniper berry, cypress, AromaTouch®	Urinary pg. 366
Uterine Bleeding	Any loss of blood from the uterus. ClaryCalm®, helichrysum, geranium, frankincense, lavender	Pregnancy, Labor & Nursing pg. 341; Women's Health pg. 374
Uvetitis	An infection of the uveal tract, which lines the inside of the eye behind the cornea. Do not drop oil directly in eye. myrrh, juniper berry, frankincense, Immortelle, sandalwood	Nervous pg. 327
Vaginal Yeast Infection	Fungal infection that causes irritation, discharge and intense itchiness of the vagina and the vulva. melaleuca, spikenard, thyme, frankincense or myrrh, DDR Prime®	Candida pg. 252; Women's Health pg. 374
Vaginitis	Vaginal inflammation. melaleuca, patchouli, spikenard, yarrow, rosemary	Candida pg. 252; Women's Health pg. 374
Varicose Veins	Tortuous, dilated, elongated superficial veins that are commonly seen in the legs. cypress, helichrysum, coriander, yarrow, bergamot	Cardiovascular pg. 256; Integumentary pg. 304
Vertigo	A feeling of whirling or irregular motion, either of oneself or of external objects, generally caused by inner ear disease. frankincense, rosemary, ylang ylang, ginger, Balance®	Brain pg. 248; Cardiovascular pg. 256
Virus	A microorganism that cannot grow or reproduce apart from a living cell. A virus invades living cells and uses their chemical machinery to keep itself alive and to replicate itself. melissa, thyme, black pepper, yarrow, oregano	Immune & Lymphatic pg. 299

* For oil usage with eyes, apply oils to temples and around eyes. Dilute as necessary. Do NOT place oils in eyes or even touch eyes when oils are on your fingers.

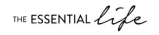

STEPS: 1 Look up ailment. 2 Choose one or more of the recommended oils. (Order of recommendation is left to right.) 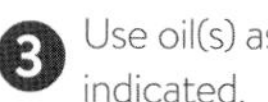 3 Use oil(s) as indicated. 4 Learn more in corresponding body system/focus area. 5 Find more solutions at essentiallife.com

AILMENT	RECOMMENDED OILS AND USAGE	BODY SYSTEM/FOCUS AREA
Vision (blurred)	The loss of sharpness of eyesight, making objects appear out of focus and hazy. Do not drop oil(s) directly in eye. DDR Prime® · lemongrass · helichrysum · frankincense · Immortelle	Nervous pg. 327
Vision (poor)	Decreased ability to see to a degree that causes problems not fixable by usual means, such as glasses. DDR Prime® · Immortelle · cypress · lemongrass · juniper berry	Nervous pg. 327
Vitiligo	A condition in which the pigment is lost from areas of the skin, causing whitish patches. Zendocrine® · Whisper® · vetiver · DDR Prime® · sandalwood	Autoimmune pg. 240; Integumentary pg. 304
Vomiting	Forcible elimination of contents of stomach through the mouth. DigestZen® or Tamer™ · peppermint · fennel · ginger · pink pepper	Digestive & Intestinal pg. 275; Immune & Lymphatic pg. 299; Eating Disorders pg. 280
Warts	Small, benign growths generated by a viral infection of the mucous or skin membrane. melissa · arborvitae · oregano · frankincense · lemongrass	Integumentary pg. 304
Wasp Sting	Painful stings or bites from bees, yellow jackets, hornets, wasps, and ants. These stings are generally harmless; however, more serious allergic reactions may occur which can be deadly. Purify · Roman chamomile · lavender · peppermint · cedarwood	First Aid pg. 291
Water Retention	Excessive buildup of fluid in the circulatory system, body tissues, or cavities in the body. lemon · celery seed or cypress · Slim & Sassy® · juniper berry · grapefruit	Urinary pg. 366; Cardiovascular pg. 256; Pregnancy, Labor & Nursing pg. 341
Weight Issues	Having more or less body fat than is optimally healthy. Slim & Sassy® · grapefruit · Zendocrine® · bergamot · DDR Prime®	Weight pg. 369
Whiplash	Neck injury due to forceful, rapid back-and-forth movement of the neck. PastTense® · Siberian fir · lemongrass · Deep Blue® · AromaTouch®	Muscular pg. 323
Withdrawal Symptoms	Unpleasant physical or mental symptoms that accompany the process of ceasing to take an addictive drug. Motivate® · frankincense · spikenard · Zendocrine® · Cheer®	Addictions pg. 230; Mood & Behavior pg. 319; Focus & Concentration pg. 295
Workout Recovery	The period of time following sustained exercise needed for the body to recuperate and for muscles tc repair. AromaTouch® · lemon · Deep Blue® · peppermint · PastTense®	Athletes pg. 237; Muscular pg. 323
Worms	A family of parasites that mainly reside in the intestinal tract, but can also live in the brain or muscles. clove · oregano · thyme · lemongrass · blue tansy	Parasites pg. 338; Digestive & Intestinal pg. 275

Aromatic: Inhale from cupped hands or diffuse into the air.

Topical: Apply directly to affected area(s) or bottom of feet.

Internal: Take in a capsule, glass of water, or on/under tongue.

TIP For adults use 2-3 drops; for children use 1-2 drops.

AILMENT	RECOMMENDED OILS AND USAGE	BODY SYSTEM/FOCUS AREA
Wounds	An injury to living tissue caused by a cut, blow, or other impact, typically one in which the skin is cut or broken. melaleuca (topical); lavender (topical); yarrow (topical); helichrysum (topical); frankincense (topical)	Integumentary pg. 304; First Aid pg. 291
Wrinkles	A fold, ridge, or crease in the skin typically appearing as a result of aging processes. Immortelle (topical); petitgrain (topical); spikenard (topical); geranium & neroli (topical); sandalwood (topical)	Integumentary pg. 304
Xenoestrogens	A type of xenohormone that imitates estrogen and creates byproduct estrogen metabolites as it is utilized by the body. lemon (internal, topical); ClaryCalm® (topical); Zendocrine® (internal, topical); thyme (internal, topical); ginger (internal, topical)	Women's Health pg. 374; Detoxification pg. 270
Xerophthalmia	Abnormal dryness of the eyes. lavender (internal, topical); sandalwood (topical, internal); lemon (internal); Immortelle (topical); Zendocrine® (internal, topical)	Respiratory pg. 349
Yeast	Overgrowth of the Candida fungi, which live on the surfaces of the body, causing systemic infection. melaleuca (internal, topical); thyme (internal, topical); oregano (internal, topical); DDR Prime® (internal, topical); lemongrass (internal, topical)	Candida pg. 252; Women's Health pg. 374; Children pg. 265

SECTION 3

NATURAL SOLUTIONS

Becoming familiar with the qualities and common benefits of essential oils is a key part of living THE ESSENTIAL LIFE. As you become versed in the powerful qualities of each oil, blend, and supplement, you will find confidence in turning to nature as your first resource for wellness. Nature's vast diversity provides answers for any health interest, be it physical, mental, or emotional.

SINGLE OILS

This section provides a detailed reference for the origins, qualities, purposes, and safety of individual essential oils. The top uses of each oil are intended to be a succinct guide, as more detailed uses are highlighted in *Body Systems*.

Please note the symbols Ⓐ=aromatic Ⓣ=topical Ⓘ=internal that specify recommended usage. While all oils are meant to be used aromatically and most topically, only verified pure therapeutic essential oils are intended for internal use. (See *Why Quality Matters* and *How to Use Essential Oils* for further detail.)

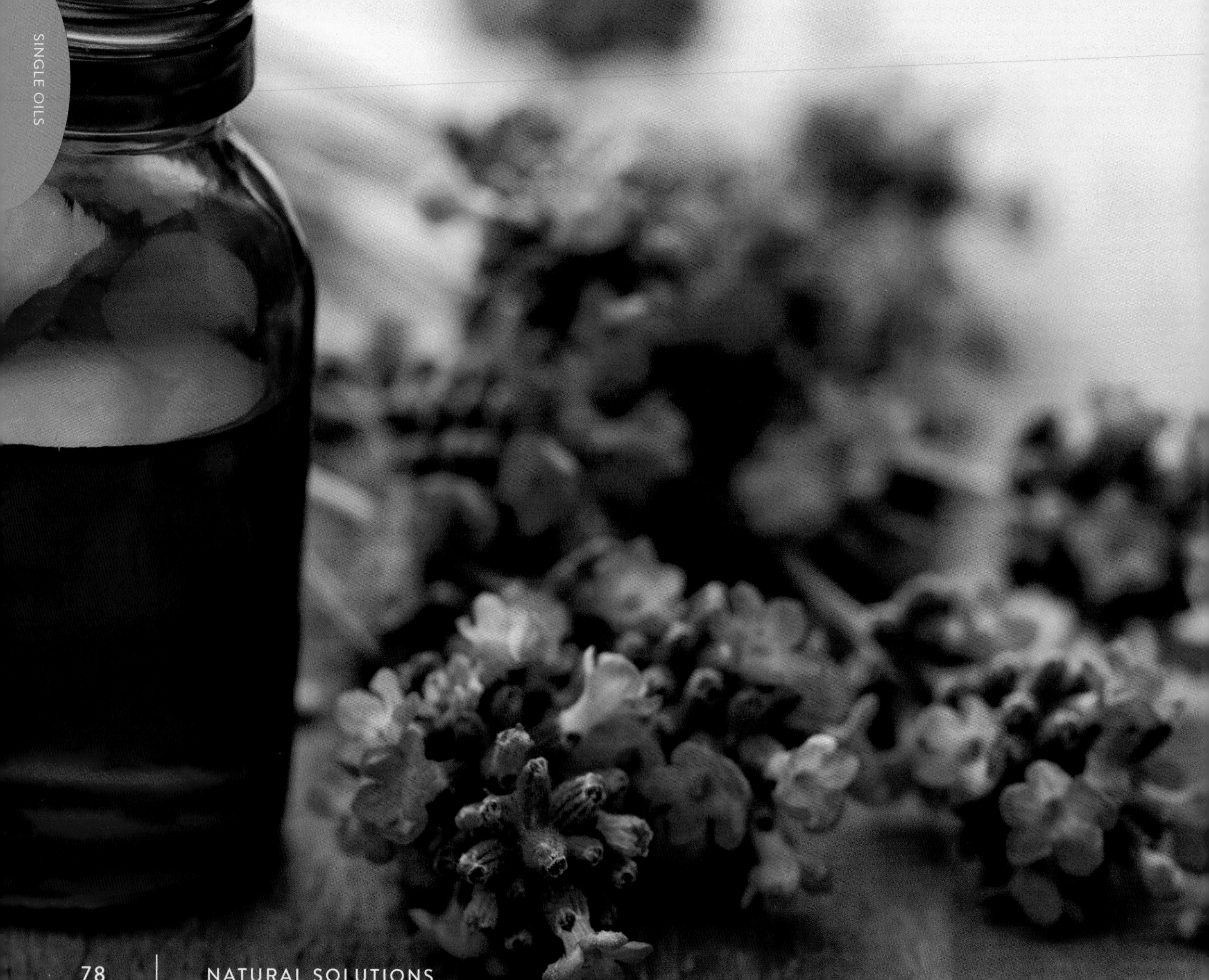

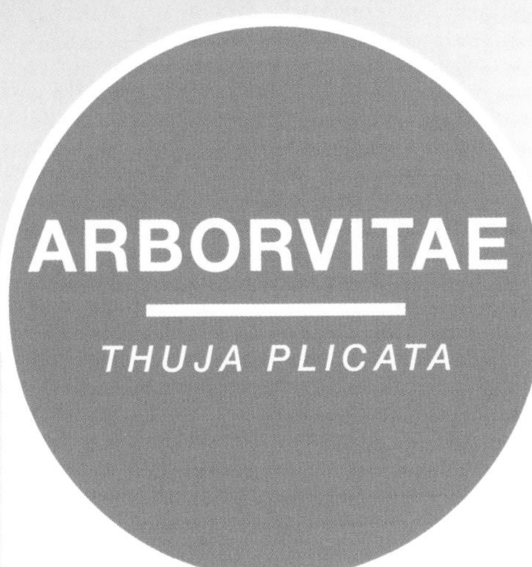

ARBORVITAE

THUJA PLICATA

woody majestic strong

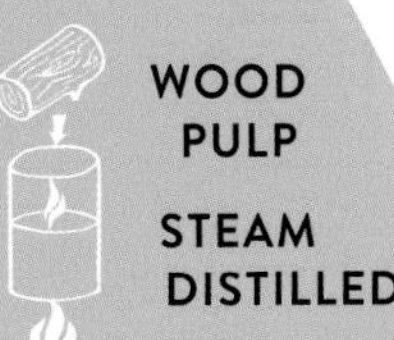

WOOD PULP

STEAM DISTILLED

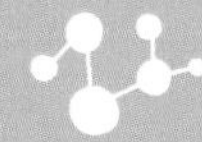

MAIN CONSTITUENTS
Methyl thujate
Hinokitiol
Thujic acid

TOP PROPERTIES
Antiviral
Antifungal
Antibacterial
Stimulant

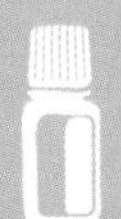

FOUND IN
TerraShield®

BLENDS WELL WITH
Birch
Cedarwood
Frankincense
Siberian fir

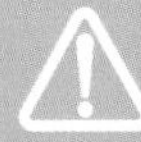

SAFETY
Dilution recommended. Possible skin sensitivity.

TOP USES

CANDIDA & FUNGAL ISSUES
Apply to bottoms of feet or area(s) of concern.

VIRUSES
Apply to bottoms of feet.

COLD SORES & WARTS
Apply to sore or wart frequently.

RESPIRATORY ISSUES
Apply to chest with fractionated coconut oil.

REPELLENT
Diffuse, spray on surfaces, or apply to repel bugs and insects.

CANCER
Apply to bottoms of feet.

STIMULANT
Apply under nose and back of neck to stimulate body systems and awareness.

BACTERIAL SUPPORT
Apply to bottoms of feet or spine with fractionated coconut oil. Spray diluted in water on surfaces or diffuse to kill airborne pathogens.

SKIN COMPLAINTS
Apply with lavender to troubled skin.

SUNSCREEN
Apply with helichrysum or lavender to protect against sun exposure.

MEDITATION
Diffuse to enhance spiritual awareness and state of calm.

EMOTIONAL BALANCE
Use aromatically and topically to get from Overzealous ———> Composed.

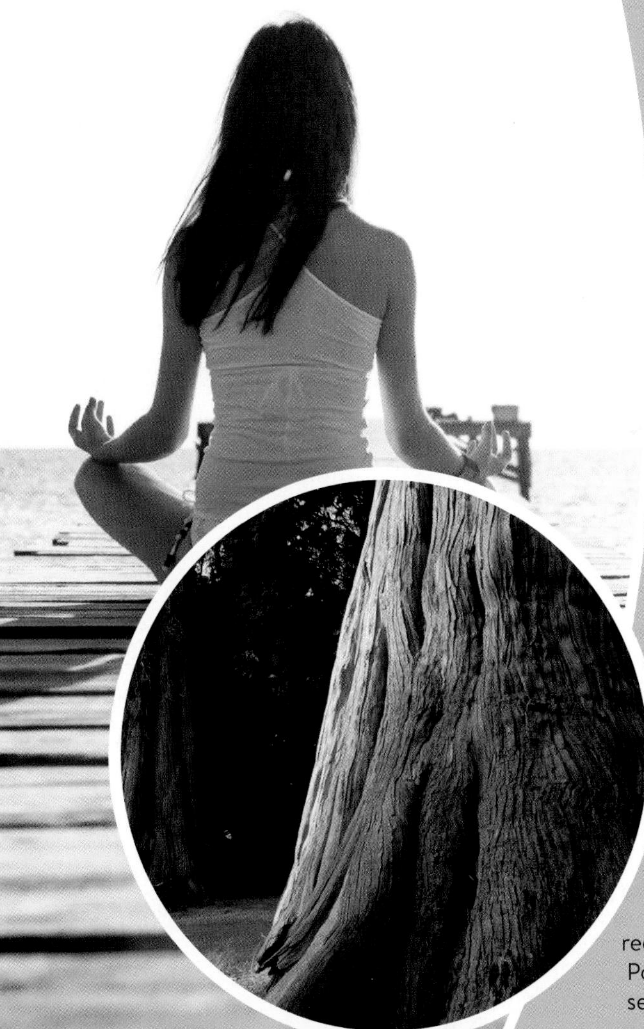

Arborvitae trees can live for over 800 years. It's no surprise that Arborvitae means "Tree of Life."

RESEARCH: Effect of arborvitae seed on cognitive function and a-7nAChR protein expression of hippocampus in model rats with Alzheimer's disease, Cheng XL, Xiong XB, Xiang MQ, *Cell Biochem Biophys*, 2013

Conservative surgical management of stage IA endometrial carcinoma for fertility preservation, Mazzon I, Corrado G, Masciullo V, Morricone D, Ferrandina G, Scambia G., *Fertil Steril*, 2010

= Aromatically = Topically = Internally

SINGLE OILS

BASIL

OCIMUM BASILICUM

regenerating
uplifting
stimulating

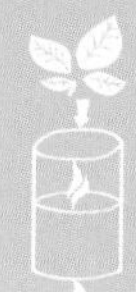

LEAVES

STEAM DISTILLED

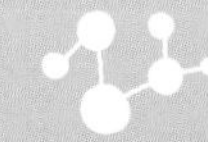

MAIN CONSTITUENTS
Linalool
Methylchavicol
Eugenol

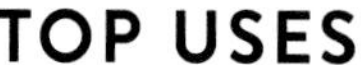

TOP USES

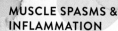

ADRENAL FATIGUE
Apply under nose, to bottoms of feet, back of neck, forehead, and/or over the adrenal area.

EARACHE
Apply behind and down beneath ear area; swab ear canal to relieve pain and infection.

LOSS OF SENSE OF SMELL
Apply under nose and to toes to regain or increase sense of smell.

MIGRAINES & DIZZINESS
Apply with wintergreen or peppermint to temples and back of neck.

MENTAL FATIGUE & FOCUS
Breathe in, diffuse or apply across forehead.

NAUSEA & CRAMPING
Take in a capsule or apply to abdomen to ease discomfort.

GOUT & RHEUMATISM
Apply to spine, bottoms of feet, ears, ankles, or area over heart.

PMS & MENSTRUAL ISSUES
Apply to lower abdomen to stimulate menstrual flow and assist with menstrual cramping.

MUSCLE SPASMS & INFLAMMATION
Apply to spine or bottoms of feet, or take in a capsule.

BUG, SNAKE & SPIDER BITES
Diffuse or spray diluted in water to repel insects. Apply topically to bite.

EMOTIONAL BALANCE
Use aromatically and topically to get from Inundated ——> Relieved.

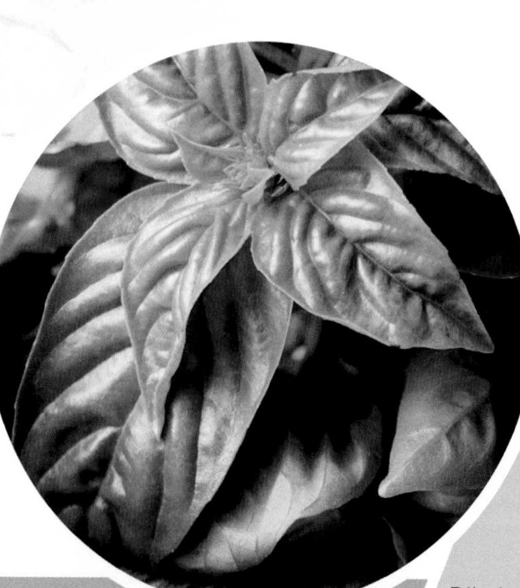

TOP PROPERTIES
Stimulant
Neurotonic
Steroidal
Regenerative
Antispasmodic
Anti-inflammatory
Antibacterial
Digestive

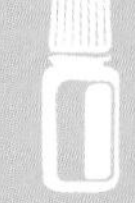

FOUND IN
Align®
AromaTouch®
PastTense®

BLENDS WELL WITH
Bergamot
Lime
Litsea
Peppermint

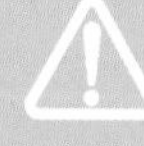

SAFETY
Dilution recommended. Possible skin sensitivity. Caution with pregnancy and epilepsy.

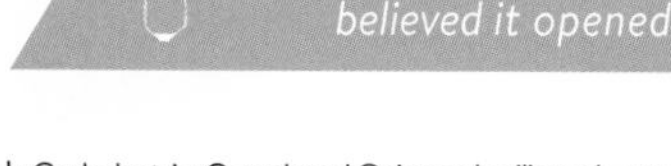

One of the most universally applicable oils, basil is from the Greek word meaning "king." Ancient Greeks believed it opened the gateways to heaven.

RESEARCH: Cyclodextrin-Complexed Ocimum basilicum Leaves Essential Oil Increases Fos Protein Expression in the Central Nervous System and Produces an Antihyperalgesic Effect in Animal Models for Fibromyalgia, Nascimento SS, *International Journal of Molecular Sciences,* 2014

Central Properties and Chemical Composition of Ocimum basilicum Essential Oil, Ismail M, *Pharmaceutical Biology,* 2006

A comparative study of antiplaque and antigingivitis effects of herbal mouthrinse containing tea tree oil, clove, and basil with commercially available essential oil mouthrinse, Kothiwale SV, Patwardhan V, Gandhi M, Sohoni R, Kumar A, *Journal of Indian Society of Periodontology,* 2014

Protective effect of basil (Ocimum basilicum L.) against oxidative DNA damage and mutagenesis, Berić T, *Food and Chemical Toxicology,* 2008

Biological effects, antioxidant and anticancer activities of marigold and basil essential oils, Mahmoud GI, *Journal of Medicinal Plants Research,* 2013

Increased seizure latency and decreased severity of pentylenetetrazol-induced seizures in mice after essential oil administration, Koutroumanidou E, *Epilepsy Research and Treatment,* 2013

Antigiardial activity of Ocimum basilicum essential oil, de Almeida I, *Parasitology Research,* 2007

Antibacterial Effects of the Essential Oils of Commonly Consumed Medicinal Herbs Using an In Vitro Model, Soković M, *Molecules,* 2010

uplifting • assuring • restoring

BERGAMOT

CITRUS BERGAMIA

TOP USES

ADDICTIONS
Apply to back of neck and bottoms of feet or diffuse.

INSOMNIA
Inhale or diffuse before sleep.

STRESS
Apply to back of neck and bottoms of feet or diffuse.

JOINT ISSUES & MUSCLE CRAMPS
Apply to affected area(s).

FUNGAL ISSUES
Apply to affected area(s) or take in a capsule.

COUGHS, INFECTIONS & BRONCHITIS
Apply to chest.

ACNE, OILY SKIN, ECZEMA & PSORIASIS
Apply diluted to affected area.

APPETITE LOSS
Breathe in and/or take in a capsule.

SELF-WORTH ISSUES
Apply to belly button and over heart to enhance feelings of worth.

EMOTIONAL BALANCE
Use aromatically and topically to get from Inadequate ———> Worthy.

= Aromatically = Topically = Internally

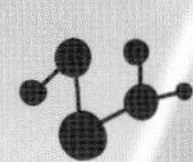

RIND

COLD PRESSED

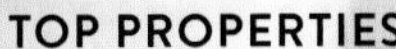

MAIN CONSTITUENTS
Limonene
Linalyl formate
Linalool

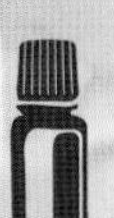

TOP PROPERTIES
Neurotonic
Anti-inflammatory
Antidepressant
Antibacterial
Antifungal
Digestive Stimulant

FOUND IN
Beautiful®
Align®
Citrus Bliss®
ClaryCalm®

BLENDS WELL WITH
Ylang ylang
Lavender
Patchouli

SAFETY
Possible skin sensitivity. Avoid sunlight or UV rays to applied area for up to 12 hours.

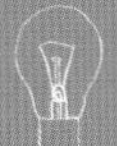

Bergamot was used in the first eau de cologne & is used to flavor Earl Grey tea.

RESEARCH: Anticancer activity of liposomal bergamot essential oil (BEO) on human neuroblastoma cells, Celia C, Trapasso E, Locatelli M, Navarra M, Ventura CA, Wolfram J, Carafa M, Morittu VM, Britti D,
Di Marzio L, Paolino D, *Colloids and Surfaces,* 2013

The essential oil of bergamot enhances the levels of amino acid neurotransmitters in the hippocampus of rat: implication of monoterpene hydrocarbons, Morrone LA, Rombolà L, Pelle C, Corasaniti MT, Zappettini S, Paudice P, Bonanno G, Bagetta G, *Pharmacological Research,* 2007

The effects of inhalation of essential oils on the body weight, food efficiency rate and serum leptin of growing SD rats, Hur MH, Kim C, Kim CH, Ahn HC, Ahn HY, *Korean Society of Nursing Science,* 2006

BIRCH

BETULA LENTA

invigorate
activate
soothe

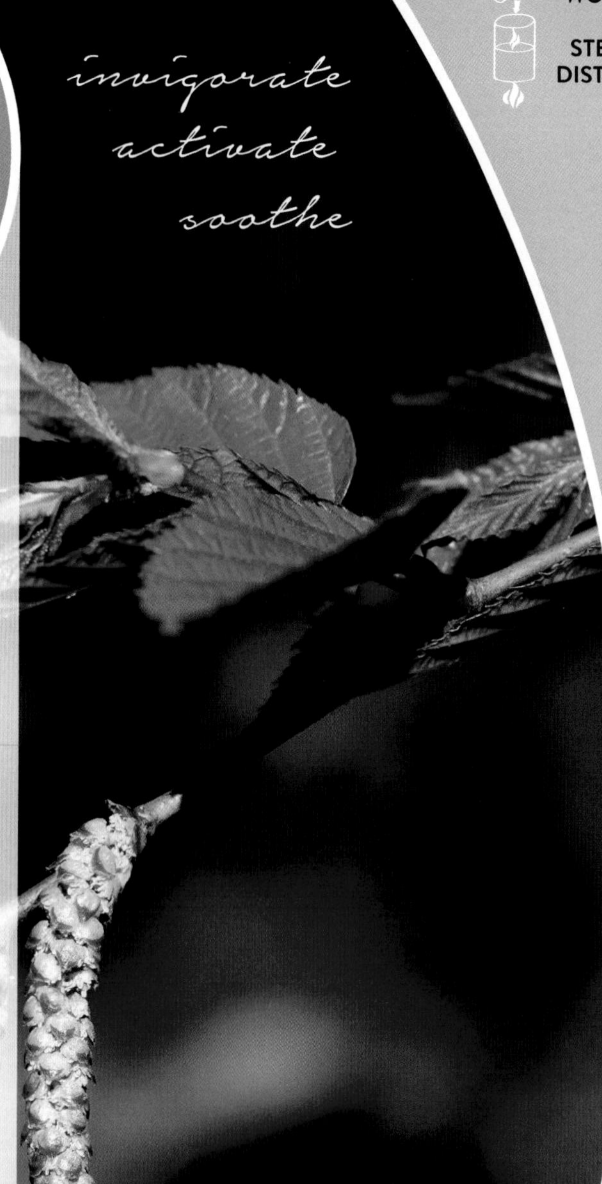

TOP USES

CONNECTIVE TISSUE & MUSCLE INJURIES
Apply to affected area.

ARTHRITIS, RHEUMATISM & GOUT
Apply to affected area.

MUSCLE PAIN & SPASMS
Apply to area(s) of concern for steroidal support.

FEVER
Apply on spine.

BONE SPURS, GALLSTONES, KIDNEY STONES & CATARACTS
Apply to bottoms of feet or area(s) of concern.

ULCERS & CRAMPS
Apply to abdomen as needed.

BROKEN BONES & TOOTH PAIN
Apply to area of concern.

EMOTIONAL BALANCE
Use aromatically and topically to get from Cowardly ——> Courageous.

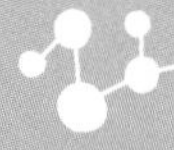

WOOD

STEAM DISTILLED

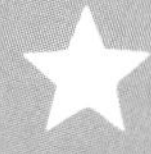

MAIN CONSTITUENT
Methyl salicylate
Betulene
Butulinol

TOP PROPERTIES
Analgesic
Neurotonic
Anti-rheumatic
Stimulant
Steroidal
Warming

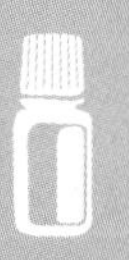

BLENDS WELL WITH
Bergamot
Cedarwood
Vetiver
Wild orange

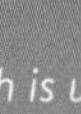

Birch is used to make root beer.

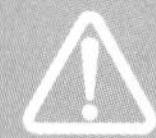

SAFETY
Not for internal use. Avoid during pregnancy. Not for use by epileptics.

RESEARCH: Repelling properties of some plant materials on the tick Ixodes ricinus L., Thorsell W, Mikiver A, Tunón H, *Phytomedicine*, 2006

SINGLE OILS

spicy • warming • circulating

BLACK PEPPER

PIPER NIGRUM

TOP USES

CONSTIPATION, DIARRHEA & GAS
Take (I) in capsule or apply (T) to abdomen.

RESPIRATORY & LYMPHATIC DRAINAGE & CLEANSING
Use a drop (I) under tongue or inhale/diffuse (A).

POOR CIRCULATION & COLD EXTREMITIES
Apply (T) with a warm compress to increase circulation and blood flow to muscles and nerves.

CATARACTS
Take 1-2 drops (I) in a capsule 1-2 times daily, apply (T) under 2nd and 3rd toes.

COLD, FLU, ACHES & CHILLS
Use (I) in a capsule or apply (T) to bottoms of feet or along spine.

CONGESTED AIRWAYS
Diffuse (A) or apply (T) to chest with eucalyptus to clear airways.

FOOD FLAVOR
Enhance favorite foods by adding a drop to add flavor and support digestion.

ANXIETY
Diffuse (A) or apply (T) under nose or to bottoms of feet.

CRAMPS, SPRAINS & MUSCLE SPASMS
Apply (T) to affected area(s).

SMOKING
Take a drop (I) under tongue & inhale (A) or diffuse to ease nicotine cravings and associated anxiety.

EMOTIONAL BALANCE
Use (A) aromatically and (T) topically to get from Repressed ———> Honest.

(A) = Aromatically (T) = Topically (I) = Internally

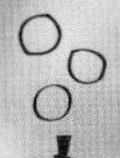

PEPPERCORN

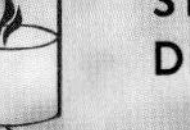

STEAM DISTILLED

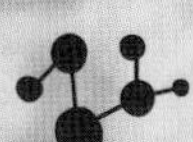

MAIN CONSTITUENTS
Caryophyllene
Limonene
Carene

TOP PROPERTIES
Antioxidant
Antispasmodic
Digestive Stimulant
Expectorant
Neutronic
Stimulant
Rubefacient

FOUND IN
Amavi®
On Guard® softgels
Anchor®

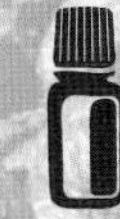

BLENDS WELL WITH
Cardamom
Copaiba
Clove
Juniper berry
Manuka

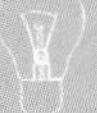

SAFETY
Dilution recommended. Possible skin sensitivity if old or oxidized.

Black pepper shares a similar chemical structure to melissa essential oil.

SINGLE OILS

RESEARCH: Black pepper and piperine reduce cholesterol uptake and enhance translocation of cholesterol transporter proteins, Duangjai A, *Journal of Natural Medicine*, 2013

Growth inhibition of pathogenic bacteria and some yeasts by selected essential oils and survival of L. monocytogenes and C. albicans in apple-carrot juice., Irkin R, *Foodborne Pathogens and Disease*, 2009

Antioxidative Properties and Inhibition of Key Enzymes Relevant to Type-2 Diabetes and Hypertension by Essential Oils from Black Pepper, Oboh G, *Advances in Pharmacological Sciences*, 2013

Black pepper essential oil to enhance intravenous catheter insertion in patients with poor vein visibility: a controlled study, Kristiniak S, *Journal of Alternative and Complementary Medicine*, 2012

Olfactory stimulation using black pepper oil facilitates oral feeding in pediatric patients receiving long-term enteral nutrition, Munakata M, *The Tohoku Journal of Experimental Medicine*, 2008

The effects of aromatherapy on nicotine craving on a U.S. campus: a small comparison study, Cordell B, Buckle J, *The Journal of Alternative and Complementary Medicine*, 2013

A randomized trial of olfactory stimulation using black pepper oil in older people with swallowing dysfunction, Ebihara T, *Journal of the American Geriatrics Society*, 2009

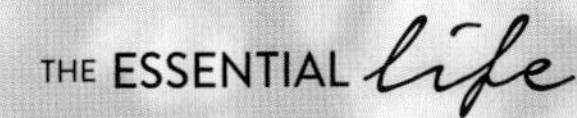

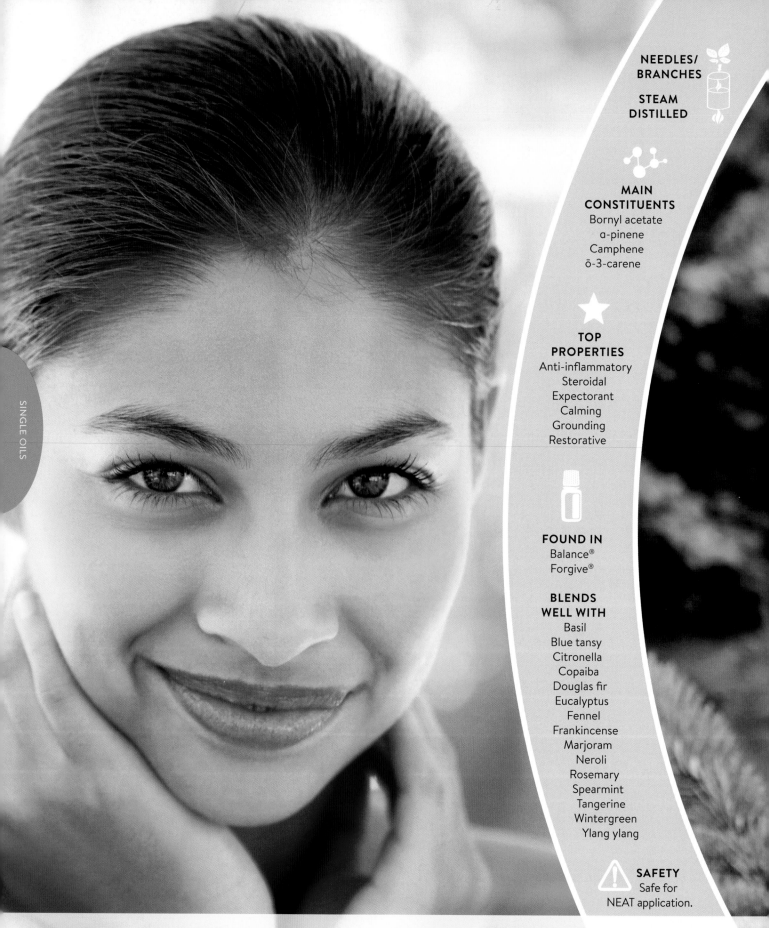

Composition, antimicrobial and antioxidant activities of seven essential oils from the North American boreal forest.

Poaty B, Lahlah J, Porqueres F, Bouafif H.

World J Microbiol Biotechnol. 2015 Jun;31(6):907-19. doi: 10.1007/s11274-015-1845-y. Epub 2015 Mar 24

Essential oils (EOs) were steam-extracted from the needles and twigs of balsam fir, black spruce, white spruce, tamarack, jack pine and eastern white cedar that remained after logging in eastern Canada. All of these oils exhibited antibacterial properties, especially when examined in closed tube assay compared to the traditional 96-well microliter format. These antimicrobial activities (minimum inhibitory concentration ≥ 0.2% w/v), comparable to those of exotic EOs, were shown against common pathogenic bacteria and fungi.

BLACK SPRUCE

PICEA MARIANA

grounding
enduring
advancing

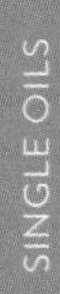

TOP USES

OVERSTRIVING, ADRENAL/NERVOUS EXHAUSTION & FATIGUE, MELANCHOLIC
Diffuse and apply to forehead, above kidney area, and/or over heart. Repeat as needed.

CHRONIC JOINT/BACK PAIN DUE TO POOR CIRCULATION & STRESS
Apply up spine, over back, to bottoms of feet and area(s) of concern. Repeat 2-4x's per day.

FEELING DISCONNECTED FROM POTENTIAL, OR THWARTED
Diffuse and apply to pulse points and over heart. Repeat as often as needed.

ASTHMA, BRONCHITIS, SINUSITIS, SPASTIC & MOIST COUGHS
Add 2-3 drops to warm/wet washcloth, place on chest; or to hot water, cover head with towel, inhale vapors.

HORMONE & STRESS-RELATED SKIN OUTBREAKS, HIGH BLOOD PRESSURE
Apply to area(s) of concern for a natural steroid-like effect. Dilute for skin sensitivity.

LACK OF SELF-ACCEPTANCE OR CONFIDENCE, INSECURE & INDECISIVE
Diffuse and apply over heart and pulse points.

HYPOTHALAMUS, PITUITARY & THYMUS IRREGULARITIES, HYPERTHYROIDISM
Apply up spine, base of skull, across forehead and bottoms of feet. Repeat 2-4x's per day.

WOUND HEALING, ESPECIALLY AFTER SURGERY, CANCER
Apply to area(s) of concern. Dilute for sensitive skin.

LOW TESTOSTERONE, PERFORMANCE & MEN'S COLOGNE
Blend with fennel and apply to wrist and reflex points.

INSATIABLE EATING DUE TO ANXIOUS FEELINGS
Diffuse and/or apply to pulse points.

PARALYZED OR OVERLY RISKY DUE TO FEAR BROUGHT ON BY MEMORIES
Diffuse and apply to forehead and back of neck. Repeat as often as necessary.

STRESS-INDUCED SHORT-TERM MEMORY LOSS & ALZHEIMER'S DISEASE
Apply to back of neck, across forehead and to toes. Repeat 2x's per day.

FEELING UNABLE TO INFLUENCE, SET BACK BY LIMITING BELIEFS OF OTHERS, UNFORGIVING
Diffuse and apply over heart and pulse points. Repeat as often as necessary.

EMOTIONAL BALANCE
Use aromatically and topically to get from Halted ⟶ Acclaimed.

Native Americans utilized black spruce for ointments, salves, and lotions made with honey and alum used to treat skin problems. The balsam was made into chewing gum, caulking or glue, and the inner bark and shoots of the tree were used as a food source.

The antioxidant potential of the boreal samples was determined by the 1,1-diphenyl-2-picrylhydrazyl radical scavenging (concentration providing 50% inhibition ≥ 7 mg/ml) and reducing power methods. Finally, this investigation revealed some boreal EOs to be potential antimicrobial and antioxidant agents that would notably benefit products in the personal hygiene and care industry.

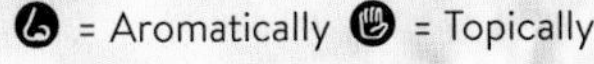
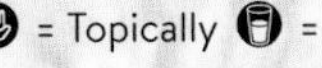
= Aromatically = Topically = Internally

BLUE TANSY

TANACETUM ANNUUM

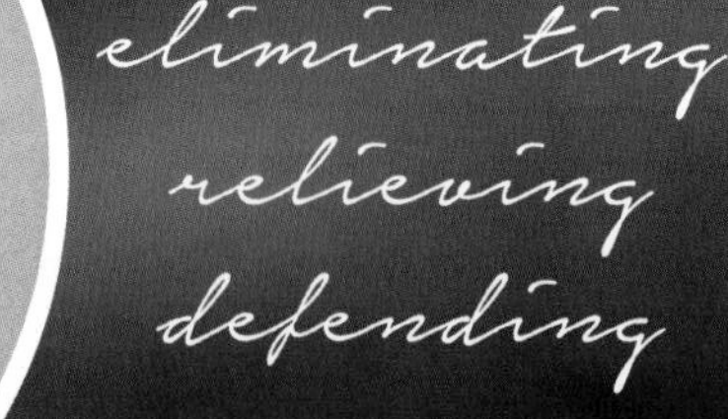

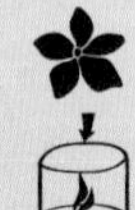

FLOWER/LEAF & STEM

STEAM DISTILLED

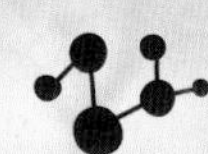

MAIN CONSTITUENT
Sabinene
Chamazulene

TOP PROPERTIES
Anti-histamine
Insect Repellent
Anti-allergenic
Antifungal
Vermicide
Antiviral
Stomachic

FOUND IN
Balance®
Deep Blue®

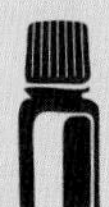

BLENDS WELL WITH
Clary sage
Marjoram
Helichrysum
Geranium
Petitgrain
Spikenard
Wintergreen

SAFETY
Can be harmful to small animals. Possible skin sensitivity. May stain surfaces, fabrics and skin.

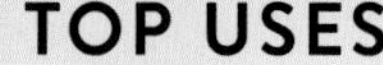

TOP USES

ALLERGIES, ITCHING, RASHES, WATERY EYES & SNEEZING
Apply to bottoms of feet and/or affected area(s).

ACNE, ECZEMA, PSORIASIS & SUNBURN
Apply to affected area(s) with helichrysum.

FIBROMYALGIA, SCIATICA, ARTHRITIS, & RHEUMATISM
Apply to affected area(s).

FUNGAL & SKIN INFECTIONS, SPORES
Apply to affected area(s).

ASTHMA & RESPIRATORY ISSUES, HICCUPS
Combine with eucalyptus or peppermint and apply to chest and/or under nose.

TENSION & SINUS HEADACHES, MIGRAINES, TOOTHACHE
Massage into temples, sides of nose, or gums.

INDIGESTION, STOMACH ULCERS & INTESTINAL WORMS
Massage into abdomen.

COLD, FLU, MUMPS, CHICKEN POX, & MUSCLE ACHES
Apply to affected area(s) or bottoms of feet.

ADDICTIONS & LOW SELF-CONFIDENCE
Diffuse or inhale from cupped hands.

BUG BITES, SCABIES & INSECT REPELLENT
Apply to affected area(s), diffuse to deter insects, or add a few drops to a spray bottle with water.

THYROID & THYMUS ISSUES
Apply over thyroid and to back of neck.

EMOTIONAL BALANCE
Use aromatically and topically to get from Overwhelmed ———> Encouraged.

Tansy comes from the Greek word "Athanaton" meaning immortal.

ː: Chemical composition, antibacterial activity and cytotoxicity of essential oils ...nparthenium in different developmental stages. Mohsenzadeh F, Chehregani ...harm Biol. 2011 Sep;49(9):920-6. doi: 10.3109/13880209.2011.556650. Epub ... PMID: 21592001

Select item 18568393 Parthenolide inhibits proliferation of fibroblast-like synoviocytes in vitro. Parada-Turska J, Mitura A, Brzana W, Jalonkski M, Majdan M, Rzeski W. Inflammation. 2008 Aug; 31(4):281-5. doi: 10.1007/s10753-008-9076-0. PMID: 18568393

CARDAMOM

ELETTARIA CARDAMOMUM

invigorate
relax
cleanse

TOP USES

CONGESTION
Apply to chest and bridge of nose or diffuse.

STOMACH ACHE & CONSTIPATION
Take in a capsule or apply to abdomen.

COLITIS & DIARRHEA
Apply to abdomen.

GASTRITIS & STOMACH ULCERS
Use in a capsule.

MENSTRUAL & MUSCULAR PAIN
Apply to area(s) of concern to relieve pain and inflammation.

SORE THROAT & FEVER
Gargle a drop in water or apply to throat and back of neck.

CATARACTS
Take 1-2 drops in a capsule 1-2 times daily, apply under 2nd and 3rd toes.

MENTAL FATIGUE & CONFUSION
Apply under nose and to back of neck to clear your mind and ease fatigue.

PANCREATITIS
Apply to area over pancreas and bottoms of feet to cleanse and restore pancreatic function.

BAD BREATH & HOUSEHOLD ODORS
Take in a capsule for breath or diffuse to clear air of odors.

COOKING
Use to season your favorite foods and enhance flavors.

EMOTIONAL BALANCE
Use aromatically and topically to get from Self-centered ——→ Charitable.

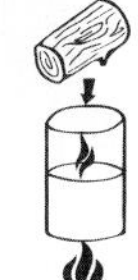

SEEDS

STEAM DISTILLED

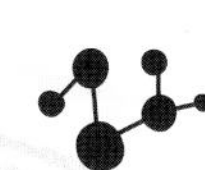

MAIN CONSTITUENTS
Terpinyl acetate
1,8-cineole
Linalool

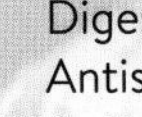

TOP PROPERTIES
Digestive Stimulant
Antispasmodic
Anti-inflammatory
Decongestant
Expectorant
Tonic
Stomachic
Carminative

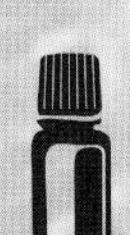

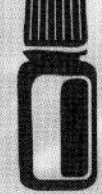

FOUND IN
Breathe®
Breathe® lozenge

BLENDS WELL WITH
Clove
Lavender
Peppermint

SAFETY
Safe for NEAT application.

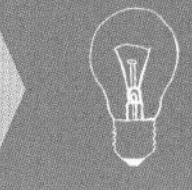

Known as one of the most expensive cooking spices, cardamom is also a close relative of ginger.

SINGLE OILS

RESEARCH: Antimicrobial activity of the bioactive components of essential oils from Pakistani spices against Salmonella and other multi-drug resistant bacteria., Naveed R, Hussain I, *BMC Complementary and Alternative Medicine*, 2013

Gastroprotective effect of cardamom, Elettaria cardamomum Maton, fruits in rats, Jamal A, *Journal of Ethnopharmacology*, 2006

Aromatherapy as a Treatment for Postoperative Nausea: A randomized trial, Hunt R, *Anesthesia and Analgesia*, 2013

Treatment of irritable bowel syndrome with herbal preparations: results of a double-blind, randomized, placebo-controlled, multi-centre trial, Madisch A, *Alimentary Pharmacology and Therapeutics*, 2004

Identification of proapoptopic, anti-inflammatory, anti-proliferative, anti-invasive and anti-angiogenic targets of essential oils in cardamom by dual reverse virtual screening and binding pose analysis, Bhattacharjee B, Asian Pacific *Journal of Cancer Prevention*, 2013 *Activity of Essential Oils Against Bacillus subtilis Spores*, Lawrence HA, *Journal of Microbiology and Biotechnology*, 2009

= Aromatically = Topically = Internally

CASSIA

CINNAMOMUM CASSIA

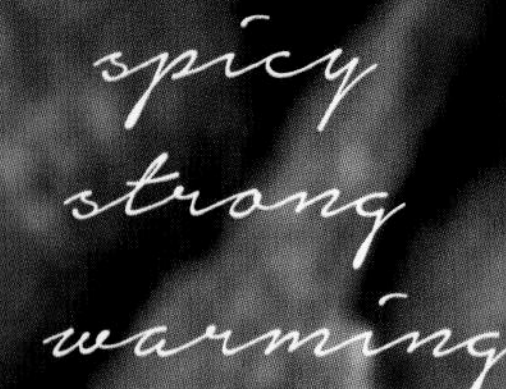

BARK

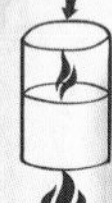

STEAM DISTILLED

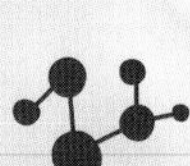

MAIN CONSTITUENT
Cinnamaldehyde
Eugenol
Chavicol

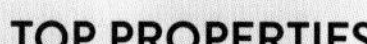

TOP PROPERTIES
Decongestant
Carminative
Detoxifier
Cardiotonic
Antimicrobial
Antiviral
Antifungal
Antispasmodic

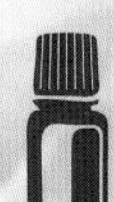

BLENDS WELL WITH
Ginger
Siberian fir
Wild orange

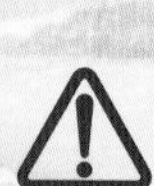

SAFETY
Dilution recommended.
Possible skin sensitivity.
Can reduce milk supply in lactating women.

TOP USES

COLD EXTREMITIES
Apply diluted to bottoms of feet to increase blood flow and bring warmth.

UPSET STOMACH & VOMITING
Take in a capsule to resolve and restore digestion.

DETOX FOR EAR, NOSE, THROAT, & LUNGS
Use in a capsule to clear yeast, phlegm and plaque.

WATER RETENTION & KIDNEY INFECTION
Take in a capsule or apply to bottoms of feet to kidney reflex points.

VIRUSES & BACTERIA
Take in a capsule and diffuse.

BLOOD SUGAR BALANCE
Take in a capsule with meals.

METABOLISM BOOST
Take in a capsule.

SEXUAL DRIVE
Diffuse or inhale aroma from bottle or apply to bottoms of feet to increase sexual desire.

COOKING
Add a drop to your favorite recipe for a sweet cinnamon-like flavor.

EMOTIONAL BALANCE
Use aromatically and topically to get from Uncertain ———> Bold.

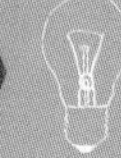

Make spicy sweet candy water by combining 1 drop cassia and 2 drops grapefruit to water.

RESEARCH: Anti-inflammatory effects of essential oil from the leaves of Cinnamomum cassia and cinnamaldehyde on lipopolysaccharide-stimulated J774A.1 cells., Pannee C, *Journal of Advanced Pharmaceutical Technology & Research*, 2014

From type 2 diabetes to antioxidant activity: a systematic review of the safety and efficacy of common and cassia cinnamon bark., Dugoua JJ, Seely D, Perri D, Cooley K, Forelli T, Mills E, Koren G, *Canadian Journal of Physiology and Pharmacology*, 2007

A review on anti-inflammatory activity of monoterpenes, de Cássia da Silveira e Sá R, Andrade LN, de Sousa DP, *Molecules*, 2013

Cinnamomum cassia essential oil inhibits MSH-induced melanin production and oxidative stress in murine B16 melanoma cells, Chou ST, Chang WL, Chang CT, Hsu SL, Lin YC, Shih Y, *International Journal of Molecular Sciences*, 2013

Randomized clinical trial of a phytotherapic compound containing Pimpinella anisum, Foeniculum vulgare, Sambucus nigra, and Cassia augustifolia for chronic constipation, Picon PD, Picon RV, Costa AF, Sander GB, Amaral KM, Aboy AL, Henriques AT, *BMC Complementary and Alternative Medicine*, 2010

Antimicrobial activities of cinnamon oil and cinnamaldehyde from the Chinese medicinal herb Cinnamomum cassia Blume, Ooi LS, Li Y, Kam SL, Wang H, Wong EY, Ooi VE, *The American Journal of Chinese Medicine*, 2006

WOOD

STEAM DISTILLED

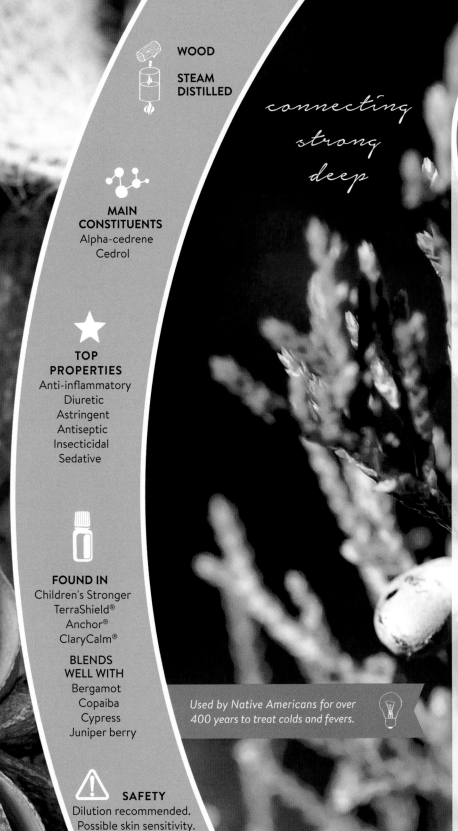

connecting strong deep

CEDARWOOD

JUNIPERUS VIRGINIANA

MAIN CONSTITUENTS
Alpha-cedrene
Cedrol

TOP PROPERTIES
Anti-inflammatory
Diuretic
Astringent
Antiseptic
Insecticidal
Sedative

FOUND IN
Children's Stronger
TerraShield®
Anchor®
ClaryCalm®

BLENDS WELL WITH
Bergamot
Copaiba
Cypress
Juniper berry

SAFETY
Dilution recommended. Possible skin sensitivity.

Used by Native Americans for over 400 years to treat colds and fevers.

TOP USES

ADD, ADHD, & LOW GABA LEVELS
Apply to back of neck, across forehead, and/or diffuse/inhale to soothe anxious feelings, and regain focus and concentration.

PSORIASIS & ECZEMA
Apply with a drop of lavender to affected area.

CALMING & ANXIETY
Put on palm of hands and inhale or apply to back of neck or bottoms of feet.

COUGH & SINUS ISSUES
Apply to chest and forehead and inhale from cupped hands.

STROKE & SEIZURES
Apply on back of neck and bottoms of feet.

URINARY TRACT, BLADDER & VAGINAL INFECTION
Apply to lower abdomen for infection support.

GUM ISSUES
Apply along jawline.

INSECT REPELLENT
Apply diluted or diffuse to deter insects.

ACNE
Apply with a drop of melaleuca to blemishes.

EMOTIONAL BALANCE
Use aromatically and topically to get from Alone ——> Connected.

RESEARCH: Repellency of Essential Oils to Mosquitoes (Diptera: Culicidae), Barnard DR, *Journal of Medical Entomology*, 1999

Repellency of essential oils to mosquitoes (Diptera: Culicidae), Barnard DR, *Journal of Medical Entomology*, 1999

Fumigant toxicity of plant essential oils against Camptomyia corticalis (Diptera: Cecidomyiidae), Kim JR, Haribalan P, Son BK, Ahn YJ, *Journal of Economic Entomology*, 2012

Bactericidal activities of plant essential oils and some of their isolated constituents against Campylobacter jejuni, Escherichia coli, Listeria monocytogenes, and Salmonella enterica, Friedman M, Henika PR, Mandrell RE, *Journal of Food Protection*, 2002

Chemical composition and antibacterial activity of selected essential oils and some of their main compounds, Wanner J, Schmidt E, Bail S, Jirovetz L, Buchbauer G, Gochev V, Girova T, Atanasova T, Stoyanova A, *Natural Product Communications*, 2010

Randomized trial of aromatherapy: successful treatment for alopecia areata, Hay IC, Jamieson M, Ormerod AD, *Archives of Dermatology*, 1998

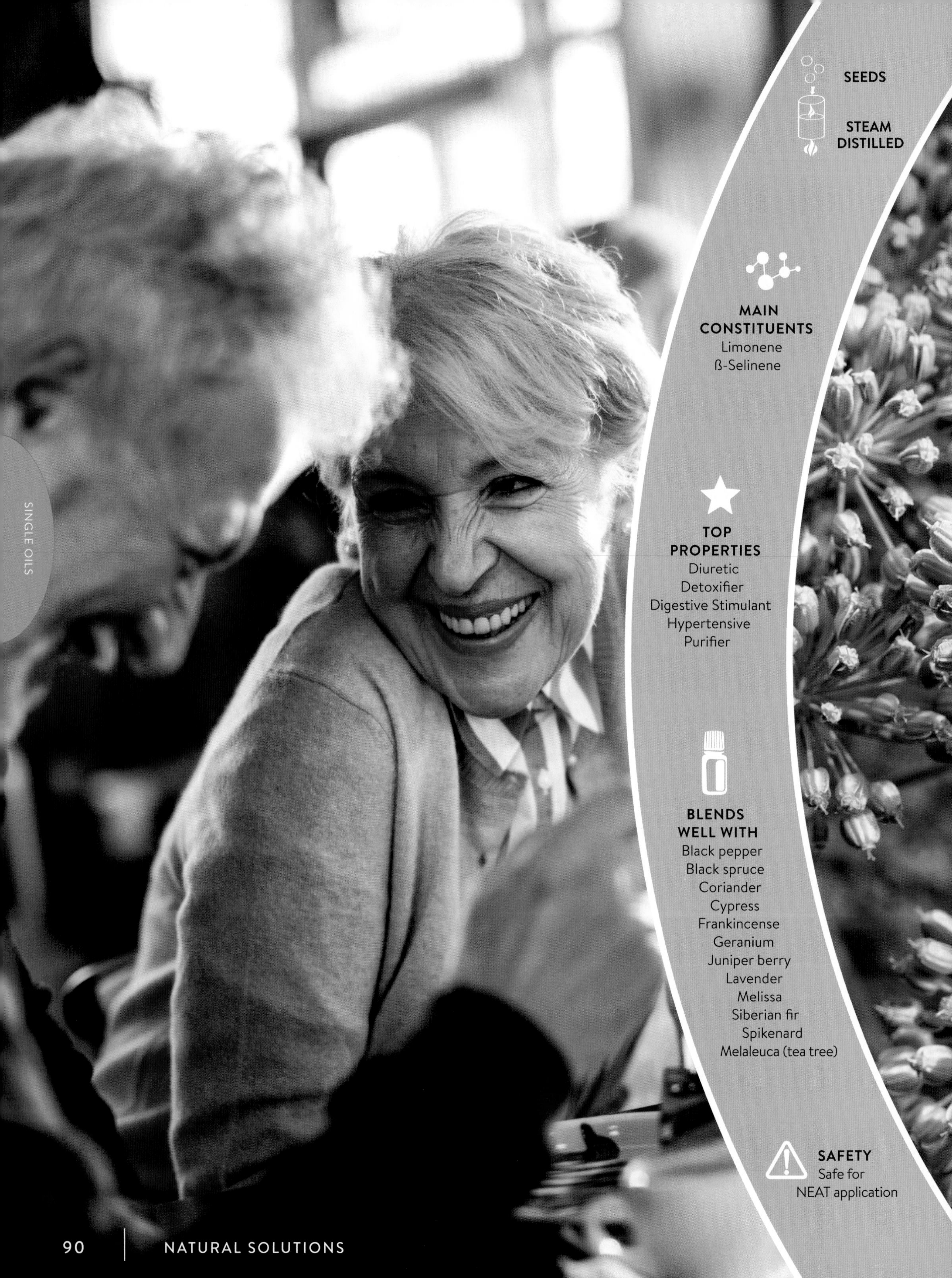
SEEDS
STEAM DISTILLED
MAIN CONSTITUENTS
Limonene
ß-Selinene
TOP PROPERTIES
Diuretic
Detoxifier
Digestive Stimulant
Hypertensive
Purifier
BLENDS WELL WITH
Black pepper
Black spruce
Coriander
Cypress
Frankincense
Geranium
Juniper berry
Lavender
Melissa
Siberian fir
Spikenard
Melaleuca (tea tree)
SAFETY
Safe for
NEAT application

detoxifing
dispersing
reinstating

CELERY SEED

APIUM GRAVEOLENS

TOP USES

CELERY JUICE ALTERNATIVE
Use (internally) with 4 drops per 8 ounces of purified water as a celery juice alternative.

WATER RETENTION & EDEMA, URINARY HEALTH
Take 1-2 drops (internally) in water or juice as needed and/or apply (topically) on lower abdomen and bottoms of feet.

BLOOD & LIVER TOXICITY, DETOX
Take (internally) 1-2 drops in capsule and apply (topically) to bottoms of feet and over liver.

WEAK & STIFF JOINTS, GOUT, ARTHRITIS & RHEUMATISM, OSTEOPOROSIS
Apply (topically) to bottoms of feet and area(s) of concern. Repeat 2-4x's per day.

HIGH BLOOD PRESSURE & RESTRICTED BLOOD FLOW
Apply (topically) over heart, liver, and bottoms of feet.

INDIGESTION, FLATULENCE, DIARRHEA, POOR APPETITE
Take 1-2 drops (internally) in capsule or apply (topically) on abdomen. Repeat as needed.

PERIPHERAL NERVE DAMAGE & NEUROPATHY, WEAKENED SPINAL DISCS
Apply (topically) to neck, up spine, back of neck, bottoms of feet, and area(s) of concern. Repeat 2-4x's per day.

KIDNEY, BLADDER OR GALLSTONES & PREVENTION
Take 2 drops (internally) in capsule and apply (topically) to area(s) of concern. Repeat 2-4x's per day until resolved.

ULCERS, GERD & STOMACH LINING ISSUES
Take 1-2 drops (internally) in capsule 2-4x's per day and apply (topically) on abdomen.

MUSCLE ACHE, CRAMPS & SPASMS
Apply (topically) to area(s) of concern. Repeat as often as needed.

HEADACHE & DIZZINESS, EPILEPSY & STROKE
Apply (topically) to area(s) of concern, up spine and across forehead.

IRREGULAR MENSTRUAL FLOW & CRAMPS, UTERINE HEALTH
Apply (topically) in clockwise motion on lower abdomen and area(s) of concern. Repeat as needed.

INSECT REPELLENT
Diffuse (aromatically). Add to glass spray bottle, and/or apply (topically) to clothing and exposed areas. Reapply every 4 hours.

PERSONAL FRAGRANCE
Combine 1 drop each with black spruce, cypress, frankincense, and/or juniper berry and apply (topically).

COOKING
Use 1-2 drops (internally) as an alternative to add celery flavoring to dishes. OR add 10-12 drops to ½ cup coarse sea salt and salt as usual to flavor foods.

EMOTIONAL BALANCE
Use (aromatically) aromatically and (topically) topically to get from Aggravated ⟶ Reconciled.

Conventionally grown celery is one of the most heavily sprayed vegetables available and has been found to contain as many as 19 pesticides, routinely exceeding government established human tolerance standards.

High quality essential oils are thoroughly screened for the presence of pesticides, although these molecules are generally too large to carry over into an essential oil during steam distillation. Screening can also detect if any pesticide contamination occurs post-distillation.

(A) = Aromatically (T) = Topically (I) = Internally

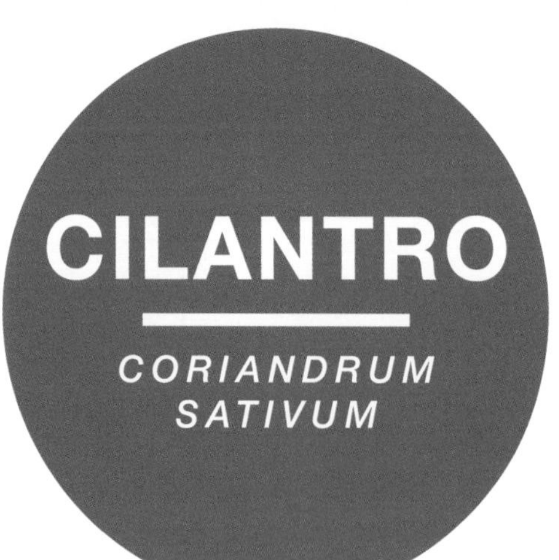

CILANTRO

CORIANDRUM SATIVUM

fresh awakening cleansing

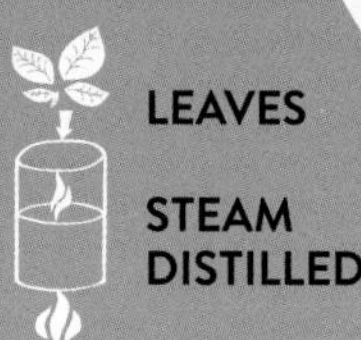

LEAVES

STEAM DISTILLED

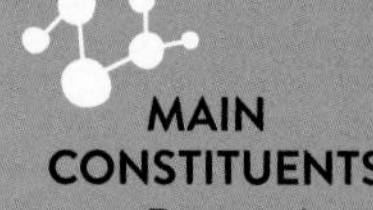

MAIN CONSTITUENTS
Decenal
Dodecenal

TOP PROPERTIES
Antioxidant
Antifungal
Detoxifying
Antibacterial

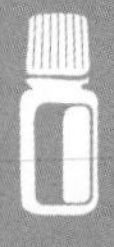

FOUND IN
Zendocrine®
PastTense®
Purify

BLENDS WELL WITH
Basil
Lemon
Melaleuca (tea tree)

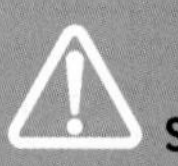

SAFETY
Safe for NEAT application.

SINGLE OILS

TOP USES

HEAVY METAL DETOX
Use in a capsule to detox from heavy metals and free radicals.

GAS, BLOATING & CONSTIPATION
Apply over abdomen.

ALLERGIES
Apply over liver or to bottoms of feet to ease allergies by reducing liver toxicity.

LIVER & KIDNEY SUPPORT
Take in a capsule or apply over liver and kidney area.

FUNGAL & BACTERIAL INFECTIONS
Use in a capsule and apply to infected area.

COOKING
Dip toothpick and add to favorite salad, dip, or guacamole.

BODY ODOR
Combine with peppermint in a capsule.

ANXIETY
Inhale or diffuse.

EMOTIONAL BALANCE
Use aromatically and topically to get from Obsessed ———> Expansive.

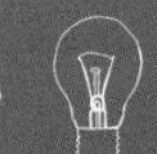

Relatives of parsley, cilantro and coriander essential oils come from the same plant. Cilantro is extracted from the leaf and coriander from the seed.

RESEARCH: Antimicrobial activity of individual and mixed fractions of dill, cilantro, coriander and eucalyptus essential oils, Delaquis PJ, Stanich K, Girard B, Mazza G, *International Journal of Food Microbiology*, 2002

protecting
spicy
awakening

CINNAMON BARK

CINNAMOMUM ZEYLANICUM

TOP USES

DIABETES & HIGH BLOOD SUGAR
Take (internally) in a capsule to balance blood sugar.

COLD & FLU
Take (internally) in a capsule or apply (aromatically) to bottoms of feet. Diffuse (topically) to cleanse air.

CHOLESTEROL & HEART ISSUES
Apply (topically) diluted to bottoms of feet or take (internally) in a capsule for increased blood flow.

ORAL HEALTH
Gargle a drop (internally) in water to combat oral infection.

FUNGUS & BACTERIA
Take (internally) in a capsule.

KIDNEY INFECTION
Take (internally) in a capsule.

VAGINAL HEALTH
Take (internally) in a capsule.

LOW LIBIDO & SEXUAL STIMULANT
Take (internally) in a capsule or dilute and apply (topically) to warm and stimulate.

MUSCLE STRAIN & PAIN
Apply (topically) diluted to relieve.

COOKING
Add (internally) to favorite baking recipe for a spicy twist.

EMOTIONAL BALANCE
Use (aromatically) aromatically and (topically) topically to get from Denied ⟶ Receptive.

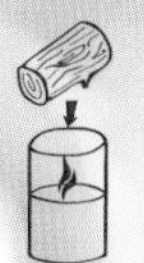

BARK

STEAM DISTILLED

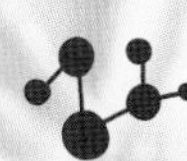

MAIN CONSTITUENTS
Cinnamaldehyde
Eugenol
Phenol

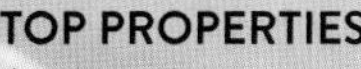

TOP PROPERTIES
Antiseptic
Antimicrobial
Antioxidant
Antifungal
Antiviral
Aphrodisiac

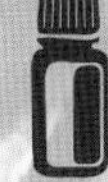

FOUND IN
Children's Brave™
ClaryCalm®
Slim & Sassy®
On Guard®
Anchor®

BLENDS WELL WITH
Copaiba
Manuka
Myrrh
Patchouli
Wild orange

SAFETY
Dilution recommended. Possible skin sensitivity.

Used in biblical times and by the ancient Egyptians, cinnamon was often traded, but its origin was a closely guarded secret.

RESEARCH: Some evidences on the mode of action of Cinnamomum verum bark essential oil, alone and in combination with piperacillin against a multi-drug resistant Escherichia coli strain., Yap PS, Krishnan T, Chan KG, Lim SH, *Journal of Microbiology and Biotechnology*, 2014

In-vitro and in-vivo anti-Trichophyton activity of essential oils by vapour contact, Inouye S, Uchida K, Yamaguchi H, *Mycoses*, 2001

Ameliorative effect of the cinnamon oil from Cinnamomum zeylanicum upon early stage diabetic nephropathy, Mishra A, Bhatti R, Singh A, Singh Ishar MP, *Planta Medica*, 2010

Cinnamon bark extract improves glucose metabolism and lipid profile in the fructose-fed rat, Kannappan S, Jayaraman T, Rajasekar P, Ravichandran MK, *Anuradha CV*, 2006

The cinnamon-derived dietary factor cinnamic aldehyde activates the Nrf2-dependent antioxidant response in human epithelial colon cells, Wondrak GT, Villeneuve NF, Lamore SD, Bause AS, Jiang T, Zhang DD, *Molecules*, 2010

Antibacterial activity of essential oils and their major constituents against respiratory tract pathogens by gaseous contact, Inouye S, Takizawa T, Yamaguchi H, *The Journal of Antimicrobial Chemotherapy*, 2001

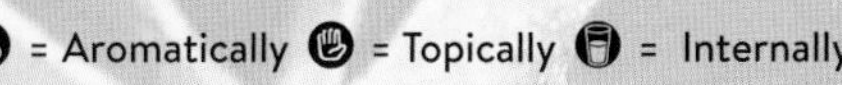

repelling • reckoning • freshening

GRASS

STEAM DISTILLED

MAIN CONSTITUENTS
Citronellal
Geraniol
Citronellol

TOP PROPERTIES
Insect Repellent
Insecticidal
Detoxifier
Cleanser
Bactericidal
Antifungal
Astringal
Astringent
Fungicidal
Deodorant

FOUND IN
Purify

BLENDS WELL WITH
Arborvitae
Black spruce
Eucalyptus
Frankincense
Geranium
Lemon
Lemongrass
Peppermint
Roman chamomile
Siberian fir
Melaleuca (tea tree)
Thyme

SAFETY
Dilution recommended for possible skin sensitivity.

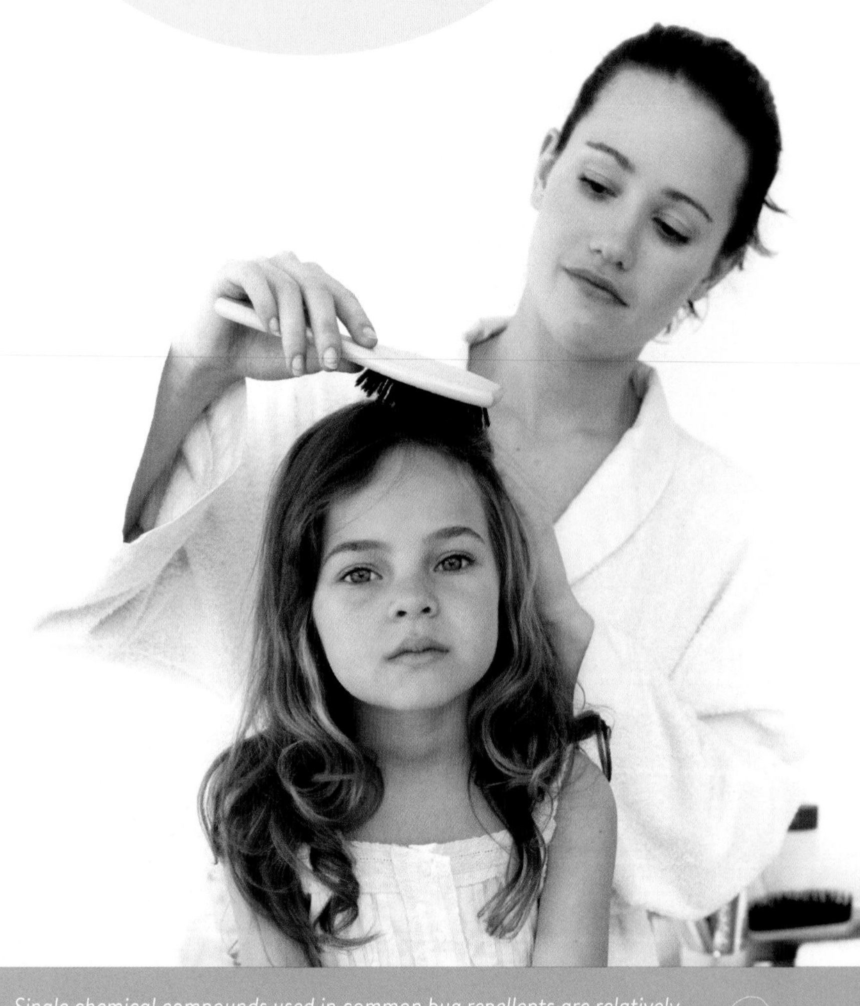

Single chemical compounds used in common bug repellents are relatively easy for insects to develop resistance to. However, it is virtually impossible to do so with an essential oil due to the chemical complexity.

SINGLE OILS

RESEARCH: Hellen Braga Martins, Nathan das Neves Selis, Clarissa Leal Silva e Souza, Flávia S. Nascimento, Suzi Pacheco de Carvalho, Lorena D'Oliveira Gusmão, Jannine dos Santos Nascimento, Anne Karoline Pereira Brito, Samira Itana de Souza, Marcio Vasconcelos de Oliveira, Jorge Timenetsky, Regiane Yatsuda, Ana Paula T. Uetanabaro, and Lucas M. Marques
Evidence-Based Complementary and Alternative Medicine Volume 2017, Article ID 2505610
2017 research paper published in the Evidence-Based Complementary and Alternative Medicine Journal states that citronella essential oil sedates inflammation, particularly those situations which pertain to the liver, stomach, intestines and other parts of the digestive system. The inflammations caused as side effects of drugs, excessive use of alcohol or narcotics, hard and spicy food, any disease, or any toxic element getting into the body can also be alleviated using this oil.

Genome wide transcriptome profiling reveals differential gene expression in secondary metabolite pathway of Cymbopogon winterianus
Devi K, Mishra SK, Sahu J, Panda D, Modi MK1, Sen P
Sci Rep. 2016 Feb 15;6:21026. doi: 10.1038/srep21026
Advances in transcriptome sequencing provide fast, cost-effective and reliable approach to generate large expression datasets especially suitable for non-model species to identify putative genes, key pathway and regulatory mechanism. Citronella (Cymbopogon winterianus) is an aromatic medicinal grass used for anti-tumoral, antibacterial, anti-fungal, antiviral, detoxifying and natural insect repellent properties. The present study is a pioneering attempt to generate an exhaustive molecular information of secondary metabolite pathway and to increase genomic resources in Citronella. Using high-throughput RNA-Seq technology, root and leaf ranscriptome was analyzed at an unprecedented depth (11.7 Gb). Targeted searches identified majority of the genes associated with metabolic pathway and other natural

CITRONELLA

CYMBOPOGON WINTERIANUS

TOP USES

INSECT REPELLENT (INCL. FLEAS, TICKS) & PARASITE EXPULSION
Diffuse and apply to exposed areas. Add to glass spray bottle to treat surfaces or apply to clothing.

GREASY HAIR & LICE, DETANGLER
Add 2-3 drops per shampooing.

DIGESTIVE & INTESTINAL INFLAMMATION, REACTION TO SPICY FOODS & CARRAGEENAN
Apply to bottoms of feet and over upper abdomen and liver.

SIDE EFFECTS CAUSED BY DRUGS, ALCOHOL, NARCOTICS & TOXINS
Diffuse and apply to bottoms of feet and affected area(s).

FUNGAL & BACTERIAL CONDITIONS OF INTESTINAL & URINARY TRACTS, PROSTATE
Apply to lower abdomen, bottoms of feet and/or reflex points.

POOR SECRETION OR RELEASE OF HORMONES, ENZYMES
Apply to lower abdomen, liver, bottoms of feet and area(s) of concern.

ACNE, ATHLETE'S FOOT & NAIL FUNGUS
Apply to area(s) of concern twice per day.

POOR PERSPIRATION OR TOXIN ELIMINATION, FEVERS
Apply to bottoms of feet, over liver, and area(s) of concern.

OXIDATIVE STRESS & CELL MUTATION, TUMORS
Diffuse and apply to bottoms of feet and over liver.

POST-SURGERY PAIN, SWOLLEN JOINTS & ARTHRITIS
Apply to area(s) of concern 2-4x's per day.

POOR CIRCULATION & HEART PALPATIONS, SEIZURES, HIGH BLOOD PRESSURE
Apply over heart, to bottoms of feet and extremities twice per day.

ANXIOUS & DEPRESSED STATES, INSOMNIA, LOW ENERGY
Diffuse and apply to neck and forehead, up spine, and bottoms of feet.

SURFACE CLEANSING & AIR FRESHENING
Diffuse. Add 6-8 drops + 1 tablespoon vinegar to glass spray bottle filled with water.

EMOTIONAL BALANCE
Use aromatically and topically to get from Punished ——> Averting.

product pathway viz. antibiotics synthesis along with many novel genes. Terpenoid biosynthesis genes comparative expression results were validated for 15 unigenes by RT-PCR and qRT-PCR.

Effects of citronella oil (Cymbopogon winterianus Jowitt ex Bor) on Spodoptera frugiperda (J. E. Smith) midgut and fat body
Silva C, Wanderley-Teixeira V, Cunha FM, Oliveira JV, Dutra KA, Navarro DF, Teixeira A
Biotech Histochem. 2018;93(1):36-48. doi: 10.1080/10520295.2017.1379612. Epub 2017 Dec 5
The armyworm, Spodoptera frugiperda, is the principal pest of corn in Brazil. Control is achieved primarily by synthetic insecticides, which cause problems for the agro-ecosystem. Alternative methods of control are under investigation and citronella (Cymbopogon winterianus) essential oil appears to be a promising agent. We investigated the effects of citronella oil using histological, histochemical and immunohistochemical methods. The midgut of larvae treated with citronella exhibited altered epithelium including cytoplasmic protrusions, columnar cell extrusion, pyknotic nuclei, and increased periodic acid-Schiff positive granules. Regenerative cells in the epithelium of the midgut increased in number, which facilitated subsequent regeneration of this tissue. After exposure to citronella, trophocytes, the principal cell type of the fat body, possessed enlarged vacuoles and mitotic bodies, and contained reduced amounts of glycogen, lipid, and protein. Citronella oil caused morphological changes of the midgut and reduction of stored resources in the fat body, which may adversely affect insect reproduction and survival.

= Aromatically = Topically = Internally

CLARY SAGE

SALVIA SCLAREA

balancing
musky
feminine

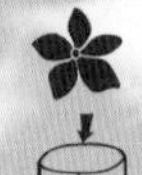

FLOWER

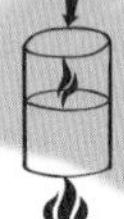

STEAM DISTILLED

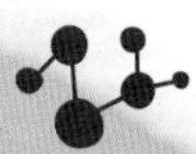

MAIN CONSTITUENT
Linalyl acetate

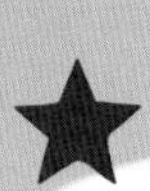

TOP PROPERTIES
Emmenagogue
Galactagogue
Neurotonic
Mucolytic
Anticoagulant
Sedative
Antispasmodic

FOUND IN
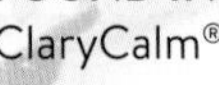
ClaryCalm®

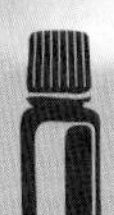

BLENDS WELL WITH
Geranium
Lavender
Manuka
Neroli
Yarrow
Ylang ylang

SAFETY
Caution during earlier stages of pregnancy.

TOP USES

ENDOMETRIOSIS & BREAST CANCER
Apply diluted to breasts or take in capsule to regulate estrogen.

BREAST ENLARGEMENT
Apply diluted to each breast for natural enlargement.

PARKINSON'S, SEIZURES & CONVULSIONS
Apply to back of neck to support healthy brain function.

CHILD BIRTH & LOW MILK SUPPLY
Apply diluted down spine or over abdomen to help bring on labor. Apply to each breast for increased lactation.

INFERTILITY & PROSTATE/UTERINE HEALTH
Use in a capsule or apply to abdomen and uterine reflex points.

PMS & MENOPAUSE
Take in a capsule or apply on abdomen or bottoms of feet.

POSTPARTUM DEPRESSION & ANXIETY
Inhale/diffuse or apply to the heart area and bottoms of feet.

HOT FLASHES
Combine with water and a few drops of peppermint in a glass spray bottle and spritz on back of neck for cooling relief.

PINK EYE & CATARACTS
Apply a drop around but not in eye. Take 1-2 drops in a capsule 1-2 times daily, apply under 2nd and 3rd toes.

INSOMNIA
Take under the tongue or apply to bottoms of the feet. Diffuse at bedtime with bergamot.

EMOTIONAL BALANCE
Use aromatically and topically to get from Limited ———> Enlightened.

Clary sage is derived from Latin meaning "clear eyes." Medieval monks favored it for eye troubles.

EARCH: Changes in 5-hydroxytryptamine and Cortisol Plasma Levels in Menopausal Women Inhalation of Clary Sage Oil, Lee KB, Cho E, Kang YS, *Phytotherapy Research*, 2014

omized controlled trial for Salvia sclarea or Lavandula angustifolia: differential effects on blood ure in female patients with urinary incontinence undergoing urodynamic examination, Seol Lee YH, Kang P, You JH, Park M, Min SS, *The Journal of Alternative and Complementary icine*, 2013

epressant-like effect of Salvia sclarea is explained by modulation of dopamine activities in rats, Seol GH, Shim HS, Kim PJ, Moon HK, Lee KH, Shim I, Suh SH, Min SS, *Journal of Ethnopharmacolo*

Aromatherapy massage on the abdomen for alleviating menstrual pain in high school girls: a pr nary controlled clinical study, Hur MH, Lee MS, Seong KY, Lee MK, *Evidence-Based Comple ry and Alternative Medicine*, 2012

Pain relief assessment by aromatic essential oil massage on outpatients with primary dysmeno a randomized, double-blind clinical trial, Ou MC, Hsu TF, Lai AC, Lin YT, Lin CC, *The Journal o Obstetrics and Gynecology Research*, 2012

CLOVE

EUGENIA CARYOPHYLLATA

warm
spicy
protective

TOP USES

LIVER & BRAIN SUPPORT
Dilute Ⓐ and apply Ⓣ to bottoms of feet or take Ⓘ in a capsule.

IMMUNE BOOST
Apply Ⓣ diluted to bottoms of feet or take Ⓘ in a capsule.

CIRCULATION & HYPERTENSION
Apply Ⓣ diluted to spine and bottoms of feet to increase blood flow.

TOOTH PAIN & CAVITIES
Dilute and apply Ⓣ to affected area to numb and ease pain.

THYROID ISSUES & METABOLISM SUPPORT
Apply Ⓣ diluted to big toe and take Ⓘ in a capsule.

INFECTION & PARASITES
Take Ⓘ in a capsule.

SMOKING ADDICTION
Take Ⓘ with black pepper along tongue to decrease nicotine cravings.

VIRUS & COLD
Apply Ⓣ diluted along spine or take Ⓘ in a capsule.

EMOTIONAL BALANCE
Use Ⓐ aromatically and Ⓣ topically to get from Dominated ———> Supported.

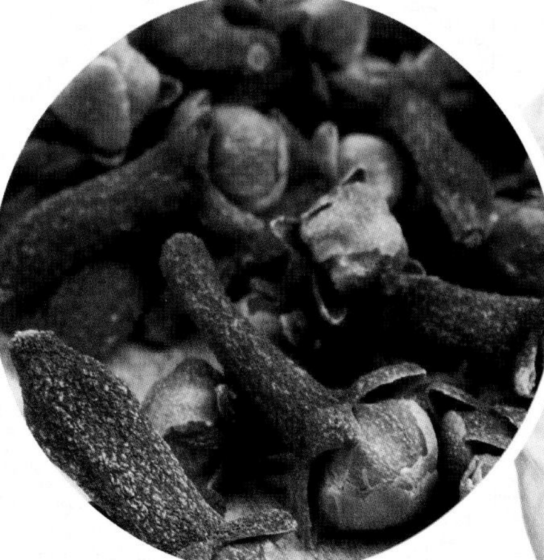

Ⓐ = Aromatically Ⓣ = Topically Ⓘ = Internally

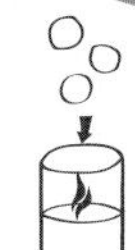

BUDS

STEAM DISTILLED

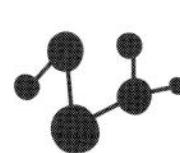

MAIN CONSTITUENTS
Eugenol

TOP PROPERTIES
Antioxidant
Antiviral
Antifungal
Expectorant
Nervine
Anti-parasitic
Vermicide

FOUND IN
On Guard®
DDR Prime®

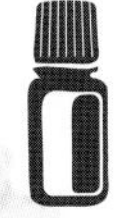

BLENDS WELL WITH
Cinnamon
Copaiba
Rosemary
Wild orange

SUBSTITUTION
Cinnamon
Clove

SAFETY
Dilution recommended. Possible skin sensitivity. To reduce liver stress, use with Zendocrine®, helichrysum, cumin, green mandarin, geranium, or Roman chamomile.

Clove is a powerful antioxidant. As a dried spice it measures 300,000 on the ORAC scale and as an essential oil, measures over 1 million.

RESEARCH: Antimicrobial Activities of Clove and Thyme Extracts, Nzeako BC, Al-Kharousi ZS, Al-Mahrooqui Z, *Sultan Qaboos University Medical Journal*, 2006

Antimicrobial activity of clove oil and its potential in the treatment of vaginal candidiasis, Ahmad N, Alam MK, Shehbaz A, Khan A, Mannan A, Hakim SR, Bisht D, Owais M, *Journal of Drug Targeting*, 2005

Eugenol (an essential oil of clove) acts as an antibacterial agent against Salmonella typhi by disrupting the cellular membrane, Devi KP, Nisha SA, Sakthivel R, Pandian SK, *Journal of Ethnopharmacology*, 2010

The effect of clove and benzocaine versus placebo as topical anesthetics, Alqareer A, Alyahya A, Andersson L, *Journal of Dentistry*, 2006

Synergistic effect between clove oil and its major compounds and antibiotics against oral bacteria, Moon SE, Kim HY, Cha JD, *Archives of Oral Biology*, 2011

Antifungal activity of clove essential oil and its volatile vapour against dermatophytic fungi, Chee HY, Lee MH, *Mycobiology*, 2007

Microbicide activity of clove essential oil (Eugenia caryophyllata), Nuñez L, Aquino MD, *Brazilian Journal of Microbiology*, 2011

Anti-arthritic effect of eugenol on collagen-induced arthritis experimental model, Grespan R, Paludo M, Lemos Hde P, Barbosa CP, Bersani-Amado CA, Dalalio MM, Cuman RK, *Biological and Pharmaceutical Bulletin*, 2012

A novel aromatic oil compound inhibits microbial overgrowth on feet: a case study, Misner BD, *Journal of the International Society of Sports Nutrition*, 2007

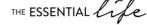

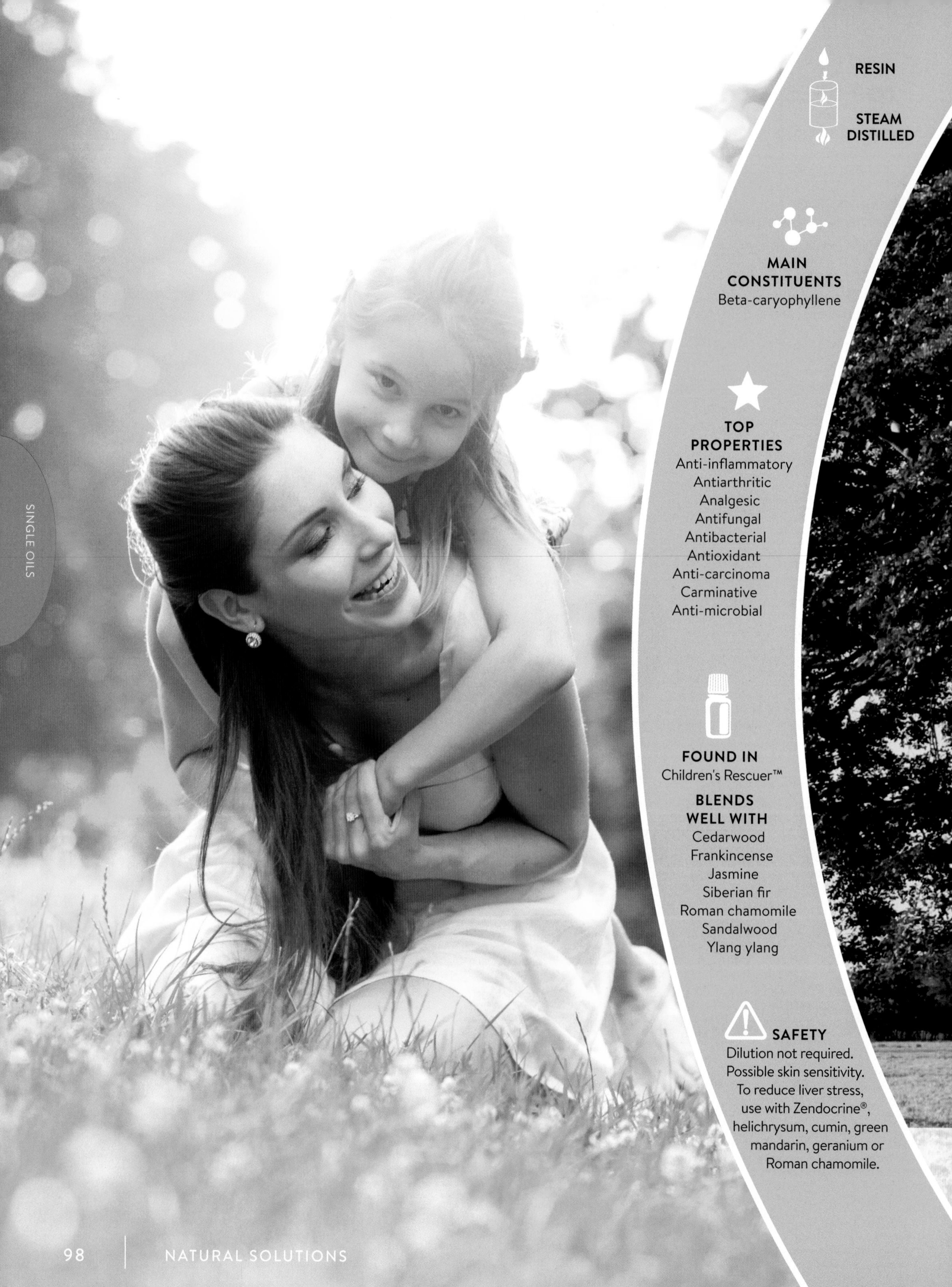

RESIN

STEAM DISTILLED

MAIN CONSTITUENTS
Beta-caryophyllene

TOP PROPERTIES
Anti-inflammatory
Antiarthritic
Analgesic
Antifungal
Antibacterial
Antioxidant
Anti-carcinoma
Carminative
Anti-microbial

FOUND IN
Children's Rescuer™

BLENDS WELL WITH
Cedarwood
Frankincense
Jasmine
Siberian fir
Roman chamomile
Sandalwood
Ylang ylang

SAFETY
Dilution not required. Possible skin sensitivity. To reduce liver stress, use with Zendocrine®, helichrysum, cumin, green mandarin, geranium or Roman chamomile.

COPAIBA

COPAIFERA OFFINCINALIS

commanding
comforting
magnifying

SINGLE OILS

TOP USES

PAIN & INFLAMMATION, ARTHRITIS, GOUT & MUSCLE CRAMPS
Diffuse A, inhale from cupped hands, and/or apply T to area of concern.

LIVER TOXICITY & ISSUES
Take I in a capsule or in water.

TENDONITIS, PLANTAR FASCIITIS & HEEL SPURS
Apply T to area of concern.

RESPIRATORY ISSUES, SORE THROAT & TONSILS
Diffuse A, inhale from cupped hands, apply T under nose, and/or to chest.

BEDWETTING & INCONTINENCE
Apply T to abdomen and/or take I in a capsule.

COLITIS & INTESTINAL INFECTIONS
Apply T to abdomen and/or take I in a capsule.

CANCER & AUTOIMMUNE DISORDERS
Take I in a capsule, apply T to bottoms of feet, and/or along spine. Combine with frankincense and Siberian fir.

FUNGAL, BACTERIAL & VIRAL INFECTIONS
Take I in a capsule, apply T to area(s) of concern, bottoms of feet, and/or along spine.

NAUSEA, VOMITING, ABDOMINAL PAIN & BLOATING
Take I in a capsule or apply T to abdomen.

DRY SKIN & HAIR, ACNE, ECZEMA, PSORIASIS
Apply T to area(s) of concern or combine with skin or hair care products. Combine with cedarwood.

AGING SKIN & COLLAGEN PRODUCTION, WOUND HEALING
Apply T to area(s) of concern to promote collagen production.

HEADACHES & MIGRAINES
Apply T to temples, forehead, and/or take I in a capsule.

ENDOMETRIOSIS & PMS
Take I in a capsule or in water.

HIGH BLOOD PRESSURE & ATHEROSCLEROSIS
Take I in a capsule or in water.

ANXIETY & SLEEP ISSUES
Diffuse A, inhale form cupped hands, apply T to bottoms of feet and/or under nose.

BLISTERS, BITES, BURNS, BRUISING & SPRAINS
Apply T to area(s) of concern.

EMOTIONAL BALANCE
Use A aromatically and T topically to get from Plagued ———> Directed.

Extracted from mature trees between 30-50 years in age and considered one of the most anti-inflammatory substances on earth.

RESEARCH: Bacteriostatic effect of copaiba oil (Copaifera officinalis) against Streptococcus mutans. Pieri FA et al. Braz Dent J. (2012)

Antimicrobial Activity of Copaiba (Copaifera officinalis) and Pracaxi (Pentaclethra macroloba) Oils against Staphylococcus Aureus: Importance in Compounding for Wound Care.Guimarães AL et al. Int J Pharm Compd. (2016)

Anti-Inflammatory and Antioxidant Actions of Copaiba Oil Are Related to Liver Cell Modifications in Arthritic Rats. Castro Ghizoni CV, Arssufi Ames AP, Lameira OA, Bersani Amado CA, Sá Nakanishi AB, Bracht L, Marçal Natali MR, Peralta RM, Bracht A, Comar JF. J Cell Biochem. 2017 Mar 21. doi: 10.1002/jcb.25998. [Epub ahead of print] PMID:28322470

Development and pharmacological evaluation of in vitro nanocarriers composed of lamellar silicates containing copaiba oil-resin for treatment of endometriosis. de Almeida Borges VR, da Silva JH, Barbosa SS, Nasciutti LE, Cabral LM, de Sousa VP. Mater Sci Eng C Mater Biol Appl. 2016 Jul 1;64:310-7. doi: 10.1016/j.msec.2016.03.094. Epub 2016 Mar 31.PMID: 27127058

A = Aromatically T = Topically I = Internally

CORIANDER

CORIANDRUM SATIVUM

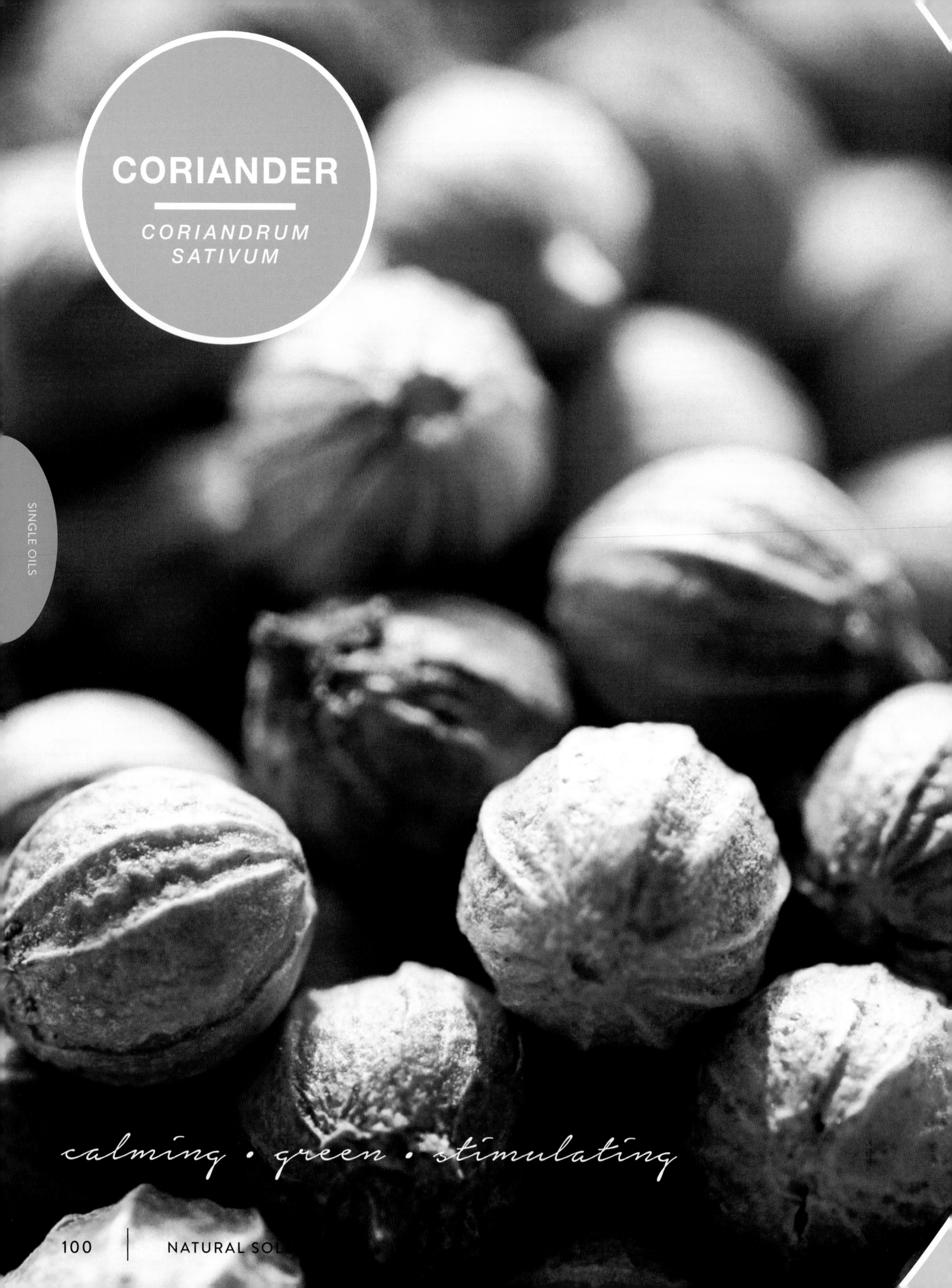

SINGLE OILS

calming • green • stimulating

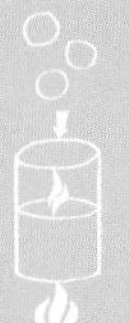

SEEDS

STEAM DISTILLED

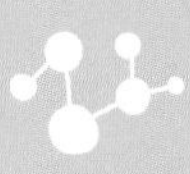

MAIN CONSTITUENTS
Linalool
Terpenes

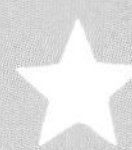

TOP PROPERTIES
Analgesic
Antioxidant
Anti-inflammatory
Digestive Stimulant
Antibacterial
Antispasmodic

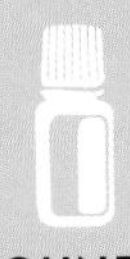

FOUND IN
DigestZen®
Align®
Children's Steady™

BLENDS WELL WITH
Clove
Ginger
Neroli
Peppermint

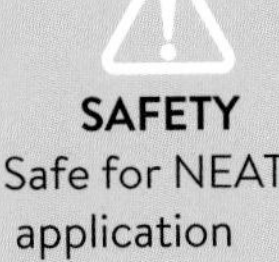

SAFETY
Safe for NEAT application

TOP USES

GAS & NAUSEA
Massage into abdomen or take in a capsule or in water.

HIGH BLOOD SUGAR & DIABETES
Use with cinnamon in a capsule with meals to help regulate blood sugar.

ITCHY SKIN & RASHES
Apply to area of concern.

JOINT PAIN
Apply directly to area of concern for soothing relief.

NEUROPATHY
Use in a capsule.

NO APPETITE
Take in a capsule or inhale from cupped hands.

FOOD POISONING & DIARRHEA
Use in a capsule or apply to abdomen.

BODY ODOR
Take in a capsule.

LOW ENERGY & NERVOUS EXHAUSTION
Inhale from cupped hands or apply to bottoms of feet.

EMOTIONAL BALANCE
Use aromatically and topically to get from Apprehensive ———> Participating.

SINGLE OILS

Coriander comes from the seeds of the cilantro herb; cilantro is from the leaf of the same plant.

RESEARCH: Coriandrum sativum L. protects human keratinocytes from oxidative stress by regulating oxidative defense systems., Park G, Kim HG, Kim YO, Park SH, Kim SY, Oh MS, *Skin Pharmacology and Physiology*, 2012

Antioxidant and Hepatoprotective Potential of Essential Oils of Coriander (Coriandrum sativum L.) and Caraway (Carum carvi L.) (Apiaceae), Samojlik I, Lakic N, Mimica-Dukic N, Dakovic-Svajcer K, Bozin B, *Journal of Agricultural and Food Chemistry*, 2010

Inhalation of coriander volatile oil increased anxiolytic-antidepressant-like behaviors and decreased oxidative status in beta-amyloid (1-42) rat model of Alzheimer's disease., Cioanca O, Hritcu L, Mihasan M, Trifan A, Hancianu M, *Physiology & Behavior*, 2014

Coriandrum sativum L. (Coriander) Essential Oil: Antifungal Activity and Mode of Action on Candida spp., and Molecular Targets Affected in Human Whole-Genome Expression, Freires Ide A, Murata RM, Furletti VF, Sartoratto A, Alencar SM, Figueira GM, de Oliveira Rodrigues JA, Duarte MC, Rosalen PL, *PLoS One*, 2014

Antimicrobial activity against bacteria with dermatological relevance and skin tolerance of the essential oil from Coriandrum sativum L. fruits, Casetti F, Bartelke S, Biehler K, Augustin M, Schempp CM, Frank U, *Phytotherapy Research*, 2012

Coriander (Coriandrum sativum L.) essential oil: its antibacterial activity and mode of action evaluated by flow cytometry, Silva F, Ferreira S, Queiroz JA, Domingues FC, *Journal of Medical Microbiology*, 2011

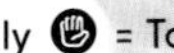
= Aromatically = Topically = Internally

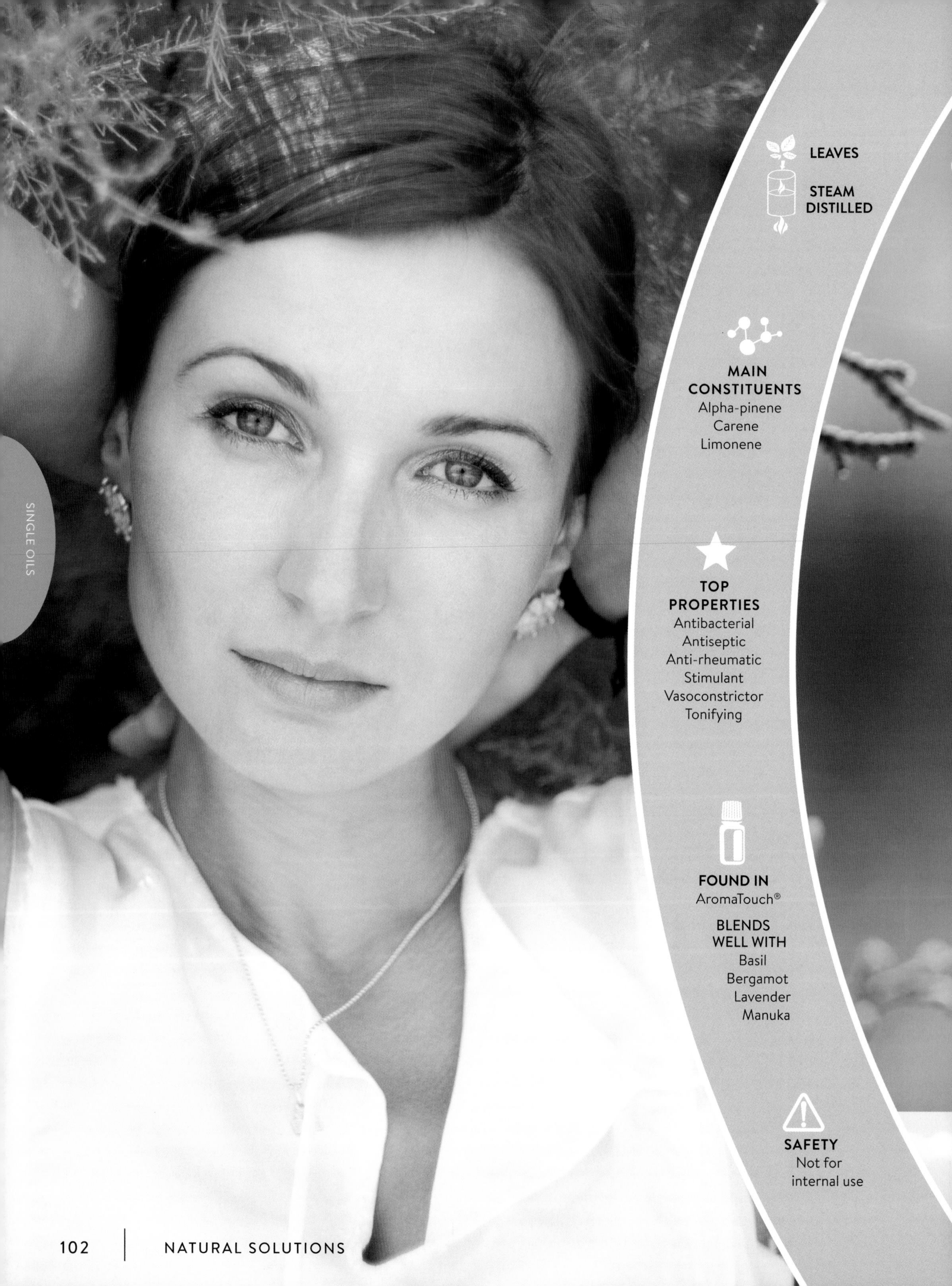
SINGLE OILS
LEAVES
STEAM DISTILLED
MAIN CONSTITUENTS
Alpha-pinene
Carene
Limonene
TOP PROPERTIES
Antibacterial
Antiseptic
Anti-rheumatic
Stimulant
Vasoconstrictor
Tonifying
FOUND IN
AromaTouch®
BLENDS WELL WITH
Basil
Bergamot
Lavender
Manuka
SAFETY
Not for internal use

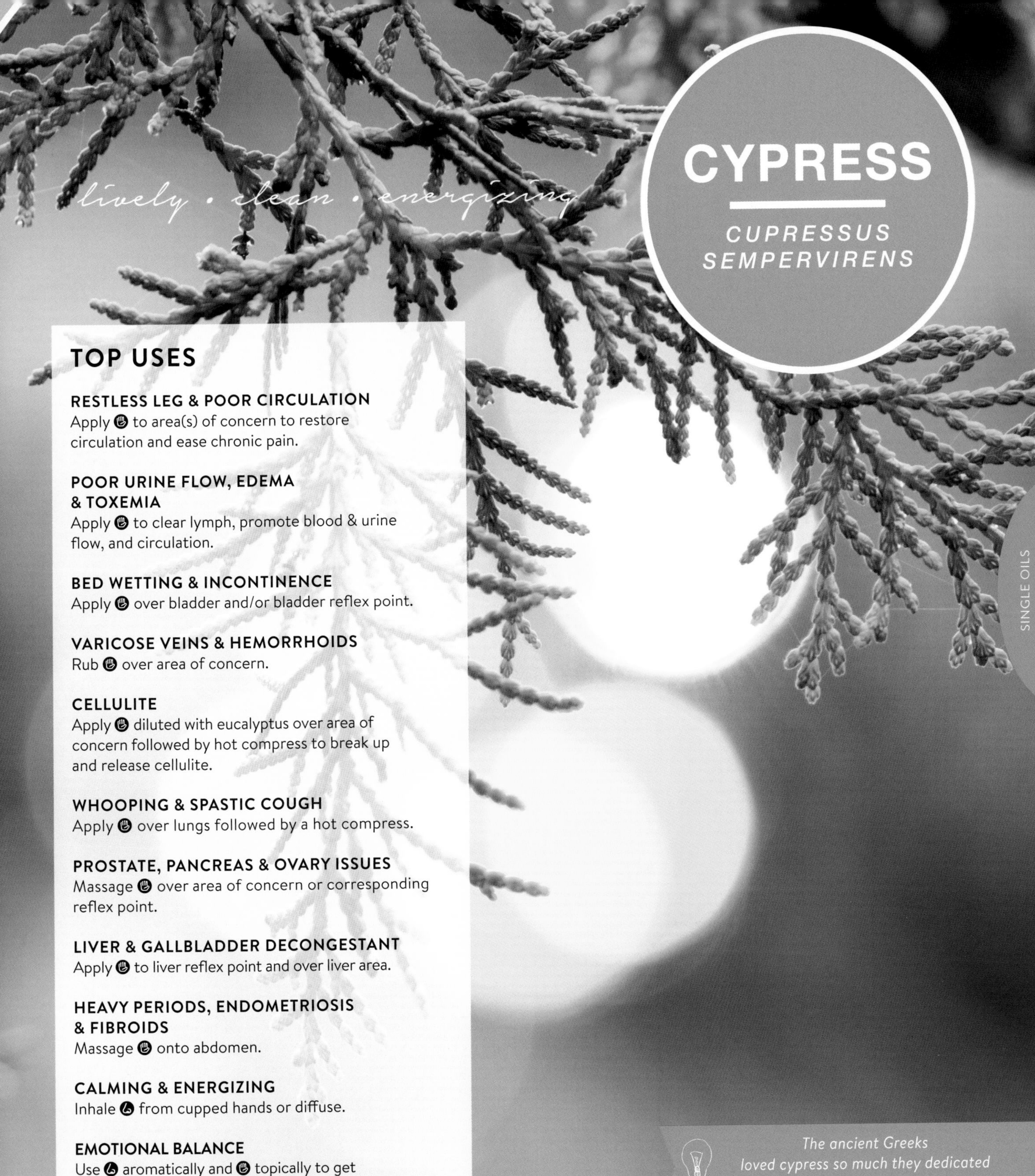

CYPRESS

CUPRESSUS SEMPERVIRENS

TOP USES

RESTLESS LEG & POOR CIRCULATION
Apply ⓣ to area(s) of concern to restore circulation and ease chronic pain.

POOR URINE FLOW, EDEMA & TOXEMIA
Apply ⓣ to clear lymph, promote blood & urine flow, and circulation.

BED WETTING & INCONTINENCE
Apply ⓣ over bladder and/or bladder reflex point.

VARICOSE VEINS & HEMORRHOIDS
Rub ⓣ over area of concern.

CELLULITE
Apply ⓣ diluted with eucalyptus over area of concern followed by hot compress to break up and release cellulite.

WHOOPING & SPASTIC COUGH
Apply ⓣ over lungs followed by a hot compress.

PROSTATE, PANCREAS & OVARY ISSUES
Massage ⓣ over area of concern or corresponding reflex point.

LIVER & GALLBLADDER DECONGESTANT
Apply ⓣ to liver reflex point and over liver area.

HEAVY PERIODS, ENDOMETRIOSIS & FIBROIDS
Massage ⓣ onto abdomen.

CALMING & ENERGIZING
Inhale ⓐ from cupped hands or diffuse.

EMOTIONAL BALANCE
Use ⓐ aromatically and ⓣ topically to get from Stalled ———> Progressing.

The ancient Greeks loved cypress so much they dedicated it to one of their gods, Pluto.

RESEARCH: Immunological and Psychological Benefits of Aromatherapy Massage, Kuriyama H, Watanabe S, Nakaya T, Shigemori I, Kita M, Yoshida N, Masaki D, Tadai T, Ozasa K, Fukui K, Imanishi J, *Evidence-based Complementary and Alternative Medicine,* 2005

Chemical composition, bio-herbicidal and antifungal activities of essential oils isolated from Tunisian common cypress (Cupressus sempervirens L.), Ismail A, Lamia H, Mohsen H, Samia G, Bassem J, *Journal of Medicinal Plants Research,* 2013

Immunological and Psychological Benefits of Aromatherapy Massage, Kuriyama H, Watanabe S, Nakaya T, Shigemori I, Kita M, Yoshida N, Masaki D, Tadai T, Ozasa K, Fukui K, Imanishi J, *Evidence-Based Complementary and Alternative Medicine,* 2005

Effect of aromatherapy massage on abdominal fat and body image in post-menopausal women, Kim HJ, *Taehan Kanho Hakhoe Chi,* 2007

Evaluation of the Effects of Plant-derived Essential Oils on Central Nervous System Function Using Discrete Shuttle-type Conditioned Avoidance Response in Mice, Umezu T., *Phytotherapy Research,* 2012

ⓐ = Aromatically ⓣ = Topically ⓘ = Internally

DILL

ANETHUM GRAVEOLENS

SINGLE OILS

detoxing • disinfecting • cleansing

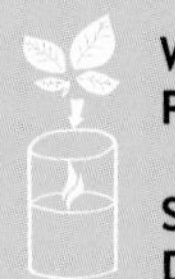

WHOLE PLANT

STEAM DISTILLED

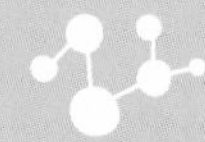

MAIN CONSTITUENTS
Monoterpenes
D-limonene
Alpha & Beta Pinenes

TOP PROPERTIES
Antispasmodic
Expectorant
Stimulant
Galactagogue
Carminative
Emmenagogue
Hypertensive
Antibacterial

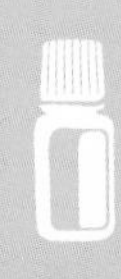

BLENDS WELL WITH
Black pepper
Cinnamon
Citrus oils
Clove
Peppermint
Spearmint

SAFETY
Safe for NEAT application.

TOP USES

MUSCLE SPASMS
Apply to calm muscles.

NERVOUSNESS
Inhale from cupped hands or apply under nose or back of neck with Roman chamomile to calm nervousness.

SUGAR ADDICTION & PANCREAS SUPPORT
Take in a capsule to decrease addiction and lower glucose levels.

LOW BREAST MILK SUPPLY
Apply to chest or take in a capsule.

DETOX & ELECTROLYTE BALANCE
Take in a capsule as part of a detox.

CHOLESTEROL & HIGH BLOOD PRESSURE
Take in a capsule.

RESPIRATORY ISSUES
Apply diluted to chest or take in a capsule to dislodge and break up mucus.

GAS, BLOATING & INDIGESTION
Take in a capsule or in water.

LACK OF MENSTRUATION
Apply diluted over abdomen.

COLIC
Apply diluted to bottoms of feet or abdomen.

EMOTIONAL BALANCE
Use aromatically and topically to get from Avoiding ——> Intentional.

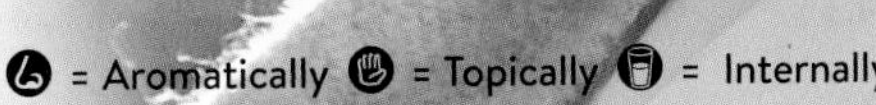

Used extensively in soft drinks and alcoholic beverages.

RESEARCH: Effects of Cd, Pb, and Cu on growth and essential oil contents in dill, peppermint, and basil, Zheljazkov VD, Craker LE, Xing B, *Environmental and Experimental Botany*, 2006

Dill (Anethum graveolens L.) seed essential oil induces Candida albicans apoptosis in a metacaspase-dependent manner, Chen Y, Zeng H, Tian J, Ban X, Ma B, Wang Y, *Fungal Biology*, 2014

Anethum graveolens: An Indian traditional medicinal herb and spice, Jana S, Shekhawat GS, *Pharmacognosy Review*, 2010

Hypolipidemic activity of Anethum graveolens in rats, Hajhashemi V, Abbasi N, *Phytotherapy Research*, 2008

Antifungal mechanism of essential oil from Anethum graveolens seeds against Candida albicans, Chen Y, Zeng H, Tian J, Ban X, Ma B, Wang Y, *Journal of Medical Microbiology*, 2013

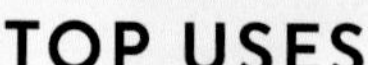

DOUGLAS FIR

PSEUDOTSUGA MENZIESII

cleansing
promoting
grounding

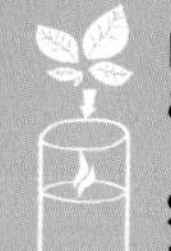

NEEDLES & BRANCH

STEAM DISTILLED

TOP USES

MENTAL FOG & LOW ENERGY
Apply to temples and forehead or diffuse to clear mind and revive enthusiasm.

DEPRESSION & TENSION
Apply to temples, forehead, and back of neck or diffuse to relax and ground.

CONGESTION & SINUS ISSUES
Apply to chest or bridge of nose.

RESPIRATORY INFECTION & COUGH
Apply to throat, chest or diffuse.

MUSCLE & JOINT SORENESS
Massage with wintergreen to affected area for soothing relief.

RHEUMATIC & ARTHRITIC CONDITIONS
Apply to affected area(s).

CONSTIPATION
Apply diluted to abdomen.

SKIN IRRITATIONS & CUTS
Apply diluted to affected area(s).

CELLULITE & SKIN CLEANSING
Massage diluted with grapefruit to desired area.

EMOTIONAL BALANCE
Use aromatically and topically to get from Upset ———> Renewed.

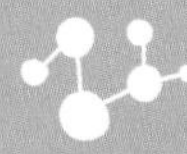

MAIN CONSTITUENTS
Beta-pinene
Alpha-pinene
3-carvene
Sabinene

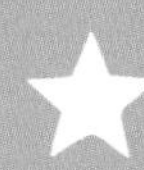

TOP PROPERTIES
Antioxidant
Analgesic
Antimicrobial
Antiseptic
Anticatarrhal
Astringent
Diuretic
Expectorant
Laxative
Sedative
Stimulant
Tonic

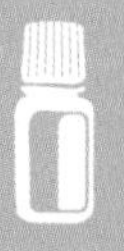

BLENDS WELL WITH
Bergamot
Cedarwood
Siberian fir
Vetiver
Wild orange

Considered to be the classic Christmas tree, the Douglas fir tree was used by Native Americans in the Pacific Northwest to heal a wide variety of ailments.

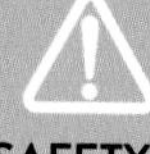

SAFETY
Not for internal use.

RESEARCH: Antimicrobial activity of some Pacific Northwest woods against anaerobic bacteria and yeast. Johnston WH, Karchesy JJ, Constantine GH, Craig AM. Phytother Res. 2001 Nov;15(7):586-8.

Douglas-fir root-associated microorganisms with inhibitory activity towards fungal plant pathogens and human bacterial pathogens. Axelrood PE, Clarke AM, Radley R, Zemcov SJ. Can J Microbiol. 1996 Jul;42(7):690-700.

Food-related odor probes of brain reward circuits during hunger: a pilot FMRI study. Bragulat V, Dzemidzic M, Bruno C, Cox CA, Talavage T, Considine RV, Kareken DA. Obesity (Silver Spring). 2010 Aug;18(8):1566-71. doi: 10.1038/oby.2010.57. Epub 2010 Mar 25.

Contemporary use of bark for medicine by two Salishan native elders of southeast Vancouver Island, Canada. Turner NJ, Hebda RJ. J Ethnopharmacol. 1990 Apr;29(1):59-72.

enlivening • fresh • clearing

EUCALYPTUS

EUCALYPTUS RADIATA

TOP USES

CONGESTION, COUGH, BRONCHITIS & PNEUMONIA
Apply to chest and over the bridge of nose. Diffuse or inhale from cupped hands.

SHINGLES, MALARIA, COLD & FLU
Apply to bottoms of feet or along spine and diffuse.

ASTHMA, SINUSITIS & RESPIRATORY
Put in palms of hands and inhale from cupped hands or apply diluted to chest and feet.

FEVERS & HEAT SENSITIVITY
Apply with peppermint down the spine for cooling effect.

MUSCLE FATIGUE & PAIN
Dilute and massage into overused muscles.

KIDNEY STONES
Gently massage over kidneys or area(s) of pain.

CELLULITE
Dilute and massage over area of concern.

EARACHES
Dilute and apply to outer ear and bone behind the ear.

BREAST ISSUES & CANCER
Dilute and massage into breast tissues.

MENTAL SLUGGISHNESS
Inhale with rosemary from cupped hands.

DUST MITES
Apply 10-15 drops to a glass spray bottle and use as a dust mite deterrent.

CLEANING DISINFECTANT
Add 10-15 drops to a glass spray bottle with water for a quick-drying disinfecting cleaner.

EMOTIONAL BALANCE
Use aromatically and topically to get from Congested ⟶ Stimulated.

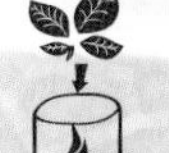

LEAVES

STEAM DISTILLED

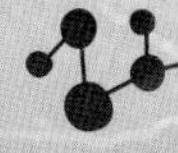

MAIN CONSTITUENTS
Eucalyptol
Alpha-terpineol

TOP PROPERTIES
Antiviral
Antibacterial
Expectorant
Analgesic
Insecticidal
Hypotensive
Disinfectant
Catalyst

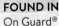

FOUND IN
On Guard®
HD Clear®
Breathe®
TerraShield®

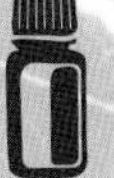

BLENDS WELL WITH
Cardamom
Peppermint
Rosemary

SAFETY
Dilution recommended. Possible skin sensitivity. Not for internal use.

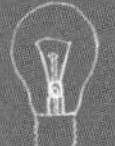

Eucalyptus was widely used in World War I to control infections and influenza.

RESEARCH: Remedies for common family ailments: 10. Nasal decongestants, Sinclair A, *Professional Care of Mother and Child*, 1996

Immune-Modifying and Antimicrobial Effects of Eucalyptus Oil and Simple Inhalation Devices, Sadlon AE, Lamson DW, *Alternative Medicine Review: A Journal of Clinical Therapeutic*, 2010

Effect of inhaled menthol on citric acid induced cough in normal subjects, Morice AH, Marshall AE, Higgins KS, Grattan TJ, *Thorax*, 1994

The effects of aromatherapy on pain, depression, and life satisfaction of arthritis patients, Kim MJ, Nam ES, Paik SI, *Taehan Kanho Hakhoe Chi*, 2005

In vitro antagonistic activity of monoterpenes and their mixtures against 'toe nail fungus' pathogens, Ramsewak RS, Nair MG, Stommel M, Selanders L, *Phytotherapy Research*, 2003

Antibacterial, antifungal, and anticancer activities of volatile oils and extracts from stems, leaves, and flowers of Eucalyptus sideroxylon and Eucalyptus torquata, Ashour HM, *Cancer Biology and Therapy*, 2008

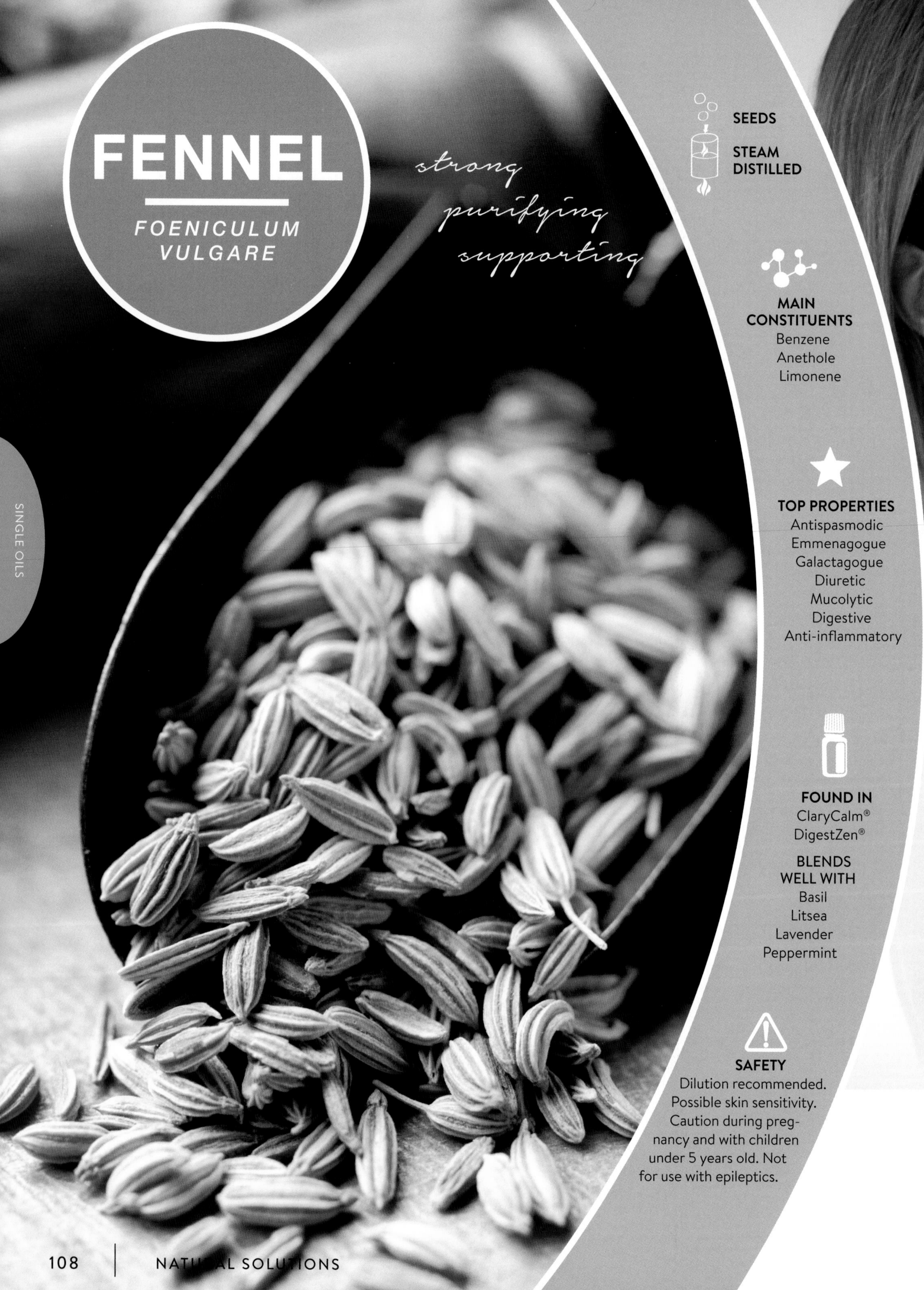

FENNEL

FOENICULUM VULGARE

strong
purifying
supporting

SEEDS

STEAM DISTILLED

MAIN CONSTITUENTS
Benzene
Anethole
Limonene

TOP PROPERTIES
Antispasmodic
Emmenagogue
Galactagogue
Diuretic
Mucolytic
Digestive
Anti-inflammatory

FOUND IN
ClaryCalm®
DigestZen®

BLENDS WELL WITH
Basil
Litsea
Lavender
Peppermint

SAFETY
Dilution recommended. Possible skin sensitivity. Caution during pregnancy and with children under 5 years old. Not for use with epileptics.

TOP USES

NAUSEA, COLIC & FLATULENCE
Take in a capsule or in water or massage into abdomen.

MENSTRUAL ISSUES & PMS
Take in a capsule or apply to abdomen to balance and tone female organs.

MENOPAUSE & PREMENOPAUSE ISSUES
Take in a capsule or massage over abdomen.

CRAMPS & SPASMS
Dilute and rub onto distressed muscles.

BREAST FEEDING OR LOW MILK SUPPLY
Use in a capsule or in water to increase milk supply.

EDEMA & FLUID RETENTION
Combine with grapefruit and massage over affected areas or take in a capsule.

COUGH & CONGESTION
Apply diluted to chest and throat.

INTESTINAL PARASITES & SLUGGISH BOWELS
Take with lemon in a capsule.

BLOOD SUGAR IMBALANCE
Take in a capsule or add to glass of water.

HUNGER PAINS
Take under tongue or in water to curb hunger as needed.

STROKE
Take in a capsule or massage on back of neck.

EMOTIONAL BALANCE
Use aromatically and topically to get from Unproductive ⟶ Flourishing.

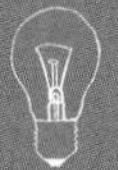

Ancient Roman warriors used fennel because it was believed it gave them strength during battle.

= Aromatically = Topically = Internally

RESEARCH: In vitro antifungal activity and mechanism of essential oil from fennel (Foeniculum vulgare L.) on dermatophyte species, Zeng H, Chen X, Liang J, *Journal of Medical Microbiology*, 2014

Antinociceptive activity of alpha-pinene and fenchone, Him A, Ozbek H, Turel I, Oner AC, *Pharmacology Online*, 2008

The palliation of nausea in hospice and palliative care patients with essential oils of Pimpinella anisum (aniseed), Foeniculum vulgare var. dulce (sweet fennel), Anthemis nobilis (Roman chamomile) and Mentha x piperita (peppermint), Gilligan NP, *International Journal of Aromatherapy*, 2005

Comparison of fennel and mefenamic acid for the treatment of primary dysmenorrhea, Namavar Jahromi B, Tartifizadeh A, Khabnadideh S, *International Journal of Gynaecology and Obstetrics: the Official Organ of the International Federation of Gynaecology and Obstetrics*, 2003

Carvacrol, a component of thyme oil, activates PPAR alpha and gamma and suppresses COX-2 expression, Hotta M, Nakata R, Katsukawa M, Hori K, Takahashi S, Inoue H., *Journal of Lipid Research*, 2010,

Effects of herbal essential oil mixture as a dietary supplement on egg production in quail, Çabuk M, Eratak S, Alçicek A, Bozkurt M., *The Scientific World Journal*, 2014

Antimicrobial and antiplasmid activities of essential oils, Schelz Z, Molnar J, Hohmann J, *Fitoterapia*, 2006

Chemical composition, antimicrobial and antioxidant activities of anethole-rich oil from leaves of selected varieties of fennel [Foeniculum vulgare Mill. ssp. vulgare var. azoricum (Mill.) Thell], Senatore F, Oliviero F, Scandolera E, Taglialatela-Scafati O, Roscigno G, Zaccardelli M, De Falco E, *Fitoterapia*, 2013

Salinity impact on yield, water use, mineral and essential oil content of fennel (Foeniculum vulgare Mill.), Semiz GD, Unlukara A, Yurtseven E, Suarez DL, Telci I, *Journal of Agricultural Science*, 2012

Efficacy of plant essential oils on postharvest control of rots caused by fungi on different stone fruits in vivo, Lopez-Reyes JG, Spadaro D, Prelle A, Garibaldi A, Gullino ML, *Journal of Food Protection*, 2013

FRANKINCENSE

BOSWELLIA FREREANA

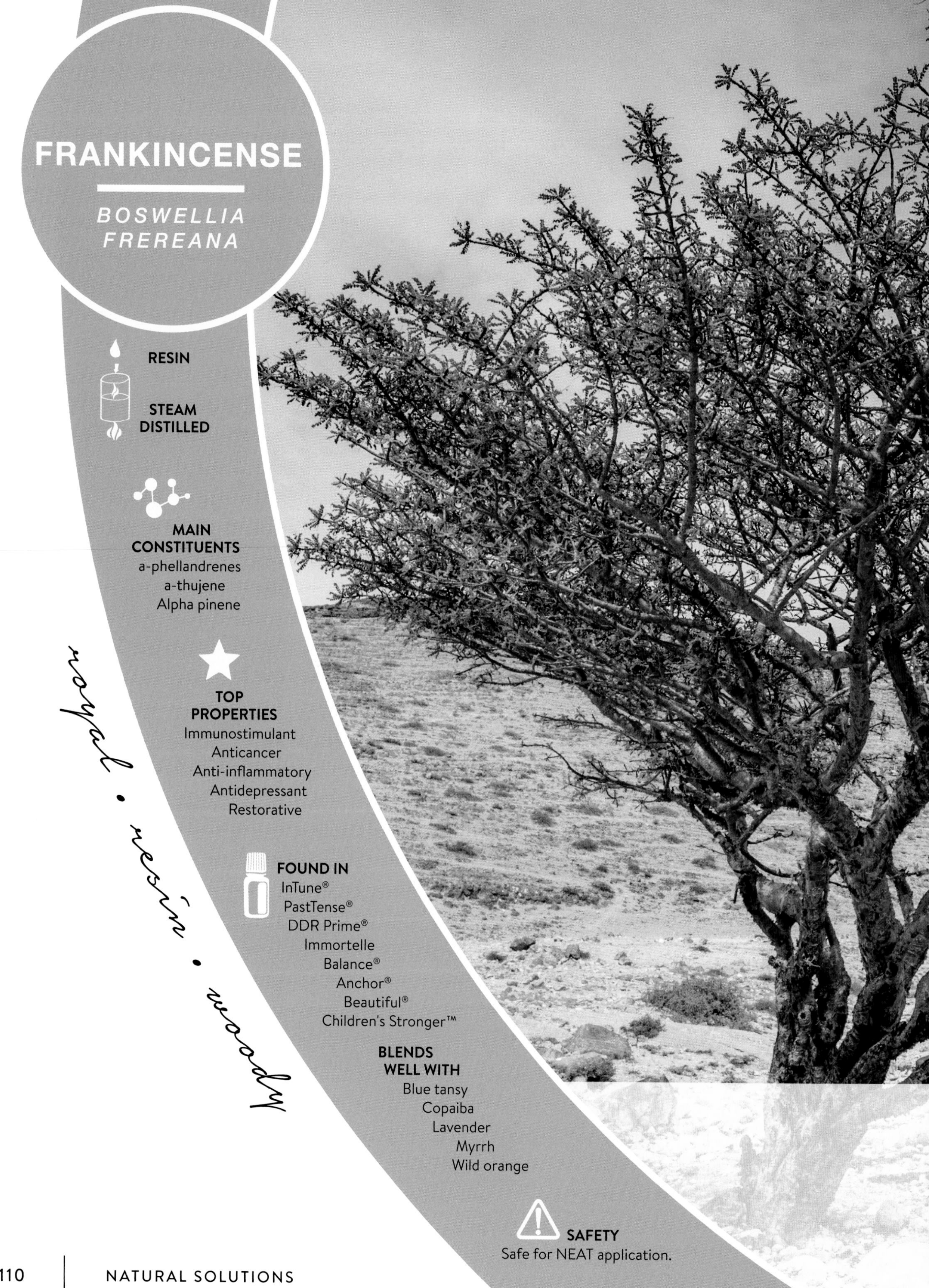

SINGLE OILS

RESIN

STEAM DISTILLED

MAIN CONSTITUENTS
a-phellandrenes
a-thujene
Alpha pinene

TOP PROPERTIES
Immunostimulant
Anticancer
Anti-inflammatory
Antidepressant
Restorative

royal • resin • woody

FOUND IN
InTune®
PastTense®
DDR Prime®
Immortelle
Balance®
Anchor®
Beautiful®
Children's Stronger™

BLENDS WELL WITH
Blue tansy
Copaiba
Lavender
Myrrh
Wild orange

SAFETY
Safe for NEAT application.

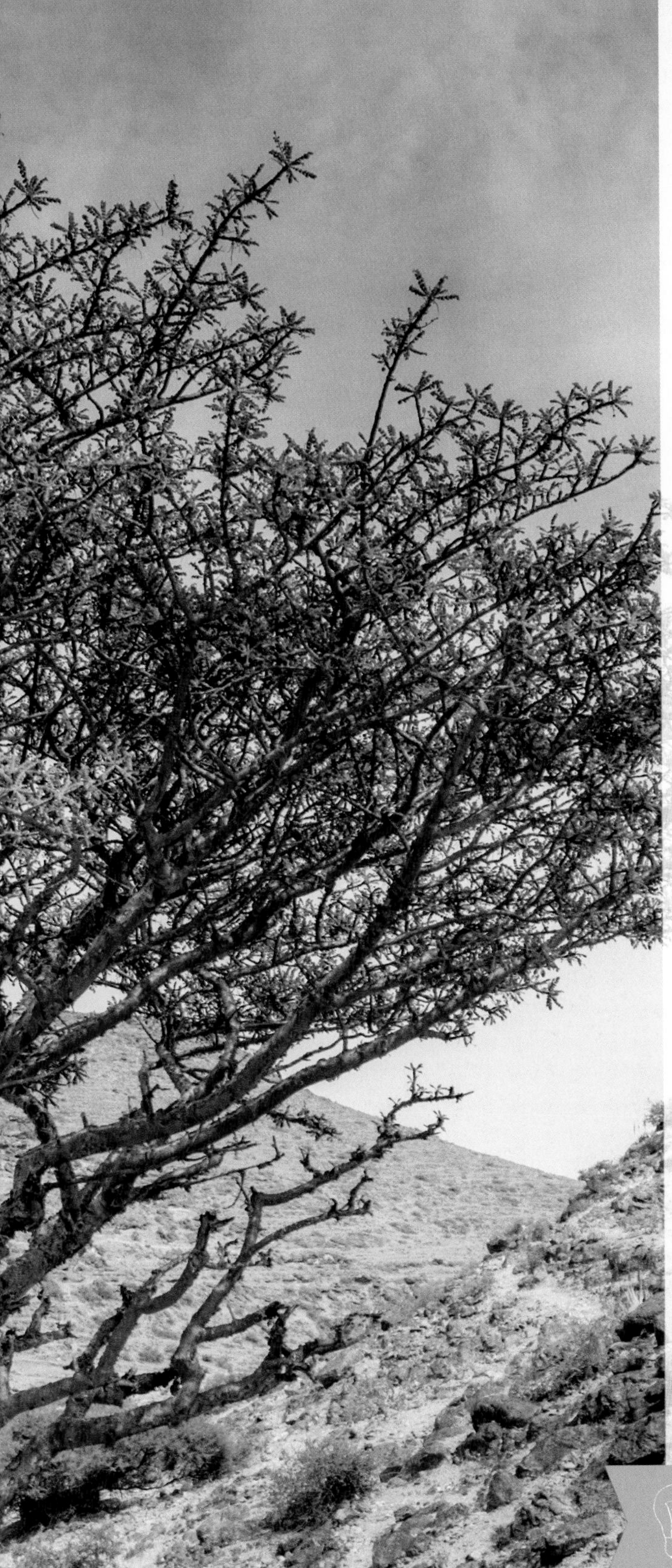

TOP USES

CANCER & TUMORS
Take in capsule with oil(s) that target area of interest or massage over affected area.

SEIZURES & TRAUMA
Put a drop under the tongue and apply along hairline.

ALZHEIMER'S DISEASE, DEMENTIA & BRAIN INJURY
Use or apply under nose and back of neck, or diffuse.

DEPRESSION
Diffuse or put under the tongue to ease the effects of depression.

WOUND HEALING & WRINKLES
Apply to wounds or wrinkles to support skin regeneration.

SCARS & STRETCH MARKS
Combine with myrrh and apply to reduce the appearance of scars and stretch marks.

SCIATICA, BACK PAIN & HEADACHES
Apply over affected area or take in a capsule to reduce inflammation.

IMMUNE SYSTEM & CELLULAR HEALTH
Take in a capsule or apply to bottoms of feet.

LIVER DETOXIFICATION & JAUNDICE
Take in a capsule or apply to abdomen or bottoms of feet.

AUTOIMMUNE DISORDERS
Take in a capsule, apply to bottoms of feet, or over spleen.

WARTS
Apply to site with oregano diluted.

CONGESTION, COUGH & ALLERGIES
For gentle relief, inhale and apply diluted combined with peppermint and rosemary to chest and throat.

BREAST CANCER PREVENTION
Apply diluted to breast to cleanse breast tissue. Apply twice per day for 30 days, 3-4 times per year.

MEDITATION, PRAYER & FOCUS
Apply under nose and back of neck or in a diffuser.

EMOTIONAL BALANCE
Use aromatically and topically to get from Separated ——→ Unified.

= Aromatically = Topically = Internally

Nearly all ancient religions have used frankincense in their spiritual practices including ancient Egyptians, Greeks, Romans, Christians, Jews, Muslims, Hindus, and Buddhists.

RESEARCH: Frankincense oil derived from Boswellia carteri induces tumor cell specific cytotoxicity, Frank MB, Yang Q, Osban J, Azzarello JT, Saban MR, Saban R, Ashley RA, Welter JC, Fung KM, Lin HK, *BMC Complementary and Alternative Medicine*, 2009

Differential effects of selective frankincense (Ru Xiang) essential oil versus non-selective sandalwood (Tan Xiang) essential oil on cultured bladder cancer cells: a microarray and bioinformatics study, Dozmorov MG, Yang Q, Wu W, Wren J, Suhail MM, Woolley CL, Young DG, Fung KM, Lin HK, 2014

Composition and potential anticancer activities of essential oils obtained from myrrh and frankincense, Chen Y, Zhou C, Ge Z, Liu Y, Liu Y, Feng W, Li S, Chen G, Wei T, *Oncology Letters*, 2013

Volatile composition and antimicrobial activity of twenty commercial frankincense essential oil samples, Van Vuurena SF, Kamatoub GPP, Viljoenb, AM, *South African Journal of Botany*, 2010

Effects of Aroma Hand Massage on Pain, State Anxiety and Depression in Hospice Patients with Terminal Cancer, Chang SY, *Journal of Korean Academy of Nursing*, 2008

Evaluation of the Effects of Plant-derived Essential Oils on Central Nervous System Function Using Discrete Shuttle-type Conditioned Avoidance Response in Mice, Umezu T., *Phytotherapy Research*, 2012

Chemistry and immunomodulatory activity of frankincense oil, Mikhaeil BR, Maatooq GT, Badria FA, Amer MM, *Zeitschrift fur Naturforschung C*, 2003

Boswellia frereana (frankincense) suppresses cytokine-induced matrix metalloproteinase expression and production of pro-inflammatory molecules in articular cartilage, Blain EJ, Ali AY, Duance VC, *Phytotherapy Research*, 2012

The additive and synergistic antimicrobial effects of select frankincense and myrrh oils – a combination from the pharaonic pharmacopoeia, de Rapper S, Van Vuuren SF, Kamatou GP, Viljoen AM, Dagne E, *Letters in Applied Microbiology*, 2012

GERANIUM

PELARGONIUM GRAVEOLENS

strengthening releasing stabilizing

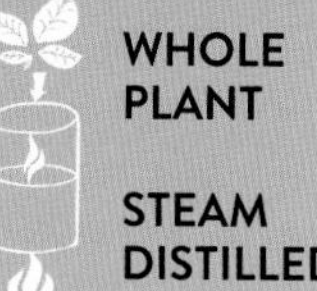

WHOLE PLANT

STEAM DISTILLED

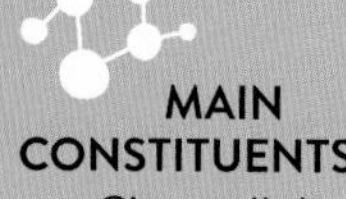

MAIN CONSTITUENTS
Citronellol
Geraniol

TOP PROPERTIES
Haemostatic
Detoxifier
Regenerative
Anti-allergenic
Antihemorrhagic
Antitoxic

FOUND IN
ClaryCalm®
Zendocrine®
Align®

BLENDS WELL WITH
Lavender
Neroli
Patchouli
Sandalwood
Tangerine

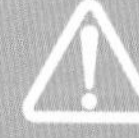

SAFETY
Dilution recommended. Possible skin sensitivity.

TOP USES

LIVER, GALLBLADDER, PANCREAS & KIDNEY ISSUES
Apply over area of concern or take in a capsule.

BLOOD ISSUES & BLEEDING
Apply to troubled area to restore healthy blood or stop bleeding.

CUTS & WOUNDS
Apply to area of concern to keep wounds clean, stop bleeding, and regenerate tissue.

PMS & HORMONE BALANCING
Massage on abdomen or take a drop under tongue.

LOW LIBIDO
Massage diluted over abdomen or take a drop under tongue to increase sexual drive.

DRY OR OILY HAIR & SKIN
Apply to scalp or troubled skin to retain oil balance.

MOISTURIZER
Apply diluted and use as a moisturizer for skin hydration and balance.

BODY ODOR
Apply under arms as a deodorant.

EMOTIONAL BALANCE
Use aromatically and topically to get from Neglected ——→ Mended.

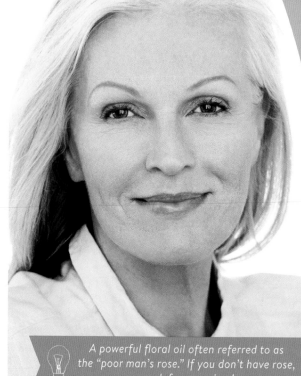

A powerful floral oil often referred to as the "poor man's rose." If you don't have rose, reach for geranium!

RESEARCH: Bioactivity-guided investigation of geranium essential oils as natural tick repellents, Tabanca N, Wang M, Avonto C, Chittiboyina AG, Parcher JF, Carroll JF, Kramer M, Khan IA, *Journal of Agricultural and Food Chemistry*, 2013

The antibacterial activity of geranium oil against Gram-negative bacteria isolated from difficult-to- heal wounds, Sienkiewicz M, Poznacska-Kurowska K, Kaszuba A, Kowalczyk E, *Burns*, 2014

Suppression of neutrophil accumulation in mice by cutaneous application of geranium essential oil, Maruyama N, Sekimoto Y, Ishibashi H, Inouye S, Oshima H, Yamaguchi H, Abe S, *Journal of Inflammation (London, England)*, 2005

Hypoglycemic and antioxidant effects of leaf essential oil of Pelargonium graveolens, L'Hér. in alloxan induced diabetic rats, Boukhris M, Bouaziz M, Feki I, Jemai H, El Feki A, Sayadi S, *Lipids in Health and Disease*, 2012

Antioxidant and Anticancer Activities of Citrus reticulate (Petitgrain Mandarin) and Pelargonium graveolens (Geranium) Essential Oils, Fayed SA, *Research Journal of Agriculture and Biological Sciences*, 2009

Aromatherapy Massage Affects Menopausal Symptoms in Korean Climacteric Women: A Pilot-Controlled Clinical Trial, Myung-HH, Yun Seok Y, Myeong SL, *Evidence-based Complementary and Alternative Medicine*, 2008

warming
accelerating
stimulating

GINGER

ZINGIBER OFFICINALE

TOP USES

SPASMS, CRAMPS & SORE MUSCLES
Dilute and massage into area of discomfort for warming relief.

NAUSEA, MORNING SICKNESS & LOSS OF APPETITE
Diffuse, take a drop in a glass with warm water, apply diluted to wrists or to bottoms of feet.

MOTION SICKNESS & VERTIGO
Inhale from cupped hands or take in a capsule.

MEMORY & BRAIN SUPPORT
Inhale from cupped hands or take in a capsule.

HEARTBURN & REFLUX
Take in a capsule with lemon.

ALCOHOL ADDICTION
Take in a capsule as needed to ease cravings.

HORMONE & BLOOD SUGAR IMBALANCES
Take in a capsule.

COLIC & CONSTIPATION
Apply diluted over abdomen or take in a glass of warm water.

NEUROTRANSMITTER DEFICIENCIES
Inhale from cupped hands or take in a capsule.

CONGESTION, SINUSITIS & LARYNGITIS
Dilute and apply over chest, bridge of nose, and throat, or diffuse or take with lemon.

COLD, FLU & SORE THROAT
Take in a capsule, gargle or apply to bottoms of feet.

SPRAINS & BROKEN BONES
Dilute and apply to sprain or break to promote healing.

EMOTIONAL BALANCE
Use aromatically and topically to get from Apathetic ———> Activated.

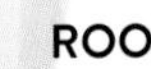

ROOT

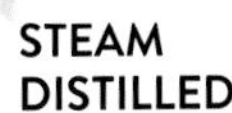

STEAM DISTILLED

MAIN CONSTITUENT
Alpha-zingiberene

TOP PROPERTIES
Anti-inflammatory
Antispasmodic
Digestive Stimulant
Laxative
Analgesic
Stimulant
Decongestant
Neurotonic

FOUND IN
Slim & Sassy®
DigestZen®

BLENDS WELL WITH
Cinnamon
Frankincense
Grapefruit
Litsea

SAFETY
Dilution recommended. Possible skin sensitivity.

Ginger has been used as a medicinal herb for centuries.

RESEARCH: Gastroprotective activity of essential oils from turmeric and ginger, Liju VB, Jeena K, Kuttan R., *Journal of Basic and Clinical Physiology and Pharmacology,* 2014

Reversal of pyrogallol-induced delay in gastric emptying in rats by ginger (Zingiber officinale), Gupta YK, Sharma M, *Methods and Findings in Experimental and Clinical Pharmacology,* 2001

The essential oil of ginger, Zingiber officinale, and anaesthesia, Geiger JL, *International Journal of Aromatherapy,* 2005

Effectiveness of aromatherapy with light thai massage for cellular immunity improvement in colorectal cancer patients receiving chemotherapy, Khiewkhern S, Promthet S, Sukprasert A, Eunhpinitpong W, Bradshaw P, *Asian Pacific Journal of Cancer Prevention,* 2013

Antioxidant, anti-inflammatory and antinociceptive activities of essential oil from ginger, Jeena K, Liju VB, Kuttan R, *Indian Journal of Physiology and Pharmacology,* 2013

A brief review of current scientific evidence involving aromatherapy use for nausea and vomiting, Lua PL, Zakaria NS, *The Journal of Alternative and Complementary Medicine,* 2012

Anti-inflammatory effects of ginger and some of its components in human bronchial epithelial (BEAS-2B) cells, Podlogar JA, Verspohl EJ, *Phytotherapy Research,* 2012

Medicinal plants as antiemetics in the treatment of cancer: a review, Haniadka R, Popouri S, Palatty PL, Arora R, Baliga MS, *Integrative Cancer Therapies,* 2012

Inhibitory potential of ginger extracts against enzymes linked to type 2 diabetes, inflammation and induced oxidative stress, Rani MP, Padmakumari KP, Sankarikutty B, Cherian OL, Nisha VM, Raghu KG, *International Journal of Food Sciences and Nutrition,* 2011

Ginger: An herbal medicinal product with broad anti-inflammatory actions, Grzanna R, Lindmark L, Frondoza CG, *Journal of Medicinal Food,* 2005

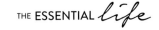

= Aromatically = Topically = Internally

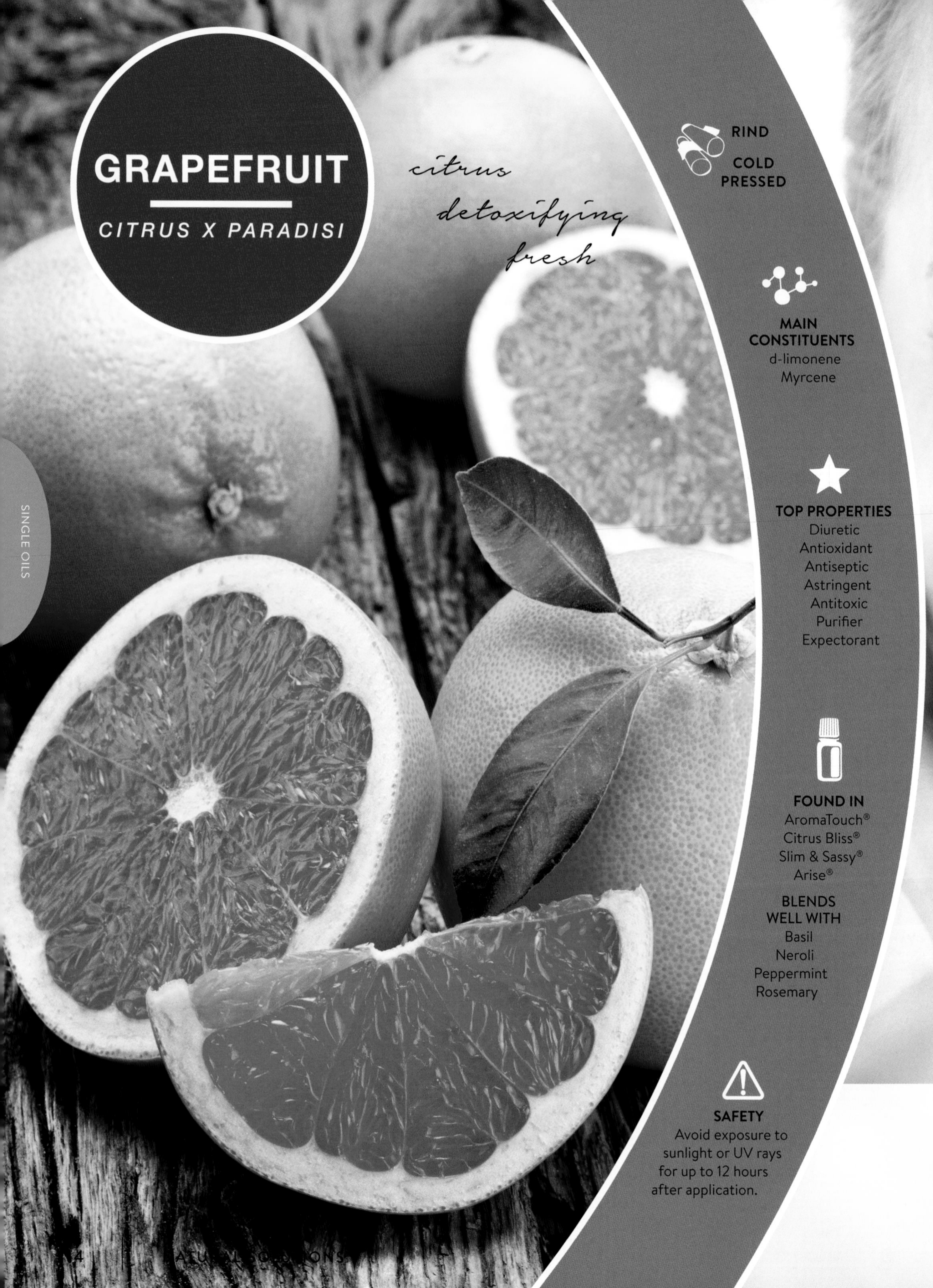
GRAPEFRUIT
CITRUS X PARADISI
citrus
detoxifying
fresh
RIND
COLD PRESSED
MAIN CONSTITUENTS
d-limonene
Myrcene
TOP PROPERTIES
Diuretic
Antioxidant
Antiseptic
Astringent
Antitoxic
Purifier
Expectorant
FOUND IN
AromaTouch®
Citrus Bliss®
Slim & Sassy®
Arise®
BLENDS WELL WITH
Basil
Neroli
Peppermint
Rosemary
SAFETY
Avoid exposure to sunlight or UV rays for up to 12 hours after application.
SINGLE OILS

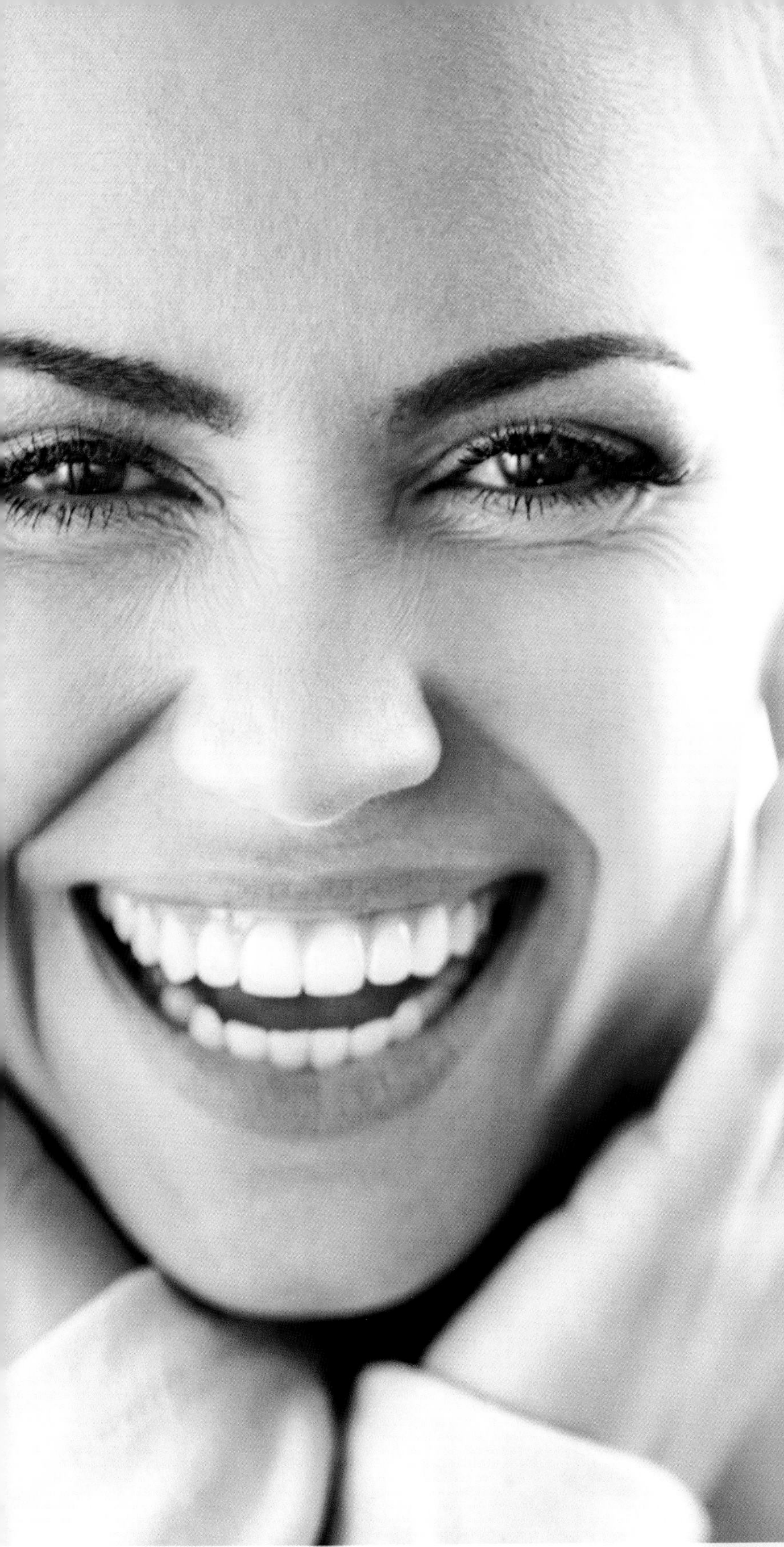

TOP USES

WEIGHT LOSS & OBESITY

Drink a few drops in water or take in a capsule. Apply to area(s) of concern to breakdown fat cells.

BREAST & UTERINE ISSUES & PROGESTERONE BALANCE

Take in a capsule or apply diluted to area of concern.

ADDICTIONS & SUGAR CRAVINGS

Diffuse or take in a capsule.

OILY SKIN & ACNE

Apply to area(s) of concern to better manage breakouts.

DETOXIFICATION & CELLULITE

Rub on bottoms of feet or drink in water for an overall detox. Apply diluted to problem area(s) to breakdown cellulite.

LYMPHATIC & KIDNEY TOXICITY

Take in water or apply diluted over lymph nodes, kidney area, or bottoms of feet.

ADRENAL FATIGUE

Apply diluted with basil over adrenal area, to bottoms of feet or back of neck. Take in a capsule.

GALLSTONES & GALLBLADDER SUPPORT

Take with geranium in a capsule.

HANGOVER & JET LAG

Take in a capsule to ease symptoms.

EMOTIONAL BALANCE

Use aromatically and topically to get from Divided ——> Validate.

SINGLE OILS

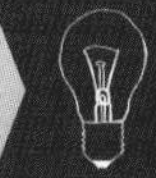

Some prescription drugs contain a warning against grapefruit. The essential oil has different chemical composition then the fruit.

= Aromatically = Topically = Internally

RESEARCH: Olfactory stimulatory with grapefruit and lavender oils change autonomic nerve activity and physiological function, Nagai K, Niijima A, Horii Y, Shen J, Tanida M, *Autonomic Neuroscience: basic & clinical*, 2014

Minor Furanocoumarins and Coumarins in Grapefruit Peel Oil as Inhibitors of Human Cytochrome P450 3A4, César TB, Manthey JA, Myung K, *Journal of Natural Products*, 2009

Antimicrobial effects of essential oils in combination with chlorhexidine digluconate, Filoche SK, Soma K, Sissons CH, *Oral Microbiology and Immunology*, 2005

Inhibition of acetylcholinesterase activity by essential oil from Citrus paradisi, Miyazawa M, Tougo H, Ishihara M, *Natural Product Letters*, 2001

Olfactory stimulation with scent of essential oil of grapefruit affects autonomic neurotransmission and blood pressure, Tanida M, Niijima A, Shen J, Nakamura T, Nagai K, *Brian Research*, 2005

Mechanism of changes induced in plasma glycerol by scent stimulation with grapefruit and lavender essential oils, Shen J, Niijima A, Tanida M, Horii Y, Nakamura T, Nagai K, *Neuroscience Letters*, 2007

Olfactory stimulation with scent of grapefruit oil affects autonomic nerves, lipolysis and appetite in rats, Shen J, Niijima A, Tanida M, Horii Y, Maeda K, Nagai K, *Neuroscience Letters*, 2005

Effects of fragrance inhalation on sympathetic activity in normal adults, Haze S, Sakai K, Gozu Y, *The Japanese Journal of Pharmacology*, 2002

Effect of olfactory stimulation with flavor of grapefruit oil and lemon oil on the activity of sympathetic branch in the white adipose tissue of the epididymis, Niijima A, Nagai K, *Experimental Biology and Medicine*, 2003

Effect of aromatherapy massage on abdominal fat and body image in post-menopausal women, Kim HJ, *Taehan Kanho Hakhoe Chi*, 2007

GREEN MANDARIN

CITRUS NOBILIS

composing
reclaiming
resolving

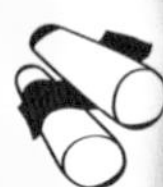

RIND OF UNRIPE FRUIT

COLD PRESSED

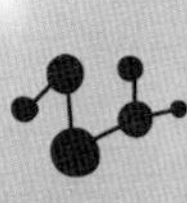

MAIN CONSTITUENTS
Limonene
y-Terpinene

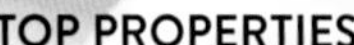

TOP PROPERTIES
Uplifting
Refreshing
Digestive Stimulant
Cleanser
Expectorant
Calming

FOUND IN
Citrus Bliss®

BLENDS WELL WITH
Black pepper
Clove
Copaiba
Juniper berry
Lemon
Sandalwood
Spearmint
Neroli

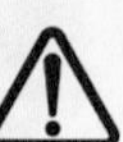

SAFETY
Avoid sunlight or UV rays to applied area for up to 12 hours to prevent mild photo toxicity.

ODOR & SURFACE CLEANING
Diffuse or spritz, diluted in water.

PERFUME
Apply with neroli to pulse points.

EMOTIONAL BALANCE
Use aromatically and topically to get from Distressed ——→ Carefree.

TOP USES

DEPRESSED, AGITATED, NERVOUS, INNER CHILD WORK
Diffuse. Take 1 drop under tongue. Apply to pulse points. Especially good for children. Combine with lavender, vetiver, rose, and/or neroli.

SITUATIONAL ANXIETY
Apply 1-2 drops under nose, diffuse or inhale, or take.

GAS, SLUGGISH DIGESTION, CONSTIPATION, HEARTBURN & ULCERS
Apply 1-2 drops over area of concern or take.

POOR CIRCULATION, CONGESTED LYMPHS, WATER RETENTION
Take 1-2 drops with black pepper 2x's daily under tongue or in a capsule.

LIVER & KIDNEY DETOX, SLUGGISH BILE FLOW
Take 1-2 drops with juniper berry and lemon 2x's daily.

ACNE, OILY SKIN, WOUNDS, SCARS
Combine with skin care products and apply to area(s) of concern.

IMBALANCED BLOOD SUGAR & FAT METABOLISM & CHOLESTEROL
Take 1-2 drops daily in a capsule with lemongrass or cinnamon.

COUGH, RESPIRATORY ISSUES
Diffuse with spearmint. Apply to chest and back. Take 1-2 drops.

SKIN & BREAST CANCER
Take 1-2 drops 2x's daily with copaiba. Apply to area(s) of concern.

LACK OF ENERGY OR ALERTNESS, MENTAL FATIGUE & DEMENTIA
Apply 1-2 drops on palms of hands, rub together, inhale deeply.

WRINKLES, FINE LINES & AGE SPOTS, STRETCH MARKS
Add to skin care products and apply to area(s) of concern.

FLAVORING & NATURAL FOOD PRESERVATIVE
Add drop to dishes, frostings, smoothies, or cut fruit.

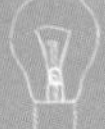

The fruit was offered to rulers in China as a show of respect, representing abundance and happiness during Chinese New Year celebrations.

HELICHRYSUM

HELICHRYSUM ITALICUM

healing
fusing
regenerating

TOP USES

WRINKLES & STRETCH MARKS
Apply with myrrh as needed.

NOSEBLEEDS, BLEEDING & HEMORRHAGING
Apply over bridge of nose or area of concern.

SCARS, WOUNDS & BRUISING
Apply to scars and wounds to support skin renewal.

SHOCK, PAIN RELIEF & NERVE DAMAGE
Apply to back of neck or area of discomfort.

ALCOHOL ADDICTION
Apply to abdomen and over liver.

PSORIASIS & SKIN CONDITIONS
Apply with geranium on area of concern.

VARICOSE VEINS
Massage diluted with cypress into affected areas.

TINNITIS & EARACHE
Massage behind the ears to calm spasms, pain, and inflammation.

SINUS CONGESTION
Combine with sandalwood and lemon, apply to forehead, swab nostrils. Diffuse.

LIVER ISSUES & HEAVY METAL TOXICITY
Take in a capsule to promote heavy metal chelation and liver cleansing.

EMOTIONAL BALANCE
Use aromatically and topically to get from
Wounded ———> Released.

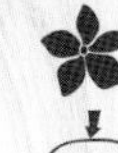

FLOWERS

STEAM DISTILLED

MAIN CONSTITUENTS
Neryl acetate
Italidione
y-curcumene
l-limonene

TOP PROPERTIES
Antispasmodic
Anticatarrhal
Neuroprotective
Neurotonic
Vasoconstrictor
Haemostatic
Nervine
Analgesic

FOUND IN
Deep Blue®
Immortelle

BLENDS WELL WITH
Clary Sage
Lavender
Rose
Yarrow

SAFETY
Safe for NEAT application.

This precious oil is often hand picked on the island of Corsica and used as "liquid stitches."

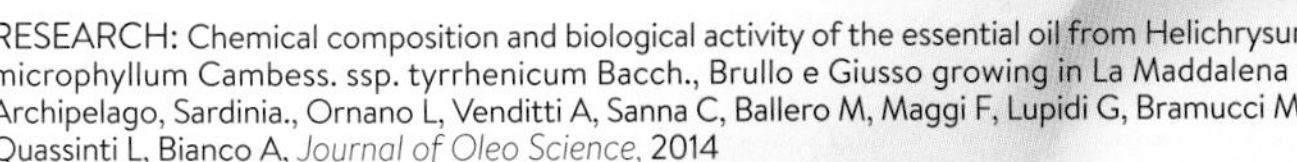

RESEARCH: Chemical composition and biological activity of the essential oil from Helichrysum microphyllum Cambess. ssp. tyrrhenicum Bacch., Brullo e Giusso growing in La Maddalena Archipelago, Sardinia., Ornano L, Venditti A, Sanna C, Ballero M, Maggi F, Lupidi G, Bramucci M, Quassinti L, Bianco A, *Journal of Oleo Science*, 2014

Arzanol, an anti-inflammatory and anti-HIV-1 phloroglucinol alpha-Pyrone from Helichrysum italicum ssp. microphyllum, Appendino G, Ottino M, Marquez N, Bianchi F, Giana A, Ballero M, Sterner O, Fiebich BL, Munoz E, *Journal of Natural Products*, 2007

Protective role of arzanol against lipid peroxidation in biological systems, Rosa A, Pollastro F, Atzeri A, Appendino G, Melis MP, Deiana M, Incani A, Loru D, Dessì MA, *Chemical and Physics of Lipids*, 2011

Arzanol, a prenylated heterodimeric phloroglucinyl pyrone, inhibits eicosanoid biosynthesis and exhibits anti-inflammatory efficacy in vivo, Bauer J, Koeberle A, Dehm F, Pollastro F, Appendino G, Northoff H, Rossi A, Sautebin L, Werz O, *Biochemical Pharmacology*, 2011

Anti-inflammatory and antioxidant properties of Helichrysum italicum, Sala A, Recio M, Giner RM, Máñez S, Tournier H, Schinella G, Ríos JL, *The Journal of Pharmacy and Pharmacology*, 2002

Effects of Helichrysum italicum extract on growth and enzymatic activity of Staphylococcus aureus, Nostro A, Bisignano G, Angela Cannatelli M, Crisafi G, Paola Germanò M, Alonzo V, *International Journal of Antimicrobial Agents*, 2001

Helichrysum italicum extract interferes with the production of enterotoxins by Staphylococcus aureus., Nostro A, Cannatelli MA, Musolino AD, Procopio F, Alonzo V, *Letters in Applied Microbiology*, 2002

Assessment of the anti-inflammatory activity and free radical scavenger activity of tiliroside., Sala A, Recio MC, Schinella GR, Máñez S, Giner RM, Cerdá-Nicolás M, Rosí JL, *European Journal of Pharmacology*, 2003

= Aromatically = Topically = Internally

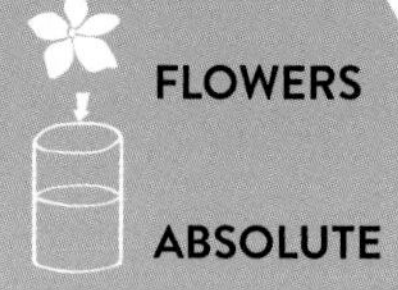

JASMINE

JASMINUM GRANDIFLORUM

euphoria
splendor
joy

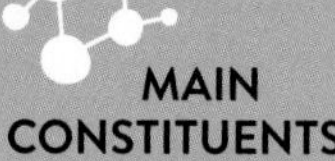

MAIN CONSTITUENTS
Benzyl acetate
Benzyl benzoate
phytol

TOP PROPERTIES
Antidepressant
Aphrodisiac
Antispasmodic
Calming
Regenerative
Carminative

FOUND IN
ClaryCalm®
Align®

BLENDS WELL WITH
Passion®
Immortelle
Neroli
Rose
Sandalwood

SAFETY
Safe for NEAT application.

SINGLE OILS

TOP USES

DEPRESSION & ANXIETY
Inhale (A) from cupped hands or apply (T) diluted under nose and back of neck.

UTERINE HEALTH, LABOR & DELIVERY
Apply (T) diluted over abdomen and to reflex points or diffuse (A).

FINE LINES & WRINKLES
Add two drops to bottle of moisturizer and apply (T) to skin nightly.

PINKEYE
Apply (T) diluted around (not in) eye.

EXHAUSTION
Apply (T) diluted to back of neck and bottoms of feet.

IRRITATED & DRY SKIN
Apply (T) diluted to affected area.

PMS & LOW LIBIDO
Apply (T) diluted to back of neck and over abdomen.

OVULATION & FERTILITY
Apply (T) diluted over abdomen to regulate hormones.

PERFUME
Combine with sandalwood or Amavi® and apply (T) as desired.

EMOTIONAL BALANCE
Use (A) aromatically and (T) topically to get from Hampered ———> Liberated.

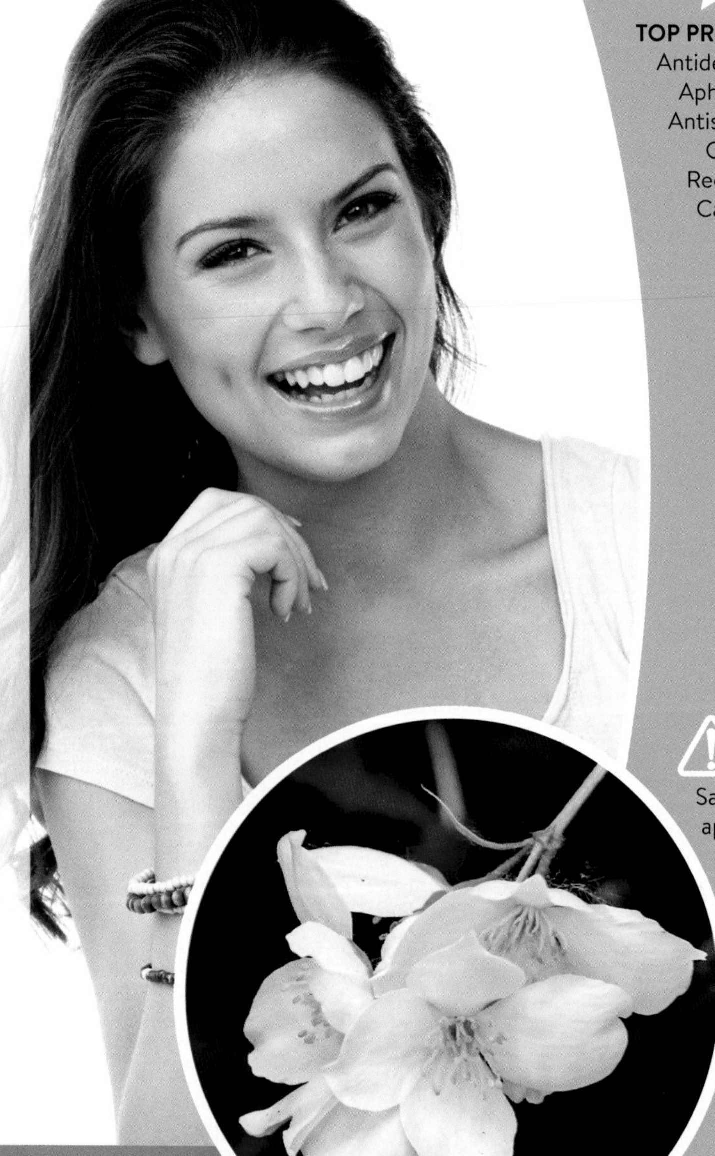

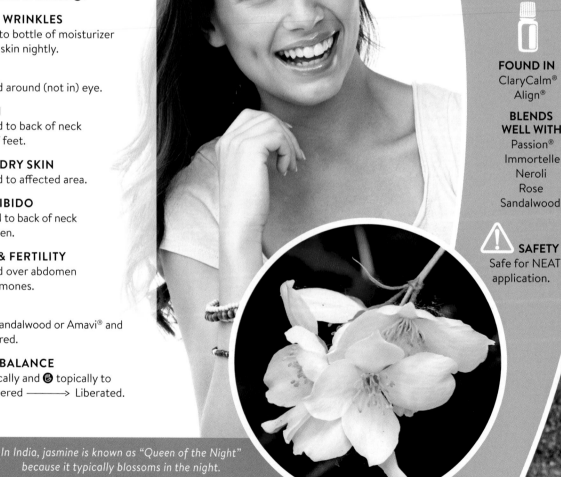

In India, jasmine is known as "Queen of the Night" because it typically blossoms in the night.

RESEARCH: The influence of essential oils on human attention and alertness, Ilmberger J, Heuberger E, Mahrhofer C, Dessovic H, Kowarik D, Buchbauer G, *Chemical Senses*, 2001

The influence of essential oils on human vigilance, Heuberger E, Ilmberger J, *Natural Product Communications*, 2010

Effects of Aromatherapy Massage on Blood Pressure and Lipid Profile in Korean Climacteric Women, Myung-HH , Heeyoung OH, Myeong SL , Chan K, Ae-na C, Gil-ran S, *International Journal of Neuroscience*, 2007

Sedative effects of the jasmine tea odor and (R)-(-)-linalool, one of its major odor components, on autonomic nerve activity and mood states, Kuroda K, Inoue N, Ito Y, Kubota K, Sugimoto A, Kakuda T, Fushiki T, *European Journal of Applied Physiology*, 2005

Aromatherapy Massage Affects Menopausal Symptoms in Korean Climacteric Women: A Pilot-Controlled Clinical Trial, Myung-HH, Yun Seok Y, Myeong SL, *Evidence-based Complementary and Alternative Medicine, 2008*

Stimulating effect of aromatherapy massage with jasmine oil, Hongratanaworakit T, *Natural Product Communications*, 2010

Activities of Ten Essential Oils towards Propionibacterium acnes and PC-3, A-549 and MCF-7 Cancer Cells, Zu Y, Yu H, Liang L, Fu Y, Efferth T, Liu X, Wu N, *Molecules*, 2010

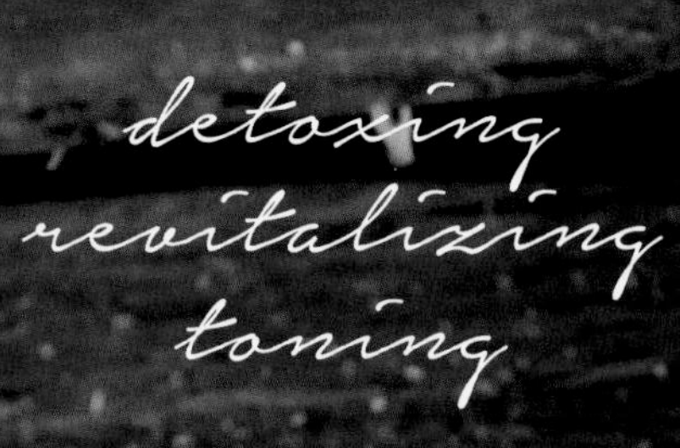

JUNIPER BERRY

JUNIPERUS COMMUNIS

TOP USES

JAUNDICE, LIVER ISSUES & DETOX
Take in a capsule to support cleansing.

KIDNEY STONES & INFECTION
Take in a capsule or apply over abdomen.

ACNE & PSORIASIS
Apply to area of concern, diluting as needed.

URINARY HEALTH & WATER RETENTION
Combine with lemon and apply over abdomen or take in a capsule.

SORE JOINTS & MUSCLES
Apply to area of concern, diluting as needed.

BACTERIA & VIRUSES
Apply down spine, bottoms of feet or take in a capsule.

HIGH CHOLESTEROL & BLOOD SUGAR LEVELS
Take in a capsule.

TENSION, STRESS & DEPRESSION
Inhale deeply from cupped hands, diffuse, and/or apply under nose or to bottoms of feet.

EMOTIONAL BALANCE
Use aromatically and topically to get from Denying ———→ Insightful.

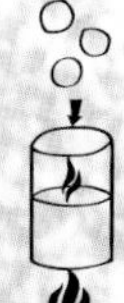

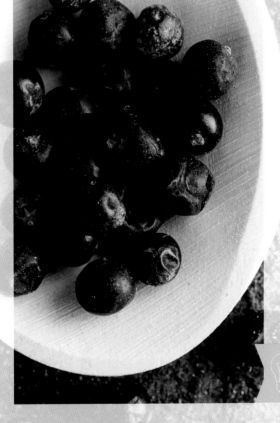

BERRIES

STEAM DISTILLED

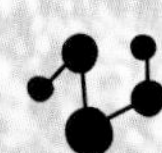

MAIN CONSTITUENTS
Alpha pinene
Sabinene

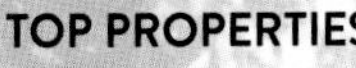

TOP PROPERTIES
Detoxifier
Diuretic
Antiseptic
Antispasmodic
Astringent
Anti-rheumatic
Carminative
Anti-parasitic

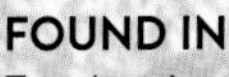

FOUND IN
Zendocrine®

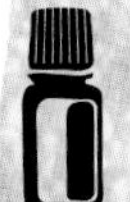

BLENDS WELL WITH
Bergamot
Blue tansy
Cypress
Grapefruit
Yarrow

SAFETY
Safe for NEAT application.

A favorite oil for its fragrance, juniper berries are also used for making gin.

RESEARCH: Fumigant toxicity of plant essential oils against Camptomyia corticalis (Diptera: Cecidomyiidae), Kim JR, Haribalan P, Son BK, Ahn YJ, *Journal of Economic Entomology*, 2012
Antimicrobial activity of juniper berry essential oil (Juniperus communis L., Cupressaceae), Pepeljnjak S, Kosalec I, Kalodera Z, Blazevic N, *Acta Pharmaceutica*, 2005
Antioxidant activities and volatile constituents of various essential oils, Wei A, Shibamoto T, *Journal of Agriculture and Food Chemistry*, 2007

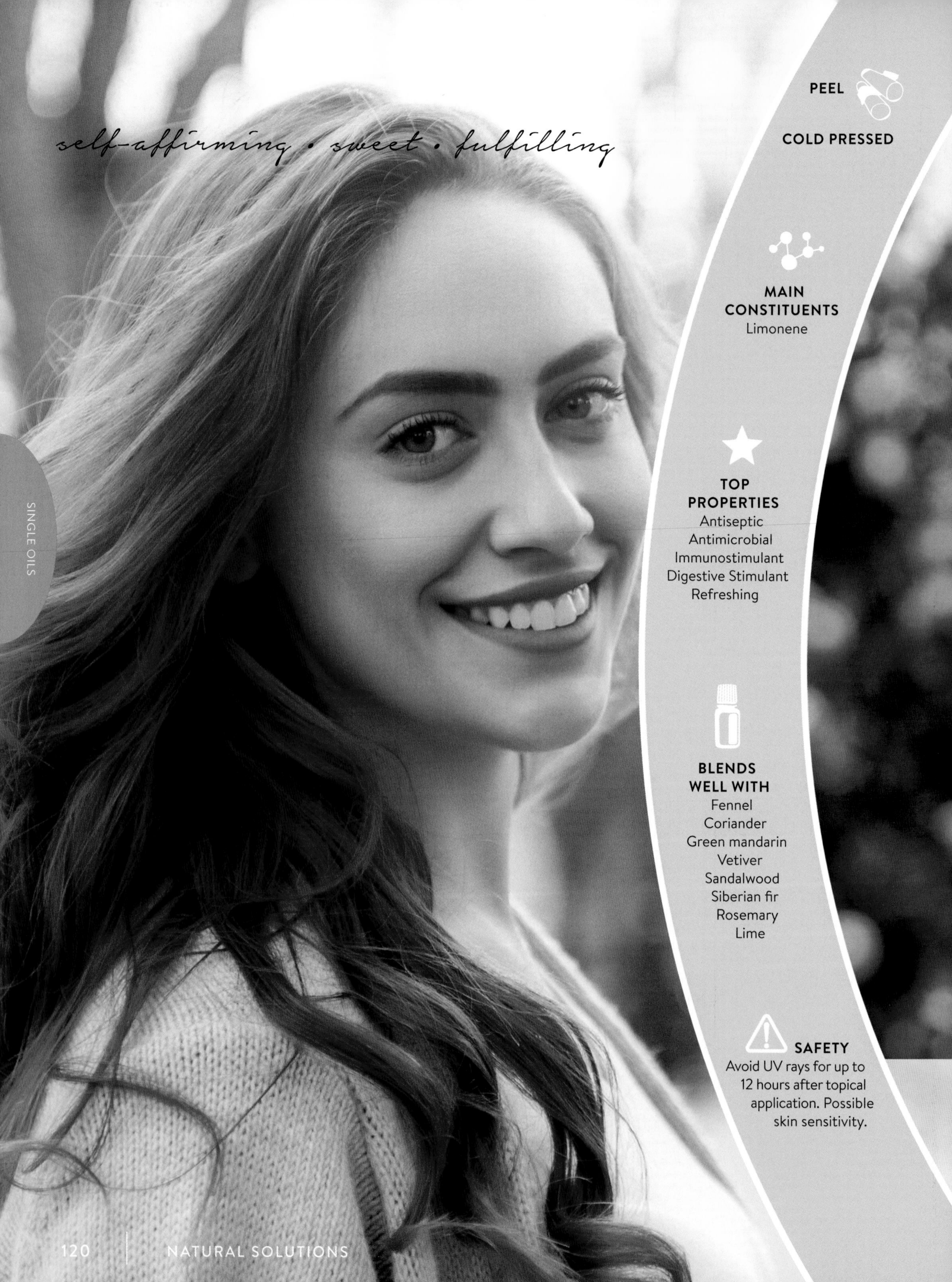
self-affirming • sweet • fulfilling
PEEL
COLD PRESSED
MAIN CONSTITUENTS
Limonene
TOP PROPERTIES
Antiseptic
Antimicrobial
Immunostimulant
Digestive Stimulant
Refreshing
BLENDS WELL WITH
Fennel
Coriander
Green mandarin
Vetiver
Sandalwood
Siberian fir
Rosemary
Lime
SAFETY
Avoid UV rays for up to 12 hours after topical application. Possible skin sensitivity.

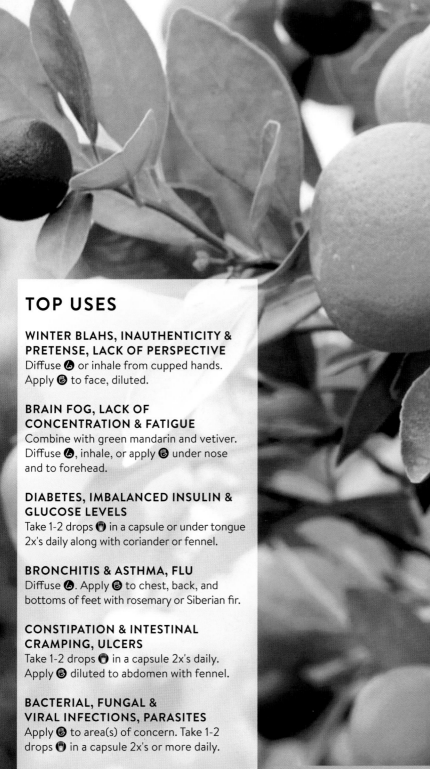

KUMQUAT

FORTUNELLA JAPONICA

TOP USES

WINTER BLAHS, INAUTHENTICITY & PRETENSE, LACK OF PERSPECTIVE
Diffuse or inhale from cupped hands. Apply to face, diluted.

BRAIN FOG, LACK OF CONCENTRATION & FATIGUE
Combine with green mandarin and vetiver. Diffuse, inhale, or apply under nose and to forehead.

DIABETES, IMBALANCED INSULIN & GLUCOSE LEVELS
Take 1-2 drops in a capsule or under tongue 2x's daily along with coriander or fennel.

BRONCHITIS & ASTHMA, FLU
Diffuse. Apply to chest, back, and bottoms of feet with rosemary or Siberian fir.

CONSTIPATION & INTESTINAL CRAMPING, ULCERS
Take 1-2 drops in a capsule 2x's daily. Apply diluted to abdomen with fennel.

BACTERIAL, FUNGAL & VIRAL INFECTIONS, PARASITES
Apply to area(s) of concern. Take 1-2 drops in a capsule 2x's or more daily.

SORE THROAT & SWOLLEN GLANDS
Diffuse. Gargle 1-2 drops every few hours and apply diluted to neck area.

HIGH BLOOD PRESSURE & CHOLESTEROL, POOR CIRCULATION
Take 1-2 drops in a capsule 2x's daily. Apply to chest and bottoms of feet.

OVERWEIGHT, EXCESSIVE APPETITE, DETOXIFICATION
Dilute and apply to area(s) of concern. Take 1-2 drops in a capsule 2x's or more daily.

MACULAR DEGENERATION & CATARACTS
Take 1-2 drops in a capsule. Dilute and apply around eyes.

WRINKLES & AGE SPOTS
Add to daily skin care products with a drop of sandalwood and apply to area(s) of concern.

ODOR & SPRING CLEANING
Diffuse 5 drops each with green mandarin and Siberian fir.

COOKING & FLAVORING
Add drop to salad dressings, baked goods, frostings, smoothies, or cut fruit.

EMOTIONAL BALANCE
Use aromatically and topically to get from Divided ——→ Integrous.

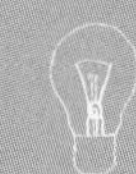

Depending on the harvesting conditions, Kumquat essential oil is anywhere from 70%-95% limonene, but of its other 105 known constituents, 46 have not been found in any other essential oil. The Kumquat peel is sweet and flesh bitter, the reverse of most citrus fruits.

RESEARCH: AInhibitory effects of Fortunella japonica var. margarita and Citrus sunki essential oils on nitric oxide production and skinpathogens.
Acta Microabiologica et immunologica Hungarica Yang EJ; Kim SS; Moon JY; Oh TH; Baik JS; Lee NH; Hyun CG in this study, the essential oils of the citrus species C. sunki (CSE) and F. japonica var. margarita (FJE), both native to the island of Jeju, Korea, were examined for their anti-inflammatory and antimicrobial activities against skin pathogens. Four human skin pathogenic microorganisms, Staphylococcus epidermidis CCARM 3709, Propionibacterium acnes CCARM 0081, Malassezia furfur KCCM 12679, and Candida albicans KCCM 11282, were studied. CSE and FJE exhibited strong antimicrobial activity against most of the pathogenic bacteria and yeast strains that were tested. Interestingly, CSE and FJE even showed antimicrobial activity against antibiotic-resistant S. epidermidis CCARM 3710, S. epidermidis CCARM 3711, P. acnes CCARM9009, and P. acnes CCARM9010 strains. In addition, CSE and FJE reduced the lipopolysaccharide (LPS)-induced secretion of nitric oxide (NO) in RAW 264.7 cells, indicating that they have anti-inflammatory effects. Taken together, these findings indicate that CSE and FJE have great potential to be used in human skin health applications.

Analysis of biologically active oxyprenylated ferulic acid derivatives in citrus fruits.
Plant Foods for Human Nutrition

Genovese S; Fiorito S; Locatelli M; Carlucci G; EpifanoF
4'-Geranyloxyferulic (GOFA) and boropinic acid have been discovered during the last decade as interesting phytochemicals having valuable pharmacological effects as cancer chemopreventive, anti-inflammatory, neuroprotective, and anti-Helicobacter pylori agents. A reverse-phase HPLC-UV/Vis method for the separation and quantification of the title oxyprenylated ferulic acid derivatives in extracts obtained from peels of nine edible Citrus and Fortunella fruits was successfully applied.

= Aromatically = Topically = Internally

LAVENDER

LAVANDULA ANGUSTIFOLIA

calming
regenerating
healing

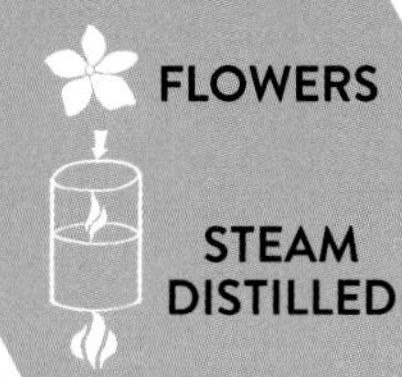

FLOWERS

STEAM DISTILLED

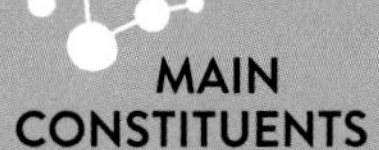

MAIN CONSTITUENTS
Linalool
a-terpineol
Linalyl acetate
b-ocimene

TOP PROPERTIES
Sedative
Antihistamine
Cytophylactic
Hypotensive
Nervine
Relaxing
Soothing
Antibacterial
Regenerative

FOUND IN
PastTense®
Serenity®
ClaryCalm®
Immortelle
AromaTouch®
Anchor®
Children's Calmer™
Children's Rescuer™

BLENDS WELL WITH
Clary sage
Frankincense
Manuka
Tangerine
Wild orange

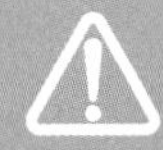

SAFETY
Safe for NEAT application.

SINGLE OILS

TOP USES

SLEEP ISSUES
Apply under nose, to bottoms of feet or diffuse to promote better sleep.

STRESS, ANXIETY & TEETH GRINDING
Apply over heart, on back of neck or inhale from cupped hands.

SUNBURNS, BURNS & SCARS
Apply to area of concern to soothe, heal, and reduce scarring.

ALLERGIES & HAY FEVER
Take in a capsule or under tongue with lemon and peppermint or rub in palms and inhale from cupped hands.

COLIC & UPSET BABY
Massage diluted along spine, abdomen or bottoms of feet to calm.

CUTS, WOUNDS & BLISTERS
Apply on site to cleanse, heal, and limit or avoid scarring.

BUG BITES & HIVES
Apply on site to soothe as a natural antihistamine.

NOSEBLEEDS & PINK EYE
Apply across bridge of nose or around eye.

HIGH BLOOD PRESSURE
Use on pulse points and over heart or take in a capsule.

MIGRAINES & HEADACHES
Inhale and apply to temples and back of neck.

EMOTIONAL BALANCE
Use aromatically and topically to get from Unheard ———> Expressed.

Lavender means "to wash" in Latin. It is likely the most used essential oil globally, and for good reason, as it serves in all things calming! When in doubt use lavender!

RESEARCH: An olfactory stimulus modifies nighttime sleep in young men and women, Goel N, Kim H, Lao RP, *Chronobiology International,* 2005

Effects of lavender aromatherapy on insomnia and depression in women college students, Lee IS, Lee GJ, *Taehan Kanho Hakhoe Chi,* 2006

Effects of lavender (lavandula angustifolia Mill.) and peppermint (Mentha cordifolia Opiz.) aromas on subjective vitality, speed, and agility, Cruz AB, Lee SE, Pagaduan JC, Kim TH, *The Asian International Journal of Life Sciences,* 2012

Topical lavender oil for the treatment of recurrent aphthous ulceration, Altaei DT, *American Journal of Dentistry,* 2012

Lavender essential oil inhalation suppresses allergic airway inflammation and mucous cell hyperplasia in a murine model of asthma, Ueno-lio T, Shibakura M, Yokota K, Aoe M, Hyoda T, Shinohata R, Kanehiro A, Tanimoto M, Kataoka M, *Life Sciences,* 2014

Lavender essential oil in the treatment of migraine headache: a placebo-controlled clinical trial, Sasannejad P, Saeedi M, Shoeibi A, Gorji A, Abbasi M, Foroughipour M, *European Neurology,* 2012

Effect of aromatherapy on symptoms of dysmenorrhea in college students: A randomized placebo-controlled clinical trial, Han SH, Hur MH, Buckle J, Choi J, Lee MS, *The Journal of Alternative and Complementary Medicine,* 2006

The effects of aromatherapy on pain, depression, and life satisfaction of arthritis patients, Kim MJ, Nam ES, Paik SI, *Taehan Kanho Hakhoe Chi,* 2005

Effect of lavender oil (Lavandula angustifolia) on cerebral edema and its possible mechanisms in an experimental model of stroke,Vakili A, Sharifat S, Akhavan MM, Bandegi AR, *Brain Research,* 2014

Two US practitioners' experience of using essential oils for wound care, Hartman D, Coetzee JC, *Journal of Wound Care,* 2002

Lavender and the nervous system, Koulivand PH, Khaleghi Ghadiri M, Gorji A, *Evidence-Based Complementary and Alternative Medicine,* 2013

LEMON

CITRUS LIMON

uplifting
invigorating
refreshing

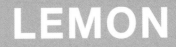

TOP USES

KIDNEY & GALLSTONES
Apply (T) diluted over area of discomfort; add a heat pack to intensify action. Ingest (I) a few drops in water or in a capsule to break up stones.

PH ISSUES & LYMPHATIC CLEANSING
Take (I) in a glass of water or apply (T) to ears and ankles to cleanse and balance pH.

EDEMA & WATER RETENTION
Take (I) in a capsule, glass of water, or massage (T) onto legs and bottoms of feet.

HEARTBURN & REFLUX
Take (I) with ginger in a capsule or glass of water.

CONGESTION & MUCUS
Rub (T) over chest or diffuse (A).

RUNNY NOSE & ALLERGIES
Inhale (A) or apply (T) over bridge of nose to relieve runny nose. Take 2-4 drops (I) with lavender and peppermint in glass of water or in capsule for allergy relief.

GOUT, RHEUMATISM & ARTHRITIS
Take (I) in a glass of water.

LIVER & KIDNEY DETOX
Take (I) in a glass of water or apply (T) to bottoms of feet.

DEGREASER & FURNITURE POLISH
Use 10-15 drops (T) mixed with water in a glass spray bottle.

VARICOSE VEINS
Apply (T) diluted with cypress.

CONCENTRATION
Inhale (A) with rosemary.

EMOTIONAL BALANCE
Use (A) aromatically and (T) topically to get from Mindless ——→ Energized.

It takes approximately 45 lemons to produce a 15 ml bottle of lemon essential oil.

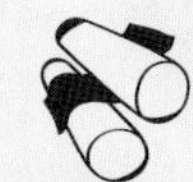
RIND

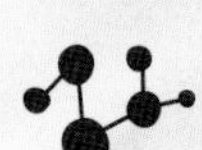
COLD PRESSED

MAIN CONSTITUENTS
d-limonene
Alpha-pinenes
Beta-pinenes

TOP PROPERTIES
Antiseptic
Diuretic
Antioxidant
Antibacterial
Detoxifier
Disinfectant
Mucolytic
Astringent
Degreaser

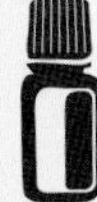
FOUND IN
Breathe®
Citrus Bliss®
Purify
Slim & Sassy®
Arise®

BLENDS WELL WITH
Basil
Manuka
Peppermint
Rosemary
Siberian fir

SAFETY
Avoid exposure to sunlight or UV rays for up to 12 hours after application.

RESEARCH: Screening of the antibacterial effects of a variety of essential oils on respiratory tract pathogens, using a modified dilution assay method, Inouye S, Yamaguchi H, Takizawa T, *Journal of Infection and Chemotherapy: Official Journal of the Japan Society of Chemotherapy*, 2001

Antioxidative effects of lemon oil and its components on copper induced oxidation of low density lipoprotein, Grassmann J, Schneider D, Weiser D, Elstner EF, *Arzneimittel-Forschung*, 2001

The effect of lemon inhalation aromatherapy on nausea and vomiting of pregnancy: a double- blinded, randomized, controlled clinical trial, Yavari Kia P, Safajou F, Shahnazi M, Nazemiyeh H, *Iranian Red Crescent Medical Journal*, 2014

Chemical composition of the essential oils of variegated pink-fleshed lemon (Citrus x limon L. Burm. f.) and their anti-inflammatory and antimicrobial activities, Hamdan D, Ashour ML, Mulyaningsih S, El-Shazly A, Wink M, *Zeitschrift Fur Naturforschung C-A Journal of Biosciences*, 2013

Essential oil from lemon peels inhibit key enzymes linked to neurodegenerative conditions and pro-oxidant induced lipid peroxidation, Oboh G, Olasehinde TA, Ademosun AO, *Journal of Oleo Science*, 2014

Effect of flavour components in lemon essential oil on physical or psychological stress, Fukumoto S, Morishita A, Furutachi K, Terashima T, Nakayama T, Yokogoshi H, *Stress and Health*, 2008

Cytological aspects on the effects of a nasal spray consisting of standardized extract of citrus lemon and essential oils in allergic rhinopathy, Ferrara L, Naviglio D, Armone Caruso A, *ISRN Pharmaceutics*, 2012

Aromatherapy as a safe and effective treatment for the management of agitation in severe dementia: the results of a double-blind, placebo-controlled trial with Melissa, Ballard CG, O'Brien JT, Reichelt K, Perry EK, *The Journal of Clinical Psychiatry*, 2002

(A) = Aromatically (T) = Topically (I) = Internally

LEMON EUCALYPTUS

EUCALYPTUS CITRIODORA

resolving
stimulating
refreshing

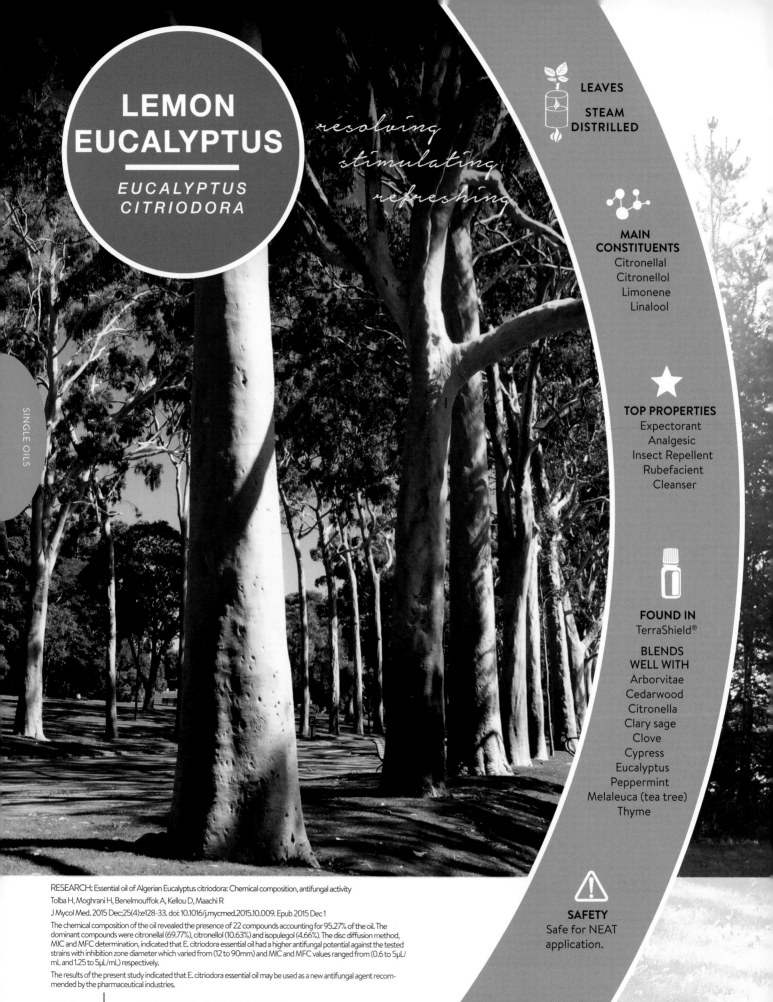

LEAVES

STEAM DISTRILLED

MAIN CONSTITUENTS
Citronellal
Citronellol
Limonene
Linalool

TOP PROPERTIES
Expectorant
Analgesic
Insect Repellent
Rubefacient
Cleanser

FOUND IN
TerraShield®

BLENDS WELL WITH
Arborvitae
Cedarwood
Citronella
Clary sage
Clove
Cypress
Eucalyptus
Peppermint
Melaleuca (tea tree)
Thyme

SAFETY
Safe for NEAT application.

RESEARCH: Essential oil of Algerian Eucalyptus citriodora: Chemical composition, antifungal activity

Tolba H, Moghrani H, Benelmouffok A, Kellou D, Maachi R

J Mycol Med. 2015 Dec;25(4):e128-33. doi: 10.1016/j.mycmed.2015.10.009. Epub 2015 Dec 1

The chemical composition of the oil revealed the presence of 22 compounds accounting for 95.27% of the oil. The dominant compounds were citronellal (69.77%), citronellol (10.63%) and isopulegol (4.66%). The disc diffusion method, MIC and MFC determination, indicated that E. citriodora essential oil had a higher antifungal potential against the tested strains with inhibition zone diameter which varied from (12 to 90mm) and MIC and MFC values ranged from (0.6 to 5μL/mL and 1.25 to 5μL/mL) respectively.

The results of the present study indicated that E. citriodora essential oil may be used as a new antifungal agent recommended by the pharmaceutical industries.

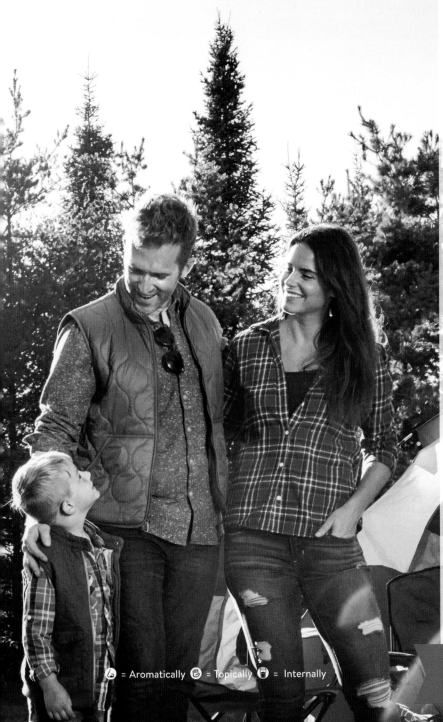

TOP USES

BRONCHITIS, ASTHMA, COUGHS, SINUSITIS, FLU & MALARIA
Diffuse (A) and/or apply (T) on chest and back. Repeat 2-4x's daily.

INSECT (INCL. TICKS & MOSQUITOES) & GERM REPELLENT
Diffuse (A), apply (T) to exposed areas, and/or add to glass spray bottle to treat surfaces or apply to clothing.

OSTEOARTHRITIS, RHEUMATIC & JOINT PAIN, HEADACHES
Apply (T) to bottoms of feet and area(s) of concern. Repeat 2-4x's per day.

BURNS, FEVERS & OVERHEATED, OVEREXERTION
Apply (T) to area(s) of concern, or up spine, across forehead, and bottoms of feet. Repeat as needed.

POOR CIRCULATION & BLOOD OXYGENATION
Apply (T) to bottoms of feet and over liver. Repeat 2-4x's daily.

DANDRUFF, ATHLETE'S FOOT & JOCK ITCH
Add 2-3 drops per shampooing or apply (T) 2x's per day to area(s) of concern.

CHRONIC CONSTIPATION, POOR DIGESTION & BLOATING, INTESTINAL CRAMPS
Apply (T) in clockwise motion on abdomen and area(s) of concern until resolved.

CUTS & WOUNDS, COLD SORES
Apply (T) to break in skin, or area(s) of concern.

BODY ODOR & HOUSEHOLD SMELLS
Diffuse (A) and use (T), add 1-2 drops to body wash.

SURFACE CLEANSING & DISINFECTING
Diffuse (A) and/or add 6-8 drops + 1 tablespoon vinegar to glass spray bottle filled with water.

EMOTIONAL BALANCE
Use (A) aromatically and (T) topically to get from Concealed ———> Revealing.

(A) = Aromatically (T) = Topically (I) = Internally

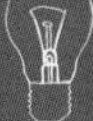

By the chemistry, it's as if lemon, citronella, and eucalyptus had a baby.

Plant-based insect repellents: a review of their efficacy, development and testing
Marta Ferreira Maia, Sarah J Moore
Malar J. 2011; 10 (Suppl 1): S11.
Published online 2011 Mar 15. doi: 10.1186/1475-2875-10-S1-S11
PMD from lemon eucalyptus (Corymbia citriodora) extract
Corymbia citriodora (Myrtaceae), also known as lemon eucalyptus, is a potent natural repellent extracted from the leaves of lemon eucalyptus trees (Table (Table1).1). It was discovered in the 1960s during mass screenings of plants used in Chinese traditional medicine. Lemon eucalyptus essential oil, comprising 85% citronellal, is used by cosmetic industries due to its fresh smell. However, it was discovered that the waste distillate remaining after hydro-distillation of the essential oil was far more effective at repelling mosquitoes than the essential oil itself. Many plant extracts and oils repel mosquitoes, with their effect lasting from several minutes to several hours (Table (Table1).1). Their active ingredients tend to be highly volatile, so although they are effective repellents for a short period after application, they rapidly evaporate leaving the user unprotected. The exception to this is para-menthane 3, 8 diol, which has a lower vapour pressure than volatile monoterpines found in most plant oils and provides very high protection from a broad range of insect vectors over several hours, whereas the essential oil is repellent for around one hour. PMD is the only plant-based repellent that has been advocated for use in disease endemic areas by the CDC (Centres for Disease Control), due to its proven clinical efficacy to prevent malaria [26] and is considered to pose no risk to human health. It should be noted that the essential oil of lemon eucalyptus does not have EPA (Environmental Protection Agency) registration for use as an insect repellent.

CREDIT: Image by Geekstreet (https://commons.wikimedia.org/wiki/File:Corymbia_citriodora_-_shedding_bark_4.jpg)

LEMONGRASS

CYMBOPOGON FLEXUOSUS

electrifying
regenerating
purifying

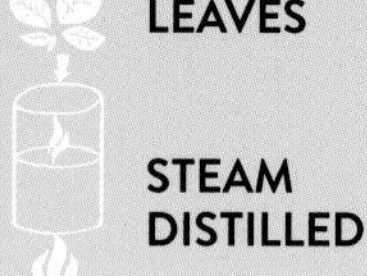

LEAVES

STEAM DISTILLED

MAIN CONSTITUENTS
Geranial
Neral
Geraniol
Farnesol

TOP PROPERTIES
Anti-inflammatory
Antimicrobial
Analgesic
Anti-carcinoma
Antimutagenic
Decongestant
Regenerative
Anti-rheumatic

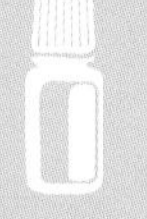

FOUND IN
DDR Prime®

BLENDS WELL WITH
Basil
Ginger
Peppermint
Siberian fir

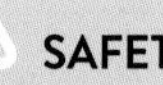

SAFETY
Dilution recommended. Possible skin sensitivity.

TOP USES

CANCER & TUMORS
Take in a capsule.

BLOOD PRESSURE & CHOLESTEROL
Take in a capsule.

HYPO- OR HYPERTHYROID
Take in a capsule.

BLADDER & KIDNEY INFECTION/STONES
Use in a capsule or apply diluted over abdomen.

CONSTIPATION & WATER RETENTION
Combine with peppermint and apply diluted over abdomen or bottoms of feet and/or take in a capsule.

CATARACTS
Take 1-2 drops in a capsule 1-2 times daily, apply under 2nd and 3rd toes.

EMOTIONAL BALANCE
Use aromatically and topically to get from Obstructed ———> Flowing.

CONNECTIVE TISSUE INJURY
Apply to affected area to soothe and repair.

JOINT, TENDON & LIGAMENT PAIN
Apply diluted to affected area.

LYMPHATIC CONGESTION
Take in a capsule or apply to bottoms of feet.

COOKING
Add a drop for more flavorful dishes.

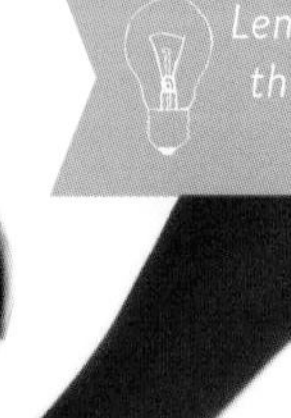

Lemongrass essential oil is used in the pharmaceutical industry for the synthesis of Vitamin A.

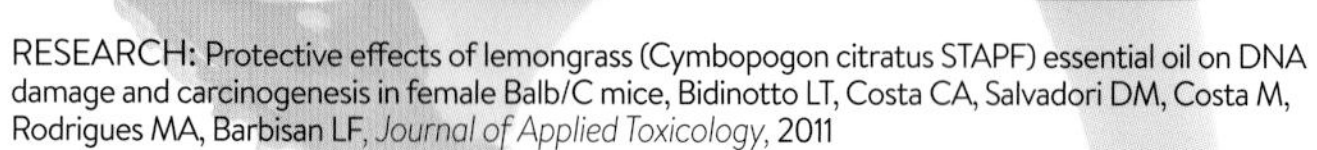

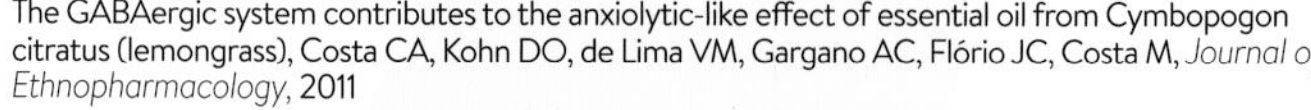

RESEARCH: Protective effects of lemongrass (Cymbopogon citratus STAPF) essential oil on DNA damage and carcinogenesis in female Balb/C mice, Bidinotto LT, Costa CA, Salvadori DM, Costa M, Rodrigues MA, Barbisan LF, *Journal of Applied Toxicology*, 2011

The anti-biofilm activity of lemongrass (Cymbopogon flexuosus) and grapefruit (Citrus paradisi) essential oils against five strains of Staphylococcus aureus, Adukwu EC, Allen SC, Phillips CA, *Journal of Applied Microbiology*, 2012

Protective effect of lemongrass oil against dexamethasone induced hyperlipidemia in rats: possible role of decreased lecithin cholesterol acetyl transferase activity, Kumar VR, Inamdar MN, Nayeemunnisa, Viswanatha GL, *Asian Pacific Journal of Tropical Medicine*, 2011

The GABAergic system contributes to the anxiolytic-like effect of essential oil from Cymbopogon citratus (lemongrass), Costa CA, Kohn DO, de Lima VM, Gargano AC, Flório JC, Costa M, *Journal of Ethnopharmacology*, 2011

The effect of lemongrass EO highlights its potential against antibiotic resistant Staph. aureus in the healthcare environment., Adukwu EC, Allen SC, Phillips CA, *Journal of Applied Microbiology*, 2012

Anticancer activity of an essential oil from Cymbopogon flexuosus (lemongrass), Sharma PR, Mondhe DM, Muthiah S, Pal HC, Shahi AK, Saxena AK, Qazi GN, *Chemico-Biological Interactions*, 2009

LIME

CITRUS AURANTIFOLIA

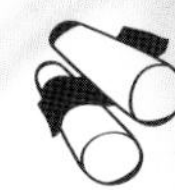

RIND

COLD PRESSED

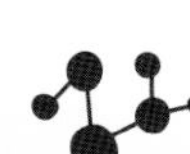

MAIN CONSTITUENTS
Limonene
Beta-pinene
Gamma terpinene

TOP PROPERTIES
Anti-inflammatory
Antiseptic
Antioxidant
Antibacterial
Tonic
Uplifting
Detoxifier
Disinfectant
Diuretic

FOUND IN
InTune®
Purify
Beautiful®

BLENDS WELL WITH
Bergamot
Black pepper
Rosemary

SAFETY
Avoid exposure to sunlight or UV rays for up to 12 hours after application.

A popular oil in perfumery for men. In times past British sailors drank lime juice to prevent scurvy.

TOP USES

SORE THROAT
Gargle a drop with water.

RESPIRATORY, LYMPH & LIVER CONGESTION
Take in a capsule or apply over area(s) of concern.

URINARY & DIGESTIVE ISSUES
Drink a few drops in a glass of water.

MEMORY & CLARITY
Inhale or diffuse.

EXHAUSTION & DEPRESSION
Apply to ears or back of neck or diffuse to energize and uplift.

HERPES & COLD SORES
Take in a capsule or apply to outbreaks.

CHICKEN POX
Use in a capsule or apply diluted to pox.

HEAD LICE
Add 20 drops with 15 drops melaleuca (tea tree) to bottle of shampoo and apply.

PAIN & INFLAMMATION
Massage over area(s) of discomfort or take in a capsule to and increase antioxidants and decrease inflammation.

EMOTIONAL BALANCE
Use aromatically and topically to get from Faint ———> Enlivened.

RESEARCH: Bactericidal activity of herbal volatile oil extracts against multidrug-resistant Acinetobacter baumannii, Intorasoot A, Chornchoem P, Sookkhee S, Intorasoot S, *Journal of Intercultural Ethnoparmacology*, 2017

Anticancer activity of Key Lime (Citrus aurantifolia), Narang N, Jiraungkoorskul W, *Pharmacognosy Review*, 2016

Anti-inflammatory properties and chemical characterization of the essential oils of four citrus species, Amorim JL, Simas DL, Pinheiro MM, Moreno DS, Alviano CS, da Silva AJ, Fernandes PD, *PLOS One*, 2016.

Essential oil from Citrus aurantifolia prevents ketotifen-induced weight-gain in mice, Asnaashari S, Delazar A, Habibi B, Vasfi R, NaharL, Hamedeyazdan S, Sarker SD, *Phytotherapy Research*, 2010.

Antioxidant effects of Citrus aurantifolia juice and peel extract on LDL oxidation, Boshtam M, Moshtaghian J, Naderi G, Asgary S, Nayeri H, *Journal of Research in Medical Sciences*, 2011.

Chemical composition and in-vitro antioxidant and antimicrobial activity of the essential oil of Citrus aurantifolia L. leaves, Al-Aamri M, Al-Abousi N, Al-Jabri Sausan, Alam T, Khan S, *Journal of Taibah University Medical Sciences*, 2018

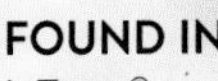

LITSEA

LITSEA CUBEBA

cleansing
refreshing
uplifting

FRUIT

STEAM DISTILLED

MAIN CONSTITUENTS
Geranial
Neral
Limonene

TOP PROPERTIES
Refreshing
Detoxifier
Uplifting
Antibacterial
Antifungal
Antispasmodic
Disinfectant
Digestive Stimulant

TOP USES

ASTHMA ATTACK, SPASTIC COUGHS, BRONCHITIS
Apply to chest or inhale from cupped hands.

ACUTE & CHRONIC BACK PAIN
Apply to affected area. Dilute as needed.

ECZEMA, ACNE & OILY SKIN
Apply to affected area(s) or add to cleanser or lotion.

HIGH BLOOD PRESSURE, IRREGULAR HEARTBEAT, ANXIETY
Apply to chest, back of neck and/or under nose.

COUGH, COLD, CHILLS & INFECTIONS
Apply to chest, back of neck or along spine.

SEASONAL BLUES, NEGATIVE THINKING OR SPEAKING
Diffuse or inhale from cupped hands.

NERVOUS TENSION, HEADACHES, STRESSED MIND
Apply across forehead, on temples, diffuse, and/or inhale from cupped hands.

NAUSEA, MOTION SICKNESS, INDIGESTION, POOR APPETITE
Massage in circular motion into abdomen. Dilute as needed.

CELLULITE, EXCESSIVE PERSPIRATION, ATHLETE'S FOOT
Apply to area of concern.

BRAIN FOG, LACK OF MOTIVATION, FATIGUE, SLEEP ISSUES
Apply across forehead, on temples, diffuse, and/or inhale from cupped hands.

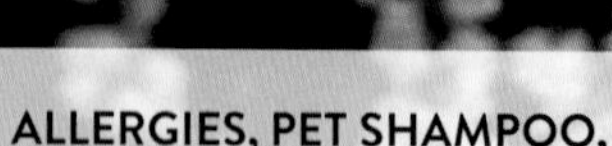

ALLERGIES, PET SHAMPOO, INSECT REPELLENT
Apply to chest, bottoms of feet, or add to shampoo and/or spray bottle of water.

LUNG CANCER & AGING
Apply to affected area or along spine.

SURFACE DISINFECTANT & AIR FRESHENER
Combine with melaleuca and water into spray bottle as a replacement for harmful chemical cleaners.

MENSTRUAL & MUSCULAR ACHES & PAINS
Apply to abdomen or area of concern.

EMOTIONAL BALANCE
Use aromatically and topically to get from Encumbered ——> Purified.

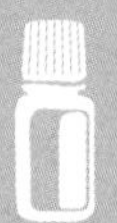

FOUND IN
HD Clear®
TerraShield®
DDR Prime®
Children's Stronger™

BLENDS WELL WITH
Basil
Cedarwood
Fennel
Geranium
Ginger
Rose
Rosemary
Sandalwood
Vetiver

Sweeter than lemongrass and without the musty note, more citrusy in its scent than melissa.

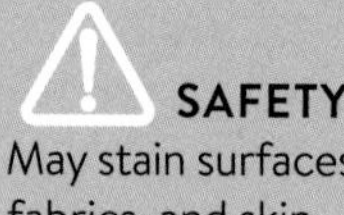

SAFETY
May stain surfaces, fabrics, and skin.

:SEARCH: Anti-Inflammatory Effects of Boldine and Reticuline Isolated from Lits- cubeba through JAK2/STAT3 and NF-ĐB Signaling Pathways. Yang X, Gao X, Cao Y, Guo Q, S, Zhu Z, Zhao Y, Tu P, Chai X. Planta Med. 2017 Jun 26. doi: 10.1055/s-0043- 113447. [Epub ead of print] PMID: 28651290

sential Oil Compositions and Antimicrobial Activities of Various Parts of Lits- cubeba from Taiwan. Su YC, Ho CL. Nat Prod Commun. 2016 Apr;11(4):515-8. PMID: 396208

Anti-inflammatory constituents from the root of Litsea cubeba in LPS-induced RAW 264.7 macrophages. Lin B, Sun LN, Xin HL, Nian H, Song HT, Jiang YP, Wei ZQ, Qin LP, Han T. Pharm Biol. 2016 Sep;54(9):1741-7. doi: 10.3109/13880209.2015.1126619. Epub 2016 Jan 5. PMID: 26731513

Antibacterial activity of Litsea cubeba (Lauraceae, May Chang) and its effects on the biological response of common carp Cyprinus carpio challenged with Aeromonas hydrophila. Nguyen HV, Caruso D, Lebrun M, Nguyen NT, Trinh TT, Meile JC, Chu-Ky S, Sarter S. J Appl Microbiol. 2016 Aug;121(2):341-51. doi: 10.1111/jam.13160. Epub 2016 Jun 30. PMID: 27124660

opening · resplendent · heavenly

MAGNOLIA

MICHELIA X ALBA

TOP USES

ANXIETY, DEPRESSION & LACK OF ENERGY
Apply to back of neck, forehead, under nose, or over heart. Inhale from cupped hands.

PMS & MENSTRUAL CRAMPS, HORMONE IMBALANCES
Apply in clockwise circulatory motion over lower abdomen, and to wrists and ankles.

IRRITABILITY, ANGER & RAGE, HYSTERIA, PANIC, GRIEF & SHOCK
Apply to back of neck, forehead, under nose, over heart, or bottoms of feet. Inhale from cupped hands.

RESPIRATORY, SINUS & LYMPHATIC CONGESTION
Apply to chest and back and/or to bottom of feet. Combine with cardamom or eucalyptus.

LIBIDO & SEX DRIVE, BREAST & PROSTATE ISSUES
Apply to wrists, chest, back of neck, or reproductive organ reflex points.

STRESSED, WORRIED, UPTIGHT & TENSE
Apply to back of neck, forehead, under nose, or bottoms of feet. Inhale from cupped hands.

LACK OF ABILITY TO RECEIVE LOVE, WEAK HEART CHAKRA
Apply over heart/chest area and to bottoms of feet. Inhale from cupped hands.

ABRASIONS & WOUNDS, SKIN IRRITATIONS, SCARS
Apply to area(s) of concern. Combine with melaleuca or frankincense.

ACNE & DRY SKIN
Add to skin care routine and apply 2x's daily.

INSOMNIA & SLEEP ISSUES
Apply to back of neck, forehead, and/or under nose.

PERFUME
Apply to pulse points, layered with jasmine or neroli.

EMOTIONAL BALANCE
Use aromatically and topically to get from Disturbed ———> Confident.

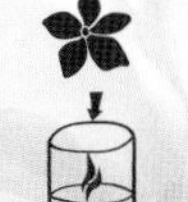

FLOWER PETALS

STEAM DISTILLED

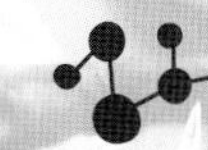

MAIN CONSTITUENTS
Linalool

TOP PROPERTIES
Sedative
Relaxant
Antidepressant
Aphrodisiac
Decongestant
Stomachic

FOUND IN
Children's Steady™

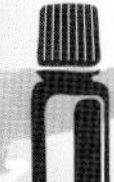

BLENDS WELL WITH
Jasmine
Neroli
Lime
Sandalwood
Roman chamomile
Kumquat
Patchouli
Rose

SAFETY
Avoid keeping in hot places (e.g. glove box of car) to prevent oxidation.

Fossilized Magnolia genus is over 20 million years old, a time prior to the presence of bees, and was pollinated by beetles. Harvested at night when blooms are most fragrant, magnolia was traditionally used in ceremonies to enhance confidence and well-being.

RESEARCH: Natural Product Research Farag, MA; Al-Mahdy, DA

The biological activities and the determined major volatile components in the Magnolia grandiflora and M. virginiana flowers extracts were compared. Volatile components were detected in the essential oil by dynamic headspace sampling (HS). 2-Phenylethanol (40% and 61%) was found as the main constituent in the essential oil and HS samples of M. virginiana, respectively. In the M. grandiflora oil sample, (E,E)-farnesol (18%) and 2-phenylethanol (10%) were found as main constituents, whereas germacrene D (17%) and [illegible]- bisabolene (17%) were the main components of the HS sample. The essential oil in M. virginiana displayed a moderate antioxidant activity relative to vitamin E, whereas both essential oils were active against human lung carcinoma and breast carcinoma cell lines, even at concentrations higher than 200 μg mL(-1).

= Aromatically = Topically = Internally

supporting
transforming
harmonizing

MANUKA

LEPTOSPERMUM SCOPARIUM

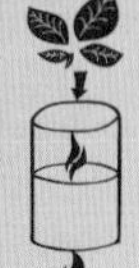

BRANCHES & LEAVES

STEAM DISTILLED

MAIN CONSTITUENTS

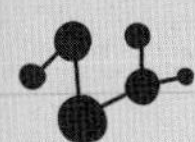

Leptospermone
E-calamenene
Alpha-pinene
Cadina-3
5-diene

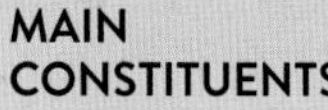

TOP PROPERTIES

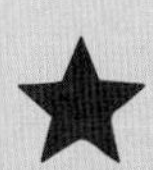

Anti-allergenic
Antibacterial
Anti-inflammatory
Antiviral
Relaxant

BLENDS WELL WITH

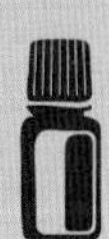

Black pepper
Clary sage
Lavender
Marjoram
Ylang ylang

SAFETY

Safe for NEAT application.

TOP USES

ACHY JOINTS & MUSCLE PAIN
Massage diluted into affected area(s).

DANDRUFF, SCALP ISSUES
Apply to scalp or add 2-3 drops to shampoo or conditioner.

ATHLETE'S FOOT, TOE FUNGUS OR FINGERNAIL ISSUES
Apply to bottoms of feet and/or drop into warm soak.

IRRITATED & CHAFFED SKIN, ACNE, RASHES
Apply to affected area(s). Dilute as needed.

INTESTINAL, RESPIRATORY, URINARY TRACT BACTERIAL INFECTION
Apply to bottoms of feet, abdomen, and/or chest.

COLD, FEVER, COUGH, SINUS CONGESTION, ASTHMA
Diffuse, inhale from cupped hands, apply to chest.

MUSCLES SPASMS & CONTRACTIONS
Apply diluted with eucalyptus over affected area.

INDIGESTION, SPICY FOOD ISSUES, & TOXICITY
Apply to abdomen.

SEASONAL ALLERGIES & SENSITIVITY TO DUST, PETS & DANDER
Diffuse, inhale from cupped hands, or apply to bottoms of feet.

BITES, STINGS, & BURNS
Apply to affected area to relieve.

EAR & FUNGAL INFECTIONS, HERPES
Apply around ears and to bottoms of feet.

DAMAGED SKIN & SCARS, WOUNDS, RADIATION TREATMENT SIDE EFFECTS
Apply to affected area(s).

MENTAL STRESS, ANXIETY, & HIGH BLOOD PRESSURE
Diffuse, inhale from cupped hands, apply to back of neck, forehead, and/or chest.

EMOTIONAL BALANCE
Use aromatically and topically to get from Bothered ——→ Revived.

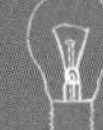

The Maori people use all parts of this plant as part of their natural medicine.

: Sub-inhibitory stress with essential oil affects enterotoxins production and essential ·bility in Staphylococcus aureus. Turchi B, Mancini S, Pistelli L, Najar B, Cerri D, Fratini F. ·s. 2017 Jun 8:1-7. doi: 10.1080/14786419.2017.1338284. [Epub ahead of print] PMID:

·l effects of Manuka honey on in vitro biofilm formation by Clostridium difficile. Piotrowski · P, Pituch H, van Belkum A, Obuch-WoszczatyÐski P. Eur J Clin Microbiol Infect Dis. 2017 ·0.1007/s10096-017- 2980-1. [Epub ahead of print] PMID:28417271

Strawberry-Tree Honey Induces Growth Inhibition of Human Colon Cancer Cells and Increases ROS Generation: A Comparison with Manuka Honey. Afrin S, Forbes-Hernandez TY, Gasparrini M, Bompadre S, Quiles JL, Sanna G, Spano N, Giampieri F, Battino M. Int J Mol Sci. 2017 Mar 11;18(3). pii: E613. doi: 10.3390/ijms18030613. PMID: 28287469

Plants and other natural products used in the management of oral infections and improvement of oral health. Chinsembu KC. Acta Trop. 2016 Feb;154:6-18. doi: 10.1016/j.actatropica.2015.10.019. Epub 2015 Oct 29. Review. PMID: 26522671

relaxing
connecting
pleasing

MARJORAM

ORIGANUM MAJORANA

TOP USES

CARPAL TUNNEL, TENDINITIS & ARTHRITIS
Use on area of discomfort to soothe and calm.

MUSCLE CRAMPS & SPRAINS
Massage diluted to relieve cramping or sprain.

HIGH BLOOD PRESSURE & HEART ISSUES
Apply over heart and to pulse points or take with 2 drops lemongrass in a capsule.

CROUP & BRONCHITIS
Apply to neck, chest, and upper back.

PANCREATITIS
Apply a drop or two over pancreas area.

OVERACTIVE SEX DRIVE
Apply to abdomen.

BOILS, COLD SORES & RINGWORM
Take in a capsule or apply to affected area.

MIGRAINES & HEADACHES
Massage onto back of neck, along hairline, and temples.

COLIC & CONSTIPATION
Take in a capsule or massage diluted over abdomen and on lower back.

CALMING & ANXIETY
Rub on back of neck and bottoms of feet or diffuse to relieve stress.

EMOTIONAL BALANCE
Use aromatically and topically to get from Doubtful ⟶ Trusting.

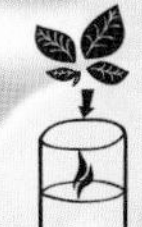

LEAVES

STEAM DISTILLED

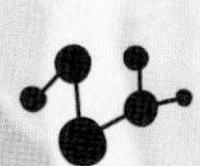

MAIN CONSTITUENTS
Linalool
Terpinen-4-ol

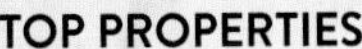

TOP PROPERTIES
Vasodilator
Antispasmodic
Digestive Stimulant
Antibacterial
Antifungal
Hypotensive
Sedative

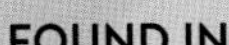

FOUND IN
AromaTouch®
PastTense®
Align®

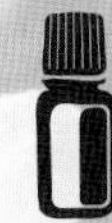

BLENDS WELL WITH
Lavender
Manuka
Rosemary
Siberian fir
Ylang ylang

SAFETY
Caution during earlier stages of pregnancy.

Also known as "Joy of the Mountains", marjoram symbolized happiness to the ancient Greeks and Romans.

SINGLE OILS

RESEARCH: Comparative effects of Artemisia dracunculus, Satureja hortensis and Origanum majorana on inhibition of blood platelet adhesion, aggregation and secretion, Yazdanparast R, Shahriyary L, *Vascular Pharmacology*, 2008

The effects of aromatherapy on pain, depression, and life satisfaction of arthritis patients, Kim MJ, Nam ES, Paik SI, *Taehan Kanho Hakhoe Chi*, 2005

Immunological and Psychological Benefits of Aromatherapy Massage, Kuriyama H, Watanabe S, Nakaya T, Shigemori I, Kita M, Yoshida N, Masaki D, Tadai T, Ozasa K, Fukui K, Imanishi J, *Evidence-Based Complementary and Alternative Medicine*, 2005

Ovicidal and adulticidal activities of Origanum majorana essential oil constituents against insecticide-susceptible and pyrethroid/malathion-resistant Pediculus humanus capitis (Anoplura: Pediculidae), Yang YC, Lee SH, Clark JM, Ahn YJ, *Journal of Agricultural and Food Chemistry*, 2009

Essential oil inhalation on blood pressure and salivary cortisol levels in prehypertensive and hypertensive subjects, Kim IH, Kim C, Seong K, Hur MH, Lim HM, Lee MS, *Evidence-Based Complementary and Alternative Medicine*, 2012

Free radical scavenging and antiacetylcholinesterase activities of Origanum majorana L. essential oil, Mossa AT, Mawwar GA, *Human & Experimental Toxicology*, 2011

Pain relief assessment by aromatic essential oil massage on outpatients with primary dysmenorrhea: a randomized, double-blind clinical trial, Ou MC, Hsu TF, Lai AC, Lin YT, Lin CC, *The Journal of Obstetrics and Gynecology Research*, 2012

= Aromatically = Topically = Internally

MELALEUCA

MELALEUCA ALTERNIFOLIA

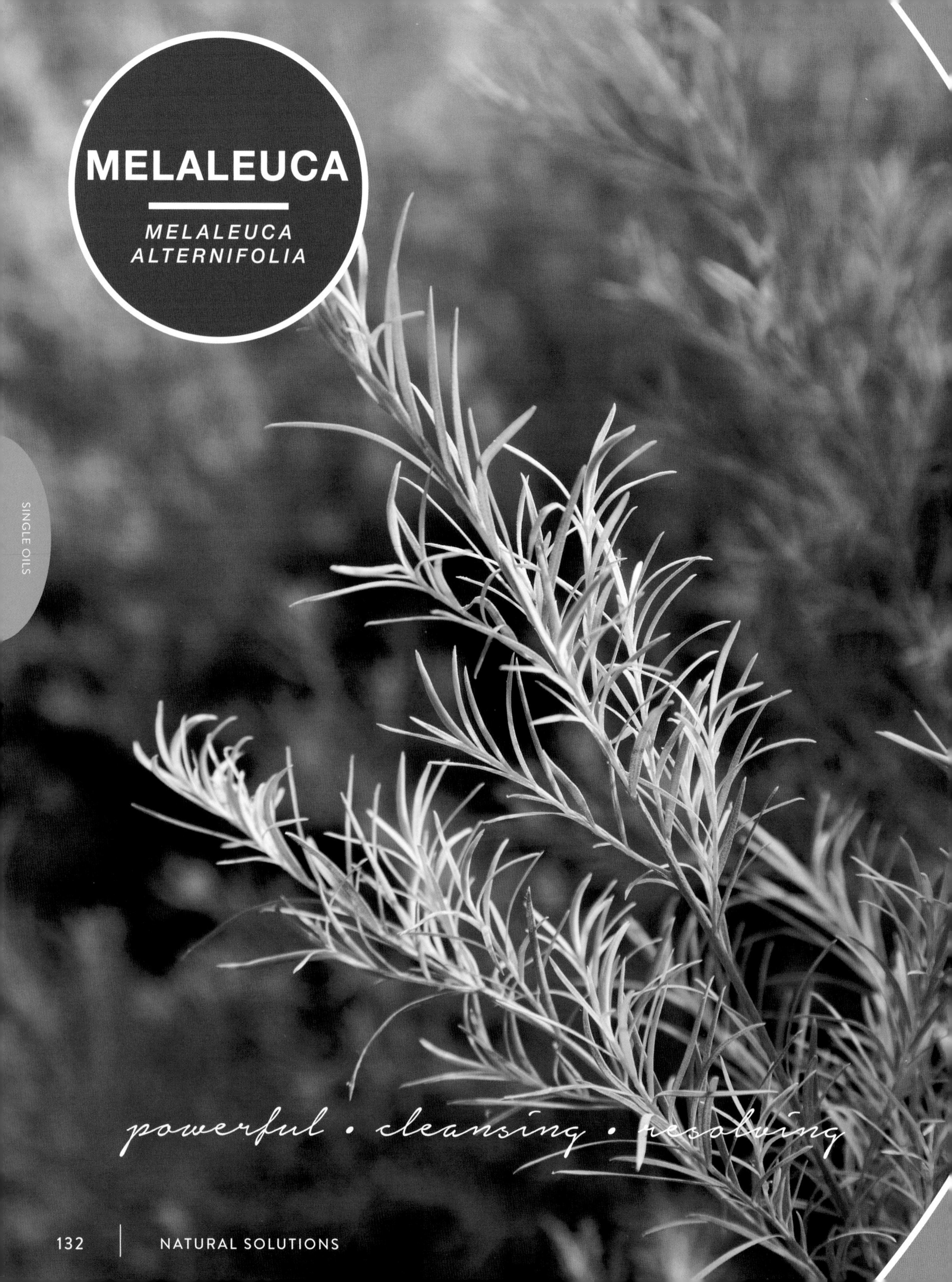

SINGLE OILS

powerful • cleansing • resolving

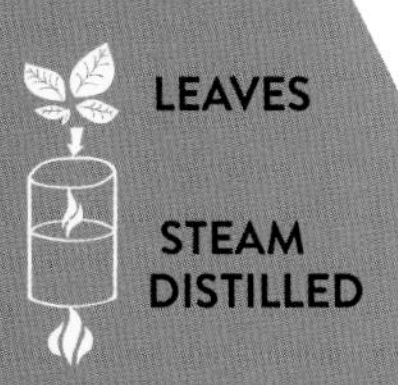

LEAVES

STEAM DISTILLED

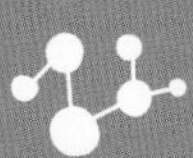

MAIN CONSTITUENTS
a-terpinenes
y-terpinenes
Terpinen-4-ol
p-cymene

TOP PROPERTIES
Antiseptic
Antibacterial
Antifungal
Anti-parasitic
Antiviral
Analgesic
Decongestant

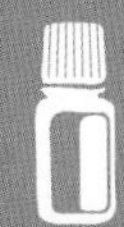

FOUND IN
Breathe®
Purify

BLENDS WELL WITH
Cypress
Lavender
Litsea
Siberian fir
Thyme

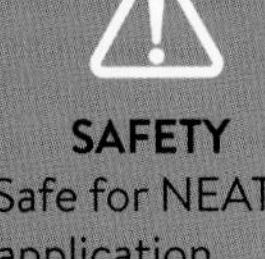

SAFETY
Safe for NEAT application.

TOP USES

CUTS & WOUNDS
Apply (T) to clean and disinfect wounds.

BACTERIA, VIRUSES & DIARRHEA
Take (I) in a capsule or apply (T) to abdomen.

CANKERS & COLD SORES
Use (T) on site to prevent and treat.

ATHLETE'S FOOT & CANDIDA ISSUES
Take (I) in a capsule or apply (T) diluted to affected area.

SORE THROAT & TONSILLITIS
Take (I) in a capsule or gargle with warm water.

DANDRUFF, SCABIES, LICE
Apply (T) to affected area or add to shampoo, lather and soak.

EAR INFECTIONS
Apply (T) behind and around ear.

SHOCK
Apply (T) under nose or along spine.

ACNE, PINKEYE, STAPH INFECTION & MRSA
Take (I) in a capsule or apply (T) on or around affected area.

BRONCHITIS, COLD & FLU
Use (I) in a capsule, rub (T) on throat or diffuse (A).

HIVES, RASHES & ITCHY EYES
Take (I) in a capsule or apply (T) to affected area or bottoms of feet.

CAVITIES & GUM DISEASE
Use (I) in a capsule or apply (T) on affected area.

EMOTIONAL BALANCE
Use (A) aromatically and (T) topically to get from Unsure ———> Collected.

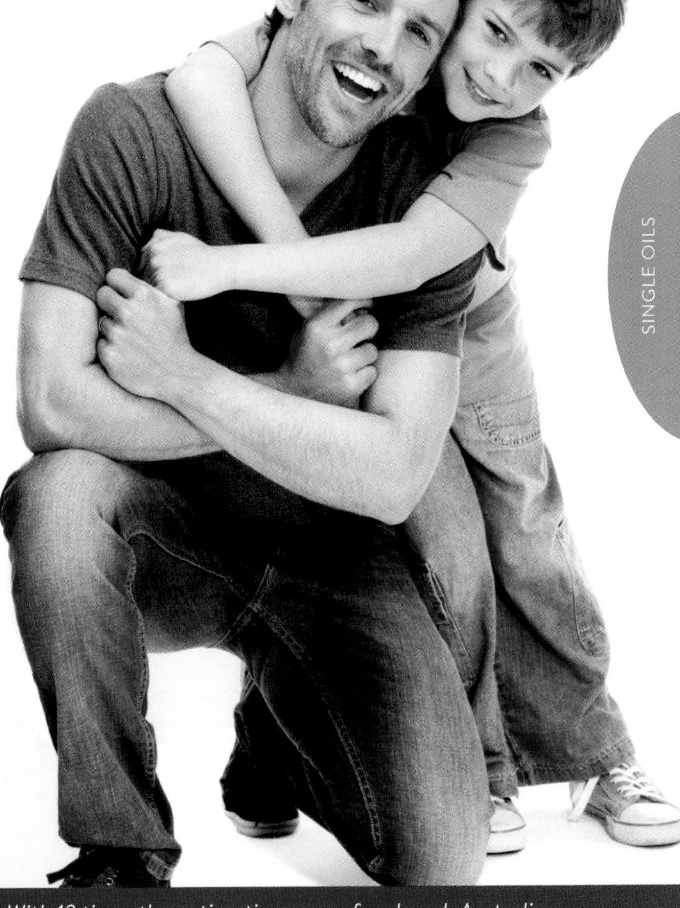

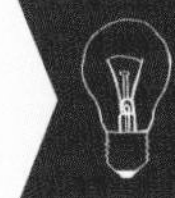

With 12 times the antiseptic power of a phenol, Australian Aborigines have used "Tea Tree" for centuries, often crushing leaves in their hands and inhaling the aroma for colds and illnesses.

RESEARCH: Essential oil of Melaleuca alternifolia for the treatment of oral candidiasis induced in an immunosuppressed mouse model, de Campos Rasteiro VM, da Costa AC, Araújo CF, de Barros PP, Rossoni RD, Anbinder AL, Jorge AO, Junqueira JC, *BMC Complementary and Alternative Medicine,* 2014

Tea tree oil-induced transcriptional alterations in Staphylococcus aureus., Cuaron JA, Dulal S, Song Y, Singh AK, Montelongo CE, Yu W, Nagarajan V, Jayaswal RK, Wilkinson BJ, Gustafson JE, *Phytotherapy Research,* 2013

Susceptibility to Melaleuca alternifolia (tea tree) oil of yeasts isolated from the mouths of patients with advanced cancer, Bagg J, Jackson MS, Petrina Sweeney M, Ramage G, Davies AN, *Oral Oncology,* 2006

Cooling the burn wound: evaluation of different modalites., Jandera V, Hudson DA, de Wet PM, Innes PM, Rode H, *Burns: Journal of the International Society for Burn Injuries,* 2000

Anti-inflammatory effects of Melaleuca alternifolia essential oil on human polymorphonuclear neutrophils and monocytes, Caldefie-Chézet F, Guerry M, Chalchat JC, Fusillier C, Vasson MP, Guillot J, *Free Radical Research,* 2004

Tea tree oil reduces histamine-induced skin inflammation, Koh KJ, Pearce AL, Marshman G, Finlay-Jones JJ, Hart PH, *British Journal of Dermatology,* 2002

Terpinen-4-ol, the main component of Melaleuca alternifolia (tea tree) oil inhibits the in vitro growth of human melanoma cells, Calcabrini A, Stringaro A, Toccacieli L, Meschini S, Marra M, Colone M, Salvatore G, Mondello F, Arancia G, Molinari A, *Journal of Investigative Dermatology,* 2004

A comparative study of tea-tree oil versus benzoylperoxide in the treatment of acne, Bassett IB, Pannowitz DL, Barnetson RS, *Medical Journal of Australia,* 1990

Topically applied Melaleuca alternifolia (tea tree) oil causes direct anti-cancer cytotoxicity in subcutaneous tumour bearing mice, Ireland DJ, Greay SJ, Hooper CM, Kissick HT, Filion P, Riley TV, Beilharz MW, *Journal of Dermatological Science,* 2012

Tea tree oil as a novel anti-psoriasis weapon, Pazyar N, Yaghoobi R, *Skin Pharmacology and Physiology, 2012*

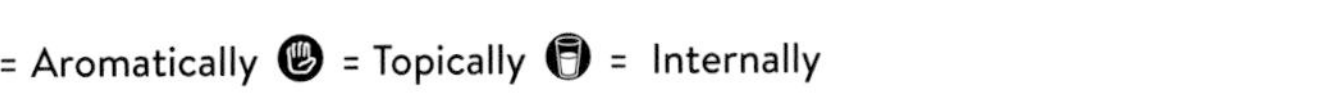
(A) = Aromatically (T) = Topically (I) = Internally

MELISSA

MELISSA OFFICINALIS

awakening
authentic
restorative

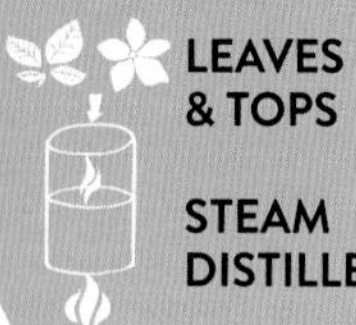

LEAVES & TOPS

STEAM DISTILLED

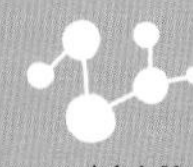

MAIN CONSTITUENTS
Geranial
Germacrene
Neral
B-Caryophyllene

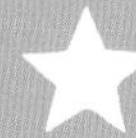

TOP PROPERTIES
Antioxidant
Antibacterial
Antidepressant
Antispasmodic
Antihistamine
Antiviral
Hypotensive
Nervine
Sedative

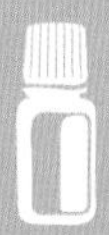

FOUND IN
Elevation™
On Guard® softgels
Arise®

BLENDS WELL WITH
Geranium
Lemon
Lavender
Neroli

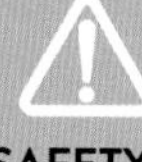

SAFETY
Safe for NEAT application.

TOP USES

FEVERS, COLDS & VIRAL INFECTIONS
Apply diluted along spine, bottoms of feet, or take in a capsule to boost anti-viral strength.

COLD SORES, HERPES & FEVER BLISTERS
Apply directly to sores or take in a capsule.

DEPRESSION, ANXIETY & SHOCK
Apply to back of neck and ears, diffuse, or apply to roof of mouth and hold for 5-10 seconds.

BITES, STINGS & WARTS
Apply directly to area of concern or to bottoms of feet.

ALLERGIES
Breathe in from cupped hands, or apply over bridge of nose and to bottoms of feet. Take in a capsule.

HYPERTENSION, PALPITATIONS & HIGH BLOOD PRESSURE
Diffuse, take in a capsule, or apply to back of neck or over heart.

VERTIGO
Take in a capsule or apply behind ears and back of neck.

ECZEMA
Massage diluted over area of discomfort for calming relief.

INFERTILITY, STERILITY & MENSTRUAL ISSUES
Gently rub over abdomen or take in a capsule to regulate hormones.

DYSENTERY & INDIGESTION
Use in a capsule or apply over abdomen.

EMOTIONAL BALANCE
Use aromatically and topically to get from Depressed ——→ Light-filled.

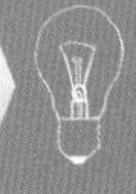

Also known as "Lemon Balm." To make this precious oil it requires 66 lbs/30 kgs of plant matter in order to fill one 5ml bottle.

RESEARCH: Low level of Lemon Balm (Melissa officinalis) essential oils showed hypoglycemic effects by altering the expression of glucose metabolism genes in db/db mice, Mi Ja Chung, Sung-Yun Cho and Sung-Joon Lee, *The Journal of the Federation of American Societies for Experimental Biology*, 2008

Apoptosis-Inducing Effects of Melissa officinalis L. Essential Oil in Glioblastoma Multiforme Cells, Queiroz RM, Takiya CM, Guimarães LP, Rocha Gda G, Alviano DS, Blank AF, Alviano CS, Gattass CR, *Cancer Investigation*, 2014

In Vivo Potential Anti-Inflammatory Activity of Melissa officinalis L. Essential Oil, Bounihi A, Hajjaj G, Alnamer R, Cherrah Y, Zellou A, *Advances in Pharmacological Sciences*, 2013

Antiviral activity of the volatile oils of Melissa officinalis L. against Herpes simplex virus type-2, Allahverdiyev A, Duran N, Ozguven M, Koltas S, *Phytomedicine*, 2004

Aromatherapy as a safe and effective treatment for the management of agitation in severe dementia: the results of a double-blind, placebo-controlled trial with Melissa, Ballard CG, O'Brien JT, Reichelt K, Perry EK, *The Journal of Clinical Psychiatry*, 2002

Chemical composition and in vitro antimicrobial activity of essential oil of Melissa officinalis L. from Romania, Hăncianu M, Aprotosoaie AC, Gille E, Poiată A, Tuchiluş C, Spac A, Stănescu U, *Revista Medico-Chirurgicala a Societatii de Medici si Naturalisti din Iasi*, 2008

Chemical composition and larvicidal evaluation of Mentha, Salvia, and Melissa essential oils against the West Nile virus mosquito Culex pipiens, Koliopoulos G, Pitarokili D, Kioulos E, Michaelakis A, Tzakou O, *Parasitology Research*, 2010

MYRRH

COMMIPHORA MYRRHA

drying • healing • nurturing

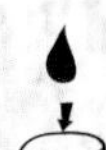

RESIN

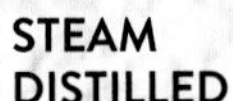

STEAM DISTILLED

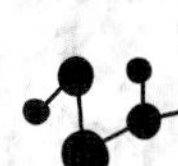

MAIN CONSTITUENTS
Furanoedudesma 1,3-diene
Curzerene

TOP PROPERTIES
Anti-inflammatory
Antiviral
Antimicrobial
Expectorant
Anti-infectious
Carminative
Antifungal

FOUND IN
Immortelle

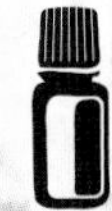

BLENDS WELL WITH
Frankincense
Lavender
Neroli
Sandalwood

SAFETY
Safe for NEAT application.

TOP USES

GUM DISEASE & BLEEDING
Apply directly to gums to soothe and repair.

FINE LINES & DRY SKIN
Apply to area(s) of concern.

THYROID & IMMUNE HEALTH
Apply to base of neck and bottoms of feet.

DIGESTIVE UPSET & CRAMPING
Apply to abdomen or take in capsule.

ECZEMA & WOUNDS
Apply to affected area, especially to weeping areas.

INFECTION & VIRUS
Take in a capsule or apply to bottoms of feet.

CONGESTION & MUCUS
Apply to chest and diffuse to clear airways and dry up congestion.

MEDITATION
Diffuse to create a sense of calm.

DEPRESSION & ANXIETY
Apply to reflex points or diffuse.

EMOTIONAL BALANCE
Use aromatically and topically to get from Disconnected ———> Nurtured.

= Aromatically = Topically 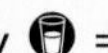 = Internally

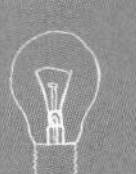

Myrrh means "bitter" and was referred to in the Bible as the balm of Gilead. It was given as a gift to the Christ child and also presented at his death to be used prior to burial.

RESEARCH: Systematic Review of Complementary and Alternative Medicine Treatments in Inflammatory Bowel Diseases., Langhorst J, Wulfert H, Lauche R, Klose P, Cramer H, Dobos GJ,Korzenik,J, *Journal of Crohn's & Colitis*, 2015

Clinical trial of aromatherapy on postpartum mother's perineal healing, Hur MH, Han SH, *Journal of Korean Academy of Nursing*, 2004

Composition and potential anticancer activities of essential oils obtained from myrrh and frankincense, Chen Y, Zhou C, Ge Z, Liu Y, Liu Y, Feng W, Li S, Chen G, Wei T, *Oncology Letters*, 2013

In vitro cytotoxic and anti-inflammatory effects of myrrh oil on human gingival fibroblasts and epithelial cells, Tipton DA, Lyle B, Babich H, Dabbous MKh, Toxicology in Vitro, 2003

Anti-inflammatory and analgesic activity of different extracts of Commiphora myrrha, Su S, Wang T, Duan JA, Zhou W, Hua YQ, Tang YP, Yu L, Qian DW, *Journal of Ethnopharmacology*, 2011

Myrrh: Medical Marvel or Myth of the Magi?, Nomicos EY, *Holistic Nursing Practice*, 2007

Chemical composition and antibacterial activity of selected essential oils and some of their main compounds, Wanner J, Schmidt E, Bail S, Jirovetz L, Buchbauer G, Gochev V, Girova T, Atanasova T, Stoyanova A, *Natural Product Communications*, 2010

The Effect of Commiphora molmol (Myrrh) in Treatment of Trichomoniasis vaginalis infection, El-Sherbiny GM, El Sherbiny ET, *Iranian Red Crescent Medical Journal*, 2011

Sesquiterpenoids from myrrh inhibit androgen receptor expression and function in human prostate cancer cells, Wang XL, Kong F, Shen T, Young CY, Lou HX, Yuan HQ, *Acta Pharmacologica Sinica*, 2011

NEROLI

CITRUS AURANTIUM

arousing
rejuvenating
tranquilizing

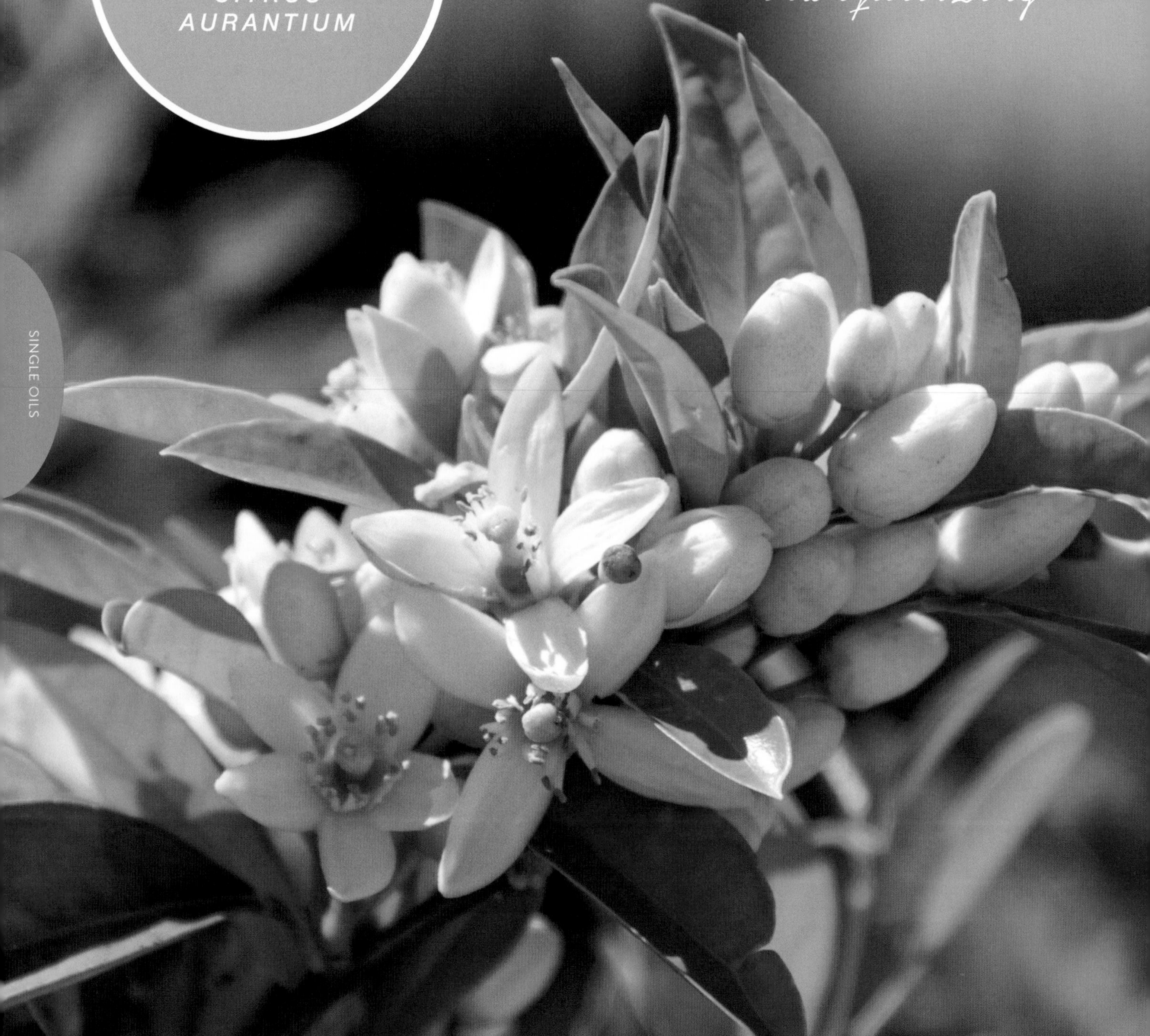

RESEARCH: Neroli oil (citrus aurantium) to have pharmacological effects on fatigue and insomnia, *Essential oils used in aromatherapy*, Babar Ali, Naser Ali Al-Wabel, Saiba Shams, Aftab Ahamand, Shah Alam Khan, Firoz Anwar, Asian Pacific Journal of Tropical Biomedicine, 2015.

Inhalation of neroli oil by postmenopausal women improved their quality of life related to menopausal symptoms, increased sexual desire, and reduced blood pressure. In addition, inhalation of neroli oil may reduce stress levels and stimulate the endocrine system. Choi, Seo Yeon et al. "Effects of Inhalation of Essential Oil of Citrus AurantiumL. Var. amara on Menopausal Symptoms, Stress, and Estrogen in Postmenopausal Women: A Randomized Controlled Trial." *Evidence-based Complementary and Alternative Medicine*, 2014

Aromatherapy with C. *aurantium* blossom oil is a simple, inexpensive, noninvasive, and effective intervention to reduce anxiety during labor. Namazi, Masoumeh et al. "Aromatherapy With Citrus Aurantium Oil and Anxiety During the First Stage of Labor." *Iranian Red Crescent Medical Journal* (2014)

Neroli EO (that is extracted from flowers of Citrus aurantium) demonstrated the capacity to reduce systolic pressure in patients undergoing colonoscopy. Stea, Susanna, Alina Beraudi, and Dalila De Pasquale. "Essential Oils for Complementary Treatment of Surgical Patients: State of the Art." *Evidence-based Complementary and Alternative Medicine*, 2014.

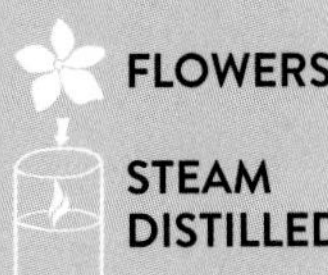

FLOWERS

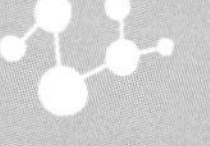

STEAM DISTILLED

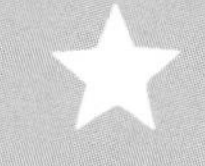

MAIN CONSTITUENTS
Linalool
Geraniol
Limonene
Alpha-Terpineol
Beta-pinene

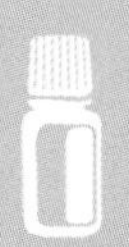

TOP PROPERTIES
Antidepressant
Anti-inflammatory
Antimutagenic
Aphrodisiac
Cytophylactic
Neurotonic
Regenerative
Sedative
Warming

BLENDS WELL WITH
Frankincense
Geranium
Ginger
Jasmine
Myrrh
Rose
Sandalwood
Spikenard
Ylang ylang
Citrus oils

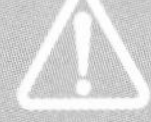

SAFETY
Dilution recommended.
Possible skin sensitivity.

LOSS OF SEXUAL AROUSAL, IMPOTENCE, ERECTILE DYSFUNCTION & FRIGIDITY
Apply Ⓣ diluted to area of concern, diffuse Ⓐ, and/or inhale from cupped hands.

CHRONIC & STRESS-RELATED OR NERVOUS DEPRESSION, ELEVATED CORTISOL LEVELS & TENSION HEADACHES
Diffuse Ⓐ, inhale from cupped hands, apply Ⓣ diluted to chest, solar plexus, back of neck, temples, and/or under nose.

DAMAGED, DRY, WRINKLED, SAGGING & SCARRED SKIN
Apply Ⓣ diluted to area of concern.

CHILDBIRTH & PREGNANCY
Apply Ⓣ under nose and/or to abdomen to soothe mother. Apply Ⓣ diluted to lower back to ease anxiety during labor.

HEART PALPITATIONS, HIGH BLOOD PRESSURE, & SEIZURES
Apply Ⓣ to heart area, area of concern, and/or back of neck.

MENOPAUSE & CHRONIC INSOMNIA, PMS, ESTROGEN IMBALANCE
Inhale Ⓐ from cupped hands, apply Ⓣ to abdomen, and/or drop into a warm bath just before bed.

HYSTERIA, PANIC, GRIEF, SHOCK, IRRITATION & ANGER
Diffuse Ⓐ, inhale from cupped hands, apply Ⓣ to bottoms of feet followed by a foot bath.

OVERTHINKING, OVERWHELM, CONFUSION & DISTRESSED THINKING
Apply Ⓣ under nose, across forehead, diffuse Ⓐ, or inhale from cupped hands.

MENSTRUAL & MUSCLE CRAMPS, SPASTIC COUGHS
Massage Ⓣ into abdomen, area of concern, or drop into warm bath water.

CRAMPING FROM INDIGESTION, COLITIS, DIARRHEA & FOOD POISONING
Massage Ⓣ diluted into abdomen.

ACNE & RELATED DARK SPOTS, ECZEMA, RASHES
Apply Ⓣ diluted to affected area(s).

WOUND DISINFECTANT, ATHLETE'S FOOT, RINGWORM, PAINFUL TETANUS INJECTION SITE
Apply Ⓣ diluted to area of concern.

DEODORANT, PERFUME & ROOM FRESHENER
Apply Ⓣ diluted to under arms, pulse points, area of concern, or diffuse/inhale Ⓐ.

EMOTIONAL BALANCE
Use Ⓐ aromatically and Ⓣ topically to get from Afflicted ——→ Released.

1 ton of blossoms is needed to produce 1 kg of neroli oil. This historically desired fragrance can be heavily diluted and remain highly effective.

RESEARCH: The results suggest that neroli possesses biologically active constituent(s) that have anticonvulsant activity which supports the ethnomedicinal claims of the use of the plant in the management of seizure. Azanchi, T, H Shafaroodi, and J Asgarpanah. "Anticonvulsant activity of Citrus aurantium blossom essential oil (neroli): involvement of the GABAergic system." *Natural Products Communication*, 2014.

Results suggest that neroli possesses biologically active constituent(s) that have significant activity against acute and especially chronic inflammation, and have central and peripheral antinociceptive effects which support the ethnomedicinal claims of the use of the plant in the management of pain and inflammation. Asgarpanah, J, P Khadobakhsh, and H Shafaroodi. "Analgesic and anti-inflammatory activities of Citrus aurantium L. blossoms essential oil (neroli): involvement of the nitric oxide/cyclic-guanosine monophostphate pathway." *Journal of Natural Medicines*, 2015.

Ⓐ = Aromatically Ⓣ = Topically Ⓘ = Internally

OREGANO

ORIGANUM VULGARE

strong resolving powerful

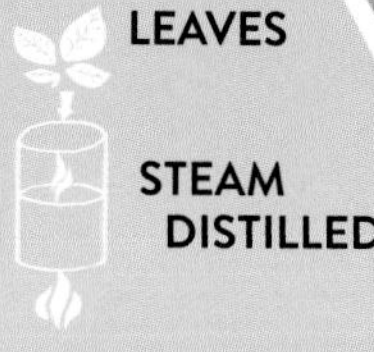

STEAM DISTILLED

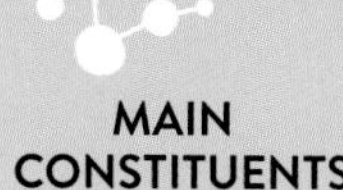

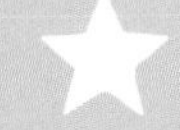

MAIN CONSTITUENTS
Carvacrol

TOP PROPERTIES
Antibacterial
Antifungal
Anti-parasitic
Antiviral
Immunostimulant

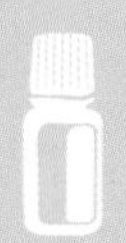

FOUND IN
On Guard® softgels

BLENDS WELL WITH
Basil
Clove
Thyme

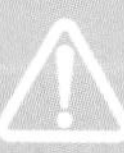

SAFETY
Dilution recommended. Possible skin sensitivity. To reduce liver stress, use with Zendocrine®, helichrysum, cumin, green mandarin, geranium or Roman chamomile.

SINGLE OILS

TOP USES

VIRUSES & BACTERIAL INFECTIONS
Take in a capsule.

STREP THROAT & TONSILLITIS
Gargle a drop as needed.

STAPH INFECTION & MRSA
Apply diluted to affected area or take in a capsule.

INTESTINAL WORMS & PARASITES
Take in a capsule.

WARTS, CALLUSES & CANKER SORES
Apply diluted with fractionated coconut oil and frankincense directly to affected area(s).

PNEUMONIA & TUBERCULOSIS
Apply diluted or neat to bottoms of feet.

BOOST PROGESTERONE
Take in a capsule.

URINARY INFECTION
Take with lemongrass in a capsule.

ATHLETE'S FOOT, RINGWORM & CANDIDA
Apply diluted to area of concern and/or take in a capsule.

CARPAL TUNNEL & RHEUMATISM
Take in a capsule.

EMOTIONAL BALANCE
Use aromatically and topically to get from Obstinate ———> Unattached.

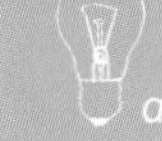

This powerful and potent essential oil packs a punch. It is helpful against antibiotic-resistant bacteria.

RESEARCH: Antiviral efficacy and mechanisms of action of oregano essential oil and its primary component carvacrol against murine norovirus, Gilling DH, Kitajima M, Torrey JR, Bright KR, *Journal of Applied Microbiology*, 2014

Origanum vulgare subsp. hirtum Essential Oil Prevented Biofilm Formation and Showed Antibacterial Activity against Planktonic and Sessile Bacterial Cells, Schillaci D, Napoli EM, Cusimano MG, Vitale M, Ruberto A, *Journal of Food Protection*, 2013

Oregano essential oil as an antimicrobial additive to detergent for hand washing and food contact surface cleaning, Rhoades J, Gialagkolidou K, Gogou M, Mavridou O, Blatsiotis N, Ritzoulis C, Likotrafiti E, *Journal of Applied Microbiology*, 2013

Evaluation of bacterial resistance to essential oils and antibiotics after exposure to oregano and cinnamon essential oils, Becerril R, Nerín C, Gómez-Lus R, *Foodborne Pathogens and Disease*, 2012

Supercritical fluid extraction of oregano (Origanum vulgare) essentials oils: anti-inflammatory properties based on cytokine response on THP-1 macrophages, Ocaña-Fuentes A, Arranz-Gutiérrez E, Señorans FJ, Reglero G, *Food and Chemical Toxicology*, 2010

Antioxidant and antimicrobial activities of essential oils obtained from oregano, Karakaya S, El SN, Karagözlü N, Sahin S, *Journal of Medicinal Food*, 2011

Anti-inflammatory and anti-ulcer activities of carvacrol, a monoterpene present in the essential oil of oregano, Silva FV, Guimarães AG, Silva ER, Sousa-Neto BP, Machado FD, Quintans-Júnior LJ, Arcanjo DD, Oliveira FA, Oliveira RC, *Journal of Medicinal Food*, 2012

PATCHOULI

POGOSTEMON CABLIN

calming · recovering · stabilizing

TOP USES

ANXIETY & DOPAMINE ISSUES
Diffuse Ⓐ or apply Ⓣ under nose and back of neck to calm emotions.

SHINGLES & HERPES
Apply Ⓣ to area of concern and bottoms of feet, and/or take Ⓘ in a capsule.

DRY SKIN & DANDRUFF
Apply Ⓣ to area of concern.

OILY HAIR & IMPETIGO
Apply Ⓣ to area of concern.

NERVE ISSUES
Apply Ⓣ to soothe and heal nerves.

BODY ODOR
Apply Ⓣ as a deodorant and take Ⓘ in a capsule.

FLUID RETENTION
Take Ⓘ with grapefruit in a capsule.

INSECT & MOSQUITO REPELLENT
Diffuse Ⓐ or apply Ⓣ to repel pests.

INSECT BITES, SNAKE BITES & STINGS
Apply Ⓣ with lavender to soothe bites or stings.

INTERNAL TOXICITY
Take Ⓘ in a capsule with ginger.

APPETITE & WEIGHT ISSUES
Take Ⓘ in a capsule with ginger.

STRETCH MARKS & SKIN ISSUES
Apply Ⓣ with myrrh to soothe troubled skin.

EMOTIONAL BALANCE
Use Ⓐ aromatically and Ⓣ topically to get from Degraded ———> Enhanced.

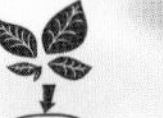

LEAVES

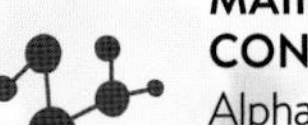

STEAM DISTILLED

MAIN CONSTITUENTS
Alpha-pinene
Sabinene

TOP PROPERTIES
Aphrodisiac
Sedative
Diuretic
Antifungal
Antispasmodic
Insecticide
Antidepressant

FOUND IN
Whisper®
InTune®
Anchor®
Amavi®

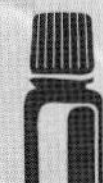

BLENDS WELL WITH
Bergamot
Clary sage
Cypress
Grapefruit
Sandalwood
Vetiver

SAFETY
Safe for NEAT application.

Patchouli has a long history in the perfume trade, but became famous from the 1960's hippie movement.

RESEARCH: Immunological and Psychological Benefits of Aromatherapy Massage, Kuriyama H, Watanabe S, Nakaya T, Shigemori I, Kita M, Yoshida N, Masaki D, Tadai T, Ozasa K, Fukui K, Imanishi J, *Evidence-based Complementary and Alternative Medicine*, 2005

Chemical composition, bio-herbicidal and antifungal activities of essential oils isolated from Tunisian common cypress (Cupressus sempervirens L.), Ismail A, Lamia H, Mohsen H, Samia G, Bassem J, *Journal of Medicinal Plants Research*, 2013

Immunological and Psychological Benefits of Aromatherapy Massage, Kuriyama H, Watanabe S, Nakaya T, Shigemori I, Kita M, Yoshida N, Masaki D, Tadai T, Ozasa K, Fukui K, Imanishi J, *Evidence-Based Complementary and Alternative Medicine*, 2005

Effect of aromatherapy massage on abdominal fat and body image in post-menopausal women, Kim HJ, *Taehan Kanho Hakhoe Chi*, 2007

Evaluation of the Effects of Plant-derived Essential Oils on Central Nervous System Function Using Discrete Shuttle-type Conditioned Avoidance Response in Mice, Umezu T., *Phytotherapy Research*, 2012

Ⓐ = Aromatically Ⓣ = Topically Ⓘ = Internally

PEPPERMINT

MENTA PIPERITA

adaptive • invigorating • cooling

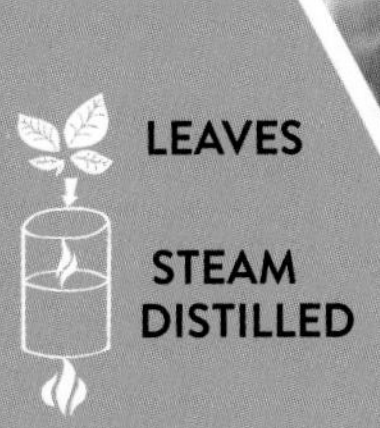

LEAVES

STEAM DISTILLED

MAIN CONSTITUENTS
Menthol
Menthone
a-pinenes
b-pinenes
Menthyl acetate

TOP PROPERTIES
Anti-inflammatory
Analgesic
Antispasmodic
Warming
Invigorating
Cooling
Expectorant
Vasoconstrictor
Stimulating

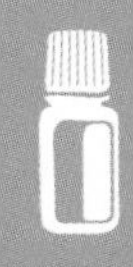

FOUND IN
PastTense®
Slim & Sassy®
Deep Blue®
DigestZen®
AromaTouch®
Breathe®
Align®
Children's Thinker™

BLENDS WELL WITH
Grapefruit
Tangerine
Wild orange

SAFETY
Because of its stimulating properties, avoid use at bedtime. Dilution recommended. Possible skin sensitivity.

TOP USES

ALERTNESS & ENERGY
Inhale or apply under nose or back of neck.

FEVERS & HOT FLASHES
Apply on back of neck, spine, or bottoms of feet for cooling effect.

BURNS & SUNBURN
Apply neat or diluted to burned skin.

MEMORY ISSUES & AUTISM
Apply on back of neck, spine, or bottoms of feet.

CRAVINGS
Inhale or apply under nose or take a drop on tongue before or in between meals to suppress appetite.

MUSCLE STIFFNESS & TENSION
Apply directly to stiff, tense, or exhausted muscles or apply pre-workout to avoid stiffness.

ALLERGIES & HIVES
Take in a capsule, in water, apply under nose, or to bottoms of feet.

HEADACHES & MIGRAINES
Apply to temples, above ears, and back of neck.

BAD BREATH & HANGOVER
Gargle with water.

ASTHMA & SINUSITIS
Apply to chest and back or bottoms of feet.

DECREASE MILK SUPPLY
Apply diluted to breasts, take in a capsule or in water.

LOSS OF SENSE OF SMELL
Inhale or apply diluted over bridge of nose.

GASTRITIS & DIGESTIVE DISCOMFORT
Take in a capsule, in water, or apply over abdomen.

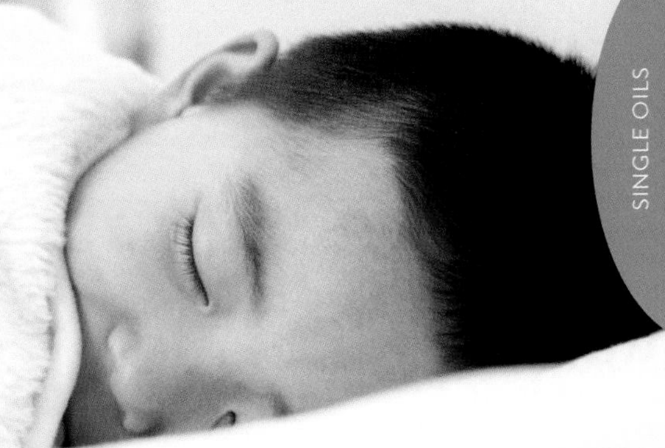

GAMMA RADIATION EXPOSURE
Take in a capsule or with water for antioxidant support.

EMOTIONAL BALANCE
Use aromatically and topically to get from Hindered ———> Invigorated.

= Aromatically = Topically = Internally

Peppermint, with its stimulant qualities, and lavender, with its sedative qualities, make a great combination.

RESEARCH: Screening of the antibacterial effects of a variety of essential oils on respiratory tract pathogens, using a modified dilution assay method, Inouye S, Yamaguchi H, Takizawa T, *Journal of Infection and Chemotherapy: Official Journal of the Japan Society of Chemotherapy*, 2001

The influence of essential oils on human attention and alertness, Ilmberger J, Heuberger E, Mahrhofer C, Dessovic H, Kowarik D, Buchbauer G, *Chemical Senses*, 2001

Enteric-coated, pH-dependent peppermint oil capsules for the treatment of irritable bowel syndrome in children, Kline RM, Kline JJ, Di Palma J, Barbero GJ, *The Journal of Pediatrics*, 2001

Cutaneous application of menthol 10% solution as an abortive treatment of migraine without aura: a randomised, double-blind, placebo-controlled, crossed-over study, Borhani Haghighi A, Motazedian S, Rezaii R, Mohammadi F, Salarian L, Pourmokhtari M, Khodaei S, Vossoughi M, Miri R, *The International Journal of Clinical Practice*, 2010

Peppermint oil for the treatment of irritable bowel syndrome: a systematic review and meta-analysis, Khanna R, MacDonald JK, Levesque BG, *Journal of Clinical Gastroenterology*, 2014

Effects of Peppermint and Cinnamon Odor Administration on Simulated Driving Alertness, Mood and Workload, Raudenbush B, Grayhem R, Sears T, Wilson I., *North American Journal of Psychology*, 2009

Preliminary investigation of the effect of peppermint oil on an objective measure of daytime sleepiness, Norrish MI, Dwyer KL, *International journal of psychophysiology: official journal of the International Organization of Psychophysiology*, 2005

Controlled breathing with or without peppermint aromatherapy for postoperative nausea and/or vomiting symptom relief: a randomized controlled trial, Sites DS, Johnson NT, Miller JA, Torbush PH, Hardin JS, Knowles SS, Nance J, Fox TH, Tart RC, *Journal of PeriAnesthesia Nursing*, 2014

Antioxidant components of naturally-occurring oils exhibit marked anti-inflammatory activity in epithelial cells of the human upper respiratory system, Gao M, Singh A, Macri K, Reynolds C, Singhal V, Biswal S, Spannhake EW, *Respiratory Research*, 2011

The effects of peppermint on exercise performance, Meamarbashi A, Rajabi A, *Journal of International Society of Sports Nutrition*, 2013

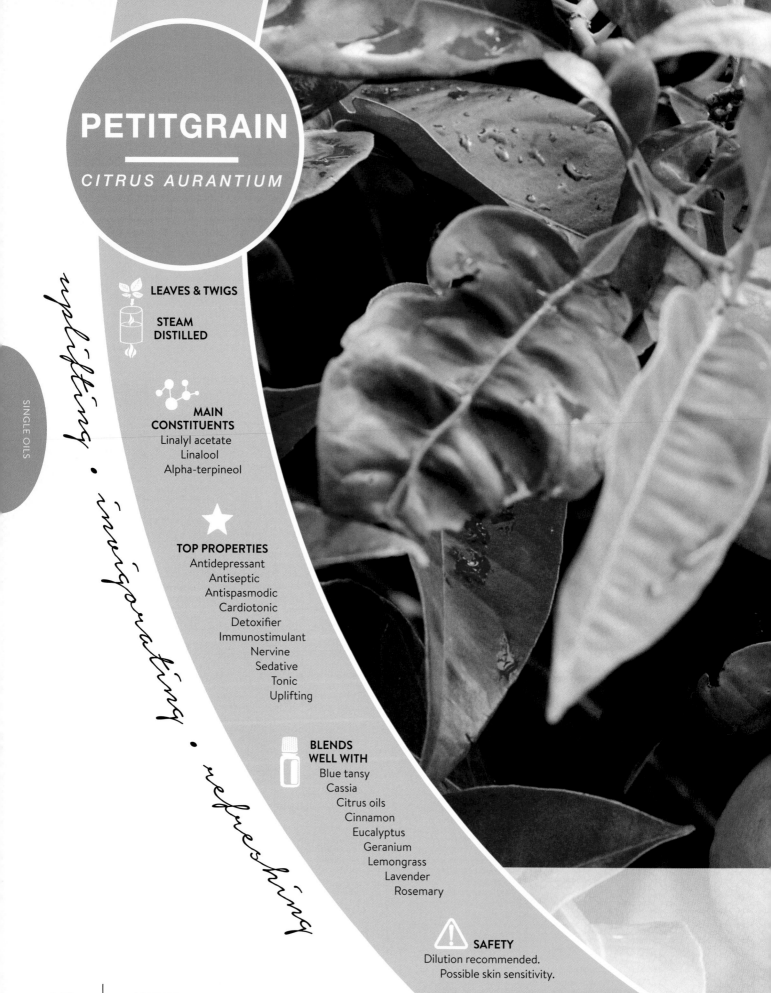

PETITGRAIN

CITRUS AURANTIUM

uplifting • invigorating • refreshing

LEAVES & TWIGS

STEAM DISTILLED

MAIN CONSTITUENTS
Linalyl acetate
Linalool
Alpha-terpineol

TOP PROPERTIES
Antidepressant
Antiseptic
Antispasmodic
Cardiotonic
Detoxifier
Immunostimulant
Nervine
Sedative
Tonic
Uplifting

BLENDS WELL WITH
Blue tansy
Cassia
Citrus oils
Cinnamon
Eucalyptus
Geranium
Lemongrass
Lavender
Rosemary

SAFETY
Dilution recommended.
Possible skin sensitivity.

TOP USES

BACTERIAL INFECTIONS & WOUNDS
Apply to affected area or take in a capsule.

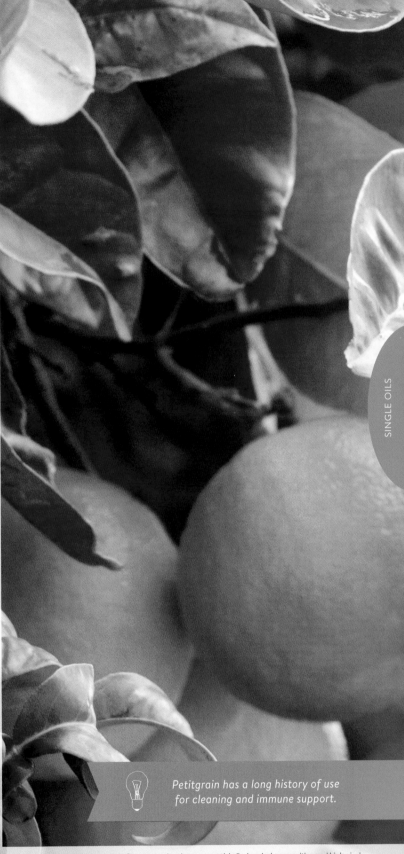

SPASTIC COUGH & CONGESTION
Apply to chest, diffuse, or take in a capsule.

ABDOMINAL & MUSCULAR CRAMPS/SPASMS
Apply diluted to affected area.

CONVULSIONS & SEIZURES
Apply to back of neck, and/or bottoms of feet.

FEARFUL & ANXIOUS THINKING
Diffuse or inhale from cupped hands.

SUDDEN ANGER, SHOCK & HYSTERIA
Diffuse or inhale from cupped hands.

WEAKENED NERVES & INSOMNIA
Diffuse before going to bed or apply a few drops with lavender or bergamot to pillows and bedding.

BODY ODOR
Blend with other oils and apply as perfume, cologne, body spray, or body lotion.

DANDRUFF & OILY HAIR
Add 2 drops to shampoo and apply, lather, soak, and rinse.

PALPITATIONS & HYPERTENSION
Apply to back of neck, forehead, or bottoms of feet.

NERVOUSNESS & EXCESSIVE SWEATING
Diffuse to calm/relax or take in a capsule to calm nervous system and ease anxiety.

CONVALESCENCE & LONELINESS
Diffuse for clarity of mind and mental wellness.

DRY, CRACKED SKIN & ACNE
Apply to area of concern and add to am/pm facial care regimen.

NAUSEA & VOMITING
Take in a capsule or apply to abdomen.

EMOTIONAL BALANCE
Use aromatically and topically to get from Conflicted ———> Harmonized.

Petitgrain has a long history of use for cleaning and immune support.

RESEARCH: Aromatherapy Improves Work Performance Through Balancing the Autonomic Nervous System, Huang L, Capdevila L, *J Altern Complement Med,* 2016

Characterization of radicals arising from oxidation of commercially-important essential oils, Mori HM, Iwahashi H., *Free Radic Res.* 2016

Determination of allergenic hydroperoxides in essential oils using gas chromatography with electron ionization mass spectrometry, Rudbäck J, Ramzy A, Karlberg AT, Nilsson U, *J Sep Sci.* 2014

Volatile constituents and antioxidant activity of peel, flowers and leaf oils of Citrus aurantium L. growing in Greece, Sarrou E, Chatzopoulou P, Dimassi-Theriou K, Therios I. *Molecules,* 2013

A sensitive method for determination of allergenic fragrance terpene hydroperoxides using liquid chromatography coupled with tandem mass spectrometry, Rudbäck J, Islam N, Nilsson U, Karlberg AT, *J Sep Sci,* 2013

Season's variation impact on Citrus aurantium leaves essential oil: chemical composition and biological activities, Ellouze I, Abderrabba M, Sabaou N, Mathieu F, Lebrihi A, Bouajila J, *J Food Sci,* 2012

Determination of petitgrain oils landmark parameters by using gas chromatography-combustion-isotope ratio mass spectrometry and enantioselective multidimensional gas chromatography, Schipilliti L, Bonaccorsi I, Sciarrone D, Dugo L, Mondello L, Dugo G., *Anal Bioanal Chem,* 2013

Chemotaxonomic investigations of peel and petitgrain essential oils from 17 citron cultivars, Venturini N, Curk F, Desjobert JM, Karp D, Costa J, Paolini J, *Chem Biodivers.* 2010

= Aromatically = Topically = Internally

PINK PEPPER

SCHINUS MOLLE

eliminating
clarifying
enlivening

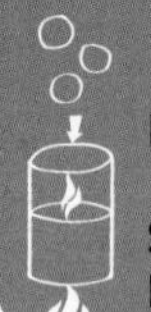

PEPPERCORN

STEAM DISTILLED

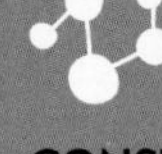

MAIN CONSTITUENTS
Limonene
α-Phellandrene
Myrcene

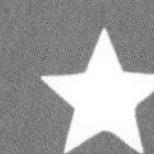

TOP PROPERTIES
Invigorating
Purifier
Anti-inflammatory
Antioxidant
Refreshing
Antimicrobial
Digestive Stimulant

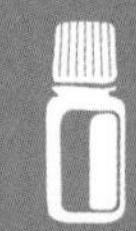

BLENDS WELL WITH
Cardamom
Clove
Grapefruit
Green mandarin
Jasmine
Roman chamomile
Vetiver

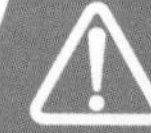

SAFETY
Because of stimulating properties, avoid use at bedtime. Dilution recommended.

SINGLE OILS

TOP USES

LYMPHATIC & CANDIDA CLEANSING, CANCER
Combine with frankincense and take 1-2 drops 2x's daily in water or capsule.

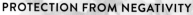

CROHN'S DISEASE, NAUSEA & VOMITING, GAS & BLOATING, POOR APPETITE
Use with cardamom and apply to area(s) of concern. Take 1-2 drops multiple times per day.

PAIN MED ADDICTION
Combine with copaiba & black pepper and take 1-2 drops 2x's daily.

GOUT, RHEUMATISM & ARTHRITIS
Apply with frankincense and copaiba to area(s) of concern and/or take.

PMS, CRAMPS, MENSTRUAL PAIN, BREAST HEALTH
Apply to area(s) of concern or related reflex points with marjoram and geranium.

RESPIRATORY ISSUES & BRONCHITIS
Apply to chest and back over lung area or take 1-2 drops. Diffuse with melaleuca (tea tree).

DEPRESSION & ANXIETY
Diffuse with green mandarin, lavender, or Roman chamomile. Apply over heart.

INFECTION & FEVER, PROMOTE PERSPIRATION
Take or apply with melaleuca (tea tree). Dilute as needed.

MUSCLE TENSION, CRAMPS, & PAIN
Apply with marjoram every hour to area(s) of concern until relief.

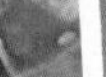

FATIGUE & LACK OF ALERTNESS
Diffuse or inhale from palms of hands. Apply to chest and bottoms of feet.

INSECT REPELLENT
Diffuse, spray on surfaces, and apply.

PROTECTION FROM NEGATIVITY
Diffuse with clove and apply over heart and/or bottoms of feet.

APHRODISIAC, EUPHORIC, WARMING & INVIGORATING
Diffuse or apply with ylang ylang and jasmine.

METABOLIC SYNDROME & OBESITY, BLOOD SUGAR, CHOLESTEROL
Take 2x's daily and/or diffuse with grapefruit and clove.

POOR CIRCULATION
Take or apply diluted with clove.

FLAVORING
Dip toothpick into oil and add to foods as a subtle pepper flavor.

EMOTIONAL BALANCE
Use aromatically and topically to get from Impeded ———> Aroused.

This powerhouse faux pepper (or fake, because it's not hot) potentizes a number of other essential oils in highly complimentary ways.

RESEARCH: Schinus molle L., native of South America, produces an active antibacterial essential oil extracted from the leaves and fruits. This work reports a complete study of its chemical composition and determines the antibacterial activity of Schinus molle L. essential oil and its main components. The results showed that the crude extract essential oil has a potent antibacterial effect on Staphylococcus aureus ATCC 25923, a strong / moderate effect on Escherichia coli ATCC 25922.

Schinus molle L. has been used in folk medicine as antibacterial, antiviral, topical antiseptic, antifungal, antioxidant, anti-inflammatory, anti-tumoural as well as antispasmodic and analgesic.

reviving
clearing
relaxing

RAVENSARA

RAVENSARA AROMATICA

TOP USES

CHILLS & FLU
Apply (topically) to affected area and bottoms of feet.

WHOOPING COUGH & BRONCHITIS
Apply (topically) to chest, upper back, and bottoms of feet, or diffuse (aromatically).

NERVOUS & MENTAL FATIGUE
Apply (topically) to back of neck and adrenal pulse points.

GERMS & BUGS
Diffuse (aromatically) to cleanse air.

MUSCLE & JOINT PAIN
Apply (topically) to affected area.

EMOTIONAL BALANCE
Use (aromatically) aromatically and (topically) topically to get from Uncommitted ———> Resolute.

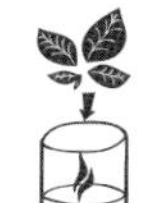

LEAVES

STEAM DISTILLED

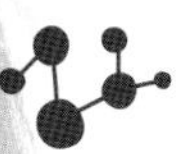

MAIN CONSTITUENTS
Alpha pinene
1,8-cineole

TOP PROPERTIES
Antiviral
Antibacterial
Immunostimulant
Expectorant
Analgesic
Muscle Relaxant
Stimulant

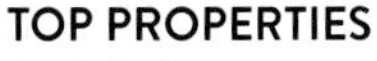

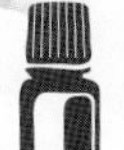

FOUND IN
On Guard® softgels

BLENDS WELL WITH
Cedarwood
Lavender
White fir

SAFETY
Safe for NEAT application.

Ravensara is indigenous to Madagascar and has grown in popularity since the '80s.

SINGLE OILS

(A) = Aromatically (T) = Topically (I) = Internally

RED MANDARIN

CITRUS RETICULATA

cleansing
guided
supported

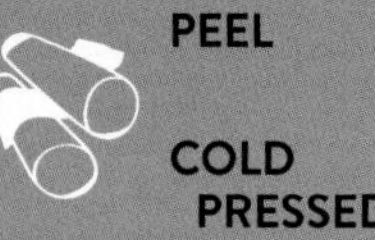

PEEL

COLD PRESSED

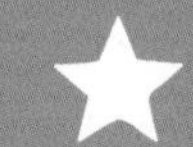

MAIN CONSTITUENTS
Limonene
gamma-Terpinene

TOP PROPERTIES
Antimicrobial
Antiseptic
Detoxifying
Digestive Stimulant
Cytophylactic
Immunostimulant
Antispasmodic
Uplifting

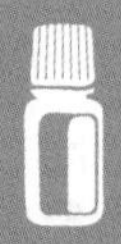

BLENDS WELL WITH
Bergamot
Cinnamon
Clove
Frankincense
Ylang ylang

SUBSTITUTION
Wild orange
Green mandarin

SAFETY
No UV precautions. Avoid keeping in hot places (e.g. glove box of car) to prevent oxidation.

TOP USES

ACNE & OILY SKIN, WOUNDS
Apply to area(s) of concern to clarify and prevent wound infection.

BLOATING, GAS, HICCUPS & INDIGESTION, IBS, COLIC, LEAKY GUT
Apply to chest, back, or forehead. Take 1-2 drops under tongue or in a capsule.

CONGESTION, SEVERE & SPASTIC COUGHS
Apply to chest , back, or forehead. Take 1-2 drops under tongue as often as needed.

WRINKLES, AGE SPOTS, SCARS, STRETCH MARKS
Add to daily skin care products and apply to area(s) of concern.

BACTERIAL, FUNGAL & VIRAL INFECTIONS
Apply to areas of concern. Take 1-2 drops in a capsule every few hours as needed.

NERVOUS AFFLICTIONS, TENSION, HYPERACTIVITY IN CHILDREN
Apply under nose and to bottoms of feet. Diffuse . Take 1-2 drops under tongue.

INCREASE APPETITE, ULCERS, UPSET STOMACH & ESOPHAGEAL SPASMS
Take 1-2 drops under tongue or in a capsule. Apply for relief.

LIVER, URINARY & LYMPHATIC TOXICITY, EDEMA & POOR BILE FLOW
Take 1-2 drops in a capsule 2x's daily. Apply to reflex points.

DEPRESSION & MENTAL FATIGUE, CONVULSIONS
Diffuse or inhale. Apply under nose and to bottoms of feet. Take 1-2 drops .

FEAR, FATIGUE, IRRITABILITY, TANTRUMS & HYSTERIA
Diffuse or apply to bottoms of feet. Take 1-2 drops under tongue as needed.

LACK OF SLEEP & RESTLESSNESS
Diffuse . Apply to back of neck and under nose. Spritz on pillowcase.

GOUT, ARTHRITIS, RHEUMATISM
Take 1-2 drops and apply multiple times per day for relief.

VARICOSE VEINS & POOR CIRCULATION
Apply to area(s) of concern. Take 1-2 drops in a capsule 2x's daily.

ODOR & SURFACE CLEANING
Diffuse 7-10 drops. Add 20 drops to 16 oz glass spray bottle with water and vinegar.

FLAVORING & PROTECT FOOD FROM BACTERIA
Add 1-2 drops to dishes, frostings, smoothies, or cut fruit.

EMOTIONAL BALANCE
Use aromatically and topically to get from Troubled ⟶ Resilient.

Mandarins are often confused with Tangerines and although their taste and tree appearance are similiar, Mandarins are lighter, smoother, and easier to peel.

RESEARCH: Methyl-N-methylanthranilate, a pungent compound from Citrus reticulata Blanco leaves. Pharmacology Biology 2016 Correa E; Quinones W; Echeverri F

Terpenes are compounds found in essential oils. The compound responsible for the pungency of mandarin and other citrus leaves was isolated, and surprisingly it was identified as a methyl-N-methylanthranilate. This kind of molecule with this activity could be used to discover new analgesics in human therapy against pain.

In vitro comparative analysis of antiproliferative activity of essential oil from mandarin peel and its principal component limonene. Natural Product Research 2013

Manassero CA; Girotti JR; Mijailovsky S; Garcia de Bravo M; Polo M

The effects of the essential oil of mandarin peel (Corrientes, Argentina) and limonene (its major component) were studied on two human tumor cell lines growth (lung adenocarcinoma A549 and hepatocarcinoma HepG2). Both mandarin essential oil and limonene tested showed a strong dose-dependent effect on the growth inhibition of these cell lines. The essential oil was more effective in A549 than in HepG2 cells and more effective than limonene in both the cases. It is likely that minor components and limonene of the oil could exert additive or synergistic effects. Hence, mandarin essential oil could lead to the development of anti-tumor agent or complementary and alternative medicines for the treatment of diverse cancers.

Decoctions from Citrus reticulata Blanco seeds protect the uroepithelium against Escherichia coli invasion.

Journal of Ethnopharmacology

Vollmerhausen TL; Ramos NL; Dzung DT; Brauner A

Citrus reticulata treatment decreased 1 integrin expression and reduced bacterial invasion while adhesion of uroepithelial cells was not affected. Results show that Citrus reticulata has a protective effect on the uroepithelium as seen by reduced bacterial invasion of uroepithelial cells. These properties suggest that seeds from Citrus reticulata may have therapeutic potential in preventing UTI.

ROMAN CHAMOMILE

ANTHEMIS NOBILIS

bright • calming • sweet

TOP USES

STRESS & SHOCK
Diffuse Ⓐ or apply Ⓣ to back of neck and inhale Ⓐ from cupped hands.

DRY, IRRITATED & AGING SKIN
Apply Ⓣ to area of concern.

LOWER BLOOD PRESSURE
Apply Ⓣ over heart, back of neck, or take Ⓘ in a capsule.

SCIATICA & LOWER BACK PAIN
Apply Ⓣ to area of concern.

INSOMNIA & OVEREXCITEMENT
Diffuse Ⓐ or apply Ⓣ to back of neck and forehead.

PMS & CRAMPS
Apply Ⓣ to abdomen or area(s) of discomfort. Reapply frequently.

FEVERS & EARACHES
Apply Ⓣ to bottoms of feet and ears as needed.

ANGER, IRRITABILITY & AGITATION
Diffuse Ⓐ or apply Ⓣ under nose or back of neck.

PARASITES & WORMS
Apply Ⓣ to abdomen or take Ⓘ in a capsule to promote expulsion.

ANOREXIA
Apply Ⓣ to back of neck or take Ⓘ in a capsule.

INSECT BITES, BEE & HORNET STINGS
Apply Ⓣ to area of concern or take Ⓘ in a capsule.

ALLERGIES & ITCHY EYES
Take Ⓘ in a capsule, apply Ⓣ near eyes, or to bottoms of feet.

EMOTIONAL BALANCE
Use Ⓐ aromatically and Ⓣ topically to get from Frustrated ———> Purposeful.

Ⓐ = Aromatically Ⓣ = Topically Ⓘ = Internally

FLOWERS

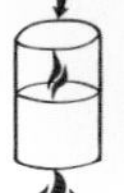

STEAM DISTILLED

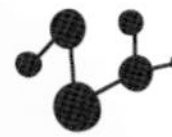

MAIN CONSTITUENTS
Geranial
Germacrene
Neral
Caryophyllene

TOP PROPERTIES
Antihistamine
Antibacterial
Antifungal
Sedative
Immunostimulant

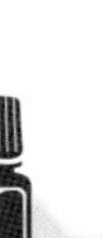

FOUND IN
InTune®
PastTense®
Serenity®
ClaryCalm®
Children's Calmer™

BLENDS WELL WITH
Copaiba
Lavender

SUBSTITUTION
Bergamot
Clary sage

SAFETY
Safe for NEAT application.

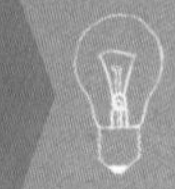

Ancient Romans used Roman chamomile before battle to empower them with courage and clear minds.

SINGLE OILS

RESEARCH: Cytological aspects on the effects of a nasal spray consisting of standardized extract of citrus lemon and essential oils in allergic rhinopathy, Ferrara L, Naviglio D, Armone Caruso A, *ISRN Pharm*, 2012

Volatiles from steam-distilled leaves of some plant species from Madagascar and New Zealand and evaluation of their biological activity, Costa R, Pizzimenti F, Marotta F, Dugo P, Santi L, Mondello L., *Nat Prod Commun*, 2010 Nov

Application of near-infrared spectroscopy in quality control and determination of adulteration of African essential oils, Juliani HR, Kapteyn J, Jones D, Koroch AR, Wang M, Charles D, Simon JE, *Phytochem Anal*, 2006 Mar-Apr

Determination of the absolute configuration of 6-alkylated alpha-pyrones from Ravensara crassifolia by LC-NMR, Queiroz EF, Wolfender JL, Raoelison G, Hostettmann K, *Phytochem Anal*, 2003 Jan-Feb

Antiviral activities in plants endemic to madagascar, Hudson JB, Lee MK, Rasoanaivo P, *Pharm Biol*, 2000

Two 6-substituted 5,6-dihydro-alpha-pyrones from Ravensara anisata, Andrianaivoravelona JO, Sahpaz S, Terreaux C, Hostettmann K, Stoeckli-Evans H, Rasolondramanitra J, *Phytochemistry 1999* Sep

Study of the antimicrobial action of various essential oils extracted from Malagasy plants. II: Lauraceae, Raharivelomanana PJ, Terrom GP, Bianchini JP, Coulanges P, *Arch Inst Pasteur Madagascar*, 1989

ROSE

ROSA DAMASCENA

intimate
connecting
radiant

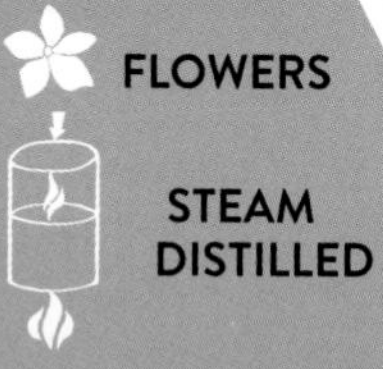

FLOWERS

STEAM DISTILLED

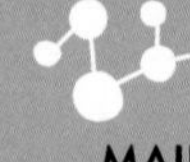

MAIN CONSTITUENTS
Cirronellol
Geranol
Nerol

TOP PROPERTIES
Antidepressant
Aphrodisiac
Antispasmodic
Emmenagogue
Sedative
Tonic

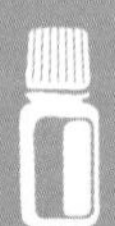

FOUND IN
Immortelle
Whisper®
Align®
Children's Stronger™

BLENDS WELL WITH
Geranium
Lavender
Neroli
Sandalwood
Console®
Passion®

TOP USES

LOW LIBIDO
Diffuse or inhale (A) from cupped hands, or apply (T) diluted to abdomen or bottoms of feet.

BACTERIAL INFECTIONS, SCARS, WOUNDS
Apply (T) a drop to area of concern.

GRIEF & DEPRESSION
Diffuse (A) and apply (T) to back of neck and over heart.

CHILDBIRTH & BABY BLUES
Diffuse (A) and apply (T) to back of neck and over heart.

IRREGULAR OVULATION & MENSTUATION
Apply (T) diluted over abdomen.

SEIZURES, BRAIN ISSUES & NERVE ISSUE
Apply (T) diluted to back of neck.

WRINKLES, FACIAL CAPILLARIES & REDNESS
Apply (T) diluted to area of concern.

SEMEN PRODUCTION, IMPOTENCY, & PROSTATE ISSUES
Apply a drop (T) to navel and to bottoms of feet.

PERFUME
Combine with jasmine or neroli and apply (T) as desired.

EMOTIONAL BALANCE
Use (A) aromatically and (T) topically to get from Isolated ———> Loved.

Known as the "Queen of Flowers", it requires about 12,000 rose blossoms to make 1 5mL bottle.

SAFETY
Safe for NEAT application.

refreshing • cooling • clearing

ROSEMARY

ROSMARINUS OFFICINALIS

TOP USES

RESPIRATORY INFECTIONS & CONDITIONS
Apply to chest and diffuse.

PROSTATE ISSUES & NIGHTTIME URINATION
Apply to bottoms of feet and in a capsule.

CANCER
Take in a capsule, and/or apply to bottoms of feet.

HAIR LOSS & DANDRUFF
Apply to scalp.

MEMORY & FOCUS
Apply under nose and across forehead or diffuse.

BELL'S PALSY & MULTIPLE SCLEROSIS
Apply to bottoms of feet or in a capsule.

MENTAL, ADRENAL & CHRONIC FATIGUE
Diffuse or apply under nose with basil or peppermint.

JAUNDICE, LIVER & KIDNEY ISSUES
Apply to bottoms of feet or in a capsule.

NERVOUSNESS, DEPRESSION, ADDICTION & DOPAMINE ISSUES
Apply under nose or diffuse.

MUSCLE & BONE PAIN
Apply to area of concern.

CELLULITE
Take in a capsule.

JET LAG
Apply under nose, back of neck or diffuse.

FAINTING
Apply under nose or inhale from cupped hands.

EMOTIONAL BALANCE
Use aromatically and topically to get from Confused ———> Open-minded.

= Aromatically = Topically = Internally

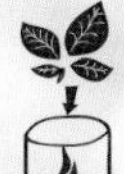

LEAVES

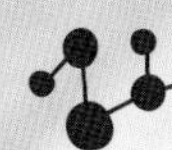

STEAM DISTILLED

MAIN CONSTITUENTS
Linalool
Terpinen-4-ol
1,8-cineole

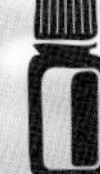

TOP PROPERTIES
Analgesic
Anticatarrhal
Stimulant
Neurotonic

FOUND IN
Zendocrine®
PastTense®
Children's Thinker™

BLENDS WELL WITH
Basil
Lavender
Peppermint
Tangerine

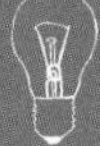

SAFETY
Caution with use with epileptics, during pregnancy and high blood pressure.

In ancient times, rosemary was a favorite oil to drive away evil spirits.

SINGLE OILS

RESEARCH: The effects of prolonged rose odor inhalation in two animal models of anxiety, Bradley BF, Starkey NJ, Brown SL, Lea RW, *Physiology & Behavior*, 2007

The metabolic responses to aerial diffusion of essential oils, Wu Y, Zhang Y, Xie G, Zhao A, Pan X, Chen T, Hu Y, Liu Y, Cheng Y, Chi Y, Yao L, Jia W, *PLOS One*, 2012

Essential oils and anxiolytic aromatherapy, Setzer WN, *Natural Product Communications*, 2009

The effects of clinical aromatherapy for anxiety and depression in the high risk postpartum woman – a pilot study, Conrad P, Adams C, *Complementary Therapies in Clinical Practice*, 2012

Anxiolytic-like effects of rose oil inhalation on the elevated plus-maze test in rats, de Almeida RN, Motta SC, de Brito Faturi C, Catallani B, Leite JR, *Pharmacology Biochemistry and Behavior*, 2004

Rose geranium essential oil as a source of new and safe anti-inflammatory drugs, Boukhatem MN, Kameli A, Ferhat MA, Saidi F, Mekarnia M, *The Libyan Journal of Medicine*, 2013

Effect of "rose essential oil" inhalation on stress-induced skin-barrier disruption in rats and humans, Fukada M, Kano E, Miyoshi M, Komaki R, Watanabe T, *Chemical Senses*, 2012

Effects of fragrance inhalation on sympathetic activity in normal adults, Haze S, Sakai K, Gozu Y, *The Japanese Journal of Pharmacology*, 2002

Relaxing effect of rose oil on humans, Hongratanaworakit T, *Natural Product Communications*, 2009

SANDALWOOD

SANTALUM ALBUM

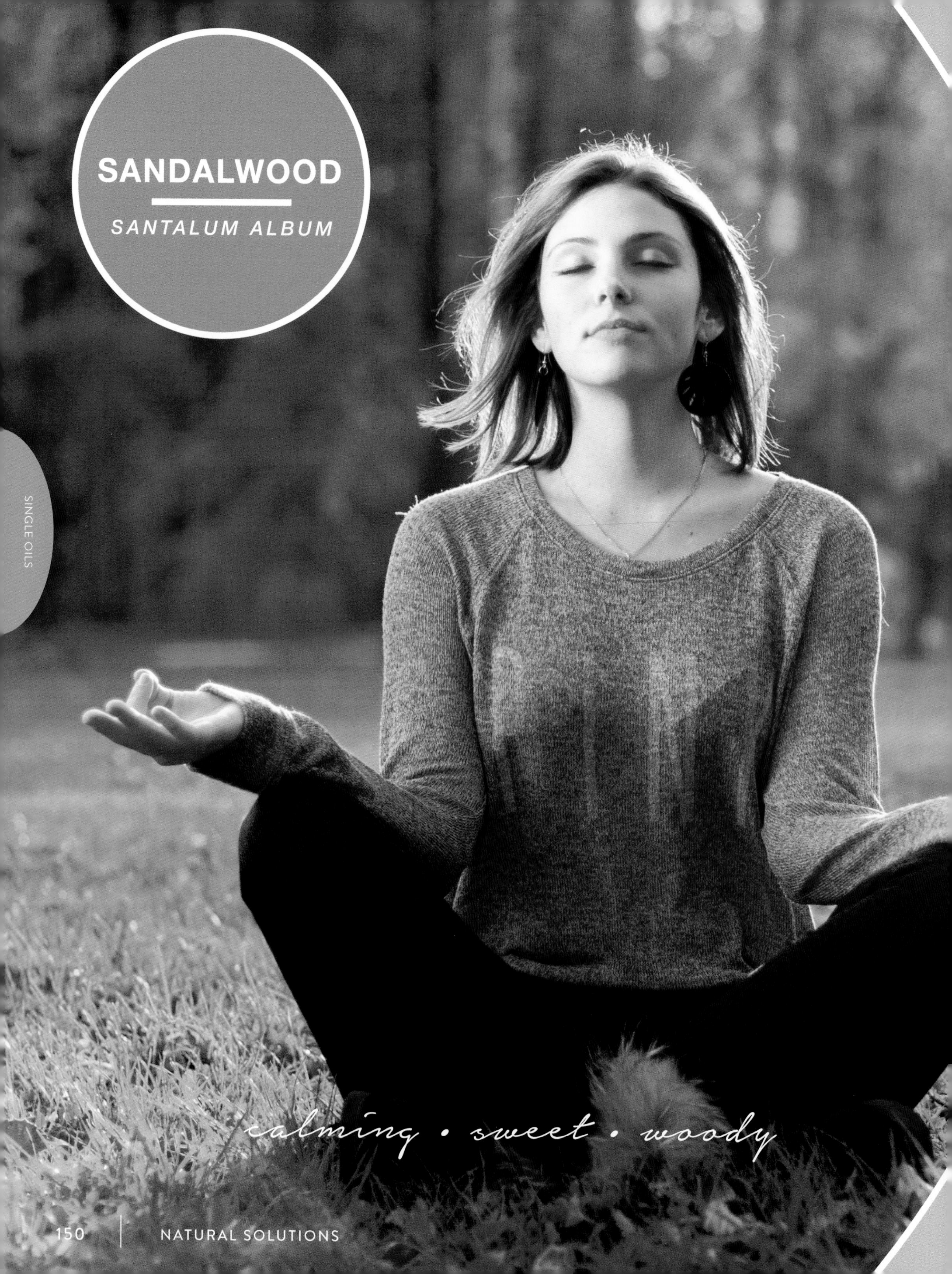

SINGLE OILS

calming • sweet • woody

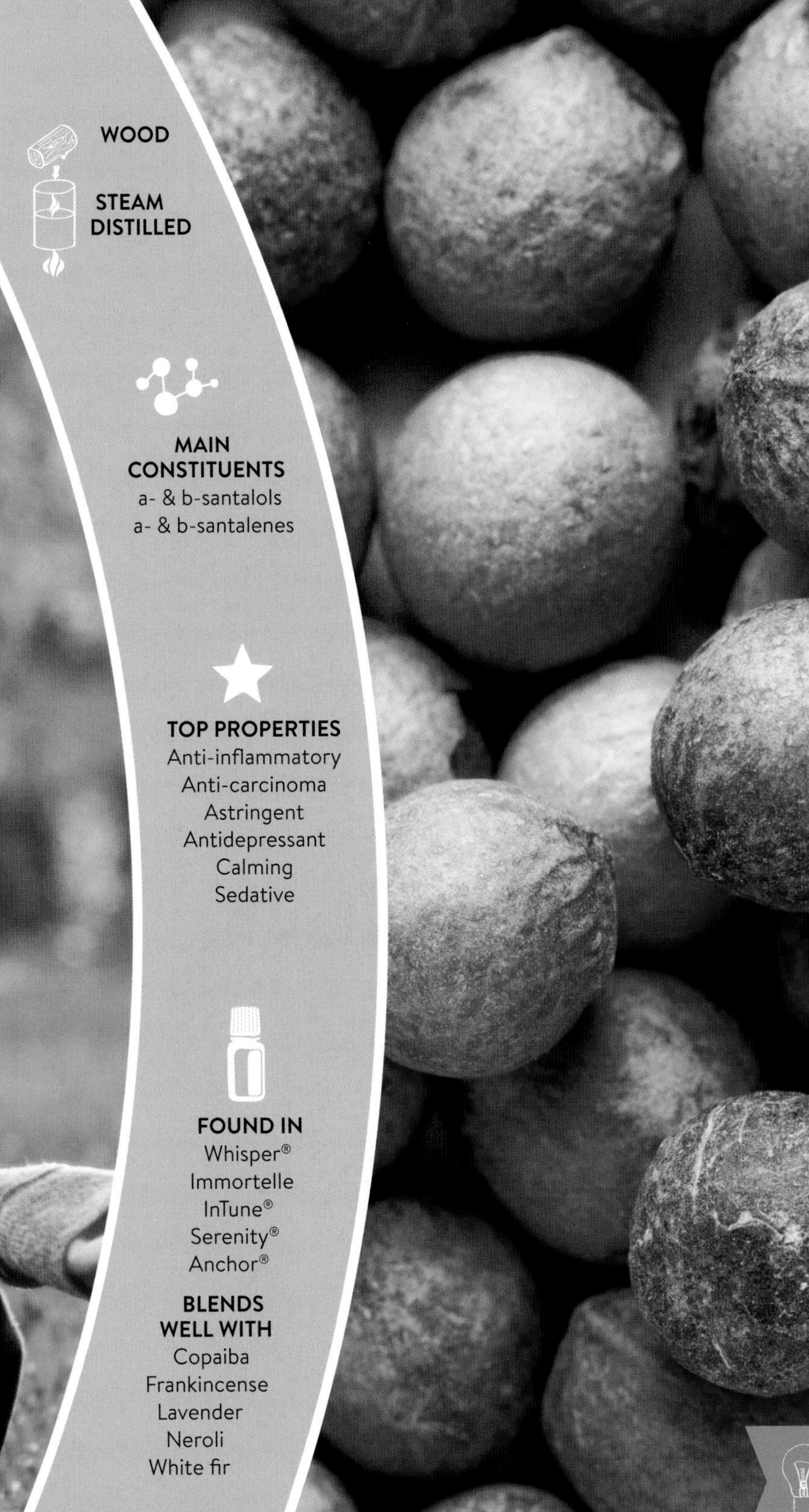

WOOD

STEAM DISTILLED

MAIN CONSTITUENTS
a- & b-santalols
a- & b-santalenes

TOP PROPERTIES
Anti-inflammatory
Anti-carcinoma
Astringent
Antidepressant
Calming
Sedative

FOUND IN
Whisper®
Immortelle
InTune®
Serenity®
Anchor®

BLENDS WELL WITH
Copaiba
Frankincense
Lavender
Neroli
White fir

SAFETY
Safe for NEAT application.

TOP USES

DRY SKIN & SCALP
Use topically or add to shampoo.

CALMING & RELAXING
Inhale or diffuse and apply under nose.

SCARS & BLEMISHES
Apply directly to affected area.

WOUND CARE & SKIN INFECTIONS
Apply to heal skin.

SPASMS & CRAMPS
Apply over area of concern.

LOW TESTOSTERONE & IMPOTENCE
Apply to area of desired results.

SINUS INFECTION
Apply over bridge of nose, inhale from cupped hands, or take in a capsule.

CANCER & TUMORS
Take in a capsule to protect against tumors.

ALZHEIMER'S DISEASE
Take in a capsule or apply to bottoms of feet and back of neck.

INSOMNIA & RESTLESSNESS
Apply under nose, to bottoms of feet, and diffuse for a restful night.

MEDITATION & YOGA
Inhale from cupped hands or diffuse to enhance meditation or yoga practice.

EMOTIONAL BALANCE
Use aromatically and topically to get from Uninspired ——→ Devoted.

Sandalwood has been used for various spiritual and religious uses. Today Hindus still use it to anoint the temple floor and walls to enhance spiritual ambiance.

RESEARCH: Olfactory receptor neuron profiling using sandalwood odorants, Bieri S, Monastyrskaia K, Schilling B, *Chemical Senses*, 2004

Differential effects of selective frankincense (Ru Xiang) essential oil versus non-selective sandalwood (Tan Xiang) essential oil on cultured bladder cancer cells: a microarray and bioinformatics study, Dozmorov MG, Yang Q, Wu W, Wren J, Suhail MM, Woolley CL, Young DG, Fung KM, Lin HK, *Chinese Medicine*, 2014

Sandalwood oil prevent skin tumour development in CD1 mice, Dwivedi C, Zhang Y, *European Journal of Cancer Prevention*, 1999

Chemopreventive effects of α-santalol on skin tumor development in CD-1 and SENCAR mice, Dwivedi C, Guan X, Harmsen WL, Voss AL, Goetz-Parten DE, Koopman EM, Johnson KM, Valluri HB, Matthees DP, Cancer Epidemiology, *Biomarkers and Prevention*, 2003

Alpha-santalol, a chemopreventive agent against skin cancer, causes G2/M cell cycle arrest in both p53-mutated human epidermoid carcinoma A431 cells and p53 wild-type human melanoma UACC-62 cells, Zhang X, Chen W, Guillermo R, Chandrasekher G, Kaushik RS, Young A, Fahmy H, Dwivedi C, *BMC Research Notes*, 2010

α-santalol, a derivative of sandalwood oil, induces apoptosis in human prostate cancer cells by causing caspase-3 activation, Bommareddy A, Rule B, VanWert AL, Santha S, Dwivedi C, *Phytomedicine*, 2012

Skin cancer chemopreventive agent, α-santalol, induces apoptotic death of human epidermoid carcinoma A431 cells via caspase activation together with dissipation of mitochondrial membrane potential and cytochrome c release, Kaur M, Agarwal C, Singh RP, Guan X, Dwivedi C, Agarwal R, *Carcinogenesis*, 2005

Evaluation of in vivo anti-hyperglycemic and antioxidant potentials of α-santalol and sandalwood oil, Misra BB, Dey S, *Phytomedicine*, 2013

= Aromatically = Topically = Internally

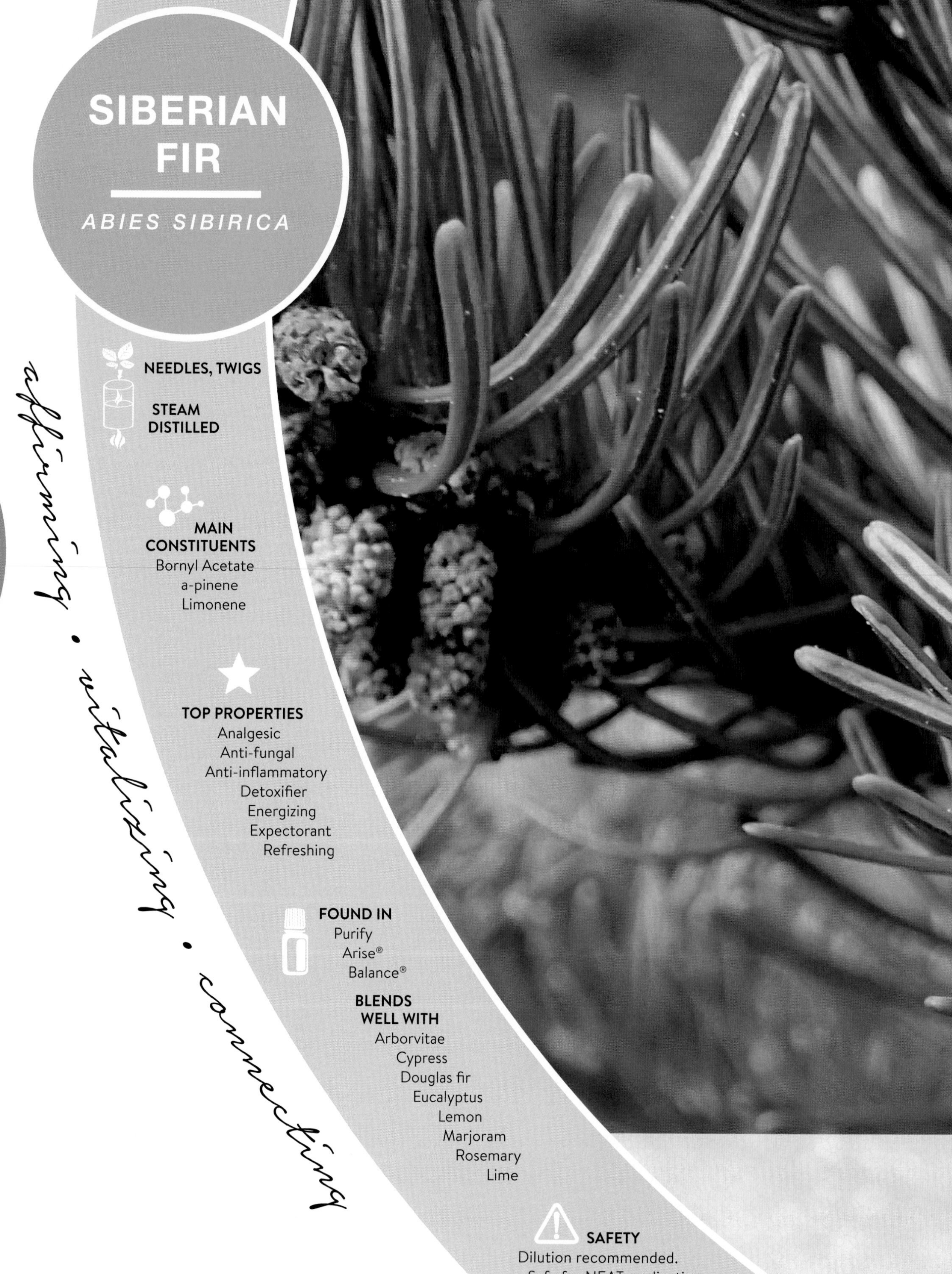

SIBERIAN FIR

ABIES SIBIRICA

affirming • vitalizing • connecting

NEEDLES, TWIGS

STEAM DISTILLED

MAIN CONSTITUENTS
Bornyl Acetate
a-pinene
Limonene

TOP PROPERTIES
Analgesic
Anti-fungal
Anti-inflammatory
Detoxifier
Energizing
Expectorant
Refreshing

FOUND IN
Purify
Arise®
Balance®

BLENDS WELL WITH
Arborvitae
Cypress
Douglas fir
Eucalyptus
Lemon
Marjoram
Rosemary
Lime

SAFETY
Dilution recommended.
Safe for NEAT application.

TOP USES

PAIN & INFLAMMATION, RHEUMATISM, ARTHRITIS & GOUT, TIRED & ACHY MUSCLES
Take in a capsule or massage into area of concern.

CONSTRICTED BREATHING, CONGESTION, COLD, FLU, FEVER & SORE THROAT
Apply to chest, bottoms of feet, along spine; diffuse and/or inhale from cupped hands.

BROKEN BONES & OSTEOPOROSIS
Apply diluted with helichrysum and cypress or take in a capsule.

CANDIDA & URINARY INFECTIONS
Take in a capsule, and/or apply to abdomen.

POOR CIRCULATION, HEMORRHOIDS & LOW BLOOD PRESSURE
Apply to area of concern and/or to bottoms of feet.

SLUGGISH DIGESTION, METABOLISM & LIVER FUNCTION
Massage into abdomen, or take in a capsule.

BODY ODOR
Apply diluted under arms, take in a capsule to detox and increase sweating.

CANCER & AUTO-IMMUNE DISORDERS
Take in a capsule, apply to area of concern, and/or bottoms of feet.

BURNS, WOUNDS, ECZEMA, DERMATITIS
Apply to area of concern. Dilute as needed.

HORMONE BALANCING & PROSTATITIS
Take in a capsule, apply on abdomen, and/or reflex points.

ANXIETY, BRAIN FOG & EXHAUSTION
Apply under nose, across forehead, bottoms of feet, diffuse, and/or inhale from cupped hands.

EMOTIONAL BALANCE
Use aromatically and topically to get from Excluded ⟶ Empowered.

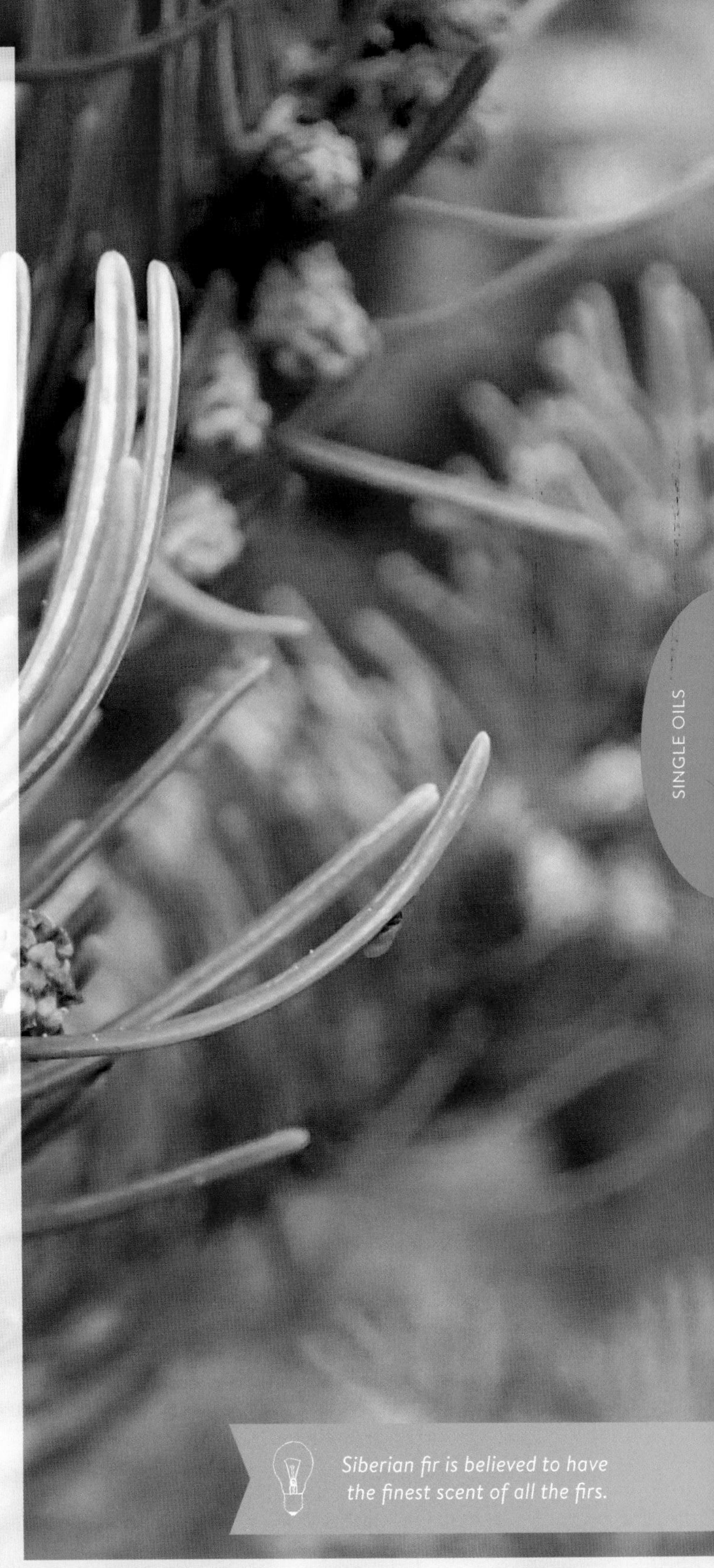

Siberian fir is believed to have the finest scent of all the firs.

RESEARCH: General Toxicity and Antifungal Activity of a New Dental Gel with Essential Oil from Abies SibiricaL.Noreikaitė A, Ayupova R, Satbayeva E, Seitaliyeva A, Amirkulova M, Pichkhadze G, Datkhayev U, Stankevičius E. Med Sci Monit. 2017 Jan 29;23:521-527. PMID: 281320653

General Toxicity and Antifungal Activity of a New Dental Gel with Essential Oil from Abies SibiricaL. Noreikaitė A, Ayupova R, Satbayeva E, Seitaliyeva A, Amirkulova M, Pichkhadze G, Datkhayev U, Stankevičius E. Med Sci Monit. 2017 Jan 29;23:521-527. PMID: 28132065

CREDIT: *Photography done by Krzysztof Ziarnek, Kenraiz*

Effects of Abies sibirica terpenes on cancer- and aging-associated pathways in human cells. Kudryavtseva A, Krasnov G, Lipatova A, Alekseev B, Maganova F, Shaposhnikov M, Fedorova M, Snezhkina A, Moskalev A. Oncotarget. 2016 Dec 13;7(50):83744-83754. doi: 10.18632/oncotarget.13467. PMID: 27888805

In vitro effect of Knotolan, a new lignan from Abies sibirica, on the growth of hormone-dependent breast cancer cells. Zhukova OS, Fetisova LV, Trishin AV, Anisimova NY, Scherbakov AM, Yashunskii DV, Tsvetkov DE, Men'shov VM, Kiselevskii MV, Nifant'ev NE. Bull Exp Biol Med. 2010 Oct;149(4):511-4. English, Russian. Erratum in: Bull Exp Biol Med. 2011 Feb;150(4):556. Shcherbakov, A E [corrected to Scherbakov, A M]. PMID: 21234454

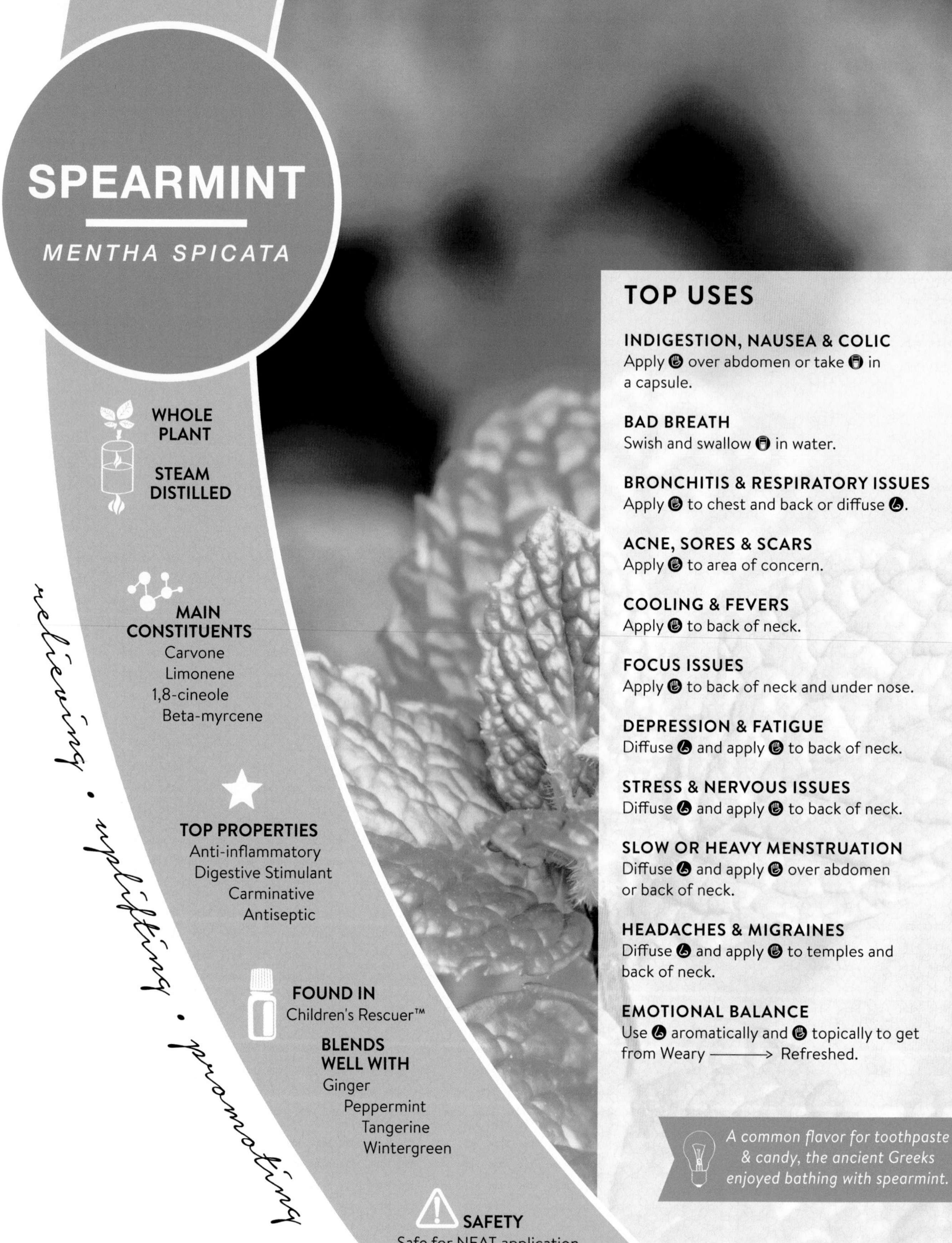

SPEARMINT

MENTHA SPICATA

relieving • uplifting • promoting

WHOLE PLANT

STEAM DISTILLED

MAIN CONSTITUENTS
Carvone
Limonene
1,8-cineole
Beta-myrcene

TOP PROPERTIES
Anti-inflammatory
Digestive Stimulant
Carminative
Antiseptic

FOUND IN
Children's Rescuer™

BLENDS WELL WITH
Ginger
Peppermint
Tangerine
Wintergreen

SAFETY
Safe for NEAT application.

TOP USES

INDIGESTION, NAUSEA & COLIC
Apply over abdomen or take in a capsule.

BAD BREATH
Swish and swallow in water.

BRONCHITIS & RESPIRATORY ISSUES
Apply to chest and back or diffuse.

ACNE, SORES & SCARS
Apply to area of concern.

COOLING & FEVERS
Apply to back of neck.

FOCUS ISSUES
Apply to back of neck and under nose.

DEPRESSION & FATIGUE
Diffuse and apply to back of neck.

STRESS & NERVOUS ISSUES
Diffuse and apply to back of neck.

SLOW OR HEAVY MENSTRUATION
Diffuse and apply over abdomen or back of neck.

HEADACHES & MIGRAINES
Diffuse and apply to temples and back of neck.

EMOTIONAL BALANCE
Use aromatically and topically to get from Weary ———→ Refreshed.

A common flavor for toothpaste & candy, the ancient Greeks enjoyed bathing with spearmint.

RESEARCH: Aromatherapy as a Treatment for Postoperative Nausea: A randomized Trial, Hunt R, Dienemann J, Norton HJ, Hartley W, Hudgens A, Stern T, Divine G, *Anesthesia and Analgesia*, 2013

Inhibition by the essential oils of peppermint and spearmint of the growth of pathogenic bacteria, Imai H, Osawa K, Yasuda H, Hamashima H, Arai T, Sasatsu M, *Microbios*, 2001

Influence of the chirality of (R)-(-)- and (S)-(+)-carvone in the central nervous system: a comparative study, de Sousa DP, de Farias Nóbrega FF, de Almeida RN, Chirality, 2007

Comparison of essential oils from three plants for enhancement of antimicrobial activity of nitrofurantoin against enterobacteria, Rafii F, Shahverdi AR, *Chemotherapy*, 2007

Botanical perspectives on health peppermint: more than just an after-dinner mint, Spirling LI, Daniels IR, *Journal for the Royal Society for the Promotion of Health*, 2001

The effect of gender and ethnicity on children's attitudes and preferences for essential oils: a pilot study, Fitzgerald M, Culbert T, Finkelstein M, Green M, Johnson A, Chen S, *Explore (New York, N.Y.)*, 2007

healing · rejuvenating · uplifting

SPIKENARD

NARDOSTACHYS JATAMANSI

TOP USES

AGING & IRRITATED SKIN
Add (T) to facial cleanser or moisturizer.

INSOMNIA, STRESS & TENSION
Diffuse (A) and apply (T) to bottoms of feet.

PMS & MENSTRUAL ISSUES, INFERTILITY
Apply (T) to abdomen, back of neck, and pulse points.

CANDIDA & VAGINAL THRUSH
Apply (T) to affected area diluted.

CONVULSIONS, SEIZURES & MUSCLE SPASMS
Apply (T) to back of neck and affected area.

DETOXING, DIURETIC & CELLULITE
Apply (T) to affected area or bottoms of feet.

TERMINALLY ILL & HOSPICE
Apply (T) to bottoms of feet and diffuse (A).

ULCERS, GAS & INDIGESTION
Apply (T) to abdomen.

PINKEYE & RASHES
Apply (T) diluted to affected area or around eye.

PERFUME
Create (T) a personalized fragrance; combine with clove, cypress, frankincense, geranium, juniper berry, lavender, myrrh, wild orange, rose, or vetiver.

ANXIETY, DEPRESSION & OLD EMOTIONAL BLOCKS
Apply (T) to pulse points and diffuse (A).

EMOTIONAL BALANCE
Use (A) aromatically and (T) topically to get from Agitated ———> Tranquil.

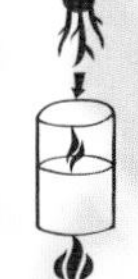

ROOTS

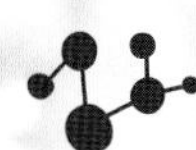

STEAM DISTILLED

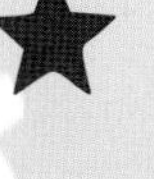

MAIN CONSTITUENTS
Jatamansone

TOP PROPERTIES
Anti-inflammatory
Antispasmodic
Sedative
Antibacterial
Antifungal
Deodorant
Laxative
Tonic

BLENDS WELL WITH
Blue tansy
Clove
Cypress
Frankincense
Geranium
Juniper berry
Lavender
Myrrh
Wild orange
Vetiver

SAFETY
Safe for NEAT application.

Spikenard, one of the Romans' favorite perfumes, and is featured in the Bible several times.

RESEARCH: Aromatherapy as a Treatment for Postoperative Nausea: A randomized Trial, Hunt R, Dienemann J, Norton HJ, Hartley W, Hudgens A, Stern T, Divine G, *Anesthesia and Analgesia*, 2013

Inhibition by the essential oils of peppermint and spearmint of the growth of pathogenic bacteria, Imai H, Osawa K, Yasuda H, Hamashima H, Arai T, Sasatsu M, *Microbios*, 2001

Influence of the chirality of (R)-(-)- and (S)-(+)-carvone in the central nervous system: a comparative study, de Sousa DP, de Farias Nóbrega FF, de Almeida RN, *Chirality*, 2007

Comparison of essential oils from three plants for enhancement of antimicrobial activity of nitrofurantoin against enterobacteria, Rafii F, Shahverdi AR, *Chemotherapy*, 2007

Botanical perspectives on health peppermint: more than just an after-dinner mint, Spirling LI, Daniels IR, *Journal for the Royal Society for the Promotion of Health*, 2001

The effect of gender and ethnicity on children's attitudes and preferences for essential oils: a pilot study, Fitzgerald M, Culbert T, Finkelstein M, Green M, Johnson A, Chen S, *Explore (New York, N.Y.)*, 2007

TANGERINE

CITRUS RETICULATA

calming · cleansing · uplifting

RIND

COLD PRESSED

MAIN CONSTITUENTS
Limonene

TOP PROPERTIES
Energizing
Sedative
Uplifting
Antioxidant
Cytophylactic
Detoxifier
Mucolytic
Stomachic

FOUND IN
Zendocrine®
Citrus Bliss®
Elevation™

BLENDS WELL WITH
Cinnamon
Frankincense
Lavender
Neroli
Peppermint
Spearmint

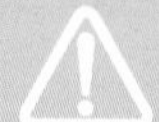

SAFETY
Avoid exposure to sunlight or UV rays for up to 12 hours after application.

TOP USES

ANTIOXIDANT, IMMUNE BOOST & CELL PROTECTION
Take in water or in a capsule.

SADNESS & IRRITABILITY, IMPULSIVENESS
Diffuse or inhale from cupped hands. Appy under nose or take in water.

SLEEP ISSUES & ANXIETY, NERVOUSNESS
Diffuse or inhale from cupped hands. Appy under nose, or take in water.

DIGESTIVE & ELIMINATIVE DISTURBANCES, PARASITES
Take in water or in a capsule and apply to abdomen.

OVERTHINKING & FEELING STUCK
Diffuse or inhale from cupped hands or apply under nose and across forehead.

EDEMA, CELLULITE, POCKET FAT
Massage into area of concern or take in water or in a capsule.

SKIN IRRITATIONS, RASHES & BURNS
Apply diluted to area of concern.

DRY, CRACKED SKIN & DANDRUFF
Apply diluted to area of concern.

CONGESTION, COUGHS, ASTHMA
Apply to chest area.

BOOST METABOLISM & WEIGHT LOSS
Massage into area of concern. Take in water or in a capsule with fennel.

POOR CIRCULATION, CONVULSIONS
Apply to area of concern, back of neck, or bottoms of feet or take in water.

ACHY FATIGUED MUSCLES & LIMBS
Massage into area of concern.

ARTHRITIS & MUSCLE PAIN, TENSION
Massage into area of concern.

EMOTIONAL BALANCE
Use aromatically and topically to get from Oppressed ——→ Restored.

Tangerine has been used for over 3000 years and remains valuable in integrative medicine.

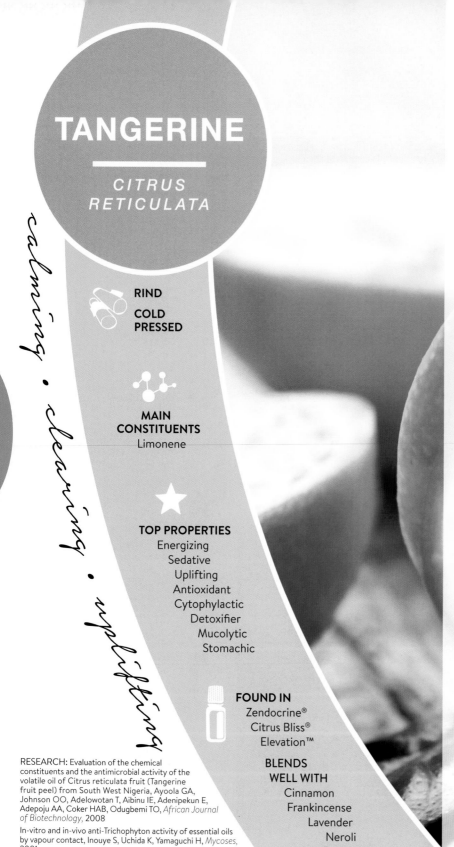

RESEARCH: Evaluation of the chemical constituents and the antimicrobial activity of the volatile oil of Citrus reticulata fruit (Tangerine fruit peel) from South West Nigeria, Ayoola GA, Johnson OO, Adelowotan T, Aibinu IE, Adenipekun E, Adepoju AA, Coker HAB, Odugbemi TO, *African Journal of Biotechnology*, 2008

In-vitro and in-vivo anti-Trichophyton activity of essential oils by vapour contact, Inouye S, Uchida K, Yamaguchi H, *Mycoses*, 2001

Antidepressant-like effect of carvacrol (5-Isopropyl-2-methylphenol) in mice: involvement of dopaminergic system, Melo FH, Moura BA, de Sousa DP, de Vasconcelos SM, Macedo DS, Fonteles MM, Viana GS, de Sousa FC, *Fundamental and Clinical Pharmacology*, 2011

Atomic force microscopy analysis shows surface structure changes in carvacrol-treated bacterial cells, La Storia A, Ercolini D, Marinello F, Di Pasqua R, Villani F, Mauriello G, *Research in Microbiology*, 2011

Screening of the antibacterial effects of a variety of essential oils on microorganisms responsible for respiratory infections, Fabio A, Cermelli C, Fabio G, Nicoletti P, Quaglio P, *Phytotherapy Research*, 2007

Stimulative and sedative effects of essential oils upon inhalation in mice, Lim WC, Seo JM, Lee CI, Pyo HB, Lee BC, *Archives of Pharmacal Research*, 2005

resolving · powerful · expelling

THYME

THYMUS VULGARIS

TOP USES

COLD, FLU & VIRUSES
Take in a capsule or inhale.

ASTHMA, CROUP & PNEUMONIA
Dilute and massage into chest, inhale from cupped hands, or take in a capsule.

CANDIDA & PARASITES
Take in a capsule or inhale.

INFERTILITY, PROGESTERONE, BREAST, OVARY & PROSTATE ISSUES
Apply to reflex points on feet and take in a capsule.

MEMORY, CONCENTRATION & DEMENTIA
Inhale and apply to back of neck to increase alertness, memory, and brain health.

LOW BLOOD PRESSURE
Apply to bottoms of feet and pulse points.

INCONTINENCE & BLADDER INFECTION
Combine with geranium and take in a capsule or apply over abdomen.

FIBROIDS & CANCER
Take in a capsule or inhale.

PAIN & SORE MUSCLES
Apply with wintergreen.

FATIGUE, STRESS & DEPRESSION
Combine with basil to apply diluted to back of neck. Inhale to de-stress and combat fatigue.

HAIR LOSS
Add a few drops to shampoo bottle and apply to stimulate hair growth.

EMOTIONAL BALANCE
Use aromatically and topically to get from Unyielding ———> Yielding.

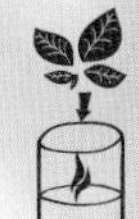

LEAVES

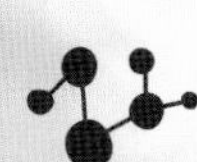

STEAM DISTILLED

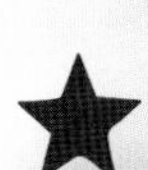

MAIN CONSTITUENTS
Thymol
Terpinen-4-ol

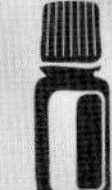

TOP PROPERTIES
Analgesic
Mucolytic
Stimulant
Antioxidant
Anti-rheumatic
Antiviral
Expectorant

FOUND IN
Zendocrine®
PastTense®

BLENDS WELL WITH
Basil
Lavender
Manuka
Rosemary

SAFETY
Caution with use with epileptics, during pregnancy and high blood pressure.

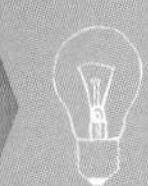

Thyme means "to fumigate" in Greek, and is one of the most potent antioxidant essential oils.

RESEARCH: Antimicrobial Activities of Clove and Thyme Extracts, Nzeako BC, Al-Kharousi ZS, Al-Mahrooqui Z, *Sultan Qaboos University Medical Journal*, 2006

Effects of Thymol and Carvacrol, Constituents of Thymus vulgaris L. Essential Oil, on the Inflammatory Response, *Evidence-Based Complementary and Alternative Medicine Volume* 2012

Encapsulated thyme (Thymus vulgaris) essential oil used as a natural preservative in bakery product, Goncalves ND, Pena FL, Sartoratto A, Derlameline C, Duarte MCT, Antune AEC, Prata AS, *Food Res Int.*, 2017

Down-regulatory effect of Thymus vulgaris L. on growth and Tri4 gene expression in Fusarium oxysporum strains, Divband K, Shokri H, Khosravi AR, *Microbial Pathogenesis*, 2017

Antifungal Activity of Essential Oils Against Candida Species Isolated from Clinical Samples, Cordoba S, Vivot W, Szusz W, Albo G, *Mycopathologia*, 2019

Activity of Thymus capitatus essential oil components against in vitro cultured Echinococcus multilocularis metacestodes and germinal layer cells, Hizem A, Lundstrom-Stadelmann, M'rad S, Souial S, *Parasitology*, 2019

Combined effect of conventional antimicrobials with essential oils and their main components against resistant Streptococcus suis strains, de Aguiar FC, Solarte, AL, Tarradas C, Gomez-Gascon L, Astorga R, Maldonado A, Huerta B, *Letters in Applied Microbiology*, 2019

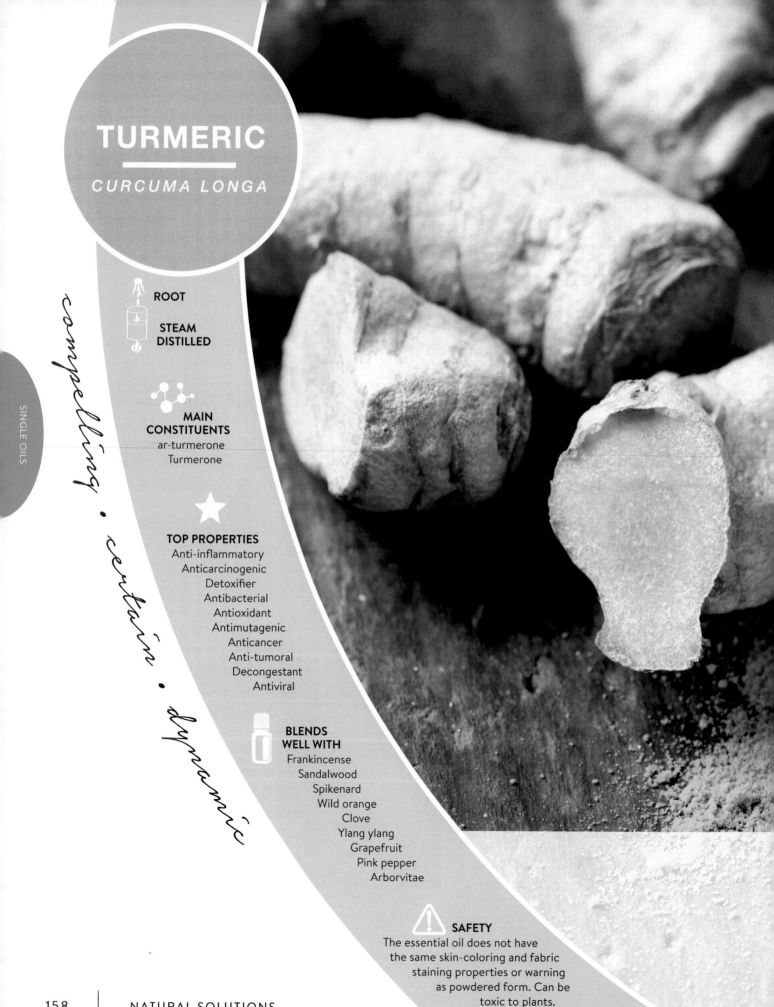

TURMERIC

CURCUMA LONGA

compelling · certain · dynamic

ROOT

STEAM DISTILLED

MAIN CONSTITUENTS
ar-turmerone
Turmerone

TOP PROPERTIES
Anti-inflammatory
Anticarcinogenic
Detoxifier
Antibacterial
Antioxidant
Antimutagenic
Anticancer
Anti-tumoral
Decongestant
Antiviral

BLENDS WELL WITH
Frankincense
Sandalwood
Spikenard
Wild orange
Clove
Ylang ylang
Grapefruit
Pink pepper
Arborvitae

SAFETY
The essential oil does not have the same skin-coloring and fabric staining properties or warning as powdered form. Can be toxic to plants.

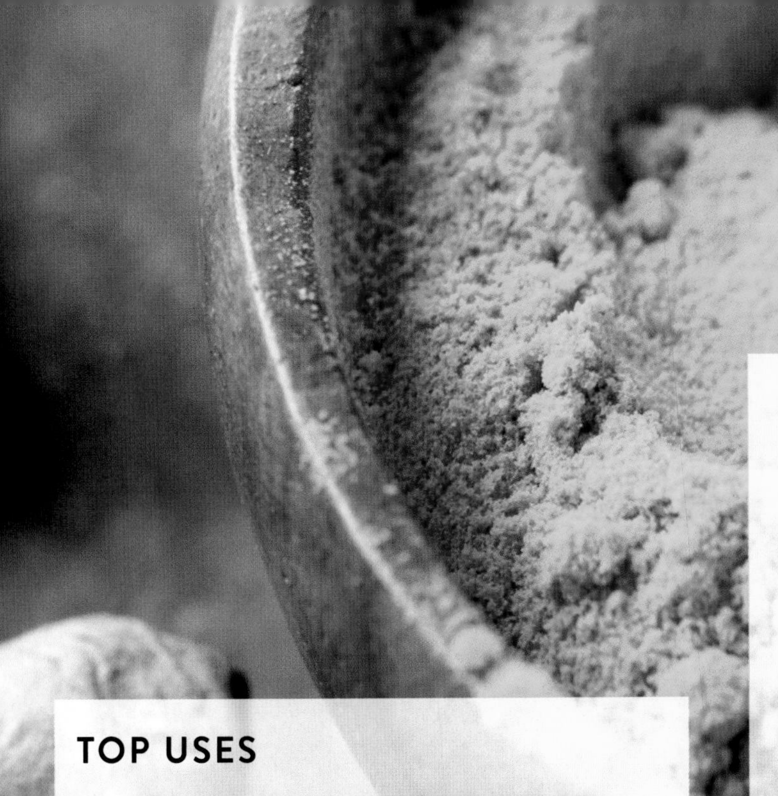

TOP USES

CANCER & TUMORS, AUTOIMMUNE DISORDERS
Take 1-2 drops (internally) multiple times daily as part of a protocol.

JOINT PAIN & SWELLING, ARTHRITIS, GOUT, RHEUMATISM
Apply (topically) to area(s) of concern. Take 1-2 drops (internally) multiple times daily.

FUNGAL, BACTERIAL OR VIRAL INFECTIONS
Take 1-2 drops (internally) multiple times daily and apply (topically) where needed until relief.

ALZHEIMERS, STROKE, POOR BLOOD SUPPLY
Take 1-2 drops (internally) multiple times daily. Inhale (aromatically) from palms. Apply (topically) to forehead, bottoms of feet, and along spine.

BLOOD & LYMPH PURIFIER, LIVER & GALLBLADDER DETOX
Take 1-2 drops (internally) multiple times daily as part of a detox program. Apply (topically) to reflex points and bottoms of feet.

INTESTINAL WORMS & PARASITES
Take 1-2 drops (internally) 2x's daily or more as needed.

ACNE, ECZEMA & PSORIASIS
Add to skin care products and apply (topically) to affected areas. Take 1-2 drops (internally) 2x's daily as part of a detox program.

DEPRESSION & DISCOURAGEMENT, TENSION & ANXIETY
Diffuse (aromatically). Apply (topically) to back of head and along spine.

ULCERS, GAS & BLOATING, INDIGESTION, COMPROMISED INTESTINAL FLORA
Take 1-2 drops (internally) repeatedly until relief. Apply (topically) to area of concern.

POOR CIRCULATION, DIABETES & METABOLISM, HIGH CHOLESTEROL
Take 1-2 drops (internally) in capsule at least 2x's daily. Apply (topically) to bottoms of feet.

COUGH, RESPIRATORY ISSUES & BRONCHITIS
Apply (topically) to chest and back. Take 1-2 drops (internally) in a capsule.

SORE MUSCLES & MENSTRUAL CRAMPS
Combine with complimentary oils and massage (topically) area(s) of concern.

CAVITIES & ORAL HEALTH
Add (internally) to toothpaste or mouthwash. Gargle, swish, and spit.

INSECT REPELLENT, BITES & STINGS
Apply (topically) or add to TerraShield® for added protection.

COOKING & NATURAL FOOD PRESERVATIVE
Add a drop (internally) to dishes for savory flavor.

EMOTIONAL BALANCE
Use (aromatically) aromatically and (topically) topically to get from Compromised ——→ Assured.

Turmeric, or "sacred earth" in Latin, is renowned for a myriad of profound properties, including its powerful action against cancer and inflammation. On an energetic level, it cleanses chakras and energy fields and promotes feelings of prosperity.

SINGLE OILS

RESEARCH: Effects of Turmeric (Curcuma longa) on Skin Health Phytotherapy Research
Vaughn AR; Branum A; Sivamani RK
Turmeric (Curcuma longa) has anti-inflammatory, anti-inflammatory, antimicrobial, antioxidant, and antineuroplastic properties, and may be used to treat a variety of dermatologic diseases. Researchers studied effects of ingestion, topical use, and concurrent ingestion and topical use, and concurrent ingestion and topical use on a variety of skin conditions. Ten studies noted statistically signicant improvement in skin disease severity in the turmeric/curcumin treatment groups compared with control groups. Overall, there is early evidence that turmeric / curcumin products and supplements, both oral and topical, may provide therapeutic beneifts for skin health.

Is Curcumin a Possibility to Treat Inflammatory Bowel Diseases? *Journal of Medicinal Food*
Mazieiro R; Frizon RR; Barbalho SM' Goulart RA
Curcumin is a natural anti-inflammatory bowel diseases (such as Crohn's disease and Ulcerative colitis) IBD due to its remarkable anti-inflammatory properties.

Curcumin suppresses the progression of laryngeal squamous cell carcinoma through the upregulation of miR-145 and inhibition of the PI3K/Akt/mTOR pathway.
Onco Targets & Therapy / Zhy X; Zhu R
The administration of curcumin markedly suppressed cell proliferation, migration and invasion and induced cell cycle arrest and apoptosis in laryngeal squamous cell carcinoma cells (LSCC).

Curcuma longa L. alleviates skin inflammation
Inflammonpharmacology
Kumar A; Agarwal K; Singh M; Yadav P; Maurya AK; Yadav A; Tandon S; Chanda D; Bawankule DU
These findings of topical anti-inflammatory properties of EOCI provide a scientific basis for medicinal use of this plant material against inflammatory disorders.

Evaluation of the Antiproliferative Activity of Some Nanoparticulate Essential Oils Formulated in Microemulsion on Selected Human Carcinoma Cell Lines.
Current Clinical Pharmacology
Abd-Rabou AA; Edros AE
Some EOs and their microemulstions may potentially be used as natural adjuvants to classical anti-cancer drugs.

(aromatically icon) = Aromatically (topically icon) = Topically (internally icon) = Internally

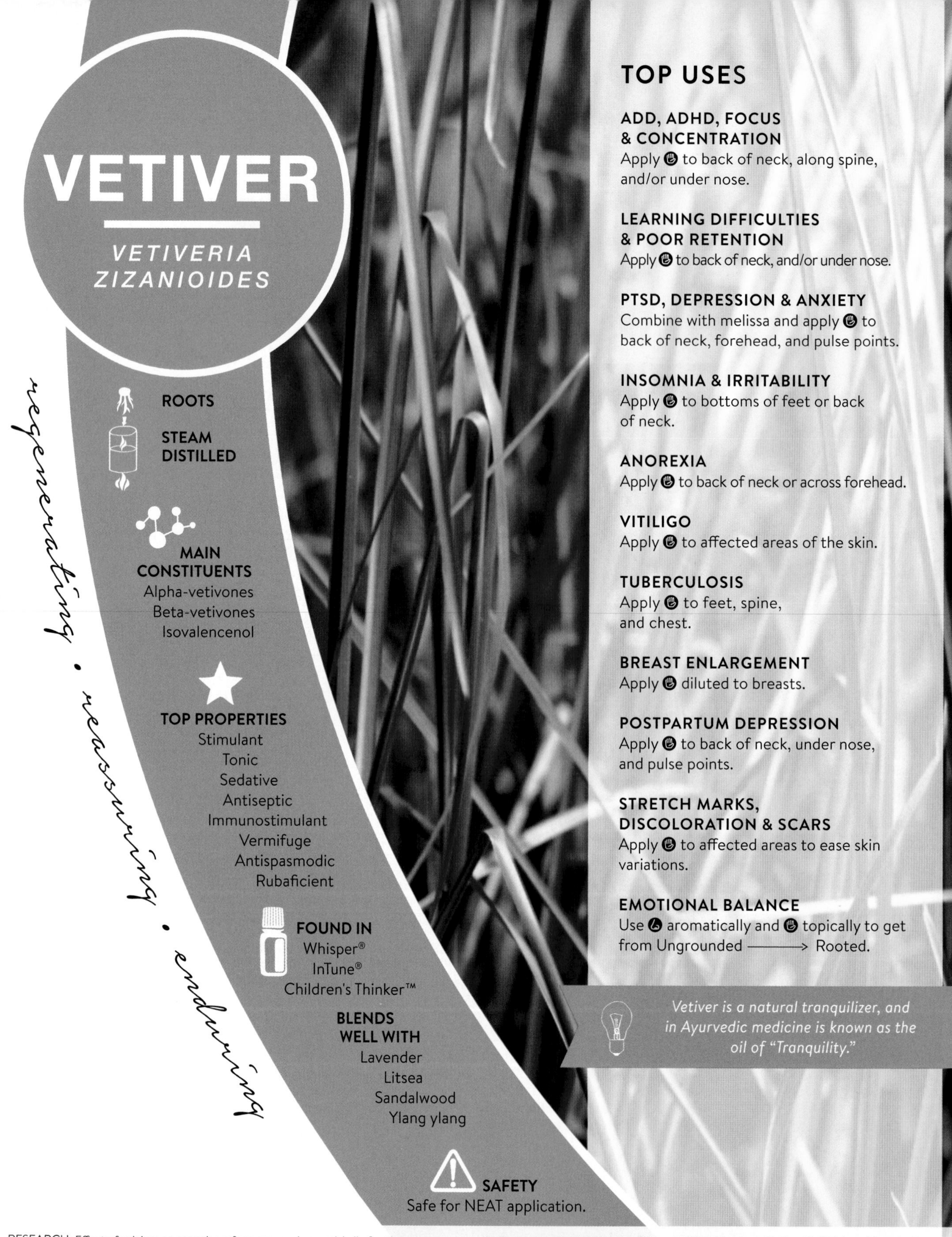

VETIVER

VETIVERIA ZIZANIOIDES

regenerating • reassuring • enduring

ROOTS

STEAM DISTILLED

MAIN CONSTITUENTS
Alpha-vetivones
Beta-vetivones
Isovalencenol

TOP PROPERTIES
Stimulant
Tonic
Sedative
Antiseptic
Immunostimulant
Vermifuge
Antispasmodic
Rubaficient

FOUND IN
Whisper®
InTune®
Children's Thinker™

BLENDS WELL WITH
Lavender
Litsea
Sandalwood
Ylang ylang

SAFETY
Safe for NEAT application.

TOP USES

ADD, ADHD, FOCUS & CONCENTRATION
Apply to back of neck, along spine, and/or under nose.

LEARNING DIFFICULTIES & POOR RETENTION
Apply to back of neck, and/or under nose.

PTSD, DEPRESSION & ANXIETY
Combine with melissa and apply to back of neck, forehead, and pulse points.

INSOMNIA & IRRITABILITY
Apply to bottoms of feet or back of neck.

ANOREXIA
Apply to back of neck or across forehead.

VITILIGO
Apply to affected areas of the skin.

TUBERCULOSIS
Apply to feet, spine, and chest.

BREAST ENLARGEMENT
Apply diluted to breasts.

POSTPARTUM DEPRESSION
Apply to back of neck, under nose, and pulse points.

STRETCH MARKS, DISCOLORATION & SCARS
Apply to affected areas to ease skin variations.

EMOTIONAL BALANCE
Use aromatically and topically to get from Ungrounded ———> Rooted.

Vetiver is a natural tranquilizer, and in Ayurvedic medicine is known as the oil of "Tranquility."

SINGLE OILS

RESEARCH: Effect of calcium on growth performance and essential oil of vetiver grass (Chrysopogon zizanioides) grown on lead contaminated soils, Danh LT, Truong P, Mammucari R, Foster N, *International Journal of Phytoremediation*, 2011

Effect of Vetiveria zizanioides Essential Oil on Melanogenesis in Melanoma Cells: Downregulation of Tyrosinase Expression and Suppression of Oxidative Stress, Peng HY, Lai CC, Lin CC, Chou ST, *The Scientific World Journal*, 2014

Constituents of south Indian vetiver oils, Mallavarapu GR, Syamasundar KV, Ramesh S, Rao BR, *Natural Product Communications*, 2012

In Vitro Antioxidant Activities of Essential Oils, Veerapan P, Khunkitti W, Isan *Journal of Pharmaceutical Sciences*, 2011

Antioxidant potential of the root of Vetiveria zizanioides (L.) Nash, Luqman S, Kumar R, Kaushik S, Srivastava S, Darokar MP, Khanuja SP, *Indian Journal of Biochemistry and Biophysics*, 2009

Volatiles emitted from the roots of Vetiveria zizanioides suppress the decline in attention during a visual display terminal taskvi, Matsubara E, Shimizu K, Fukagawa M, Ishizi Y, Kakoi C, Hatayama T, Nagano J, Okamoto T, Ohnuki K, Kondo R, *Biomedical Research*, 2012

Evaluation of the Effects of Plant-derived Essential Oils on Central Nervous System Function Using Discrete Shuttle-type Conditioned Avoidance Response in Mice, Umezu T, *Phytotherapy Research*, 2012

stimulating · clearing · calming

WHITE FIR

ABIES ALBA

TOP USES

SINUSITIS & ASTHMA
Apply topically to bridge of nose and chest or diffuse aromatically to ease breathing.

MUSCLE & JOINT PAIN
Massage topically diluted on affected area for soothing relief.

MUSCLE FATIGUE & REGENERATION
Apply topically diluted to area of concern.

BURSITIS & RHEUMATISM
Apply topically to affected area(s).

AIRBORNE PATHOGENS
Diffuse aromatically to fight germs.

CIRCULATION ISSUES & BRUISING
Massage topically into affected areas to increase circulation and healing.

STRESS & FOGGY MIND
Diffuse aromatically with frankincense for increased focus and clarity.

BRONCHITIS & CONGESTION
Apply topically to chest or bridge of nose.

COLDS & FLU
Apply topically to chest and diffuse aromatically.

URINARY INFECTION & EDEMA
Apply topically over lower abdomen.

FURNITURE POLISH
Apply topically to surface using a cloth.

EMOTIONAL BALANCE
Use aromatically and topically to get from Blocked ——> Receiving.

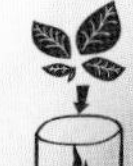

NEEDLES

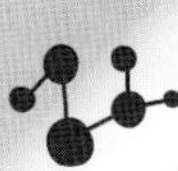

STEAM DISTILLED

MAIN CONSTITUENTS
l-limonene
b-pinene
Camphene

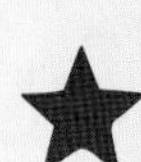

TOP PROPERTIES
Analgesic
Antiarthritic
Antiseptic
Stimulant
Antioxidant

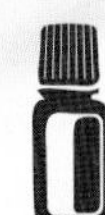

BLENDS WELL WITH
Bergamot
Frankincense
Lavender
Siberian fir

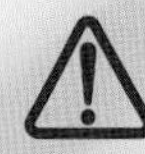

SAFETY
Safe for NEAT application.

Used to decorate homes as Christmas trees. Native Americans used this tree to clear respiratory problems.

SINGLE OILS

RESEARCH: Repellency to Stomoxys calcitrans (Diptera: Muscidae) of Plant Essential Oils Alone or in Combination with Calophyllum inophyllum Nut Oil, Hieu TT, Kim SI, Lee SG, Ahn YJ, *Journal of Medical Etomology*, 2010

The battle against multi-resistant strains: Renaissance of antimicrobial essential oils as a promising force to fight hospital-acquired infections, Warnke PH, Becker ST, Podschun R, Sivananthan S, Springer IN, Russo PA, Wiltfang J, Fickenscher H, Sherry E, *Journal of Cranio-Maxillo-Facial Surgery*, 2009

WILD ORANGE

CITRUS SINENSIS

uplifting
invigorating
renewing

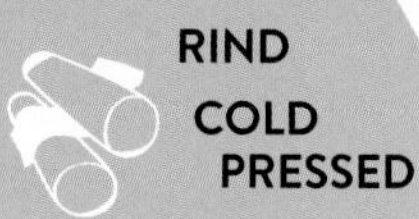

RIND
COLD PRESSED

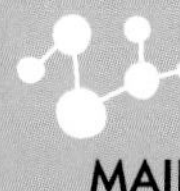

MAIN CONSTITUENTS
d-limonene
Terpinolene
Myrcene

TOP PROPERTIES
Energizing
Sedative
Anti-carcinoma
Carminative
Antiseptic
Antidepressant
Immunostimulant

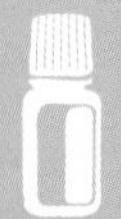

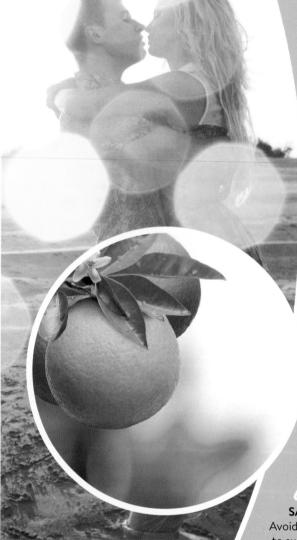

FOUND IN
Citrus Bliss®
TerraShield®
DDR Prime®
On Guard®
Children's Brave™

BLENDS WELL WITH
Cinnamon
Lavender
Neroli
Peppermint
Siberian fir

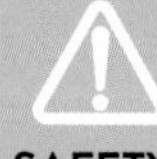

SAFETY
Avoid exposure to sunlight or UV rays for up to 12 hours after application.

TOP USES

INSOMNIA & STRESS
Diffuse or inhale from cupped hands or take a few drops under tongue at bedtime.

HEARTBURN & SLUGGISH BOWELS
Take in a capsule with ginger.

SCURVY & COLDS
Diffuse or apply to bottoms of feet.

MENOPAUSE
Apply to abdomen, pulse points, and diffuse.

DEPRESSION, FEAR, ANXIETY & IRRITABILITY
Apply under nose, across forehead, or pulse points. Diffuse or inhale from cupped hands.

LACK OF ENERGY, CREATIVITY & PRODUCTIVITY
Take in a capsule, apply under nose, or diffuse.

CONCENTRATION
Combine with peppermint and diffuse or inhale from cupped hands.

DETOX & REGENERATION
Take in a glass of water or capsule.

DIGESTIVE UPSET DUE TO ANXIETY
Take in a capsule and inhale from cupped hands.

COOKING
Add a drop to dishes, frostings, and smoothies for a sweet, rich citrus flavor.

EMOTIONAL BALANCE
Use aromatically and topically to get from Drained ———> Productive.

The Chinese first recognized the value of the peel of an orange for treating coughs and colds.

RESEARCH: Antimicrobial Effect and Mode of Action of Terpeneless Cold Pressed Valencia Orange Essential Oil on Methicillin-Resistant Staphylococcus aureus, Muthaiyan A, Martin EM, Natesan S, Crandall PG, Wilkinson BJ, Ricke SC, Journal of Applied Microbiology, 2012

Insecticidal properties of volatile extracts of orange peels, Ezeonu FC, Chidume GI, Udedi SC, Bioresource Technology, 2001

An experimental study on the effectiveness of massage with aromatic ginger and orange essential oil for moderate-to-severe knee pain among the elderly in Hong Kong, Yip YB, Tam AC, Complementary Therapies in Medicine, 2008

Oil of bitter orange: new topical antifungal agent, Ramadan W, Mourad B, Ibrahim S, Sonbol F, International Journal of Dermatology, 1996

Ambient odor of orange in a dental office reduces anxiety and improves mood in female patients, Lehrner J, Eckersberger C, Walla P, Pötsch G, Deecke L, Physiology and Behavior, 2000

Effect of sweet orange aroma on experimental anxiety in humans., Goes TC, Antunes FD, Alves PB, Teixeira-Silva F, The Journal of Alternative and Complementary Medicine

Effect of aromatherapy on patients with Alzheimer's disease, Jimbo D, Kimura Y, Taniguchi M, Inoue M, Urakami K, Psychogeriatrics, 2009

warming
relieving
repairing

WINTERGREEN

GAULTHERIA FRAGRANTISSIMA

TOP USES

GOUT & RHEUMATISM
Dilute and apply (T) to affected area to soothe discomfort.

WARMING & CIRCULATION TO EXTREMITIES
Dilute and apply (T) to affected area(s).

ARTHRITIS & JOINTS
Dilute and apply (T) to ease pain.

NEURALGIA & CRAMPS
Dilute and apply (T) to relieve cramps.

BONE SPURS & PAIN
Dilute and apply (T) to affected area.

CARTILAGE INJURY & BRUISING
Dilute and apply (T).

ROTATOR CUFF ISSUES & FROZEN SHOULDER
Dilute and apply (T) to affected area to ease pain and inflammation.

DANDRUFF
Mix a few drops with shampoo and apply (T) to scalp.

DERMATITIS
Dilute and apply (T) to affected areas to reduce irritation.

BLADDER INFECTION & KIDNEY STONES
Dilute and apply (T) over abdomen with a hot pack.

EMOTIONAL BALANCE
Use (A) aromatically and (T) topically to get from Stubborn ——> Accepting.

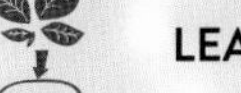
LEAVES

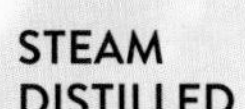
STEAM DISTILLED

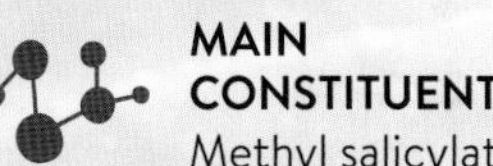
MAIN CONSTITUENT
Methyl salicylate

TOP PROPERTIES
Anti-inflammatory
Analgesic
Anti-rheumatic

FOUND IN
Deep Blue®
PastTense®

BLENDS WELL WITH
Blue tansy
Copaiba
Helichrysum
Siberian fir
Yarrow

SAFETY
Dilution recommended. Possible skin sensitivity.

A naturally occurring compound found in wintergreen, "methyl salicylate" is related to the chemical that makes aspirin.

SINGLE OILS

RESEARCH: Comparison of oral aspirin versus topical applied methyl salicylate for platelet inhibition, Tanen DA, Danish DC, Reardon JM, Chisholm CB, Matteucci MJ, Riffenburgh RH, *Annals of Pharmacotherapy*, 2008

Fumigant toxicity of plant essential oils against Camptomyia corticalis (Diptera: Cecidomyiidae), Kim JR, Haribalan P, Son BK, Ahn YJ, *Journal of Economic Entomology*, 2012

Field evaluation of essential oils for reducing attraction by the Japanese beetle (Coleoptera: Scarabaeidae), Youssef NN, Oliver JB, Ranger CM, Reding ME, Moyseenko JJ, Klein MG, Pappas RS, *Journal of Economic Entomology*, 2009

Essential oils and their compositions as spatial repellents for pestiferous social wasps, Zhang QH, Schnidmiller RG, Hoover DR, *Pest Management Science*, 2013

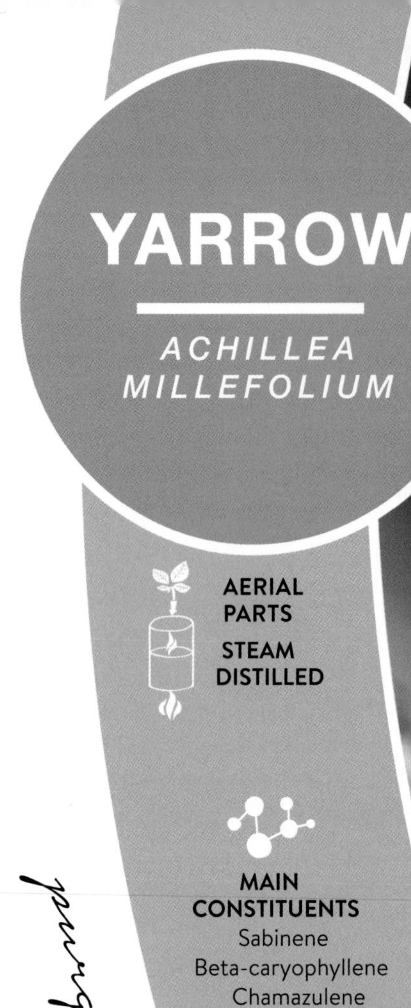

YARROW

ACHILLEA MILLEFOLIUM

AERIAL PARTS

STEAM DISTILLED

MAIN CONSTITUENTS
Sabinene
Beta-caryophyllene
Chamazulene

TOP PROPERTIES
Antihemorrhagic
Anti-rheumatic
Antiviral
Emmenagogue
Regenerative

purging • relieving • mending

SINGLE OILS

TOP USES

BLEEDING, HEMORRHAGING, INTERNAL WOUNDS & SCARRING
Take in a capsule or in water.

VARICOSE VEINS & HEMORRHOIDS, SAGGING & AGING SKIN
Apply with carrier oil to affected area. Add a hot compress to take deeper.

IRREGULAR OR ABSENT MENSTRUATION & EARLY MENOPAUSE
Apply to abdomen, drop in a sitz bath, and/or take in a capsule.

DEPRESSION, ANXIETY & FATIGUE
Inhale from cupped hands, apply under nose, and/or bottoms of feet.

PAIN & INFLAMMATION, ARTHRITIS, RHEUMATISM
Apply to area of concern, or take in a capsule.

FEVER, VIRAL INFECTION & ALLERGIES
Take in a capsule, apply to bottoms of feet and/or along spine.

LOW PERSPIRATION & POOR CIRCULATION
Apply to bottoms of feet or area of concern. Use in a steam bath to promote sweating and release toxins.

CANCER, FREE RADICAL DAMAGE, CELLULAR OVARIAN HEALTH
Take in a capsule or in water for antioxidant qualities.

ACNE, ECZEMA, HAIR LOSS & SCALP ISSUES
Apply to area of concern or add to skin or hair care products.

SLUGGISH LIVER, STOMACH & INTESTINES
Take in a capsule or massage into abdomen.

TOOTHACHE & LOOSENED TEETH
Apply to gums and teeth.

INDIGESTION, BELCHING, BLOATING, & ULCERS
Take in a capsule or massage into abdomen.

MUSCLE & RESPIRATORY SPASMS
Apply to area of concern.

METABOLIC DISORDERS & BLOOD SUGAR IMBALANCE
Take 1-2 drops am and pm.

EMOTIONAL BALANCE
Use aromatically and topically to get from Invaded ⟶ Shielded.

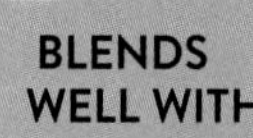

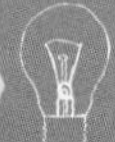

In ancient Greece, Achilles was said to use yarrow to ease a painful Achilles tendon.

BLENDS WELL WITH
Clary sage
Cypress
Helichrysum
Rosemary
Ylang ylang

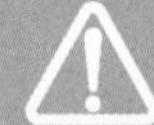

SAFETY
Dilution recommended. Possible skin sensitivity. May stain surfaces, fabric, and skin.

RESEARCH: Chamazulene carboxylic acid and matricin: a natural profen and its natural prodrug, identified through similarity to synthetic drug substances, Ramadan M, Goeters S, Watzer B, Krause E, Lohmann K, Bauer R, Hempel B, Imming P, *Journal of Natural Products,* 2006

Comparative evaluation of 11 essential oils of different origin as functional antioxidants, antiradicals and antimicrobials in foods, Sacchetti G, Maietti S, Muzzoli M, Scaglianti M, Manfredini S, Radice M, Bruni R, *Food Chemistry,* 2005

calming · floral · soothing

YLANG YLANG

CANANGA ODORATA

TOP USES

LOW LIBIDO, IMPOTENCE, INFERTILITY & HORMONE IMBALANCE
Apply (T) to abdomen, pulse points, or take (I) under tongue, or in a capsule.

EQUILIBRIUM & HIGH BLOOD PRESSURE,
Apply (T) to back of neck, across forehead, and behind ears. Inhale (A) from cupped hands, take (I) under tongue, or in a capsule.

IRREGULAR HEARTBEAT & PALPITATIONS
Apply (T) to bottoms of feet and over the heart. Inhale (A) from cupped hands.

ADRENAL, MENTAL, OR HEART FATIGUE/ LOSS OF WILL OR APATHY
Apply (T) on affected area or take (I) in a capsule.

ANXIETY, FRUSTRATION, STRESS & FEAR
Diffuse or inhale (A) from cupped hands and apply (T) under nose or to bottoms of feet.

HAIR LOSS
Massage (T) into scalp to stimulate hair growth.

COLIC & STOMACH ACHE
Apply (T) diluted to abdomen or take (I) in a capsule.

OILY SKIN
Apply (T) to oily skin or take (I) in a capsule.

EMOTIONAL BALANCE
Use (A) aromatically and (T) topically to get from Burdened ———> Exuberant.

(A) = Aromatically (T) = Topically (I) = Internally

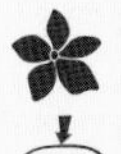

FLOWERS

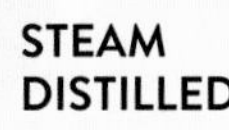

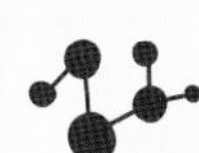

STEAM DISTILLED

MAIN CONSTITUENTS
Germacrene
Caryophyllene
a-farnesene

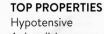

TOP PROPERTIES
Hypotensive
Aphrodisiac
Antispasmodic
Sedative

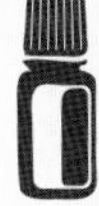

FOUND IN
InTune®
Serenity®
Elevation™
ClaryCalm®
Whisper®
TerraShield®

BLENDS WELL WITH
Bergamot
Frankincense
Manuka
Sandalwood
Yarrow

SAFETY
Safe for NEAT application.

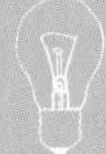

In Java, ylang ylang flowers adorn the newlyweds' bed and are often used as an aphrodisiac.

RESEARCH: Relaxing Effect of Ylang ylang Oil on Humans after Transdermal Absorption, Hongratanaworakit T, Buchbauer G, *Phytotherapy Research*, 2006

Safety assessment of Ylang-Ylang (Cananga spp.) as a food ingredient., Burdock GA, Carabin IG, *Food and Chemical Toxicology*, 2008

Effects of Ylang-Ylang aroma on blood pressure and heart rate in healthy men, Jung DJ, Cha JY, Kim SE, Ko IG, Jee YS, *Journal of Exercise Rehabilitation*, 2013

Evaluation of the harmonizing effect of ylang-ylang oil on humans after inhalation, Hongratanaworakit T, Buchbauer G, *Planta Medica*, 2004

Essential oil inhalation on blood pressure and salivary cortisol levels in prehypertensive and hypertensive subjects, Kim IH, Kim C, Seong K, Hur MH, Lim HM, Lee MS, *Evidence-Based Complementary and Alternative Medicine*, 2012

The Effects of Herbal Essential Oils on the Oviposition-deterrent and Ovicidal Activities of Aedes aegypti (Linn.), Anopheles dirus (Peyton and Harrison) and Culex quinquefasciatus (Say), Siriporn P, Mayura S, *Tropical Biomedicine*, 2012

Evaluation of the Effects of Plant-derived Essential Oils on Central Nervous System Function Using Discrete Shuttle-type Conditioned Avoidance Response in Mice, Umezu T., *Phytotherapy Research*, 2012

Effects of aromatherapy on changes in the autonomic nervous system, aortic pulse wave velocity and aortic augmentation index in patients with essential hypertension, Cha JH, Lee SH, Yoo YS, *Journal of Korean Academy of Nursing*, 2010

OIL BLENDS

While many companies provide blends of essential oils, the proprietary blends found in this book have been carefully and artistically crafted to offer superior efficacy and therapeutic benefits. Because natural chemistry is a crucial point of attention in the art of blending essential oils, it is important to turn to blends that possess qualities of highest purity, potency, and complementary relationships between the individual oils that comprise the blend.

Please note the symbols (=aromatic =topical =internal) that specify recommended usage. While all oils are meant to be used aromatically, and most topically, only verified pure therapeutic essential oils are intended for internal use. (See *"Why Quality Matters,"* pg. 13 and *"How to Use Essential Oils"* pg. 16 for further detail.)

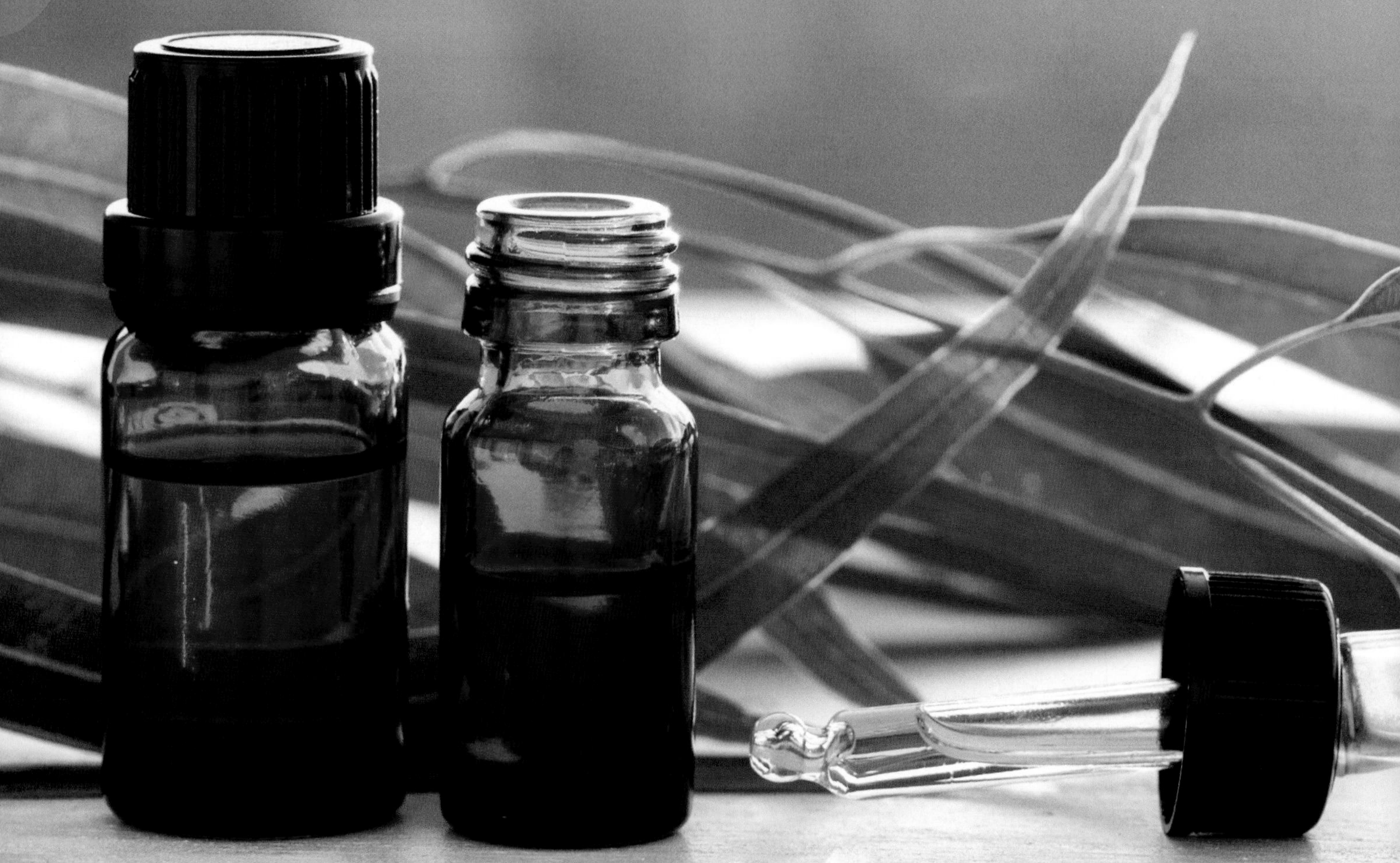

relieving • centering • enlivening

ADAPTIV®

CALMING BLEND

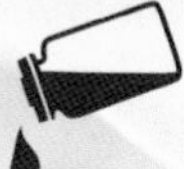

MAIN INGREDIENTS
Wild orange
Lavender
Copaiba
Spearmint
Magnolia
Rosemary
Neroli
Sweetgum

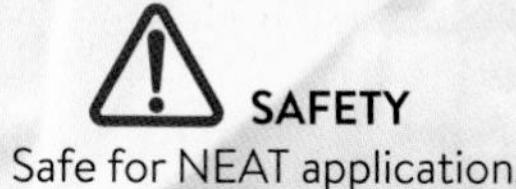

Safe for NEAT application.

TOP USES

CHAOTIC ENVIRONMENTS & SITUATIONS, LACK OF TRANQUILITY
Diffuse and apply to bottoms of feet.

LOSS OF COMPOSURE, POOR COPING CAPACITY & ANXIETY
Diffuse and apply up spine and back of neck, and to bottoms of feet.

MENSTRUATION & MENOPAUSE-RELATED MOODINESS & DEPRESSION
Apply to abdomen, reflex points for ovaries, and to bottoms of feet.

ADDICTIVE & COMPULSIVE OR OBSESSIVE BEHAVIORS, OVERTHINKING
Diffuse and apply over liver and to bottoms of feet.

LACK OF MOTIVATION & MENTAL FATIGUE
Diffuse and apply to back of neck.

LACK OF FOCUS & CONCENTRATION, INABILITY TO STAY ON TASK, RESTLESSNESS
Apply to back of neck, across forehead, and to bottoms of feet as needed.

UPSET BABY, COLIC
Diffuse and apply diluted in circular motion on abdomen and/or to bottoms of feet.

TIRED, ACHY OR WEAKENED MUSCLES, GROWING PAINS
Apply on area(s) of concern. Repeat 2-4x's per day.

LOSS OF SENSE OF SMELL
Apply to back of neck and across forehead.

WRINKLES, SKIN BREAKOUTS & IRRITATIONS
Apply to area(s) of concern and/or add to moisturizer for daily use.

BRAIN, ALZHEIMER'S DISEASE, ELEVATED CORTISOL LEVELS
Apply to back of neck, bottoms of feet and area(s) of concern.

PERFUME
Wear to enhance mood and promote relaxation and euphoria.

Sweet gum, a lesser known essential oil with its sweet forest-like aroma, has a chemical composition reminiscent of a mixture of copaiba, frankincense, and Douglas fir.

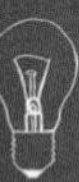

= Aromatically = Topically = Internally

strengthening • woody • fearless

AMAVI®

MEN'S FORTIFYING BLEND

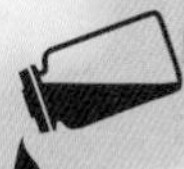

MAIN INGREDIENTS
Buddha wood
Balsam fir
Black pepper
Hinoki
Patchouli
Cocoa extract

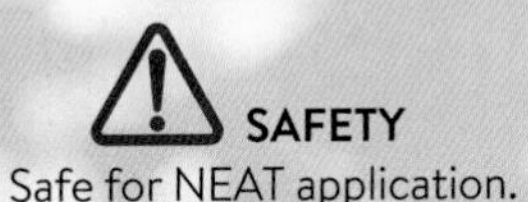

Safe for NEAT application.

TOP USES

DISCOURAGED, ENRAGED, AGITATED & IRRITATED
Diffuse. Apply over heart, to back of neck, spine, and/or bottoms of feet.

CALM, GROUNDED & RELAXED
Diffuse. Apply to pulse points and/or bottoms of feet.

FOCUSED HEART, MIND & BODY
Diffuse. Apply over heart, to forehead, and/or bottoms of feet.

MENTAL CLARITY, MEDITATION & TRANQUILITY
Diffuse. Apply to forehead, over heart, and bottoms of feet.

COLOGNE
Apply to pulse points, neck, and behind ears.

WOMEN'S PERFUME
Blend with jasmine or Beautiful®. Apply to pulse points, back of neck, or behind ears.

Replacing colognes that are made using synthetic chemicals with essential oils is a great way to choose to live a healthier lifestyle.

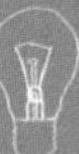

relieving
renewing
circulating

AROMATOUCH®

MASSAGE BLEND

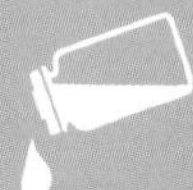

MAIN INGREDIENTS
Cypress
Peppermint
Marjoram
Basil
Grapefruit
Lavender

SAFETY
Avoid exposure to sunlight or UV rays for up to 12 hours after application.

TOP USES

MUSCLE ACHES & ARTHRITIS
Apply Ⓣ to area(s) of concern.

HEADACHE, NECK & BACK PAIN
Apply Ⓣ to neck, shoulders, and along spine.

NEUROPATHY & RESTLESS LEG SYNDROME
Apply Ⓣ to area(s) of concern to stimulate nerves and circulation.

CONNECTIVE TISSUE & LIGAMENT SUPPORT
Apply Ⓣ to area(s) of concern.

LYMPHATIC SUPPORT
Apply Ⓣ to bottoms of feet.

HIGH BLOOD PRESSURE
Apply Ⓣ to bottoms of feet.

POOR CIRCULATION & COLD EXTREMITIES
Apply Ⓣ to area(s) of concern.

MUSCLE TENSION, SORENESS & CRAMPS
Apply Ⓐ to area(s) of concern.

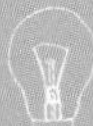

This blend encourages muscle tissue healing, relaxes and soothes muscles, and enhances blood flow.

Ⓐ = Aromatically Ⓣ = Topically Ⓘ = Internally

BALANCE®

GROUNDING BLEND

stabilizing • centering • sweet

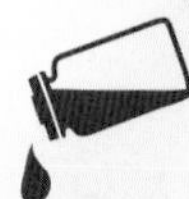

MAIN INGREDIENTS
Spruce
Ho wood
Frankincense
Blue tansy
Blue chamomile
Osmanthus

SAFETY
Safe for NEAT application.

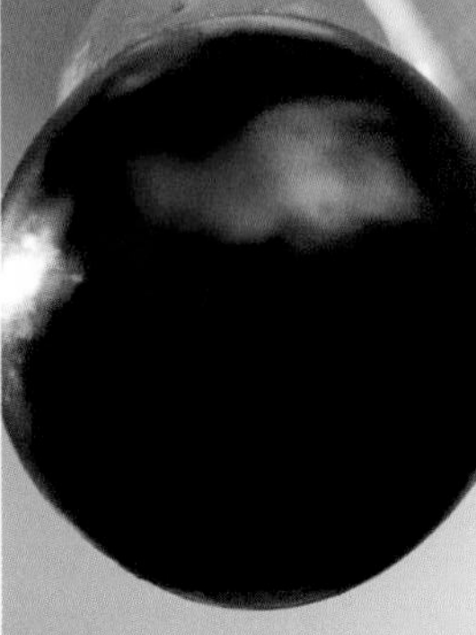

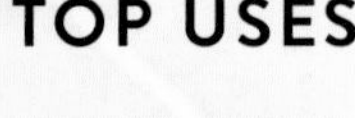

TOP USES

STRESS & ANXIETY
Apply to bottoms of feet and diffuse or inhale from cupped hands.

JET LAG & TRAVEL ANXIETY
Inhale from cupped hands or apply under nose.

MOOD SWINGS & STRESS
Diffuse, apply under nose, and/or back of neck.

NEUROLOGICAL CONDITIONS
Apply to back of neck, pulse points, or bottoms of feet.

CONVULSIONS, EPILEPSY & PARKINSON'S
Apply to back of neck, along spine, and/or bottoms of feet.

TRANQUILITY & MEDITATION
Apply under nose, across forehead or inhale from cupped hands.

ANGER & RAGE
Diffuse, apply under nose, or back of neck.

FEAR, GRIEF & TRAUMA
Diffuse, apply under nose or back of neck.

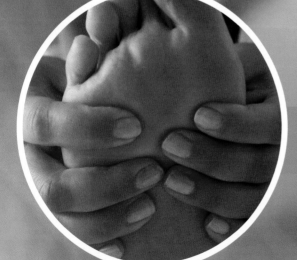

Life's little surprises and stress can leave us off guard and unbalanced. This blend helps to restore and ground us.

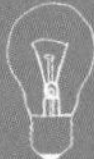

BEAUTIFUL®

CAPTIVATING BLEND

alluring
exquisite
lovely

TOP USES

ENERGIZING, UPLIFTING MOOD & ENVIRONMENT
Diffuse. Apply to pulse points, back of neck, along spine, and/or bottoms of feet.

CALM, SUPPORTED & RELAXED
Diffuse. Apply to pulse points, back of neck, along spine, and/or bottoms of feet.

FOCUSED HEART, MIND & BODY
Diffuse. Apply to pulse points, back of neck, along spine, and/or bottoms of feet.

EMPOWERED, MEDITATION & TRANQUILITY
Diffuse. Apply to pulse points, back of neck, along spine, and/or bottoms of feet.

BE TRUE TO SELF
Diffuse. Apply to pulse points, back of neck, along spine, and/or bottoms of feet.

MAGNIFY YOUR RADIANCE IN FEMININE ENERGY
Diffuse. Apply to pulse points, back of neck, along spine, and/or bottoms of feet.

PERFUME
Apply to pulse points, chest, back of neck, and behind ears.

Replace synthetic perfumes with natural essential oils to support a healthier lifestyle and hormones.

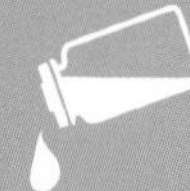

MAIN INGREDIENTS
Lime
Osmanthus
Bergamot
Frankincense

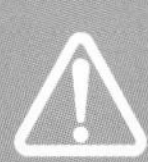

SAFETY
Safe for NEAT application. Avoid exposure to sunlight or UV rays for up to 12 hours after application.

OIL BLENDS

= Aromatically = Topically = Internally

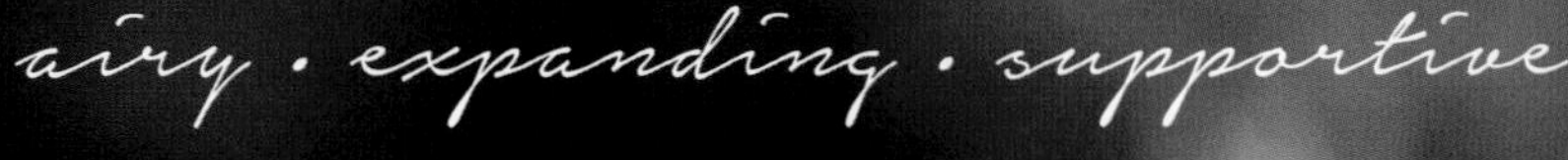

BREATHE®

RESPIRATION BLEND

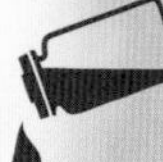

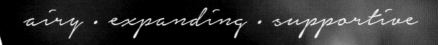

MAIN INGREDIENTS
Laurel
Peppermint
Eucalyptus
Melaleuca (Tea tree)
Lemon
Cardamom
Ravintsara
Ravensara

SAFETY
Dilution recommended. Possible skin sensitivity. Avoid exposure to sunlight or UV rays for up to 12 hours after application.

TOP USES

PNEUMONIA & ASTHMA
Diffuse or apply under nose and on chest.

ALLERGIES
Inhale from cupped hands or apply under nose.

COUGH & CONGESTION
Diffuse or apply under or over bridge of nose, and to chest.

BRONCHITIS & INFLUENZA
Diffuse and/or apply to chest.

SINUSITIS & NASAL POLYPS
Apply across or under nose.

SLEEP ISSUES
Diffuse with lavender and/or apply to bottoms of feet.

CONSTRICTED BREATHING
Diffuse and apply to chest.

EXERCISE-INDUCED ASTHMA
Diffuse and apply to chest.

Healthy airflow and oxygen supply bring life and energy with each breath. Enjoy a restful sleep with this blend.

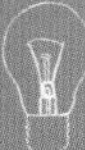

gladdening
illuminating
resilient

CHEER®

UPLIFTING BLEND

TOP USES

DEPRESSION & DISCOURAGEMENT
Diffuse (A), inhale from cupped hands, apply (T) to pulse points, under nose and/or across forehead.

HYSTERIA & ANXIETY
Diffuse (A), inhale from cupped hands, apply (T) to pulse points, under nose and/or across forehead.

DISCONNECTION
Diffuse (A), inhale from cupped hands, apply (T) to pulse points, under nose and/or across forehead.

PMS
Diffuse (A), inhale from cupped hands, apply (T) to pulse points, under nose and/or across forehead.

CELLULAR HEALTH
Apply (T) to bottoms of feet.

INFLAMMATION & STIFFNESS
Apply (T) diluted to affected area.

INDIGESTION & IRRITABLE BOWELS
Apply (T) diluted to abdomen and bottoms of feet.

BLOOD SUGAR & CHOLESTEROL
Apply (T) diluted to bottoms of feet, back of neck, or chest.

Go from discouraged, distressed or disinterested to an uplifted and resilient state of mind with this blend.

MAIN INGREDIENTS
Wild orange
Clove
Star anise
Lemon myrtle
Nutmeg
Vanilla bean extract
Ginger
Cinnamon
Zdravetz

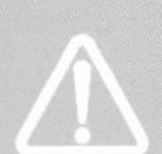

SAFETY
Safe for NEAT application. Avoid exposure to sunlight or UV rays for up to 12 hours after application.

CHILDREN'S BRAVE™

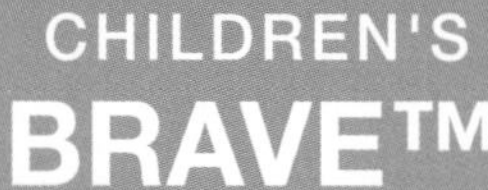

COURAGE BLEND

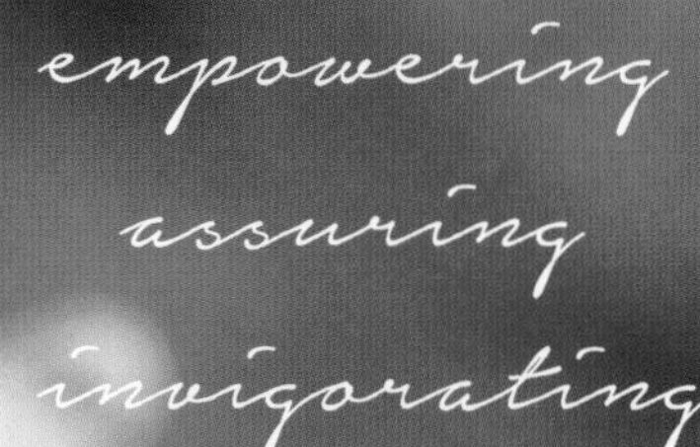

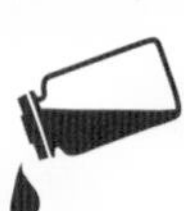

MAIN INGREDIENTS
Wild orange
Amyris
Osmanthus
Cinnamon

SAFETY
Safe for NEAT application. Avoid sunlight or UV rays to applied area for up to 12 hours.

TOP USES

DISCOURAGED & UNENTHUSED
Apply under nose, to back of neck, over heart, and/or bottoms of feet.

TIRED & WEARY
Apply under nose, to back of neck, forehead, and/or bottoms of feet.

LACK OF DETERMINATION & CONVICTION
Apply under nose, along spine, over heart, and/or bottoms of feet.

AFRAID & SCARED
Apply under nose, to back of neck, along spine, and/or bottoms of feet.

LACK OF CONFIDENCE & MOTIVATION
Apply under nose, to chest, back, and/or bottoms of feet.

CONFUSED & OVERWHELMED
Apply under nose, to back of neck, and forehead.

DIGESTIVE UPSET, NERVOUS & AGITATED
Apply to abdomen, forehead, and/or bottoms of feet.

ACHES & PAINS
Apply to area(s) of concern.

Children's blends are uniquely formulated to offer younger users a positive essential oil introduction by using m aromas and careful plant selection to avoid unnecessary sensitiza immature, thin skin and smaller bodies. Intentional early introduc the perfect way to empower children to safely learn personal appl methods and experience the power of healthy, nurturing tc and gentle massage with caregivers.

pacifying
relaxing
unwinding

CHILDREN'S

CALMER™

RESTFUL BLEND

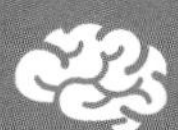

TOP USES

UNSETTLED & RESTLESS, SLEEP ISSUES
Apply (T) under nose and to bottoms of feet.

STRESSED & ANXIOUS
Apply (T) under nose, to back of neck, and forehead.

FUSSY, EASILY UPSET & STARTLED
Apply (T) to chest, and/or bottoms of feet.

UPTIGHT & WOUND UP, MOODY
Apply (T) under nose and across forehead or inhale (A) deeply from cupped hands.

MUSCLE ACHES & GROWING PAINS
Apply (T) to area(s) of concern.

ANGRY, AGITATED & IRRITABLE
Apply (T) to bottoms of feet and spine.

BATH & BEDTIME ROUTINE
Apply (T) under nose, to forehead, and bottoms of feet. Relax in warm bath.

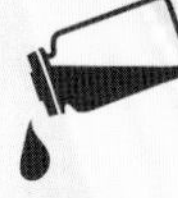

MAIN INGREDIENTS
Lavender
Cananga
Buddha wood
Roman chamomile

SAFETY
Safe for NEAT application.

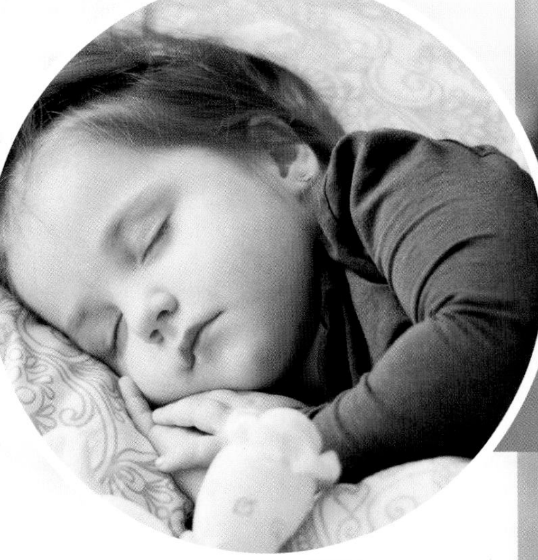

Children's blends are uniquely formulated to offer younger users a positive essential oil introduction by using milder aromas and careful plant selection to avoid unnecessary sensitization in immature, thin skin and smaller bodies. Intentional early introduction is the perfect way to empower children to safely learn personal application methods and experience the power of healthy, nurturing touch and gentle massage with caregivers.

(A) = Aromatically (T) = Topically (I) = Internally

CHILDREN'S

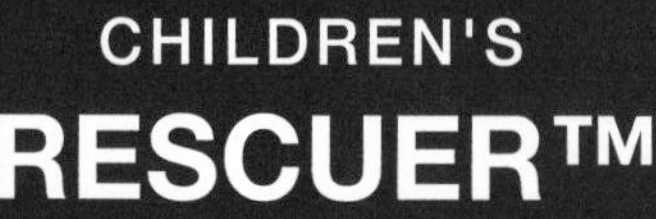

RESCUER™

SOOTHING BLEND

alleviating
calming
comforting

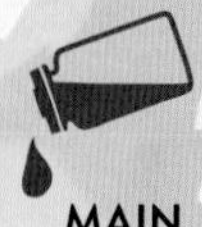

MAIN INGREDIENTS
Copaiba
Lavender
Spearmint
Zanthoxylum

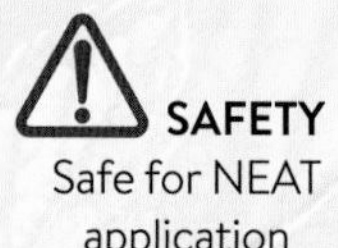

SAFETY
Safe for NEAT application

TOP USES

SHOCK, DISTRESS & FEAR
Apply under nose, back of neck, forehead, and/or bottoms of feet.

MUSCLE ACHES & TENSION
Apply to area(s) of concern.

GROWING PAINS
Apply to area(s) of concern.

HEADACHE, MIGRAINES & NECK PAIN
Apply to back of neck, forehead/temples, and shoulders.

BRUISES & INJURIES
Apply to area(s) of concern.

BATH & BEDTIME ROUTINE
Apply to area(s) of concern and bottoms of feet. Relax in warm bath.

Children's blends are uniquely formulated to offer younger users a positive essential oil introduction by using milder aromas and careful plant selection to avoid unnecessary sensitization in immature, thin skin and smaller bodies. Intentional early introduction is the perfect way to empower children to safely learn personal application methods and experience the power of healthy, nurturing touch and gentle massage with caregivers.

balancing
steadying
quieting

CHILDREN'S STEADY™

GROUNDING BLEND

TOP USES

UNCOOPERATIVE & OBSTINATE, OUT OF CONTROL
Apply to chest, forehead, and/or bottoms of feet.

OVERSTIMULATED & OVERWHELMED
Apply under nose, to back of neck, and forehead.

DISCONNECTED FROM THE EARTH & REALITY
Apply under nose, and/or to bottoms of feet.

FOCUS ISSUES & MOOD SWINGS
Apply under nose, over heart, and/or to forehead.

RESTLESS & WOUND UP
Apply under nose, to back of neck, along spine, and/or bottoms of feet.

ANGER & FRUSTRATION, TANTRUMS
Apply under nose, to back of neck, along spine, over heart, and/or bottoms of feet.

GRIEF & SADNESS, DISAPPOINTMENT
Apply under nose, to chest, forehead, and/or bottoms of feet.

BATH & BEDTIME ROUTINE
Apply to bottoms of feet. Relax in warm bath.

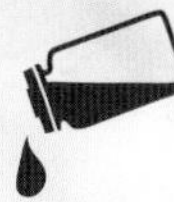

MAIN INGREDIENTS
Amyris
Balsam fir
Coriander
Magnolia

SAFETY
Safe for NEAT application.

Children's blends are uniquely formulated to offer younger users a positive essential oil introduction by using milder aromas and careful plant selection to avoid unnecessary sensitization in immature, thin skin and smaller bodies. Intentional early introduction is the perfect way to empower children to safely learn personal application methods and experience the power of healthy, nurturing touch and gentle massage with caregivers.

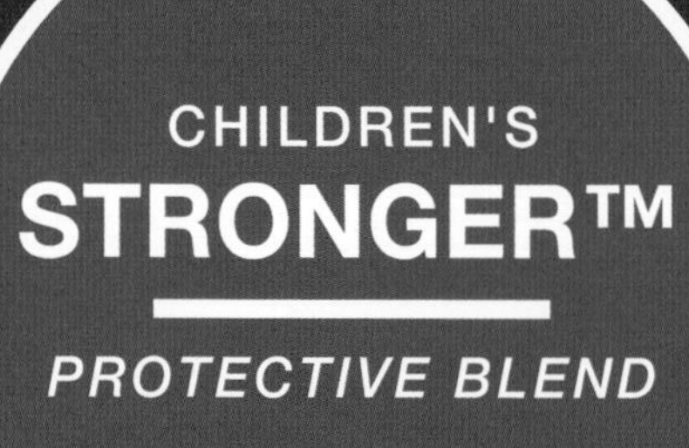

CHILDREN'S STRONGER™

PROTECTIVE BLEND

fortifying • shielding • b

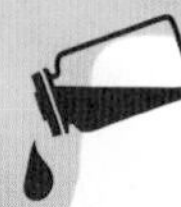

MAIN INGREDIENTS
Cedarwood
Litsea
Frankincense
Rose

SAFETY
Safe for NEAT application.

TOP USES

BACTERIA & VIRUSES, AIRBORNE PATHOGENS
Apply to areas of concern and bottoms of feet.

FLU, WEAK IMMUNITY, POOR RECOVERY
Apply under nose, over heart, along spine, and/or bottoms of feet.

EMOTIONAL DISTRESS & POOR BOUNDARIES
Inhale deeply from cupped hands. Apply to bottoms of feet.

STAPH, STREP THROAT & COUGH
Apply to throat/neck, chest, along spine, and/or bottoms of feet.

COLD SORES, WARTS & INFECTED WOUNDS
Apply to area(s) of concern.

CUTS & SCRAPES
Apply to area(s) of concern.

FUNGUS & PARASITES
Apply to area(s) of concern, over abdomen, along spine, and bottoms of feet.

CHRONIC FATIGUE & AUTOIMMUNE DISEASE
Apply to chest, back, and/or bottoms of feet.

Children's blends are uniquely formulated to offer younger users a positive essential oil introduction by using mi aromas and careful plant selection to avoid unnecessary sensitiza immature, thin skin and smaller bodies. Intentional early introduc the perfect way to empower children to safely learn personal appli methods and experience the power of healthy, nurturing to and gentle massage with caregivers.

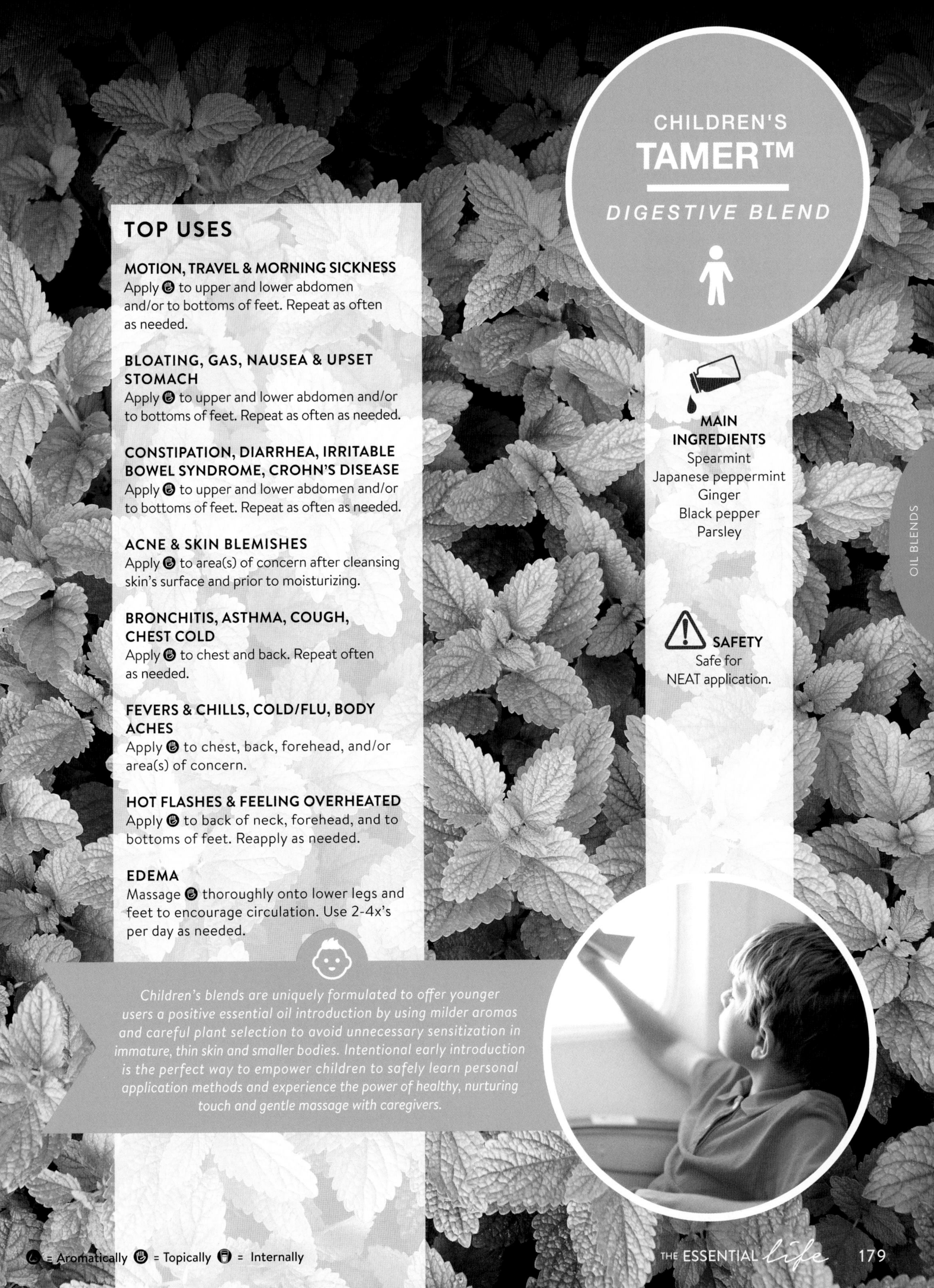

CHILDREN'S
TAMER™
DIGESTIVE BLEND

TOP USES

MOTION, TRAVEL & MORNING SICKNESS
Apply to upper and lower abdomen and/or to bottoms of feet. Repeat as often as needed.

BLOATING, GAS, NAUSEA & UPSET STOMACH
Apply to upper and lower abdomen and/or to bottoms of feet. Repeat as often as needed.

CONSTIPATION, DIARRHEA, IRRITABLE BOWEL SYNDROME, CROHN'S DISEASE
Apply to upper and lower abdomen and/or to bottoms of feet. Repeat as often as needed.

ACNE & SKIN BLEMISHES
Apply to area(s) of concern after cleansing skin's surface and prior to moisturizing.

BRONCHITIS, ASTHMA, COUGH, CHEST COLD
Apply to chest and back. Repeat often as needed.

FEVERS & CHILLS, COLD/FLU, BODY ACHES
Apply to chest, back, forehead, and/or area(s) of concern.

HOT FLASHES & FEELING OVERHEATED
Apply to back of neck, forehead, and to bottoms of feet. Reapply as needed.

EDEMA
Massage thoroughly onto lower legs and feet to encourage circulation. Use 2-4x's per day as needed.

MAIN INGREDIENTS
Spearmint
Japanese peppermint
Ginger
Black pepper
Parsley

SAFETY
Safe for NEAT application.

OIL BLENDS

Children's blends are uniquely formulated to offer younger users a positive essential oil introduction by using milder aromas and careful plant selection to avoid unnecessary sensitization in immature, thin skin and smaller bodies. Intentional early introduction is the perfect way to empower children to safely learn personal application methods and experience the power of healthy, nurturing touch and gentle massage with caregivers.

= Aromatically = Topically = Internally

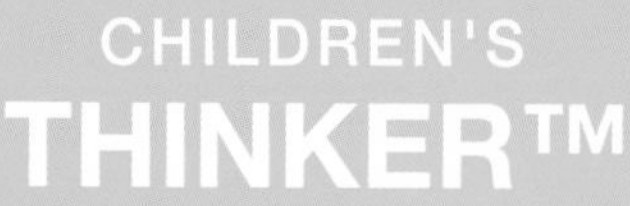

CHILDREN'S THINKER™

FOCUS BLEND

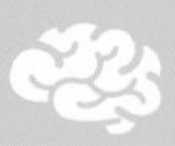

Children's blends are uniquely formulated to offer younger users a positive essential oil introduction by using milder aromas and careful plant selection to avoid unnecessary sensitization in immature, thin skin and smaller bodies. Intentional early introduction is the perfect way to empower children to safely learn personal application methods and experience the power of healthy, nurturing touch and gentle massage with caregivers.

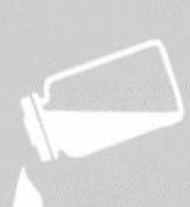

MAIN INGREDIENTS
Vetiver
Peppermint
Clementine
Rosemary

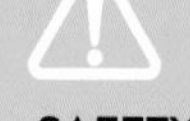

SAFETY
Safe for NEAT application. Avoid sunlight or UV rays to applied area for up to 12 hours.

anchoring · enlivening · signaling

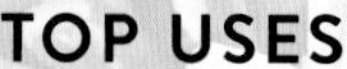

TOP USES

ADD / ADHD, HYPERACTIVITY
Apply under nose, to forehead, along spine, back of neck, and/or bottoms of feet.

OVER & UNDERACTIVE BRAIN
Apply under nose, to forehead, along spine, back of neck, and/or bottoms of feet.

LACK OF MENTAL CLARITY, FOCUS & CONCENTRATION
Apply under nose, to forehead, along spine, back of neck, and/or bottoms of feet.

OVERWHELMED & OVERTHINKING
Apply under nose, to forehead, along spine, back of neck, and/or bottoms of feet.

STRESSED OUT & UNGROUNDED
Apply under nose, to forehead, along spine, back of neck, and/or bottoms of feet.

NERVOUS, ANXIOUS & MOODY
Apply under nose, to chest, along spine, back of neck, and/or bottoms of feet.

AFTERNOON SLUMP & DISCONNECTED
Apply under nose, to chest, along spine, and/or bottoms of feet.

SEIZURES
Apply under nose, to forehead, along spine, back of neck, and/or bottoms of feet.

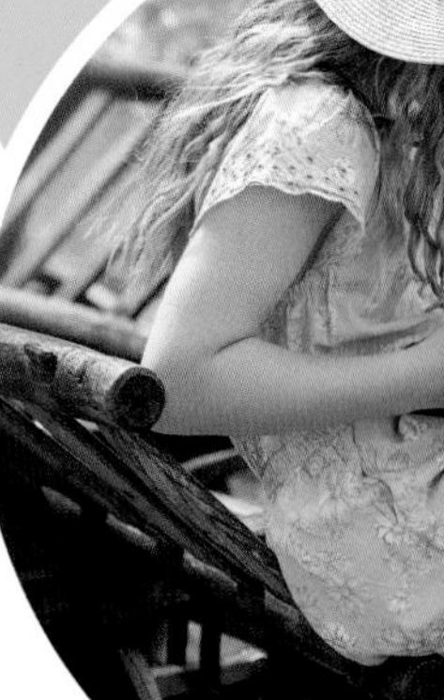

alleviating
pacifying
easing

CITRUS BLISS®

INVIGORATING BLEND

TOP USES

LOW ENERGY & EXHAUSTION
Diffuse Ⓐ, apply Ⓣ under nose, and/or back of neck to energize and uplift.

STRESS, ANXIETY & DEPRESSION
Diffuse Ⓐ, apply Ⓣ under nose, and/or back of neck.

AIR FRESHENER
Diffuse Ⓐ to clear air of odors and uplift.

ANTISEPTIC CLEANER
Mix with water in a glass bottle and apply to surfaces.

EATING DISORDERS
Diffuse Ⓐ, or inhale from cupped hands, or apply Ⓣ to abdomen.

PERFUME
Apply Ⓣ to pulse points as desired.

LAUNDRY
Add 2-4 drops to rinse cycle to freshen and kill germs.

LYMPHATIC & IMMUNE BOOST
Diffuse Ⓐ, apply Ⓣ under nose, and/or back of neck.

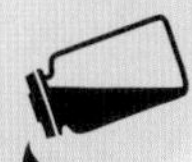

MAIN INGREDIENTS
Wild orange
Lemon
Grapefruit
Mandarin
Bergamot
Tangerine
Clementine
Vanilla bean absolute

SAFETY
Avoid exposure to sunlight or UV rays for up to 12 hours after application.

When you pause to uplift and invigorate your senses with this blend of citrus essential oils, you will find increased energy and zest for life.

Ⓐ = Aromatically Ⓣ = Topically Ⓘ = Internally

CLARYCALM®

WOMEN'S MONTHLY BLEND

floral • warm • calming

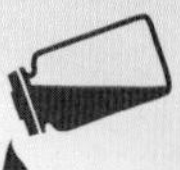

MAIN INGREDIENTS
Clary sage
Lavender
Bergamot
Roman chamomile
Ylang ylang
Cedarwood
Geranium
Fennel
Carrot
Palmarosa
Vitex

SAFETY
Safe for NEAT application. Avoid exposure to sunlight or UV rays for up to 12 hours after application.

This gentle and safe blend brings harmony by balancing and stabilizing hormones.

TOP USES

HORMONE BALANCING
Apply to back of neck, abdomen, and/or bottoms of feet.

HEAVY PERIODS, PMS & CRAMPS
Apply to abdomen, back of neck, and/or bottoms of feet.

PRE & PERIMENOPAUSE
Apply to abdomen, back of neck, and/or bottoms of feet.

HOT FLASHES
Apply to abdomen and/or back of neck.

MOOD SWINGS
Apply to abdomen, back of neck, chest, and/or bottoms of feet.

SKIN ISSUES & WOUNDS
Apply to area(s) of concern.

SEX DRIVE & LOW LIBIDO
Apply to abdomen.

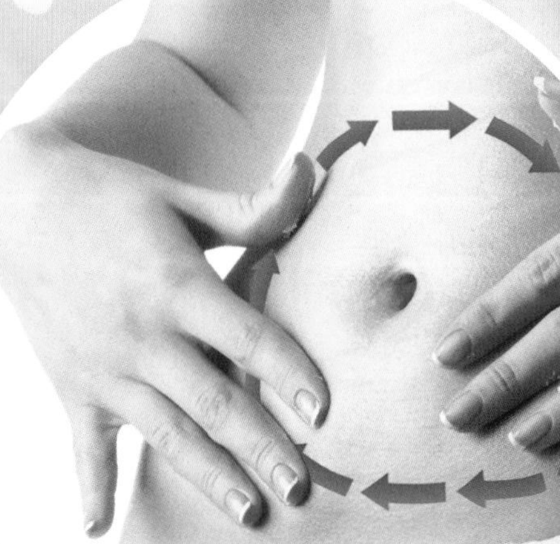

asustaining
reconciling
alleviatin

CONSOLE®

COMFORTING BLEND

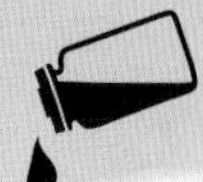

MAIN INGREDIENTS
Frankincense
Patchouli
Ylang ylang
Laudanum
Amyris
Sandalwood
Rose
Osmanthus

SAFETY
Avoid exposure to sunlight or UV rays for up to 12 hours after application.

TOP USES

GRIEF & SADNESS
Diffuse or apply under nose and to chest.

EMOTIONAL RELEASE & REASSURANCE
Diffuse and apply under nose and over heart.

FEAR & EMOTIONAL PAIN RELIEF
Diffuse or apply under nose and to chest.

BRAIN IMPAIRMENT
Apply to forehead, back of neck, and toes.

SPIRITUAL CONNECTIVITY & MEDITATION
Apply to forehead and chest and inhale from cupped hands.

LOW LIBIDO
Diffuse or apply to abdomen.

SKIN REPAIR & ANTI-AGING
Apply to affected area with carrier oil.

LUNG & BRONCHIAL INFECTION
Apply to chest, bottoms of feet, and/or diffuse.

URINARY INFECTION, EDEMA & CONSTIPATION
Apply over abdomen or to bottoms of feet.

IRREGULAR & RACING HEARTBEAT
Apply under nose and to chest.

When the loss of something loved or treasured occurs, use this blend to comfort through sadness or grief and move forward in life.

= Aromatically = Topically = Internally

OIL BLENDS

DDR® PRIME

CELLULAR COMPLEX BLEND

regenerating
corrective
repairing

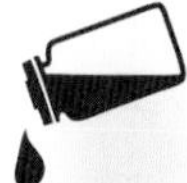

MAIN INGREDIENTS
Frankincense
Wild orange
Litsea
Thyme
Clove
Summer savory
Niaouli
Lemongrass

SAFETY
Dilution recommended. Possible skin sensitivity. Avoid exposure to sunlight or UV rays for up to 12 hours after application.

TOP USES

CANCER & TUMORS
Apply diluted to back of neck, along spine, or bottoms of feet. Take in a capsule.

ESTROGEN, PROGESTERONE, & THYROID ISSUES
Take in a capsule or apply to bottoms of feet.

CANDIDA & FUNGAL ISSUES
Apply to bottoms of feet or take in a capsule.

NERVE DAMAGE
Apply diluted to back of neck, along spine, or bottoms of feet. Take in a capsule.

AUTOIMMUNE DISORDERS
Apply diluted to back of neck, along spine, or bottoms of feet. Take in a capsule.

SEIZURES & AGING BRAIN
Apply diluted to back of neck, along spine, or bottoms of feet. Take in a capsule for antioxidant power.

BREAST ISSUES
Apply diluted to breasts, bottoms of feet, or take in a capsule.

HOT FLASHES & NIGHT SWEATS
Apply to bottoms of feet or take in a capsule.

DETOX & VIRUSES
Apply to bottoms of feet or take in a capsule.

INFLAMMATION ISSUES
Apply diluted to area of concern.

Cellular damage from free radicals is an underlying contributor to many of today's illnesses. This powerful antioxidant blend will protect your cellular health as it protects your long-term wellness.

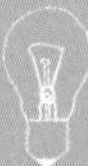

minty
athletic
cooling

DEEP BLUE®

SOOTHING BLEND

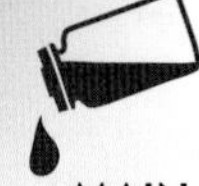

MAIN INGREDIENTS
Wintergreen
Camphor
Peppermint
Ylang ylang
Helichrysum
Blue tansy
Blue chamomile
Osmanthus

SAFETY
Safe for NEAT application.
Possible skin sensitivity.

TOP USES

MUSCLE, BACK & JOINT PAIN
Apply Ⓣ to area(s) of discomfort.

ARTHRITIS & ACHES
Apply Ⓣ to area(s) of discomfort.

NEUROPATHY & CARPAL TUNNEL
Apply Ⓣ to area(s) of discomfort.

FIBROMYALGIA & LUPUS
Apply Ⓣ to area(s) of concern.

WHIPLASH & MUSCLE TENSION
Apply Ⓣ to area(s) of discomfort.

PRE- & POST-WORKOUT
Apply Ⓣ to area(s) of discomfort.

GROWING PAINS
Apply Ⓣ to affected area.

HEADACHE & NECK PAIN
Apply Ⓣ to back of neck, shoulders, and temples.

BRUISES & INJURIES
Apply Ⓣ to affected area to reduce inflammation and scar tissue.

A toxic-free substitute for topical ointments and creams. This blend naturally reduces pain and inflammation.

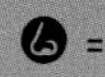 = Aromatically 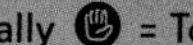 = Topically 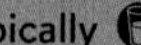 = Internally

supportive • soothing • settling

DIGESTZEN®

DIGESTION BLEND

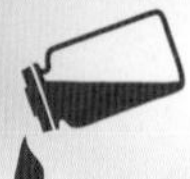

MAIN INGREDIENTS
Anise
Peppermint
Ginger
Caraway
Coriander
Tarragon
Fennel

SAFETY
Safe for NEAT application.

TOP USES

BLOATING, GAS, HEARTBURN, NAUSEA & INDIGESTION
Apply over abdomen and take in a capsule.

REFLUX & COLIC
Take in water or in a capsule with lemon.

DRY OR SORE THROAT
Drop directly onto back of throat.

MORNING SICKNESS & HEARTBURN
Apply to chest, pulse points, abdomen, and/or take in a glass of water.

MOTION & TRAVEL SICKNESS
Inhale, apply under nose or drink in water.

COLITIS & IRRITABLE BOWEL
Take in a capsule, in water, and/or massage into abdomen daily.

DIARRHEA & CONSTIPATION
Take in a capsule or in water until symptoms subside.

CROHN'S DISEASE & CHRONIC FATIGUE
Take in a capsule or rub on abdomen.

FOOD POISONING
Take in a capsule or in water frequently.

COUGH & SINUS CONGESTION
Apply diluted to navel and over bridge of nose or drink in water.

A regular cleansing regime helps ensure healthy kidney and liver function. Take 1-3 drops in a capsule, juice, or tea during first week of weight loss program.

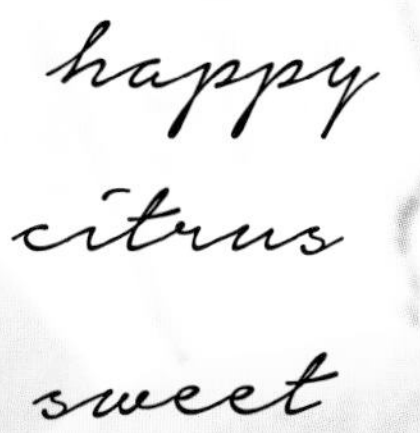

ELEVATION™

JOYFUL BLEND

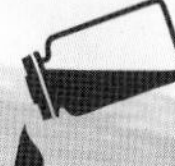

MAIN INGREDIENTS

Lavandin
Tangerine
Lavender
Amyris
Clary sage
Hawaiian sandalwood
Ylang ylang
Ho wood
Osmanthus
Lemon myrtle
Melissa

SAFETY

Avoid exposure to sunlight or UV rays for up to 12 hours after application.

TOP USES

ELEVATE MOOD & MIND
Diffuse, apply under nose, or pulse points.

ENERGIZE & REFRESH
Diffuse, apply under nose, and/or pulse points.

STRESS & ANXIETY
Apply under nose, ears, back of neck and inhale from cupped hands.

DEPRESSION & MOOD DISORDERS
Apply to back of neck and inhale.

GRIEF & SORROW
Diffuse, apply to chest, and/or pulse points.

STIMULATING & UPLIFTING
Apply under nose, back of neck, and/or inhale from cupped hands.

IMMUNITY
Apply to bottoms of feet.

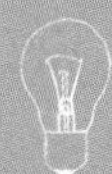

Use this blend to energize both body and mind.

= Aromatically = Topically = Internally

OIL BLENDS

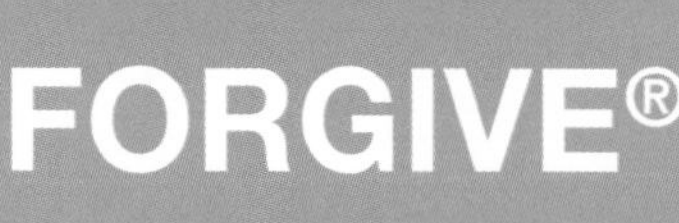

FORGIVE®

RENEWING BLEND

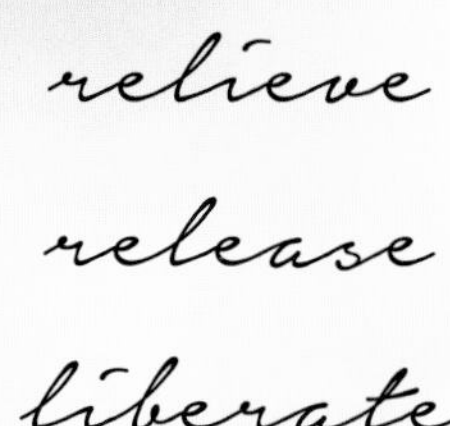

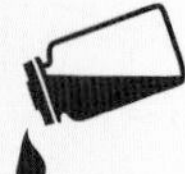

MAIN INGREDIENTS

Spruce
Bergamot
Juniper berry
Myrrh
Arborvitae
Nootka
Thyme
Citronella

SAFETY

Dilution recommended. Possible skin sensitivity. Avoid exposure to sunlight or UV rays for up to 12 hours after application.

TOP USES

FORGIVENESS, ATTACHMENT & HOLDING ON
Apply to temples, back of neck and/or diffuse.

ANXIETY
Apply under nose, across forehead, and/or back of neck to soothe and ground.

ULCERS & LIVER ISSUES
Apply over abdomen and affected areas.

SKIN INFECTION & DAMAGE
Apply to affected areas.

ADDICTIONS & IRRITABILITY
Diffuse and apply to wrist pulse points.

CIRCULATION
Apply to chest or diffuse.

FUNGUS & PARASITES
Apply to bottoms of feet.

SPIRITUAL & EMOTIONAL TOXICITY
Diffuse and apply under nose and/or to chest.

HAIR LOSS, PROSTATE ISSUES & LIBIDO
Apply to affected areas, abdomen, or bottoms of feet.

INCONTINENCE
Apply over abdomen or bottoms of feet.

EMOTIONAL REPRESSION
Diffuse or inhale from cupped hands to get from fear or frigidity to passion or intimacy.

Whether you are feeling stubborn, attached, guilty, bitter, angry or judgmental, this blend invites you to let go, trust the process of life, and be renewed.

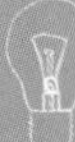

cleansing
clear
sweet

HD CLEAR®

SKIN CLEARING BLEND

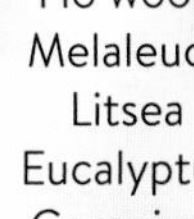

MAIN INGREDIENTS
Black cumin
Ho wood
Melaleuca
Litsea
Eucalyptus
Geranium

SAFETY
Safe for NEAT application. Possible skin sensitivity.

OIL BLENDS

TOP USES

ACNE & PIMPLES
Apply (Topically) to area(s) of concern.

OILY SKIN & OVERACTIVE SEBACEOUS GLANDS
Apply (Topically) to area(s) of concern.

SKIN BLEMISHES & IRRITATIONS
Apply (Topically) to area(s) of concern.

DERMATITIS & ECZEMA
Apply (Topically) to area(s) of concern.

FUNGAL & BACTERIAL ISSUES
Apply (Topically) to area(s) of concern.

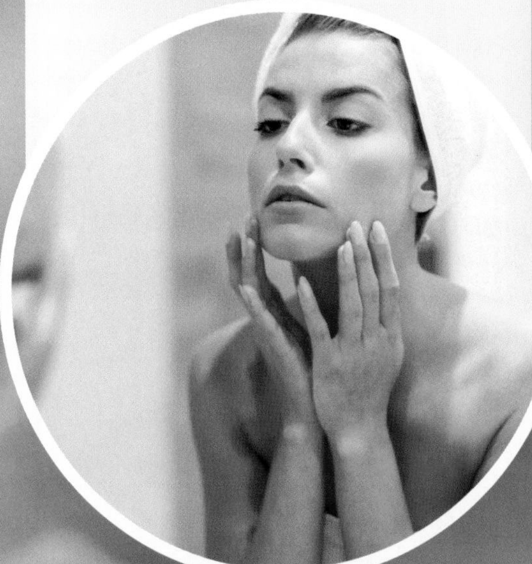

This blend is cleansing and calming to the skin. It reduces two components that encourage acne: bacteria and inflammation.

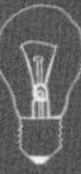

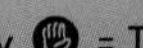 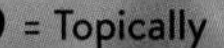 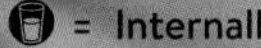
= Aromatically = Topically = Internally

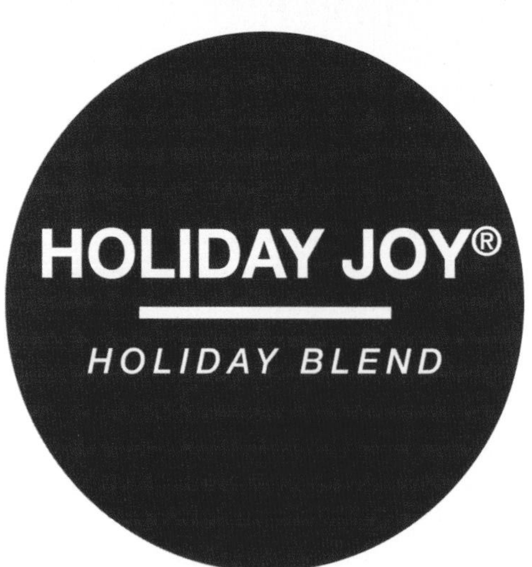

festive

warming

spicy

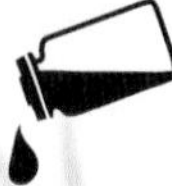

MAIN INGREDIENTS
Siberian fir
Wild orange
Clove
Cinnamon
Cassia
Douglas fir
Nutmeg
Vanilla bean absolute

SAFETY
Dilution recommended. Possible skin sensitivity. Avoid exposure to sunlight or UV rays for up to 12 hours after application.

OIL BLENDS

TOP USES

REFRESHING & JOYFUL
Diffuse or inhale from cupped hands.

IMMUNE BOOST
Diffuse or inhale from cupped hands.

COLD & FLU PREVENTION
Diffuse or inhale from cupped hands.

HEADACHE & MIGRAINE
Apply to temples and back of neck.

TENSION & STRESS
Apply to pulse points and diffuse.

NECK & SHOULDER DISCOMFORT
Apply to area(s) of discomfort.

ARTHRITIS
Apply to area(s) of discomfort.

PROTECTING & WARMING
Apply to back of neck and/or pulse points.

This blend inspires the joy of the holidays while also stimulating immunity.

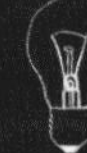

regenerating
youthful
replenishing

IMMORTELLE

ANTI-AGING BLEND

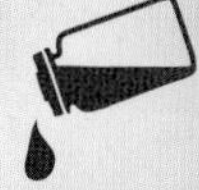

MAIN INGREDIENTS
Frankincense
Hawaiian sandalwood
Lavender
Myrrh
Helichrysum
Rose

SAFETY
Safe for NEAT application

TOP USES

WRINKLES & FINE LINES
Apply to face, neck, and hands.

SUN DAMAGE & SKIN CANCER
Apply to affected area to promote renewal and healing.

SCARS & STRETCH MARKS
Apply to affected area(s).

BLEMISHES
Apply to affected area(s).

TENSION & MOOD BALANCE
Apply to heart, back of neck, forehead, pulse points, and/or under nose.

MEDITATION
Apply under nose or to pulse points.

CATARACTS
Add 1-2 drops in a capsule 1-2x daily, under 2nd & 3rd toes.

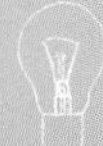

A beautiful blend with time-honored essential oils for radiant skin.

OIL BLENDS

= Aromatically = Topically

INTUNE®

FOCUS BLEND

grounding
earthy
clarifying

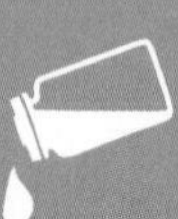

MAIN INGREDIENTS
Amyris
Patchouli
Frankincense
Lime
Ylang ylang
Hawaiian sandalwood
Roman chamomile

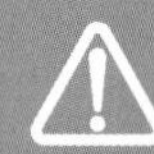

SAFETY
Avoid exposure to sunlight or UV rays for 12 hours after application.

TOP USES

ADD/ADHD
Apply to back of neck, spine, or bottoms of feet.

OVER- & UNDER- ACTIVE BRAIN ACTIVITY
Apply to back of neck or spine to balance activity.

MENTAL CLARITY, FOCUS & CONCENTRATION
Apply under nose and back of neck.

CALMING & GROUNDING
Apply under nose, back of neck or to pulse points.

NERVOUSNESS, ANXIETY & DEPRESSION
Apply under nose to bottoms of feet and back of neck.

STRESS & HYPERACTIVITY
Apply to back of neck and pulse points.

MID-AFTERNOON SLUMP
Diffuse, apply under nose and/or back of neck.

SEIZURES
Apply to back of neck, spine, up to or bottoms of feet.

Everyone needs extra help to focus from time to time. This blend of essential oils works together to enhance mental focus.

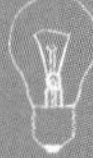

motivating
energizing
believing

MOTIVATE®

ENCOURAGING BLEND

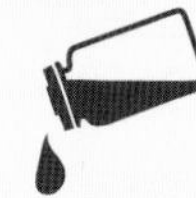

MAIN INGREDIENTS
Peppermint
Clementine
Coriander
Basil
Yuzu
Melissa
Rosemary
Vanilla bean absolute

TOP USES

LACK OF CONFIDENCE, COURAGE OR MOTIVATION
Diffuse 🅐 and apply 🅣 under nose, on forehead, back of neck, or chest.

CONFUSION & OVERWHELM
Inhale 🅐 or apply 🅣 under nose, on forehead, back of neck, or chest.

MENTAL FATIGUE & EXHAUSTION
Diffuse 🅐 or apply 🅣 to temples and back of neck.

DEPLETION & STAGNATION
Inhale 🅐 from cupped hands and apply 🅣 to pulse points.

DEPRESSION
Diffuse 🅐 or apply 🅣 to chest, forehead, and back of neck.

PHYSICAL EXHAUSTION
Inhale 🅐 from cupped hands, apply 🅣 under nose, over adrenals, or to bottoms of feet to enhance endurance.

DIGESTIVE ISSUES
Apply 🅣 over abdomen, on pulse points, or to bottoms of feet.

BRONCHITIS & ASTHMA
Diffuse 🅐 or apply 🅣 to neck and chest.

ACHES & PAINS
Apply 🅣 to affected area(s).

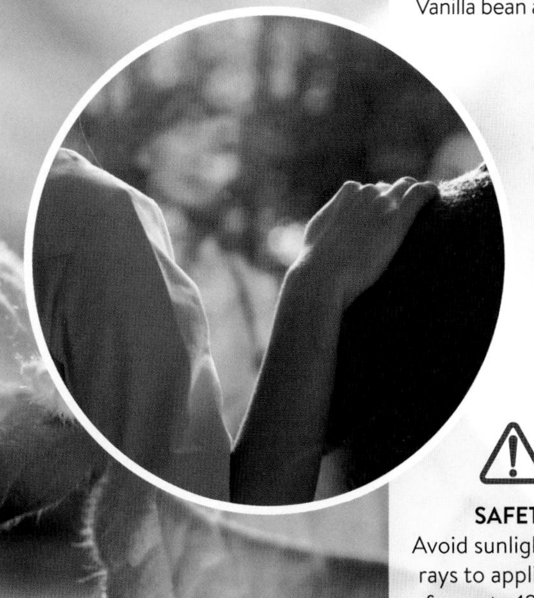

SAFETY
Avoid sunlight or UV rays to applied area for up to 12 hours.

Squelch the frustration and doubt that can halt progress with this blend's ability to encourage productivity, creativity, and confidence.

🅐 = Aromatically 🅣 = Topically 🅘 = Internally

ON GUARD®

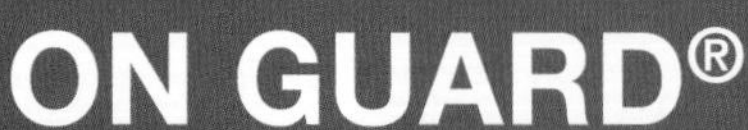

PROTECTIVE BLEND

spicy
supportive
warming

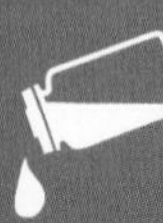

MAIN INGREDIENTS
Wild orange
Clove
Cinnamon leaf/bark
Eucalyptus
Rosemary

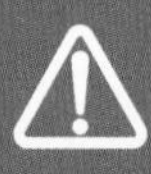

SAFETY
Dilution recommended. Possible skin sensitivity. Avoid exposure to sunlight or UV rays for up to 12 hours after application.

TOP USES

KILLING GERMS & AIRBORNE PATHOGENS
Take in a capsule, apply to bottoms of feet, or diffuse.

SEASONAL IMMUNE BOOST
Diffuse and take in water or in a capsule.

COLDS & FLU
Take in a capsule or apply to bottoms of feet.

STAPH, STREP THROAT & COUGH
Gargle a drop in water and swallow. Apply to chest, throat, or take in a capsule or with water.

COLD SORES, WARTS & INFECTED WOUNDS
Apply diluted to affected area(s).

ORAL HEALTH
Gargle a drop in water.

FUNGAL & PARASITE ISSUES
Apply to affected area or take in a capsule.

URINARY TRACT ISSUES
Take in a capsule or apply to lower abdomen.

ANTISEPTIC & LAUNDRY CLEANER
Diffuse or dilute with water and apply to surfaces.

CHRONIC FATIGUE & AUTOIMMUNE DISEASE
Take in a capsule or apply to bottoms of feet.

A strong immunity combats viral and bacterial threats to the body. Use this blend to keep your family healthy.

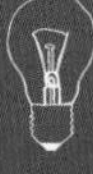

spontaneous

enlivening

daring

PASSION®

INSPIRING BLEND

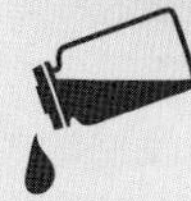

MAIN INGREDIENTS
Cardamom
Cinnamon
Ginger
Clove
Sandalwood
Jasmine
Vanilla bean absolute
Damiana

TOP USES

APATHY, DEPRESSION & ENERGY ISSUES
Diffuse or inhale from cupped hands to energize and uplift.

LOW LIBIDO & SEXUAL PERFORMANCE
Diffuse, inhale from cupped hands, apply to bottoms of feet, and/or abdomen.

MENTAL FOG & MEMORY ISSUES
Apply to toes or diffuse.

STIMULATING
Apply under nose or to bottoms of feet.

SLUGGISH DIGESTION & ELIMINATION
Apply diluted to lower abdomen.

LUNG & SINUS CONGESTION
Diffuse or inhale from hands.

FRIGIDITY & POOR CIRCULATION
Apply to bottoms of feet to warm and stimulate blood flow.

MENSTRUATION & MENOPAUSE ISSUES
Apply diluted to lower abdomen or pressure points below inside and outside of ankles.

INFECTIONS
Apply to bottoms of feet.

PERFUME
Apply diluted to wrists or neck.

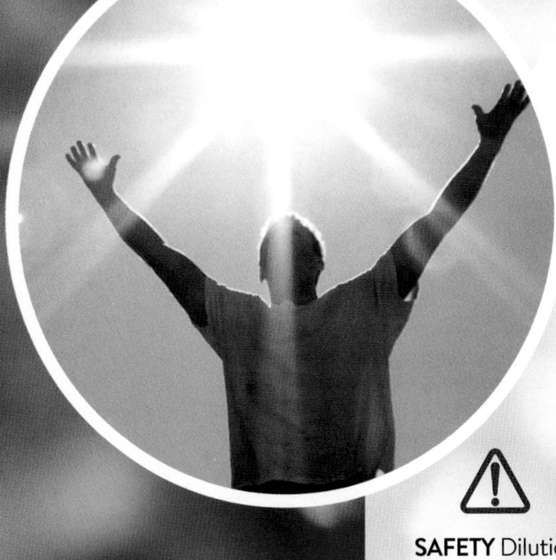

SAFETY Dilution recommended. Possible skin sensitivity.

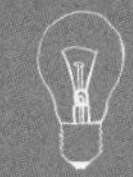

This blend can nurture the natural desire to embrace new and exciting experiences in life with passion and courage.

= Aromatically = Topically = Internally

PASTTENSE®

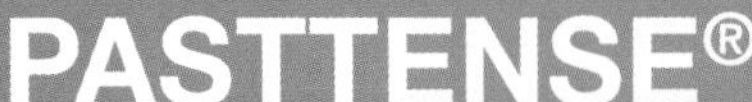

TENSION BLEND

relieving
renewing
awakening

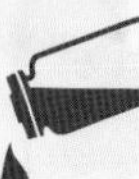

MAIN INGREDIENTS
Wintergreen
Lavender
Peppermint
Frankincense
Cilantro
Marjoram
Roman chamomile
Basil
Rosemary

SAFETY
Safe for NEAT application.Possible skin sensitivity.

TOP USES

HEADACHES & MIGRAINES
Apply to temples, forehead, and back of neck.

MUSCLE ACHES, SWELLING & CRAMPING
Apply to area(s) of concern.

HANGOVER
Apply under nose and to back of neck.

HOT FLASHES & COOLING
Apply to abdomen and back of neck to cool and calm.

BRUISES & BURNS
Apply to area(s) of concern. Dilute as needed.

JOINT PAIN
Apply to area(s) of concern.

TENSION & STRESS
Apply to pulse points and inhale from cupped hands.

NECK & SHOULDER PAIN
Apply to area(s) of discomfort.

ARTHRITIS
Apply to area(s) of discomfort.

RESTFUL SLEEP
Apply to back of neck.

Tension is the cause of many neurological complaints including headaches. This blend relieves tension and increases blood flow.

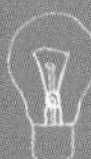

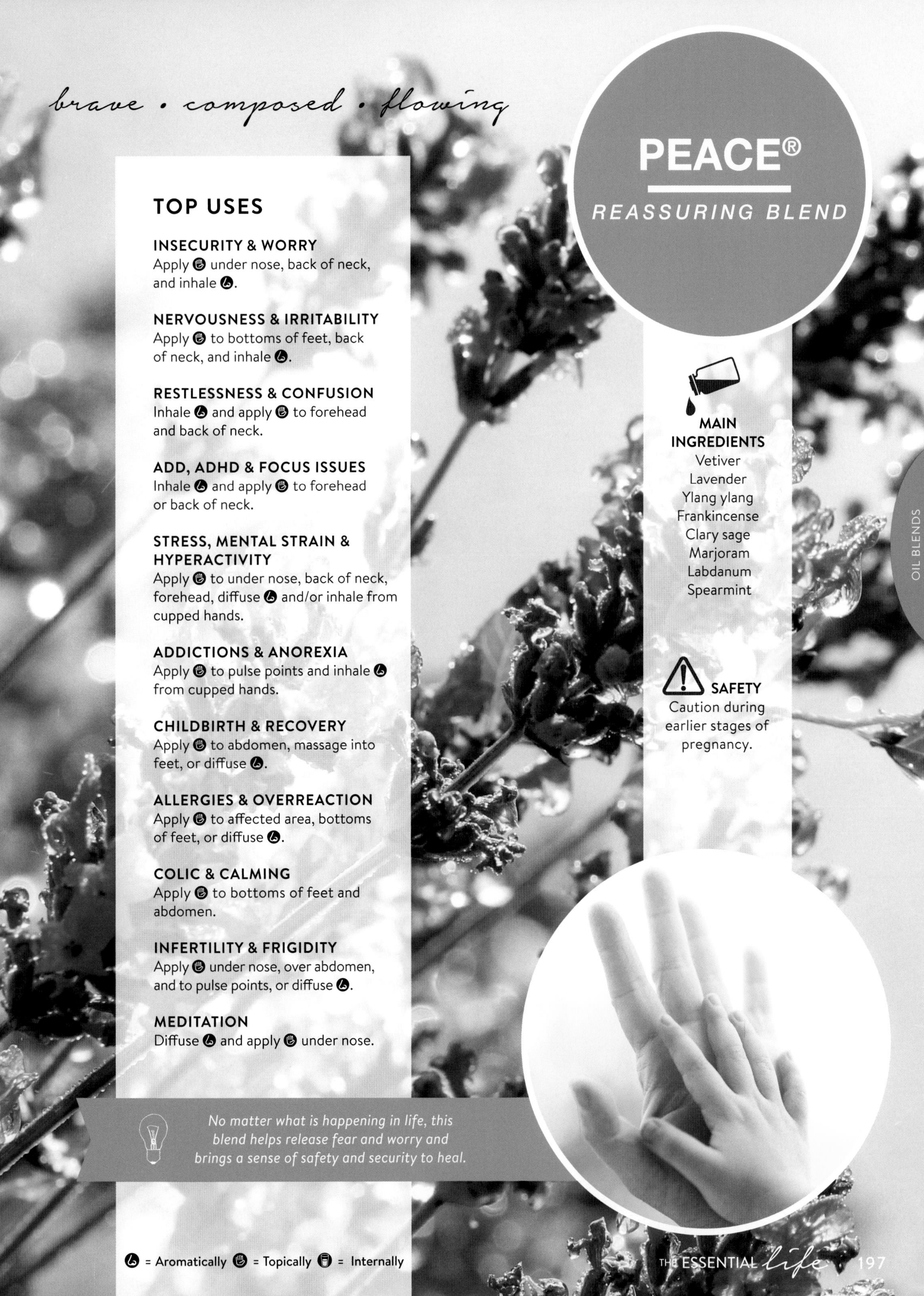

brave • composed • flowing

PEACE®

REASSURING BLEND

MAIN INGREDIENTS
Vetiver
Lavender
Ylang ylang
Frankincense
Clary sage
Marjoram
Labdanum
Spearmint

SAFETY
Caution during earlier stages of pregnancy.

TOP USES

INSECURITY & WORRY
Apply under nose, back of neck, and inhale.

NERVOUSNESS & IRRITABILITY
Apply to bottoms of feet, back of neck, and inhale.

RESTLESSNESS & CONFUSION
Inhale and apply to forehead and back of neck.

ADD, ADHD & FOCUS ISSUES
Inhale and apply to forehead or back of neck.

STRESS, MENTAL STRAIN & HYPERACTIVITY
Apply to under nose, back of neck, forehead, diffuse and/or inhale from cupped hands.

ADDICTIONS & ANOREXIA
Apply to pulse points and inhale from cupped hands.

CHILDBIRTH & RECOVERY
Apply to abdomen, massage into feet, or diffuse.

ALLERGIES & OVERREACTION
Apply to affected area, bottoms of feet, or diffuse.

COLIC & CALMING
Apply to bottoms of feet and abdomen.

INFERTILITY & FRIGIDITY
Apply under nose, over abdomen, and to pulse points, or diffuse.

MEDITATION
Diffuse and apply under nose.

No matter what is happening in life, this blend helps release fear and worry and brings a sense of safety and security to heal.

= Aromatically = Topically = Internally

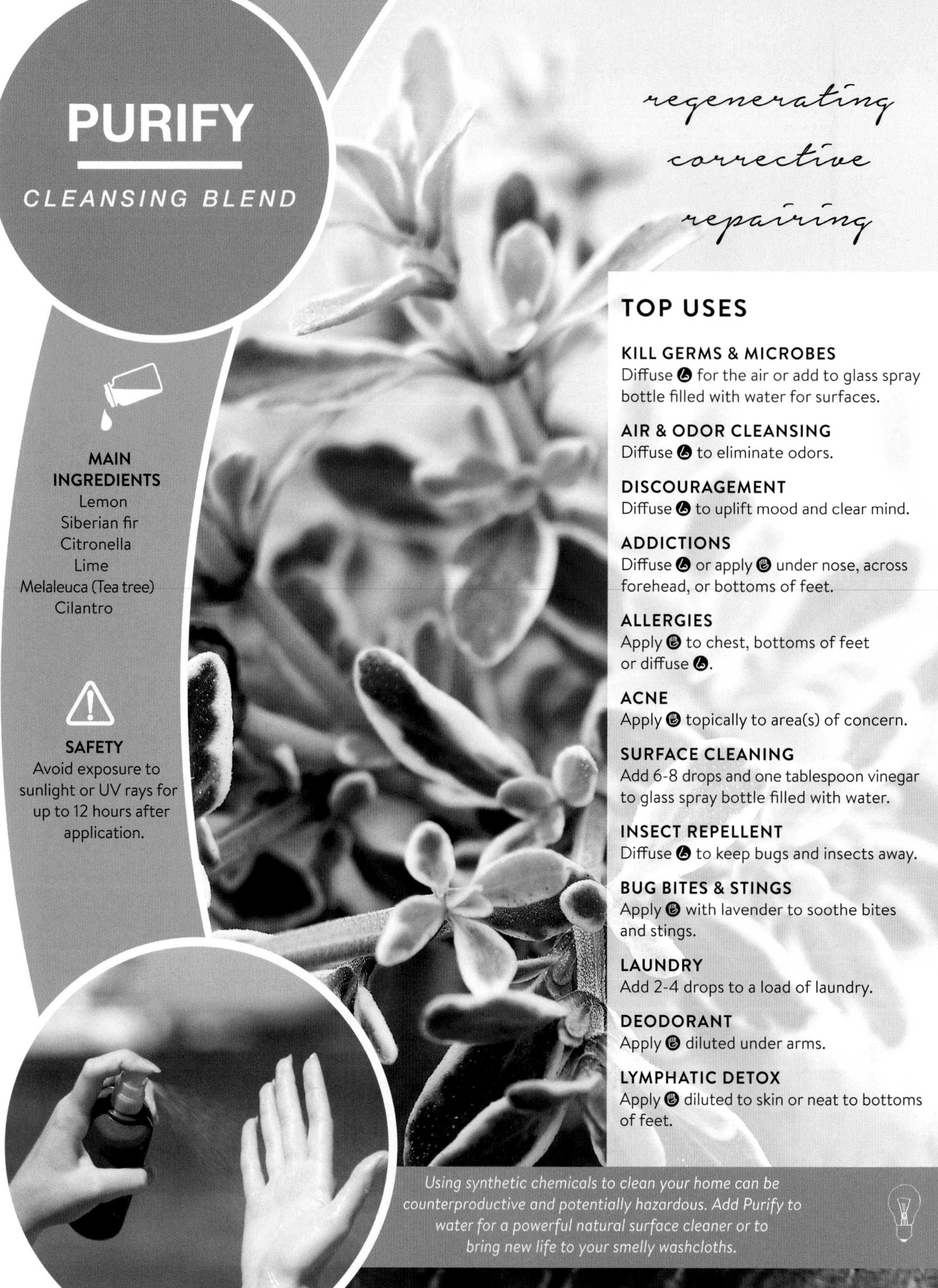

PURIFY

CLEANSING BLEND

regenerating
corrective
repairing

MAIN INGREDIENTS
Lemon
Siberian fir
Citronella
Lime
Melaleuca (Tea tree)
Cilantro

SAFETY
Avoid exposure to sunlight or UV rays for up to 12 hours after application.

TOP USES

KILL GERMS & MICROBES
Diffuse for the air or add to glass spray bottle filled with water for surfaces.

AIR & ODOR CLEANSING
Diffuse to eliminate odors.

DISCOURAGEMENT
Diffuse to uplift mood and clear mind.

ADDICTIONS
Diffuse or apply under nose, across forehead, or bottoms of feet.

ALLERGIES
Apply to chest, bottoms of feet or diffuse.

ACNE
Apply topically to area(s) of concern.

SURFACE CLEANING
Add 6-8 drops and one tablespoon vinegar to glass spray bottle filled with water.

INSECT REPELLENT
Diffuse to keep bugs and insects away.

BUG BITES & STINGS
Apply with lavender to soothe bites and stings.

LAUNDRY
Add 2-4 drops to a load of laundry.

DEODORANT
Apply diluted under arms.

LYMPHATIC DETOX
Apply diluted to skin or neat to bottoms of feet.

Using synthetic chemicals to clean your home can be counterproductive and potentially hazardous. Add Purify to water for a powerful natural surface cleaner or to bring new life to your smelly washcloths.

sweet

warm

calming

SERENITY®

RESTFUL BLEND

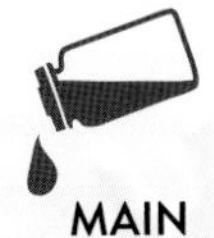

MAIN INGREDIENTS
Lavender
Cedarwood
Ho wood
Ylang ylang
Marjoram
Roman chamomile
Vetiver
Vanilla bean absolute
Hawaiian sandalwood

TOP USES

INSOMNIA & SLEEP ISSUES
Diffuse, apply under nose; bottoms of feet.

STRESS & ANXIETY
Apply under nose, to back of neck, and/or diffuse.

FUSSY BABY & RESTLESS CHILD
Diffuse, apply, to bottoms of feet; or up spine to calm. Dilute as needed.

TENSION & MOOD SWINGS
Diffuse, inhale from cupped hands. Apply to back of neck and/or over chest.

SKINCARE
Apply to area(s) of concern.

MUSCLE TENSION
Apply to area(s) of concern.

PERFUME
Apply to pulse points.

CALM FEARS & NERVOUSNESS
Apply to back of neck, diffuse, and/or inhale from cupped hands.

BATH & BEDTIME ROUTINE
Use in baths or apply to bottoms of feet to relax and unwind.

ANGER, AGITATION & IRRITABILITY
Diffuse, apply, under nose; to bottoms of feet to calm.

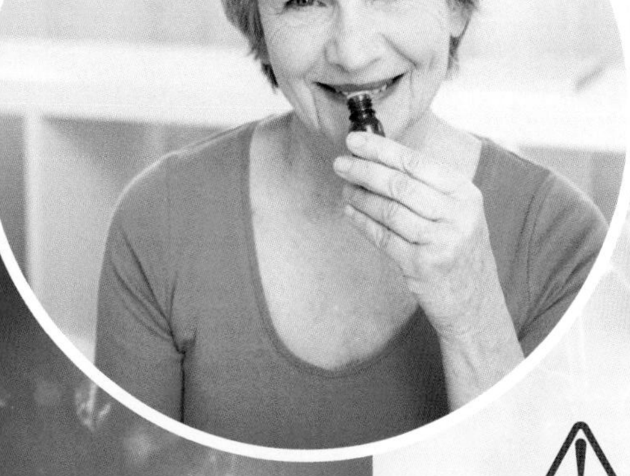

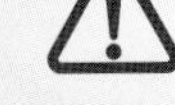

SAFETY
Safe for NEAT application. Possible skin sensitivity.

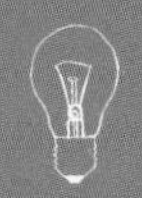

Create a tranquil feeling and immediately transport yourself to a state of blissful repose by calming the mind and emotions, soothing the senses, and supporting a restful sleep with this grounding aroma.

= Aromatically = Topically = Internally

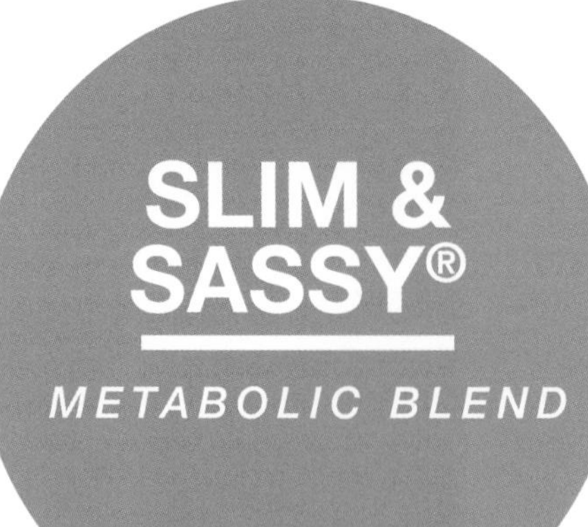

SLIM & SASSY®

METABOLIC BLEND

cleansing • spicy • refreshing

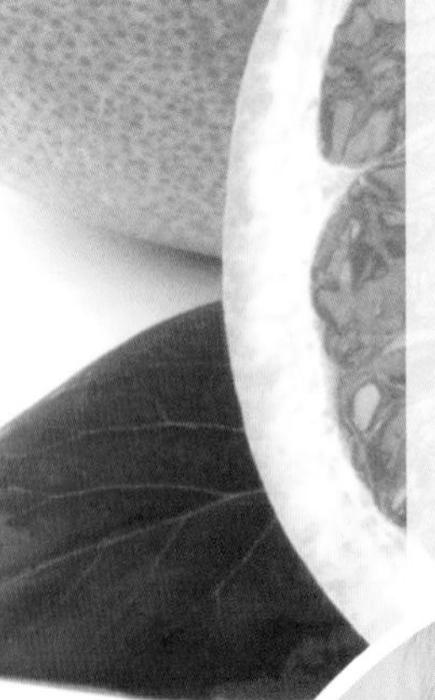

OIL BLENDS

MAIN INGREDIENTS
Grapefruit
Lemon
Peppermint
Ginger
Cinnamon

SAFETY
Avoid exposure to sunlight or UV rays for up to 12 hours after application.

TOP USES

WEIGHT LOSS, OBESITY & LOW METABOLISM
Take 5 drops up to 5 times daily in capsule or water.

CELLULITE
Apply diluted to area(s) of concern. Add patchouli if desired.

OVER-FATIGUE & EATING DISORDERS
Take in a capsule or with water or apply to bottoms of feet or diffuse.

APPETITE & CRAVINGS
Take a drop under tongue and inhale from bottle or apply under nose to balance appetite.

LYMPHATIC STIMULANT & SUPPORT
Diffuse or apply to bottoms of feet.

CONGESTION & COLDS
Take in a capsule or in water.

URINARY TRACT SUPPORT
Take in a capsule or in water.

BLOOD SUGAR BALANCE
Take in a capsule or in water.

DETOXIFICATION & CLEANSING
Take in a capsule or in water.

DIGESTIVE STIMULANT & CALMING
Take in a capsule or in water.

HIGH CHOLESTEROL
Take in a capsule or in water.

GALLBLADDER ISSUES & STONES
Take in a capsule or in water.

INFLAMMATION ISSUES
Apply to bottoms of feet or take in a capsule.

Reducing cravings and balancing blood sugar are important steps for weight loss.

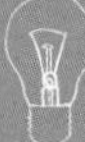

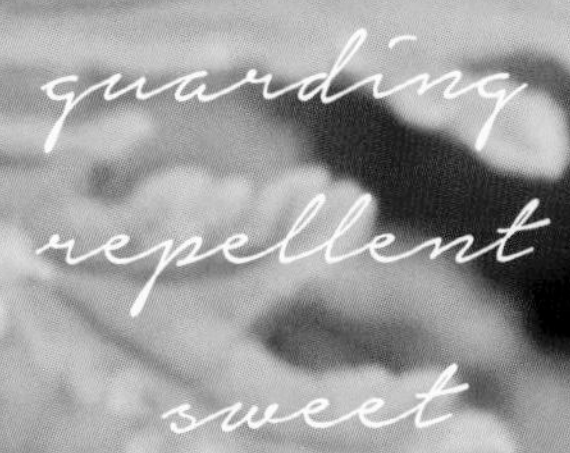

TERRASHIELD®

REPELLENT BLEND

TOP USES

INSECT REPELLENT
Diffuse, spray on surfaces, or apply to exposed areas to repel bugs and insects.

CELLULAR HEALTH
Apply to pulse points and bottoms of feet to promote healthy cell function.

SUNSCREEN
Apply to exposed skin with helichrysum or lavender to protect against sun exposure.

SKIN COMPLAINTS
Apply with lavender to troubled skin.

HEALTHY BOUNDARIES
Diffuse or apply to strengthen resolve and boundaries.

WOOD POLISH
Mix 4 drops with fractionated coconut oil to polish and preserve wood.

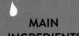

MAIN INGREDIENTS
Ylang ylang
Tamanu
Nootka
Cedarwood
Catnip
Lemon eucalyptus
Litsea
Vanilla bean absolute
Arborvitae

OIL BLENDS

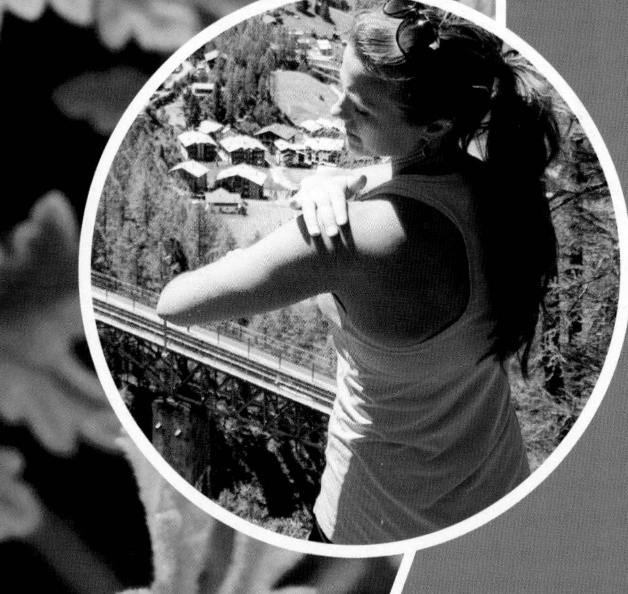

SAFETY
Safe for NEAT application.

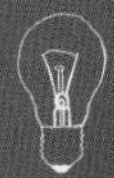

A toxic-free alternative to guard against bugs and pests. Fractionated coconut oil helps the blend stay on the skin longer, prolonging its effect.

= Aromatically = Topically = Internally

YOGA
ALIGN®
CENTERING BLEND

trusting • fluid • accepting

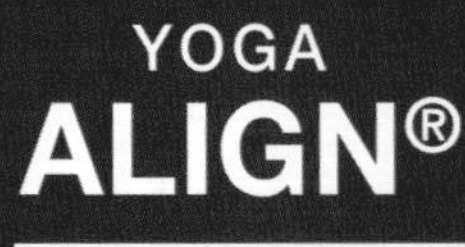

MAIN INGREDIENTS
Bergamot
Coriander
Marjoram
Peppermint
Jasmine
Rose

SAFETY
Safe for NEAT application. Avoid exposure to sunlight or UV rays for up to 12 hours after application.

TOP USES

COMPLIMENTARY YOGA POSES
Seated Meditation, Warrior II, Triangle, and Gate Pose.

SCATTERED & OVERWHELMED
Apply under nose and across forehead. Inhale deeply from cupped hands.

ALIGNED, SINGLEMINDED, TRANQUIL & FOCUSED
Diffuse. Apply to crown, neck area, and forehead.

ACCEPTED & WORTHY
Diffuse. Apply under nose, over heart, spleen, and solar plexus.

MEDITATION & PRAYER
Diffuse. Apply over heart, to forehead, and inhale deeply.

APATHETIC & LOW ENERGY
Diffuse. Apply to pulse points, over heart, and bottoms of feet.

ANGER, RAGE & IMBALANCED MOOD
Diffuse. Apply 1-2 drops in palm of hands, rub together, inhale deeply.

PERFUME
Apply to pulse points, chest, behind ears, and on ankles.

AFFIRMATION STATEMENT:
I know, accept and am true to myself.

OIL BLENDS

stabilizing
harmonizing
centering

YOGA
ANCHOR®
STEADYING BLEND

TOP USES

COMPLIMENTARY YOGA POSES
Seated Meditation, Seated Twist, and Bhu Mudra.

MEDITATION, PRAYER & FOCUS
Diffuse . Apply to forehead, behind ears, along spine, and/or bottoms of feet.

ANCHORED, COURAGEOUS & AUTHENTIC
Diffuse . Apply to ankles, along spine, and/or bottoms of feet.

COMPOSED, CALM & RESTED
Diffuse . Apply to back of neck, along spine, and/or bottoms of feet.

ROOTED TO THE EARTH, SPEAKING TRUTH
Diffuse . Apply to throat area, along spine, and/or bottoms of feet.

FEARFUL & DISCONNECTED
Diffuse . Apply 1-2 drops in palm of hands, rub together, inhale deeply.

PERFUME
Apply to pulse points, chest, and behind ears.

AFFIRMATION STATEMENT:
I am living who I really am.

MAIN INGREDIENTS
Lavender
Cedarwood
Frankincense
Cinnamon
Sandalwood
Black pepper
Patchouli

SAFETY
Safe for NEAT application.

= Aromatically = Topically = Internally

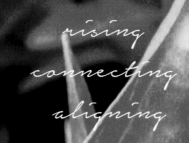

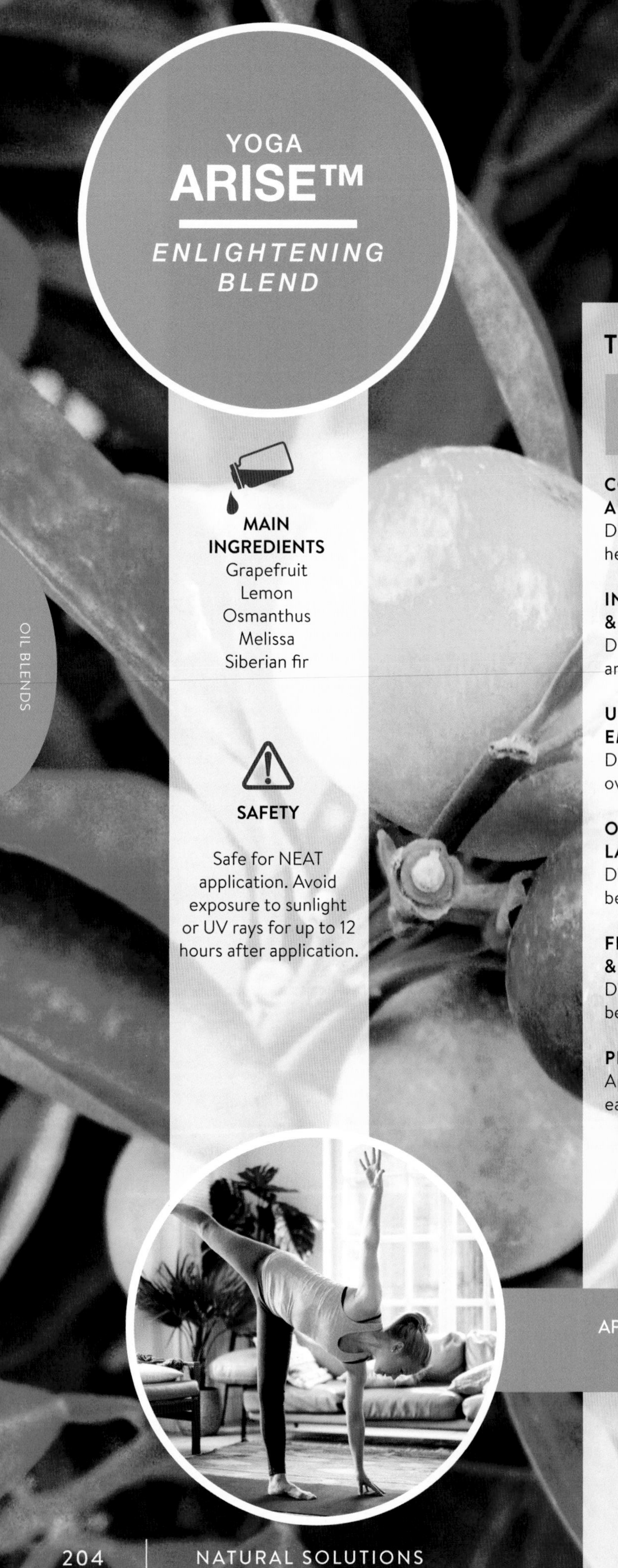

YOGA ARISE™

ENLIGHTENING BLEND

rising
connecting
aligning

MAIN INGREDIENTS
Grapefruit
Lemon
Osmanthus
Melissa
Siberian fir

SAFETY

Safe for NEAT application. Avoid exposure to sunlight or UV rays for up to 12 hours after application.

TOP USES

COMPLIMENTARY YOGA POSES
Volcano, Standing Side Stretch, and Half Moon.

CONNECTEDNESS WITH SELF AND HIGHER POWER
Diffuse. Apply to crown, over heart, and along spine.

INTENTIONAL, ACTION-ORIENTED & MANIFESTING
Diffuse. Apply to ankles, along spine, and bottoms of feet.

UPLIFTED, COURAGEOUS & EMPOWERED
Diffuse. Apply to forehead, over heart, and bottoms of feet.

OVERWHELMED, MENTAL CHATTER, LACK OF CLARITY & FOCUS
Diffuse. Apply to forehead, heels, and behind ears.

FEELING CHALLENGED, DEPRESSION & MOOD SWINGS
Diffuse. Apply to crown, over heart, behind ears, bottoms of feet, and pulse points.

PERFUME
Apply to pulse points, chest, behind ears, and on ankles.

AFFIRMATION STATEMENT:
I am one with the Divine.

fresh
balancing
cleansing

WHISPER®

WOMEN'S PERFUME BLEND

TOP USES

BALANCE HORMONES
Apply to pulse points and back of neck.

PERFUME
Apply to pulse points and/or chest.

HOT FLASHES
Apply to back of neck and/or abdomen.

LIBIDO & SEX DRIVE
Apply to pulse points and/or abdomen.

ANGER
Diffuse, inhale from cupped hands, and/or apply to pulse points to release and calm.

SELF-EXPRESSION & PRESENCE
Diffuse, inhale from cupped hands, or apply under nose and/or to pulse points.

SELF-CONFIDENCE & CREATIVITY
Diffuse, inhale from cupped hands, and/or apply to pulse points.

MAIN INGREDIENTS
Patchouli
Bergamot
Hawaiian Sandalwood
Rose
Vanilla bean absolute
Jasmine
Cinnamon
Vetiver
Labdanum
Cocoa bean
Ylang ylang

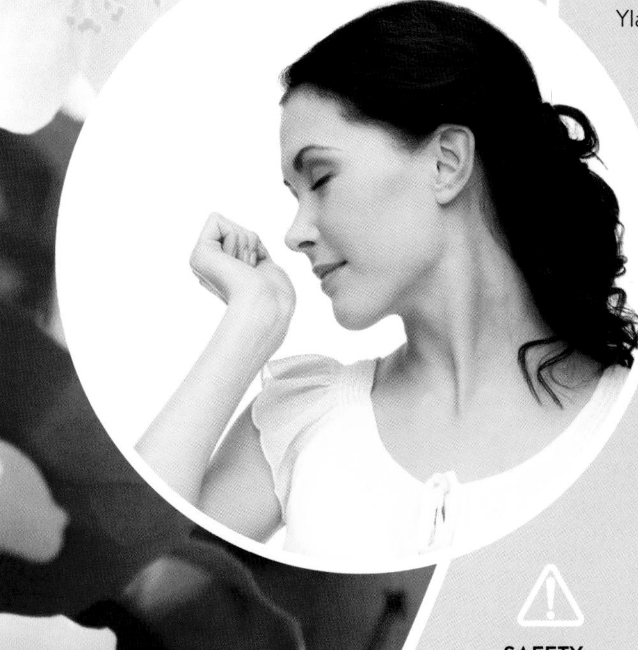

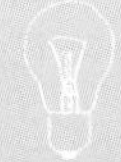

Each woman's unique body chemistry makes the scent of this blend her own.

SAFETY
Safe for NEAT application. Avoid exposure to sunlight or UV rays for up to 12 hours after application.

= Aromatically = Topically = Internally

refreshing • detoxing • clearing

ZENDOCRINE®

DETOXIFICATION BLEND

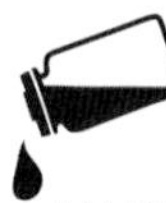

MAIN INGREDIENTS
Tangerine
Rosemary
Geranium
Juniper berry
Cilantro

SAFETY
Avoid exposure to sunlight or UV rays for up to 12 hours after application.

TOP USES

KIDNEY, GALLBLADDER & LIVER CLEANSING
Take (internally) in a capsule or apply (topically) diluted to lower abdomen.

HEAVY METAL DETOXIFICATION
Take (internally) in a capsule.

CONSTIPATION & URINARY TRACT INFECTION
Take (internally) or apply (topically) diluted over abdomen.

WEIGHT LOSS & DETOXIFICATION
Take (internally) in a capsule.

COLITIS & JAUNDICE
Take (internally) in a capsule or apply (topically) to abdomen or bottoms of feet.

ENDOCRINE & HORMONE IMBALANCE
Take (internally) in a capsule or apply (topically) to abdomen or bottoms of feet.

ADRENAL FATIGUE & EXHAUSTION
Take (internally) in a capsule or apply (topically) diluted to abdomen, back of neck, or bottoms of feet.

HANGOVER
Take (internally) in a capsule or apply (topically) to bottoms of feet.

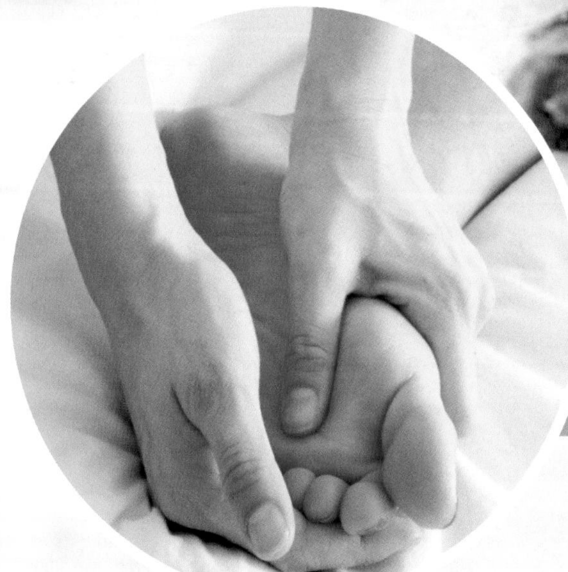

A regular cleansing regime helps ensure healthy kidney and liver function. Take 1-3 drops in a capsule, juice, or tea during first week of weight loss program.

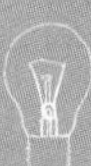

(A) = Aromatically (T) = Topically (I) = Internally

SUPPLEMENTARY PRODUCTS

Is your energy low? Do you experience chronic pain or discomfort in your body? Dealing with challenges in sustaining energy and concentration throughout the day, along with maintaining adequate immune and physical health, are the norm for many. However, virtually any health compromise or issue can be traced to some kind of underlying deficiency or toxicity. Numerous studies have been conducted over decades to determine the optimal nutritional state for the human body. The scientific community agrees that virtually everyone falls short in obtaining the bare minimum of recommended daily nutritional requirements in at least some areas.

These declines can be attributed to two main factors. The first is the increasing level of compromises in farming practices and the rising interest by food growers to genetically modify foods. Even those eating a wholesome, balanced diet find it challenging to consume adequate levels of certain nutrients. The second factor contributing to decline is our consumption of refined, processed, nutrient-void foods loaded with empty calories, which has been on the increase globally for decades. Similarly, adults and children alike are consuming excessive amounts of animal protein while consuming far too few fresh fruits and vegetables.

With these drastic changes in both food supply and consumption, examining one's own nutritional status is a worthy course of action. Consider asking yourself if you have any diet, health, or lifestyle habits or compromises that contribute to a lack in health and vitality and make adjustments accordingly. Whether feeling healthy or not, anyone can benefit from commitment to a daily supplemental program.

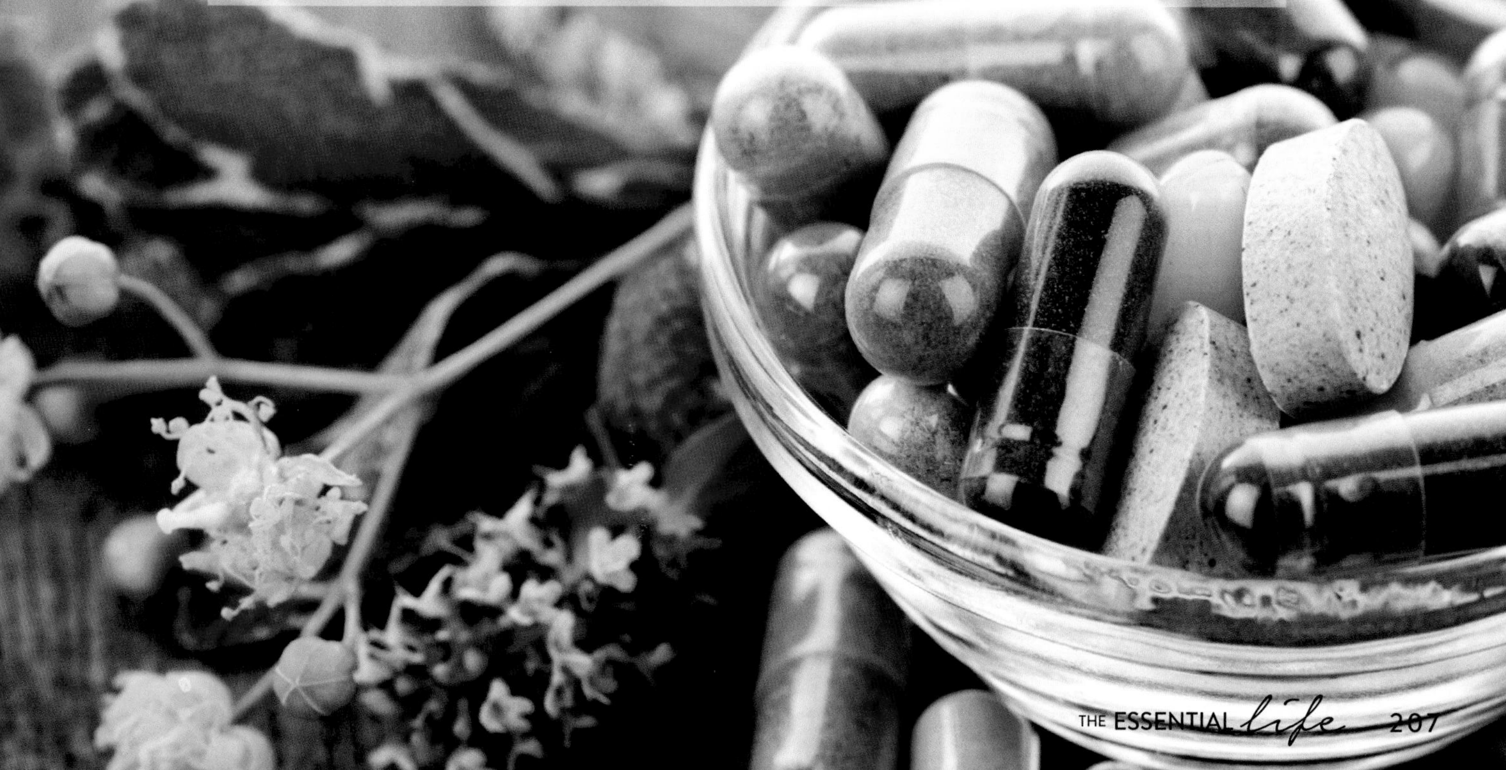

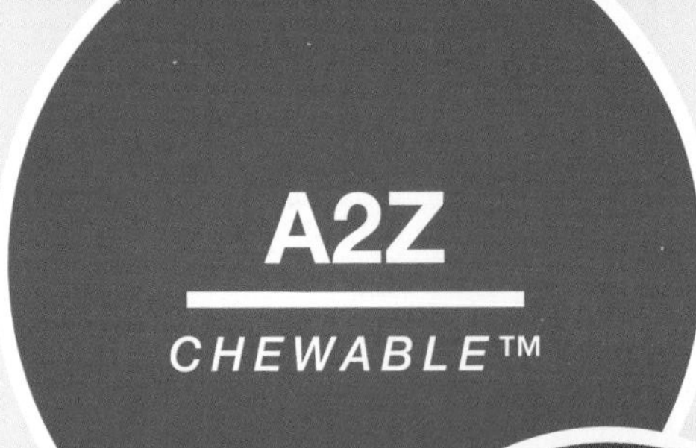

A2Z

CHEWABLE™

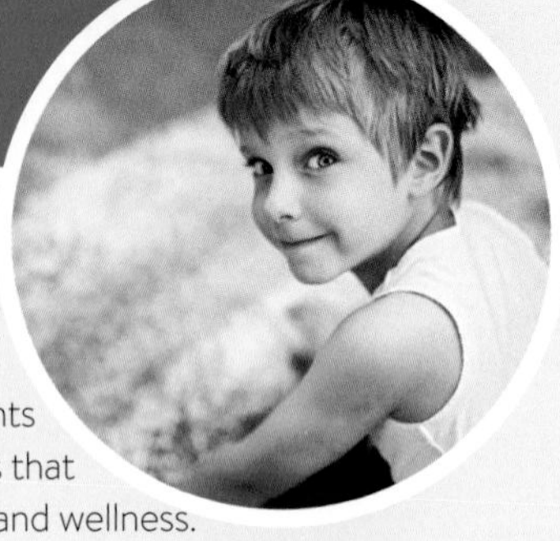

Multivitamin, mineral and botanical chewable for children and adults that have difficulty swallowing. Blended with antioxidants and herbal compounds that increase overall health and wellness.

TOP USES

Low energy and fatigue, compromised digestion and immunity, brain fog, oxidative cell damage, malnutrition, and poor health.

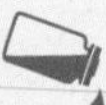

INGREDIENTS

- Vitamins A, C, D3, E, K, and full B-complex: Antioxidants and cellular energy, bringing synergy and vital nutrients to the cells of the body and brain. Also supports a healthy immune function.
- Calcium, copper, iron, iodine, magnesium, manganese, potassium and zinc: Bioavailable minerals which lay the foundation for bone health and nerve cell functions. Also supports fluid transportation and utilization by the cells.
- Superfood blend of pineapple, pomegranate extract, lemon bioflavonoids, spirulina, sunflower oil, rice bran, beet greens, broccoli, brown rice, carrot, mango, cranberry, rose hips, acerola cherry extract, spinach: Blend of antioxidants and whole food nutrients to support healthy cell function and increase utilization of other nutrients throughout the body.
- Cellular vitality complex of tomato extract, turmeric extract, boswellia serrata extract, grape seed extract, marigold flower extract: Synergistic blend of natural anti-inflammatories, antioxidants and cellular repair compounds.

SAFETY

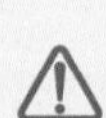

No gluten, wheat, dairy, soy or nut products. Pregnant or lactating women should consult a physician or health care provider before use. Do not use if safety seal is broken or missing.

Selected vitamins and trace elements support immune function by strengthening epithelial barriers and cellular and humoral immune responses, Maggini S, Wintergerst ES, Beveridge S, Hornig DH, British Journal of Nutrition, 2007

Contribution of selected vitamins and trace elements to immune function, Wintergerst ES, Maggini S, Hornig DH, Ann Nutr Met, 2007

Minerals and vitamins in bone health: The potential value of dietary enhancement, Bonjour JP, Gueguen L, Palacios C, et al, Bri J Nutr, 2009

The immunological functions of the vitamin D endocrine system, Hayes CE, Nashold FE, Spach KM & Pedersen LB, Cell Molec Biol, 2003

Possible role for dietary lutein and zeaxanthin in visual development, Hammond BR, Nutr Rev, 2008

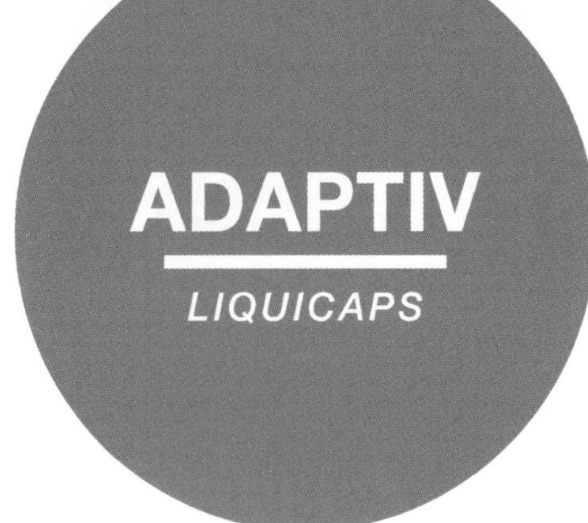

ADAPTIV

LIQUICAPS

A blend of essential oils and botanicals combined to both relax, and empower and encourage when adapting to stressful situations or acclimating to new surroundings. Intended as a tool to help manage effects of stress, tension, uneasiness, and worry that come during everyday life.

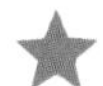

TOP USES

Manage stress, boost mood, balance mind and body, promotes positive attitude and feelings, improve state of mind, encourage relaxation and mental well-being.

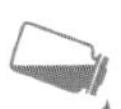

INGREDIENTS

- Lavender oil: Highly versatile, best known for calming and relaxing properties; major uses include promoting peaceful sleep, easing emotional and physical tension.
- Coriander oil: Eases stomach upset and balances blood sugar (both of which are aggravated by states of stress), while promoting feelings of relaxation.
- Wild orange oil: Stress-protective antioxidants and anti-inflammatory properties, calms emotionally-based digestive upset, energizes and uplifts mind and body.
- Fennel oil: Curbs cravings for sweets, soothes digestive upset, addresses blood sugar imbalances all due to prolonged stress, helps move a person out of emotionally-paralyzed inactivity with relaxing properties.
- Sceletium root extract: Unique phytochemical, stirs "alert serenity," supports healthy emotional responses to everyday stressors, stimulates production of mood stabilizing hormones, improves cognitive function while combating occasional nervousness, promotes sense of well-being and euphoria.
- GABA: Quieting neurotransmitter, promotes relaxation through natural comforting effects, helps reduce feelings of apprehension and fear by decreasing neuronal excitability, moving the brain and body into a lower gear by lowering activity of neural cells and central nervous system.
- Ahiflower seeds: Superior omega-rich oil, contains higher quality and quantity of omegas than any other seed oils, known for capacity to help maintain self-confidence, emotional stability, positive attitude while reducing restlessness.

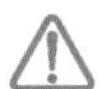

SAFETY

Keep out of reach of children. If pregnant, nursing, or under a doctor's care, consult physician. Do not use if safety seal is broken or missing. Store in cool, dry place.

ALPHA CRS®+

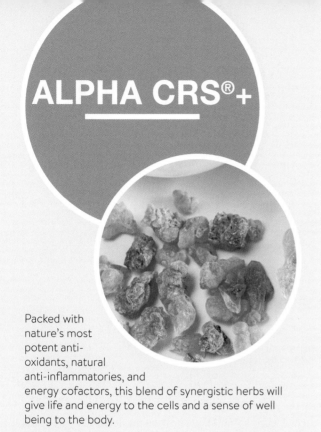

Packed with nature's most potent antioxidants, natural anti-inflammatories, and energy cofactors, this blend of synergistic herbs will give life and energy to the cells and a sense of well being to the body.

TOP USES

Pain and inflammation, arthritis, osteoarthritis, fibromyalgia, foggy brain, cirrhosis, jaundice, cellular repair, fatigue, mood, and cancer prevention.

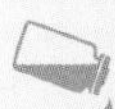

INGREDIENTS

- Boswellia serrata gum resin: Inflammatory modulator (helps regulate and decrease inflammation and pain).
- Scutellaria root (baicalin): Inflammatory modulator and cellular damage repair, supports liver and kidney health.
- Milk thistle (silymarin): Powerful liver protectant and free radical scavenger.
- Polygonum cuspidatum (resveratrol): Increases healthy cell proliferation and decreases free radical damage from cells.
- Green tea leaf (EGCG): Powerful antioxidant, free radical scavenger, and anticancer properties.
- Pomegranate fruit extract: Antioxidant shown to lower LDL cholesterol, blood pressure, and increase heart health.
- Pineapple (bromelain): An enzyme shown to decrease pain and inflammation.
- Turmeric extract (curcumin): Powerful anti-inflammatory and anticancer compound.
- Grape seed extract: Proanthocyanidins shown to decrease free radical damage and increase cellular repair.
- Sesame seed extract: Antioxidant shown to protect liver from oxidative damage.
- Pine bark extract (pycnogenol): Antioxidant shown to increase vasodilation of the arteries and decrease free radical damage.
- Gingko Biloba leaf: Increases circulation to the brain and brings mental clarity.
- Acetyl-L-Carnitine: Increases energy production by the mitochondria and increases glutathione (internal antioxidant) levels in the body.
- Alpha-Lipoic acid: Antioxidant vital for cellular energy and neutralizing free radicals.
- Coenzyme Q10: Plays a significant role in energy production for the heart and muscle cells.
- Quercetin: Potent antioxidant flavonoid known to decrease cell damage and increase recovery.
- Stomach comfort blend of peppermint, ginger and caraway: Calms and soothes the digestive processs.

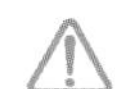

SAFETY

For men, women and teens. Pregnant or lactating women should consult a physician or health care provider before use. Do not use if safety seal is broken or missing.

OIL BLENDS

Gene Expression Profiling of Aging in Multiple Mouse Strains: Identification of Aging Biomarkers and Impact of Dietary Antioxidants, Park SK, Kim K, Page GP, Allison DB, Weindruch R, Prolla TA, Aging Cell, 2009

Antioxidative and anti-inflammatory activities of polyhydroxyflavonoids of Scutellaria baicalensis GEORGI, Huang WH, Lee AR, Yang CH, Biosci Biotechnol Biochem, 2006 Oct

New therapeutic aspects of flavones: the anticancer properties of Scutellaria and its main active constituents Wogonin, Baicalein and Baicalin, Li-Weber M, Cancer Treat Rev, 2009 Feb

The SIRT1 activator resveratrol protects SK-N-BE cells from oxidative stress and against toxicity caused by alpha-synuclein or amyloid-beta (1-42) peptide, Albani D, Polito L, Batelli S, De Mauro S, Fracasso C, Martelli G, Colombo L, Manzoni C, Salmona M, Caccia S, Negro A, Forloni G, J Neurochem, 2009

Resveratrol induces mitochondrial biogenesis in endothelial cells, Csiszar A, Labinskyy N, Pinto JT, Ballabh P, Zhang H, Losonczy G, Pearson K, de Cabo R, Pacher P, Zhang C, Ungvari Z, Am J Physiol Heart Circ Physiol, 2009 Jul

In vitro effects of tea polyphenols on redox metabolism, oxidative stress, and apoptosis in PC12 cells, Raza H, John A, Ann N Y Acad Sci, 2008 Sep

Orally administered green tea polyphenols prevent ultraviolet radiation-induced skin cancer in mice through activation of cytotoxic T cells and inhibition of angiogenesis in tumors, Mantena SK, Meeran SM, Elmets CA, Katiyar SK, J Nutr, 2005 Dec

Grape seed and red wine polyphenol extracts inhibit cellular cholesterol uptake, cell proliferation, and 5-lipoxygenase activity, Leifert WR, Abeywardena MY, Nutr Res, 2008 Dec

Quercetin increases brain and muscle mitochondrial biogenesis and exercise tolerance, Davis JM, Murphy EA, Carmichael MD, Davis B, Am J Physiol Regul Integr Comp Physiol, 2009 Apr

Mineral and vitamin deficiencies can accelerate the mitochondrial decay of aging, Ames BN, Atamna H, Killilea DW, Mol Aspects Med, 2005 Aug-Oct

Boswellic acid inhibits growth and metastasis of human colorectal cancer in orthotopic mouse model by downregulating inflammatory, proliferative, invasive and angiogenic biomarkers, Yadav, VR, Prasad S, Sung, B, Gelovani, JG, Guha, S, Krishnan, S, Aggarwal, BB Int. J. Cancer, 2012

Plant food supplements with anti-inflammatory properties: A systematic review, Di Lorenzo C, Dell'agli M, Badea M, et al, Critical Reviews in Food Science and Nutrition, 2013

Polyphenols, inflammation, and cardiovascular disease, Tangney CC, Rasmussen HE, Curr Atheroscler Rep, 2013

Bioavailability and activity of phytosome complexes from botanical polyphenols: The silymarin, curcumin, green tea, and grape seed extracts, Kidd PM, Alternative Medicine Review, 2009

Open, randomized controlled clinical trial of Boswellia serrata extract as compared to valdecoxib in osteoarthritis of knee, Sontakke S, Thawani V, Pimpalkhute S, Kapra P, Babhulkar S, Hingorani L, Indian Journal of Pharmacology. 2007

Baicalin, an emerging multi-therapeutic agent: pharmacodynamics, pharmacokinetics, and considerations from drug development perspectives, Srinivas NR, Xenobiotica, 2010

BONE

NUTRIENT COMPLEX

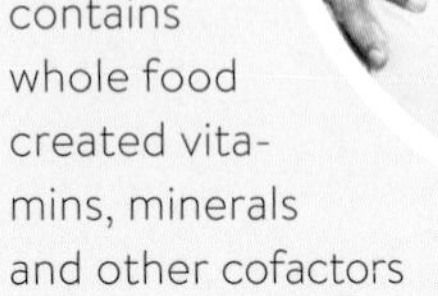

This blend contains whole food created vitamins, minerals and other cofactors necessary for bone integrity, strength and overall health. Not just for women, this complex is bioavailable to the body so the cells not only will recognize, but also utilize the compounds for bone reformation.

TOP USES

Weak or fragile bones, osteopenia and osteoporosis prone individuals, bone fractures, growing individuals, and anyone needing more bone density.

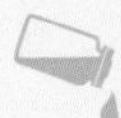

INGREDIENTS

- Vitamin C: Protective role in building strong bones and preventing fractures.
- Vitamin D2 and D3: Increases the absorption of calcium and other minerals by the intestines, increasing utilization of minerals for bone density.
- Biotin: Increase efficiency of bone marrow cell function as well as plays a role in the growth of hair, skin, and nails.
- Calcium, magnesium, zinc, copper, manganese, and boron: Work synergistically to build the foundation of bone tissue and integrity.

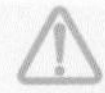

SAFETY

Safe for use by women, teens and men. Pregnant or lactating women should consult a physician or health care provider before use. Do not use if safety seal is broken or missing.

Association between serum 25-hydroxyvitamin d levels, bone geometry, and bone mineral density in healthy older adults, Mosele M, Coin A, Manzato E, et al, The Journals of Gerontology Series A: Biological Sciences and Medical Sciences. 2013

Nutritional aspects of the prevention and treatment of osteoporosis, Peters BS, Martini LA, Arquivos Brasileiros de Endocrinologia & Metabologia, 2010

Minerals and vitamins in bone health: the potential value of dietary enhancement, Bonjour JP, Gueguen L, Palacios C, et al, 2009

Magnesium and osteoporosis: current state of knowledge and future research directions, Castiglioni S, Cazzaniga A, Albisetti W, Maier JA, Nutrients, 2013

The physiological effects of dietary boron, Devirian TA, Volpe SL, Critical Reviews in Food Science and Nutrition, 2003

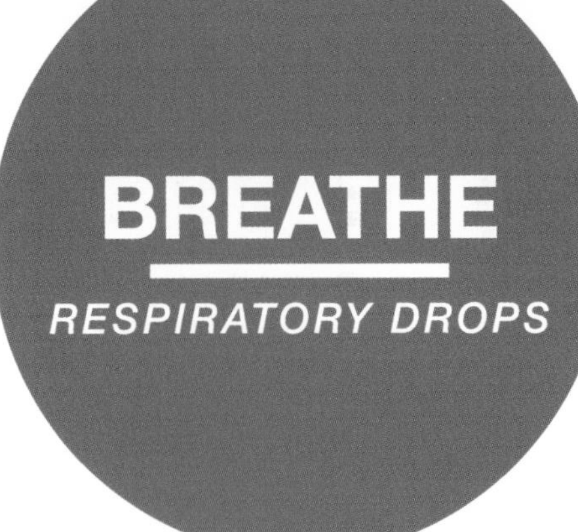

BREATHE

RESPIRATORY DROPS

A blend of essential oils in a convenient, organically sweetened throat lozenge for the use of opening the airways a supporting the respiratory system.

TOP USES

Congestion, head cold, sore throat, bronchitis, asthma, allergies, cough, sinusitis, bad breath, and motion sickness.

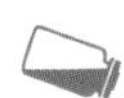

INGREDIENTS

- Cardamom oil: Clears and opens respiratory system, promotes digestion, decreases nausea and motion sickness.
- Peppermint oil: Bronchodilator, soothes digestion, anti-inflammatory, and stimulates brain.
- Eucalyptus oil: Decreases fevers, congestion and body pains; and antiviral effects on the respiratory system.
- Lemon oil: Antioxidant, antiseptic, promotes physical energy, health and cleansing.
- Thyme oil: Strong antioxidant and antiseptic, and supports healthy immune system.
- Melissa oil: Antiviral properties and supports against respiratory ailments.

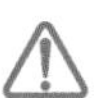

SAFETY

Be aware with small children that are prone to choking.

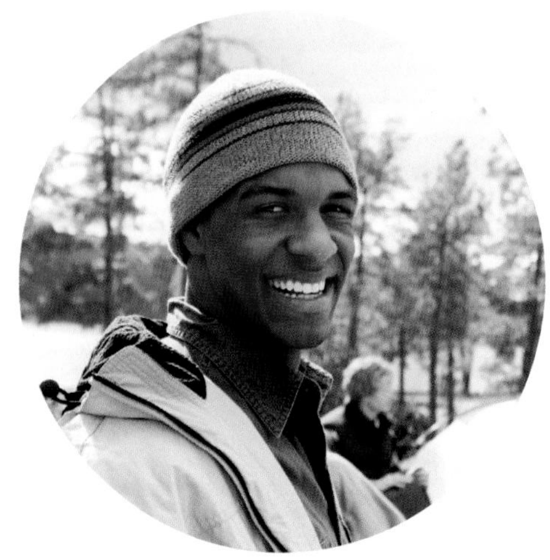

OIL BLENDS

CELLULAR BEAUTY

COMPLEX CAPSULES

A blend of essential oils and extracts designed to combat oxidative stress and help maintain skin's youthful appearance from the inside out. Outstanding for anti-aging, vitality, overall wellness, and skin health with powerful antioxidants and anti-inflammatory compounds.

TOP USES

Cellular, skin, immune and nervous system support; metabolic health, improve skin firmness, reduce skin imperfections, illuminate and brighten complexion, and calm mind and body.

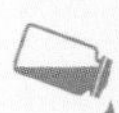

INGREDIENTS

- Yarrow oil: Skin healing accelerator; sagging, aging skin and surface veins; scars, acne, eczema.
- Pomegranate oil: Superior moisturizing ability, nourishing and softening skin.
- Celery seed oil: Promote detoxification, blood purification; facilitate elimination of toxins, excess fluid.
- Frankincense oil: Lift, tighten skin, slow signs of aging; help reduce acne blemishes, appearance of large pores; prevent wrinkles, repair cellular damage.
- Palmarosa oil: Cell renewal benefits; nourish, restore skin health, harmony; regulate skin moisture and oil production.
- Turmeric oil: Skin lightening, reduce facial hyperpigmentation, fine lines, wrinkles, acne.
- Melissa oil: Tighten and hydrate skin, improve elasticity, smooth wrinkles, overcome sensitive skin.
- Grape seed extract: Increase cellular repair, help reverse or reduce aging and wrinkling effects.
- Zinc citrate: Vital to collagen formation and healthy tissue development.
- Vitamin C: Prevent UV skin damage; even skin tone, reverse damage caused by sun exposure; boost cellular energy and nutrient absorption.
- Melon extract: Extremely hydrating, helps reduce signs and progression of aging, wrinkles; improve skin radiance.

SAFETY

Keep out of reach of children. If pregnant, nursing, or under a doctor's care, consult physician. Do not use if safety seal is broken or missing. Store in cool, dry place.

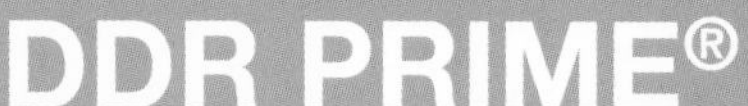

DDR PRIME®

SOFTGELS

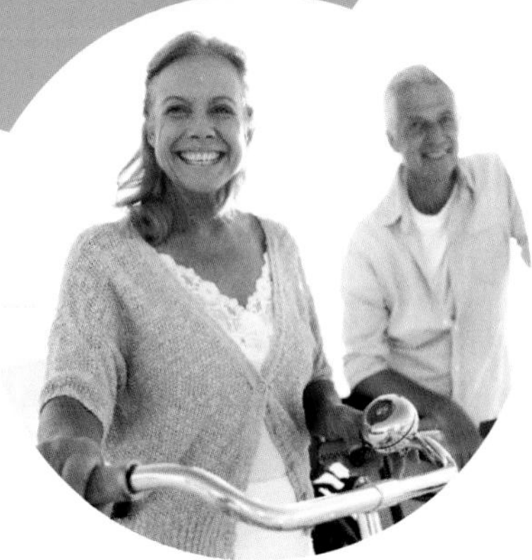

A blend of essential oils that have been shown in clinical studies to help protect cells against free radical damage while supporting cellular function through apoptosis of damaged and mutated cells, and proliferation of healthy cells.

TOP USES

Damaged or mutated cellular diseases, oxidative stress, autoimmune diseases and anything that requires cellular regeneration and healthy cellular function.

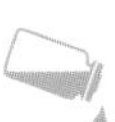

INGREDIENTS

- Frankincense oil: Anti-inflammatory and immune-stimulant properties. Is often used to help support the body's response to cancer and other cellular diseases.
- Wild orange oil: High levels of d-Limonene, which helps inhibit cancer tumor growth and reduction of cholesterol.
- Lemongrass oil: Anti-inflammatory and antiseptic and has the ability to inhibit cancer cell growth and to induce apoptosis (cellular death).
- Thyme oil: Strong antioxidant and antiseptic. Supports the brain as it ages.
- Summer savory oil: Antifungal and anti-inflammatory properties. Shows ability to reduce DNA damage from oxidative stress.
- Clove oil: Powerful antioxidant and anti-infectious and helps support healthy liver and thyroid function.
- Niaouli oil: Powerful antifungal and anti-inflammatory, helps protect against radiation, and helps to regenerate damaged tissues.
- Litsea oil: High in geranial, neral and limonene; helps with multi-tasking.

SAFETY

Not for small children. If pregnant or lactating, women should consult a physician or health care provider before use. Do not use if safety seal is missing or broken

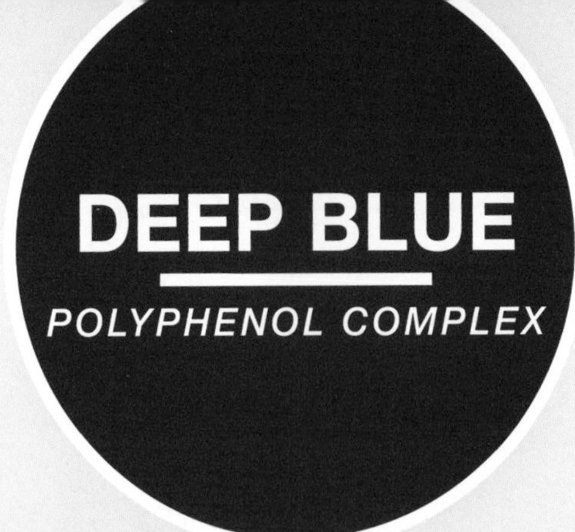

A blend of powerful polyphenols clinically tested to help soreness and discomfort from physical activities and daily life.

TOP USES

Joint pain, inflammation, arthritis, rheumatoid arthritis and anything "itis", fibromyalgia, sore muscles, Alzheimer's disease, and cancer prevention.

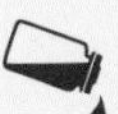

INGREDIENTS

- Frankincense (boswellia serrata) gum resin extract: Inflammatory modulator which helps regulate and decrease inflammation and pain.
- Curcumin: Extract from turmeric, has been shown to inhibit amyloid beta plaque formation and decrease risk of Alzheimer's Disease. Also shows powerful anti-inflammatory properties.
- Ginger root extract: Reduces pain and inflammation, warming effect and increases circulation.
- Green tea leaf extract (caffeine-free): Powerful antioxidant, free radical scavenger, and anticancer properties.
- Pomegranate fruit extract: Antioxidant shown to lower LDL cholesterol, blood pressure, and increase heart health.
- Grape seed extract: 95% polyphenols shown to decrease free radical damage and increase cellular repair.
- Resveratrol: Increases healthy cell proliferation and inhibits proliferation of damaged and mutated cells.
- Stomach comfort blend of peppermint, ginger, caraway: Helps soothe the digestive process and tames the stomach.

SAFETY

Not for use for children. If pregnant or lactating, women should consult a physician or health care provider before use. Do not use if safety seal is broken or missing.

J Biol Chem. 2005 Feb 18;280(7):5892-901. Epub 2004 Dec 7.Curcumin inhibits formation of amyloid beta oligomers and fibrils, binds plaques, and reduces amyloid in vivo.Yang F1, Lim GP, Begum AN, Ubeda OJ, Simmons MR, Ambegaokar SS, Chen PP, Kayed R, Glabe CG, Frautschy SA, Cole GM.
BMC Cancer. 2015;15(1):1119. doi: 10.1186/s12885-015-1119-y. Epub 2015 Mar 5. Resveratrol suppresses epithelial-to-mesenchymal transition in colorectal cancer through TGF-1/Smads signaling pathway mediated Snail/E-cadherin expression. Ji Q1, Liu X, Han Z, Zhou L, Sui H, Yan L, Jiang H, Ren J, Cai J, Li Q.
Yadav, V.R., Prasad S., Sung, B., Gelovani, J. G., Guha, S., Krishnan, S. and Aggarwal, B.B. Boswellic acid inhibits growth and metastasis of human colorectal cancer in orthotopic mouse model by downregulating inflammatory, proliferative, invasive and angiogenic biomarkers. Int. J. Cancer: 2012 130: 2176–2184.
Di Lorenzo C, Dell'agli M, Badea M, et al. Plant food supplements with anti-inflammatory properties: A systematic review. Critical Reviews in Food Science and Nutrition. 2013;53(5):507-516.
Int J Rheum Dis. 2013 Apr;16(2):219-29. doi: 10.1111/1756-185X.12054. Epub 2013 Apr 4. Protective effects of ginger-turmeric rhizomes mixture on joint inflammation, atherogenesis, kidney dysfunction and other complications in a rat model of human rheumatoid arthritis.
Ramadan G1, El-Menshawy O.
Tangney CC, Rasmussen HE. Polyphenols, inflammation, and cardiovascular disease. Curr Atheroscler Rep. 2013;15:324-334.
Kidd PM. Bioavailability and activity of phytosome complexes from botanical polyphenols: The silymarin, curcumin, green tea, and grape seed extracts. Alternative Medicine Review. 2009;14(3):226-246
Sontakke S, Thawani V, Pimpalkhute S, Kapra P, Babhulkar S, Hingorani L. Open, randomized controlled clinical trial of Boswellia serrata extract as compared to valdecoxib in osteoarthritis of knee. Indian Journal of Pharmacology. 2007;39:27-29.

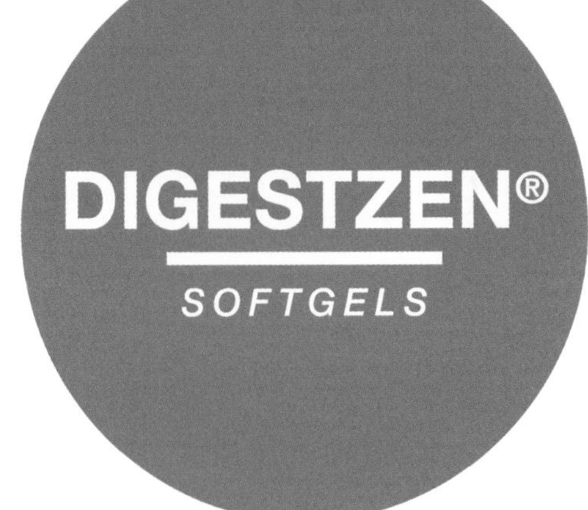

A synergistic blend of essential oils that help ease digestion and increase digestive health.

TOP USES

Upset stomach, constipation, diarrhea, IBS, vomiting, heartburn and acid indigestion/reflux.

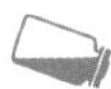

INGREDIENTS

- Ginger oil: Renowned for its ability to soothe stomach upset and ease indigestion.
- Peppermint oil: Supports healthy gastrointestinal function and aids in digestion.
- Tarragon oil: Promotes healthy digestion.
- Fennel oil: Helps relieve indigestion and a myriad of stomach issues.
- Caraway oil: Acts as a natural carminative while supporting a healthy gastrointestinal tract.
- Coriander oil: Eases occasional stomach upset.
- Anise oil: Promotes healthy digestion.

SAFETY

Can be taken by all ages that can swallow capsules. Keep out of reach of small children. Do not use if safety seal is broken or missing.

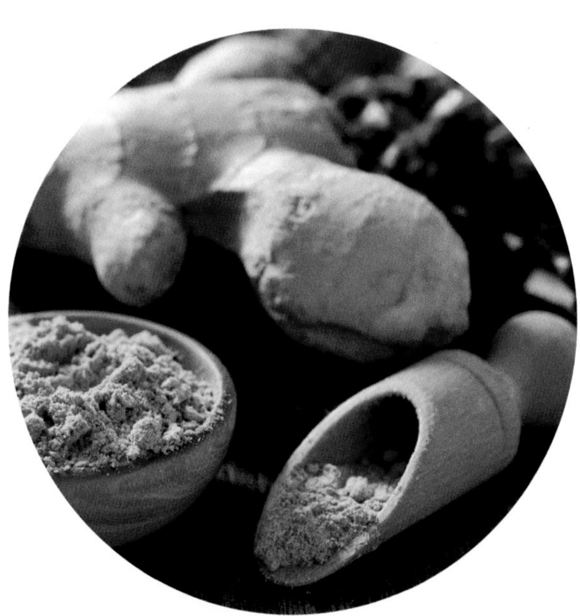

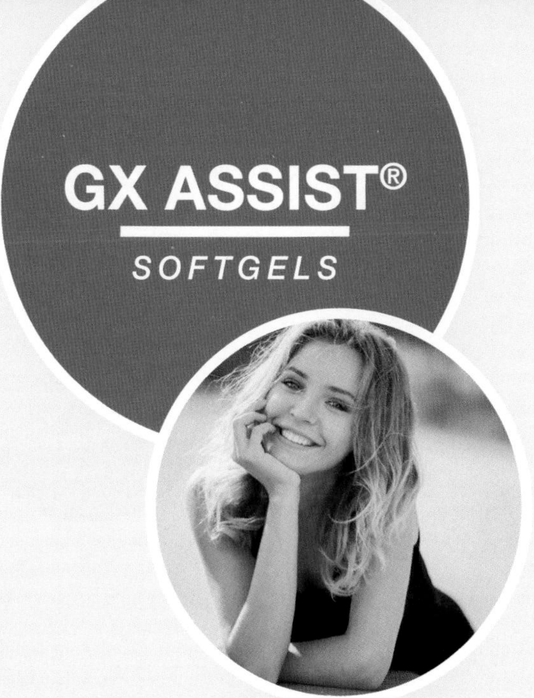

A blend of essential oils that support a healthy gastrointestinal (GI) tract by decreasing the overgrowth of pathogens in the gut; thereby increasing gut integrity and creating a healthy environment for new, good bacteria to thrive.

TOP USES

For overgrowth of candida albicans and other negative pathogens, autoimmune diseases, compromised digestive system, brain fog, illness and infections.

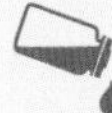

INGREDIENTS

- Oregano oil: Anti-fungal, anti-bacterial, anti-parasitic, decreases allergies, heartburn and bloating.
- Melaleuca (Tea tree) oil: Fights bad bacteria, fungus, and yeast infections and supports the immune system.
- Lemon oil: Antioxidant, anti-microbial, increases liver health and glutathione (internal antioxidant) production.
- Lemongrass oil: Anti-inflammatory, anti-microbial, supports immunity and digestive health.
- Peppermint oil: Soothes digestion, decreases heartburn and upset stomach.
- Thyme oil: Decreases inflammation, nausea and fatigue, anti-parasitic and fights bad bacteria.

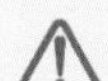

SAFETY

Keep out of reach of small children. If pregnant or lactating, women should consult a physician or health care provider before use. Do not use if safety seal is broken or missing.

Effect of thyme oil on small intestine integrity and antioxidant status, phagocytic activity and gastrointestinal microbiota in rabbits, Placha I, Chrastinova L, Laukova A, et al, Acta Veterinaria Hungarica. 2013

Antimicrobial activity of essential oils against Helicobacter pylori, Ohno T, Kita M, Yamaoka Y, et al, Helicobacter, 2003

Inhibition of enteric parasites by emulsified oil of oregano in vivo, Force M, Sparks WS, Ronzio RA, Phytotherapy Research, 2000

Antimicrobial activity of five essential oils against origin strains of the Enterobacteriaceae family, Penalver P, Huerta B, Borge C, et al, APMIS, 2005

In vitro antibacterial activity of some plant essential oils, Prabuseenivasan S, Jayakumar M, Ignacimuthu S, BMC Complementary and Alternative Medicine, 2006

Antimicrobial and antioxidant activities of three Mentha species essential oils, Mimica-Dukic N, Bozin B, Sokovic M, et al, Planta Med, 2003

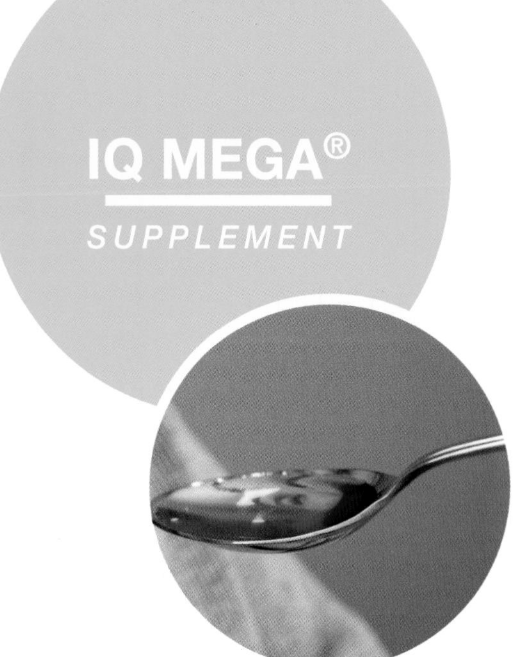

This product has both eicosapentaenoic acid (EPA) and docosahexaenoic acid (DHA) which combine to make up a balance of omega-3 essential fatty acids in fish oil form. Blended with essential oils to bring a less fishy flavor and a more pleasant one.

TOP USES

Brain fog, ADD/ADHD, cardiovascular disease, dry skin, joint pain and arthritis, anything "itis", weak muscles, and compromised immune system.

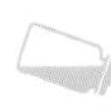

INGREDIENTS

- Fish oil (from cod, saithe, haddock) concentrate: High content omega-3 fatty acids extensively tested to ensure the oils are free of toxins and heavy metals. Supports brain function, increase mood, heart and cardiovascular function, increase attention, memory, concentration and skin health.
- DHA: Essential fatty acid shown to increase brain function, concentration, attention, memory, joint health, cell membrane integrity, nerve cell function, immunity and decrease inflammation.
- EPA: Essential fatty acid shown to increase mood, well being, cognitive function, nerve cell function and overall health of joints and inflammation in the body.
- Essential oils (wild orange and rosemary): For flavor, energy, concentration and memory.

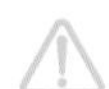

SAFETY

Keep out of reach of small children, keep refrigerated after opening. Do not use if safety seal is broken or missing.

Omega-3 fatty acid intakes are inversely related to elevated depressive symptoms among United States women, Beydoun MA, Kuczmarski MTF, Beydoun HA, et a, J Nutr 2013

Low blood long chain omega-3 fatty acids in UK children are associated with poor cognitive performance and behavior: A cross-sectional analysis from the DOLAB study, Montgomery P, Burton JR, Sewell RP, et al, PLoS ONE. 2013

Omega-3 fatty acids; Their beneficial role in cardiovascular health, Schwalfenberg G, Can Fam Physician. 2006

Omega-3 polyunsaturated fatty acids and the treatment of rheumatoid arthritis; a meta-analysis, Lee YH, Bae SC, Song GG, Arch Med Res, 2012

Effect of omega-3 fatty acids supplementation on endothelial function: A meta-analysis of randomized controlled trials, Wang Q, Liang X, Wang L, et al, Atherosclerosis. 2012

The importance of the ratio of omega-6/omega-3 essential fatty acids, Simopoulos AP, Biomed Pharmacother, 2002

MICROPLEX

VMz

Revolutionary micronutrient supplement providing naturally balanced amounts of all vitamins, minerals, trace elements, phytonutrients and antioxidants that give your body the most beneficial and safe amounts needed for long term health and vitality.

TOP USES

Low energy and fatigue, compromised digestion and immunity, oxidative cell damage, malnutrition, poor health and imbalanced nutrition.

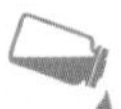

INGREDIENTS

- Water soluble vitamins, B-complex and C: Support energy and enhances macronutrient metabolism, transportation and elimination; enhances immunity and cognitive function, and strengthens the viscosity of the mucosa membranes lining the smooth muscle of the GI tract.
- Fat soluble vitamins A, E and K: Increases free radical scavenging, enhances utilization of macro-minerals and increases immune function.
- Vitamin D3: Immune system regulator. Enhances maro-mineral absorption, hormone balance, muscle health. Increases cognitive function.
- Macro-minerals (calcium, iron, iodine, magnesium, zinc, selenium, copper, manganese and chromium): Supports and enhances bone strength and density, proper bowel health, muscle contraction and release, fluid balance, nervous system health, cell function, immunity, anti-oxidation and hormone health.
- Polyphenol blend (grape seed extract, quercetin, rutin, pomegranate fruit extract, citrus fruit polyphenol extract, resveratrol, Indian Kino tree wood extract): enhances free radical scavenging, decreases inflammation, increases proper cellular function and proliferation.
- Whole foods blend (kale leaf extract, dandelion leaf powder, parsley leaf powder, spinach leaf powder, broccoli aerial parts powder, cabbage leaf extract, Brussels sprout immature inflorescences powder): A blend of whole foods and phytonutrients which enhance digestion and absorption of micronutrients and give balanced nutrition.
- Stomach comfort blend of ginger, peppermint extract and caraway: Calms and soothes the digestive process.

SAFETY

Can be taken by all ages that can swallow capsules. Do not use if safety seal is broken or missing.

Selected vitamins and trace elements support immune function by strengthening epithelial barriers and cellular and humoral immune responses, Maggini S, Wintergerst ES, Beveridge S, Hornig DH, British Journal of Nutrition. 2007

Contribution of selected vitamins and trace elements to immune function, Wintergerst ES, Maggini S, Hornig DH, Ann Nutr Met, 2007

Efficacy and tolerability of a fixed combination of peppermint oil and caraway oil in patients suffering from functional dyspepsia, May B, Kohler S, Schneider B, Aliment Pharmacol Therapy. 2000

The immunological functions of the vitamin D endocrine system, Hayes CE, Nashold FE, Spach KM & Pedersen LB, Cell Molec Biol, 2003

Use of calcium or calcium in combination with vitamin D supplementation to prevent fractures and bone loss in people aged 50 years and older: a meta-analysis, Tang BMP, Eslick GD, Nowson C, et al, The Lancet, 2007

MITO2MAX®

COMPLEX

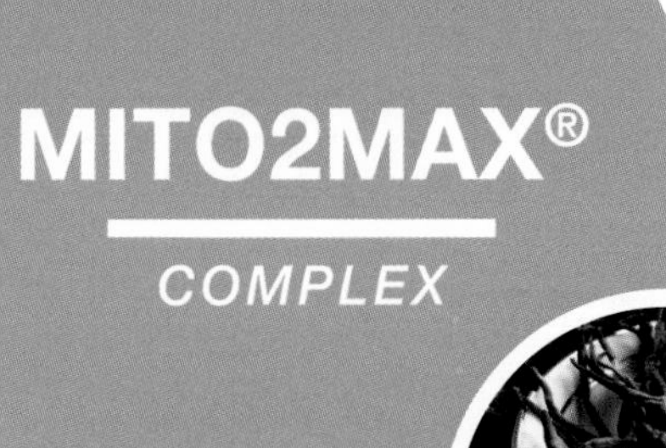

A blend of adaptogenic herbs and extracts with energy co-factors made to increase mitochondrial biogenesis and overall energy while decreasing the stress response due to physical activity and daily life.

TOP USES

Body fatigue and tiredness, adrenal fatigue, hormonal imbalance, libido, physical stress, anxiety, and poor circulation.

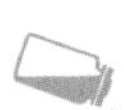

INGREDIENTS

- Acetyl-l-carnitine HCL: Increases energy production by the mitochondria and increases glutathione (internal antioxidant) levels in the body.
- Alpha-lipoic acid: Antioxidant vital for cellular energy and neutralizing free radicals.
- Coenzyme Q10: Plays a significant role in energy production for the heart and muscle cells.
- Lychee fruit extract and green tea leaf polyphenol extract: Increases circulation, decreases inflammation, and decreases oxidative stress.
- Quercetin dihydrate: Potent antioxidant flavonoid known to decrease cell damage and increase recovery.
- Cordyceps mycelium: An Adaptogen which enhances respiratory health and physical endurance, hormonal health, increased libido and liver function.
- Ginseng (panax quinquefolius) root extract: Increases energy and adaption to stress as well as stimulates the immune system by increasing the amount of white blood cells in the blood.
- Ashwagandha (withania somnifera) root extract: Powerful adaptogen that lowers cortisol by decreasing the mental and physical stress response. Also gives energy and vitality to the body.

SAFETY

Not for children. Keep out of reach of small children. If pregnant or lactating, women should consult a physician or health care provider before use. Do not use if safety seal is broken or missing.

Ginkgo biloba special extract EGb 761 in generalized anxiety disorder and adjustment disorder with anxious mood: A randomized, double-blind, placebo-controlled trial, Woelk H, Arnoldt KH, Kieser M, Hoerr R, Journal of Psychiatric Research 2007

Effects of ginkgo biloba on mental functioning in healthy volunteers, Cieza A, Maier P, Poppel E, Archives of Medical Research, 2002

Translating the basic knowledge of mitochondrial functions to metabolic therapy: role of L-carnitine, Marcovina SM, Sirtori C, Peracino A, et al, Translational Research 2013

Effects of lipoic acid on mtDNA damage following isolated muscle contractions, Fogarty MC, Deviot G, Hughes CM, et al, Med Sci Sports Exerc, 2013

The effects and mechanisms of mitochondrial nutrient a-lipoic acid on improved age-associated mitochondrial and cognitive dysfunction: An overview, Liu J, Neurochem Res, 2008

Effect of Cs-4 (Cordyceps sinensis) on exercise performance in healthy older subjects: A double-blind, placebo controlled trial, Chen S, Li Z, Krochmal R, et al, The Journal of Alternative and Complementary Medicine. 2010

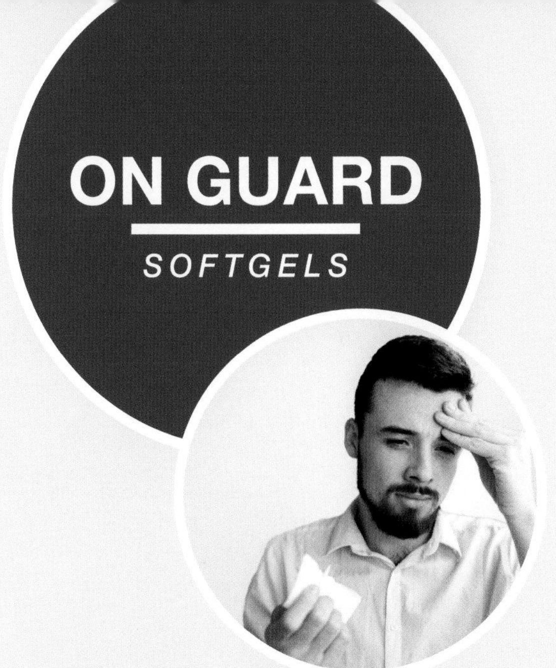

ON GUARD SOFTGELS

A blend of several essential oils in a convenient softgel that protect the immune system from foreign invaders (pathogens).

TOP USES

Sore or dry throat, cough, colds and flus, illness, laryngitis, preventative care, and compromised immunity.

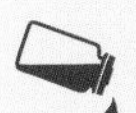

INGREDIENTS

- Wild orange oil: Antioxidant and anti-inflammatory properties, antimicrobial and promotes healthy digestion.
- Clove oil: Powerful antioxidant, anti-parasitic and anti-fungal properties, improves blood circulation, decreases pain (numbing agent) and inflammation, and inhibits pathogenic activity.
- Black pepper oil: Antiseptic, anti-catarrhal, and expectorant properties. Helps respiratory system by promoting blood flow and circulation.
- Cinnamon oil: Highly anti-bacterial, anti-fungal, and anti-microbial, promotes healthy blood sugar and insulin balance.
- Eucalyptus oil: Decreases fevers, congestion and body pains, and has anti-viral effects on the respiratory system.
- Oregano oil: Powerful antibacterial, antiviral, and antifungal properties. Helps support the immune system against ailments.
- Rosemary oil: Great expectorant/decongestant, increases memory and concentration, inflammation and has a balancing effect on the endocrine system.
- Melissa oil: Antiviral properties and supports against respiratory ailments.

SAFETY

Not for children. Keep out of reach of small children. If pregnant or lactating, women should consult a physician or health care provider before use. Do not use if safety seal is broken or missing.

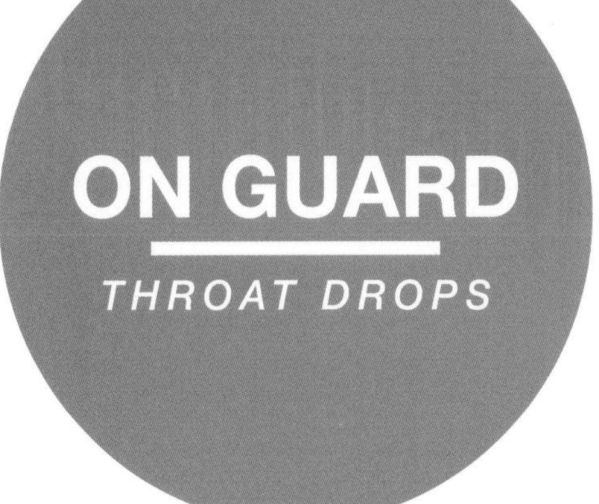

ON GUARD THROAT DROPS

A blend of several essential oils in a convenient, organically sweetened throat lozenge that soothe the throat and protect the immune system from foreign invaders. (pathogens).

TOP USES

Sore or dry throat, cough, colds and flu, illness, laryngitis, preventative care, and compromised immunity.

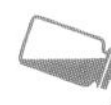

INGREDIENTS

- Wild orange oil: Antioxidant and anti-inflammatory properties, antimicrobial and promotes healthy digestion.
- Clove oil: Powerful antioxidant, anti-parasitic and anti-fungal properties, improves blood circulation, decreases pain (numbing agent) and inflammation, and inhibits pathogenic activity.
- Cinnamon oil: Highly anti-bacterial, anti-fungal, and anti-microbial, promotes healthy blood sugar and insulin balance.
- Eucalyptus oil: Decreases fevers, congestion and body pains, and has anti-viral effects on the respiratory system.
- Rosemary oil: Great expectorant/decongestant, increases memory and concentration, inflammation and has a balancing effect on the endocrine system.
- Myrrh oil: Supports blood flow to gums and teeth, antioxidant properties.
- Organic cane juice: Natural sweetener.
- Organic brown rice syrup: Natural sweetener.

SAFETY

Be aware with small children that are prone to choking.

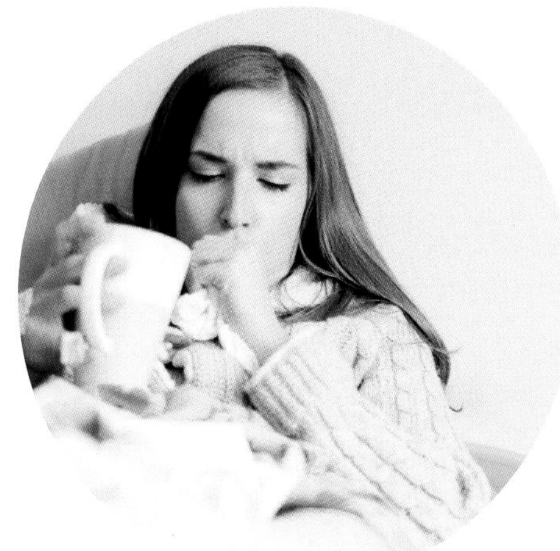

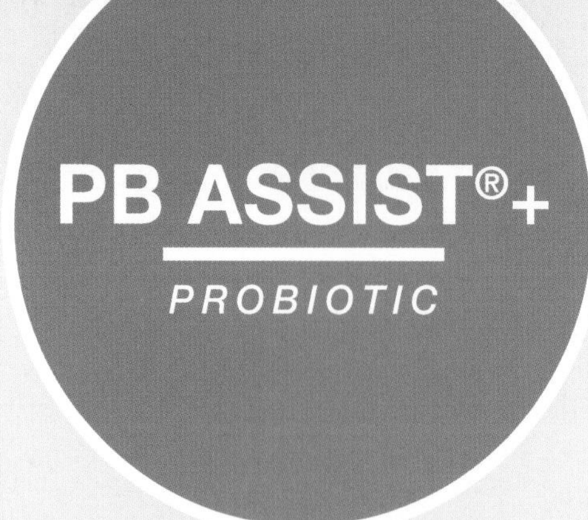

PB ASSIST®+

PROBIOTIC

A double-encapsulated, time-release probiotic capsule or powdered encapsulated probiotic supplement (for children or adults who have trouble swallowing pills) with six different strains of good bacteria and prebiotic fiber for maximum delivery and cultivation of healthy gut flora.

TOP USES

Flatulence, constipation or diarrhea, malabsorption, irritable bowel, compromised immune system, leaky gut, allergies, autoimmune diseases, anxiety and depression, mental disorders, and infections.

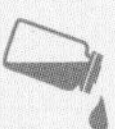

INGREDIENTS (capsule)

- L. acidophilus, L. salivarius, L. casei: Lactobacillus strains of bacteria which increase the integrity of the villi of the upper intestinal tract to improve the absorption of other nutrients. Also enhancing immunity and the gut-brain connection increasing proper neurotransmitter and brain function.
- B. lactis, B. bifidum, B. longum: Bifidobacterium strains that help digestion and immunity of the large intestines and enhance overall colon health. Also increasing the functions of the brain and improving mood.
- FOS (fructo-oligosaccharides) prebiotic: Indigestible fibers that enhance the growth and cultivation of good bacteria while decreasing growth of bad bacteria.

INGREDIENTS (powder)

- L. rhamnosus. L. salivarius, L. plantarum (LP01, LP02), B. breve, B. lactic strains selected for unique stability at room temperature, ability to survive harsh extremes of digestive system, reach the intestines safely, and benefits among children. Also to maintain healthy intestinal microflora balance and support healthy function of digestive, immune, female reproductive systems, and GI tract (particularly the intestines and colon), kidneys, bladder, and urinary tract. Promotes optimal metabolism and absorption of nutrients and healthy lung and respiratory tract function. Also enhancing healthy brain and nervous system function and establishing health benefits for long-term well-being.
- FOS prebiotic to help sustain a healthy balance of beneficial friendly flora.

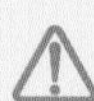

SAFETY

For all ages. NOTE: Do not mix with hot water.

PEPPERMINT

SOFTGELS

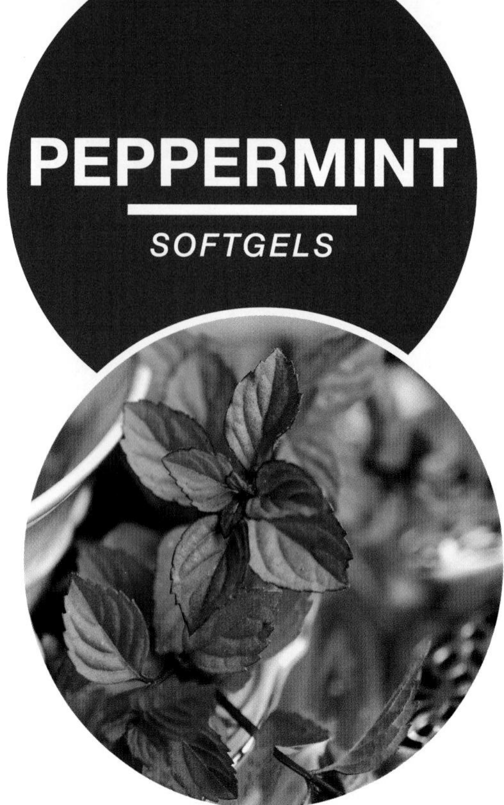

Highly versatile with a long history in herbal preparations and as a food additive, an enteric coated capsule ensures peppermint essential oil passes through the stomach undissolved for small intestine delivery where its most effective for specific and intended purposes.

TOP USES

Help ease and relax gastrointestinal muscles, while calming stomach and intestinal tract; helpful to an irritable bowel or spastic colon with conditions such as IBS, Crohn's disease, and colitis.

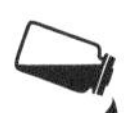

INGREDIENTS

- Peppermint oil: With high menthol content, gastrointestinal applications include appetite reduction, relief of gas, bloating, and stomach upset, soothing digestion and heartburn. Other internal use benefits can include helping ease respiratory congestion, improve alertness, stimulate brain, decrease breast milk supply, overcome loss of sense of smell.

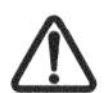

SAFETY

Keep out of reach of children. If pregnant, nursing, or under a doctor's care, consult physician. Do not use if safety seal is broken or missing. Store in cool, dry place.

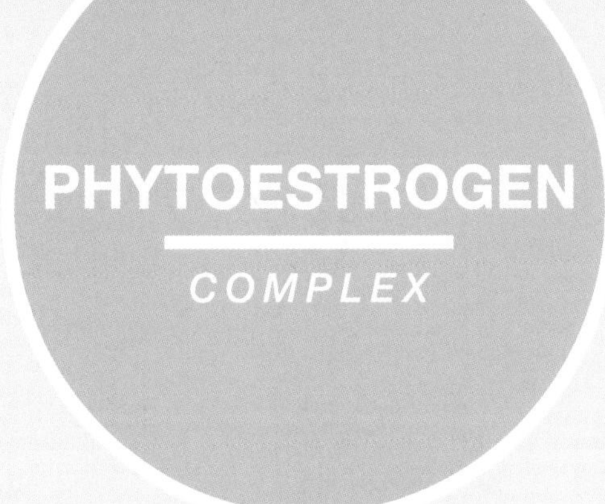

PHYTOESTROGEN

COMPLEX

Blend of standardized extracts of plant (phyto) estrogens and lignans to help create a balance of hormones throughout the body and eliminate unwanted metabolites.

TOP USES

Menopause, perimenopause, andropause, hormonal imbalances and mood swings (PMS).

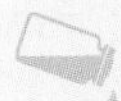

INGREDIENTS

- Genistein (soy extract): An isoflavone antioxidant that promotes healthy breast and uterine tissue and brings balance to hormones in both men and women. Also shown to help prevent prostate cancer in men and ovarian and breast cancer in women.
- Flax seed extract (lignans): Decreases estrogen metabolites for further hormone balance and protection of the sex organ tissues and cells.
- Pomegranate extract: Powerful antioxidant shown to help the reduction of free radical damage to the cells.

SAFETY

Not for children. Keep out of reach of small children.Okay for men and women. If pregnant or lactating, women should consult a physician or health care provider before use. Do not use if safety seal is broken or missing.

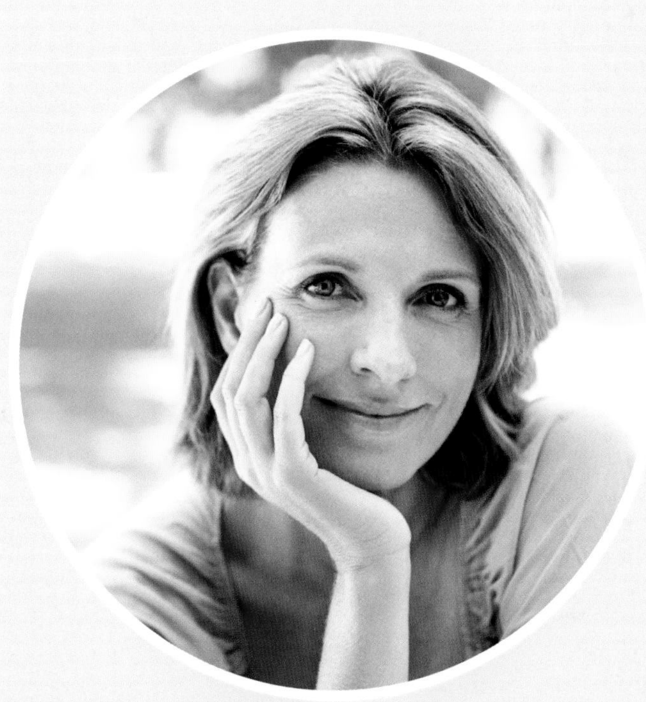

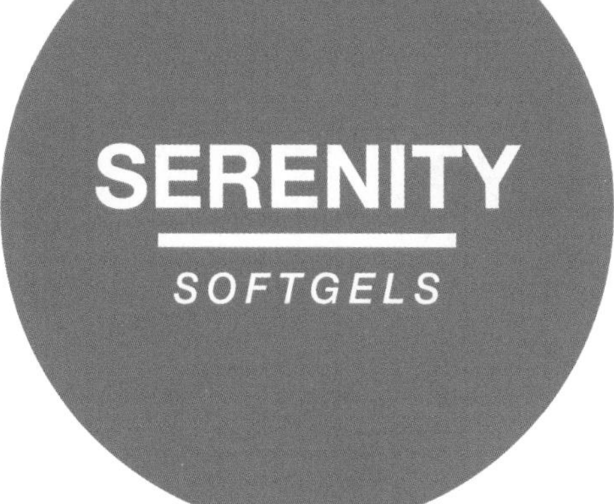

SERENITY

SOFTGELS

A blend of lavender essential oil and natural plant extracts to enhance a restful night's sleep by promoting relaxation without feeling groggy or sleepy the next day.

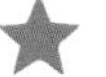

TOP USES

Insomnia, inability to fall asleep or wake up easily, groggy feelings upon rising in morning, lack of adequate sleep, negative impact due to lack of sleep: decreased ability to lose weight, learn, or control emotions; poor reaction time, increased presence of stress hormones, decreased sense of well-being, negative impact on cardiovascular health and body's natural ability to recuperate and restore.

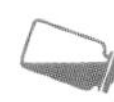

INGREDIENTS

- Lavender oil: Long history of traditional internal use to encourage restful sleep, calm the nervous system, reduce stress.
- L-Theanine (non-protein amino acid found in green tea [camellia sinensis]): Promotes pre-sleep relaxation and quality sleep without feeling groggy or drowsy the next day. Improves mood, calmness, and general relaxation.
- Lemon balm oil: Calming effects for anxiety, sleep problems, restlessness. Used for attention deficit, hyperactivity, hysteria, tension headaches, and rapid heartbeat due to nervousness. Boosts alertness upon waking, improves memory, problem-solving, brain protection, and mood.
- Passionflower oil: Used for insomnia, nervous stomach/ ulcers, anxiety, nervousness, drug withdrawal, hysteria, attention deficit, hyperactivity, excitability, heart palpitations, an overactive mind, stress.
- German chamomile oil: Acts as a mild sedative, promotes healthy serotonin levels. Used traditionally to treat nervous stomach or bowels, anxiety, tension headaches, and at bedtime for insomnia. Promotes body's healing and restorative capacity and ability to get rid of dark circles under eyes.

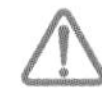

SAFETY

Keep out of reach of children. If you are pregnant, nursing, or under a doctor's care, consult your physician. Do not use if safety seal is broken or missing.

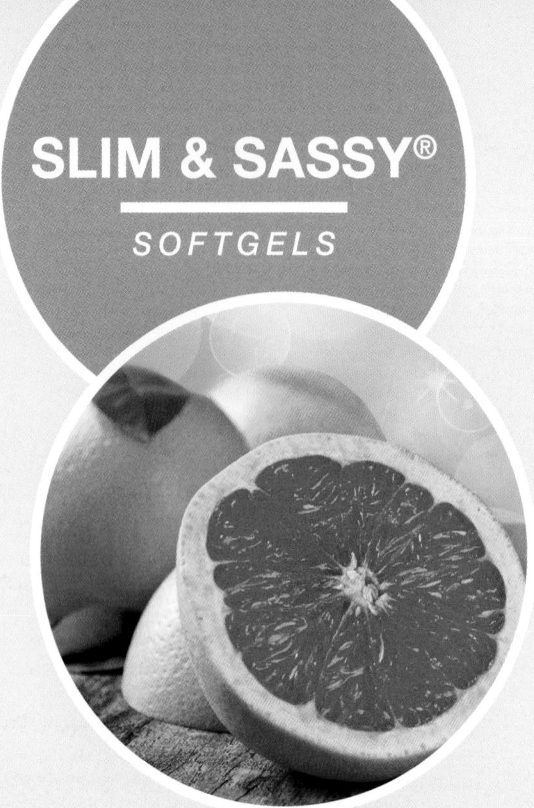

A blend of essential oils in convenient softgels to help manage hunger throughout the day while boosting metabolism and promoting a positive mood, cleanse the body, aide digestion, curb the appetite, provide a stimulating and positive effect on the endocrine system and to assist with weight loss.

TOP USES

Slow metabolism, overweight or obese individuals, lack of energy (fatigue), diabetes, toxic liver, and compromised endocrine system.

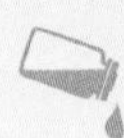

INGREDIENTS

- Grapefruit oil: Promotes cleansing, detoxifying, decreases appetite, and induces lipolysis (mobilization of fat cells from stored fat).
- Lemon oil: Cleansing, aids digestion, powerful antioxidant, increases lipolysis, and elevates the mood.
- Peppermint oil: Helps manage hunger cravings, soothes digestion, and invigorates the mind.
- Ginger oil: Promotes healthy digestion and enhances metabolism and thermogenesis (increased heat through metabolic stimulation).
- Cinnamon oil: Has a positive effect on the endocrine system to assist with weight loss, lowers blood sugar, and balances insulin response. Also inhibits adipogenesis (fat storage).

SAFETY

Not for children. Keep out of reach of small children. If pregnant or lactating, women should consult a physician or health care provider before use. Do not use if safety seal is broken or missing.

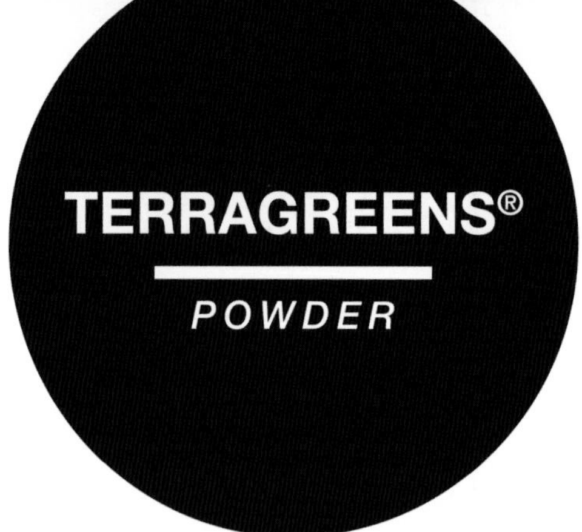

TOP USES

For people with poor nutrition, busy and stressful lifestyle habits, weight management, compromised digestion and immunity.

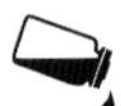

INGREDIENTS

- Green powder blend (kale, dandelion greens, spinach, parsley, collard greens leaf, broccoli, cabbage): Phytonutrients, which are cleansing to the body and immune building. Also anticancer and antioxidant properties.
- Grass powder blend (wheat grass, alfalfa juice, oat grass, barley grass, oat grass juice and barley grass juice): High in chlorophyll and other phytonutrients which have powerful blood-cleansing and -strengthening properties as well as enhancing immune function.
- Fruit powder blend (pineapple juice, guava fruit, mango juice, goji berry, mangosteen, and acerola cherry): Powerful antioxidant and free radical scavenging properties.
- Lemon and ginger oils: Aids in digestive and metabolic functions.

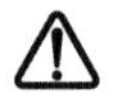

SAFETY

For all ages. Gluten-free and non-GMO. Vegan-friendly. Do not use if safety seal is broken or missing.

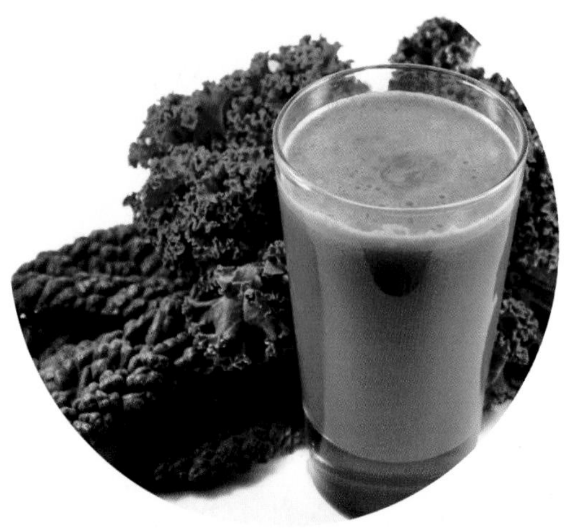

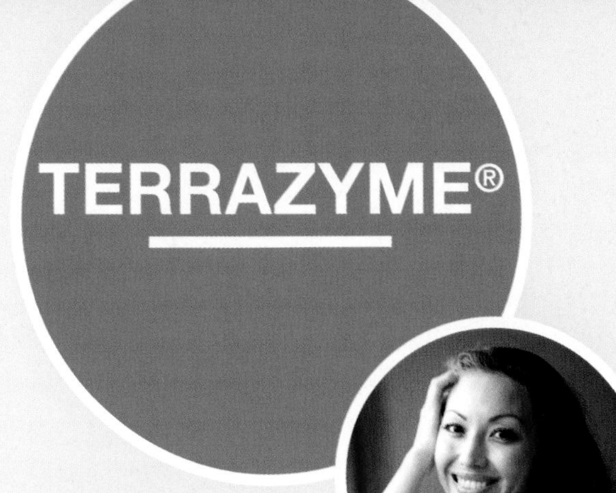

TERRAZYME®

A blend of several, active, whole-food enzymes and mineral cofactors that help the breakdown of proteins, fats, complex carbohydrates, sugars, and fiber, giving the body better digestion nutrients readily available by for absorption and utilization.

TOP USES

Poor nutrition, heartburn or indigestion, slow metabolism, upset stomach, bloating, and flatulence.

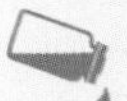

INGREDIENTS

- Protease: Breaks down protein to peptides and amino acids.
- Papain: Breaks down protein.
- Amylase: Breaks down carbohydrates, starches, and sugars.
- Lipase: Breaks down fats and oils to be absorbed in the intestine.
- Lactase: Breaks down lactose in milk sugars.
- Alpha galactosidase: Breaks down complex polysaccharide sugars in legumes and cruciferous vegetables that can cause bloating and gas.
- Cellulase: Breaks down fiber to help digest fruits and vegetables.
- Sucrase: Breaks down sucrose to fructose and glucose for energy.
- Anti-gluten enzyme blend: Assists in breaking down gluten.
- Glucoamylase: Breaks down starch.
- Betaine HCL: Aids in protein digestion.
- Stomach comfort peppermint, ginger, caraway: Helps soothe the digestive process and tames the stomach.

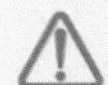

SAFETY

Can be taken by all ages that can swallow capsules. If pregnant or lactating, women should consult a physician or health care provider before use. Do not use if safety seal is broken or missing.

A broader view: Microbial enzymes and their relevance in industries, medicine, and beyond, Gurung N, Ray S, Bose S, Rai V, Biomed Res Int 2013

Enzyme replacement therapy for pancreatic insufficiency: Present and future, Fieker A, philpott J, Armand M, Clinical and Experimental Gastroenterology, 2011

Randomised clinical trial: A 1-week, double-blind, placebo-controlled study of pancreatin 25000 Ph. Eur. Minimicrospheres for pancreatic exocrine insufficiency after pancreatic surgery, with a 1-year open-label extension, Seiler Cm, Izbicki J, Varga-Szabo L, et al, Aliment Pharmacol Ther, 2013

Fate of pancreatic enzymes during small intestinal aboral transit in humans, Layer P, Go VLW, DiMagno EP, Intraluminal Fate of Pancreatic Enzymes, 1986

Effects of different levels of supplementary alpha-amylase on digestive enzyme activities and pancreatic amylase mRNA expression of young broilers, Jiang Z, Zhou Y, Lu F, et al, Asian-Aust J Anim Sci. 2008

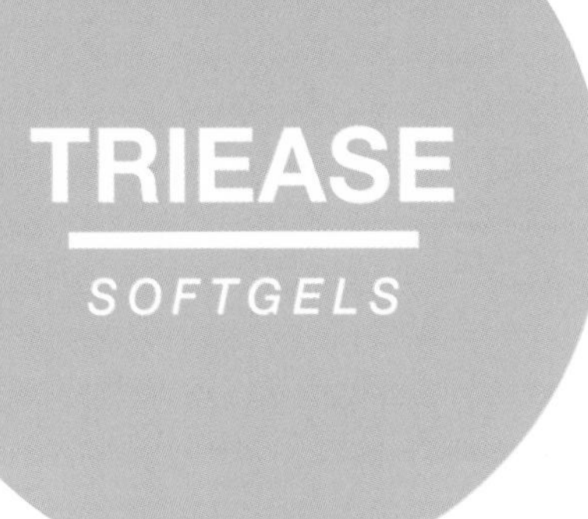

TRIEASE

SOFTGELS

A blend of essential oils in a convenient softgel to be consumed quickly and easily when traveling, attending outdoor events, or when seasonal or environmental elements are particularly high, or on a daily basis during times of seasonal discomfort to promote clear breathing and overall respiratory health.

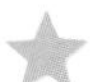

TOP USES

Seasonal allergies, hay fever, congestion, head colds and headaches, bronchitis, asthma, and sinusitis.

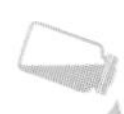

INGREDIENTS

- Lemon oil: Antioxidant, antiseptic, promotes respiratory health and cleansing.
- Lavender oil: Renowned for its calming and balancing effects, both internally and externally.
- Peppermint oil: Bronchodilator, soothes digestion, stimulates brain and helps decrease allergy symptoms.

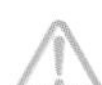

SAFETY

Be aware with small children that are prone to choking. Do not use if safety seal is broken or missing.

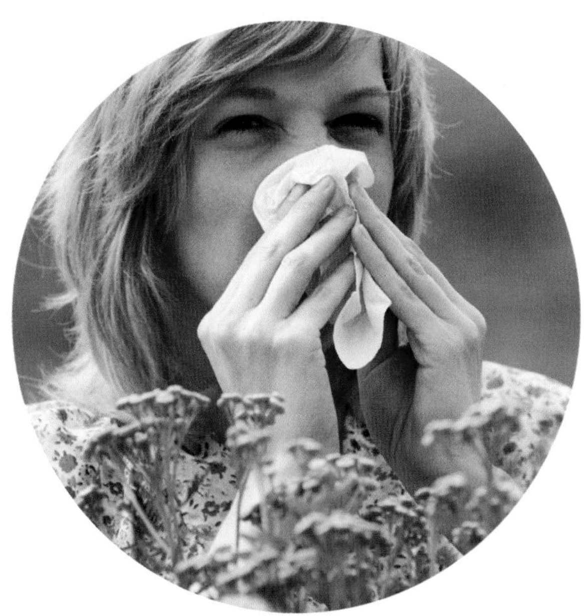

TRIMSHAKE®

REPLACEMENT SHAKE

A convenient and delicious weight management shake mix that provides low-fat, low-calorie, high-protein, high-fiber, nutrients as a lean alternative for individuals trying to lose fat or maintain a lean body composition through calorie reduction and exercise.

TOP USES

Weight management, poor nutrition, slow metabolism, and stressful lifestyle habits.

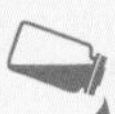

INGREDIENTS

- Protein blend (whey protein isolate and egg white protein): Proteins necessary for lean muscle recovery and development while promoting a healthy lifestyle through diet and exercise.
- Fiber blend (non-GMO soluble corn fiber, xanthan gum, citrus fiber, tara gum, oligofructose): A mixture of insoluble and prebiotic soluble fiber that promotes beneficial bacterial function and elimination.
- Ashwagandha root/leaf extract: An adaptogen for energy production, helps control the release of the stress hormone cortisol, which is associated with the accumulation of fat, particularly around the stomach, hips, and thighs. Has also been demonstrated to help control stress induced appetite, overeating, and carbohydrate cravings, helps support blood sugar levels, enhances energy, and alleviates fatigue.
- Potato protein powder: Supports an increased feeling of satiety, and helps to control snacking between meals, portion control, and feeling full faster and longer.
- Vitamin and mineral blend: Creates a synergy of nutrients similar to whole foods.

SAFETY

For all ages. Gluten free and non GMO. Do not use if safety seal is broken or missing.

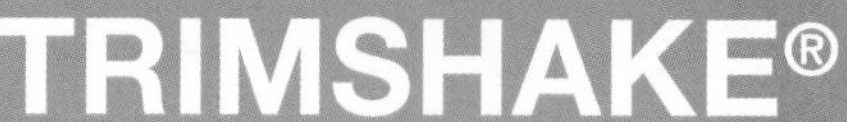

TRIMSHAKE®

REPLACEMENT SHAKE - VEGAN

A convenient and delicious weight management vegan shake mix that provides low-fat, low-calorie, high-protein, high-fiber, nutrients as a lean alternative for individuals trying to lose fat or maintain a lean body composition through calorie reduction and exercise.

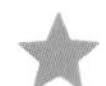

TOP USES

Weight management, poor nutrition, slow metabolism, stressful lifestyle habits, and vegan alternative.

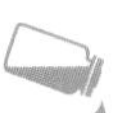

INGREDIENTS

- Protein blend (pea protein, quinoa, and amaranth): Proteins necessary for lean muscle recovery and development while promoting a healthy lifestyle through diet and exercise.
- Fiber blend (non-GMO soluble corn fiber, xanthan gum, citrus fiber, tara gum, oligofructose): A mixture of insoluble and prebiotic soluble fiber that promotes beneficial bacterial function and elimination.
- Ashwagandha root/leaf extract: An adaptogen for energy production, helps control the release of the stress hormone cortisol, which is associated with the accumulation of fat, particularly around the stomach, hips, and thighs. Has also been demonstrated to help control stress induced appetite, overeating, and carbohydrate cravings, helps support blood sugar levels, enhances energy, and alleviates fatigue.
- Potato protein powder: Supports an increased feeling of satiety, and helps to control snacking between meals, portion control, and feeling full faster and longer.
- Vitamin and mineral blend: Creates a synergy of nutrients similar to whole foods.

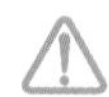

SAFETY

For all ages. Gluten-free and non-GMO. Do not use if safety seal is broken or missing.

Slows gastric emptying, reducing postprandial levels of insulin and glucose Schwartz JG, Guan D, Green GM, Phillips WT, Diabetes Care, 1994

Protease inhibitor concentrate derived from potato reduced food intake and weight gain in healthy rats by increasing CCK levels, Komarnytsky S, Cook A, Raskin I, International Journal of Obesity, 2011

Taking two capsules a day of 300 mg ashwagandha root extract each for 60 days resulted in a significant reduction in cortisol levels, Chandrasekhar K, Kapoor J, Anishetty S, Indian Journal of Psychological Medicine, 2012

A low-fat, high-protein diet seems to enhance weight loss and provide a better long term maintenance of reduced intra-abdominal fat stores, Due A, Toubro S, Skov AR, Astrup A, International Journal of Obesity. 2004

An energy-restricted, high-protein, low-fat diet provides nutritional and metabolic benefits that are equal to and sometimes greater than those observed with a high-carbohydrate diet, Noakes M, Keogh JB, Foster PR, Clifton PM, American Journal of Clinical Nutrition, 2005

A standardized withania somnifera extract significantly reduces stress-related parameters in chronically stressed humans: A double-blind, randomized, placebo controlled study, Auddy B, Hazra J, Mitra A, et al, The Journal of the American Nutraceutical Association, 2008

TURMERIC

DUAL CHAMBER CAPSULES

A unique dual chamber, providing an inner layer of botanical extract and outer layer of essential oil, intended to promote better absorption in a convenient delivery system. Turmeric is chemically diverse in composition, with more than 235 chemical constituents identified.

TOP USES

Cancer, tumors, leukemia, cellular and immune health, autoimmune conditions, joint pain and swelling, arthritis, gout, rheumatism; neurological diseases, fungal, bacterial, viral infections; cognitive dysfunction, stroke, poor circulation and blood supply to brain, epilepsy; high blood sugar and cholesterol, poor metabolism; blood, liver and lymph toxicity; intestinal worms and parasites, acne, eczema, psoriasis, ulcers, gas, bloating, cough, bronchitis, menstrual cramps, cavities, oral health, bites, stings, skin health.

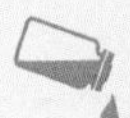

INGREDIENTS

- Turmeric oil: Increases bioavailability of curcuminoids for better potency and absorption, supports healthy nervous, glucose, immune response, helps prevent cancer cells from forming, multiplying.
  - ar-Turmerone and Turmerone: Antioxidant, anti-inflammatory, inhibits reception of pain, promotes stem cell proliferation and differentiation in brain for self-repair and recovery of brain function, stomach, liver ailments; reproductive problems, infectious diseases, blood disorders.
- Turmeric extract: Anti-inflammatory, anticancer compounds, help fight foreign invaders, heart disease, cancer, metabolic syndrome, Alzheimer's, degenerative conditions.
  - Curlone: Antioxidant, antifungal, antibacterial, clogged arteries, strokes or heart attacks, blood sugar control.
  - Curcumin extract: Antioxidant, stimulates body's own antioxidant enzymes, decreases risk of Alzheimer's disease, helping to improve learning and memory; boosts growth and development of new neurons, improving symptoms related to neurodegenerative and psychiatric disorders.

SAFETY

Keep out of reach of children. If pregnant, nursing, or under a doctor's care, consult physician. Do not use if safety seal is broken or missing. Store in cool, dry place.

vEO MEGA

COMPLEX VEGAN

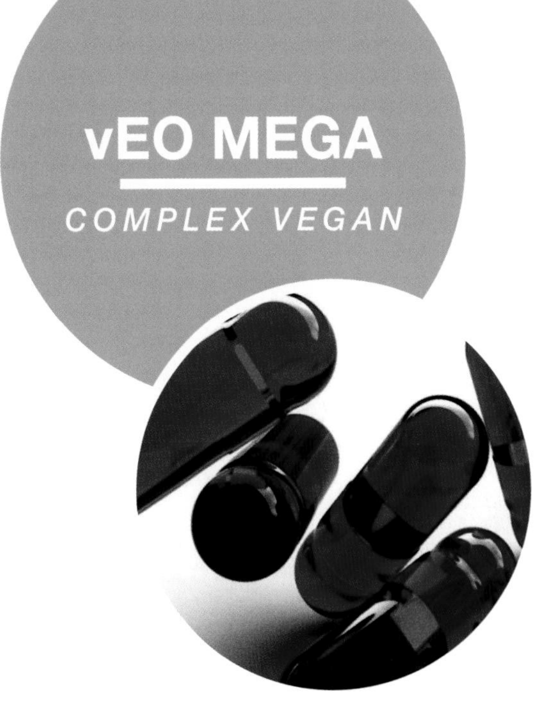

A blend of marine base and land base omega essential fatty acids in a unique assimilation capsule with essential oils and fat-soluble vitamins.

TOP USES

Inflammation and pain, arthritis, anything "itis", compromised immune system, brain fog, concentration, ADD/ADHD, aging skin, PMS, postpartum depression, depression and anxiety, cardiovascular disease, dry skin and skin issues.

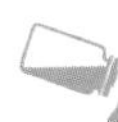

INGREDIENTS

- Flax seed oil: ALA essential fatty acid that support the production of EPA and DHA in the body increasing all the benefits of omega-3 fatty acids.
- Algae oil (DHA): Essential fatty acid that support brain function and increase mood, heart, and cardiovascular function, decreases LDL and triglyceride levels, increased attention, memory, concentration, joint health, skin health, immunity and decreases inflammation.
- Inca Inchi seed oil: Essential fatty acid that promotes inflammatory modulation and decreases oxidative stress.
- Borage oil: GLA essential fatty acid that supports inflammatory markers in the body, clears skin, and balances out the mood and hormones.
- Cranberry oil: Shown to decrease LDL and triglyceride levels, enhances mood and concentration as well as provides beneficial fats for skin health.
- Pomegranate oil: Antioxidant oil that increases skin health and decreases inflammation in the skin.
- Pumpkin oil: Helps to increase HDL (good) cholesterol and can promotes energy in the brain.
- Grape oil: Promotes a reduction in LDL (bad) cholesterol and triglyceride levels.

- Natural vitamin E: Protects cell membranes against oxidative damage and promotes eye health.
- Astaxanthin: Powerful carotenoid that promotes cellular regeneration, heart and cardiovascular strength, decreases macular degeneration and strengthens the eyes.
- Lutein: Shown to increase strength of the eyes, heart and cells.
- Zeaxanthin: Potent antioxidant good for the eyes and cardiovascular system.
- Lycopene: Fights free radicals and strengthens the integrity of the cell membranes.
- Alpha and beta carotene: Antioxidants that promote eye health and fight free radicals.
- Essential oil blend of caraway, clove, cumin, frankincense, German chamomile, ginger, peppermint, thyme, and wild orange: Powerful antioxidant properties, immune system properties, promotes healthy digestion, cellular function, and anti-inflammation.

SAFETY

Can be taken by all ages that can swallow capsules. If pregnant or lactating, women should consult a physician or health care provider before use. Do not use if safety seal is broken or missing.

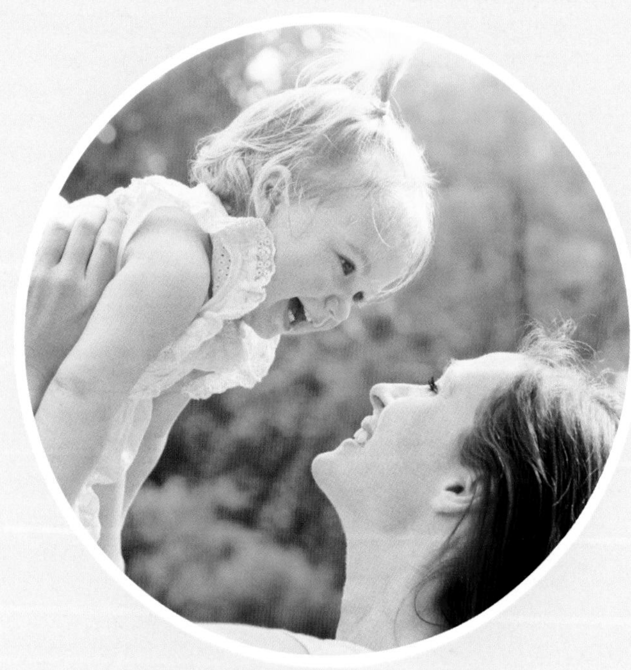

A meta-analysis shows that docosahexaenoic acid from algal oil reduces serum triglycerides and increases HDL-cholesterol and LDL-cholesterol in person without coronary heart disease, Bernstein AM, Ding EL, Willett WC, Rimm EB, The Journal of Nutrition, 2012

Astaxanthin, cell membrane nutrient with diverse clinical benefits and anti-aging potential, Kidd P, Alternative Medicine Review, 2011

a-Linolenic acid and risk of cardiovascular disease: a systematic review and meta-analysis, Pan A, Chen M, Chowdhury R, et al, The American Journal of Clinical Nutrition, 2012

The cardiovascular effects of flaxseed and its omega-3 fatty acid, alpha-linolenic acid, Rodriguez-Leyva D, Bassett CMC, McCullough R, Pierce GN, Can J Cardiol, 2010

Macular pigment optical density and eye health, Alexander DE, Kemin Technical Literature, 2010

xE0 MEGA

COMPLEX

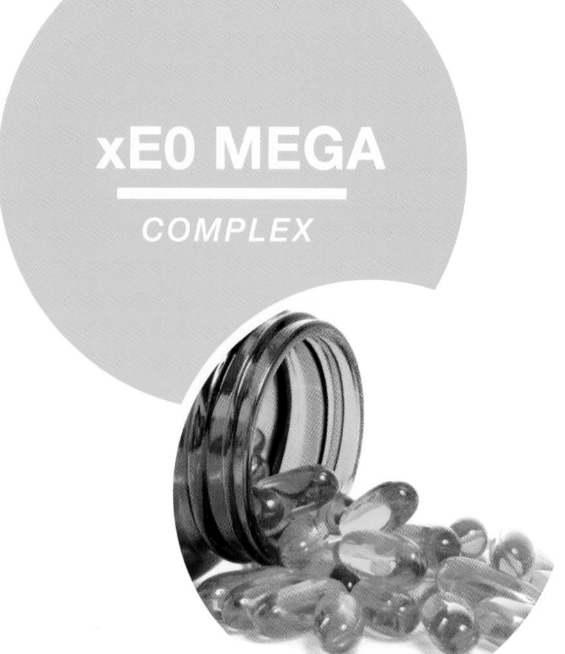

A blend of marine base and land base omega essential fatty acids in a unique assimilation capsule with essential oils and fat-soluble vitamins.

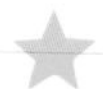

TOP USES

Inflammation and pain, arthritis, anything “itis”, compromised immune system, brain fog, concentration, ADD/ADHD, aging skin, PMS, post-partum depression, anxiety and depression, cardiovascular disease, dry skin and skin issues.

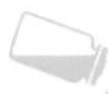

INGREDIENTS

- Fish oil (from anchovy, sardine, mackerel, and calamari) concentrate: EPA and DHA essential fatty acids that support brain function and increase mood, heart and cardiovascular function, decrease LDL and triglyceride levels, increase attention, memory, concentration, joint health, skin health, immunity and decrease inflammation.
- Echium plantagineum seed oil: a blend of ALA, SDA, and GLA essential fatty acids that support the cardiovascular system, decrease LDL and increase HDL triglyceride levels, balances inflammatory markers, enhances mood, brain, and skin health.
- Pomegranate oil: Antioxidant oil that increases skin health and decreases inflammation in the skin.
- Vitamin A (as alpha and beta carotene): Antioxidants that promote eye health and fight free radicals.
- Vitamin D3 (as natural cholecalciferol): Supports immune system function, enhances macro-mineral absorption, hormone balance, muscle health, and increases cognitive function.
- Vitamin E: Protects cell membranes against oxidative damage and promotes eye health.
- Astaxanthin: Powerful carotenoid that promotes cellular regeneration, heart and cardiovascular strength, decreases macular degeneration and strengthens the eyes.
- Lutein: Shown to increase strength of the eyes, heart and cells.

- Zeaxanthin: Potent antioxidant good for the eyes and cardiovascular system.
- Essential oil blend of caraway, clove, cumin, frankincense, German chamomile, ginger, peppermint, thyme, and wild orange: Powerful antioxidant properties, immune system properties, promotes healthy digestion, cellular function, and anti-inflammation.

SAFETY

Can be taken by all ages that can swallow capsules. If pregnant or lactating, women should consult a physician or health care provider before use. Do not use if safety seal is broken or missing.

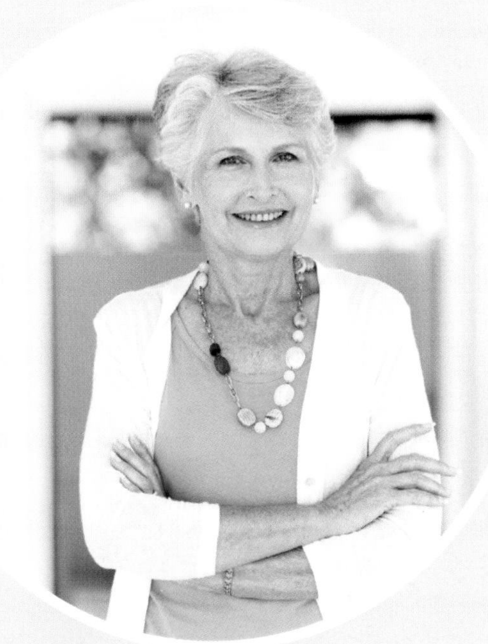

Serum and macular responses to multiple xanthophyll supplements in patients with early age-related macular degeneration, Huang YM, Yan SF, Ma L, et al, Nutrition, 2013
a-Linolenic acid and risk of cardiovascular disease: a systematic review and meta-analysis, Pan A, Chen M, Chowdhury R, et al, The American Journal of Clinical Nutrition, 2012
Protective effect of borage seed oil and gamma linolenic acid on DNA: In Vivo and In Vitro Studies, Tasset-Cuevas I, Fernandez-Bedmar Z, Lozano-Baena MD, et al, PLoS ONE, 2013
Fish oil omega-3 fatty acids and cardio-metabolic health, alone or with statins, Minihane AM, European Journal of Clinical Nutrition, 2013
Essential fatty acids as potential anti-inflammatory agents in the treatment of affective disorders, Song C, Mod Trends Pharmacopsychiatry, 2013

ZENDOCRINE®

COMPLEX

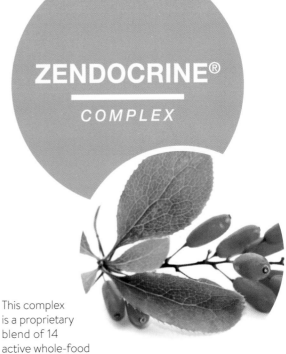

This complex is a proprietary blend of 14 active whole-food extracts in a patented enzyme delivery system that supports healthy cleansing and filtering functions of the liver, kidneys, colon, lungs, and skin.

TOP USES

Toxic liver, jaundice, cirrhosis, bloating, toxic gallbladder, pancreatitis, kidney damage, respiratory issues, colon issues and constipation.

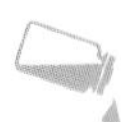

INGREDIENTS

- Barberry leaf, milk thistle seed, burdock root, clove bud, dandelion root, garlic fruit, red clover leaf: Targets the cleansing and support of the liver and helps filter the blood of toxins.
- Turkish rhubarb stem, burdock root, clove bud, dandelion root: Targets the cleansing of the kidneys while bringing strength and integrity to it.
- Psyllium seed husk, turkish rhubarb stem, acacia gum bark, marshmallow root: Helps to strengthen the elimination process of the colon and colon health.
- Osha root, safflower petals: Helps to strengthen and cleanse the lungs from environmental and other toxins.
- Kelp, milk thistle seed, burdock root, clove bud, garlic fruit: Helps support the cleansing of toxins from the skin.
- Enzyme assimilation system of amylase and cellulase their natural mineral cofactors magnesium and manganese: Increases digestion and utilization of the rest of the ingredients.

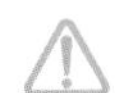

SAFETY

Not for children. Keep out of reach of small children. If pregnant or lactating, women should consult a physician or health care provider before use. Do not use if safety seal is broken or missing.

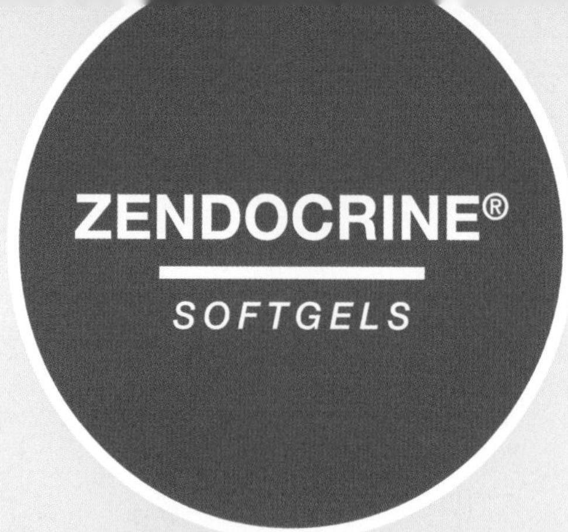

A blend of essential oils that support natural detoxification of the body to help cleanse it of toxins and free radicals that can slow your systems down, leaving a heavy, weighted feeling.

TOP USES

Toxic liver, jaundice, cirrhosis, bloating, toxic gallbladder, pancreatitis, kidney damage, and hormonal imbalances.

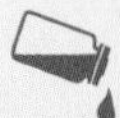

INGREDIENTS

- Tangerine oil: Antioxidant and cleansing properties of the liver and kidneys.
- Rosemary oil: Supports a healthy liver and gallbladder as well as reduces xenoestrogens (foreign estrogens form plastics, growth hormones and environmental toxins).
- Geranium oil: Cleanses liver, gallbladder and balances hormones and rids the body of unwanted estrogens.
- Juniper berry oil: Powerful detoxifier of the kidneys and decreases water retention.
- Cilantro oil: Powerful cleansing agent that eliminates toxins from the body, including heavy metals.

SAFETY

Not for children. Keep out of reach of small children. If pregnant or lactating, women should consult a physician or health care provider before use. Do not use if safety seal is broken or missing.

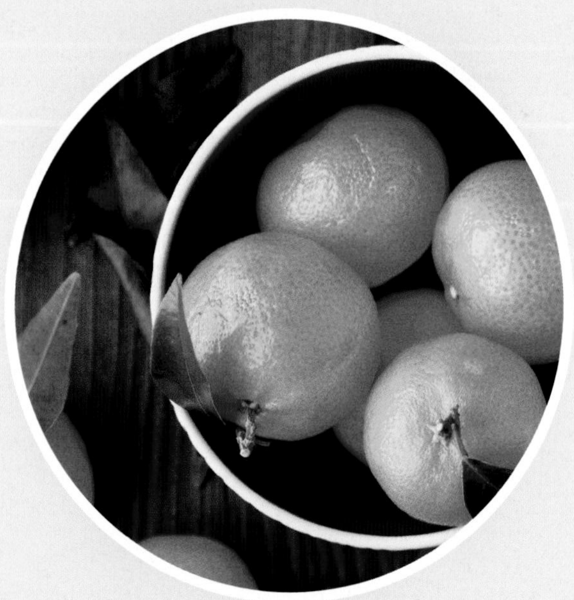

Tips for Taking Supplements

- **Partner with quality.** Use supplements with optimal, not exaggerated or deficient, levels of nutrients by buying from a reputable source.
- **Dose diligence.** All products provide dose recommendations. Maximal benefit comes from the consistent use of a variety of specific and complementary supplements. When first starting a program, some individuals may choose to start with a lower dose and work up. The basic recommendations may be adequate or even excessive for a healthy person who has implemented a healthy diet, lifestyle, and regular supplementation program. However, someone with longstanding health issues may require an extensive regimen that may include consumption beyond label recommendations.
- **Start slowly.** Over the course of the first week, start with a few supplements at lower doses and then add from there. This will support awareness of how individual supplements make you feel. Gradually add others and increase doses of each supplement. Synergy between supplements coupled with using the proper therapeutic dose is generally required to achieve optimal benefit. Most supplements can be taken at the same time.
- **Time it right.** Most people do better taking supplements with food while digestive processes are in action. Use on an empty stomach (except at bedtime) can trigger nausea. Just a few bites of food can be enough (e.g. half a banana). Avoid taking with tea, coffee, soda, or even some dairy products as this can interfere with absorption. Dinner and bedtime are also excellent times of day as the body's repair mode and hormone secretions are at their highest capacity while sleeping. Most products recommend dividing doses, say two or three times during the day. Spreading consumption over the course of the day maximizes absorption.
- **Make it a habit.** Consider targeting two set times per day to establish routine or ritual for basic daily nutrition habits. This is what most people can handle and remember. Add additional times for other supplemental needs. In the beginning, or as needed, place reminders in line of sight or set alarms.
- Be practical. Keep your supplements in locations that provide easy access. Most do not require refrigeration, so keeping them out on kitchen and bathroom counters creates visibility and supports routine use. Many people find it useful to purchase some kind of pill box or container

that allows a week's worth of supplements to be pre-counted and organized for each day. This way, consumption can be accomplished quickly or supplements easily placed in a pocket or small container to consume later. Marking on lids with markers or posting a sheet on the inside of a cupboard door for dose instruction can also be helpful. Use a small cup or glass to put the capsules in before you take them. Keep it close by for reuse.

- **Stay the course.** Most people experience an increased sense of well being when beginning a supplementation program. Some individuals are an exception and feel worse before starting to feel better. A few common causes of discomfort are the elimination of microbes or dealing with chronic illness or disease. In Lyme disease treatment, this phenomenon is referred to as a Herxheimer reaction, but it can occur with any microbial infection. If a new symptom occurs that can be specifically defined as a side effect to a particular supplement (such as nausea after taking a certain supplement), consider first if it was taken with food. If an exacerbation of symptoms occurs, reduce the dose of supplements until symptoms ease and then gradually increase the dose again over time. If adverse reactions occur that seem beyond these parameters, consider discontinuing use until issues can be addressed or a more suitable choice can be made.
- **Make supplements part of your lifestyle.** Supplements to support general health can be continued indefinitely and are an excellent component of a healthy lifestyle. Supplements that support immune function, reduce inflammation, and provide antimicrobial properties should be continued at the higher doses recommended until symptoms subside, when doses may be reduced or supplements discontinued completely. Rotate different supplements over time as needed. Consider intermittent programs to maintain health results. For example, engage in a quarterly detox program for the duration of fourteen to thirty days as a complementary commitment to a basic daily routine.
- **Take them along.** When you travel, take your supplements with you. Get a pill box that contains specific, marked sections for different times of the day. Most allow for a week's worth of doses. Plastic baggies can hold capsules for single use or to contain individual products. Use a permanent marker to label the baggies "am" or "pm" or identify the product contained.
- **Store them right.** Keep supplements out of windowsills or away from other sources of bright light. Store in dark or opaque bottles away from microwaves and other electromagnetic sources.

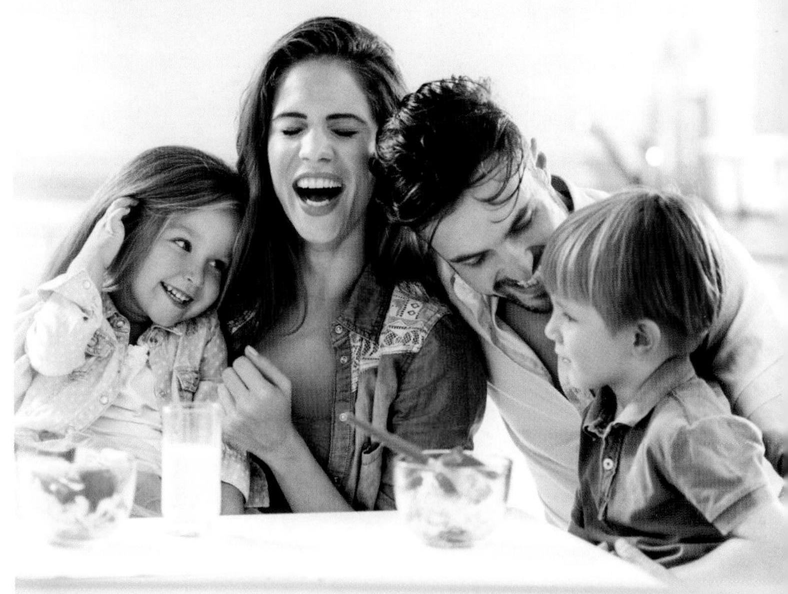

Additional Information

- **Herxheimer reactions.** Die-off of bacteria can intensify symptoms of fatigue, muscle pain, and feeling flu-like. Generally, herxheimer reactions are more common and more intense with conventional antibiotic therapy, but they can still occur with natural supplements. If you feel that you are having herxheimer reactions, back off on dose and then increase gradually and slowly.
- **Excessive stimulation.** One of the greatest benefits of natural supplementation is an increased energy and reserves. Generally this is welcomed during the day but can be a problem at night while trying to sleep. If you notice an effect, take primary supplements in the morning and afternoon.
- **Dealing with adverse effects:** Adverse effects associated with taking natural supplements are uncommon, but possible. Fortunately, most are mild and transient, and you should be able to work around them.
- **Upset stomach.** The most common adverse effects are an upset stomach, indigestion, mild nausea, and discomfort mid-chest or on the left side under the lower rib cage (where the stomach is located). First consider if consumption occurred on an empty or overly full stomach and adjust accordingly. Otherwise, if necessary, take a break from the supplements for a few days to a week. Consider adding an essential oil such as ginger, peppermint, or digestive blend to soothe upset. If chronic digestive issues already existed, additional considerations may need to be made.

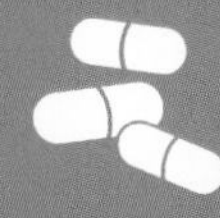

SECTION 4

BODY SYSTEMS & FOCUS AREAS

Take a holistic approach to wellness by learning to address wellness in terms of body systems. Think beyond the disease-symptom model, and instead focus on systems that govern the function of your entire body.

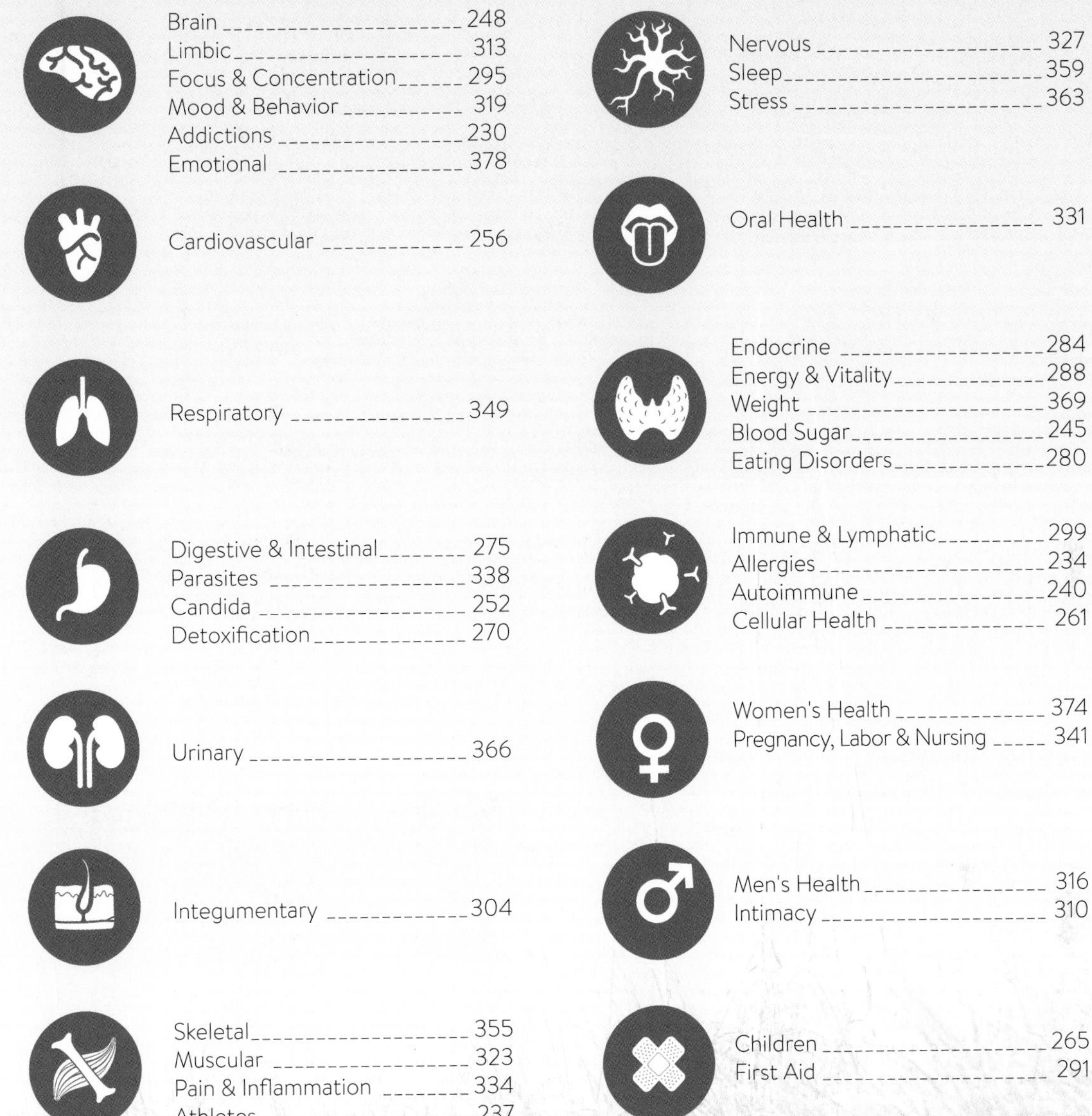

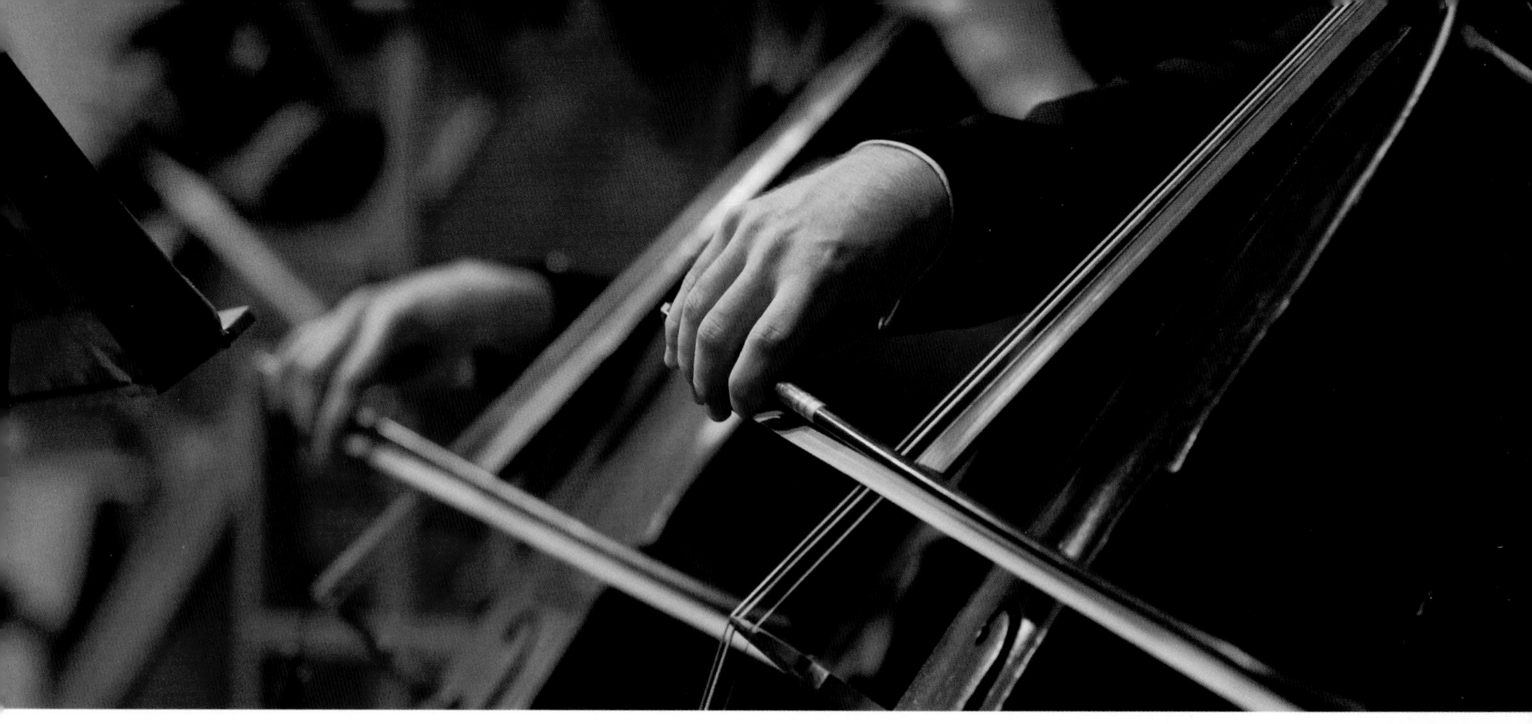

A HEALTHY BODY is like a finely tuned symphony orchestra. An orchestra is divided into sections, and sections are comprised of individual instruments. Similarly, the body is divided into sections called body systems that are comprised of individual organs. During a musical performance when out-of-tune sounds come from a single instrument, it affects not only that section, but the quality of music coming from entire orchestra. The conductor's role is to identify the underlying cause behind the affected sound, tuning and refining where necessary. So, too, is every individual the conductor of their own body's orchestrations and internal harmony in partnership with the body itself.

Take a Holistic Approach

By addressing wellness in terms of body systems, each individual is taking a holistic approach to wellness. Thinking beyond a disease-symptom model and focusing on the systems that govern the function of the entire body allows one to shift away from an ambulance mentality of "if it ain't broke don't fix it" to true whole-body thinking and a prevention mindset.

A holistic approach to wellness promotes living with a prevention mindset and addressing root causes when symptoms arise by providing support to entire body systems.

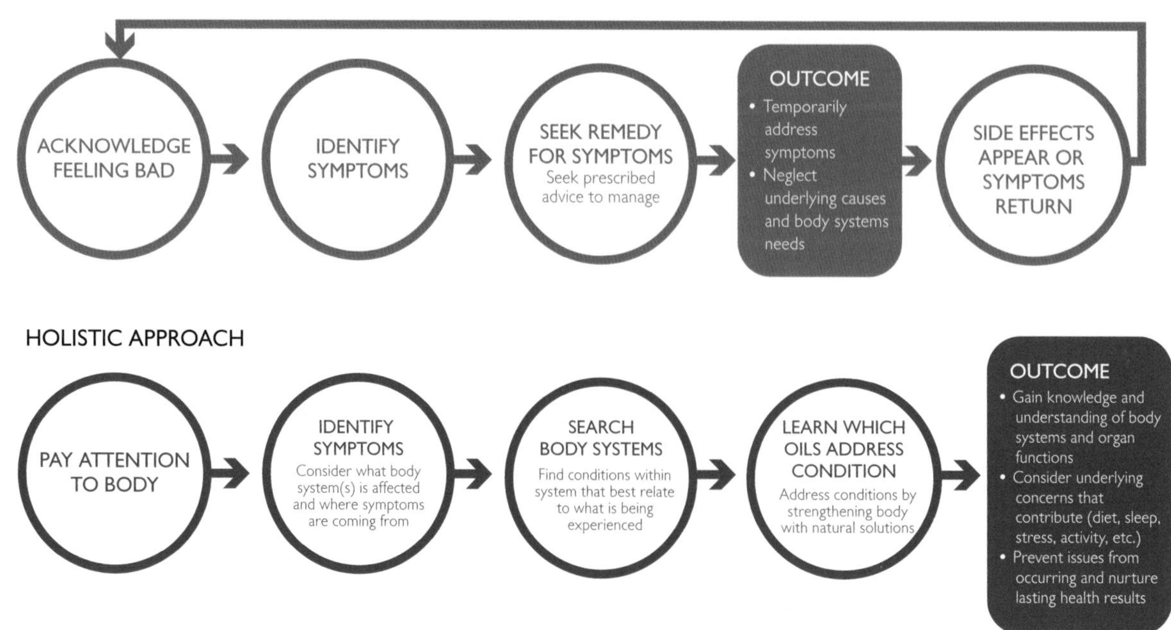
AMBULANCE APPROACH
ACKNOWLEDGE FEELING BAD
IDENTIFY SYMPTOMS
SEEK REMEDY FOR SYMPTOMS
Seek prescribed advice to manage
OUTCOME
• Temporarily address symptoms
• Neglect underlying causes and body systems needs
SIDE EFFECTS APPEAR OR SYMPTOMS RETURN
HOLISTIC APPROACH
PAY ATTENTION TO BODY
IDENTIFY SYMPTOMS
Consider what body system(s) is affected and where symptoms are coming from
SEARCH BODY SYSTEMS
Find conditions within system that best relate to what is being experienced
LEARN WHICH OILS ADDRESS CONDITION
Address conditions by strengthening body with natural solutions
OUTCOME
• Gain knowledge and understanding of body systems and organ functions
• Consider underlying concerns that contribute (diet, sleep, stress, activity, etc.)
• Prevent issues from occurring and nurture lasting health results

Interconnectivity of All Body Systems

All body systems are interconnected. When one system is hindered or malfunctions other systems are impacted. Likewise, when one system is repaired and strengthened the whole body benefits and functions can be restored. For best success, think in terms of body systems to create true wellness, and learn to use natural healing tools to aid in this process.

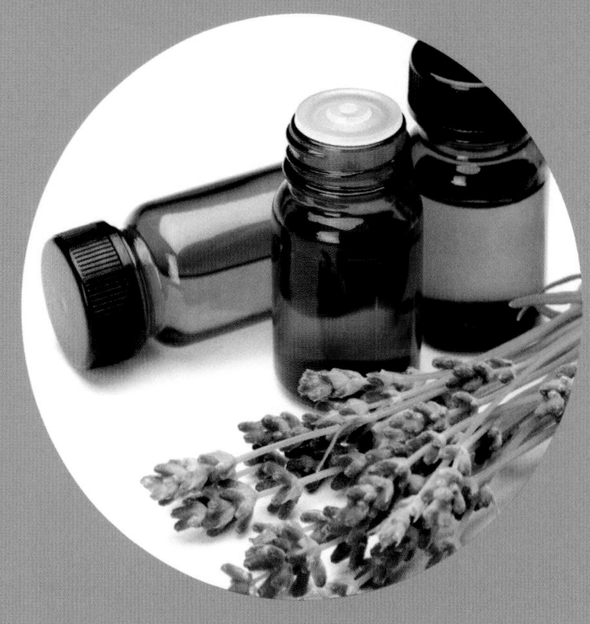

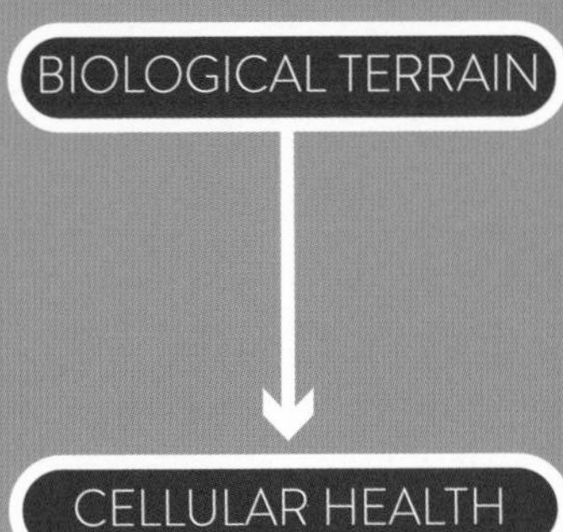

- Quality nutrients
- Water
- Oxygen
- Waste removal
- Chemical and temperature regulation
- Healthy cells are at the core of wellness.

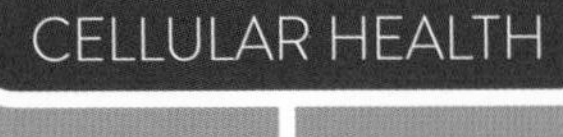

- Unhealthy cells, caused by deficiencies and toxicities, result in ailments or a diseased body.

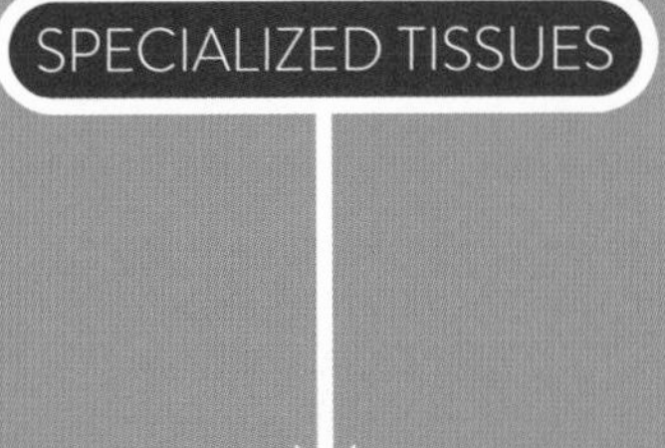

- The needs of healthy cells are met by groups of specialized tissues. These tissues form organs and body systems. They perform functions to support cellular health, and consequently, the health of the whole body.

BODY SYSTEMS

- As body systems operate normally, they function synergistically together to create overall well being. Conditions form as specialized tissues and body systems fail to perform their normal functions. Failure to function eventually gives rise to ailments, the level where most people become conscious of their health.

tips

The Body Talks
Use the *Body Systems* sections to search conditions for solutions. The body uses specific symptoms to communicate it has unmet needs.

The Long and the Short of It
Oils provide support to systems and organs for resolving current conditions and root causes as well as long-term prevention.

The Multi-Taskers
While essential oil use is supporting one system, their complex chemistry supports other systems and organs simultaneously.

Using the Body Systems Effectively

The Body Systems section of this book is designed to create an opportunity to learn, first, about a body system itself and gain a basic understanding of its purpose or role, its workingparts, and what can potentially go wrong. Second, each section contains common ailments that can occur (solutions located in the Quick Reference A-Z), key oils and supplements to be learned as go-to solutions, usage tips, additional solutions to numerous conditions, and user recommended remedies.

One additional component of each section is "By Related Properties." This section allows the user to search for solutions by related properties to certain oils. For example, if one wanted to sleep better, one would search for a properties category such as "Calming" and find an oil of choice such as lavender or Roman chamomile. To take this process to a "Power Oil User" (462) level, discover the properties chart in the back of the book and learn numerous properties of each single oil. This is the best way to comprehend and learn the multiplicity of actions an oil is capable of.

In conclusion, the desired outcome from use of *Body Systems* is to become a more experienced oil user, knowing how to "think for yourself," taking attention from symptoms to root causes, solutions, and preventative actions.

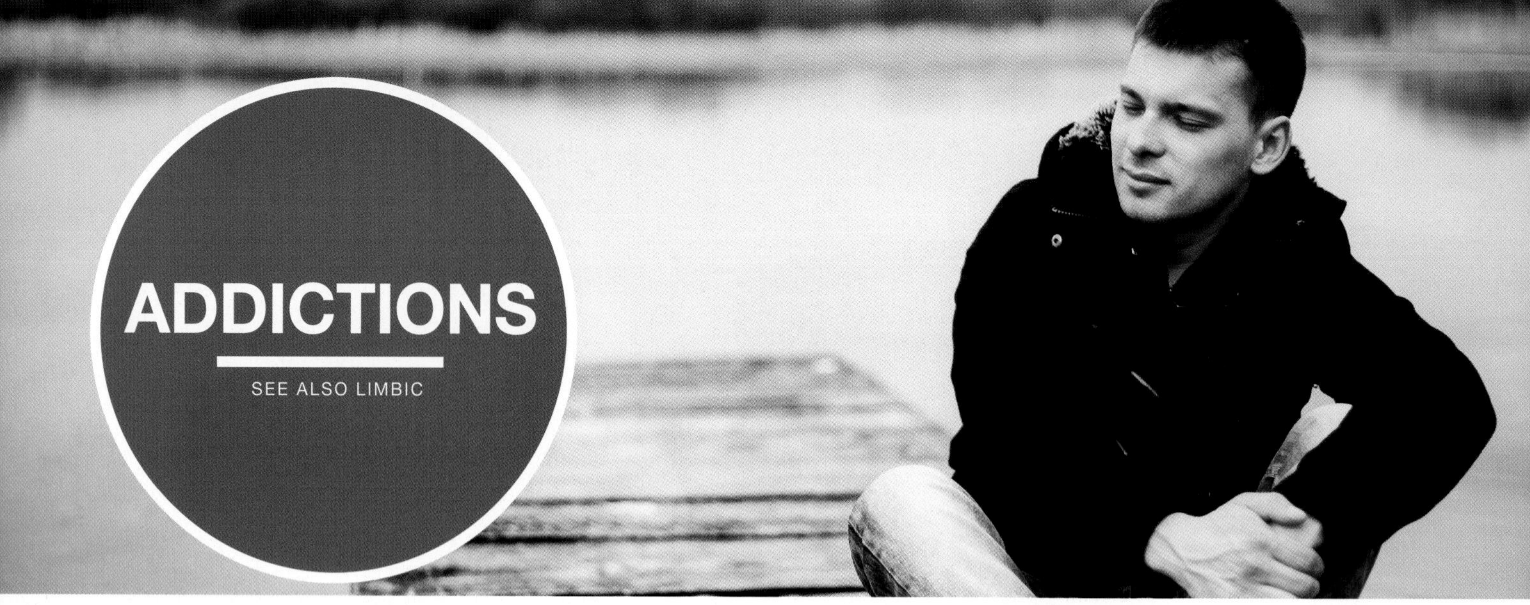

THE WORD "ADDICT" has a negative connotation, leading people to think of base individuals living among the dregs of society. But anyone can develop an addiction. To the brain, all addictions, regardless of the type, have similar damaging effects. The only difference is to the degree to which they occur. Although the substance or the body releases chemicals which enhance a "high," or feeling of euphoria, the pleasure response or relief from pain is only temporary.

Drug addiction is a powerful force that can take control of the lives of users. In the past, addiction was thought to be a weakness of character, but now research is proving that addiction is a matter of brain chemistry.

Dr. Nora Volkow, the director of the National Institute on Drug Abuse, says "the way a brain becomes addicted to a drug is related to how a drug increases levels of the naturally occurring neurotransmitter dopamine, which modulates the brain's ability to perceive reward reinforcement. The pleasure sensation that the brain gets when dopamine levels are elevated creates the motivation for us to proactively perform actions that are indispensable to our survival (like eating or procreation). Dopamine is what conditions us to do the things we need to do.

"Using addictive drugs floods the limbic brain with dopamine—taking it up to as much as five or ten times the normal level. With these levels elevated, the user's brain begins to associate the drug with an outsize neurochemical reward. Over time, by artificially raising the amount of dopamine our brains think is "normal," the drugs create a need that only they can meet." *

When the body starts to expect and incorporate this extra chemical release as part of normal body function, the addict experiences chemical addiction and will suffer from withdrawal symptoms if he or she tries to stop. To make matters worse, most addicts suffer from worsening problems in interpersonal relationships, since their psychological and physical need for relief takes over and replaces all other responsibilities that would enable them to lead a healthy, normal life (such as working, fully participating in family and social relationships, etc.). The results of addiction are typically nothing short of debilitating and eventually devastating.

There are many types of addiction, including but not limited to: alcohol, drugs, food, sugar, exercise, computer (including computer games and social media), pornography (online or other), sex, shopping, gambling, emotional intimacy (including unreasonable expectations and compulsive patterns of Romance, sexuality, and relationships), texting, risky behaviors or thrill seeking ("adrenaline junkies"), and more.

Addictions that center on ingested substances (known as exogenous addictions) change body chemistry; addictions to activities or behaviors (known as endogenous addictions) cause the body to produce extra endorphins and other chemicals that make a person feel good temporarily. Either way, changes in body chemistry create a dependency on the activity or substance. The greater the exposure, the more the body becomes desensitized to the excess chemicals.

Individuals who are addicted to substances or activities often feel helpless, frustrated, and ashamed of their situation. Often, most don't realize or admit they are addicted until they try to stop, only to find that they keep regressing to participation in the addictive behavior. Until an addict is ready to be honest and take responsibility for his or her choices, ask for help, and fully participate in successful rehabilitation programs (such as treatment programs, counseling, and twelve step programs), he or she faces a downward spiral that can include marital/family ruin or dissolution, financial devastation, criminal activity, and/or sickness or death.

Because they are chemical in nature, essential oils can assist recovering addicts with emotional and chemical support for the brain as they are seeking to get their lives under control again. To gain additional insight on how they powerfully affect the brain, read the introduction to *Limbic*.

There are essential oils that can help reprogram the body's cravings for specific substances and that can strengthen the resolution to abstain. Essential oils are also able to support and strengthen the very emotional areas of pain that caused the individual to participate in the addictive behavior in the first place, leading the individual to adopt a healthier lifestyle. Loved ones often suffer alongside the addict, as they feel helpless to prevent the collateral damage they see happening right in front of their eyes; essential oils can be a tremendous emotional support for these individuals as well.

TOP SOLUTIONS

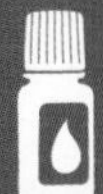

SINGLE OILS

Copaiba, Helichrysum - boosts dopamine levels (pg. 99), (pg. 117)

Grapefruit - dissipates cravings; supports detoxification, renewed energy (pg. 114)

Basil - clears negative thought patterns that block change; restores mental energy (pg. 80)

Bergamot - gives sense of empowerment and self-worth (pg. 81)

Peppermint - supports sense of buoyancy and recovery, reprieve from painful emotions (pg. 140)

By Related Properties

For more, See Oil Properties on pages 477 - 481

Anaphrodisiac - arborvitae, marjoram

Analgesic - bergamot, birch, black pepper, blue tansy, clary sage, clove, copaiba, eucalyptus, fennel, frankincense, helichrysum, juniper berry, lavender, litsea, marjoram, melaleuca, oregano, peppermint, pink pepper, Siberian fir, turmeric, wild orange, wintergreen, yarrow

Antidepressant - bergamot, cinnamon, clary sage, frankincense, geranium, lavender, lemongrass, magnolia, melissa, neroli, oregano, patchouli, pink pepper, ravensara, sandalwood, tangerine, wild orange

Anti-parasitic - bergamot, blue tansy, cinnamon, clove, frankincense, lavender, melaleuca, oregano, rosemary, tangerine, thyme, turmeric

Antitoxic - bergamot, black pepper, cinnamon, citronella, coriander, fennel, geranium, grapefruit, juniper berry, lavender, lemon, lemongrass, patchouli, thyme

Calming - bergamot, black pepper, black spruce, blue tansy, cassia, clary sage, copaiba, coriander, frankincense, geranium, juniper berry, lavender, litsea, magnolia, oregano, patchouli, Roman chamomile, sandalwood, tangerine, vetiver, yarrow

Regenerative - cedarwood, clove, coriander, geranium, jasmine, lemongrass, manuka, myrrh, neroli, patchouli, sandalwood, wild orange, yarrow

Relaxing - basil, blue tansy, cassia, cedarwood, clary sage, cypress, fennel, geranium, green mandarin, jasmine, lime, manuka, neroli, patchouli, rosemary, sandalwood, spearmint

Restorative - basil, black spruce, frankincense, lime, patchouli, rosemary, sandalwood, spearmint

Sedative - bergamot, blue tansy, cedarwood, clary sage, frankincense, geranium, juniper berry, lavender, magnolia, marjoram, melissa, neroli, patchouli, Roman chamomile, rose, spikenard, tangerine, yarrow, ylang ylang

Stimulant - basil, bergamot, black pepper, blue tansy, cardamom, clove, coriander, dill, fennel, grapefruit, juniper berry, lime, melaleuca, patchouli, pink pepper, rosemary, Siberian fir, tangerine, thyme

Stomachic - blue tansy, cardamom, cinnamon, clary sage, coriander, fennel, ginger, juniper berry, marjoram, melissa, peppermint, rosemary, tangerine, wild orange, yarrow

Uplifting - cardamom, cedarwood, clary sage, cypress, grapefruit, green mandarin, lemon, lime, litsea, melissa, pink pepper, tangerine, wild orange

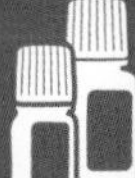

BLENDS

Serenity® - promotes calm, peaceful, tranquil state of being; quiets mind

Zendocrine® - promotes elimination, detoxification of toxins (pg. 206)

Motivate® - promotes self-belief, confidence, trust (pg. 193)

Balance® - restores sense of solidity/feeling grounded in life (pg. 170)

Purify - cleanses and detoxifies (pg. 198)

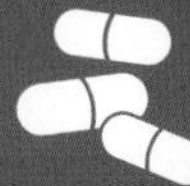

SUPPLEMENTS

Alpha CRS®+, **Mito2Max® (pg. 214)**, DDR Prime® Softgels, **xEO Mega (pg. 222)**, Zendrocrine® Complex, TerraZyme®, **IQ Mega® (pg. 213)**, Slim & Sassy® softgels, MicroPlex VMz supplement

Related Ailments: Adrenaline, Alcohol Addition, Drug Addiction, Food Addiction, Smoking Addiction, Video Game Addiction, Withdrawal Symptoms, Work Addiction

USAGE TIPS: For best support for addiction recovery

- **Aromatic:** Choose an oil(s) to diffuse or inhale from a bottle or hands, or whatever method seems most effective at the time. Wear an oil(s) as perfume/cologne.
- **Topical:** Apply under nose, behind ears, to base of skull (especially in suboccipital triangles) and forehead, and on roof of mouth (closest location to the amygdala; place on pad of thumb, then suck on thumb); place oil that is best match to emotional state over heart area. Use a carrier oil as needed for sensitive skin or "hot" oils. Use to prevent and eliminate urges.
- **Internal:** For immediate impact, in addition to inhalation, place a drop or two of chosen oil under tongue, hold for 30 seconds, swallow; take oils in capsule or in glass of water. Consider detoxification products/oils or a program - see *Detoxification*.

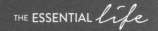

Conditions

Accountability, lack of - fennel, ginger, Balance®
Anesthetize pain, attempting to - birch, clove, helichrysum, wintergreen, Deep Blue®
Anguish - helichrysum, melissa, Elevation™
Antisocial - cardamom, cedarwood, marjoram, Balance®
Anxiety - basil, bergamot, black spruce, cedarwood, frankincense, juniper berry, lavender, magnolia, vetiver, ylang ylang, Adaptiv®, Balance®, Elevation™, Motivate®, Peace®, Serenity®
Appetite stimulant - blue tansy, ginger, wild orange, Slim & Sassy®; see *Digestive & Intestinal*
Appetite, excessive - cassia, cinnamon, ginger, grapefruit, peppermint, Slim & Sassy®; see *Digestive & Intestinal, Eating Disorders, Weight*
Checked out - basil, cedarwood, clary sage, frankincense, patchouli, sandalwood, Balance®, InTune® or Passion®
Control, loss of - blue tansy, clove, Balance®
Cravings - cilantro, cinnamon, clove, grapefruit, peppermint, Balance®, Serenity®, Slim & Sassy®,
Deceptive/lying/secretive - clary sage
Despairing/hopeless - bergamot, clary sage, lemongrass, melissa, Elevation™, Forgive®, Motivate®, Peace®
Dishonest - black pepper, clary sage, frankincense, lavender, melissa, ClaryCalm®, Purify, Serenity®
Dopamine levels, low - basil, bergamot, cedarwood, copaiba, frankincense, jasmine, lemon, patchouli, Roman chamomile, rosemary, sandalwood, wild orange, Cheer®
Financial issues - wild orange, Motivate®
Guilt - bergamot, lemon, peppermint, Forgive®, HD Clear®
Hangover - cassia, cinnamon, geranium, grapefruit, lemon, PastTense®, Slim & Sassy®, Zendocrine®
Irrational - cedarwood, lemon, Adaptiv®, InTune®
Irresponsible - fennel, ginger, Balance®
Irritable - cardamom, Forgive®, Serenity®
Obsession/fixation with drug of choice - cypress, patchouli, ylang ylang, Adaptiv®, Balance®; see *Limbic "Obsessive/compulsive thoughts/behaviors"*
Relapsing - clove, ginger, lavender, melissa, InTune®, Motivate®, Passion®, Zendocrine®,
Stealing - black pepper, cassia, clary sage, frankincense, geranium, lavender, vetiver, ylang ylang, ClaryCalm®, Purify, Serenity®, Zendocrine®
Stress management, poor - lavender, Serenity®; see *Stress*
Thrill seeking, excessive - birch, clove, frankincense, helichrysum, oregano, peppermint, white fir, wintergreen, Deep Blue®
Urges, intense - black spruce, cedarwood, patchouli
Withdrawal - cilantro, cinnamon, copaiba, frankincense, grapefruit, juniper berry, lavender, marjoram, sandalwood, spikenard, wild orange, Adaptiv®, DDR Prime®, Elevation™, Motivate®, Passion®, Peace®, citrus essential oils

*http://bigthink.com/going-mental/your-brain-on-drugs-dopamine-and-addiction

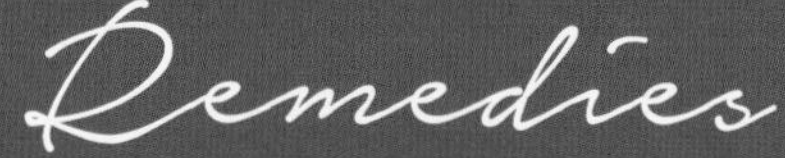

DOPAMINE BOOST: 1 drop cinnamon, 1 drop bergamot, 1 drop copaiba in a capsule or under tongue. The cinnamon burns.

ALCOHOL CRAVINGS
- 1 or 2 drops of copaiba on the tongue when cravings hit.
- Consume 2 drops twice per day of helichrysum in a capsule or under tongue.

CHEWING TOBACCO CRAVINGS: Apply coriander outside of lip, thumb to roof of mouth, and a few drops in a cotton ball in snuff container.

TOBACCO/NICOTINE CRAVINGS (top oils: black pepper, clove, On Guard®) - Suggestions:
- Aromatically use black pepper to alleviate cravings; diffuse, inhale.
- Clary sage, patchouli, spikenard - use topically, internally, aromatically.
- Put a drop of On Guard® or cinnamon oil on toothbrush, brush teeth.
- Combine 2 drops each of clove, frankincense, peppermint oils. Inhale in palms, apply to bottom of feet, or drink one drop of mixture with water.
- Use On Guard® on the tongue or in water when the urge strikes; additional considerations: cassia, cinnamon.

PORNOGRAPHY ADDICTION RECOVERY SUPPORT: Use 1-2 drops frankincense under tongue one to two times per day. Apply helichrysum or vetiver over lower abdomen as least once per day. Determine which aromas (basil, cardamom, frankincense, grapefruit, helichrysum, Purify, Balance®, On Guard®) are preferred and utilize both preventatively (e.g. wear as cologne/perfume) and when urges arise.

WORK ADDICTION: Diffuse 5-10 drops oil(s) in work space for a minimum of 2-3 hours per day as needed. Use any of following oils alone or combined as desired: basil, geranium, wild orange, and/or ylang ylang or Serenity® to create the 10 drops for diffuser. Experiment with what combination best serves needs. Here are some suggested combinations:
- 3 drops wild orange and 2 drops ylang ylang.
- 2 drops geranium, 2 drops ylang ylang, and 3 drops Whisper®.
- 2 drops basil, 3 drops wild orange, and 2 drops ylang ylang.
- 6 drops Serenity® and1-2 drops ylang ylang.

ENERGY DRINK & CAFFEINE ADDICTION: Place 3 drops basil oil on bottom of each foot and inhale regularly throughout the day. Drink 5 drops of Slim & Sassy® in water or a capsule three to five times daily. Place one drop grapefruit oil under tongue, hold for 30 seconds, swallow anytime experiencing cravings.

DRUG & ALCOHOL ADDICTION: Place 2-3 drops of any one or more oil listed on bottoms of feet, abdomen (specifically over liver area), and forehead. Choose from basil, frankincense, Roman chamomile and/or Zendocrine®. Dilute with fractionated coconut oil as needed or desired.

OILS TO ADDRESS EMOTIONAL STATES FOR ADDICTION RECOVERY

For emotional states associated with addictions - see *Mood & Behavior*

SINGLES

Basil - overcomes chronic fatigue (creates desire for stimulants); release toxins
Bergamot - encourages self-love, restores sense of self worth
Cardamom - helps overcoming objectifying (common problem with addictions)
Cedarwood - supports healthy GABA (anti-excitatory), serotonin levels
Clary sage - dispels darkness and illusion
Clove - restores healthy boundaries
Copaiba - boosts dopamine levels
Coriander - effective with any addiction
Frankincense - connects to divine love/acceptance, purpose, higher brain function
Geranium - assists with love and acceptance
Ginger - supports being fully present, taking full responsibility
Grapefruit - reduces cravings; restores relationship with body's natural energy
Helichrysum - supports healing from deep, intense pain, trauma
Juniper berry - supports accessing, releasing unaccessed/unresolved fears
Lemon - supports restoration of logical thinking; clears generational patterns
Melissa - restores connection to reality, truth, light; instills courage
Patchouli - grounds and stabilizes; get the "guts" to take a leap of faith
Peppermint - promotes sense of recovery
Roman chamomile - helps one live true to one's self
Thyme - releases and resolves toxic emotions
Vetiver - gets to "root" cause and face it head on; supports amygdala
White fir - clears inherited/passed on addictions; tendencies in families
Wild orange - supports creative thoughts, expression; restores playfulness
Ylang ylang - releases trauma; recovers connection to the heart, to feel/trust again

BLENDS

Adaptiv® - brings transquility and motivation and stirs a coping capacity
Balance® - restores sense of solidity/feeling grounded in life; brings electrical balance to body and focus to mind
DDR Prime® - supports knowing what's worth keeping vs. releasing
Deep Blue® - supports deep emotional healing; restores normal endorphin levels
Elevation™ - soothes heart, balances emotions; stabilizes mood, supports serotonin
InTune® - normalizes, stabilizes brain activity; invites acceptance of reality
PastTense® - invites releasing fears, relaxing and enjoying life again
Purify - supports detoxification; provides freedom from past habits/patterns
Serenity® - quiets mind; encourages facing issues; helps balance expectations
Slim & Sassy® - supports restoration of a positive relationship to one's body and natural sources of energy
Zendocrine® - supports detox processes; detoxing old habits, beliefs

SOLUTIONS FOR SPECIFIC ADDICTIONS:

Adrenaline - basil, bergamot, black spruce, clary sage, oregano, patchouli, rosemary, Adaptiv®, Balance®, Console®, InTune®, Motivate®, Serenity®
Alcohol* - basil, cassia, citronella, copaiba, eucalyptus, frankincense, ginger, grapefruit, helichrysum, juniper berry, lavender, lemon, marjoram, melissa, Roman chamomile, rosemary, Balance®, Cheer®, Forgive®, Peace®, Serenity®
Anger - black spruce, geranium, helichrysum, magnolia, marjoram, rosemary, thyme, wintergreen, Cheer®, Elevation™, Forgive®, Motivate®, Peace®, Purify, Serenity®, Whisper®; see *Mood & Behavior*
Caffeine* - basil, grapefruit, patchouli, Passion®, Peace®, Slim & Sassy®
Controlling, overly/"control freak" - cilantro, cinnamon, cypress, patchouli, sandalwood, wintergreen, Passion®, Citrus Bliss®, Slim & Sassy®
Cutting/self harm/self inflicted pain - bergamot, geranium, myrrh, rose, wintergreen, ClaryCalm®, Console®, Elevation™, Forgive®, HD Clear®, Immortelle, On Guard®, Peace®, Whisper®
Drugs* - basil, citronella, clary sage, copaiba, grapefruit, patchouli, Roman chamomile, Cheer®, Console®, Motivate®, Passion®, Peace®
Eating Disorders (anorexia, bulimia) - bergamot, cardamom, cinnamon, grapefruit, melissa, patchouli, Breathe Respiratory Drops, Citrus Bliss®, Console®, Elevation™, Forgive®, Passion®, Peace®; see *Eating Disorders*
Entertainment - peppermint, vetiver, Balance®, Console®, Elevation™, Passion®, Serenity®
Fear - black spruce, cassia, cinnamon, ginger, juniper berry, myrrh, patchouli, Peace®; see *Mood & Behavior*
Food - basil, cardamom, ginger, grapefruit, peppermint, myrrh, Console®, Motivate®, Passion®, Peace®, Slim & Sassy® ; see *Eating Disorders*
Gaming - Cheer®, Console®, Deep Blue®, Elevation™, HD Clear®, TerraShield®, Whisper®
Irritable - rose, ClaryCalm®, Serenity®, Whisper®
Marijuana - basil, patchouli, Passion®, Peace®
Nicotine - bergamot, black pepper, cassia, cinnamon (on tongue), clove, eucalyptus, ginger, Adaptiv®, Passion®, Peace®, On Guard®, On Guard® lozenges; see "Tobacco" below
Pain meds - birch, clove, eucalyptus, patchouli, pink pepper, wintergreen, Deep Blue®, Console®, Passion®, Peace®
Pornography* - basil, cardamom, frankincense, grapefruit, helichrysum, Balance®, Console®, On Guard®, Purify
Sex - arborvitae, basil, cardamom, geranium, marjoram, sandalwood, Passion®, Peace®, Motivate®, Whisper®
Sugar - cardamom, cassia, cinnamon, clove, dill, grapefruit, helichrysum, Cheer®, Motivate®, Passion®, Peace®, Slim & Sassy®
Technology - patchouli, peppermint, Cheer®, InTune®, Forgive®, Motivate®, Passion® ; see "Entertainment" above
Tobacco/chewing* - bergamot, cassia, cinnamon, clove, coriander, frankincense, Cheer®, Forgive®, On Guard®, On Guard® lozenges, Passion®, Peace®
Tobacco/smoking* - basil, bergamot, black pepper, cassia, cinnamon, clove, eucalyptus, frankincense, patchouli, peppermint, spikenard, Breathe®, Breathe Respiratory Drops, Cheer®, Forgive®, On Guard® lozenges, Passion®, Peace®
Work* - arborvitae, basil, cedarwood, geranium, lavender, marjoram, wild orange, ylang ylang, Adaptiv®, Cheer®, Forgive®, Peace®

* See remedy on pg. 232

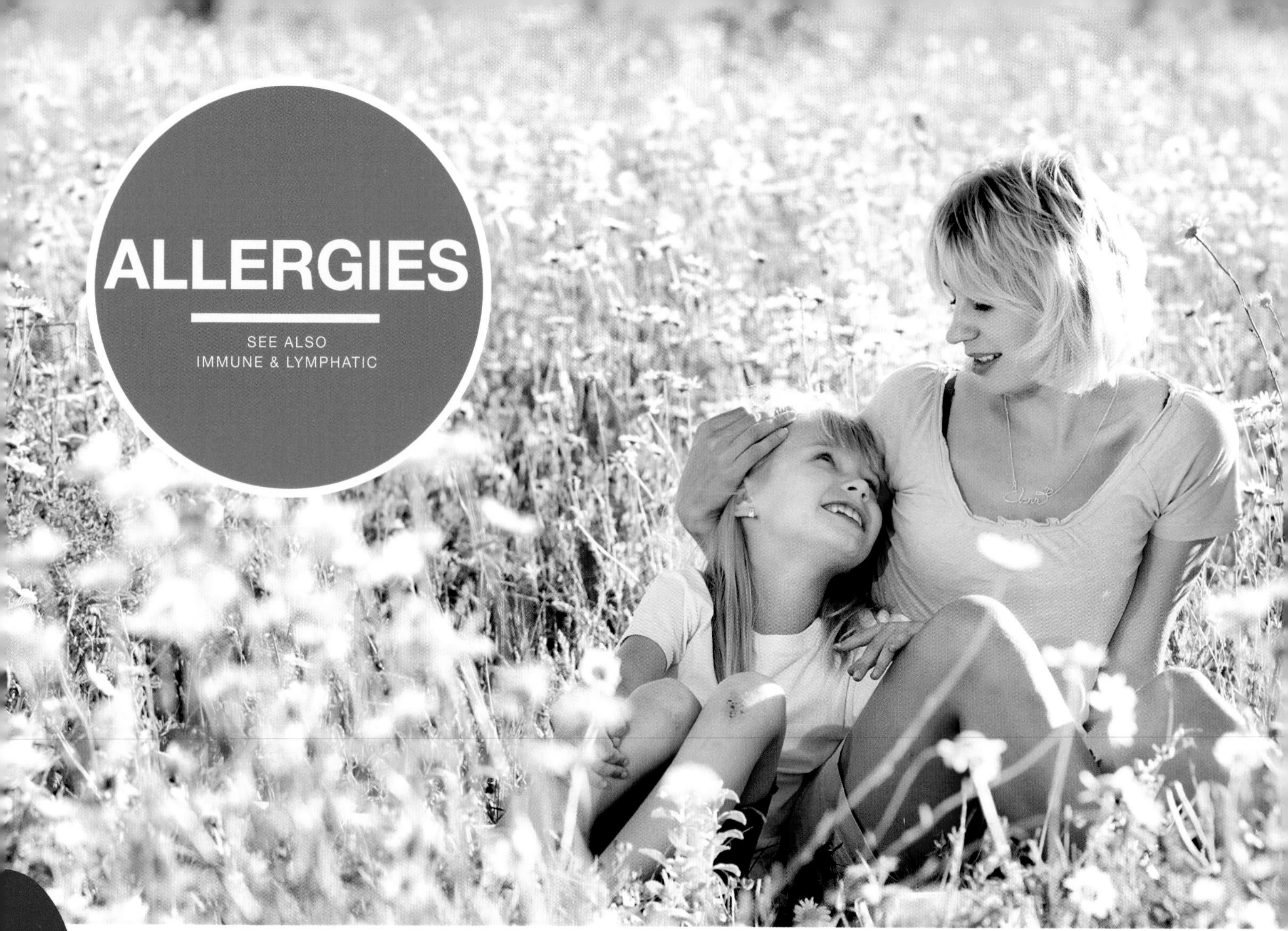

ALLERGIES

SEE ALSO
IMMUNE & LYMPHATIC

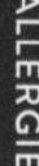

ALLERGIC REACTIONS occur when the immune system reacts to foreign substances in the environment that are normally harmless to most people, such as pollen, bee venom, or pet dander. A substance that causes a reaction is called an allergen. These reactions are generally considered to be acquired. A true allergic reaction is an immediate form of hypersensitivity and is distinctive because the immune response over-activates specific white blood cells that are triggered by antibodies.

When allergies occur, the immune system identifies a particular allergen as harmful—even if it isn't—and creates antibodies to fight it. When contact is made with the allergen, the immune system's reaction will typically inflame skin, sinuses, airways or digestive system. This reaction is known as an inflammatory response.

The severity of allergies varies from person to person and can range from minor irritation to anaphylaxis, which is a severe reaction to an allergen that can be a life-threatening emergency. Common triggers for severe reactions include insect bites or stings (wasps, bees) and certain food allergies (e.g. peanuts, shellfish). It is important to note that not all reactions or intolerances are forms of allergic responses.

Allergy symptoms depend on the allergens/substances involved and can impact the airways, sinuses and nasal passages, skin, the digestive system, and other parts of the body. Allergies are typically categorized as either respiratory or systemic (involving multiple organs - esp. digestive, respiratory, circulatory).

Common allergens include airborne particles (e.g. animal hair, car exhaust, cigarette smoke, dust, dust mites, fragrances, fungi, herbicides, mold, paint fumes, perfume, pesticides, pet dander, pollens, weeds); chemicals, latex, petroleum and automotive products; foods (e.g. peanuts, genetically modified soy products); insect stings and bites; insect or reptile venom; medications (e.g. aspirin, antibiotics such as penicillin or sulfa drugs).

Traditional treatments for allergies include avoiding known allergens or administering steroids that modify the immune system in general and medications such as antihistamines and decongestants to reduce symptoms. Essential oils have the ability to chemically support the body in its capacity to reduce and overcome acute or chronic hypersensitivity. For allergy support specifically, it is especially important to be familiar with three properties of oils and the particular oils associated with the related actions: anti-allergenic (e.g. geranium, helichrysum), antihistamine (e.g. lavender, melissa, Roman chamomile), and steroidal (e.g. basil, rosemary). See "By Related Properties" for more information. Additional, for numerous related respiratory needs refer to *Respiratory* section of this book.

TOP SOLUTIONS

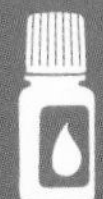

SINGLE OILS

Basil, rosemary - reduces inflammatory response and supports adrenal glands (pgs. 80 & 149)

Blue tansy, lavender - acts as an antihistamine and calms irritation (pgs. 86 & 122)

Lemon - decongests and reduces mucus (pg. 123)

Peppermint - discharges phlegm and reduces inflammation (pg. 140)

By Related Properties

For more, See Oil Properties on pages 477 - 481

Anti-allergenic - blue tansy, geranium, helichrysum, turmeric
Antihistamine - blue tansy, lavender, manuka, melissa, Roman chamomile, yarrow
Anti-inflammatory - arborvitae, basil, bergamot, birch, black pepper, blue tansy, cardamom, cassia, cedarwood, cinnamon, copaiba, coriander, cypress, eucalyptus, fennel, frankincense, geranium, ginger, helichrysum, lavender, lemongrass, lime, manuka, melaleuca, myrrh, neroli, oregano, patchouli, peppermint, Roman chamomile, rosemary, sandalwood, Siberian fir, tangerine, turmeric, yarrow
Antitoxic - bergamot, black pepper, coriander, grapefruit, juniper berry, lavender, lemon, lemongrass, thyme
Calming - basil, bergamot, black pepper, blue tansy, cassia, clary sage, copaiba, coriander, fennel, frankincense, geranium, jasmine, juniper berry, lavender, litsea, magnolia, patchouli, Roman chamomile, sandalwood, tangerine, vetiver, yarrow
Cleanser - arborvitae, cilantro, eucalyptus, grapefruit, green mandarin, juniper berry, lemon, thyme, wild orange
Detoxifier - cilantro, green mandarin, juniper berry, lime, litsea, patchouli, tangerine, turmeric, wild orange, yarrow
Steroidal - basil, bergamot, birch, cedarwood, clove, fennel, patchouli, rosemary, thyme

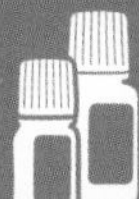

BLENDS

Breathe® - supports reduction and recovery from allergic responses (pg. 172)

Zendocrine® - supports permanent reduction of reactivity (pg. 206)

Purify - alleviates allergic responses to bites and stings (pg. 198)

DigestZen® - supports digestion to calm food allergy responses (pg. 186)

On Guard® - supports immune system (pg. 194)

Serenity® - acts as an antihistamine (pg. 199)

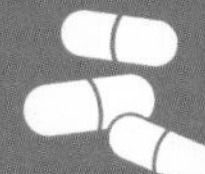

SUPPLEMENTS

Alpha CRS®+, Zendrocrine® Complex, Zendocrine® softgels, Mito2Max®, **TerraZyme® (pg. 219)**, Phytoestrogen Complex, **Breathe Respiratory Drops (pg. 210)**, **TriEase Softgels (pg. 219)**, MicroPlex VMz supplement

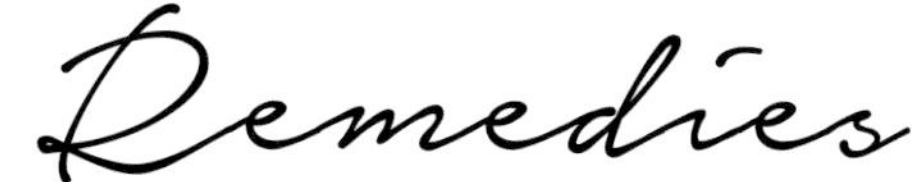

Remedies

EYE ALLERGIES: Layer 2 drops lavender and melaleuca under the pads of the index toe and middle toe and then rub in. Use a few drops of lavender at the temples and gently rubbed in. Take care to stay close to the hairline to avoid eye contact.

ALLERGY POWER TRIO: Take 2 drops lavender, 2 drops lemon, 2 drops peppermint one of three ways:
- Under the tongue, wait thirty seconds, swallow; repeat as necessary.
- Mix in 1/8 to ½ cup water, drink; repeat as necessary until symptoms subside.
- Consume blend in a capsule; repeat as necessary.
- OR Take TriEase Softgels

SKIN RASH/HIVES: Dilute lavender or melaleuca with carrier oil and rub into skin. A toxic, burdened, sluggish liver is a major culprit of allergic response. Layering oils over the liver area supports its ability to flush toxins that burden other organs, including skin and kidneys. The skin is a secondary pathway of elimination for the liver, and rashes can be indicative of its toxicity.

THE ALLERGY BOMB: Take 2-3 drops each of cilantro, melaleuca and lavender in a capsule.

ALLERGY RELIEF COMBINATION: Lemon, lavender, and Roman chamomile - use in equal parts in a capsule (for example, 1 drop of each). This blend of essential oils has been effective for relieving hay fever and other airborne, allergy-type symptoms that result in sneezing, runny nose, watery eyes, and so on.

ALLERGIES
6 drops lavender
6 drops Roman chamomile
2 drops myrrh
1 drop peppermint
Blend and apply one drop behind ears, temples, and thymus.

For more ideas, download the app at app.essentiallife.com

Related Ailments: Chemical Sensitivity Reaction [Detoxification, Immune & Lymphatic], Hay Fever [Immune & Lymphatic, Respiratory], Hives [Integumentary], Lactose Intolerance, Loss of Smell, Multiple Chemical Sensitivity Reaction, Olfactory Loss, Pet Dander

Conditions

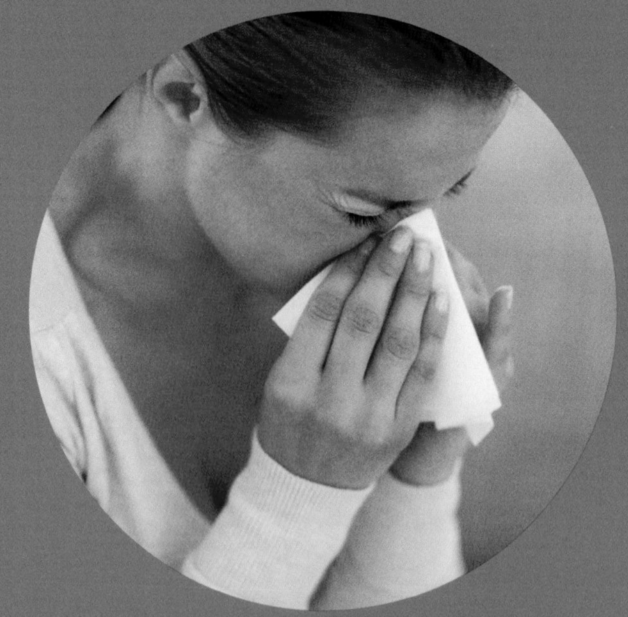

Abdominal cramping/spasms - See *Digestive & Intestinal*
Adrenal fatigue - See *Endocrine*
Airways, narrowing/constriction - birch, blue tansy, cinnamon, Douglas fir, eucalyptus, frankincense, helichrysum, lavender, lemon, marjoram, myrrh, peppermint, rosemary, thyme, white fir, wintergreen, Breathe®, Breathe Respiratory Drops, DDR Prime®, Motivate®, Serenity®
Allergies, chronic - basil, ginger, lemon, lemongrass, thyme
Allergies, general* - cilantro, frankincense, lavender, melaleuca, peppermint, yarrow, Console®, Peace®, Zendocrine®
Anxiety - See *Mood & Behavior*
Blood pressure, high or low - See *Cardiovascular*
Chemical sensitivity - arborvitae, cilantro, coriander, Douglas fir, eucalyptus, lemon, peppermint, sandalwood, wild orange, DDR Prime®, Purify, Zendocrine®
Congestion - See *Respiratory*
Cough - See *Respiratory*
Energy, loss of/fatigue, chronic - See *Energy & Vitality*
Facial pressure and pain - helichrysum, myrrh, DDR Prime®, DigestZen®
Glands, enlarged/swollen - arborvitae, cilantro, lemon, lime, oregano, Roman chamomile, wintergreen, On Guard®
Hay fever* - cilantro, lavender, lemon, melaleuca, yarrow, Breathe®, Motivate®, Purify
Headache - see *Pain & Inflammation*
Hives* - basil, cilantro, frankincense, lavender, lemongrass, melaleuca, peppermint, Roman chamomile, rosemary, DDR Prime®
Inflammation, joints - See *Skeletal*
Inflammation, skin - See *Integumentary*
Immune system, overactive - peppermint, rosemary, Elevation™
Insect bite - See *First Aid*
Itching/urge to scratch, burning - See *Integumentary*
Itchy eyes/mouth/throat* - blue tansy, cilantro, lavender, lemon, melaleuca, peppermint, Motivate®, Purify, Slim & Sassy®, Zendocrine®, TriEase Softgels
Joint pain - See *Skeletal*
Liver - See *Digestive & Intestinal*
Liver, toxic load - See *Digestive & Intestinal*; see "Anti-allergenic" property
Mold sensitivity - arborvitae, melaleuca, oregano, thyme, Purify, Zendocrine®
Nasal congestion/drip - See *Respiratory*
Nausea - See *Digestive & Intestinal*
Poison oak - See *First Aid*
Pollen sensitivity - blue tansy, cilantro, juniper berry, lavender, Purify, Zendocrine®
Rapid pulse - cardamom, cedarwood, frankincense, rosemary, ylang ylang, Elevation™, Motivate®, Purify, Serenity®; see *Cardiovascular*
Rash* - arborvitae, blue tansy, cedarwood, frankincense, lavender, lemon, melaleuca, neroli, Roman chamomile, sandalwood, tangerine, ClaryCalm®, Immortelle, Purify, Serenity®, Slim & Sassy®, Zendocrine®
Reaction - Roman chamomile
Runny nose - grapefruit, lavender, lemon, myrrh, peppermint, DigestZen®, Motivate®, Zendocrine®
Shock - See *First Aid*
Skin bumps - See *Integumentary*
Skin cracking/peeling/scaling - See *Integumentary*
Skin flushed - See *Integumentary*
Skin irritation - blue tansy, melaleuca, neroli, peppermint, yarrow, DigestZen®, Purify, Serenity®, Slim & Sassy® corrective ointment
Skin reddening - See *Integumentary*
Smoke sensitivity - black pepper, lavender, peppermint, Serenity®, Zendocrine®
Sneezing - blue tansy, Douglas fir, lavender, lemon, peppermint, Breathe®, Motivate®, Purify
Swallowing, difficulty - lavender, Motivate®, Zendocrine®
Swelling of lips, face, tongue, throat, etc. - lavender, wintergreen, Purify, Zendocrine®
Throat, dry or sore - See *Respiratory*
Voice, loss of/raspy/hoarseness - See *Respiratory*
Vomiting - See *Digestive & Intestinal*
Watery/itchy/red eyes* - blue tansy, eucalyptus, lavender, lemon, melaleuca, Roman chamomile, Purify, Zendocrine®
Welts - arborvitae, myrrh, vetiver, Purify
Wheezing - birch, lavender, wintergreen, Breathe®

USAGE TIPS: For best support in overcoming allergies:

- **Internal:** Take drops of oils in water and drink, take oil(s) in a capsule, or place a drop on or under tongue.
- **Aromatic:** Diffuse chosen oils; apply to chest, clothing, bedding, or other to inhale.
- **Topical:** Apply oils topically to forehead, cheeks (avoid eyes), chest, bottoms of feet.

* *See remedy on pg. 235*

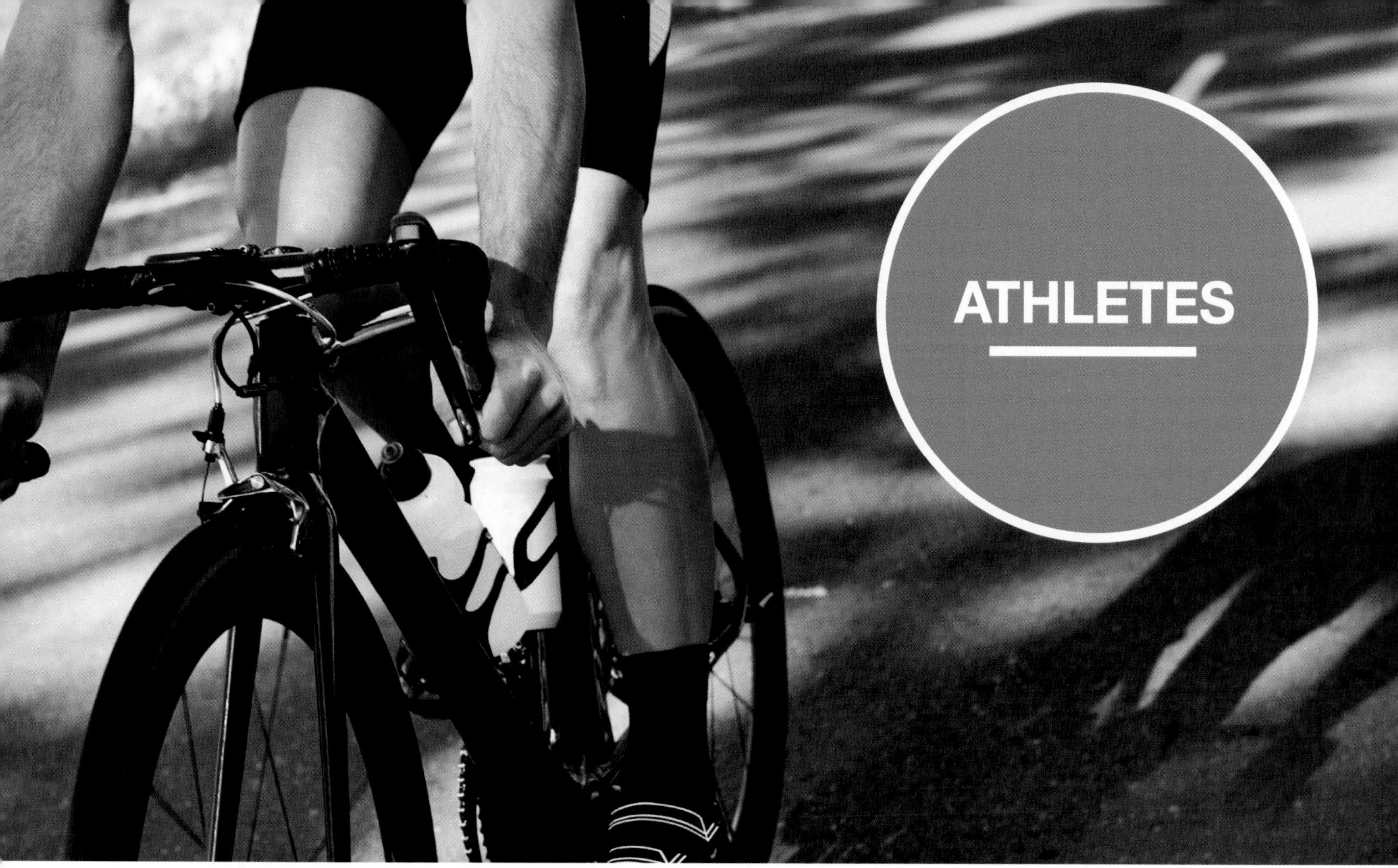

AS THEY PREPARE for their sport of preference, many athletes participate in one or more training programs that can include (but is not limited to): circuit training (develops a broad range of skills by providing stations with various exercises); interval training (short periods of vigorous activity interspersed with shorter resting periods; helps build speed endurance); Plyometrics (bounding exercises to help improve strength and speed); tempo training (the athlete maintains a faster pace than is comfortable to increase endurance ability); strength training (the use of various pieces of equipment increases muscle resistance and inspires faster conditioning); resisted and/or assisted training (helps develop faster speed as the athlete uses resistance equipment, such as bands, or participates in assistance-based exercise, such as running downhill).

As athletes push their bodies for greater conditioning and/or endurance in fitness training or sports, the potential for injury is present. Often these injuries are a result of inadequate recovery (rest) time for muscles/body tissues to adequately rebuild or repair.

Some of these injuries include:
- Muscle pain and soreness
- Overusing tendons
- "Runner's Knee" -- a generic term to describe anterior knee pain
- IT Band (iliotibial band) stress/injury -- affects approximately 12 percent of runners
- Shin splints
- Pain in Achilles tendon
- Stress fracture

Other common conditions athletes may experience during training/sports:
- Exercise-induced asthma
- Exercise-associated collapse
- Effects resulting from over training - concentration, lack of; depression, heart rate (resting) changes, injuries (increased), insomnia/restless sleep, insatiable thirst, motivation and/or self esteem diminished, muscle soreness lasting more than 72 hours, personality changes, progress hindered, sick more often

Athletes can combine sound principles of sports medicine (icing, heating, resting, etc., as appropriate) with natural remedies to increase the body's recovery time. There are oils known specifically for their ability to support connective tissue (involved in all sports injuries), to reduce inflammation, to support cellular regeneration for faster recovery time, and/or to help warm up/cool down muscle groups for better overall performance.

Adding whole-food, bio-available supplements gives cells the support they need to enhance restorative and repairing activities. Supplementation can also increase energy levels during a workout to reduce fatigue. An easily digestible protein drink consumed just after a cardio workout gives the body readily accessible protein so it doesn't have to break down proteins in the body. All these good practices help to minimize breakdown and overuse injuries in the first place, help provide energy, and increase the body's capacity to restore tissues to good health quickly.

TOP SOLUTIONS

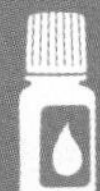

SINGLE OILS

Peppermint - pre-exercise support (pg. 140)
Lemongrass - connective tissue support (pg. 126)
Marjoram - muscle support (pg. 131)

By Related Properties

For more, See Oil Properties on pages 477 - 481

Analgesic - basil, bergamot, birch, black pepper, blue tansy, clove, copaiba, eucalyptus, ginger, helichrysum, juniper berry, lavender, lemongrass, litsea, melaleuca, oregano, peppermint, pink pepper, rosemary, Siberian fir, turmeric, wintergreen, yarrow
Anti-inflammatory - arborvitae, basil, birch, black pepper, blue tansy, cardamom, cassia, cedarwood, cinnamon, copaiba, cypress, frankincense, geranium, ginger, helichrysum, lavender, lemongrass, lime, litsea, manuka, melaleuca, neroli, oregano, patchouli, peppermint, rosemary, sandalwood, Siberian fir, spearmint, spikenard, tangerine, turmeric, wild orange, wintergreen, yarrow
Energizing - basil, cypress, ginger, grapefruit, lemongrass, lime, Siberian fir, tangerine, wild orange, yarrow
Regenerative - basil, clove, frankincense, geranium, helichrysum, lavender, lemongrass, manuka, melaleuca, myrrh, neroli, patchouli, wild orange, yarrow, ylang ylang
Relaxing - basil, blue tansy, cedarwood, cypress, geranium, helichrysum, lavender, litsea, manuka, marjoram, neroli, Roman chamomile, wild orange, ylang ylang
Steroidal - basil, bergamot, birch, cedarwood, clove, fennel, patchouli, rosemary, thyme
Vasodilator - lemongrass, marjoram, peppermint, rosemary, Siberian fir, thyme
Warming - birch, black pepper, cassia, cinnamon, ginger, marjoram, neroli, peppermint, pink pepper wintergreen

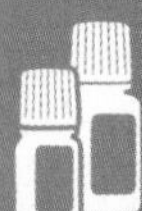

BLENDS

AromaTouch® - post-exercise recovery (pg. 169)
Deep Blue®, Deep Blue® rub - post-exercise recovery (pg. 185)

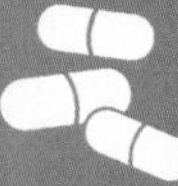

SUPPLEMENTS

Bone Nutrient Lifetime Complex (pg. 210), Alpha CRS®+, Zendrocrine® Complex, DigestZen® softgels, DDR Prime® Softgels, xEO Mega, **Mito2Max® (pg. 214)**, TerraZyme®, **Deep Blue Polyphenol Complex (pg. 212)**, MicroPlex VMz supplement, **TrimShake® (pg. 220), Slim & Sassy® softgels (pg. 218)**

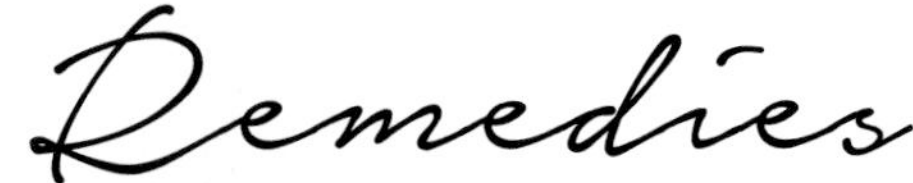

Remedies

PRE/POST-WORKOUT TIPS

- Sniff peppermint or an Citrus Bliss® before your workout to give you a boost to get you going, better your mood, and reduce fatigue.
- Add 2 drops of lemon or Slim & Sassy® to your water to keep you hydrated.
- Apply peppermint alone or with cypress, lemongrass, and/or marjoram, peppermint, or pink pepper before your workout routine to increase circulation, warm muscles (reduce possibility of injury), and oxygenate muscles.
- After your workout, apply Deep Blue® rub and copaiba
- For a more intense post-workout treatment, layer fractionated coconut oil, lemongrass, and/or marjoram, and then top off with soothing rub blend to aching muscles to reduce inflammation, improve recovery, and support injury repair.

FOR OVERHEATED/HEAT STROKE/HEAT EXHAUSTION: Place peppermint in a spritzer bottle with water and spray back of neck; massage a drop of peppermint on back of neck for cooling.

FOR OXYGEN UPTAKE: Place a few drops of peppermint or Slim & Sassy® in water and sip/drink; swipe a drop of frankincense under nose.

FOR NAUSEA: Place a few drops of peppermint in water, or use peppermint beadlets.

FOR INFLAMMATION/PAIN/STIFFNESS: Mix together 30 drops of Deep Blue® and 25 drops of frankincense in a 10ml roller bottle; fill the rest with fractionated coconut oil and shake to blend; rub onto affected area as needed.

AFTER-SPORTS MASSAGE OR BATH: 2 drops turmeric, 1 drop lavender, 1 drop Roman chamomile, 1 drop helichrysum, 2 drops marjoram, 1 drop black pepper; Combine wtih 1-2 teaspoons carrier oil and massage on area of concern; Or add to 1 cup epsom salt, stir to dissolve and add to a bath and soak.

SHIN SPLINTS AND RUNNER'S KNEE REMEDIES

- Step One: In a 10ml roller bottle, combine one of following recipes. Add fractionated coconut oil to fill remainder of bottle after essential oils are added. Shake to blend. Apply frequently. Massage oil into both the front and the back of the leg in area(s) of concern.
  - Recipe #1: 45 drops each lemongrass and rosemary oils
  - Recipe #2: 50 drops lemongrass oil, 30 drops marjoram oil, 35 drops wintergreen oil
- Optional - Step 2: Layer Deep Blue® or rub on top of either recipe and massage into tissue.

MUSCLE RELAXANT BATH SALTS: 1 drop copaiba, 3 drops frankincense, 1 drop peppermint, 1tbsp jojoba oil, ½ c Epsom salt. Combine and add to bath water for relaxation and relief.

LINIMENT: Combine the following in a 2 ounce bottle: 10 drops copaiba, 5 drops peppermint and 5 drops frankincense, then fill with fractionated coconut oil.

FIRST AID: In a 1 oz glass bottle, combine 11 drops copaiba, 2 drops helichrysum, 3 drops lavender, 1 oz aloe vera gel. Shake to blend. Apply 2-3 times a day or as needed to assist the body's natural process of healing.

For more ideas, download the app at app.essentiallife.com

Conditions

Appetite, excessive - bergamot, cassia, cinnamon, ginger, grapefruit, lemon, Slim & Sassy®; see *Weight*
Appetite, imbalanced - wild orange, Slim & Sassy®; see *Weight*
Appetite, loss of - bergamot, black pepper, ginger, lemon, Slim & Sassy®; see *Weight*
Athlete's foot - arborvitae, cardamom, cinnamon, clove, copaiba, lavender, lemon eucalyptus, lemongrass, melaleuca, myrrh, oregano, DDR Prime®, HD Clear®; see *Candida*
Blood pressure, low - See *Cardiovascular*
Body temperature, too cool - cinnamon, ginger, oregano, wintergreen
Body temperature, too high - bergamot, black pepper, lemon, peppermint, Deep Blue®, PastTense®; see "Warming" property
Bone, pain - birch, eucalyptus, helichrysum, white fir, wintergreen, Deep Blue®; see *Skeletal*
Breathing, constricted - Douglas fir, AromaTouch®, Breathe®, Deep Blue®; see *Respiratory*
Breathing, labored - ravensara, Breathe®; see *Respiratory*
Cartilage injury - basil, birch, helichrysum, marjoram, lemongrass, peppermint, white fir, wintergreen, Deep Blue®; see *Skeletal*
Circulation, poor - basil, cypress, Douglas fir, ginger, marjoram, pink pepper, turmeric, yarrow, AromaTouch®; see *Cardiovascular*
Concussion - bergamot, cedarwood, clove, cypress, frankincense, sandalwood, Balance®, InTune®; see *Brain*
Consciousness, loss of - basil, frankincense, peppermint, rosemary; see *Brain*
Dehydration - lemon, peppermint, Slim & Sassy®
Dizziness - See *Brain*
Fatigue/Exhaustion - basil, bergamot, cinnamon, cypress, Douglas fir, eucalyptus, frankincense, green mandarin, lavender, lemon, peppermint, pink pepper, ravensara, rosemary, sandalwood, wild orange, yarrow, ylang ylang, Adaptiv®, Citrus Bliss®, DDR Prime®, Elevation™, Slim & Sassy® Zendocrine® ; see *Energy & Vitality*
Feet, sore - lemongrass, marjoram, AromaTouch®
Headache - See *Pain & Inflammation*
Heat exhaustion/stroke* - bergamot, black pepper, dill, lemon, peppermint, petitgrain, spearmint, PastTense®, Zendocrine®
Inflammation* - birch, copaiba, cypress, frankincense, lavender, peppermint, rosemary, turmeric, wintergreen, Alpha CRS®+, DDR Prime®, Deep Blue®; see "Anti-inflammatory" property
Injury - birch, helichrysum, lemongrass, white fir, wintergreen, AromaTouch®; see the area of injury - muscles, bones, connective tissue, bruising/skin, etc.; see *Skeletal, Muscular*
Involuntary muscle contractions - clary sage, geranium, lavender, marjoram; see *Nervous*
Jock itch - See *Men's Health*
Joint, inflammation/stiffness* - arborvitae, basil, birch, cinnamon, clove, cypress, Douglas fir, eucalyptus, frankincense, ginger, lavender, marjoram, peppermint, rosemary, thyme, white fir, wintergreen, DDR Prime®, Deep Blue®, Deep Blue® rub, Zendocrine®; see *Skeletal*
Lactic acid buildup - dill, juniper berry, lemon, lemongrass
Ligaments/tendons/connective tissue - basil, clove (dilute for topical use), eucalyptus, helichrysum, lemongrass, white fir, see "Tendonitis" below, *Skeletal*
Lower back pain - birch, eucalyptus, frankincense, lavender, lemongrass, ginger, marjoram, peppermint, white fir, wintergreen, AromaTouch®, DDR Prime®, Deep Blue®, Deep Blue® rub, PastTense®; see *Skeletal*
Lymphatic, congestion - ginger, grapefruit, lavender, lemon, lemongrass, sandalwood, AromaTouch®, Purify; see *Immune & Lymphatic*
Mental strength/clarity - basil, patchouli, peppermint, vetiver, Adaptiv®, Balance®, InTune®; see *Focus & Concentration*
Muscle, cramps/charley horse - basil, cypress, lemongrass, marjoram, peppermint, spikenard, white fir, wintergreen, AromaTouch®, Deep Blue®, PastTense®; see *Muscular*
Muscle, fatigue/overworked - basil, black pepper, cypress, Douglas fir, eucalyptus, marjoram, rosemary, Siberian fir, white fir, AromaTouch®; see *Muscular*
Muscle, pain/sprain/strain/injury* - clove (dilute for topical use), copaiba, Douglas fir, eucalyptus, ginger, lavender, lemongrass, marjoram, peppermint, rosemary, thyme, vetiver, white fir, wintergreen, AromaTouch®, Deep Blue®; see *Muscular*
Muscle spasms - arborvitae, basil, birch, black pepper, cardamom, coriander, cypress, eucalyptus, frankincense, ginger, lavender, lemongrass, marjoram, myrrh, oregano, patchouli, peppermint, Roman chamomile, rosemary, spearmint, wild orange, wintergreen, yarrow; see *Muscular*
Muscle, stiffness/tension* - basil, Douglas fir, ginger, grapefruit, rosemary, white fir, AromaTouch®, Deep Blue®, Deep Blue® rub, PastTense®; see *Muscular*
Muscle, weak - basil, bergamot, birch, black pepper, clary sage, clove, coriander, cypress, frankincense, ginger, helichrysum, lavender, lemongrass, jasmine, marjoram, patchouli, rosemary, wintergreen; see *Muscular*
Nausea/Vomiting* - See *Digestive & Intestinal*
Nerve damage - bergamot, frankincense, helichrysum, peppermint, Serenity®; see *Nervous*
Nerve pain - basil, birch, ginger, helichrysum, wintergreen, Deep Blue®; see *Nervous*
Pain* - birch, cypress, eucalyptus, helichrysum, lemongrass, peppermint, wintergreen, Deep Blue®; see *Pain & Inflammation*
Perspiration, excess - cypress, lemongrass, peppermint, petitgrain; see *Detoxification, Integumentary*
Perspiration, lack of - black pepper, cilantro, coriander, cypress, ginger, yarrow; see *Detoxification*
Pulse, rapid - cedarwood, lavender, rosemary, ylang ylang, Serenity®; see *Cardiovascular*
Pulse, weak - cinnamon, coriander, ginger; see *Cardiovascular*
Sciatica, issues with - basil, birch, cardamom, cypress, Douglas fir, frankincense, helichrysum, lavender, peppermint, sandalwood, thyme, white fir, wintergreen, Deep Blue®, Deep Blue® rub; see *Skeletal*
Stamina, lack of - peppermint, rosemary; see *Energy & Vitality*
Stress, performance - bergamot, clary sage, sandalwood, Balance®, Peace®, Serenity®; see *Stress*
Tendonitis - basil, birch, cardamom, cypress, eucalyptus, helichrysum, lavender, lemon, lemongrass, marjoram, oregano, peppermint, rosemary, wintergreen, AromaTouch®, Deep Blue®; see *Skeletal*

ATHLETES

USAGE TIPS: For best methods of use for athletes:
- **Topical:** Use oils topically is for muscle/joint pain and injuries.
- **Aromatic:** Inhaling certain oils before and during workouts can invigorate, energize, and improve respiration.

* *See remedy on pg. 238*

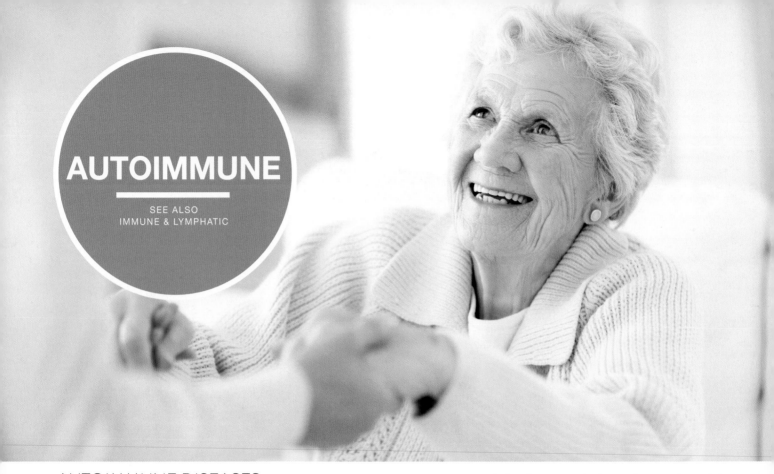

AUTOIMMUNE DISEASES occur when the body has either an abnormally low immune response to pathogens, or when the body's immune system fails to distinguish the difference between pathogens and healthy body tissues. When normal body tissue is identified as a pathogen, or invader, the adaptive immune system creates antibodies that target the destruction of these tissues.

Because they attack the body's organs in a similar manner, many autoimmune disorders tend to have similar symptoms, making it difficult to diagnose them. It is possible for individuals to have multiple conditions simultaneously. There are no known medical cures for autoimmune conditions, so treatment focuses on using medications to suppress the immune response, leaving the individual vulnerable to sickness and disease, and to manage symptoms.

Approximately 75 percent of those suffering from autoimmune disorders are women. Autoimmune disorders are among the top ten causes of death in women. A number of factors contribute to conditions leading to an autoimmune disorder. These factors include genetics, toxins from heavy metals, candida, Epstein-Barr, herpes simplex virus, nerve damage due to excessive exposure to neurotoxins, and chronic inflammation related to food sensitivities, particularly gluten intolerance.

Some of the symptoms characteristic of autoimmune conditions include: joint and/or muscle pain, weakness, tremors, weight loss, insomnia, heat intolerance, rapid heartbeat, recurrent rashes or hives, sun sensitivity, difficulty concentrating or focusing, glandular imbalances such as hypothyroidism or hyperthyroidism, fatigue, weight gain, cold intolerance, hair loss, white patches on skin or inside mouth, abdominal pain, blood or mucus in stool, diarrhea, mouth ulcers, dry eyes/mouth/skin, numbness or tingling in the extremities, blood clots, and multiple miscarriages.

Eighty percent of the immune system is directly connected to gut health, making it a vital area of focus to restore health. Using natural remedies together with a healthy diet can be an effective, non-invasive way to improve gut health. By using a consist program such as a MicroPlex VMz supplement, xEO Mega, and Alpha CRS®+ in a consistent program, along with TerraZyme®, a Zendrocrine® Complex, lemon oil, GX Assist®, and a defensive probiotic, an individual can nourish and support the body in an effort to reclaim health.

Repeating a healthy cleanse the first three to four months in a row can also help the body improve its capacity to take care of itself. Targeted support using natural remedies for certain conditions individualizes a program and targets symptoms of discomfort and disease. It is empowering to exercise options for natural solutions to target root causes, since most modern medical approaches to autoimmune conditions seek to only manage symptoms.

Additionally, a great way to help the immune system function optimally and to reduce environmental stress on the body is to perform the Oil Touch technique as it is explained in the introduction to this book. The technique is a systematic application of eight different essential oils that serves to strengthen the immune system, eliminate pathogens, reduce stress, and bring the body into homeostasis, enabling the body to function more optimally. A weekly application for three to four months is ideal. See Oil Touch technique, page 19.

TOP SOLUTIONS

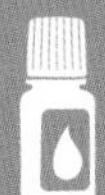

SINGLE OILS

Lemongrass - stimulates nerves and supports digestion (pg. 126)

Juniper berry - antioxidant and supports digestion (pg. 119)

Copaiba - anti-inflammatory, anti-infectious, pain reliever (pg. 99)

Ginger - invigorates nerves and cleanses (pg. 113)

Clary sage - invigorates nerves and supports endocrine system (pg. 96)

Turmeric - antioxidant and anti-inflammatory (pg. 158)

By Related Properties

For more, See Oil Properties on pages 477 - 481

Analgesic - basil, birch, blue tansy, cassia, cinnamon, clary sage, clove, copaiba, coriander, eucalyptus, fennel, frankincense, helichrysum, lavender, litsea, melaleuca, peppermint, Siberian fir, tumeric, wintergreen, yarrow
Antiarthritic - arborvitae, basil, birch, blue tansy, cassia, copaiba, cypress, ginger, manuka, turmeric, wintergreen
Antidepressant - bergamot, clary sage, frankincense, geranium, jasmine, lavender, lemon, magnolia, melissa, neroli, pink pepper, rose, tangerine, ylang ylang
Anti-infectious - basil, bergamot, cedarwood, cinnamon, clove, copaiba, cypress, frankincense, geranium, lavender, litsea, marjoram, melaleuca, patchouli, rosemary, turmeric
Anti-inflammatory - basil, birch, blue tansy, cardamom, cassia, cedarwood, cinnamon, copaiba, coriander, cypress, eucalyptus, frankincense, geranium, helichrysum, lemongrass, lime, litsea, manuka, melissa, myrrh, neroli, peppermint, rosemary, sandalwood, Siberian fir, spikenard, tangerine, turmeric, wintergreen, yarrow
Antioxidant - basil, black pepper, cassia, cilantro, cinnamon, clove, copaiba, frankincense, ginger, grapefruit, helichrysum, juniper berry, lemongrass, lime, melaleuca, neroli, oregano, tangerine, thyme, turmeric, vetiver, wild orange, yarrow
Anti-parasitic - blue tansy, cinnamon, clove, frankincense, juniper berry, lavender, melaleuca, oregano, rosemary, tangerine, thyme
Regenerative - cedarwood, clove, coriander, frankincense, geranium, helichrysum, jasmine, manuka, myrrh, neroli, patchouli, sandalwood, turmeric, wild orange, yarrow
Stomachic - blue tansy, cardamom, cinnamon, clary sage, coriander, fennel, ginger, juniper berry, marjoram, melissa, peppermint, pink pepper, rose, rosemary, tangerine, turmeric, wild orange, yarrow
Tonic - arborvitae, basil, birch, cardamom, cedarwood, clary sage, coriander, cypress, fennel, frankincense, geranium, ginger, grapefruit, green mandarin, lavender, lemon, marjoram, melissa, myrrh, neroli, patchouli, Roman chamomile, rose, rosemary, sandalwood, Siberian fir, tangerine, thyme, vetiver, wild orange, ylang ylang, yarrow
Uplifting - bergamot, cardamom, cedarwood, clary sage, cypress, grapefruit, green mandarin, lime, litsea, melissa, sandalwood, tangerine, wild orange, ylang ylang

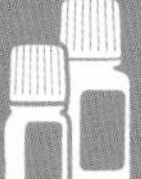

BLENDS

DDR Prime® - supports nerves and glands (pg. 184)

Zendocrine® - detoxifies and supports proper digestive function (pg. 206)

Slim & Sassy® - antioxidant and improves digestion (pg. 218)

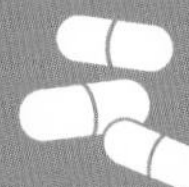

SUPPLEMENTS

Bone Nutrient Lifetime Complex, **Alpha CRS®+ (pg. 209), PB Assist®+(pg. 216)**, DigestZen® softgels, Mito2Max®, **DDR Prime® Softgels (pg. 211), xEO Mega (pg. 222), TerraZyme® (pg. 219)**, IQ Mega®, **Deep Blue Polyphenol Complex (pg. 212)**, On Guard® lozenges, On Guard® softgels (use with Balance®), MicroPlex VMz

CRITICAL AUTOIMMUNE SUPPLEMENTATION PROGRAM

- **Alpha CRS®+** with antioxidants, flavonoids, additional cellular support
- **MicroPlex VMz** as a high potency multivitamin/mineral
- **TerraZyme®** for proper digestion; add DigestZen® softgels as needed
- **XEO Mega** with land and sea omega sources, astaxanthin (use a IQ Mega® for children and elderly who can't swallow pills)

Add as needed for desired target support:

- **Bone Nutrient Lifetime Complex** necessary for numerous cellular, structural functions
- **DDR Prime® Softgels** to establish and maintain healthy cell vitality and apoptosis
- **Deep Blue Polyphenol Complex** to reduce or eliminate pain/inflammation, inflammatory responses
- **PB Assist®+**to establish and maintain healthy gut flora, eliminate harmful microorganisms
- **Mito2Max®** with CoQ10 for energy, improve circulation
- **Zendrocrine® Complex** and **Zendocrine®** to promote detoxification, proper elimination, turmeric

Remedies

For ALL autoimmune diseases consider the following:

- Critical Supplemental Program - see above
- See *Digestive & Intestinal* for digestive/intestinal issues, leaky gut
- See *Immune & Lymphatic* to manage/eliminate/prevent microorganisms
- See *Candida* to manage/eliminate/prevent candida
- Oil Touch technique or other massage techniques and heat treatments - see page 19

For the following specific autoimmune conditions, all suggestions below are recommended in addition to using the suggested critical supplements daily program and the Oil Touch technique weekly.

CELIAC DISEASE PROTOCOL

Combine in a capsule or in 12 ounces water:
2 drops lemon (tonic for the liver)
2 drops grapefruit (dissolves toxins stored in fat cells)
2 drops ginger (digestive support)
1 drop cinnamon (regulates blood sugar levels)
OR
6-7 drops of Slim & Sassy® (Includes lemon, grapefruit, ginger, cinnamon)
Take two times daily for ongoing support.

Additional Support

- Rub DigestZen® on stomach **OR** take 2-4 drops in capsule **OR** use 1-2 DigestZen® softgels during digestive discomfort or upset stomach.
- Diffuse frankincense, Elevation™, or Citrus Bliss® to combat depression or irritability.
- Take 2-3 food enzyme capsules daily.

CROHN'S DISEASE

In addition to a MicroPlex VMz supplement and xEO Mega Critical Autoimmune Supplemental Program (see above), additional specific targeted support suggestions are:

- PB Assist®+three times daily for six months
- Take 2-3 food enzyme capsules daily (at least one per meal)
- Rub DigestZen® on abdomen two times daily for 2 months
- Rub DigestZen® and ginger on bottoms of feet daily for six months
- Place 2 drops DigestZen®, 2 drops frankincense, and fractionated coconut oil (if desired) in a capsule. Take twice a day for two weeks. Then change formula to 5 drops ginger, 5 drops peppermint or marjoram, and 4 drops frankincense for two weeks.
- Topically apply pink pepper (dilute with a carrier oil), DigestZen®, or peppermint for abdominal pain
- Topically apply or diffuse lavender or Serenity® to manage stress

Consider a candida cleanse. See *Candida* section for details.

SJOGREN'S

In addition to Critical Autoimmune Supplementation Program (including the Alpha CRS®+) twice per day, take 2 -3 drops of frankincense two to four times daily under the tongue or in a capsule. Use additional oils as symptoms occur; Deep Blue® for painful joints, DigestZen® for digestive problems, lavender or geranium for skin problems, etc.

Additional suggestions:
Candida cleanse and other detoxing programs - see *Candida; Detoxification*

Chronic Dry Eye
Gently dab lavender (frankincense, myrrh, sandalwood are additional options) on the facial bones surrounding the eye, being careful to avoid the eye itself. Within minutes the dry, irritated eyes will soothe and feel better. Should you accidentally get too close to eye with any essential oil, dilute with carrier oil, never water!

Chronic Dry Mouth
Try oil pulling (see *Detoxification - Oil Pulling*) for a week and see if it helps the salivary glands to kick in.
Here is one oil pulling recipe:
1 tablespoon fractionated coconut oil
2 drop clove
2 drops oregano
Put mixture in mouth, swish in mouth for twenty minutes, then spit into the sink; repeat daily.

HASHIMOTO'S

Choose from the following protocols or use progressively over time.

- **Protocol 1:**
  40 drops each Balance® and geranium placed in 10ml roller bottle with carrier oil.
  34 drops lemongrass and 40 myrrh placed in a different 10ml roller bottle with carrier oil.
  Shake each blend after adding to roller bottle. Alternate the above two combinations weekly. Apply them directly to thyroid area and reflex points on big toe, thumb multiple times per day.

- **Protocol 2:**
  25 drops lemongrass
  25 drops clove
  10 drops frankincense
  4 drops peppermint
  Prepare the above blend in a 10ml roller bottle, fill with fractionated coconut oil, and apply topically to thyroid and reflexology points three times daily.

- **Protocol 3:**
  Apply 2-3 drops of frankincense and 1 drop peppermint topically to thyroid and reflexology points three times daily to reduce goiter size.

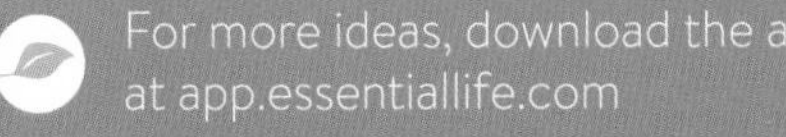

Conditions

Abdominal pain - marjoram, turmeric, AromaTouch®; see *Digestive & Intestinal, Muscles*

Blood clots - Deep Blue®, Motivate®, On Guard®, PastTense®; see *Cardiovascular*

Blood in stool - birch (ulcer), geranium (bleeding), helichrysum, (bleeding), yarrow, wintergreen (ulcer); see *Digestive & Intestinal (Ulcers)*

Blood pressure changes - celery seed, clary sage, ylang ylang (if too high); rosemary, Siberian fir, thyme (if too low); see *Cardiovascular*

Cold intolerance - black pepper, cinnamon, eucalyptus, DDR Prime®; see *Endocrine (Thyroid), Cardiovascular (Poor circulation; Warming property)*

Diarrhea or constipation - black pepper, cardamom, Douglas fir, ginger, DigestZen®, Motivate®; see *Digestive & Intestinal*

Dry eyes, mouth, or skin* - See *Respiratory, Oral Health, Integumentary*

Hair loss - clary sage, eucalyptus, rosemary, yarrow, Motivate®; see *Integumentary*

Heat intolerance - eucalyptus, peppermint; see *Endocrine (Thyroid)*

Inflammation - birch, copaiba, cypress, peppermint, turmeric, wintergreen, Motivate®; see *Pain & Inflammation*

Insomnia - lavender, frankincense, neroli, vetiver, wild orange, InTune®, Peace®, Serenity®; see *Sleep*

Joint pain - celery seed, copaiba, lemongrass, turmeric, AromaTouch®, Deep Blue®; see *Skeletal, Pain & Inflammation*

Lack of concentration or focus - basil, rosemary, InTune®, Motivate®; see *Focus & Concentration*

Mucus in stool - cardamom, ginger, DigestZen®, Motivate®; see *Digestive & Intestinal*

Muscle pain, weakness, tremor, or cramps - copaiba, marjoram, AromaTouch®, Deep Blue®, Passion®; see *Muscular, Pain & Inflammation*

Mouth ulcers - clove, myrrh, wild orange; see *Oral Health*

Multiple miscarriages - blue tansy, clary sage, grapefruit, thyme, Motivate®; see *Women's Health*

Numbness or tingling in the hands or feet - cypress, peppermint, AromaTouch®, Deep Blue®; see *Nervous*

Overactive immune system - basil, frankincense, helichrysum, lavender, neroli, Balance®

Paralysis, facial - helichrysum, patchouli, peppermint, Motivate®; see *Nervous*

Rapid heartbeat - frankincense, sandalwood, ylang ylang; see *Cardiovascular*

Rashes or hives - blue tansy, lavender, Roman chamomile; see *Allergies*

Salt cravings - celery seed; see "Critical Autoimmune Supplementation Program" above"

Skin pigmentation - cedarwood, sandalwood, Immortelle; see *Integumentary*

Sore throat, chronic - basil, cassia, cinnamon, eucalyptus, fennel, ginger, lemon, oregano, thyme, Breathe®, On Guard®

Sun sensitivity - lavender, myrrh, xEO Mega with astaxanthin; see *Integumentary*

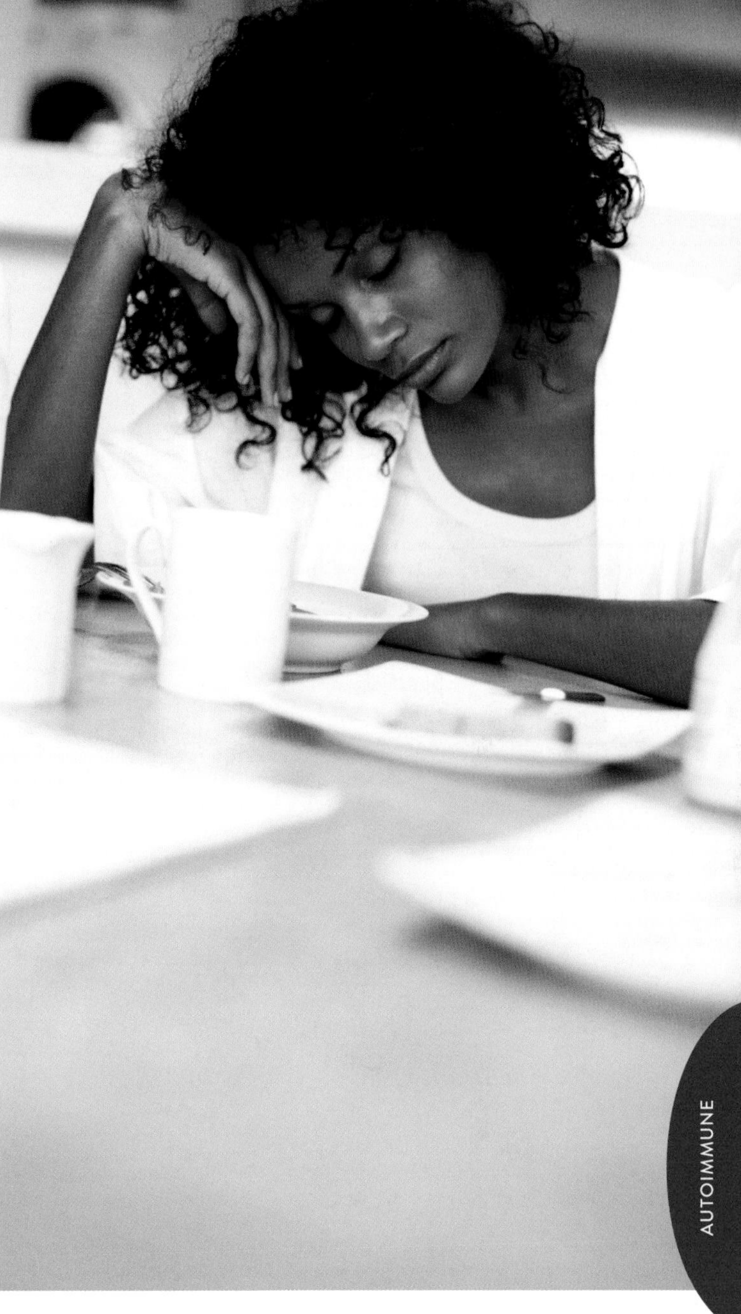

AUTOIMMUNE

Tiredness or fatigue - cinnamon, cypress, Douglas fir, peppermint, Cheer®, Motivate®; see *Energy & Vitality*

Weight gain or loss - cinnamon, ginger, Slim & Sassy®; see *Weight*

White patches on skin, inside mouth - myrrh, sandalwood; see *Integumentary*

USAGE TIPS: For best support in resolving autoimmune conditions:

- **Internal:** Take oils in a capsule, drop under tongue (hold 30 seconds; swallow).
- **Topical:** Use Oil Touch technique at least one to two times monthly; weekly if possible; apply oils on bottoms of feet, rub oils down spine and on any specific area of concern.
- **Aromatic:** Diffuse chosen oils

* See remedy on pg. 242

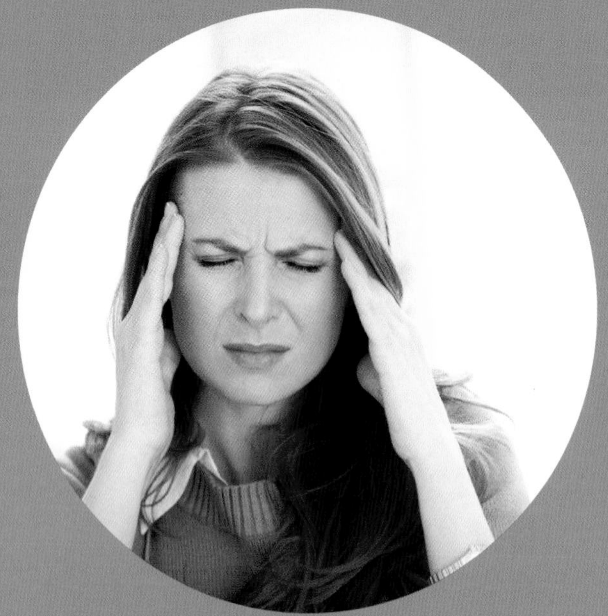

LUPUS

Cleanse (in addition to basic critical supplementation):
Do a candida cleanse. See *Immune & Lymphatic - Candida* section for details.

Address Inflammation
- Ingest citrus oils as a daily priority. Use your favorite 3-5 drops three times per day in water or veggie capsule.
- For liver and anti-inflammatory support:
  - Place 4 drops each geranium, helichrysum or lemongrass, rosemary oils in a capsule and take daily.
  - Use Zendocrine®.

For localized pain, use Deep Blue®, wintergreen, or birch topically.

For systemic pain, combine (in capsule), consume every four hours or as needed:
- 2-4 drops lavender
- 2-4 drops helichrysum
- 2-4 drops clove or thyme
- 2-4 drops turmeric

  Additionally, for a soothing bath, add above oils to: 1-2 cups Epsom salt (4 drops of oil per cup Epsom salt). Mix oils in salt prior to placing in tub water as hot as is tolerated. Dissolve the salt mixture in the water and soak for twenty minutes. Other oils to consider: cinnamon, clove, coriander, frankincense, geranium, ginger, lavender, lemongrass, myrrh, roman chamomile, wintergreen. Change oil choices/combinations as needed and desired.

SCLERODERMA

Initial Cleanse
- The Critical Supplementation Program is a must.
- Do a candida cleanse. See *Candida* section for details. Repeat the cleanse twice; take a 10 day break in between the first and second; then repeat every other month as needed. Be sure to follow up each round with five days of increased amounts of defensive probiotic.
- Drop 2-3 drops of frankincense under the tongue four times a day for two weeks.
- Pain Relief blend - use at least two times per day:
  - 3 drops each lavender, Deep Blue®, and birch OR wintergreen
  - 4 drops each myrrh and sandalwood
  - Apply topically to bottoms of feet, along spine, and outside of ears, alternating daily between blends.

Ongoing Support
Continue supplementation program.
- Daily - apply Deep Blue® to areas of concern morning, midday, evening, and anytime intense pain occurs.
- Morning:
  - Topically apply peppermint to the bottoms of feet.
  - Take 3-4 drops of peppermint, DigestZen®, frankincense, basil in capsule.
- During the day:
  - Add 1-3 drops of lemon to each glass of water. Drink lots of water. Glass containers only.
- Evening:
  - Take 3-4 drops each of peppermint, lemongrass, marjoram in capsule.
- Topically apply 2-3 drops of frankincense to bottoms of feet. Layer 2-4 drops geranium oil, AromaTouch®.

Specific Issues:
- Breathing issues - rub 2-4 drops of peppermint and/or Breathe® on chest, on/in nasal passages.
- Digestive issues - rub 3-4 drops of DigestZen® over abdomen

Related Ailments: Addison's Disease (adrenals) [Endocrine], Autoimmune Hepatitis (liver) [Digestive & Intestinal], Celiac Sprue Disease (GI tract) [Digestive & Intestinal], Crohn's Disease [Digestive & Intestinal], Diabetes Type 1 [Blood Sugar], Glomerulonephritis (kidneys) [Urinary], Grave Disease (thyroid) [Endocrine], Gout (joints, big toe) [Skeletal], Hashimoto's (thyroid) [Endocrine], Huntington's Disease (nerve cells in brain) [Brain, Nervous], Inflammatory Bowel Disease, Inflammatory Myopathies [Muscles], Lou Gehrig's/ALS (nerve cells in brain, spinal cord) [Brain, Nervous], Lupus (any part of the body such as skin, joints, and/or organs), Multiple Sclerosis (myelin sheath) [Nervous], Myasthenia Gravis, Pernicious Anemia (failure to produce red blood cells [Cardiovascular] and failure to absorb vitamin B12 - liver) [Digestive & Intestinal], Rheumatoid Arthritis (joints in hands, feet) [Skeletal], Sarcoidosis/Sarcoid (primarily lungs, lymph nodes) [Respiratory, Immune & Lymphatic; Digestive & Intestinal (leaky gut)], Schmidt's Syndrome, Scleroderma (connective tissue) [Muscles, Skeletal], Sjogrens (salivary, tear duct glands) [Oral Health, Respiratory], Vitiligo (skin pigment cells) [Integumentary, Endocrine (thyroid), Women's Health, Stress]

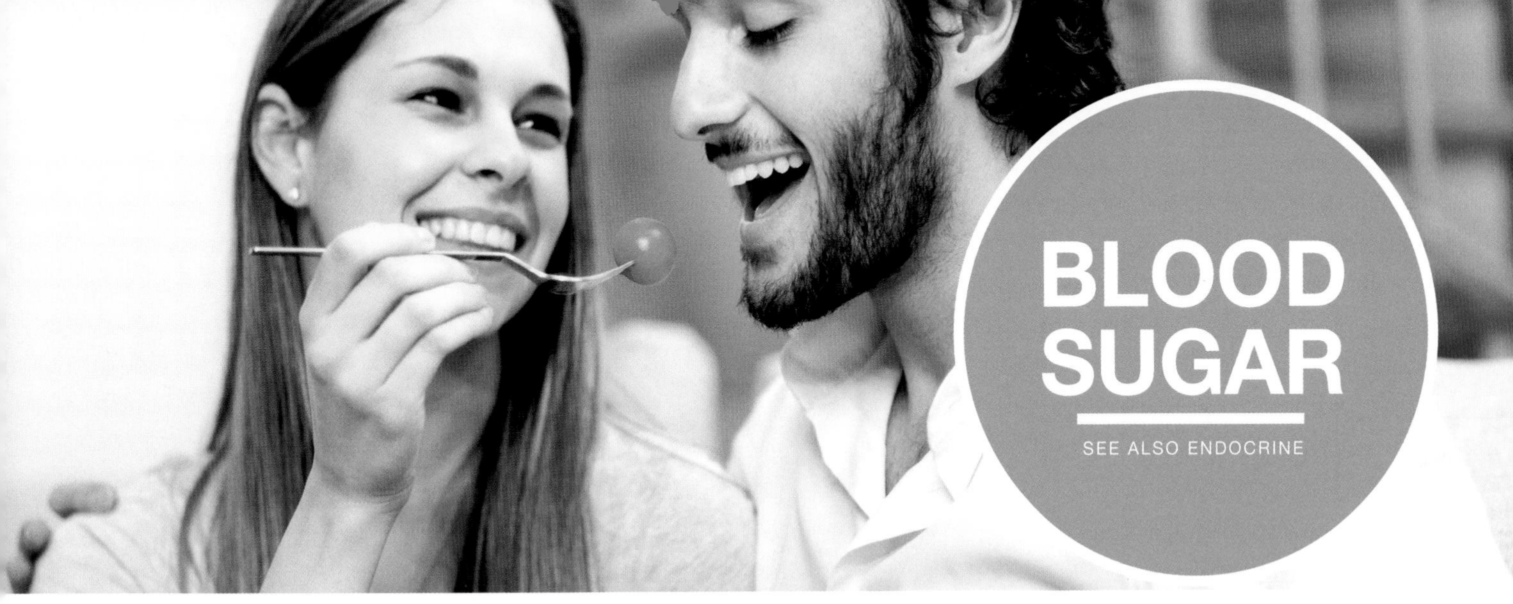

BLOOD SUGAR

INSULIN is a hormone that regulates blood sugar levels, shuttling the right amount of glucose into the cells where it is used for energy. When the body doesn't have enough insulin, blood-sugar levels become too high and cells don't have enough energy to function properly.

Diabetes is the most common endocrine disorder; it occurs when pancreas doesn't produce enough insulin (type 1 - typical onset is before age 20), or if the body is unable to use insulin (type 2 - typically over age 40). The onset age for type 2 is decreasing with an increasingly younger population suffering from what is a preventable disease. A third type, gestational diabetes, can occur during pregnancy and create potential long-term issues for both mother and child.

Hypoglycemia is a condition characterized by too little glucose in the blood. When severe, is also called "insulin reaction" or "insulin shock" and can lead to accidents, injuries, even coma and death.

When we consume healthy sources of carbohydrates with plenty of good fats and protein, the glucose from the meal enters the blood slowly and the pancreas responds by secreting a measured amount of insulin. Keeping blood sugar balanced throughout the day is the best way to avoid "sugar highs" and "sugar lows." A healthy individual can easily go three hours or more between meals without experiencing sugar cravings or feeling shaky, irritable, or tired.

Eating habits can influence the likelihood of developing blood sugar issues. When individuals consume foods too high in sugar or refined carbohydrates, these simple carbs enter the bloodstream almost immediately through the intestines, resulting in higher-than-normal blood sugar levels. The body then needs to produce more insulin to process the excess glucose. As the presence of elevated insulin levels becomes chronic, the body's sensitivity to insulin decreases (known as insulin resistance), forcing blood glucose levels to rise. Insulin is also an inflammatory agent.

Additionally, blood sugar imbalances and elevated insulin levels affect a number of functions, from hormones to heart to mood to cellular health to fertility... as well as perpetuate inflammation, which is considered to be a prime contributor to disease. One lesser known fact is that high blood pressure is another common symptom which is caused by high circulating levels of insulin in the blood. Common conditions resulting from blood sugar issues can be found in *Endocrine* and *Cardiovascular*.

Insulin and glucose levels are easily improved by positive changes in lifestyle, exercise, and diet. One of the benefits of stable blood sugar is the natural reduction of inflammation and the resulting balance of hormones. Healthy dietary changes (elimination of harmful sugars and refined carbohydrates), commitments, and consistencies are therefore significant. A study reported in the Journal of the American Medical Association (JAMA) stated, "Duration and degree of sugar exposure correlated significantly with diabetes prevalence while declines in sugar exposure correlated with significant subsequent declines in diabetes rates." *

Natural solutions can be incredibly effective in supporting the body to generate a healthy insulin response and blood-sugar regulation. Because stable blood sugar levels diminish or eliminate sugar and carb cravings, even stubborn weight can melt away and longevity may be extended.

In addition to necessary dietary and lifestyle commitments, essential oils are powerful allies in achieving and maintaining healthy blood sugar and insulin levels, improving insulin receptivity, and resolving a surprising number of related health concerns. Additionally, essential oils support bringing other body systems into balance, which is particularly helpful given the number of diabetes-related disorders. Essential oils positively impact blood sugar management. For example, coriander oil lowers glucose levels by normalizing insulin levels and supporting pancreatic function. Cinnamon oil aids in managing blood glucose levels and strengthens the circulatory and immune systems.

NOTE: Every condition listed below is considered potentially related to or associated with imbalanced blood sugar and/or insulin levels. Addressing both blood sugar and insulin levels through diet, supplementation, and the use of essential oils is critical to success. The use of suggestions below to manage symptoms is intended to be paired with these critical diet and lifestyle changes.

TOP SOLUTIONS

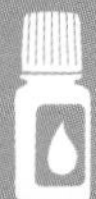

SINGLE OILS

Coriander - promotes a healthy insulin response (pg. 100)
Cinnamon - balances blood sugar levels (pg. 93)
Cassia - balances blood sugar levels (pg. 88)
Turmeric - (pg. 158)

By Related Properties

For more, See Oil Properties on pages 477 - 479

Antifungal - bergamot, blue tansy, cinnamon, clove, copaiba, coriander, fennel, helichrysum, lemongrass, litsea, manuka, melaleuca, oregano, Siberian fir, thyme, turmeric
Anti-inflammatory - birch, blue tansy, cardamom, cassia, cinnamon, clove, copaiba, coriander, frankincense, ginger, lavender, lemongrass, litsea, manuka, myrrh, neroli, oregano, patchouli, pink pepper, rosemary, Siberian fir, spikenard, tangerine, turmeric, yarrow
Antioxidant - black pepper, cinnamon, copaiba, coriander, frankincense, ginger, helichrysum, juniper berry, lemon, lemongrass, neroli, oregano, tangerine, turmeric vetiver, wild orange, yarrow
Detoxifier - arborvitae, cassia, cilantro, geranium, juniper berry, lemon, lime, litsea, patchouli, tangerine, yarrow
Invigorating - grapefruit, lemon, litsea, peppermint, pink pepper, Siberian fir, wild orange
Stimulant - basil, blue tansy, cedarwood, cinnamon, coriander, Siberian fir, tangerine, thyme, wintergreen
Stomachic - blue tansy, cardamom, cinnamon, clary sage, coriander, eucalyptus, juniper berry, marjoram, melissa, peppermint, rosemary, tangerine, wild orange, yarrow
Vasodilator - blue tansy, copaiba, lemongrass, litsea, manuka, marjoram, neroli, rosemary, thyme

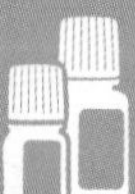

BLENDS

Slim & Sassy® - helps control blood sugar (pg. 200)
Zendocrine® - improves insulin receptivity (pg. 206)
On Guard® - balances blood sugar levels (pg. 194)

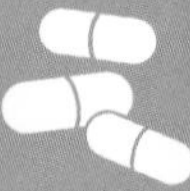

SUPPLEMENTS

Alpha CRS®+ (pg. 209), DigestZen® softgels, essential oil xEO Mega, **Slim & Sassy® softgels (pg. 218)**, MicroPlex VMz supplement

Related Ailments: Blood Sugar Headaches, Blood Sugar Imbalance, Diabetes, Diabetic Sores, Hypoglycemia, Insulin, Insulin Imbalances, Insulin Resistance, Low Blood Sugar, Sugar Headache

BLOOD SUGAR

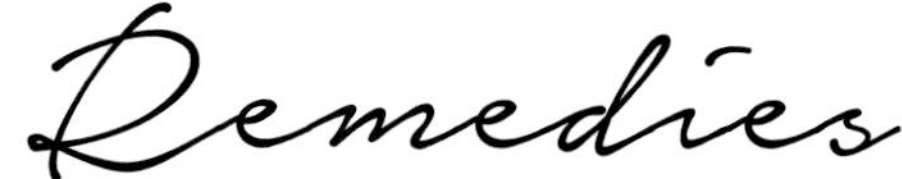

Remedies

HIGH BLOOD SUGAR REDUCER
3 drops coriander or basil
3 drops Slim & Sassy®
1 drop oregano
Taken two to three times per day in capsule.

LOW BLOOD SUGAR (use to improve)
2 drops rosemary
1 drop geranium
1 drop cypress
Apply to chest and reflexology points on feet and hands (dilute if needed), or diffuse.

BLOOD SUGAR BALANCE BLEND
- Recipe #1: 2 drops cinnamon, 2 drops clove, 4 drops rosemary, 3 drops thyme oils;
  Combine in 10ml roller bottle; fill remainder with carrier oil; apply to bottoms of feet, massage; focus on arch of foot to target pancreas reflex point(s).
- Recipe #2: 2 drops cinnamon + 5 drops cypress
  Combine in palm of one hand then distribute across bottoms of feet, center of abdomen just below the ribs (over the pancreas).

DAILY ROUTINE FOR SUPPORTING HEALTHY BLOOD SUGAR
- Rub 1-2 drops of Balance® on bottoms of feet in morning
- Use "High Blood Sugar" remedy three times daily
- Rub 1-2 drops of lavender on feet at night prior to sleep

CLEAR AND BALANCE
Combine 1 drop each cinnamon, bergamot, Siberian fir, and pink pepper to a capsule and take internally or combine 2 drops each and diffuse. Variations: consider substituting or adding fennel or coriander.

NEUROPATHY NEUTRALIZER
Apply 3-4 drops of cypress, coriander, and/or Deep Blue® to legs below knees all the way to bottoms of feet; massage. Use at least morning and night.

BLOOD SUGAR BALANCING CINNAMON TEA
Place 1-2 drops of cinnamon bark in ½ cup warm water, sweeten with 1 teaspoon raw honey or agave nectar if needed.

GRAPEFRUIT DETOX DELIGHT
1-2 drops cassia or cinnamon + 3 drops grapefruit in a 24-ounce water bottle. Shake, do not stir. Drink throughout day.

EMOTIONAL RELIEF AND PANCREAS SUPPORT
Apply 1-2 drops of geranium to bottoms of feet.

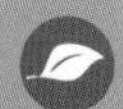

For more ideas, download the app at app.essentiallife.com

Conditions

Anxiety - cilantro, coriander, melaleuca, peppermint, Balance®, PastTense®, Serenity®, Zendocrine®; see *Mood & Behavior*

Apple-shaped body/abdominal excess weight - See *"Insulin resistance," "Insulin, excessive," "Glucose levels, high," Weight*

Blood sugar, high (hyperglycemia)* - basil, cinnamon, coriander, dill, eucalyptus, fennel, geranium, ginger, juniper berry, lemon, oregano, pink pepper, rosemary, turmeric, ylang ylang, Slim & Sassy®, Zendocrine®

Blood sugar, low (hypoglycemia)* - cassia, cypress, eucalyptus, geranium, juniper berry, lavender, lemongrass, rosemary, Zendocrine®

Blurred/compromised vision - cilantro, coriander, helichrysum, lemongrass, melissa, rose, thyme, DDR Prime®, Elevation™, Immortelle, Zendocrine®

Circulation issues/foot issues/gangrene - See *Cardiovascular*

Cravings for sweets - cassia, cinnamon, grapefruit, Slim & Sassy®; see *Eating Disorders, Weight*

Concentration, poor/Brain fog - See *Focus & Concentration*

Depression - bergamot, geranium, wild orange, ylang ylang, Elevation™; see *Mood & Behavior*

Digestive issues/chronic constipation or diarrhea - See *Digestion & Intestinal*

Dizziness - dill, helichrysum, DDR Prime®, Zendocrine®; see "Glucose levels, low (Hypoglycemia)" below

Energy dips/fatigue/drowsiness - basil, cinnamon, ginger, lemon, lime, peppermint, rosemary, wild orange, wintergreen, Cheer®, Slim & Sassy®; see *Energy & Vitality*

Feeling frequent urination - Zendocrine®; see *Urinary*

Headache - frankincense, lavender, peppermint, wintergreen, PastTense®, Slim & Sassy®, Zendrocrine®; see *Pain & Inflammation*

Heart palpitations/irregular/rapid heartbeat - See *Cardiovascular*

High blood pressure (due to the circulation of excessive insulin) - See "Glucose levels, high (Hyperglycemia)"

Hunger/excessive hunger - See *Weight*

Infections, skin/vaginal - melaleuca, On Guard®

Insulin, excessive - coriander, fennel, lemongrass, turmeric

Insulin, insufficient - dill, wild orange

Insulin resistance or poor response to - cassia, coriander, cypress, juniper berry, lavender, lemongrass, oregano, rosemary, turmeric, ylang ylang, DDR Prime®, On Guard®, Purify, Slim & Sassy®, Zendocrine®

Irritability - See *Mood & Behavior*

Kidney/urinary issues - See *Urinary*

Mood swings - geranium, patchouli, Balance®, Elevation™, InTune®, Serenity®; see *Mood & Behavior*

Nausea - basil, bergamot, ginger, juniper berry, DigestZen®; see *Digestion & Intestinal*

Nerve damage* (e.g. neuropathy, painful cold or insensitive feet, loss of hair on the lower extremities, or erectile dysfunction, tingling skin) - basil; see *Nervous*

Nervousness, sudden - cedarwood, frankincense, petitgrain, Balance®, Serenity®; see *Mood & Behavior*

Shaky/weak - black pepper, frankincense, vetiver, Elevation™, PastTense®, Serenity®

Skin, pale - cypress, wild orange, AromaTouch®

Sleep, difficulty - geranium, lavender, marjoram, patchouli, Roman chamomile, ylang ylang; see *Sleep*

Sleep, want excessive amount - geranium, wild orange

Sweating/hot flashes (blood sugar imbalance) - eucalyptus, peppermint

Thirst, excessive/increased - grapefruit, lemon, Slim & Sassy®

Urination, frequent - basil, cinnamon, cypress, AromaTouch®, On Guard®, Zendocrine®; see *Urinary*

Weight loss, sudden/excessive - cinnamon, Slim & Sassy®; see *Weight*

Wound healing, poor/slow - cypress, frankincense, helichrysum, lavender, myrrh, white fir, Immortelle; see *First Aid*

* *See remedy on pg. 246*

USAGE TIPS: For best success at targeting blood sugar and insulin levels:

- **Internal:** Place 1-5 drops in water to drink, take oil(s) in a capsule, place a drop(s) on or under tongue, or lick them off back of hand.
- **Topical:** Apply oils topically on bottoms of feet targeting reflex points for pancreas and other endocrine partners such as adrenal and thyroid locations; see Reflexology.

*JAMA, 2004; Diabetes Care, 2010; PLOS ONE, 2013. Reported by Business Insider: www.businessinsider.com/effects-of-eating-too-much-sugar-2014-3#ixzz3UKTXOpuy

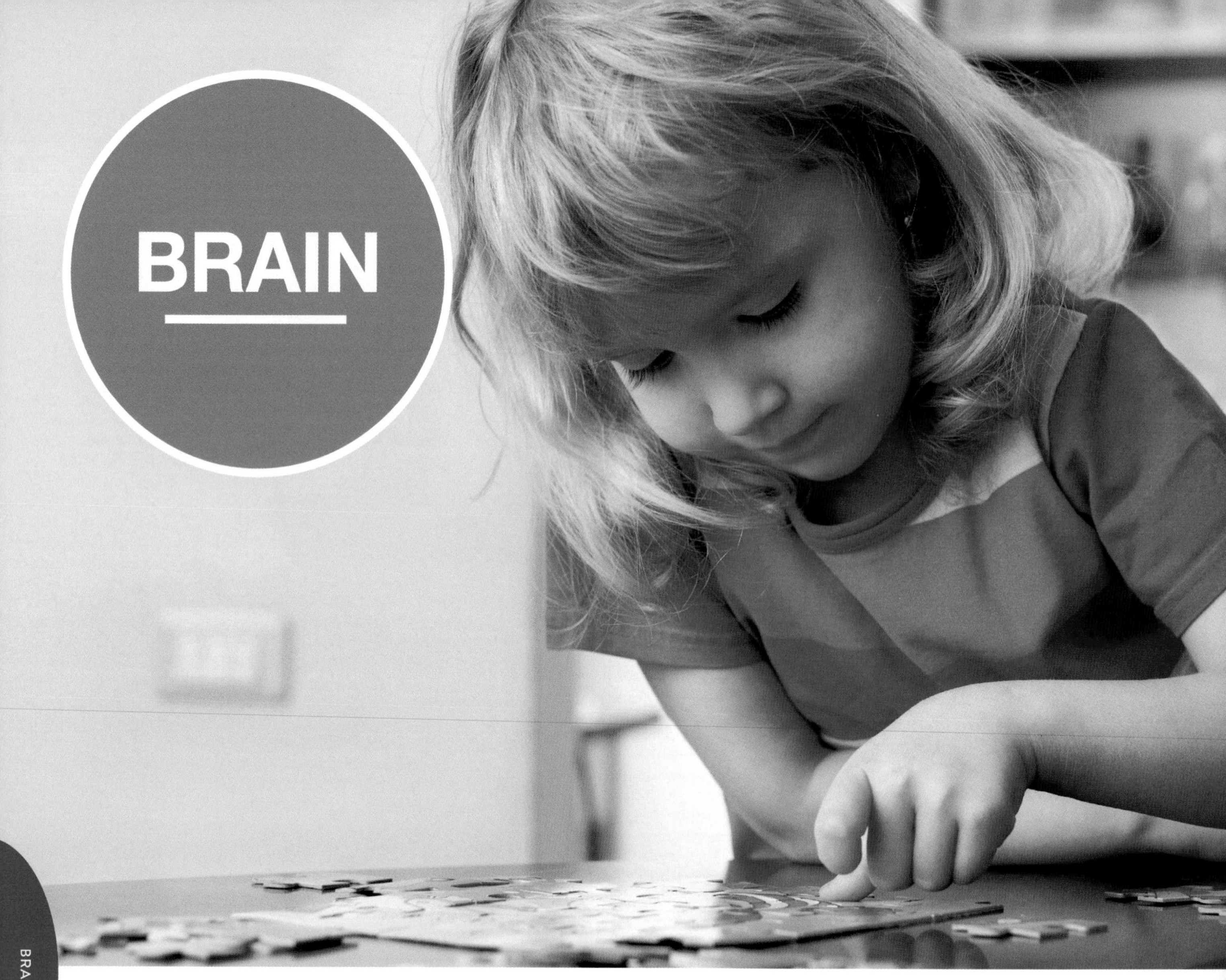

THE BRAIN, an organ the size of a small head of cauliflower, resides in the skull and is the control center of the body. The brain is the most vital organ to everyday life functioning and, together with the spinal cord and peripheral nerves, makes up the central nervous system, which directs, coordinates, and regulates voluntary (conscious) and involuntary (unconscious) processes. Sensory nerves throughout the body constantly gather information from the environment and send it to the brain via the spinal cord. The brain rapidly interprets the data and responds by sending messages with motor neurons to the rest of the body.

Scientists have found that certain parts of the brain perform certain functions. The frontal lobe, where the limbic system is located, helps regulate emotions and trauma, assists with reasoning, planning, and problem solving, and is involved with some language skills. The parietal lobe aids with recognition and interpreting data, orientation, and movement. The occipital lobe is connected to visual processing, and the temporal lobe supports perception, auditory processing, memory, and speech.

Due to its important role in managing and directing all organs, systems, and body processes, the brain has several layers of protection including the skull, the meninges (thin membranes), and cerebrospinal fluid. The brain also has what has come to be called the "blood-brain barrier," which keeps cells of the nervous system separate from cells throughout the vascular system (the rest of the body).

Essential oils powerfully benefit brain function and processes. When used aromatically, such as diffusing oils into the air or inhaling oils directly from bottle or palms of the hands, essential oils directly access the brain through the olfactory bulb and are able to initiate almost immediate physical and emotional responses in the brain.

Due to their unique chemical constituents and the fact that they are carbon based, essential oils are able to permeate the protective blood-brain barrier and provide support for such things as headaches, migraines, vertigo or other balance issues, emotions, and mood. Certain essential oils that are comprised of specific chemical constituents like sesquiterpenes, such as frankincense and sandalwood, have a particular affinity for supporting the brain. Essential oils with antioxidant and anti-inflammatory properties are also particularly important for maintaining a healthy brain.

TOP SOLUTIONS

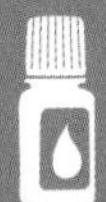

SINGLE OILS

Sandalwood - promotes optimal brain function, repair; crosses blood-brain barrier (pg. 150)

Frankincense - crosses blood-brain barrier; anti-aging brain support (pg. 110)

Cedarwood, Arborvitae - calms, stimulates, and protects brain (pg. 89, pg. 79)

Rosemary - enhances brain, cognitive performance; relieves mental fatigue (pg. 149)

Clove and thyme - provides brain protective antioxidants (pgs. 97 & 157)

Petitgrain - calms and soothes the brain (pg. 142)

Turmeric - brain protection and antioxidant (pg. 158)

By Related Properties

For more, See Oil Properties on pages 477 - 481

Anticonvulsant - clary sage, fennel, geranium, lavender, neroli, tangerine

Anti-inflammatory - basil, bergamot, birch, black pepper, blue tansy, cardamom, cedarwood, celery seed, cinnamon, clove, copaiba, coriander, dill, eucalyptus, fennel, frankincense, geranium, helichrysum, jasmine, lavender, lemongrass, lime, litsea, manuka, melaleuca, melissa, myrrh, oregano, neroli, patchouli, peppermint, pink pepper, Roman chamomile, rosemary, sandalwood, Siberian fir, spearmint, tangerine, turmeric, wild orange, wintergreen, yarrow

Antioxidant - arborvitae, basil, black pepper, black spruce, cassia, celery seed, cilantro, cinnamon, clove, copaiba, coriander, eucalyptus, frankincense, ginger, grapefruit, helichrysum, juniper berry, lemon, lemongrass, lime, melaleuca, oregano, neroli, rosemary, tangerine, thyme, turmeric, vetiver, wild orange, yarrow

Anti-parasitic - bergamot, blue tansy, cinnamon, clove, fennel, frankincense, juniper berry, melaleuca, oregano, Roman chamomile, rosemary, tangerine, thyme, turmeric

Nervine - basil, clary sage, clove, helichrysum, green mandarin, juniper berry, lavender, lemongrass, melissa, patchouli, peppermint, rosemary, thyme

Neuroprotective - frankincense, lavender, magnolia, Roman chamomile, thyme, turmeric, vetiver

Neurotonic - arborvitae, basil, bergamot, black pepper, clary sage, cypress, ginger, melaleuca, neroli

Regenerative - frankincense, geranium, helichrysum, manuka, melaleuca, neroli, patchouli, rose, sandalwood, wild orange, yarrow

Stimulant - arborvitae, basil, bergamot, birch, black pepper, blue tansy, cardamom, cedarwood, cinnamon, clove, coriander, cypress, dill, eucalyptus, fennel, ginger, grapefruit, juniper berry, lime, melaleuca, patchouli, pink pepper, rosemary, Siberian fir, spearmint, tangerine, thyme, vetiver, white fir, wintergreen, ylang ylang

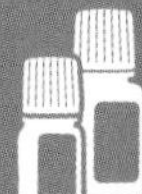

BLENDS

DDR Prime® - provides antioxidants and brain protection (pg. 184)

Zendocrine® - supports relief from mental fatigue and toxins (pg. 206)

InTune® - supports oxygen and blood flow to brain, blood brain barrier (pg. 192)

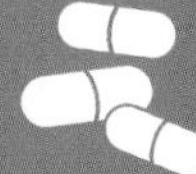

SUPPLEMENTS

Alpha CRS®+ (pg. 209), DDR Prime® Softgels, **xEO Mega (pg. 222)**, Zendrocrine® Complex, **IQ Mega® (pg. 213)**, MicroPlex VMz complex

USAGE TIPS: Some best ways to apply oils for brain health are where there's more direct access to the brain:

- **Topically:** Apply to forehead, back of skull (especially in occipital triangles), under nose, roof of mouth (place oil on pad of thumb, place on roof, "suck")
  Use reflex points on foot for brain, namely big toe, underside pad.
- **Aromatically:** Diffuse oils of choice to stimulate brain allowing entry through nose to olfactory system.

Related Ailments: Absentmindedness, Alertness, Alzheimer's Disease, Amnesia, Ataxia, Autism [Focus & Concentration], Balance Problems, Bipolar Disorder [Mood & Behavior], Body Dysmorphic Disorder, Brain Fog, Brain Injury/Focal Brain Dysfunction, Chemical Imbalance [Endocrine], Coma, Concussion, Creutzfeldt-Jakob Disease [Immune & Lymphatic], Dementia, Down Syndrome, Epilepsy, Huntington's Disease [Nervous], Hydrocephalus, Learning Difficulties, Lou Gehrig's Disease, Meniere's Disease, Memory (poor), Mental Fatigue, Narcolepsy, Obsessive-Compulsive Disorder, Parkinson's Disease, Schizophrenia, Seizures, Social Anxiety Disorder [Mood & Behavior], Stroke, Vertigo

Remedies

ALZHEIMER'S PROTOCOL

Internal:

- Take 4-5 drops each frankincense, thyme, patchouli and turmeric in a capsule daily.
- Take 4-5 drops each clove, melissa, vetiver in a capsule weekly.
- Eat 1 teaspoon of virgin coconut oil a day. Work up to 3 tablespoons a day. Great on toast.
- Take Mito2Max® and Alpha CRS®+ daily.
- Blood sugar support: Drop Slim & Sassy® under the tongue three to five times per day.

Topical:

Rub frankincense on base of skull and neck twice daily.

Brain support: Rub Immortelle on spine and suboccipital triangle area at the base of the skull at least twice daily, occasionally rotate with InTune® and patchouli. Diffuse these oils as well.

BRAIN-FOG BUSTER: (good for overall brain support): Layer 1 drop of each cedarwood, frankincense, patchouli, sandalwood, and vetiver on back of neck with a few drops of carrier oil to enhance circulation to the brain. Note: A carrier oil can be applied before, mixed with, or after essential oils are applied. If carrier oil is applied before or mixed with the essential oil, it slows the absorption. If the carrier oil is applied after, it enhances accelerates absorption.

COGNITIVE IMPROVEMENT: Place 1-2 drops melissa, frankincense, patchouli on suboccipital triangle area at the base of the skull, the bottoms of the feet, and under tongue twice daily to support improvement of cognitive impairment and help dispel agitation and depression.

AUTISM SUPPORT PROTOCOL

- **Overall detox**
  - Layer 1 drop of rosemary and wild orange on each foot at bedtime
  - Apply 2 drops Zendocrine® on each foot on top of the single oils at bedtime
- **Cleanse gut**
  - Take 2 a2z Chewable™ vitamins daily
  - Take 1 GX Assist® daily if child can swallow capsules, if not, use a good quality powder or liquid GI cleansing supplement
  - Follow up with defensive probiotics as recommended, or if not able to swallow capsules, then use a good quality powder or liquid probiotic supplement
- **Brain repair**

  Take IQ Mega® twice daily

  Apply 1 drop DDR Prime® on the base of the skull at least morning and evening, up to five times daily
- **Emotional support** - use the following aromatically in hands or in a diffuser unless otherwise directed, apply to spine or bottoms of feet if the aroma is not tolerated.
  - Use cypress, oregano (with a carrier oil), or wintergreen as needed for inflexibility
  - Use juniper berry or wintergreen morning and night to lift mood and instill courage
  - Use lime as needed for overstimulation or feelings of being overwhelmed
  - Use patchouli as needed when agitated
  - Use Roman chamomile morning and night to soothe nerves and excessive reactions
  - Use 1 drop On Guard® or TerraShield® every morning on bottom of each foot to increase sense of security

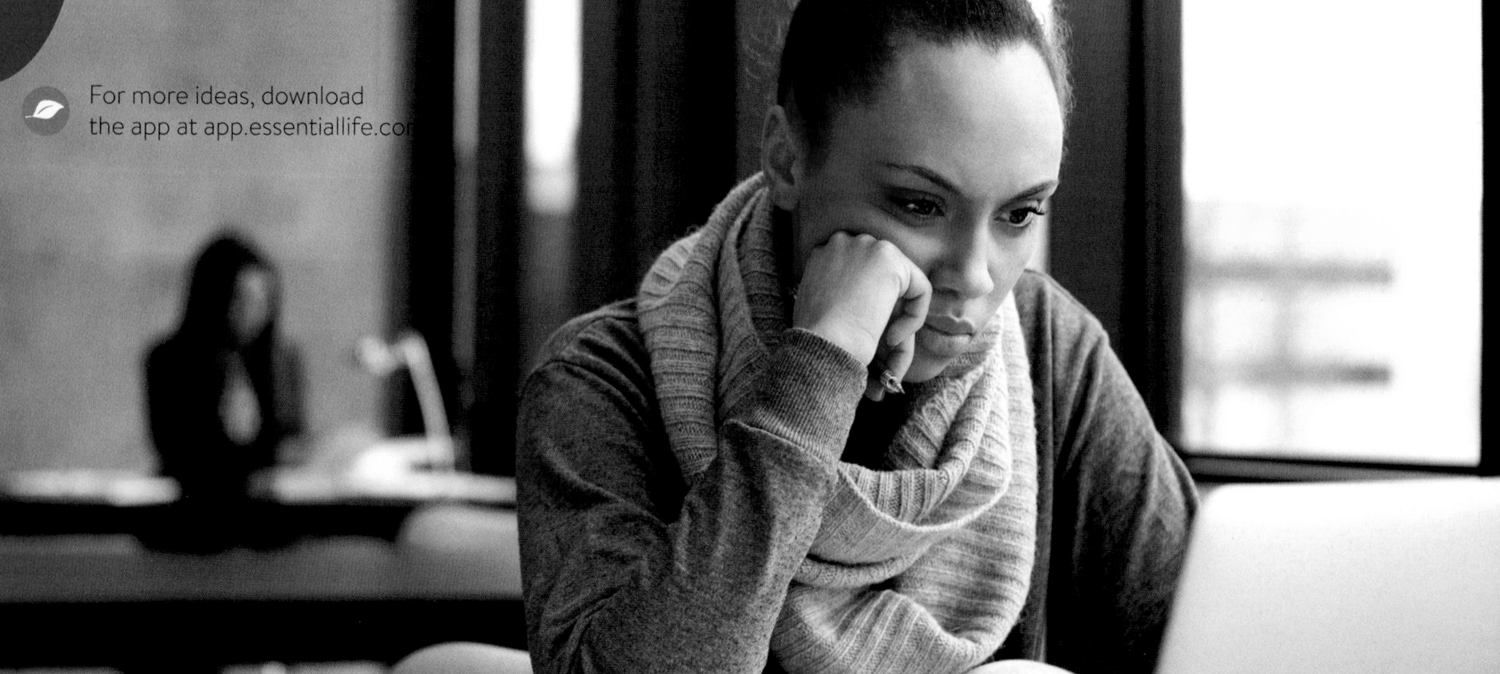

For more ideas, download the app at app.essentiallife.com

Conditions

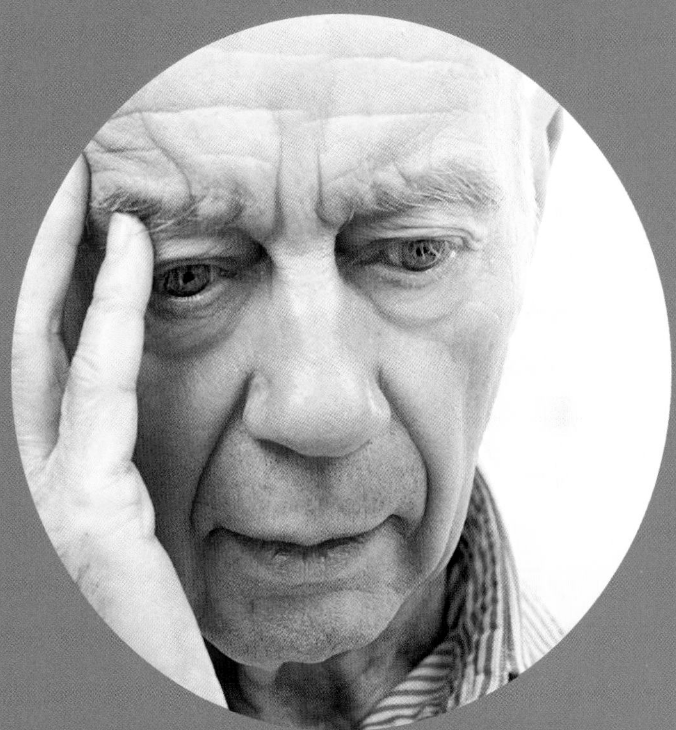

Alzheimer's* - black spruce, cilantro, clove, frankincense, lemon, melissa, oregano, sandalwood, thyme, turmeric, vetiver, Adaptiv®, Balance®, Console®, DDR Prime®, Forgive®, InTune®; see *Focus & Concentration*

Autism* - basil, bergamot, clary sage, frankincense, geranium, peppermint, rosemary, vetiver, Balance®, DDR Prime®, InTune®, Serenity®, Zendrocrine®

Balance/equilibrium - See "Dizziness" and "Vertigo" below

Blood-brain barrier - cedarwood, frankincense, ginger, myrrh, patchouli, sandalwood, Siberian fir, vetiver, ylang ylang, Balance®, DDR Prime®, InTune®, Whisper®

Brain - arborvitae, cedarwood, clove, eucalyptus, frankincense, ginger, patchouli, rosemary, sandalwood, thyme, turmeric vetiver, yarrow, Balance®, DDR Prime®, Motivate®, InTune®, On Guard®, Zendocrine®

Brain, aging - clove, copaiba, Douglas fir, frankincense, neroli, oregano, thyme, Adaptiv®, Alpha CRS®+, Balance®, Console®, InTune®, On Guard®, Peace®; see "Brain" above

Brain, aneurysm - bergamot, frankincense, helichrysum, myrrh, yarrow, DDR Prime®

Brain, blood flow - basil, black spruce, cedarwood, cypress, eucalyptus, ginger, lemongrass, oregano, patchouli, peppermint, rosemary, sandalwood, tangerine, thyme, AromaTouch®, DDR Prime®, Whisper®, Mito2Max®

Brain, injury - arborvitae, bergamot, frankincense, helichrysum, lemon, myrrh, peppermint, spikenard, Balance®, Console®, DDR Prime®, Forgive®

Brain, lesions - frankincense, peppermint, rosemary, sandalwood, Balance®, DDR Prime®

Central nervous system - bergamot, black pepper, myrrh, patchouli, rosemary, sandalwood

Chemical imbalance - cilantro, cinnamon, frankincense, geranium, melissa, patchouli, wild orange, Cheer®, DDR Prime®, Elevation™, InTune®, Zendocrine®

Coma - cedarwood, clove, frankincense, ginger, helichrysum, myrrh, sandalwood, spikenard, vetiver, Balance®, DDR Prime®, Motivate®

Concussion - bergamot, cedarwood, clove, cypress, frankincense, petitgrain, sandalwood, Balance®, InTune®

Dizziness - arborvitae, cedarwood, Douglas fir, frankincense, ginger, lavender, spearmint, rosemary, Balance®, Citrus Bliss®, Console®, DDR Prime®, InTune®, Zendocrine®

Free radicals, neutralization of - black spruce, cilantro, cinnamon, clove, coriander, ginger, lemongrass, rosemary, any citrus oil; see oils with "Antioxidant" properties

GABA, lack of - basil, black spruce, cedarwood, rosemary, thyme, ylang ylang, Balance®, Citrus Bliss®, InTune®, Motivate®, Serenity®; see *Endocrine (adrenals)*

Heat stroke - bergamot, black pepper, dill, lemon, peppermint, Deep Blue®, PastTense®, Zendocrine®

Heavy metal toxicity - cilantro; see *Detoxification*

Mental fatigue* - basil, bergamot, cardamom, frankincense, lavender, lemon, lemongrass, peppermint, pink pepper, ravensara, rose, rosemary, sandalwood, spearmint, white fir, ylang ylang, Adaptiv®, Breathe®, Citrus Bliss®, Console®, Forgive®, Motivate®, Peace®

Memory loss - arborvitae, black spruce, myrrh, Siberian fir, thyme

Memory, poor - black spruce, clove, Douglas fir, frankincense, ginger, rosemary, peppermint, sandalwood, Siberian fir, InTune®

Oxygen, lack of - cedarwood, cypress, eucalyptus, frankincense, ginger, patchouli, sandalwood, Siberian fir, vetiver; see oils with "Antioxidant" properties

Parasites - See oils under "Anti-parasitic"; see *Parasites*

Parkinson's - basil, bergamot, cedarwood, clary sage, clove, cypress, frankincense, geranium, helichrysum, jasmine, juniper berry, lemon, marjoram, melissa, patchouli, peppermint, Roman chamomile, rosemary, sandalwood, Siberian fir, thyme, vetiver, wild orange, Balance®, Cheer®, Console®, DDR Prime®, Serenity®, Zendocrine®; see *Addictions (oils to support dopamine levels)*

Seizures/convulsions, involuntary - basil, cardamom, cedarwood, celery seed, clary sage, Douglas fir, fennel, frankincense, geranium, lavender, myrrh, neroli, peppermint, petitgrain, rose (delay onset), sandalwood, spikenard, tangerine, Cheer®; see oils with "Anticonvulsant" properties

Senility/Dementia - frankincense, sandalwood; see oils with "Stimulant" properties

Sensory systems, closed/blocked - birch, wintergreen

Speech, slurred words/trouble speaking/difficulty understanding speech - arborvitae, patchouli, Whisper®, Zendocrine®

Stroke - basil, bergamot, cassia, cedarwood, celery seed, cypress, fennel, frankincense, helichrysum, turmeric, wintergreen, DDR Prime®, Purify, On Guard®; see oils with "Anti-inflammatory" and "Antioxidant" properties

Vertigo - cedarwood, frankincense, ginger, helichrysum, lavender, melissa, rosemary, Balance®, Citrus Bliss®, DDR Prime®, InTune®, Peace®

* See remedy on pg. 250

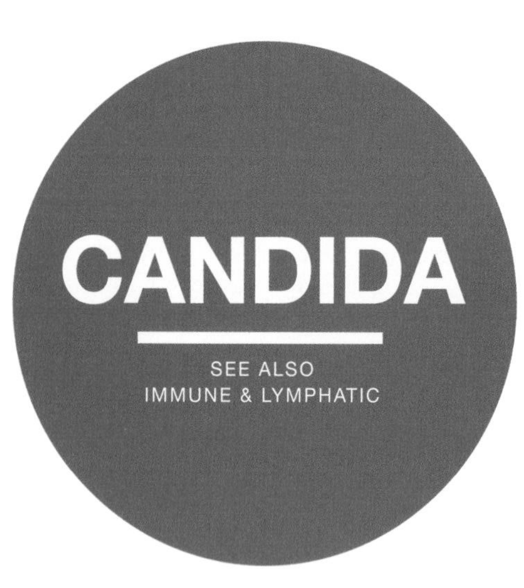

CANDIDA

SEE ALSO
IMMUNE & LYMPHATIC

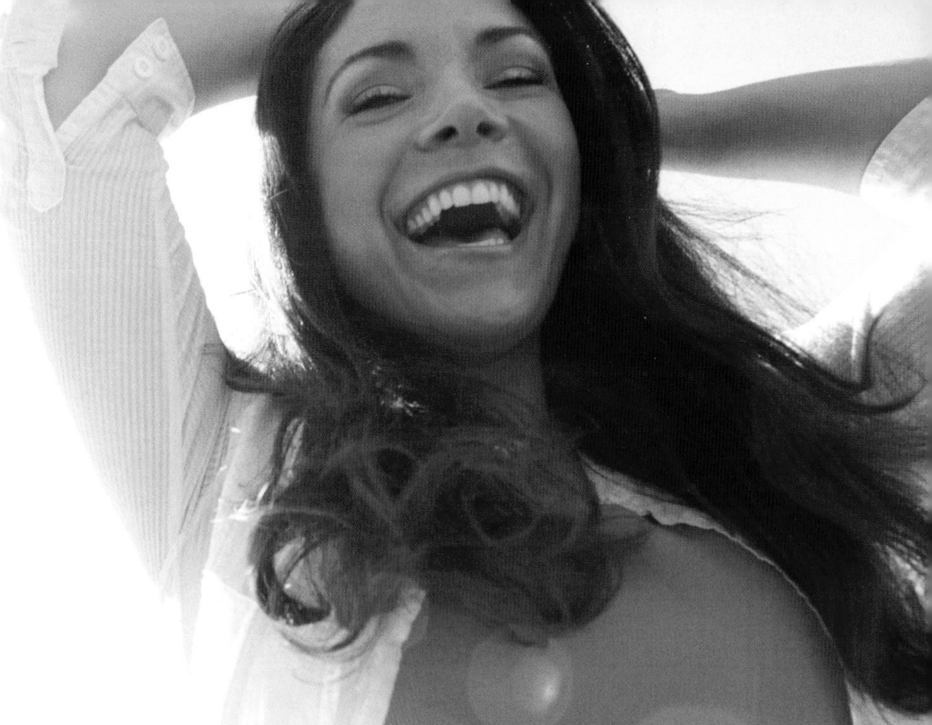

CANDIDA ALBICANS is a type of yeast that grows on the warm interior membranes of the body such as the digestive, respiratory, gastrointestinal, and female and uro-genital tracts. Candidiasis, the overgrowth of candida, can cause detrimental effects throughout the body and occurs when the balance between candida organisms and helpful bacteria in the gastrointestinal tract is disrupted. Candida mutates and grows rapidly in such situations and can cause frustrating and/or dangerous conditions in the body as it flourishes out of control.

Conditions that can result from candidiasis include headaches, autoimmune diseases, allergies, fatigue, digestive disorders (including IBS), yeast infections, infertility, skin and nail conditions/infections (such as toenail fungus or psoriasis), and strong sugar cravings or addiction.

Certain factors increase the risk of candidiasis. When these are acknowledged, awareness increases, and it becomes easier to remedy and avoid such situations:

- Candida and other microorganisms thrive when there is a lack of competing healthy organisms; a lack of friendly bacteria predisposes one to candidiasis.
- Diets high in sugar, high-fructose corn syrup, processed foods, yeast, or alcohol can depress the immune system and/or offset the delicate bacterial balance in the gut, allowing opportunity for candida to multiply.
- A single round of antibiotics is enough to kill both good and bad bacteria, leaving opportunity for harmful candida organisms to encroach. Prolonged or repeated use of antibiotics or other medications (e.g. contraceptive pills, steroidal drugs) increases risk dramatically.

Use of probiotic supplements is one of the most effective ways to restore gut flora when compromised.

- Poorly digested food particles, especially proteins, are known irritants that often stimulate mucus production as a defense or coping mechanism from the body; these affected areas can become feasting ground for microorganisms like candida albicans.

A diet rich in raw, live food as well supplementing with digestive enzymes assists in restoring proper digestion. Utilizing these enzymes as well as essential oils like a DigestZen® helps to clear both unwanted food particles and mucus accumulation.

- Stress can lead to candida in one of two ways: first, the body can respond to stressful situations by releasing cortisol, a hormone that elicits the same responses as does excess sugar. Second, stress can weaken the immune system and adrenal glands leading to exhaustion or lack of energy. Individuals in this weakened state typically don't eat well, further decreasing the body's ability to respond to pathogens such as candida.

Use of immune boosting essential oil blends such as a On Guard® as well as caring for adrenal gland health with proper rest, nutrition, and essential oils such as rosemary or basil helps preserve the body's defense system.

- One of candida albicans' toxic byproducts is estrogenic, and its presence "tricks" the body, influencing delicate hormonal states in both men and women. This toxic state undermines important functions such as fertility, negatively affects weight, and impacts prostate inflammation. This kind of activity can go undetected for years and is a culprit of many other health issues.

Use of essential oils such as clary sage and thyme combined supports the body's ability to correct exaggerated estrogen and deficient progesterone levels. Grapefruit, oregano, and thyme essential oils have demonstrated positive effects on healthy progesterone levels.

While it is important to work with expert medical professionals, especially when candidiasis has caused extensive system upset in the body, restoring the body's bio terrain to a balanced state can be done very effectively with natural remedies. Essential oils help clear toxins and harmful microorganisms gently and effectively from the gastrointestinal tract, address improved insulin response, and support digestion. Probiotics help restore balance and immune support.

TOP SOLUTIONS

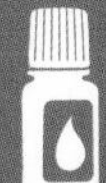

SINGLE OILS

Melaleuca - eliminates candida yeast and prevents mutation (pg. 132)

Oregano - eliminates and prevents candida yeast and fungus (pg. 138)

Pink Pepper - (pg. 144)

Thyme - eliminates and prevents candida yeast and fungus (pg. 157)

Turmeric - (pg. 158)

By Related Properties

For more, See Oil Properties on pages 477 - 481

Anti-carcinogenic - arborvitae, clove, frankincense, lemongrass, myrrh, tangerine, turmeric, wild orange, yarrow

Antifungal - arborvitae, blue tansy, cardamom, cassia, cedarwood, cilantro, cinnamon, clary sage, clove, copaiba, coriander, ginger, helichrysum, lemongrass, marjoram, melaleuca, melissa, myrrh, oregano, patchouli, pink pepper, ravensara, rosemary, Siberian fir, spearmint, tangerine, thyme, turmeric, yarrow

Antimicrobial - arborvitae, blue tansy, cassia, cilantro, cinnamon, copaiba, dill, fennel, lemongrass, litsea, manuka, myrrh, neroli, oregano, Siberian fir, spearmint;

Antimutagenic - ginger, lavender, lemongrass, turmeric

Antioxidant - basil, cassia, cinnamon, clove, copaiba, coriander, juniper berry, lemongrass, melaleuca, neroli, tangerine, thyme, turmeric

Vermifuge - arborvitae, black pepper, fennel, frankincense, geranium, lavender, lemon, Roman chamomile, turmeric

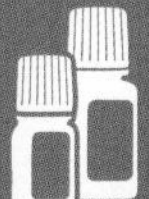

BLENDS

DDR Prime® - restores health of cells (pg. 184)

Zendocrine® - detoxifies and eliminates free radicals (pg. 206)

On Guard® - helps eliminate candida/fungus (pg. 194)

HD Clear® - cleanses skin (pg. 189)

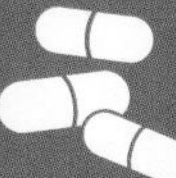

SUPPLEMENTS

PB Assist®+(pg. 216), Zendrocrine® Complex, xEO Mega, **TerraZyme® (pg. 219)**, MicroPlex VMz supplement, **GX Assist® (pg. 213)**

Related Ailments: Athlete's foot, Candidiasis, Fungal Skin Infection, Fungus, Yeast

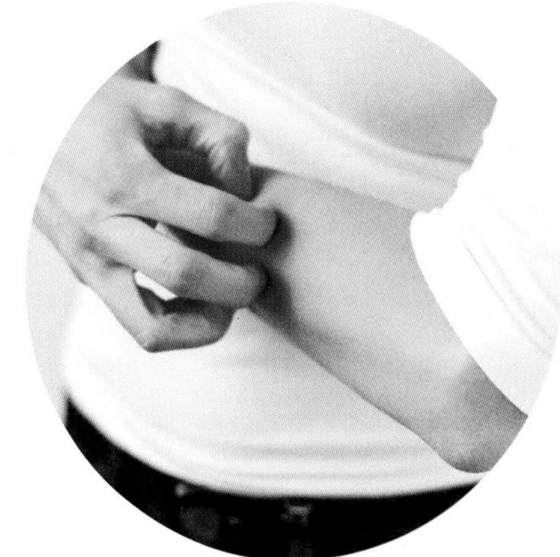

Conditions

Athlete's foot - arborvitae, cardamom, clove, copaiba, lavender, lemon eucalyptus, lemongrass, melaleuca, myrrh, neroli, oregano, AromaTouch®; see "Antifungal" property

Autoimmune disease - See *Autoimmune*

Brain fog - See *Focus & Concentration*

Concentration, poor - See *Focus & Concentration*

Cravings, sugar/refined carbohydrate - See *Weight*

Fatigue - See *Energy & Vitality*

Focus, lack of - See *Focus & Concentration*

Intestinal Flora, restore - Turmeric

Memory, poor - See *Focus & Concentration*

Moodiness - depression/irritability - See *Mood & Behavior*

Severe seasonal allergies - See *Allergies*

Sinus infection, chronic - arborvitae, cardamom, melissa, myrrh, oregano, rosemary, Siberian fir (diluted) ; consider a chronic fungal condition; see "Antifungal" property

Skin or nail infection - see *Integumentary*

Skin, eczema/psoriasis* - arborvitae, bergamot, birch, blue tansy, cedarwood, copaiba, geranium, helichrysum, juniper berry, melissa, myrrh, neroli, patchouli, peppermint, Roman chamomile, rosemary, Siberian fir, spearmint, thyme, wintergreen, yarrow

Thrush - arborvitae, bergamot, clary sage, clove (diluted), dill, fennel, lavender, lemon, melaleuca, oregano (diluted), turmeric, wild orange, On Guard® (diluted), Slim & Sassy®

Urinary infection/fungal - basil, blue tansy, cypress, eucalyptus, juniper berry, lemon, lemongrass, melaleuca, pink pepper, Siberian fir, thyme, Forgive®, On Guard®, Purify, Zendocrine®; consider a chronic fungal condition; see "Antifungal" property

Vagina, mild discharge - bergamot, spikenard

Vaginal inflammation/infection* - cinnamon (internal or diluted on bottoms of feet only), spearmint, spikenard, On Guard® (internal or diluted on bottoms of feet only), Whisper®; see *Women's Health*

Vaginal itching* - bergamot, frankincense, melaleuca, neroli, spikenard, Whisper®; see *Women's Health*

Vaginal thrush* - blue tansy, frankincense (topical, internal), melaleuca (topical - diluted, internal), oregano (internal or diluted on bottoms of feet only), spikenard, Whisper®; see *Women's Health*

Weak immune system - cinnamon, Siberian fir, On Guard®; see *Immune & Lymphatic*

Weakness, chronic - copaiba, frankincense, rosemary, Motivate®, On Guard®; see *Energy & Vitality*

** See remedy on pg. 254*

Remedies

CANDIDA SIMPLE TREATMENT
Combine basil and melaleuca and massage onto bottoms of feet.

CANDIDA MONTHLY PROTOCOL
- Step 1: 1 GI cleansing softgel three times per day with meals for ten days.
- Step 2: 1 capsule PB Assist®+each meal daily for at least next ten days.
- Step 3: Continue PB Assist®+if desired; rest for ten days.
- Step 4: Repeat steps one and two monthly as needed.
- For the entire 30 days consume:
  - 1-3 capsules TerraZyme® with meals and/or on an empty stomach
  - 1-2 Zendrocrine® Complex with AM and PM meals
  - 2 drops Zendocrine® in capsule two times per day with meals
  - 2 drops lemon three times per day in a capsule or in drinking water

CANDIDA QUARTERLY MAINTENANCE CLEANSE
- Step One: Place 5 drops each melaleuca, lemon, and choose from lemongrass, thyme or oregano in a capsule; take two capsules per day for two weeks. If oregano was utilized, after two weeks of usage, take a break for two weeks and replace in capsule with thyme or lemongrass.
- Step Two: After two weeks of usage, reduce consumption to one capsule of above combination per day for two weeks.
- Step Three: Take 2-4 PB Assist®+per day for at least one week.
- Step Four: Repeat cleanse every three months or more frequently as needed.

CANDIDA SUPPOSITORY
1 drop melaleuca
1 drop oregano
1 drop thyme
Combine essential oil(s) with virgin coconut oil and roll into the shape of a large pill. Refrigerate or freeze until solid; insert into the vagina.

CANDIDA FACIAL & SKIN OIL
3 drops clary sage
2 drops frankincense
2 drops geranium
2 drops myrrh
1 drop patchouli
Combine oils in 30ml glass bottle; fill remainder of bottle with fractionated coconut oil. Apply to affected areas to soothe and relieve irritated skin until symptoms subside.

CANDIDA SKIN RELIEF
Create a paste with ½ cup of aluminum-free baking soda and a few tablespoons of fractionated coconut oil. Then add the following essential oils:
4 drops lavender
3 drops melaleuca
3 drops rosemary
Use paste in shower as cleanser and exfoliator. Apply all over body; gently scrub for a few minutes. Repeat at least twice a week to kill the candida living on the skin.

CANDIDA RELIEF TOPICAL BLEND
9 drops cassia
8 drops clove
6 drops cinnamon
4 drops oregano
Blend oils into a 10ml roller bottle; fill remainder with carrier oil. Use topically as needed.

CANDIDA RELIEF INTERNAL BLEND
2 drops cinnamon
2 drops clove
Place oil drops in an empty capsule; ingest three times per day.

ECZEMA AND PSORIASIS
4 drops bergamot
3 drops Roman chamomile
3 drops geranium
2 drops turmeric
2 drops rosemary
1-2 teaspoons carrier oil
Apply to skin twice per day; massage in as tolerated. Additionally, use TerraZyme®.

VAGINAL THRUSH/YEAST TREATMENT
Apply a few drops of frankincense, myrrh, and/or melaleuca to tip of tampon. Insert.

CANDIDA RASH
12 drops white fir
6 drops geranium
6 drops patchouli
6 drops thyme
5 drops frankincense
Blend oils; add carrier oil. Store in a 10ml glass bottle and distribute from there. Apply to areas where candida rash is expressing. Consider some kind of candida detox.

CANDIDA TAMPON VAGINAL SUPPOSITORY
2 tablespoons of carrier oil (fractionated coconut oil or extra-virgin olive oil)
10 drops clove OR 9 drops lemongrass for a more intense treatment.
OR 15 drops frankincense, melaleuca or myrrh for a more mild treatment.
Dip tampon in oil mixture about halfway up from the insertion tip. Squeeze out excess. Insert. Wear a panty liner. Up to four fresh applications daily are appropriate. Alternate oils: four days of one, then four days of the other. This keeps pathogens from adapting. With the stronger oils it may sting intensely, especially during initial treatments, for about 15 minutes. Quantity of essential oil used can be reduced so as to reduce intensity. Response should calm over time. Use a probiotic simultaneously. Replace lid. Store for future use. Repeat nightly.

CANDIDA BOMB
3 drops cassia
2 drops oregano
Place oils in a capsule; take with meals twice a day for up to ten days. Add 1 drop of melissa or 4 drops of On Guard® as needed for more chronic cases where conditions have lasted for long periods of time or are stubborn to resolve.

CANDIDA DOUCHE
1 drop lavender
1 drop melaleuca
1 teaspoon vinegar
1 cup warm water
Combine into squeeze bottle. Douche daily for three days a week.

Candida program

Daily Program to support a balanced system and optimal capacity to experience a successful detox program

STEP ONE

Take daily:

- **MicroPlex VMz supplement** (basic core nutrition for body's daily needs)
- **PB Assist®+**- use for the first two weeks (to populate the gut with friendly bacteria)
- **TerraZyme®** (digestion of food and elimination of waste)
- **XEO Mega** (vital essential fatty acids)
- **Lemon essential oil in drinking water** (to balance and maintain healthy pH; antioxidant and detox support)
- **Optional as needed:** DigestZen® (take if experiencing unresolved digestive upset)

STEP TWO

Add detox supplement - day 14: (to support optimal function and detoxification of eliminative pathways). Length of use of detoxification supplements can vary from one person to another. Some individuals may benefit from brief use, such as two weeks; others will require longer usage, such as 90 days, to obtain desired long-term results.

- **Zendrocrine® Complex** (add to program sooner if bowels tend to be sluggish and TerraZyme® are inadequate to resolve)
- **Zendocrine® softgels**

STEP THREE

Choose one: (core antifungal supplement) - day 14 (for 7-10 days)

- DDR Prime® Softgels
- GX Assist®

STEP FOUR

Choose optional additional antifungal target support - day 21 or later

Consider an additional antifungal oil or two to target a specific area(s) of concern. This support can be added at week three or later as determined by tolerance and desired results. Although specific oils are sited for specific areas or organs of the body, all oils listed in this section are antifungal and assist the body in restoring and balancing the bio terrain. It is important for each individual to choose whatever oil feel is best for them. Intuition is a tremendous asset in decision making.

- **Adrenals** - rosemary, ginger, geranium, Zendocrine®
- **Brain** - cedarwood, clary sage, frankincense, rosemary, sandalwood
- **Heavy Metals** - cilantro, frankincense, Purify (topical only), Zendocrine®
- **Intestinal** - marjoram, melaleuca, oregano, thyme, Zendocrine®, On Guard®
- **Liver** - helichrysum, lemon, lemongrass, geranium, Zendocrine®
- **Mouth** - bergamot, lavender, melaleuca, oregano, Slim & Sassy®, On Guard®
- **Mucous membrane** (e.g. stomach, intestines, uro-genital) - melaleuca, lemon, fennel
- **Pancreas** - cassia, cinnamon, coriander, dill, Slim & Sassy®
- **Reproductive** - female/infertility - clary sage, fennel, geranium, oregano, rose, thyme, frankincense, rosemary
- **Reproductive** - male/infertility/prostate - clary sage, cypress, frankincense, geranium, thyme, ginger
- **Respiratory** - arborvitae, cardamom, myrrh, oregano, rosemary, melissa, eucalyptus
- **Skin** (e.g. eczema, psoriasis) - arborvitae, birch, bergamot, cedarwood, geranium, helichrysum, juniper berry, lavender, melissa, myrrh, oregano, patchouli, peppermint, Roman chamomile, rosemary, spearmint, thyme, wintergreen
- **Thyroid** - clove, lemongrass, myrrh, rosemary, frankincense, DDR Prime®, On Guard®
- **Urinary** - cypress, eucalyptus, juniper berry, lemon, lemongrass, basil, cinnamon, Purify, Zendocrine®
- **Vaginal** - cinnamon, thyme, melaleuca, basil, marjoram, spearmint
- **Weight, excessive** - oregano, ginger, grapefruit, Slim & Sassy®

STEP FIVE

Probiotic

After using detoxing supplements for the length of time that is appropriate, a probiotic will further assist in populating the gut with healthy bacteria.

CANDIDA

BONUS option: Choose oils by emotional state
Another method of selecting target oils is to search for oils that most closely relate to both the physical and emotional states that are being experienced and choose from there. There are resources available to discover what oils are related to what emotions. Below are a few suggestions that relate candida specifically.

Oils that support empowerment such as ginger are excellent for candida overgrowth. The body is being invaded and overpowered by microorganisms and fungi, promoting an emotional state of feeling powerless along with other states such as anger, blame, defensiveness, feeling out of control, resentment, unprotected.

The following oils may address candida-related emotions:

For more Candida ideas, downlaod the app at app.essentiallife.com

Bitterness, resentment	thyme, geranium
Blame/victim mentality/defensive	melaleuca
Deprived	myrrh
Used, betrayed	coriander, rose
Feeling out of control/invaded	oregano
Parasitical/co-dependent relationships	clove
Powerless/unprotected	cassia/cinnamon, frankincense, turmeric

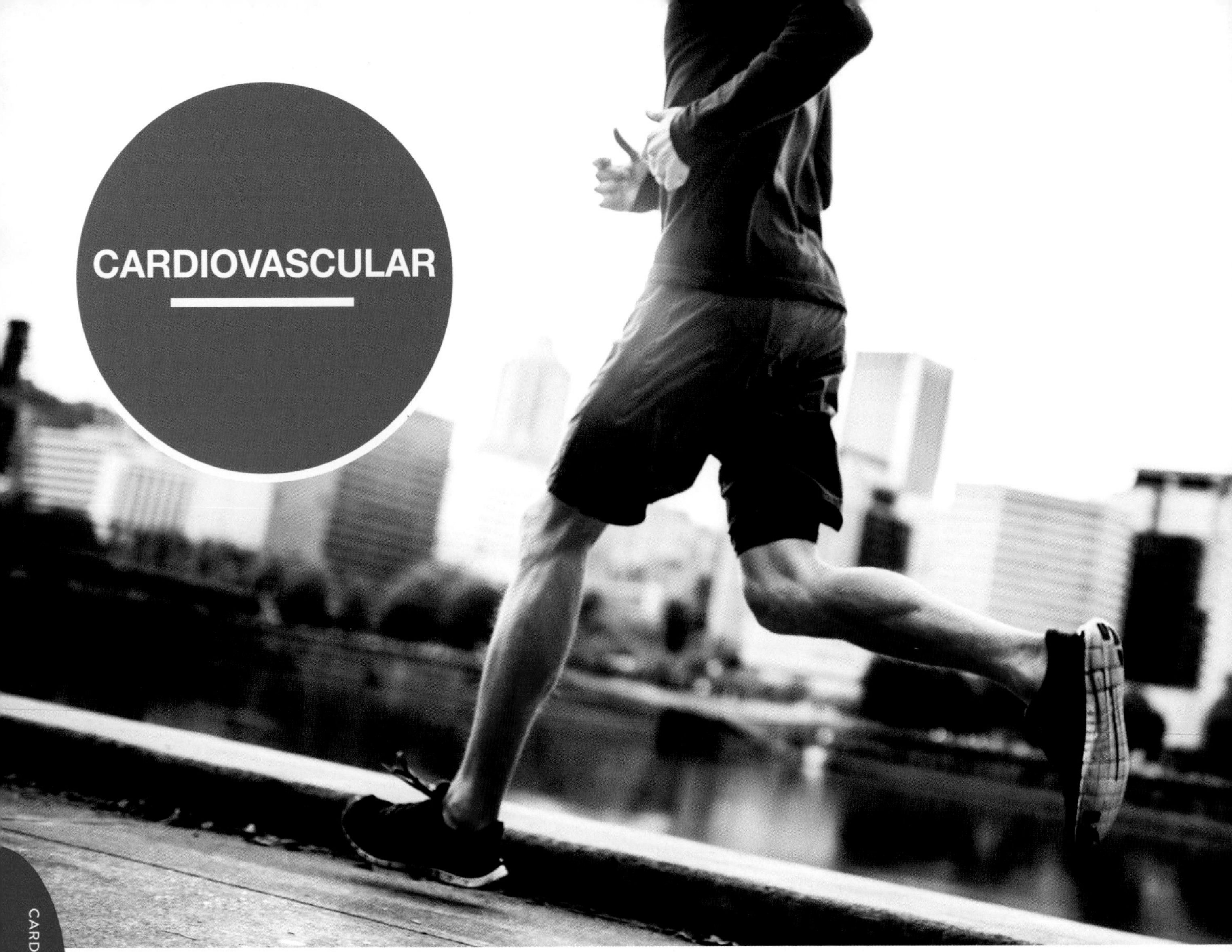

THE HEART and circulatory system make up the cardiovascular system. The heart works as a pump that pushes blood to the organs, tissues, and cells of the body. Blood delivers oxygen and nutrients to every cell and removes carbon dioxide and waste products made by those cells. Blood is carried from the heart to the rest of the body through a complex network of arteries, arterioles, and capillaries. Blood is returned to the heart through venules and veins. Many of vessels are smaller than a hair and only allow one blood cell at a time to circulate. If all the vessels of this network were laid end to end, they would extend for about 60,000 miles (more than 96,500 kilometers), which is far enough to circle the planet more than twice.

In pulmonary circulation, the roles are reversed. The pulmonary artery brings oxygen-poor blood into the lungs, and the pulmonary vein sends oxygen-rich blood back to the heart.

The oxygen and nutrient-rich blood that bring life and health to all the cells and tissues of the body, also transport essential oils. When applied topically, essential oils are absorbed through the skin. They move through the circulatory system within thirty seconds, and are then able to permeate cells and tissues throughout the body for targeted support within fourteen to twenty minutes.

Cardiovascular diseases comprise the leading cause of death globally and can refer to any disease involving the heart or blood vessels. The most common cardiovascular disease is related to arteriosclerosis/atherosclerosis, a process by which plaque causes the blood vessels to harden, stiffen, suffer a loss of elasticity, and narrow. The narrower vessels make blood flow more difficult, and blood clots can more easily block blood flow and cause serious conditions, including death. The good news is that 90% of cardiovascular disease is preventable with good lifestyle choices, including adequate rest, exercise, and nutrition. Risk factors are vast and include stress, excessive use of alcohol or caffeine, high blood pressure, smoking, diabetes, poor diet, obesity, and certain medications.

Any serious issue involving the cardiovascular system should immediately be seen by a qualified medical professional. It should be noted that natural solutions can support heart health, both preventatively and restoratively. Using certain essential oils has been shown to reduce blood pressure and heart rate. As heart disease, one of the leading causes of death, is almost entirely preventable, solutions offered with essential oils and the shifting from an ambulance mentality to a prevention mindset is most prudent.

TOP SOLUTIONS

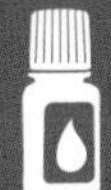

SINGLE OILS

Cypress - promotes proper circulation and blood flow throughout body (pg. 103)

Ylang ylang - balances heart rate and reduces high blood pressure (pg. 165)

Marjoram - supports the heart muscle (pg. 131)

Helichrysum, yarrow - repairs damaged blood vessels; stops bleeding; (pgs. 117 & 164)

Black pepper - warms and tones blood vessels; decongests circulatory/lymphatic (pg. 83)

Geranium - supports heart, blood, and blood vessel integrity (pg. 112)

By Related Properties

For more, See Oil Properties on pages 477 - 481

Anticoagulant - clary sage, helichrysum, lavender
Antihemorrhagic - geranium, helichrysum, lavender, lemon, lemongrass, melaleuca, myrrh, oregano, patchouli, rosemary, sandalwood, spearmint, thyme, yarrow
Anti-inflammatory - arborvitae, basil, bergamot, black pepper, blue tansy, cinnamon, clary sage, copaiba, coriander, cypress, dill, eucalyptus, frankincense, geranium, helichrysum, lavender, lemongrass, lime, litsea, manuka, melissa, neroli, patchouli, peppermint, Siberian fir, spikenard, tangerine, turmeric, wintergreen, yarrow
Antitoxic - bergamot, black pepper, cinnamon, coriander, fennel, geranium, grapefruit, juniper berry, lavender, lemon, lemongrass, patchouli, thyme
Calming - basil, blue tansy, celery seed, clary sage, copaiba, coriander, frankincense, jasmine, lavender, litsea, magnolia, oregano, patchouli, Roman chamomile, sandalwood, tangerine, vetiver, yarrow
Cardiotonic - cassia, copiaba, cypress, ginger, lavender, litsea, marjoram, pink pepper, tangerine, turmeric, yarrow
Decongestant - basil, black pepper, cardamom, copaiba, cypress, eucalyptus, ginger, grapefruit, lemon, lemongrass, litsea, melaleuca, patchouli, pink pepper, tangerine, turmeric, yarrow
Detoxifier - arborvitae, cassia, celery seed, cilantro, cypress, geranium, juniper berry, lemon, lime, litsea, patchouli, tangerine, yarrow
Hypertensive - celery seed, melissa, rosemary, Siberian fir, thyme
Hypotensive - blue tansy, clary sage, copaiba, dill, eucalyptus, lavender, lemon, litsea, manuka, marjoram, neroli, white fir, yarrow, ylang ylang
Regenerative - basil, cedarwood, clove, frankincense, geranium, helichrysum, jasmine, lavender, lemongrass, manuka, melaleuca, myrrh, neroli, patchouli, wild orange, yarrow
Relaxing - basil, blue tansy, cypress, geranium, lavender, litsea, manuka, marjoram, neroli, Roman chamomile, ylang ylang
Rubefacient - Bergamot, Birch, Black pepper, Black spruce, Eucalyptus, Ginger, Green mandarin, Helichrysum, Juniper berry, Lavender, Lemon, Lemon eucalyptus, Magnolia, Pink pepper, Red mandarin, Rosemary, Siberian fir, Thyme, Vetiver, White fir
Tonic - basil, bergamot, cypress, fennel, frankincense, geranium, lavender, lemon, lemongrass, melissa, neroli, patchouli, rose, sandalwood, Siberian fir, tangerine, thyme, vetiver, wild orange, yarrow
Vasoconstrictor - cypress, helichrysum, peppermint, Siberian fir, white fir, ylang ylang
Vasodilator - blue tansy, copaiba, lemongrass, litsea, manuka, marjoram, neroli, rosemary, thyme
Warming - birch, black pepper, cassia, cinnamon, clary sage, clove, eucalyptus, ginger, lemongrass, marjoram, neroli, oregano, peppermint, pink pepper, thyme, turmeric, wintergreen

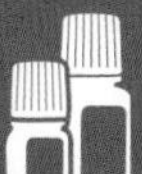

BLENDS

Purify - decongests circulatory/lymphatic congestion (pg. 198)

Passion® - promotes healthy blood flow (pg. 195)

AromaTouch® - stimulates circulation and blood flow, especially to extremities (pg. 169)

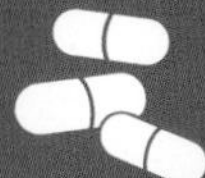

SUPPLEMENTS

Alpha CRS®+ (pg. 209), Mito2Max® (pg. 214), DDR Prime® Softgels, Phytoestrogen Complex, Deep Blue Polyphenol Complex, PB Assist®+, MicroPlex VMz supplement

USAGE TIPS: For best methods of use for cardiovascular and circulatory support consider:

- **Topical:** Apply oils directly to chest, bottoms of feet, down spine, and/or on specific areas of concern for direct affect as needed.
- **Aromatic:** Diffuse 5-10 drops of oils of choice, inhale from product bottle or self-made blend, apply a few drops to clothing, or any other method that supports inhalation for oils especially for supporting reducing stress
- **Internal:** Place 1-5 drops in water to drink, take drops in capsule, or place drop(s) under tongue to affect internal activities that impact circulation and heart activity.

Related Ailments: Anemia (iron deficiency), Aneurysm, Angina, Arrhythmia, Arteriosclerosis, Atherosclerosis, Balance Problems, Bleeding, Blood Clot, Body Temperature issues, Broken Capillaries, Broken Heart Syndrome [Mood & Behavior], Bruise [Integumentary], Cardiomyopathy, Cardiovascular Disease, Cholesterol, Circulation (poor), Cold [Endocrine (Thyroid)], Cold Hands/Feet/Nose, Congenital Heart Disease, Deep Vein Thrombosis (blood clot in vein), Dizziness, Edema (water retention), Fainting [First Aid], Fibrillation (atrial), Fibrillation (ventricular), Gangrene [Immune & Lymphatic], Hardening of Arteries, Hematoma, Hemophilia, Hemorrhage, Hemorrhoids, Hypertension (high blood pressure), Hypotension (low blood pressure), Long QT Syndrome, Marfan Syndrome (connective tissue disorder), Mitral Valve Prolapse, Palpitations, Pericardial Disease, Phlebitis (inflammation of the vein), Pulmonary Embolism, Raynaud's Disease, Renal Artery Stenosis, Restless Leg, Syndrome, Sickle Cell, Tachycardia, Thrombosis, Varicose Veins [Integumentary], Vertigo

Conditions

Anemia (iron deficiency)* - basil, cinnamon, geranium, helichrysum, lemon, rosemary, DDR Prime®, OnGuard®, Zendocrine®, MicroPlex VMz
Aneurysm* - cypress, frankincense, helichrysum, marjoram, DDR Prime®
Bleeding/hemorrhaging - arborvitae, cypress, frankincense, geranium, helichrysum, lavender, myrrh, yarrow, ylang ylang, DDR Prime®, Purify, Zendocrine®
Blood clot* - clary sage, clove, coriander, fennel, frankincense, helichrysum, marjoram, melaleuca, myrrh, patchouli, peppermint, thyme, wintergreen, AromaTouch®, DDR Prime®, Deep Blue®, Motivate®, Purify
- **Pain** - ylang ylang, AromaTouch®, Deep Blue®
- **Significant swelling** - clary sage, DDR Prime®, OnGuard®, Purify
- **Redness** - melaleuca, melissa, ylang ylang, OnGuard®, Zendocrine®
- **Warmth** - fennel, melissa, ylang ylang, AromaTouch®, PastTense®, Whisper®, Zendocrine®

Blood, dirty/toxic - basil, cassia, clove, frankincense, geranium, grapefruit, helichrysum, lime, Roman chamomile, turmeric, white fir, DDR Prime®, Zendocrine®
Blood flow, blocked* - celery seed, cypress, fennel, lavender (arteries), lemon (arteries), ylang ylang, AromaTouch®, DDR Prime®, Motivate®, Purify, Zendocrine®, Mito2Max®
Blood pressure, high (hypertension)* - birch, blue tansy, celery seed, copaiba, clove, cypress, dill, eucalyptus, lavender, lemon, lime, marjoram, melissa, neroli, patchouli, Roman chamomile, spearmint, thyme, wintergreen, ylang ylang, Breathe®, Cheer®, Citrus Bliss®
Blood pressure, low (hypotension) - basil, cardamom, helichrysum, lime, rosemary, Siberian fir, thyme, DDR Prime®, Purify, Zendocrine®
Blood vessels, blocked/obstructed - arborvitae, cinnamon, cypress, lemongrass, marjoram, Motivate®, OnGuard®
Blood vessels /capillaries, broken - cypress, frankincense, geranium, helichrysum, lavender, lemon, lime, Zendocrine®
Blood vessel integrity, lack of - black pepper, helichrysum, lemongrass, marjoram, Zendocrine®
Breathing problems - See *Respiratory*
Bruising - arborvitae, blue tansy, copaiba, cypress, fennel, geranium, helichrysum, lavender, neroli, oregano, Roman chamomile, white fir, ylang ylang, DDR Prime®, Purify, Zendocrine®
Chest pain/pressure (angina) - basil, cinnamon, ginger, marjoram, rosemary, thyme, wild orange (for false angina), DDR Prime®, OnGuard®, Purify; see *Stress*
Cholesterol/triglycerides, elevated or imbalanced* - cinnamon, coriander, cypress, green mandarin, helichrysum, juniper berry, lemon, lemongrass, marjoram, pink pepper, rosemary, turmeric, thyme, Cheer®, Slim & Sassy®
Circulation, poor/cold extremities* - arborvitae, basil, black pepper, black spruce, cassia, cedarwood, cinnamon, citronella, clove, cypress, eucalyptus, geranium, ginger, lemon eucalyptus, neroli, peppermint, pink pepper, rose, rosemary, Siberian fir, turmeric, wintergreen, yarrow, AromaTouch®, Cheer®, Console®, DDR Prime®, Motivate®, OnGuard®, Passion®, Peace®, Whisper®, Mito2Max®
Circulatory system tonic* - basil, cypress, fennel, lemon, melaleuca, rosemary, turmeric, wild orange, AromaTouch®, Deep Blue®, Forgive®, Immortelle, PastTense®
Cold, need localized warming - birch, black pepper, cinnamon, eucalyptus, pink pepper, turmeric, AromaTouch®
Cold, need overall or systemic warming - black pepper, birch, cassia, cinnamon, cypress, eucalyptus, ginger, lemongrass, pink pepper, turmeric, wintergreen, AromaTouch®, Forgive®, Passion®
Confusion or trouble walking - arborvitae, Douglas fir, eucalyptus, frankincense, myrrh, peppermint, rosemary, wild orange, Motivate®, InTune®, Purify; see *Brain*
Dizziness/loss of balance/unsteady/lightheaded - black pepper, celery seed, Douglas fir, grapefruit, marjoram, melaleuca, oregano, patchouli, rosemary, tangerine, ylang ylang, Breathe®, DDR Prime®, On Guard®, PastTense®, Whisper®, Zendocrine®
Edema (water retention, swelling in hands/ankles/feet) - basil, blue tansy, celery seed, cypress, ginger, green mandarin, juniper berry, lemon, lemongrass, rosemary, spikenard, Siberian fir, tangerine, PastTense®; see *Urinary, Detoxification*
Fainting/near fainting - basil, bergamot, cinnamon, cypress, frankincense, lavender, patchouli, peppermint, rosemary, sandalwood, wintergreen, Citrus Bliss®, Motivate®
Fibrillation/atrial fibrillation - arborvitae, black pepper, Douglas fir, ginger, lime, marjoram, ylang ylang, AromaTouch®, Breathe®, DDR Prime®, Purify
Gangrene - arborvitae, cinnamon, cypress, geranium, melaleuca, melissa, myrrh, patchouli, AromaTouch®, DDR Prime®, OnGuard®, Slim & Sassy®, Zendocrine®
Hardening of the arteries (arteriosclerosis) - arborvitae, basil, black pepper, cardamom, cinnamon, cypress, juniper berry, lavender, lemongrass, marjoram, rosemary, sandalwood, wild orange, InTune®, OnGuard®, Forgive®, Slim & Sassy®
Heart - blue tansy, copaiba, cinnamon, frankincense, geranium, lime, patchouli, sandalwood, ylang ylang, AromaTouch®, Purify, Zendocrine®
Heart attack, prevention - cassia
Heart, broken - geranium, lime, rose, ylang ylang, comfort blend
Heart infection - oregano; see *Immune & Lymphatic*
Heart murmur - Douglas fir, patchouli, peppermint, thyme, white fir, AromaTouch®, Purify, Whisper®
Heart muscle, thickening (cardiomyopathy) - basil, marjoram, rose, rosemary, ylang ylang, Purify
Heart muscle, lack of tone - cassia, helichrysum, rose, Forgive®
Heart, weak - cinnamon, coriander, ginger, rosemary, AromaTouch®
Heartbeat, irregular (arrhythmia) - basil, cedarwood, cinnamon, citronella, lavender, lemon, melissa, rosemary, ylang ylang, Console®, DDR Prime®, Peace®, OnGuard®
Heartbeat, rapid/racing (tachycardia) - arborvitae, blue tansy, cardamom, cedarwood, lavender, melissa, neroli, oregano, rosemary, wild orange, ylang ylang, Serenity®, Zendocrine®
Heartbeat, slow (bradycardia) - Douglas fir, patchouli, AromaTouch®, Motivate®, Zendocrine®
Hematoma - basil, cypress, frankincense, geranium, helichrysum, marjoram, myrrh, lemongrass, AromaTouch®, Forgive®, Immortelle
Hemorrhoids* - cypress, frankincense, geranium, helichrysum, juniper berry, myrrh, patchouli, Roman chamomile, rosemary, Siberian fir, yarrow, DigestZen®, Forgive®, Zendocrine®

CARDIOVASCULAR

* See remedy on pg. 260

Numbness/tingling/paralysis in arm, face, leg - arborvitae, basil, cardamom, cypress, frankincense, geranium, ginger, patchouli, peppermint, AromaTouch®, DDR Prime®, PastTense®, Purify, Zendocrine®
Palpitations - blue tansy, cardamom, cedarwood, cinnamon, frankincense, lavender, neroli, oregano, petitgrain, rose, rosemary, thyme, ylang ylang, AromaTouch®, On Guard®, Peace®, Serenity®, Zendocrine®
Phlebitis - basil, cypress, helichrysum, lavender, lemon, lemongrass, marjoram, Zendocrine®
Plaque, clogged arteries (atherosclerosis) - basil, clove, copaiba, ginger, lemon, lemongrass, marjoram, patchouli, rosemary, thyme, wintergreen, AromaTouch®, DDR Prime®, Motivate®, On Guard®, Purify, Zendocrine®
Prolapsed mitral valve - marjoram, myrrh, patchouli, AromaTouch®, PastTense®
Red blood cells, poor production - lemon
Redness on tip of nose - patchouli, ylang ylang, TerraShield®
Redness on tip of tongue - arborvitae, ylang ylang, Purify, Whisper®
Restless leg syndrome - arborvitae, basil, cardamom, cypress, wintergreen, AromaTouch®, Deep Blue®, PastTense®; see *Sleep*
Ringing in ears (see tinnitus) - arborvitae, cypress, TerraShield®, Zendocrine®,
Stenosis (vessel narrowing) - arborvitae, lemon, oregano, patchouli, rosemary, DDR Prime®, Purify, Zendocrine®
Stroke - See *Brain*
Skin, cold/clammy/cold sweats - patchouli, ylang ylang, AromaTouch®
Skin, color changes to skin on face, feet, hands (bluish cyanosis, grayish, pale/white) - cypress, Douglas fir, lemon, patchouli, ylang ylang, Purify
Thrombosis, deep vein:
· **narrowing (stenosis)** - patchouli, Zendocrine®
· **leaking (regurgitation/insufficiency)** - grapefruit, ylang ylang, On Guard®
· **improper closing (prolapse)** - melissa, Zendocrine®
Tongue, inflamed/red/sore - See *Heart*
Ulcers, leg/varicose - clove, cypress, frankincense, geranium, helichrysum, lavender, marjoram, AromaTouch®, DDR Prime®, PastTense®, Slim & Sassy®, Zendocrine®
Varicose veins* - bergamot, cardamom, coriander, cypress, geranium, helichrysum, lemon, lemongrass, marjoram, melaleuca, patchouli, peppermint, rosemary, yarrow, PastTense®, Peace®, Zendocrine®
Vein inflammation (phlebitis) - cypress, frankincense, marjoram, myrrh, DDR Prime®, PastTense®, Zendocrine®
Vertigo/sense room is spinning/sense of falling/loss of equilibrium (disequilibrium) - melissa, peppermint, rosemary, Balance®, Citrus Bliss®, DDR Prime®, Peace®; see *Brain*
Vision, abnormal or jerking eye movements (nystagmus) - DDR Prime®
Vision, blurred - arborvitae, Douglas fir, juniper berry, lemongrass, peppermint, DDR Prime®, Purify, Zendocrine®
Vision, trouble with seeing in one or both eyes - arborvitae, cypress, Douglas fir, lemongrass, DDR Prime®
Vision, see spots (consider low blood pressure) - arborvitae, rosemary, thyme; see *Nervous*
Weakness in arms/muscles; reduced ability to exercise - coriander, ginger, helichrysum, lemongrass, rosemary, tangerine

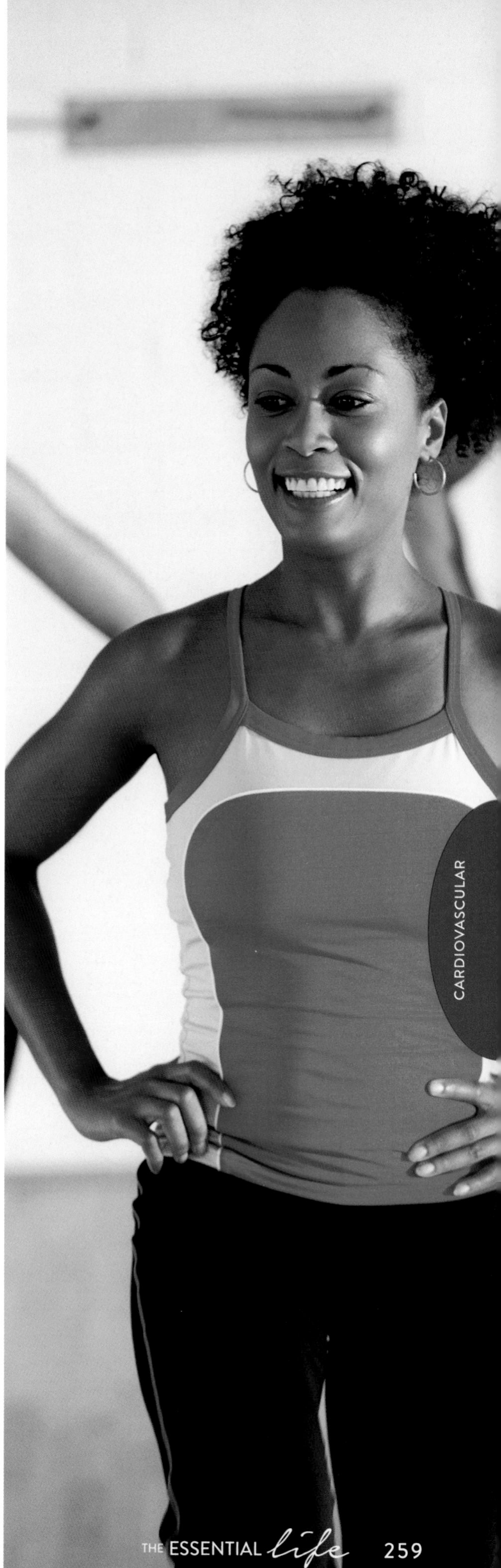

** See remedy on pg. 260*

Remedies

CHOLESTEROL FIGHTER: Combine and ingest frankincense, turmeric and lemongrass in a capsule two times per day.

CIRCULATION MOVER: Apply essential oils of choice; cover with a warm, moist towel to help drive oils into area and increase circulation.

PROMOTE CIRCULATION AND OXYGENATION
Use AromaTouch® twice per day on legs and feet.

VARICOSE VEIN SOOTHER: Use a warm compress with 3 drops cypress on affected areas at least once per day.

VARICOSE VEIN REPAIR: Apply cypress and helichrysum to veins to encourage supporting tissue to "show up."

ANEMIA RESOLVE
6 drops lavender
4 drops lemon
Combine with 1 teaspoon carrier oil and apply to bottoms of feet and stomach.

ANEURYSM SUPPORT & PREVENTION
5 drops frankincense
1 drop helichrysum
1 drop peppermint
Combine and apply to temples, heart, and feet. Dilute as needed.

CARDIOVASCULAR

BLOOD CLOT SUPPORT
4 drops grapefruit
3 drops clove
3 drops lemon
2 drops helichrysum
Combine and ingest in capsule or apply NEAT to bottoms of feet to support blood flow. Dilute if desired.

HEMORRHOID SUPPORT
10 drops cypress
10 drops helichrysum
10 drops lavender
5 drops basil
5 drops geranium
2 drops peppermint
Place oils in 2 ounce bottle with orifice reducer seal, mix; fill remainder with fractionated coconut oil. Apply 10 drops of mixture to affected areas at least twice per day and/or following bowel movement. Additionally, keep a witch hazel bottle with 5 drops of lavender in it beside toilet area; spray on affected area and use with last wipe when using bathroom. A spritzer may also be made and sprayed to affected area as needed.

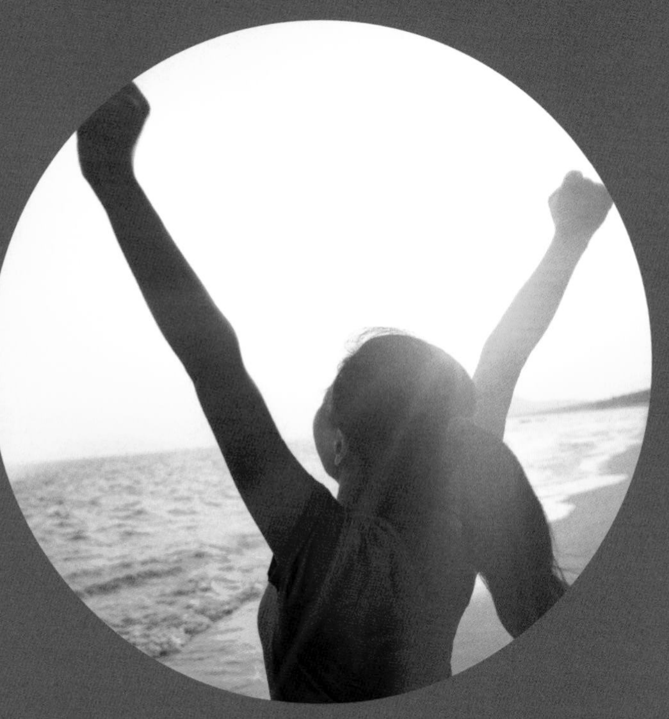

CHOLESTEROL BUILD UP BUSTER
2 drops lemongrass
2 drops marjoram
Place in capsule; take two times per day.

HIGH BLOOD PRESSURE RELIEVER
12 drops helichrysum
12 drops ylang ylang
8 drops cassia
8 drops frankincense
8 drops marjoram
Combine in 10ml roller bottle; fill remainder with fractionated coconut oil. Apply blend to the bottoms of feet, wrists, along breastbone, massage over heart, carotid arteries, and/or back of neck as needed at least two times per day.

RAYNAUD'S DISEASE REMEDY
11 drops cypress
5 drops lavender
2 tablespoons carrier oil
Combine in a glass bottle with a dropper top. Drop 6-8 drops of blend into bath. Bathe twice daily (morning and evening). Water is best hot, yet comfortable. While in the bath, massage fingers and toes. After bath, apply blend over whole body except face. If possible, have blend massaged onto back.

For more ideas, download the app at app.essentiallife.com

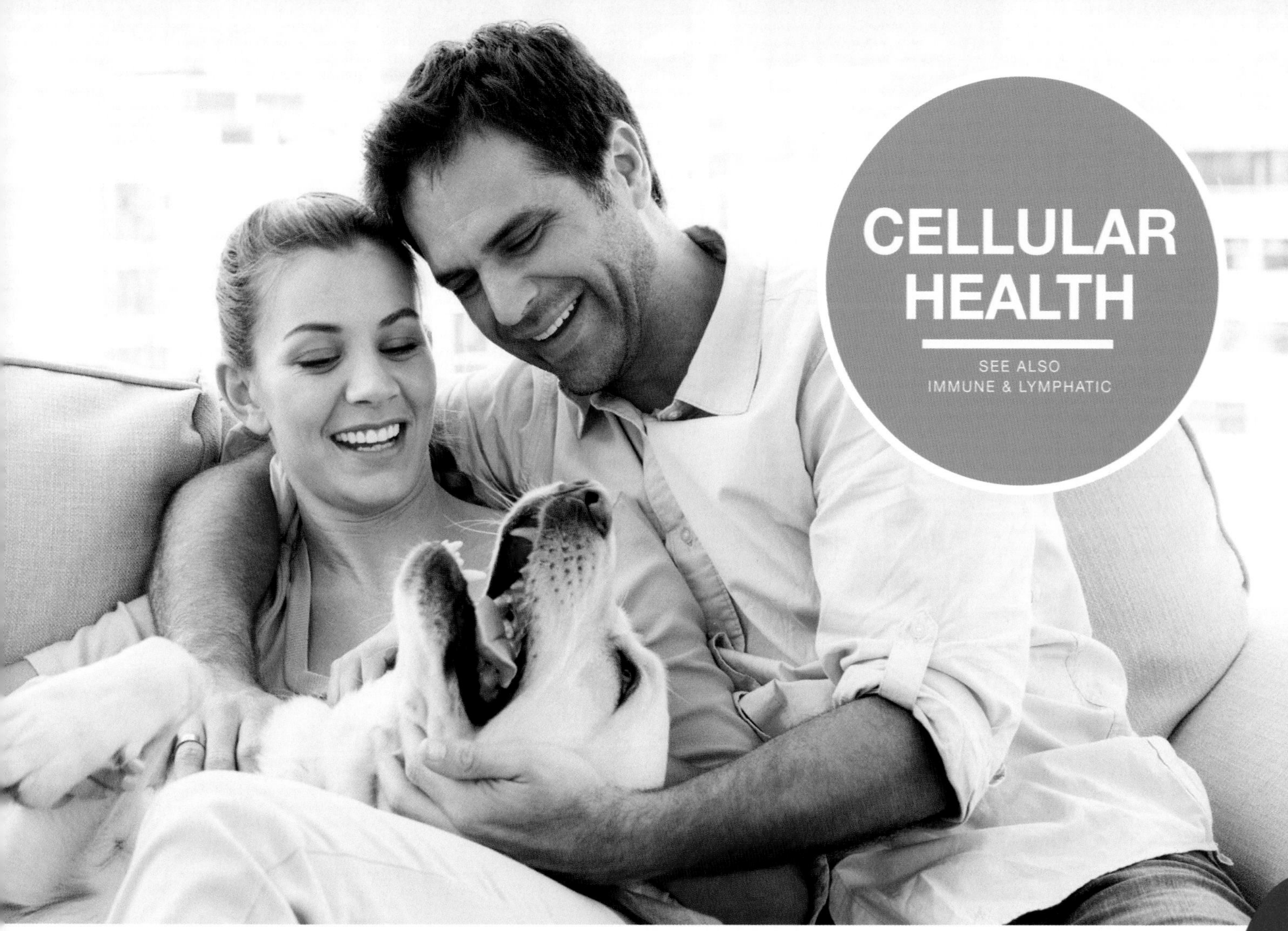

CELLULAR HEALTH

SEE ALSO
IMMUNE & LYMPHATIC

CELLS are the smallest units of life for all living organisms, and they have a lifespan consisting of three primary functions. Cells replicate themselves through a process called mitosis. They perform different specialized functions, such as epithelial, sensory, blood, hormone secreting, etc. Apoptosis, their final function, is a pre-programmed, healthy, cellular death. To achieve optimal health, it is important to nourish and support the cells throughout each stage.

In his book, *Never Be Sick Again*, Dr. Raymond Francis teaches that there's only one disease--a malfunctioning cell; there are two causes of disease--deficiency and toxicity; and there are six pathways to health and disease--nutrition, toxins, psychological/emotional state, physical, genetic, and medical. These ideas certainly simplify, and highlight, the most important areas on which to focus to achieve a healthy body. When cells do not operate efficiently, tissue and organ function is compromised, which in turn can diminish physical well being and invite a host of health conditions and diseases. By nourishing the cells, the entire body system is supported.

Safeguarding the DNA (located in the cell's nucleus) and providing energy for all body processes are two of the most critical cellular activities. Research has shown that a diet low in antioxidants and other important phytonutrients, and environmental exposure to toxins such as pesticides, can damage DNA. This damage, called "mutation," can affect the cells' ability to produce energy. It can cause cells to die early, resulting in weakened tissue or inflammation, or even worse. And it can also cause cells to replicate themselves in their mutated form.

When using essential oils to support cellular function, it is important to remember that essential oils operate chemically within the body; they do not provide nutrition. When essential oils enter the body, they bring powerful instructions to help "remind" and support cells of their healthy function -- but unless the cells are properly nourished, they won't have the energy necessary to perform their desired functions. Eating nutrient-dense raw foods is always a top priority, but many individuals have difficulty eating the quantities and types of quality food that assist cellular health. If this is the case, it's a good idea to find high-quality, bioavailable supplements, such as a whole-food nutrient supplement and xEO Mega, to assist with keeping cells well-nourished and safeguarded.

Essential oils are a powerful addition to any regimen targeting cellular health, because they are actually able to permeate the cell membrane and provide powerful support to the structures found within the cell, including safeguarding against inside threats such as viruses. Synthetic or adulterated essential oils are not able to bypass the cell membrane, and therefore are unable to assist on a cellular level in the body.

TOP SOLUTIONS

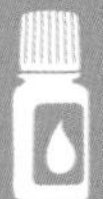

SINGLE OILS

Turmeric - cellular health and antioxidant (pg. 158)

Sandalwood - promotes healthy apoptosis and cellular health (pg. 150)

Frankincense - promotes healthy apoptosis and cellular health (pg. 110)

Lemongrass - cellular detoxifier (pg. 126)

Tangerine, wild orange - encourages healthy DNA and optimal glutathione levels (pgs. 156 & 162)

Cinnamon - promotes healthy cellular response to glucose and inflammation (pg. 93)

Patchouli, yarrow - supports the cell in eliminating harmful toxins (pgs. 139 & 164)

Clove - powerful antioxidant; supports cellular repair (pg. 97)

Thyme - cellular health and DNA repair (pg. 157)

Arborvitae - stimulates immune support and cellular repair (pg. 79)

By Related Properties

For more, See Oil Properties on pages 477 - 481

Anticarcinogenic - arborvitae, black spruce, frankincense, myrrh, peppermint, tangerine, turmeric, yarrow
Anti-carcinoma - arborvitae, copaiba, frankincense, grapefruit, lemon, lemongrass, litsea, myrrh, rosemary, sandalwood, tangerine, turmeric, wild orange
Anti-inflammatory - basil, bergamot, black pepper, blue tansy, cassia, cinnamon, clove, copaiba, coriander, cypress, eucalyptus, frankincense, geranium, ginger, lavender, lemongrass, litsea, manuka, melissa, neroli, oregano, patchouli, peppermint, pink pepper, Siberian fir, Roman chamomile, spearmint, tangerine, turmeric, white fir, yarrow
Antimutagenic - cinnamon, copaiba, ginger, lavender, lemongrass, neroli, tangerine, turmeric
Antioxidant - arborvitae, basil, black pepper, cassia, cilantro, cinnamon, clove, copaiba, coriander, eucalyptus, frankincense, ginger, grapefruit, green mandarin, helichrysum, juniper berry, lemon, lemongrass, lime, melaleuca, neroli, oregano, patchouli, peppermint, pink pepper, rosemary, tangerine, thyme, turmeric, vetiver, wild orange, yarrow
Antitoxic - black pepper, cinnamon, coriander, fennel, geranium, grapefruit, lemongrass, patchouli, thyme
Anti-tumoral - arborvitae, clove, copaiba, frankincense, lavender, myrrh, turmeric, sandalwood
Cleanser - cilantro, grapefruit, lemon, thyme, wild orange
Cytophylactic - arborvitae, frankincense, geranium, lavender, manuka, neroli, red mandarin, rosemary, tangerine
Detoxifier - cassia, cilantro, geranium, green mandarin, litsea, juniper berry, patchouli, tangerine, turmeric, yarrow
Purifier - cinnamon, eucalyptus, grapefruit, lime, marjoram, melaleuca, manuka, Siberian fir, tangerine, wild orange, yarrow
Regenerative - basil, cedarwood, citronella, clove, coriander, frankincense, geranium, helichrysum, jasmine, lavender, lemongrass, manuka, melaleuca, myrrh, neroli, patchouli, sandalwood, wild orange, yarrow
Tonic - arborvitae, basil, birch, cardamom, coriander, frankincense, geranium, lemon, lemongrass, melissa, Roman chamomile, sandalwood, Siberian fir, ylang ylang, yarrow

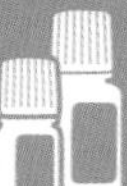

BLENDS

DDR Prime® - promotes cellular health and DNA repair (pg. 184)

Zendocrine® - helps eliminate free radicals and heavy metals (pg. 206)

Cheer® - antioxidant; neutralizes free radicals and supports cells (pg. 173)

Purify - detoxifies cells and lymphatic system (pg. 198)

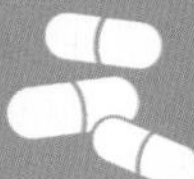

SUPPLEMENTS

Alpha CRS®+ (pg. 209), defensive probiotic, DigestZen® softgels, Mito2Max®, **DDR® Prime (pg. 211)**, xEO Mega, GX Assist®, Deep Blue Polyphenol Complex, MicroPlex VMz supplement

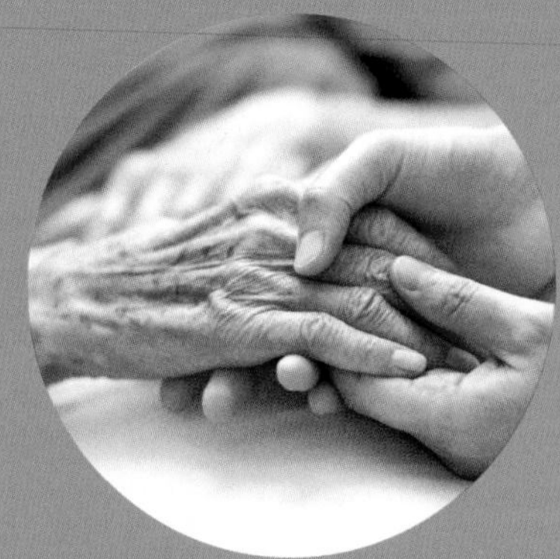

Related Ailments: Basal Cell Carcinoma, Benign Prostatic Hyperplasia, Bone Cancer, Brain Cancer, Breast Cancer, Cells [Integumentary], Cervical Cancer, Colon Cancer, Endometrial Cancer, Hodgkin's Disease, Leukemia, Lipoma, Liver Cancer, Lung Cancer, Lymphoma (Non-Hodgkin's), Melanoma, Mesothelioma, Mouth Cancer, Ovarian Cancer, Paget's Disease, Pancreatic Cancer, Polyps, Prostate Cancer, Radiation Damage [Immune & Lymphatic], Skin Cancer, Throat Cancer, Tongue Cancer, Tumor, Uterine Cancer

USAGE TIPS: For best success at supporting cellular health:

- **Topical:** Apply oils on bottoms of feet, spine, and/or on any specific area of concern. Use Oil Touch technique regularly as desired or able.
- **Internal:** Consume oils in capsules, drop under tongue, or sip in water.

Conditions

CELLULAR HEALTH:

Acidic, overly - arborvitae, dill, fennel, frankincense, lemon, lime, rosemary, wild orange, Balance®, DDR Prime®, Slim & Sassy®, Zendocrine®
Activity, poor - cinnamon, clove, frankincense, geranium, ginger, rosemary, DDR Prime®, DigestZen®, Immortelle, On Guard®, Zendocrine®
Cellular health, poor/premature aging - neroli, tangerine, Console®, DDR Prime®, Immortelle, Peace®; see "Antioxidant" property
Cellular malfunction* - arborvitae, black pepper, cedarwood, citronella, clove, frankincense, geranium, lavender, lemongrass, rosemary, Siberian fir, tangerine, thyme, turmeric, wild orange, DDR Prime®, Forgive®, Immortelle, On Guard®
Free radicals, excess damage - arborvitae, basil, cassia, cardamom, cilantro, cinnamon, clove, frankincense, ginger, grapefruit, lemon, lemongrass, lime, melaleuca, rosemary, tangerine, thyme, turmeric, yarrow, Citrus Bliss®, DDR Prime®, Forgive®, Immortelle, On Guard®; see "Antioxidant" property
Hardening of cell membrane - arborvitae, cinnamon, clove, frankincense, rosemary, sandalwood, tangerine, thyme, vetiver, Breathe®, DDR Prime®, Immortelle; see "Antioxidant" property
Inflammation - basil, bergamot, birch, black pepper, black spruce, cinnamon, clove, copaiba, coriander, cypress, Douglas fir, eucalyptus, frankincense, geranium, lavender, melissa, patchouli, peppermint, Roman chamomile, rosemary, thyme, turmeric, wintergreen, Console®, DDR Prime®, Deep Blue®; see "Anti-inflammatory" property, *Pain & Inflammation*
Nutrient absorption, poor/cellular starvation - cinnamon, ginger, Slim & Sassy®
Oxygen flow to cell, poor - black pepper, cilantro, cypress, frankincense, peppermint, sandalwood, Siberian fir, Breathe®, Slim & Sassy®
Radiation damage - arborvitae, cilantro, clove, copaiba, geranium, patchouli, peppermint, sandalwood, DDR Prime® Zendocrine®
Toxic/autointoxication - arborvitae, bergamot, copaiba, Douglas fir, frankincense, grapefruit, lemon, lime, sandalwood, Siberian fir, turmeric, wild orange, DDR Prime®, Immortelle, InTune®, Purify, Slim & Sassy®, Zendocrine®
Vitality, lack of - bergamot, cedarwood Douglas fir, wild orange, yarrow, ylang ylang, Citrus Bliss®, DDR Prime®, Purify, Zendocrine®

** See remedy on pg. 264*

SUPPORT BY BODY PARTS OR AREAS:

Bladder - basil, cinnamon, cypress, frankincense, juniper berry, lemongrass, rosemary, turmeric, AromaTouch®, DDR Prime®, Slim & Sassy®
Blood - basil, clary sage, clove, frankincense, geranium, lavender, lemongrass, myrrh, rosemary, thyme, turmeric, DDR Prime®, On Guard®, Purify, Zendocrine®
Bone - clary sage, clove, frankincense, helichrysum, lemon, lemongrass, sandalwood, thyme, turmeric, Siberian fir, DDR Prime®
Brain - arborvitae, cedarwood, clove, frankincense, grapefruit, green mandarin, helichrysum, melissa, myrrh, patchouli, pink pepper, rosemary, sandalwood, thyme, wild orange, DDR Prime®, Immortelle
Breast* - arborvitae, cinnamon, clary sage, frankincense, grapefruit, lavender, lemongrass, marjoram, oregano, pink pepper, rosemary, sandalwood, thyme, DDR Prime®, Immortelle, Whisper®
Cervix - clary sage, frankincense, geranium, lemon, patchouli, rosemary, sandalwood, thyme, vetiver, white fir, DDR Prime®, Immortelle, On Guard®, Whisper®, Zendocrine®
Fatty tissue - frankincense, grapefruit, helichrysum, lemon, lemongrass, Slim & Sassy®
General - arborvitae, basil, clary sage, clove, eucalyptus, frankincense, geranium, grapefruit, lavender, lemongrass, myrrh, rose, rosemary, sandalwood, tangerine, wild orange, DDR Prime®, Immortelle, On Guard®, Purify, Whisper®, Zendocrine®
Large intestines/colon/rectum - arborvitae, basil, cardamom, clove, frankincense, geranium, ginger, lavender, lemongrass, oregano, rosemary, sandalwood, thyme, turmeric, wild orange, anti-aging, DDR Prime®, Purify, Whisper®, Zendocrine®
Liver - clove, copaiba, frankincense, geranium, grapefruit, helichrysum, lavender, lemon, lemongrass, rosemary, tangerine, thyme, turmeric, wild orange, DDR Prime®, Zendocrine®
Lung - blue tansy, cinnamon, eucalyptus, frankincense, lavender, lemon, litsea, melissa, ravensara, rosemary, sandalwood, thyme, wild orange, Breathe®, DDR Prime®, On Guard®, Purify, Whisper®, Zendocrine®
Lymphatic system/lymph/nodes - basil, bergamot, cardamom, cilantro, cinnamon, clary sage, clove, frankincense, lavender, lemon, lemongrass, melaleuca, myrrh, rosemary, sandalwood, thyme, turmeric, DDR Prime®, Elevation™, On Guard®, Purify, Zendocrine®
Mouth - bergamot, black pepper, frankincense, geranium, melaleuca, myrrh, peppermint, thyme, turmeric, DDR Prime®
Mucus membrane - arborvitae, frankincense, geranium, lavender, lemongrass, peppermint
Ovaries - clary sage, frankincense, geranium, lemon, myrrh, rosemary, sandalwood, turmeric, vetiver, wild orange, Balance®, DDR Prime®, Immortelle, Slim & Sassy®, Whisper®, Zendocrine®
Pancreas - cinnamon, coriander, frankincense, rosemary, turmeric, DDR Prime®, On Guard®, Purify, Slim & Sassy®, Zendocrine®
Prostate - arborvitae, basil, cardamom, cassia, cedarwood, cinnamon, clary sage, cypress, frankincense, juniper berry, oregano, neroli, rose, rosemary, sandalwood, thyme, turmeric, DDR Prime®, Immortelle, InTune®, On Guard®, Slim & Sassy®, Zendocrine®
Skin - arborvitae, Douglas fir, frankincense, geranium, grapefruit, green mandarin, lavender, lemon, melaleuca, melissa, myrrh, rosemary, sandalwood, tangerine, thyme, turmeric, wild orange, DDR Prime®, Immortelle, On Guard®, Whisper®, Zendocrine®
Throat - cinnamon, frankincense, lavender, lemon, lime, myrrh, rosemary, thyme, turmeric, DDR Prime®, On Guard®, Whisper®, Zendocrine®
Thyroid - blue tansy, clary sage, frankincense, lemon, melissa, rosemary, sandalwood, thyme, DDR Prime®, Forgive®, Passion®
Tongue - bergamot, cassia, cinnamon, clove, frankincense, geranium, ginger, lavender, melaleuca, myrrh, peppermint, thyme, turmeric, DDR Prime®, DigestZen®, Zendocrine®
Tissue - clove, frankincense, geranium, grapefruit, melissa, myrrh, patchouli, sandalwood, wild orange, DDR Prime®, On Guard®, Purify, Whisper®, Zendocrine®
Uterus - clary sage, cypress, frankincense, geranium, ginger, grapefruit, lemon, lemongrass, rosemary, sandalwood, turmeric, DDR Prime®, Immortelle, Purify, On Guard®, Whisper®, Zendocrine®

Remedies

NOTE: Diet, exercise, stress, emotional and spiritual issues all contribute to the development of any degenerative disease including cancer. They must all be dealt with in order to truly heal this condition. Any efforts are best conducted with the support and care of a professional health care provider.

CELLULAR HEALTH PROGRAM - choose from the following:

- **Dietary changes** are imperative - research best options
  - Optional: add TerraGreens® to smoothies or in water
- **Use nutritional supplements** for basic and vital nutrient needs
  - MicroPlex VMz supplement - take 2 capsules am and pm with food
  - Alpha CRS®+ - take 2 capsules am and pm with food; add as needed
  - XEO Mega - take 2 capsules am and pm with food
- **Support healthy digestion & elimination** - consider the following basics
  - TerraZyme® - take 1-2 capsules with meals
  - PB Assist®+- take 2 capsules at bedtime; add as needed
  - DigestZen® if needed for digestive/intestinal upset or sluggishness
- **Use a citrus oil(s) daily** to raise glutathione levels in body
  Choose citrus oil according to needs; add to drinking water or take in capsule
  - 2-3 drops grapefruit, lemon, tangerine, and/or wild orange two times per day
- **Engage in detoxification & natural chelation**
  - **Remove toxins** from diet/lifestyle; reduce exposure to chemicals and toxins
  - **Open channels of elimination:**
    - Use Zendrocrine® Complex - take 1-2 capsules am and pm with food
    - See *Detoxification* section in this book for further ideas
  - **Support liver and rid body of heavy metal toxicity**
    Choose one of following based on what is best match for condition(s):
    - Recipe #1: Use Zendocrine®, take 4 drops two times per day
    - Recipe #2: Use 2-3 drops each cilantro, geranium, grapefruit, rosemary oil in a capsule once or twice per day
    - Recipe #3: Use 2 drops helichrysum and 2 drops Zendocrine® in capsule two times per day
- **Focus on cellular health, DNA repair, & promoting healthy apoptosis**
  Choose one or two of following:
  - Use DDR Prime® on bottoms of feet - 4 drops per foot two times per day
  - Use DDR Prime® Softgels as a supplement - 2 softgels with meals two to three times per day
  - 2 drops frankincense under tongue two times daily; hold thirty seconds; swallow
  - 2 drops clove in capsule each day with meals
  - 2-3 drops each clove, grapefruit, lavender oil, DDR Prime® in capsule two to three times per day
  - Research and create own blend using oils that are specific to condition(s)
- **Heal and maintain a healthy emotional state**
  See *Mood & Behavior* section
- **Support a healthy immune system** - consider:
  - Use On Guard® or see *Immune & Lymphatic* section
  - Consider candida detox program - see Candida section
- **Manage pain** - choose from:
  - Use Deep Blue Polyphenol Complex
  - See *Pain & Inflammation, Muscular, Nervous, Skeletal* sections
- **Maintain energy levels**
  - Use Mito2Max®
  - See *Energy & Vitality* section
- **Use a specified topical application** once or more per day
  Choose from the following:
  - Conduct the Basic Application Technique once daily - see below
  - Choose a topical application recipe or create one - see below

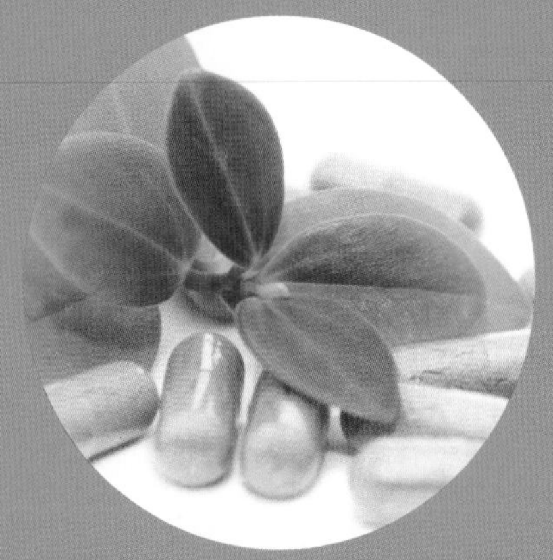

OPTIONAL TOPICAL APPLICATION RECIPES

Apply blends below to affected area(s) one to two times daily. Also apply to spine one time per day and bottoms of feet two times per day. Blends may be multiplied and stored in a glass bottle with lid to create reserves for future applications. Mix in a glass bowl or container.

- **Breast**
  2 drops frankincense + 3 drops white fir + 3 drops wild orange + 2 drops grapefruit blended into 10 drops skin clearing oil; IF lymph gland involvement, add 2 drops lemongrass; place oils in 1 ounce glass bottle; fill remainder with high quality aloe vera gel. Mix thoroughly. Apply blend to entire breast area, and underarms (if area is affected). Use twice per day.
- **Lung**
  6 drops Breathe® + 4 drops clove + 4 drops myrrh + 5 drops frankincense, 2 drops sage + 1 tablespoon carrier oil
- **Lymph**
  15 drops frankincense + 6 drops clove + 1 tablespoon carrier oil
- **Ovaries**
  15 drops frankincense + 5 drops myrrh + 6 drops geranium + 1 tablespoon carrier oil
- **Skin**
  3 drops lavender + 4 drops frankincense + 1 tablespoon carrier oil

BREAST DETOX SALVE

Melt 2 tablespoons shea butter over low heat; removed from heat as soon as butter has liquefied. Cool to room temperature, then add essential oils listed below. When salve begins to solidify, stir well. Cover and use within about two weeks.

4 drops cinnamon
4 drops Roman chamomile
3 drops thyme
2 drops frankincense
2 drops jasmine or ylang ylang

CELLULAR HEALTH LAYERING APPLICATION TECHNIQUE

1. Apply a base coat using 1-2 teaspoons fractionated coconut oil
2. Once daily, layer following oils, one at a time, on back. First drip 5-6 drops of one oil up spine; distribute across back; massage lightly. Repeat until all oils are applied:
   - clove or thyme - frankincense - lemongrass - rosemary - sandalwood
3. Alter recipe according to needs and conditions. Choose oils from particular cancer lists.

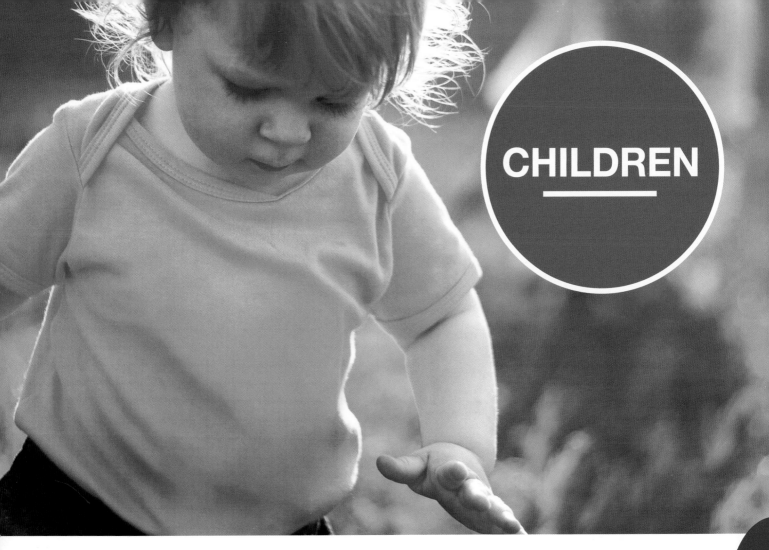

CHILDREN'S HEALTH involves both physical and mental well being. Physical health concerns range from irritating (e.g. diaper rash, crying, colic) to concerns that can quickly become serious if not addressed (e.g. scarlet fever, strep throat). Once a child begins socializing outside the home, exposure to bacterial and viral infections becomes commonplace. Since their immune systems are immature, children can more easily succumb to infectious diseases. They are also exposed to a number of compromising situations that increase risk for injury. See the *First Aid* section for tips on addressing issues resulting while engaged in typical childhood play.

Just like adults, children have mental health needs and are affected by perceived stress and trauma, responding with typical emotions such as fear, sadness, and anger. Parents and caregivers often feel poorly equipped with the knowledge and tools they need to properly care for their children. It is difficult and frustrating to have limited resources when trying to help a child resolve emotional upset, stress, hyperactivity, sadness, illness, injury, and any other potential concern.

Children are particularly responsive to aromas and healthy touch. Simply smelling or experiencing the application of an essential oil followed by a simple massage technique is very comforting to a child and can support rapid changes in behavior and responsiveness to trauma or difficult situations. Many real life situations have demonstrated that a room full of children under a variety of circumstances have a nearly universal positive response in mood, outlook, and behavior through the diffusing or dispersing of essential oils into the air.

Most children naturally love essential oils, and many seem to know what they need and when to use them. They respond particularly well to opportunities to discover their favorite oils and make their own personalized roller-bottle blend (see *Blending and Layering* for further information). For further ideas for mood support, see *Mood & Behavior*.

While proper medical care is always advised when needed, there are many situations in the home and family when natural solutions can be used as a first line of defense. Parents and caregivers are more intimately acquainted with their children than anyone else, and typically have excellent insight into the nature or causes of many issues their children encounter. It is empowering to know a few natural remedy basics that may help prevent potential issues and that will support health and wellness.

Teaching children self-care at an early age creates an empowering environment in which they may grow and advance as confident and balanced individuals. Essential oils offer an excellent opportunity to participate in this self-care process. When partnered with children's nutritional supplements and a healthy diet, a foundation of health is laid that positively affects a young person's health status for decades to come.

TOP SOLUTIONS

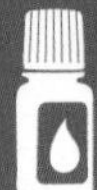

SINGLE OILS

Lavender - most used essential oil for children; all things calming (pg. 122)

Wild orange - gentle/powerful calming/uplifting; digestive support; boost immune/anti-infectious; promotes sense of abundance "there is enough for me!" (pg. 162)

Frankincense - supports brain, mood, wound healing, feeling grounded and safe/secure (pg. 110)

Roman chamomile - supports sense of calm/ relaxation; sedative effect; diffuses agitated negative thoughts/moods; detoxifying (pg. 147)

By Related Properties

For more, See Oil Properties on pages 477 - 481

Antibacterial - arborvitae, bergamot, black pepper, blue tansy, cardamom, cedarwood, cinnamon, copaiba, eucalyptus, ginger, lemongrass, litsea, manuka, marjoram, melaleuca, myrrh, oregano, patchouli, rosemary, Siberian fir, tangerine, thyme, turmeric

Anticatarrhal - black pepper, frankincense, helichrysum, myrrh, neroli, rosemary, spearmint, white fir

Antidepressant - basil, bergamot, clary sage, coriander, frankincense, geranium, lemon, lemongrass, neroli, rose, sandalwood, tangerine, wild orange

Anti-inflammatory - arborvitae, basil, bergamot, blue tansy, cedarwood, copaiba, coriander, cypress, eucalyptus, frankincense, geranium, ginger, helichrysum, lavender, lemongrass, lime, litsea, manuka, marjoram, melaleuca, myrrh, neroli, peppermint, Roman chamomile, rosemary, sandalwood, Siberian fir, tangerine, turmeric, wintergreen, yarrow

Antiseptic - basil, bergamot, black pepper, cardamom, cedarwood, clary sage, copaiba, cypress, geranium, helichrysum, jasmine, lavender, lemon, lime, manuka, marjoram, melaleuca, melissa, neroli, oregano, patchouli, ravensara, rosemary, sandalwood, Siberian fir, tangerine, thyme, white fir, wild orange, yarrow, ylang ylang

Antiviral - arborvitae, blue tansy, cassia, cinnamon, clove, copaiba, eucalyptus, lime, litsea, manuka, melaleuca, melissa, oregano, Siberian fir, thyme, turmeric, white fir, yarrow

Calming - basil, black spruce, blue tansy, copaiba, lavender, litsea, magnolia, patchouli, Roman chamomile, tangerine, vetiver, yarrow

Decongestant - copaiba, cypress, eucalyptus, lemon, melissa, rosemary, Siberian fir, white fir, yarrow

Expectorant - cardamom, dill, eucalyptus, fennel, helichrysum, jasmine, lemongrass, marjoram, melaleuca, oregano, rosemary, sandalwood, Siberian fir, thyme, white fir

Immunostimulant - arborvitae, cassia, cinnamon, clove, copaiba, eucalyptus, frankincense, lime, melissa, rosemary, Siberian fir, white fir, wild orange, yarrow

Invigorating - grapefruit, lemon, litsea, peppermint, pink pepper, Siberian fir, spearmint, wild orange, wintergreen

Mucolytic - basil, cedarwood, clary sage, copaiba, cypress, fennel, helichrysum, lemon, myrrh, tangerine, yarrow

Regenerative - basil, cedarwood, clove, cypress, frankincense, geranium, helichrysum, lavender, lemongrass, manuka, melaleuca, neroli, patchouli, sandalwood, yarrow

Relaxing - basil, blue tansy, cassia, cedarwood, geranium, jasmine, lavender, litsea, manuka, marjoram, myrrh, neroli, ravensara, Roman chamomile, ylang ylang

Sedative - basil, bergamot, blue tansy, cedarwood, coriander, frankincense, juniper berry, lavender, magnolia, neroli, patchouli, Roman chamomile, sandalwood, tangerine, vetiver, ylang ylang, yarrow

Stomachic - basil, cardamom, fennel, ginger, juniper berry, peppermint, pink pepper, rosemary, turmeric, yarrow

Uplifting - bergamot, cardamom, cedarwood, clary sage, cypress, grapefruit, litsea, sandalwood, tangerine, wild orange

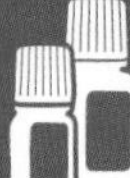

BLENDS

Calmer™ - supports sense of peace and calm (pg. 175)

Steady™ - supports feeling grounded and stable (pg. 177)

DigestZen® - supports digestion and elimination (pg. 186)

Stronger™ - boosts immune system (pg. 178)

Thinker™ - supports optimal focus and concentration (pg. 180)

Rescuer™ - (pg. 176)

Brave™ - (pg. 174)

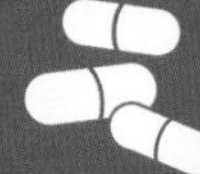

SUPPLEMENTS

A2z Chewable™ (pg. 208), PB Assist®+, **IQ Mega® supplement (pg. 213)**, TrimShake®, Breathe® lozenges

Related Ailments: Colic, Crying Baby, Diaper Rash, Fifth's Disease (human parvovirus B19), Gastroenteritis (stomach flu) [Digestive & Intestinal; Immune & Lymphatic], Growing Pains, Hand, Foot and Mouth Disease [Immune & Lymphatic - Viral], Infant Reflux, Legg-Calve-Perthes Disease [Skeletal], Roseola, RSV, Scarlet Fever, Thrush [Candida]

USAGE TIPS: Children are wonderfully responsive to the use of essential oils. They love to learn about them and be involved in the process of selecting what oils are used on their behalf. They love to nurture others with the oils as well and participate in making their own personalized roller bottle blend. Allowing a child to smell an oil prior to use creates a sense of safety.

- **Aromatic:** Use of oils at bedtime with a diffuser or smelling oils from some kind of sealed container during school can bring both peace and calming, also mental focus and concentration support. Oils supply a vast variety of emotional support.
- **Topical:** Use of oils with children is most effective when oils are combined with a carrier oil and are massaged on back, abdomen or feet (NEAT - undiluted - application on feet with 1-2 drops depending on body weight is acceptable in older children; for infants and toddlers, dilute oils with a carrier oil prior to application in most cases).

Conditions

EMOTIONAL/MENTAL STATES*

Children naturally experience any number of emotional states, as do adults. Common expressions can be anxious or stressed, defiant, excessive crying, willful, grumpy, overly reactive or over-sensitive, shy, sad, whiny, and excessively wound-up or hyperactive. See *Mood & Behavior* for suggested solutions. For attention deficits or issues with focus and concentration, see *Focus & Concentration*

PHYSICAL STATES

Acne, baby - melaleuca, HD Clear® (dilute); see *Integumentary*
Allergies - blue tansy, cilantro, lavender, lemon, melaleuca, peppermint, Zendocrine®; see *Allergies*
Antibiotic recovery - cilantro, Zendocrine®, defensive probiotic; see *Candida*
Bed-wetting* - black pepper, cilantro, cinnamon, copaiba, cypress, juniper berry, rosemary, spearmint, Peace®, Rescuer™, Zendocrine®
Birth - arborvitae, clary sage, frankincense, melaleuca, melissa, myrrh, neroli, sandalwood, patchouli, wild orange, Calmer™, Motivate®, Steady™, Thinker™; see *Pregnancy, Labor & Nursing*
Bronchitis - cardamom, clary sage, copaiba, eucalyptus, pink pepper, Siberian fir, Breathe®, Motivate®, On Guard®; see *Respiratory*
Bug bites/stings - blue tansy, copaiba, lavender, Purify; see *First Aid*
Bumps/bruises - fennel, geranium, helichrysum, lavender, Deep Blue®; see *First Aid*
Colic* - bergamot, black pepper, cardamom, cilantro, clove, coriander, cypress, dill, fennel, ginger, lavender, marjoram, Roman chamomile, rosemary, spearmint, wild orange, ylang ylang, Adaptiv®, Calmer™, DigestZen®; see *Digestive & Intestinal*
Common cold/flu* - cardamom, cedarwood, lemon, melaleuca, melissa, rose, rosemary, sandalwood, tangerine, thyme, Breathe®, Stronger™; see *Immune & Lymphatic*
Constipation - cardamom, cilantro, Douglas fir, ginger, lemongrass, marjoram, rosemary, wild orange, DigestZen®, Tamer™, Zendocrine®; see *Digestive & Intestinal*
Cradle cap* - clary sage, frankincense, geranium, lavender, lemon, melaleuca, sandalwood, Immortelle, corrective ointment; see *Integumentary*
Croup - arborvitae, Douglas fir, eucalyptus, lemon, marjoram, patchouli, sandalwood, thyme, wild orange, Breathe®, Stronger™; see *Respiratory*
Cuts - copaiba, frankincense, lavender, magnolia, melaleuca, myrrh, sandalwood, yarrow, corrective ointment; see *First Aid*
Diaper rash* - dilute: frankincense, lavender, melaleuca, patchouli, Roman chamomile, ylang ylang; see *Integumentary*
Dry lips/above lips - cedarwood, jasmine, myrrh, sandalwood, corrective ointment, fractionated coconut oil; see *Integumentary*
Dry skin - arborvitae, black spruce, copaiba, lavender, lemon (skin cleansing), melaleuca, myrrh, neroli, sandalwood, Immortelle, diluted; see *Integumentary*
Earache* - basil, clary sage, cypress, fennel, ginger, helichrysum, lavender, melaleuca, neroli, Roman chamomile, thyme, wild orange, Rescuer™; see *Respiratory*
Eczema/Psoriasis - arborvitae, black spruce, cedarwood, Douglas fir, geranium, helichrysum, myrrh, neroli, patchouli, Roman chamomile, sandalwood, Siberian fir, turmeric, yarrow, ylang ylang, corrective ointment, fractionated coconut oil; see *Integumentary*
Fever* - birch, eucalyptus, juniper berry, lavender, lemon eucalyptus, lime, peppermint, pink pepper, Roman chamomile, Siberian fir, spearmint, wintergreen, yarrow, Citrus Bliss®, PastTense®; see *Immune & Lymphatic*
Growing Pains - see *Leg Aches* below
Foot fungus (Athlete's foot) - basil, copaiba, melaleuca, neroli, On Guard®; see *Candida*
Hand, foot and mouth - arborvitae, cassia, cinnamon, clove, helichrysum, lemongrass, melaleuca, melissa, oregano, rosemary, thyme, turmeric, wild orange, wintergreen, On Guard®, Stronger™; see *Immune & Lymphatic*
Headache - lavender, peppermint, frankincense, wintergreen, Rescuer™, Zendocrine®; see *Pain & Inflammation*
Hiccups - arborvitae, basil, blue tansy, clary sage, fennel, helichrysum, lemon, peppermint, sandalwood, wild orange, Serenity®, Zendocrine®
Hives - basil, cilantro, frankincense, lavender, melaleuca, peppermint, Roman chamomile, rosemary; see *Allergies*
Immune system boost - Stronger™; see *Immune & Lymphatic*
Infant reflux - dill, lavender, peppermint, Roman chamomile, DigestZen®; Tamer™; see *Digestive & Intestinal*
Jaundice* - frankincense, geranium, helichrysum, juniper berry, lemon, lemongrass, lime, rosemary, wild orange, Zendocrine®; see *Digestive & Intestinal*
Leg aches/growing pains - arborvitae, birch, cypress, ginger, lavender, lemongrass, marjoram, melissa, rosemary, Siberian fir, white fir, wintergreen, Adaptiv®, AromaTouch®, Rescuer™; see *Pain & Inflammation*
Pinkeye (conjunctivitis) - clary sage, Douglas fir, frankincense, lavender, melaleuca, spikenard, corrective ointment; see *Immune & Lymphatic*
Rash - arborvitae, cedarwood, lavender, lemon, melaleuca, Roman chamomile, rose, sandalwood, Rescuer™, Zendocrine®; see *Integumentary*
Respiratory support - eucalyptus, rosemary, Breathe®; see *Respiratory*
Runny nose - basil, cedarwood, lemon/lavender/peppermint (use together), Breathe®, Stronger™; see *Allergies, Immune & Lymphatic, Respiratory*
Seizures - cedarwood, celery seed, Douglas fir, frankincense, petitgrain, rose (will delay onset), sandalwood, spikenard; see *Brain*
Sleep, disturbed/irregular/nighttime waking* - lavender, tangerine, vetiver, Balance®, Calmer™; see *Sleep*
Sleep, trouble getting to* - lavender, neroli, Roman chamomile, Calmer™, Steady™; see *Sleep*
Stomach flu* (Gastroenteritis) - basil, bergamot, cardamom, clove, dill, ginger, thyme, DigestZen®, Stronger™, Tamer™; see *Digestive & Intestinal*
Stuffy nose - Douglas fir, lemon, sandalwood, Breathe®, DigestZen®; see *Allergies, Immune & Lymphatic, Respiratory*
Sunburn - blue tansy, frankincense, helichrysum, lavender, peppermint, sandalwood, Immortelle; see *Integumentary*
Teeth grinding - black spruce, frankincense, geranium, marjoram, lavender, Roman chamomile, wild orange, Calmer™, Serenity®; see *Parasites*
Teething pain - blue tansy, clove, frankincense, helichrysum, lavender, Roman chamomile, sandalwood, yarrow; dilute and apply directly to gums, Rescuer™
Thumb sucking - clove or any other internally safe, unpleasant-tasting oil (diluted)
Thrush* - bergamot, clary sage, clove, dill, geranium, fennel, lavender, lemon, melaleuca, oregano, thyme, wild orange, On Guard®, Slim & Sassy®; see *Candida*
Tired, overly - lavender, neroli, Roman chamomile, yarrow, Calmer™, Forgive®, Motivate®, Serenity®, Steady™; see *Sleep*
Tooth decay - clove, copaiba, helichrysum, melaleuca; see *Oral Health*
Tooth infection - clove, helichrysum, melaleuca, Stronger™; see *Oral Health*
Tummy ache - blue tansy, cardamom, fennel, ginger, peppermint, yarrow, DigestZen®, Tamer™; see *Digestive & Intestinal*
Vomiting - bergamot, cardamom, clove, dill, ginger, pink pepper, On Guard®(dilute), DigestZen®, Purify, Tamer™, Zendocrine®; see *Digestive & Intestinal*
Warts - arborvitae, cinnamon, clove, frankincense, lemon, lemongrass, lime, melissa, oregano, thyme, On Guard®; see *Integumentary*
Whooping Cough, spastic/persistent cough - cardamom, clary sage, cypress, Douglas fir, eucalyptus, frankincense, lavender, neroli, petitgrain, Roman chamomile, rosemary, yarrow, Breathe®, Purify, Serenity®, Stronger™; see *Respiratory*

** See remedy on pg. 268*

Remedies

AID KIDS IN GOING TO SLEEP AND STAYING ASLEEP
Diffuse eight drops lavender or Serenity® and three drops wild orange.

ANGER MANAGEMENT FOR LITTLE ONES
Use Citrus Bliss®, magnolia, and Balance®; place a drop of each on palms of hands, rub together, cup over face (without making contact with skin) and inhale; then rub oils on back of neck. Other optional oils: Children's grounding and Serenity®s.

BED-WETTING For older children who can swallow capsules, 1-2 drops cilantro oil in a capsule one time per day
Increase number of times per day as needed for results.
Apply cypress as needed.
For younger children, apply 1-2 drops cypress to bottoms of feet (dilute with a carrier oil).

CHILL OUT
14 drops cypress
10 drops frankincense
25 drops lavender
12 drops vetiver
18 drops Roman chamomile
5 drops ylang ylang
5 drops cedarwood
Mix in a 50/50 ratio of essential oils to carrier oil for children and a 75/25 ratio for adults. Apply to back of neck, inside of wrists, base of skull, along spinal cord. Other optional oils: Children's grounding and Serenity®s.

COLIC BLEND
Combine 2 tablespoons almond oil with 1 drop Roman chamomile, 1 drop lavender, and 1 drop geranium or dill. Mix and apply to stomach and back. Note: Burping the baby and keeping the abdomen warm with a warm (not hot) water bottle will often bring relief.

COMMON COLD BLEND
Combine 2 tablespoons of a carrier oil with 2 drops melaleuca, 1 drop lemon, and 1 drop On Guard®. Massage a little of the blend on neck and chest. Other optional oils: Stronger™.

CRADLE CAP
Combine 2 tablespoons almond oil with 1 drop of melaleuca or lemon oil with 1 drop geranium, OR or 1 drop cedarwood and 1 drop sandalwood. Mix and apply a small amount on scalp.

For more ideas, download the app at app.essentiallife.com

DIAPER RASH BLEND
Combine 1 drop Roman chamomile and 1 drop lavender with fractionated coconut oil and apply directly to the bottom.
If skin is patchy, add melaleuca to the mixture. Diaper rash may be caused by irritation from stool/urine, reaction to new foods or products, bacterial or yeast/fungal infection, sensitive skin, chafing or rubbing, or use of antibiotics resulting in a lack of friendly bacteria.

EARACHE BLEND
Apply 1 drop of basil or melaleuca oil and carrier oil on a cotton ball and place on the surface of the ear. Avoid the ear canal; rub a little bit of diluted oil behind the ear.

FEVER
Dilute 1 drop lavender in carrier oil and massage baby or child (back of neck, feet, behind ear, etc.). Dilute 1 drop peppermint in a carrier oil and rub into bottoms of feet.

FLU
Diffuse 2 drops of cypress, lemon, and melaleuca. OR add 1 drop of each to ½ cup Epsom salts for a bath treatment.

JAUNDICE
Dilute geranium and frankincense in a carrier oil and apply on the liver area and to the liver reflex points on feet.

LIGHTS OUT! (nighty night in minutes)
2 vetiver
2 cedarwood
2 patchouli
2 Serenity®
3 ylang ylang
Blend in a 10 ml roller bottle; fill remainder of bottle with a carrier oil. Roll on feet and/or along the spine at bedtime.

THRUSH BLEND
8 drops lemon
8 drops melaleuca
2 tablespoons garlic oil
1 ml Vitamin E oil
Combine. Apply a small amount of the mixture to nipples just before nursing, or with a clean finger into baby's mouth and on tongue.

TRANSITION BLEND Helpful for children facing stressful social environment changes, like going to daycare or school. Apply 2-3 drops of Balance® and vetiver, or Brave™, on back of neck. (Focus on occipital triangle area and bottoms of feet, especially the big toes.) Apply the night before and the morning of any significant event.

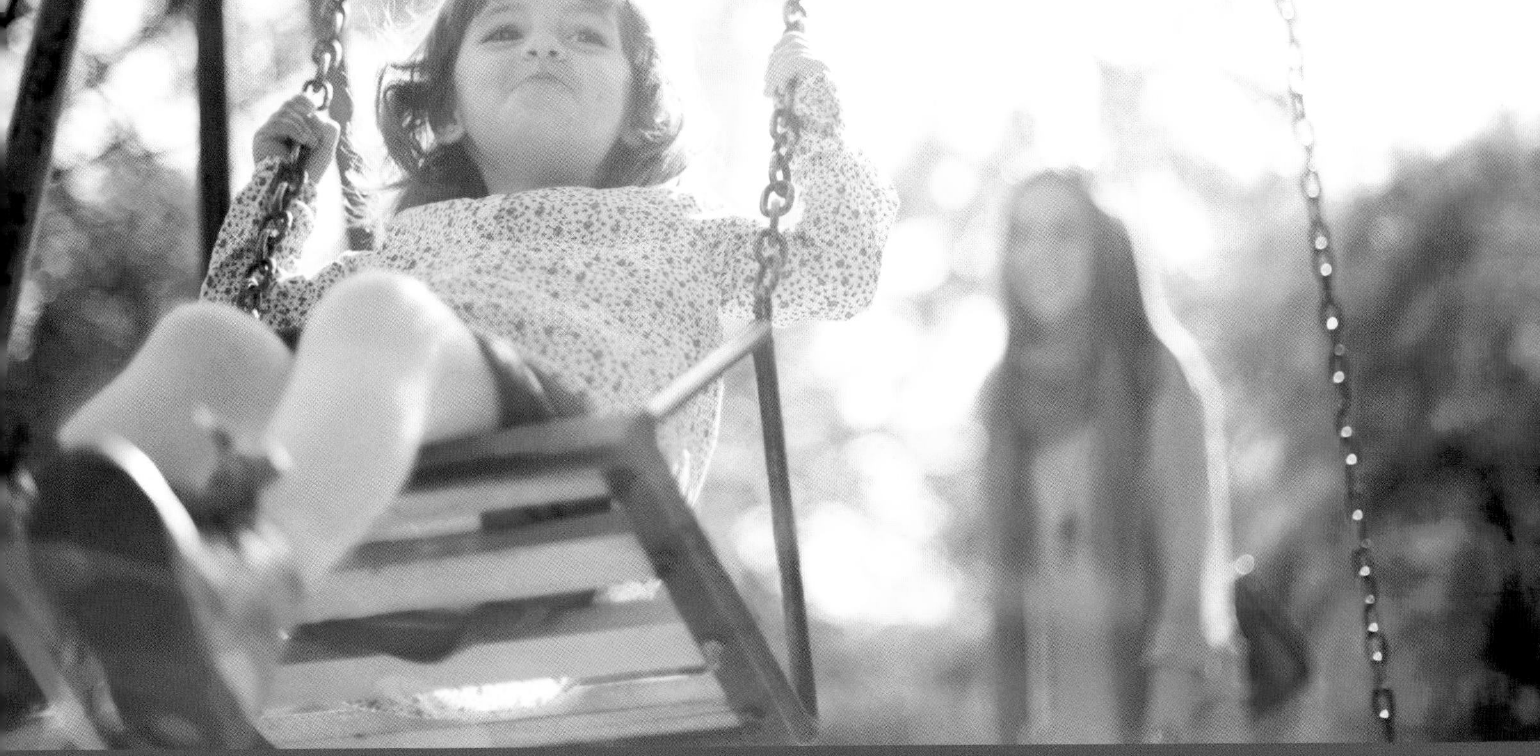

USAGE INFORMATION & NOTE TO PARENTS

Parents and caretakers bear a profound stewardship for the child's health that deserves to be taken seriously and managed responsibly. This involves educating oneself about nutrition, supplementation, preventative care options, and treatment of illnesses and injuries.

Doctors bring a wealth of medical skills and deep knowledge of disease to their work. Few have more than a cursory understanding of health maintenance essentials like supplements and nutrition. Most have no knowledge whatsoever about effective natural health care solutions like essential oils.

A parent who educates herself appropriately can choose a health care provider for her family who is open to natural solutions. Together, they can partner intelligently to provide the child an effective health maintenance program and powerful natural remedies when needed, particularly the implementation of essential oils.

Caution must be taken when researching solutions online. Most information available about aromatherapy reflects the assumption that the product used will contain synthetic ingredients. In the case of these adulterated products, warnings should be heeded as legitimate.

But when pure, unadulterated, genuine essential oils are selected, a parent can treat the family with confidence. In fact, when quality oils are used, parents can experiment much like experimenting with healthy options in the kitchen. One child might thrive on a particular grain; another might find it upsets the tummy and prefer a different selection. But no harm is done. That is what this section is designed to provide: appropriate information to encourage confidence and educated experimentation to have a healthy family.

The invitation to parents and caretakers is to know it isn't about being perfect. It is about being present. Give up the idea of doing it perfectly for the idea of being flexible and teachable. If something isn't generating the desired results, change it up, try something different, diversify efforts. Obtain fearless confidence by freely playing with the oils until you (and your children) figure them out and discover what is right for you.

Safety Rules for Essential Oil Use with Children

Generally speaking, use prudence when applying essential oils to children. Keep oils away from eyes and out of reach of children. Generally, dilution of oils with a carrier oil is recommended. When using an oil NEAT (undiluted), it is best applied on the bottoms of a child's feet.

To determine quantities, consider the child's body weight and apply a fraction of the adult recommended dosage. For example, if an adult were to apply 1-2 drops topically of an oil directly to the skin, those same number of drops could be placed in a roller bottle, highly diluted with a carrier oil, and applied repeatedly on an infant. Any oil that contains cineole such as cardamom, eucalyptus, rosemary, myrtle, laurel leaf, or niaouli should be diluted with a carrier oil, used in small amounts, or used in a blend (which changes the nature of an oil) especially with children under the age of two.

Avoid putting undiluted peppermint oil on the chest, face, or throat area of a young child (under 30 months), as the sensation and effect can startle the infant and cause them to hold their breath or stop breathing momentarily. Use peppermint diluted on the bottoms of the feet or in a blend, such as in a Breathe®.

As indicated in the safety section of this book, birch, cassia, cinnamon, clove, eucalyptus, ginger, lemongrass, oregano, peppermint, thyme, and wintergreen are all considered to be "hot" essential oils that deserve more caution and care when used in the presence of or on children. Dilution and proper storage (away from children) are essential. Avoid contact with eyes and other sensitive parts of the body.

Premature babies: Since premature babies have very thin and sensitive skin, a very conservative and highly diluted use of essential oils is recommended.

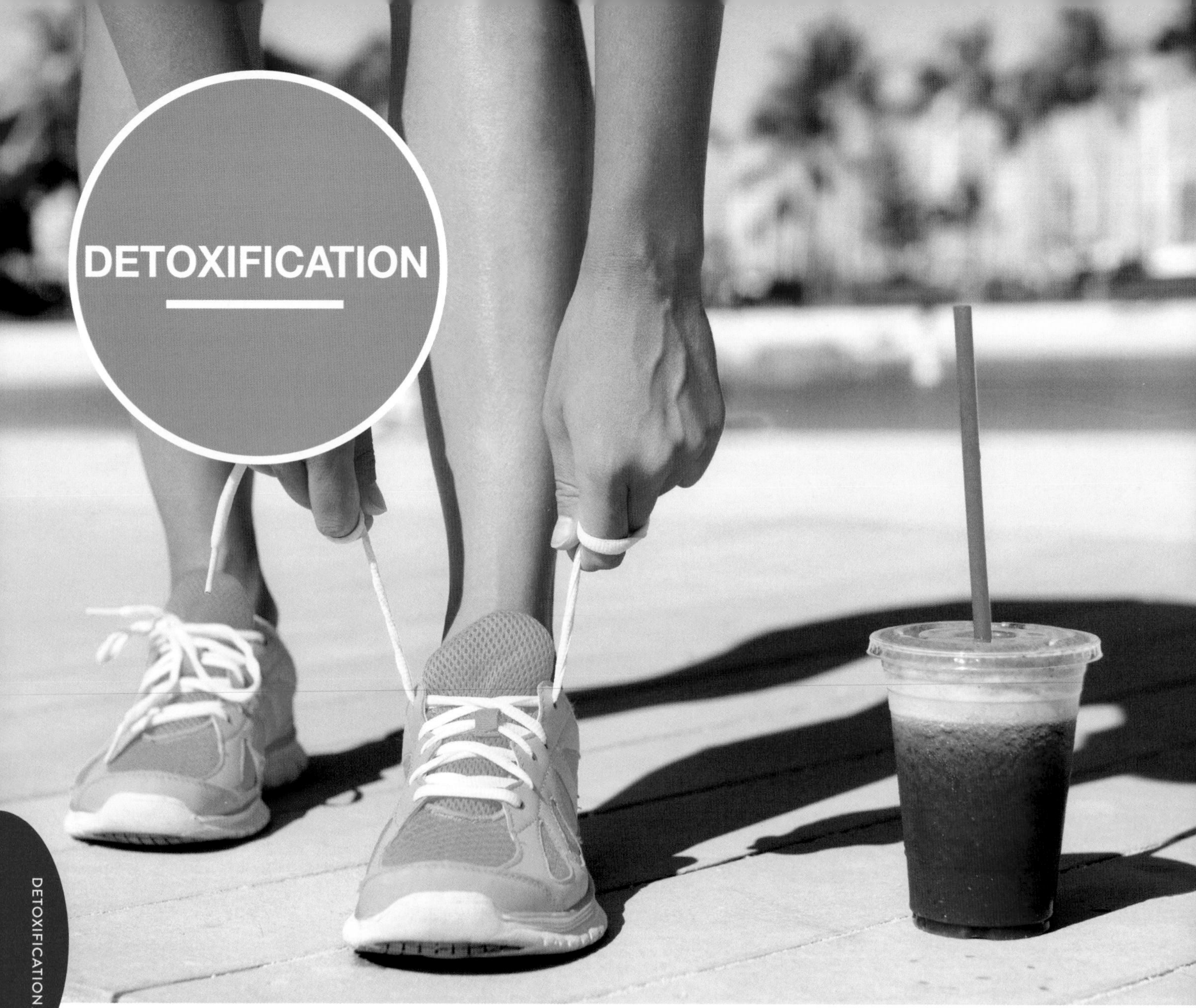

DETOXIFICATION (detoxing or cleansing) is the term used to describe the deliberate use of programs, products, dietary, and lifestyle changes to support the body in the elimination of unwanted substances and circumstances. Releasing toxins allows the body, heart, and mind to dedicate greater amounts of energy to thriving rather than just coping and surviving.

We live, eat, and breathe toxic substances every day. Consider the paint on the walls, the carpet, laundry and cleaning products, pesticides, extermination products, preservatives and chemicals in foods, the "stuff" that goes in and out of cars; personal care products and makeup also contribute to higher toxicity levels in the body. Toxicity must be dealt with even when trying to limit exposure to toxins, since contact with chemicals and other toxic agents occurs every day by eating, breathing, living, and sleeping.

When overwhelmed by toxins, the body cannot properly perform its many functions with full efficiency. Metabolism, immunity, elimination of waste, absorption of nutrients, production of important brain chemicals, reproduction, circulation, respiration, etc., are affected. Even hydration can be compromised. Toxic overload may reveal itself as fevers, headaches, acne, fatigue or lack of energy, sneezing, coughing, vomiting, diarrhea, rashes, allergies, excess weight, cellulite, brain fog or lack of mental clarity, decreased immunity, chronic pain, poor moods, and much more. Sometimes these symptoms are interpreted as sickness, when in reality the body may be trying to eliminate toxins through different systems—and the symptoms are mere side effects. Avoiding toxins and detoxifying are necessary to be healthy, happy, and free of disease.

Essential oils have unique properties that support health on a cellular level, including detoxing. When the body is overwhelmed by excess toxins, the liver will safeguard vital organs by insulating toxins in fat cells. There are oils that help release toxins from fat cells, break them down, and flush them out of the body with good hydration. Other oils stimulate cell receptor sites to greater, more efficient activity. And there are oils that are helpful in clearing the gut of harmful bacteria and restoring balance for healthy digestion and immunity. Consider what actions can reduce the intake of toxins, and how to consistently detox to maintain optimal health.

TOP SOLUTIONS

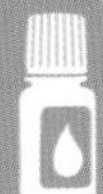

SINGLE OILS

Grapefruit - antioxidant; superb detoxifier of fat, liver, gallbladder (pg. 114)

Lemon - antioxidant; superb detoxifier of fat, chemicals, urinary, liver, lymph (pg. 123)

Lemongrass - powerhouse decongestant for any system of the body (pg. 126)

Clove - powerful antioxidant, blood and cellular cleanser (pg. 97)

By Related Properties

For more, See Oil Properties on pages 477 - 481

Antitoxic - bergamot, black pepper, cinnamon, coriander, fennel, geranium, grapefruit, juniper berry, lavender, lemon, lemongrass, patchouli, thyme

Detoxifier - arborvitae, cassia, celery seed, cilantro, citronella, cypress, geranium, green mandarin, juniper berry, lemon, lime, litsea, patchouli, rosemary, tangerine, turmeric, wild orange, yarrow

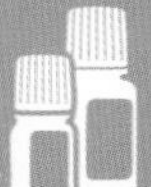

BLENDS

Zendrocrine® - detox liver, gallbladder, gut, kidneys, lungs, skin (pg. 206)

Purify - detox lymph, blood, kidneys, skin (pg. 198)

DDR Prime® - detox lymph, cells, gut, brain (pg. 184)

Slim & Sassy® - detox fat, liver, gallbladder (pg. 200)

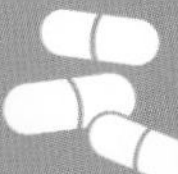

SUPPLEMENTS

Alpha CRS®+, **Zendocrine® Softgels (pg. 224), Zendocrine® Complex (pg. 223)**, Mito2Max®, DDR Prime® Softgels, xEO Mega, TerraZyme®, GX Assist®, MicroPlex VMz

Related Ailments: Acidosis, Alkalosis, Autointoxication, Blood Detoxification, Body Odor, Hangover, Lead Poisoning, Metal Toxicity, Xenoestrogens

Conditions

Blood toxicity - basil, cassia, cinnamon, clove, frankincense, geranium, grapefruit, helichrysum, lemongrass, Roman chamomile, thyme, turmeric, white fir, DDR Prime®, Zendrocrine®; see *Cardiovascular*

Brain - arborvitae, basil, bergamot, cedarwood, clove, frankincense, melissa, rosemary, sandalwood, thyme, turmeric, DDR Prime®

Candida toxicity - arborvitae, basil, lemongrass, melaleuca, oregano, Siberian fir, thyme, yarrow; see *Candida*

Cellular toxicity - arborvitae, clove, frankincense, helichrysum, lemongrass, tangerine, wild orange, yarrow, DDR Prime®; see *Cellular Health*

Cellulite - birch, cypress, Douglas fir, eucalyptus, ginger, grapefruit, lemon, lemongrass, spikenard, thyme, white fir, wild orange, Slim & Sassy®; see *Weight*

Gallbladder toxicity - geranium, grapefruit, lemongrass, lime, tangerine, turmeric, DDR Prime®, Slim & Sassy®, Zendrocrine®; see *Digestive & Intestinal*

Gut toxicity - bergamot, black pepper, cardamom, cinnamon, fennel, ginger, Roman chamomile, tangerine, wild orange, Zendrocrine®, DigestZen®; see *Digestive & Intestinal*

Heavy metal toxicity* - arborvitae, black pepper, cilantro, clove, coriander, frankincense, geranium, grapefruit, helichrysum, juniper berry, rosemary, thyme, Purify, Zendrocrine®

Kidney/urinary toxicity - bergamot, blue tansy, cardamom, cassia, cilantro, coriander, eucalyptus, fennel, geranium, green mandarin, juniper berry, lemon, lemongrass, rosemary, Siberian fir, thyme, Citrus Bliss®, Motivate®; see *Urinary*

Liver toxicity - basil, bergamot, citronella, clove, copaiba, cypress, dill, geranium, grapefruit, green mandarin, helichrysum, juniper berry, lemon, lemongrass, marjoram, peppermint, Roman chamomile, rose, rosemary, turmeric, yarrow, Slim & Sassy®, Zendrocrine®; see *Digestive & Intestinal*

Lymphatic toxicity - arborvitae, cypress, lemon, lemongrass, melaleuca, myrrh, pink pepper, rosemary, tangerine, AromaTouch®, Motivate®, Purify; see *Immune & Lymphatic*

Lung/respiratory toxicity - arborvitae, blue tansy, cardamom, cedarwood, cinnamon, Douglas fir, eucalyptus, lemon, lemongrass, lime, Breathe®, Motivate®, On Guard®, Purify, Zendrocrine®; see *Respiratory*

Nerve toxicity - arborvitae, basil, bergamot, black pepper, cypress, frankincense, ginger, helichrysum, lemongrass, myrrh, patchouli, peppermint, Balance®; see *Nervous*

Pancreas toxicity - cilantro, cinnamon, citronella, coriander, lemongrass, rosemary

Parasite, intestinal toxicity - blue tansy, clove, fennel, oregano, Roman chamomile, thyme, turmeric, On Guard®; see *Parasites*

Skin toxicity* - cedarwood, frankincense, geranium, lavender, lemon, myrrh, sandalwood, vetiver, turmeric, yarrow, ylang ylang, HD Clear®, Immortelle; see *Integumentary*

Xenoestrogen toxicity - clary sage, ginger, grapefruit, lemon, neroli, oregano, thyme, ClaryCalm®, DDR Prime®, Zendrocrine®; see *Men's or Women's Health*

DETOXIFICATION

* *See remedy on pg. 273*

Why Detox?

The body stores toxins in fat to keep harmful substances away from critical organs and functions whenever possible. During a detox program, when nutrients are provided and proper dietary parameters are observed, the body releases toxins and excess fat. Long-lasting results can be achieved when diet and lifestyle habits are supportive.

Detox Response Too Intense?

The most common detox discomfort is diarrhea, which often indicates a lack of probiotics and fiber or simply pushing the body too fast. Solutions may include increased consumption of dietary or supplemental fiber and/or probiotics, and if necessary, cut back on detox products. For example, to ease diarrhea, cut back on Zendrocrine® or DDR Prime® Softgels; if constipation is an issue, increase the same products along with TerraZyme®. If additional adverse symptoms occur - congestion, skin eruptions, etc., see the correlating section of this book for suggested solutions - *Respiratory, Integumentary*, etc.

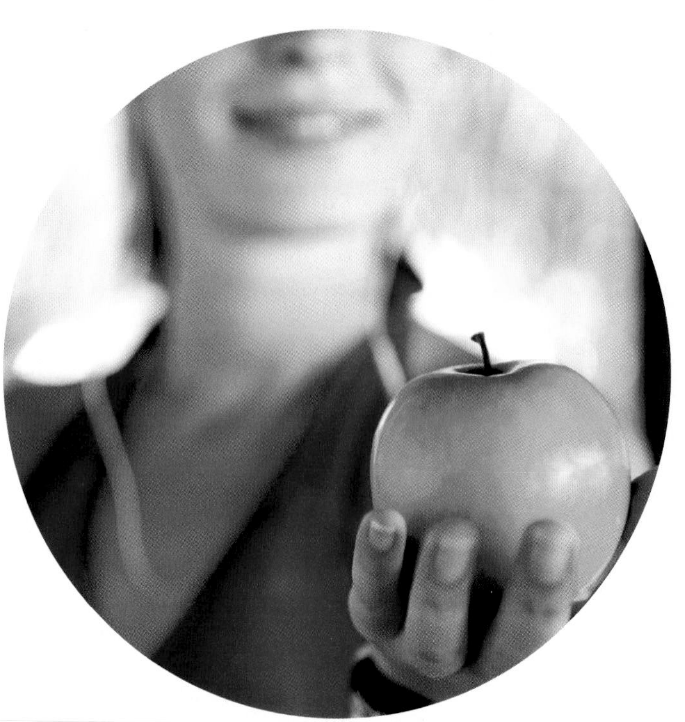

DETOXIFICATION

Basic Detox Program

TWO-WEEK PROGRAM	
CLEAN UP DIET	
Make necessary dietary adjustments to achieve results. If desired detox results are not being achieved, make additional dietary adjustments. Eliminate refined sugars, junk foods, and dairy. Increase consumption of fruits and vegetables. Eat a high-fiber diet.	
PROVIDE IMPORTANT NUTRIENTS AND SUPPORT GUT HEALTH	
MicroPlex VMz	1-2 capsules AM and PM
xEO Mega	1-2 capsules AM and PM
Alpha CRS®+	1-2 capsules AM and PM
TerraZyme®	1-2 capsules with meals BONUS: 1-2 capsules on empty stomach in AM
PB Assist®+	2 at bedtime
USE DETOX TOOLS	
Lemon oil	3 drops in 24 ounces water three times a day
Zendocrine® Complex	1-2 capsules AM and PM
Zendocrine®	5-8 drops in capsule with dinner or 1-2 softgels

BONUS	
SUPERCHARGE CLEANSE	
DDR Prime® Softgels	5-10 drops in capsule or 1-2 softgels twice daily
DAILY ENERGY SUPPORT	
Mito2Max®	1-2 capsules AM and afternoon as needed
TISSUE RELEASE	
Oil Touch technique	Weekly
TARGET EMOTIONS	
When negative emotions are retained, so are toxins. They are inextricably and chemically connected. Consider targeting toxic emotional states during a program. Use grounding blend or choose your own. See *Mood & Behavior* to select emotion(s) and oil(s) for program.	

Dosage levels are determined by body weight, tolerance, and results. Adjust accordingly.

*To take a detox commitment to the next level, see *Weight* or *Candida* for additional detox, weight management, and candida clearing programs.

Remedies

HEAVY METAL DETOX
2 drops geranium
4 drops helichrysum
2 drops lavender
3 drops cilantro
2 drops cypress
2 drops frankincense
Combine oils in a roller bottle. Fill with fractionated coconut oil. Apply to eustachian tubes and neck in downward motion.

FOOT SOAK DETOX
1 cup Epsom salt
1 cup baking soda
⅓ cup sea salt
⅓ cup Redmond Clay powder
Selected essential oil(s)
- Mix the dry ingredients only in a mason jar and store with a lid. When a foot soak is desired, put ¼ cup of dry ingredients in foot bath tub, then mix in oils.
- Add enough warm-to-hot (100-115 degrees F) water to cover feet completely.
- Choose 3-4 drops of one or more of selected oils to direct detox to a specific areas of focus. See "Conditions" list for suggestions.

DETOX BODY SCRUB
2 cups salt or sugar (e.g. sea salt, mineral salts, organic sugar)
1 cup almond oil
4 drop wild orange
4 drops basil
4 drops lemongrass
4 drops lime
4 drops thyme
4 drops rosemary
4 drops grapefruit
4 drops lavender
Combine ingredients and store in a glass jar. Apply desired amount and gently massage into skin for exfoliation; rinse.

EVERYDAY MORNING DETOX
1 tablespoon organic apple cider vinegar
1 teaspoon honey
2 drops lemon
2 drops ginger
1 drop cinnamon
10 ounces warm water
Combine in a glass and drink.

SKIN DETOX
½ cup of aluminum-free baking soda
A few tablespoons of fractionated coconut oil
4 drops lavender
3 drops rosemary
3 drops melaleuca
Create a paste; add more or less coconut oil to achieve desired consistency. Use in shower as cleanser and exfoliator. Apply all over the body and gently scrub for a few minutes; then rinse. Repeat at least twice a week. The skin naturally serves as a pathway for detoxification. Keeping the skin clean and open will aid the body in the detoxification process.

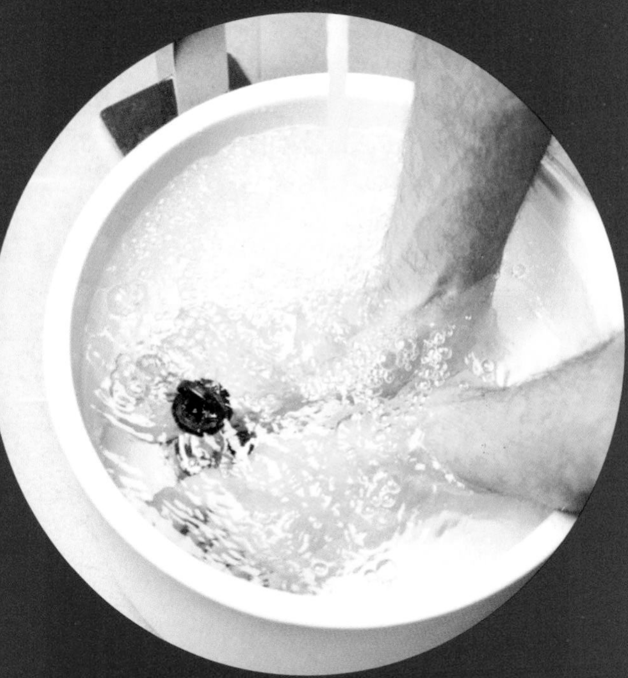

For more Detoxification ideas download the app at app.essentiallife.com

USAGE TIPS: For detoxification, various methods will contribute to success. Here are a few to focus on:
- **Internal:** Taking essential oils and supplements internally is one of the most effective ways to deliver detox "instructions" to specific organs and tissues. Consume oils in a capsule, place under tongue, or in water to drink to accomplish these targeted efforts.
- **Topical:** Invite tissue and organs to release fat and toxins by directly applying oils to specific areas of focus. Massage after application to ensure absorption. Applying oils to the bottoms of the feet will have a direct impact on blood and lymphatic fluids of the body, which is vital to detoxification. Additionally, use the Oil Touch technique to increase the success of a detox program.
- **Aromatic:** Consider addressing toxic emotional states during a program, as mood directly impacts health. Negative emotions and toxins are inextricably and chemically connected. Aromatic application immediately and directly impacts the amygdala, the center of emotions in the brain. See *Mood & Behavior* to select emotion(s) and oils that will best support a detox program.

Oil pulling

Oil pulling is an ancient practice and cleansing technique that involves the simple swishing of a specific oil in the mouth for a few minutes each day. One of the main purposes for the habit is "pulling" a variety of toxins from the bloodstream. Some of the benefits include improved gum health, whiter teeth, clear skin, elimination of bad breath, and a healthy complexion. A wide range of additional benefits have been reported that include positive changes in cellular health, immunity, and the ridding of unwanted toxins such as heavy metals and microorganisms, resulting in more energy, and much more. To increase benefits, add an essential oil that targets an area of interest. For example, add frankincense or lemon to support blood cleansing or detoxification respectively or clove for teeth health.

INSTRUCTIONS

- Oil pulling is to be done first thing in the morning on an empty stomach prior to consumption of any liquids (including water) or foods. It is not recommended to be done at any other time of day.
- Choose a "swishing" oil. Some of the top choices include: sesame, sunflower, olive (cold-pressed, extra virgin), coconut, cod liver, cedar nut, avocado, walnut, castor, black cumin, safflower. Each oil has particular properties that bring specific results. There is a lot of information available on oil pulling and the various oils both online and in written resources.
- Choose an essential oil that supports your particular health concern. Use suggestions in "By Related Properties" or "Conditions" sections of any body system for ideas.

STEP ONE

Pour one tablespoon of selected "swishing" oil in mouth. Add 1-2 drops of chosen essential oil(s) - up to 5 if desired. Older children can also do pulling with less quantity of oil provided they have the ability to not swallow it.

STEP TWO

Swish oil around in mouth. DO NOT swallow it. Move it around in mouth and through teeth, using the tongue to create the movement. Do not tilt head back. The oil will begin to get watery as it mixes with saliva. Keep swishing. If jaw muscles get sore while swishing, relax jaw and use tongue more to help move liquid. This is a gentle and relaxed process that lasts for about twenty minutes. When done correctly, it feels comfortable, especially with repeated practice. As the oil/saliva mixture is saturated with toxins, it may become more whitish or milk-like in consistency, depending on oil used. Each session varies in results and timing for such an effect. Again, twenty minutes is the general rule.

STEP THREE

As the end of the oil pulling session approaches, spit the oil out in a trash can - not down the drain (can clog the drain). Rinse mouth with warm water. Adding salt to the water (use a good quality sea salt or such) adds antimicrobial action, can soothe any inflammation or irritation, and is effective in rinsing out any residual mouth toxins.

TIP: If experiencing an urge to swallow during pulling session prior to the twenty minute mark (for example, its become too unpleasant), spit the oil out and begin again and resume the session until the above described change in the liquid has occurred to indicate completion. With practice, these urges, if present, diminish over time.

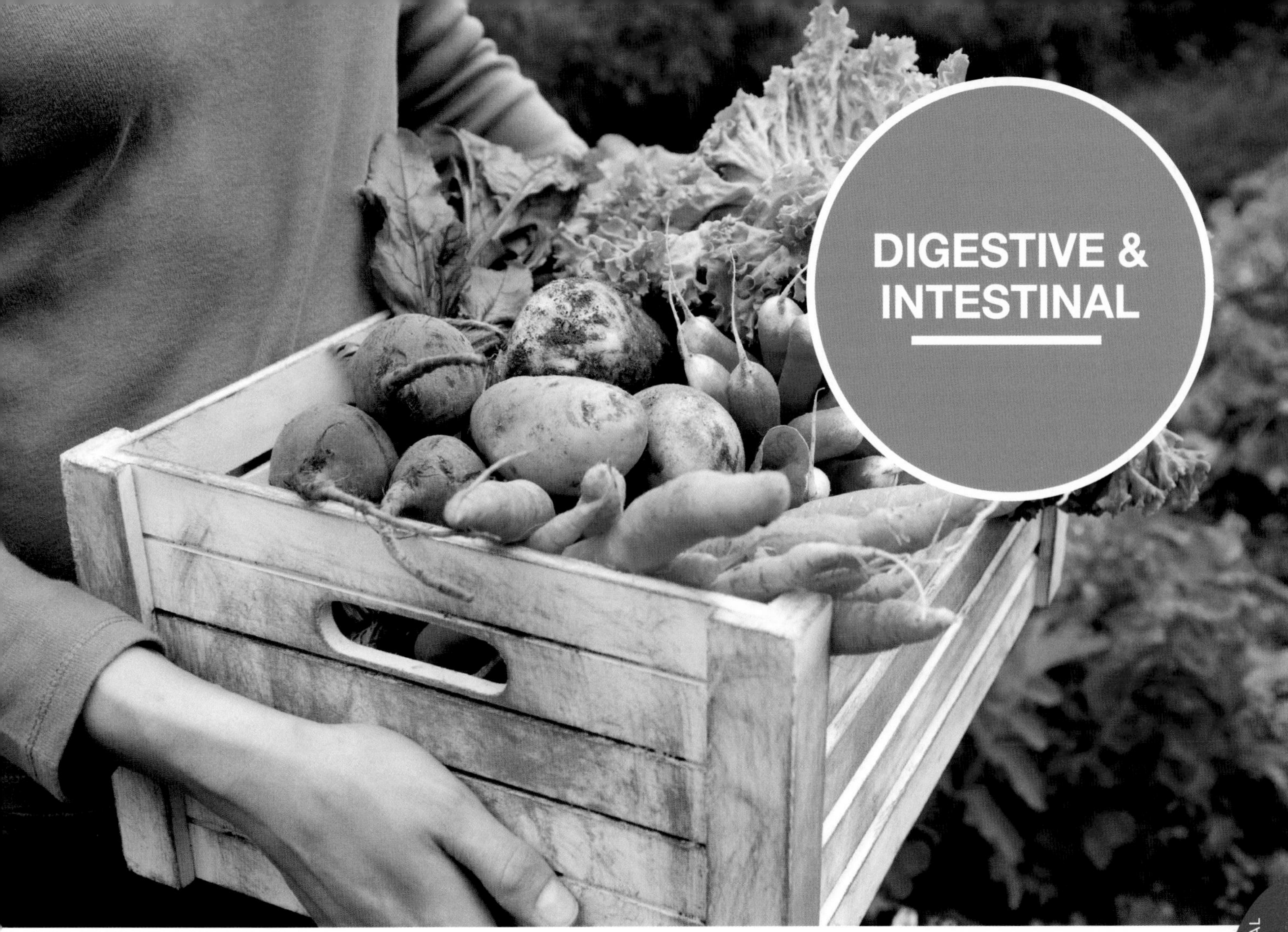

THE DIGESTIVE SYSTEM is comprised of the gastrointestinal (GI) tract and is a series of connected organs along a thirty-foot pathway responsible for chewing food, digesting and absorbing nutrients, and expelling waste. The organs involved in the digestive process are the mouth (chewing), the esophagus (swallowing), the stomach (mixing food with digestive juices), small intestine (mixing food with digestive juices of the pancreas, liver/gallbladder, and intestine, and pushing food forward for further digestion), large intestine (absorbing water and nutrients, changing remaining waste into stool), and the rectum (storing and expelling stool from the body).

The digestive tract works closely with the immune system to protect the body from pathogens and invaders. The GI tract is exposed to high quantities of outside substances including bacteria and viruses and can almost be considered to be an exterior body surface. Without the immune system (lymphoid tissue in the GI produces about 60 percent of the total immunoglobulin produced daily), the long, dark, moist GI tract would be ideal for pathogenic colonization. In return, the digestive system assists the immune system in protecting the rest of the body by breaking down bacteria and pathogens at various stages, starting with lysozyme in the saliva.

There are over one hundred million neurons embedded in the gut, which is more than exist in the spinal column or peripheral nervous system. This mesh-like network of neurons, known as the enteric nervous system (sometimes called the second brain) works together with the central nervous system to oversee every aspect of digestion. It follows then, that brain-gut interactions are highly connected to emotional health; there is a proven correlation between stress, anxiety, and gut disorders such as Crohn's disease and irritable bowel syndrome.

Digestive and eliminative problems are becoming increasingly more prevalent. They create pain, gas, bloating, excessive diarrhea, inability to absorb nutrients, and more. Mood management and emotional health issues are also on the rise. How can the neurons embedded in the gut influence healthy emotions when inflammation, blockages, candida, and other harmful bacteria are overpopulated and system imbalances are standard? They can't.

When digestive system problems are present, natural remedies offer ample opportunity for balance and restoration (see *Candida* section for additional understanding of GI tract imbalances). Start with good nutrition, clear the primary pathways of elimination so waste and toxins can be eliminated, use essential oils specifically targeted to help remove harmful bacteria, take a good prebiotic to encourage growth of good bacteria, and ingest a probiotic to repopulate the gut with live strains of helpful bacteria. Re-establishing health and balance in the gut can literally be a life-changing experience.

TOP SOLUTIONS

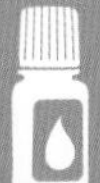

SINGLE OILS

(sorted by ailment)

Stomach - black pepper, cardamom, fennel, ginger, wild orange

Stomach/intestinal lining - grapefruit, peppermint

Intestines - basil, cardamom, ginger, green mandarin, marjoram, peppermint

Liver - basil, cilantro, geranium, grapefruit, helichrysum, lemon, rosemary

Gallbladder - geranium, grapefruit, turmeric

Pancreas - dill, fennel, geranium, ginger, thyme

By Related Properties

For more, See Oil Properties on pages 477 - 481

Calming - basil, blue tansy, celery seed, copaiba, coriander, jasmine, litsea, oregano, Roman chamomile, sandalwood, tangerine, vetiver, yarrow
Carminative - basil, bergamot, blue tansy, cardamom, cassia, cilantro, cinnamon, clary sage, clove, copaiba, coriander, cypress, dill, fennel, ginger, jasmine, juniper berry, lavender, lemon, lemongrass, litsea, melissa, myrrh, neroli, oregano, patchouli, peppermint, Roman chamomile, rose, rosemary, sandalwood, spearmint, tangerine, thyme, vetiver, wild orange, wintergreen, yarrow
Detoxifier - arborvitae, cassia, cilantro, citronella, cypress, dill, geranium, green mandarin, lavender, lime, litsea, patchouli, tangerine, turmeric, yarrow
Digestive Stimulant - basil, bergamot, black pepper, cardamom, celery seed, cinnamon, clary sage, coriander, dill, fennel, frankincense, grapefruit, helichrysum, juniper berry, lemon eucalyptus, lemongrass, litsea, marjoram, melaleuca, myrrh, oregano, patchouli, spearmint, tangerine, wild orange, yarrow
Laxative - bergamot, black pepper, blue tansy, cilantro, copaiba, fennel, ginger, lemongrass, tangerine, yarrow
Regenerative - basil, frankincense, geranium, helichrysum, lavender, manuka, myrrh, neroli, wild orange, yarrow
Stimulant - arborvitae, basil, birch, black pepper, blue tansy, cardamom, cedarwood, cinnamon, dill, fennel, ginger, grapefruit, juniper berry, Siberian fir, spearmint, tangerine, thyme, vetiver, white fir, wintergreen
Stomachic - basil, blue tansy, cardamom, celery seed, cinnamon, clary sage, coriander, fennel, ginger, green mandarin, juniper berry, marjoram, melissa, peppermint, pink pepper, rose, rosemary, tangerine, turmeric, wild orange, yarrow

USAGE TIPS: for best effect on digestive and intestinal activity:

- **Internal:** Place 1-5 drops in water and drink, take in capsule, lick off back of hand, or place drop(s) on or under tongue to allow impact directly in stomach and intestines.
- **Topical:** Apply oils topically on abdomen and/or bottoms of feet for relief.

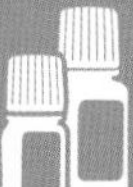

BLENDS

DigestZen® - supports digestion and elimination (pg. 186)

Slim & Sassy® - supports stomach, intestines, pancreas, liver, gallbladder, fat digestion and satiation (pg. 200)

AromaTouch® - supports peristalsis and bowel tone (pg. 169)

Zendrocrine® - supports gallbladder, liver, and pancreas (pg. 206)

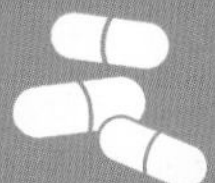

SUPPLEMENTS

Bone Nutrient Lifetime Complex, **PB Assist®+ (pg. 216)**, Zendocrine® Softgels, Zendocrine® Complex, **DigestZen® Softgels (pg. 212)**, DDR Prime® Softgels, xEO Mega, **TerraZyme® (pg. 219)**, **GX Assist® (pg. 213)**, IQ Mega®, MicroPlex VMz

Related Ailments:

- **Digestive:** Abdominal Cramps, Acid Reflux, Bloating, Esophagitis, Flatulence, Food Poisoning [Immune & Lymphatic], Gastritis, GERD, Heartburn, Hemochromatosis, Hernia(Hiatal), Indigestion, Inflammatory Bowel Disease, Metabolism, Motion Sickness, Nausea, Ulcers - Duodenal and Gastric and Peptic, Stomach ache, Vomiting [Detoxification]

- **Intestinal:** Appendicitis, Celiac, Colitis, Constipation, Crohn's Disease, Diarrhea, Dumping Syndrome, Diverticulitis, Dysentery, Giardia [Immune & Lymphatic], Irritable Bowel Syndrome, Leaky Gut Syndrome, Malabsorption Syndrome

- **Liver And Gallbladder:** Cirrhosis, Liver Disease, Gallbladder Infection, Gallbladder Stones, Jaundice [Children]

Remedies

DIGEST-EASE: Combine DigestZen®, Zendrocrine®, and oregano in a capsule; consume to ease digestive discomfort, stomach pain, and bloating.

HOT BATH: Add 10-15 drops of favorite digestive/intestinal soothing oil(s) to bath salts (e.g. Epsom); stir oils into salts; place salts in hot (as is tolerable) bathwater and soak for 20 minutes.

HOT COMPRESS: Apply digestive/intestinal soothing oil(s) with carrier oil to abdomen. Place warm, moist cloth over top to create soothing compress. Repeat as needed.

INTERNALIZE: Consume favorite digestive/intestinal soothing oil(s) internally: drop 1-2 drops under tongue and hold for thirty seconds before swallowing; sip a few drops of oil(s) in a glass of water; take a few drops in a capsule and consume every twenty to thirty minutes until symptoms subside, then reduce exposure to every two to six hours as needed.

MASSAGE MAGIC FOR RELIEF

- Apply oil(s) to abdomen, over stomach or intestinal area depending on location of discomfort.
- Apply oil(s) to bottoms of feet using the reflexology points provided on charts in *Reflexology*.

NAVEL DROP: Drop a single drop of a selected oil into navel for digestive/intestinal relief.

NO MORE NAUSEA: Aromatic use of an oil can reduce influence of nausea-triggering smells:

- Diffuse essential oil(s) of choice to dispel offensive smells or toxic fumes
- Swipe an oil under nose so unpleasant odors are overridden by the essential oil aroma
- Apply a few drops to a cotton handkerchief or such and inhale as needed

TUMMYACHE SOOTHER: Place 1 drop arborvitae in bellybutton to eliminate gas and pain or other digestive discomfort.

CIRRHOSIS OF THE LIVER
4 drops Roman chamomile
2 drops frankincense
2 drops geranium
2 drops lavender
1 drop myrrh
1 drop rosemary
1 drop rose
Place oils in 10ml roller bottle; fill remainder with fractionated coconut oil. Apply to liver area twice per day.

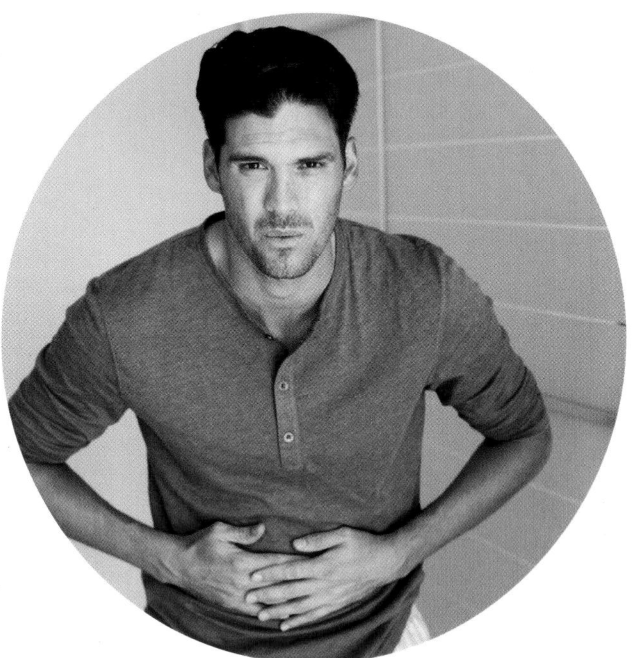

IBS RELIEF
4 drops frankincense
2 drops peppermint
2 drops fennel
2 drops ginger
Combine oils in a capsule; consume three times a day with meals. Also add GX Assist®, PB Assist®+, and a MicroPlex VMz to cleanse and rebuild the gut and to build nutritional strength.

TRAVELER'S DIARRHEA: 3-4 drops DigestZen® in a capsule or in water three times a day.
OR
1 drop each melaleuca and DigestZen® dropped under tongue every thirty minutes until symptoms subside; usually takes about four doses.

CONSTIPATION REMEDY
7 drops wild orange
5 drops coriander
4 drops green mandarin
4 drops DigestZen®
2 drops ginger
Combine in 2-ounce spray bottle; fill about 1/ 2 full of carrier oil. Spray on belly and rub in clockwise motion for three to five minutes.

GUT SUPPORT
2T fractionated coconut oil
2 drops grapefruit or tangerine
2 drops ginger
2 drops blue tansy
1 drop helichrysum
Combine in a roller bottle. Shake gently to blend. Apply to abdomen or inhale to relieve discomfort.

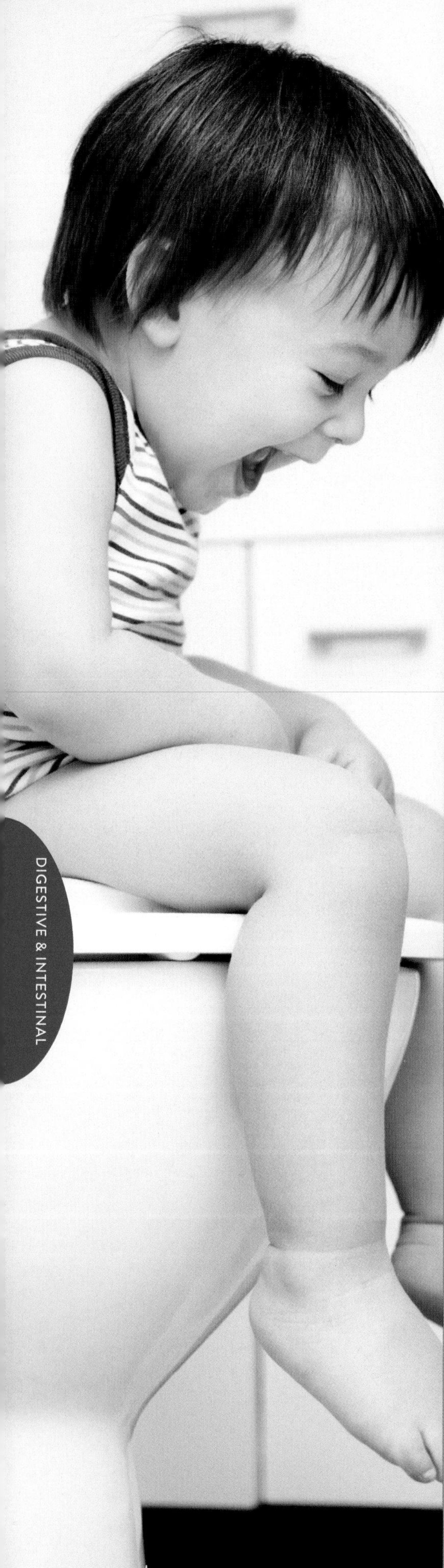

Conditions

Abdominal cramps/pain* - basil, birch, cardamom, cinnamon, clove, copaiba, dill, fennel, ginger, lavender, lemon eucalyptus, lemongrass, marjoram, melissa, patchouli, peppermint, petitgrain, AromaTouch®, DigestZen®, Forgive®, Passion®, Tamer™, Zendrocrine®
Acid reflux/regurgitation - cardamom, dill, fennel, ginger, lemon, peppermint, thyme, DigestZen®
Alcohol-related conditions - See *Addictions*
Anus, itching - cypress, geranium, helichrysum, lavender, oregano (internal), DDR Prime®, Immortelle
Anus, prolapsed - thyme, wild orange
Appendix - basil, ginger, DigestZen®, Zendrocrine®
Appetite, exaggerated - cassia, cinnamon, fennel, ginger, grapefruit, peppermint, Slim & Sassy®
Appetite, reduced/loss of - cardamom, celery seed, ginger, grapefruit, lavender, lemon, wild orange, Motivate®, PastTense®, Peace®, Slim & Sassy®
Belching/burping - cardamom, fennel, ginger, lavender, thyme, vetiver, yarrow, DigestZen®, Zendrocrine®
Bloating/swollen belly - cedarwood, cilantro, dill, ginger, melissa, myrrh, peppermint, pink pepper, tangerine, turmeric, DigestZen®; see *Gaseousness* next page
Bowel constrictions/obstructions - basil, marjoram, rosemary, thyme, Motivate®, Passion®, Zendrocrine®
Bowel inflammation - basil, ginger, peppermint, thyme, DDR Prime®, Zendrocrine®
Bowel, lack of tone - cardamom, ginger, lemongrass, marjoram
Bowel, lining (hyperpermeability/ulcerations) - basil, celery seed, frankincense, geranium, helichrysum, lavender, lemongrass, myrrh, wild orange, DDR Prime®
Bowel, pockets (diverticula) - arborvitae (topical), black pepper, cedarwood (topical), geranium, tangerine, wild orange, Zendrocrine®
Breath, bad (halitosis) - bergamot, cardamom, cilantro, juniper berry, lavender, patchouli, peppermint, spearmint, Cheer®, DDR Prime®, DigestZen®, Slim & Sassy®, Zendrocrine®
Burp, need to - dill, ginger, peppermint
Cirrhosis - frankincense, geranium, helichrysum, lemon, marjoram, myrrh, Roman chamomile, Passion®, Zendrocrine®
Colic - bergamot, black pepper, cardamom, cilantro, clove (dilute), coriander, cypress (topical only), dill, fennel, ginger, lavender, marjoram, Roman chamomile, rosemary, spearmint, wild orange, ylang ylang, Adaptiv®, Cheer®, Console®, DigestZen®, Serenity®, Tamer™
Colon polyps - arborvitae, basil, cardamom, coriander, eucalyptus, frankincense, ginger, lemongrass, peppermint, rosemary, DigestZen®
Constipation/sluggish bowels/inability to defecate despite urgency* - arborvitae, black pepper, cardamom, cilantro, copaiba, dill, Douglas fir, fennel, ginger, green mandarin, kumquat, lemon, lemon eucalyptus, lemongrass, marjoram, patchouli, peppermint, rosemary, spearmint, tangerine, vetiver, ylang ylang, Console®, DigestZen®, Forgive®, Motivate®, Tamer™, Zendrocrine®
Dehydration - green mandarin, lemon, wild orange, Slim & Sassy®
Diarrhea/urgency to pass stool* - arborvitae, black pepper, cardamom, celery seed, cinnamon, clove, coriander, cypress, frankincense, geranium, ginger, jasmine, lemon, lemongrass, melissa, myrrh, patchouli, peppermint, Roman chamomile, spearmint, tangerine, vetiver, wild orange, Cheer®, Console®, DigestZen®, Forgive®, Tamer™, Zendrocrine®
Digestive disorders* - coriander, fennel, ginger, green mandarin, peppermint, tangerine, DigestZen®, Tamer™, Zendrocrine®
Digestion, poor/sluggish* - cassia, cinnamon, coriander, geranium, green mandarin, lemon, lemon eucalyptus, spearmint, Motivate®, Tamer™
Distended abdomen (many possible contributors) - cardamom, fennel, ginger, DigestZen®, Zendrocrine®
Diverticulitis - arborvitae, basil, cedarwood, cilantro, cinnamon, ginger, lavender, DDR Prime®, DigestZen®, Slim & Sassy®, Zendrocrine®
Failure to thrive - patchouli, DDR Prime®
Fat digestion - grapefruit, lemon, tangerine, Slim & Sassy®
Flatulence - black pepper, celery seed, cilantro, coriander, dill, fennel, ginger, lavender, melissa, myrrh, Roman chamomile, rosemary, sandalwood, spearmint, tangerine, DigestZen®, Slim & Sassy®, Zendrocrine®
Food poisoning - black pepper, cinnamon, clove, coriander, juniper berry, lemon, melaleuca, peppermint, oregano, rosemary, thyme, DDR Prime®, DigestZen®, Tamer™, Zendrocrine®
Fullness, uncomfortable (lasts longer than it should) - arborvitae, DigestZen®
Gallbladder, disease - juniper berry, grapefruit, helichrysum, lemongrass
Gallbladder - basil, cypress, geranium,

** See remedy on pg. 277*

grapefruit, helichrysum, lime, rosemary, tangerine, turmeric, DDR Prime®, Slim & Sassy®, Zendrocrine®
Gallstones - bergamot, birch, celery seed, cilantro, clove, geranium, grapefruit, juniper berry, lavender, lemon, lime, patchouli, rosemary, wild orange, wintergreen, DDR Prime®, Forgive®, Peace®, Zendrocrine®
Gaseousness/bloating - black pepper, blue tansy, cardamom, cilantro, cinnamon, clove, dill, fennel, frankincense, geranium, ginger, green mandarin, lavender, lemongrass, lime, melissa, neroli, peppermint, pink pepper, turmeric, DigestZen®, Peace®, Tamer™
Gastric juices, poor production of - cinnamon
Heartburn - black pepper, cardamom, cedarwood (topical), dill, fennel, ginger, green mandarin, lemon, peppermint, wild orange, DDR Prime®, DigestZen®, Slim & Sassy®, Zendrocrine®
Hemorrhoids - cypress, geranium, helichrysum, myrrh, patchouli, Roman chamomile, yarrow, DDR Prime®, DigestZen®, Zendrocrine®
Hiatal hernia - arborvitae, basil, cypress, ginger, helichrysum, melissa, patchouli, peppermint, Zendrocrine®
Hunger pains - fennel, lavender, Slim & Sassy®
Indigestion* - arborvitae, black pepper, blue tansy, dill, ginger, lavender, lemon, lemongrass, melissa, neroli, peppermint, spearmint, thyme, turmeric, ylang ylang, DigestZen®, Passion®, Slim & Sassy®, Tamer™
Indigestion, nervous - cardamom, Tamer™
Inflammation, gut/intestinal - copaiba, fennel, ginger, lemongrass, peppermint, Roman chamomile, spearmint, thyme, turmeric, DigestZen®, Passion®
Intestinal parasites - blue tansy, citronella, clove, fennel, lemon eucalyptus, oregano, thyme
Intestinal peristalsis, lack of/spastic - marjoram, neroli, AromaTouch®, DigestZen®
Jaundice/excess bilirubin - basil, frankincense, geranium, helichrysum, juniper berry, lemon, lemongrass, lime, rosemary, wild orange, Purify, Slim & Sassy®, Zendrocrine®
Lactose issues - cardamom, coriander, dill, lemongrass, DDR Prime®, DigestZen®, TerraZyme®, Zendrocrine®
Leaky gut/gut permeability/weak intestinal lining/malabsorption - arborvitae, cardamom, dill, ginger, grapefruit, lemongrass, myrrh, patchouli, DDR Prime®, DigestZen®
Liver - basil, cilantro, clove, copaiba, cypress, frankincense, geranium, ginger, grapefruit, helichrysum, jasmine, juniper berry, lemon, rosemary, Cheer®, Console®, DDR Prime®, Forgive®, Zendrocrine®
Liver, blocked bile duct/obstruction - cumin, cypress, geranium, marjoram, patchouli, Zendrocrine®
Liver congestion - geranium, helichrysum, peppermint, rose, rosemary, Motivate®
Liver, fatty - grapefruit, lemon, rosemary, turmeric, Slim & Sassy®
Liver headaches/migraines - grapefruit, helichrysum, Zendrocrine®
Liver, hepatitis - copaiba, frankincense, geranium, helichrysum, jasmine, lemon, melaleuca, myrrh, Zendrocrine®
Liver, low bile production - geranium, green mandarin, helichrysum, lavender, peppermint, Roman chamomile, rosemary, Zendrocrine®
Liver, overloaded/sluggish/toxic- celery seed, cilantro, clove, helichrysum, lemon, Motivate®, Zendrocrine®
Liver, scarring - helichrysum, myrrh
Liver, weak - celery seed, dill, geranium, lemon, lime, Roman chamomile, rose
Nausea/motion sickness* - basil, black pepper, cardamom, cassia, clove, coriander, fennel, ginger, lavender, melissa, patchouli, peppermint, petitgrain, pink pepper, Roman chamomile, rosemary, sandalwood, spearmint, DigestZen®, Forgive®, Peace®, Slim & Sassy®, Zendrocrine®
Pancreas* - basil, cinnamon, coriander, dill, fennel, frankincense, geranium, ginger, DDR Prime®, On Guard®, Slim & Sassy®,
Pancreatic, duct blocked - cardamom, helichrysum, Zendrocrine®
Rectal bleeding - geranium, helichrysum, DDR Prime®
Rectal, fissures - geranium, helichrysum, Zendrocrine®
Rectal pain - frankincense, geranium, helichrysum, Zendrocrine®
Saliva, lack of - cardamom
Spasms, digestive - cardamom, cassia, cinnamon, clove, coriander, dill, fennel, spearmint, tangerine, wild orange, Forgive®, Passion®, Tamer™
Spasms, esophageal - wild orange
Stomach, ache/cramp/pain/inflammation* - basil, cardamom, cinnamon, coriander, ginger, helichrysum, peppermint, Roman chamomile, sandalwood, ylang ylang, Citrus Bliss®, Console®, DDR Prime®, DigestZen®, Tamer™, Zendrocrine®
Stomach flu (viral gastroenteritis) - arborvitae, melaleuca, oregano, thyme, Citrus Bliss® (topical), On Guard®, Zendrocrine®
Stomach, lack of tone - black pepper, rose, tangerine
Stomach lining - celery seed
Stomach, nervous (due to worry/anxiety/stress) - black spruce, cardamom, wild orange, Balance®, Serenity®
Stomach, upset (indigestion)* - cardamom, cinnamon, clove, dill, fennel, frankincense, ginger, grapefruit, jasmine, lavender, thyme, wild orange, Citrus Bliss® (topical), Forgive®, Tamer™
Stools, bloody - frankincense, geranium, helichrysum (bleeding); birch, wild orange, wintergreen (ulcer)
Stools, mucus - black pepper, On Guard®, Zendrocrine®
Stools, pale in color/clay-like - Zendrocrine®, DigestZen® Softgels
Swallowing, difficulty (dysphagia) - arborvitae, black pepper, frankincense, lavender, peppermint, wild orange, DDR Prime®, Serenity®
Swallowing, painful/tight throat - cardamom, wild orange, On Guard®, Zendrocrine®
Ulcer, duodenal (located in duodenum/upper intestines) - birch, bergamot, ginger, fennel, frankincense, geranium, myrrh, wintergreen, Adaptiv®, Deep Blue®, DDR Prime®, DigestZen®, Purify, Zendrocrine®
Ulcer, gastric (located in stomach) - bergamot, birch, blue tansy, celery seed, frankincense, geranium, green mandarin, myrrh, peppermint, rose, turmeric, wintergreen, yarrow, Adaptiv®, Console®, DDR Prime®, DigestZen®, Zendrocrine®
Vomiting - basil, black pepper, cardamom, cassia, clove, fennel, geranium, ginger, melaleuca, melissa, patchouli, peppermint, pink pepper, sandalwood, Console®, DigestZen®, Purify, Tamer™, Zendrocrine®
Yeast - See *Candida*

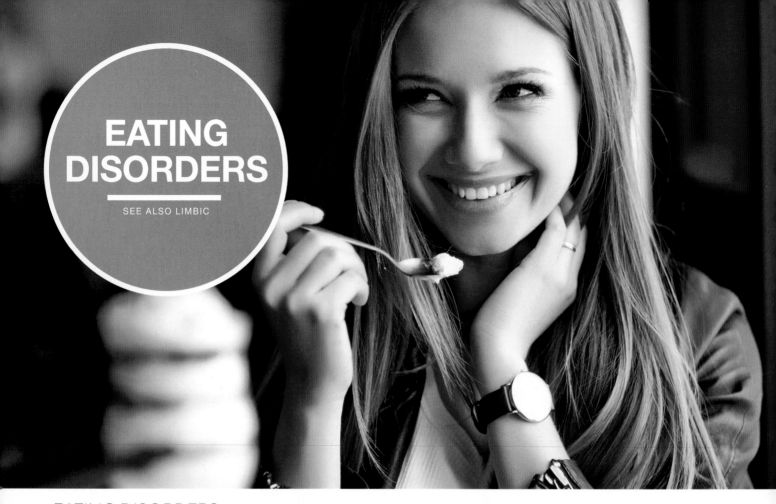

EATING DISORDERS

SEE ALSO LIMBIC

EATING DISORDERS

EATING DISORDERS comprise a group of serious disruptions in eating behavior and weight regulation that adversely impact physical, psychological, and social well being. The most common are anorexia nervosa, bulimia nervosa, and binge-eating disorder. While an individual may start by simply eating more or less food than normal, the tendency increases until he or she is eating portions outside of a healthy range and the urge to manage weight or food intake spirals out of control. While the majority of those with eating disorders are women, men have them also. An exception is binge-eating disorder, which appears to affect almost as many men as women.

Eating disorders are often accompanied by depression, substance abuse, or anxiety disorders. While they can become life-threatening if proper care is not received, it is important to remember that they are treatable medical illnesses. Such treatments usually involve psychotherapy, nutrition education, family counseling, medications, and may include hospitalization.

Anorexia nervosa is characterized by an obsession with food and being thin, even to the point of near starvation. Symptoms of this disorder may include refusal to eat and denial of hunger, intense fear of weight gain, excessive exercising, flat mood or lack of emotion, irritability, fear of eating in public, social withdrawal, trouble sleeping, menstrual irregularities or loss of menstruation (amenorrhea), constipation, abdominal pain, dry skin, irregular heart rhythms.

Alternating episodes of binging and purging are the primary symptoms of bulimia nervosa. During these episodes, an individual typically eats a large amount of food in a short duration and then tries to expel the extra calories through vomiting or excessive exercise. Additional symptoms may include eating to the point of discomfort or pain, laxative use, an unhealthy focus on body shape and weight, going to the bathroom after eating or during meals, abnormal bowel function, damaged teeth and gums, and swollen salivary glands in the cheeks.

Even though eating disorders manifest as a physical condition with physical consequences, many experts in the field believe that they actually originate from an individual's mental or emotional state. Many individuals with eating disorders may suffer from low self-esteem or self-worth or even feel helpless and thus choose to control something that is in their immediate control (the food that does or does not go into their body). Due to the unique direct relationship between emotional and physical well being with eating disorders, natural remedies can be a very effective part of treatment, since they can support individuals emotionally as they work with professionals to learn new habits and ways of coping.

Essential oils have a powerful effect in the brain. Aromas have direct access through the olfactory senses which connect directly to glands and areas such as the hypothalamus and amygdala, allowing oils to initiate rapid responses both physically and emotionally in the brain and the rest of the body. Inhalation and aromatic exposure are powerful methods of impacting the brain with essential oils. Oils offer an extremely effective way of supporting the body with eating disorders.

TOP SOLUTIONS

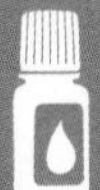

SINGLE OILS

Grapefruit - helps heal relationship with body and curb emotional eating (pg. 114)
Patchouli - supports restoring connection to and acceptance of body (pg. 139)
Bergamot - balances hormones and promotes sense of self-worth (pg. 81)
Cinnamon - balances glucose levels and metabolism; promotes sense of safety (pg. 93)

By Related Properties

For more, See Oil Properties on pages 477 - 481

Analgesic - basil, birch, blue tansy, cinnamon, clary sage, copaiba, cypress, eucalyptus, frankincense, ginger, helichrysum, jasmine, lavender, lemongrass, litsea, melaleuca, oregano, ravensara, Siberian fir, turmeric, wintergreen, yarrow
Antidepressant - bergamot, cinnamon, clary sage, frankincense, geranium, lavender, lemon, lemongrass, neroli, patchouli, pink pepper, rose, sandalwood, tangerine, wild orange, ylang ylang
Antispasmodic - black pepper, blue tansy, cardamom, cassia, clary sage, clove, cypress, fennel, ginger, helichrysum, jasmine, lavender, lemon, litsea, marjoram, melissa, neroli, peppermint, ravensara, rosemary, sandalwood, Siberian fir, spearmint, tangerine, vetiver, wintergreen, yarrow
Calming - bergamot, black pepper, blue tansy, clary sage, copaiba, coriander, geranium, juniper berry, lavender, litsea, oregano, Roman chamomile, tangerine, vetiver, yarrow
Carminative - bergamot, blue tansy, cassia, clary sage, clove, copaiba, dill, fennel, green mandarin, jasmine, juniper berry, lemongrass, litsea, neroli, patchouli, peppermint, sandalwood, spearmint, tangerine, turmeric, wintergreen, yarrow
Energizing - basil, clove, grapefruit, lemongrass, peppermint, rosemary, Siberian fir, tangerine, wild orange, yarrow
Grounding - black spruce, blue tansy, clary sage, cypress, magnolia, melaleuca, Siberian fir, vetiver
Relaxing - blue tansy, cassia, cedarwood, clary sage, cypress, lavender, litsea, manuka, magnolia, marjoram, neroli, ravensara, Roman chamomile, ylang ylang
Stomachic - blue tansy, cardamom, cinnamon, clary sage, fennel, ginger, melissa, pink pepper, rosemary, tangerine, turmeric, wild orange, yarrow

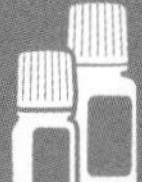

BLENDS

Slim & Sassy® - balances metabolism and insulin (pg. 200)
Balance® - balances emotions and promotes a feeling of tranquility (pg. 170)
Purify - encourages release of toxic emotions (pg. 198)

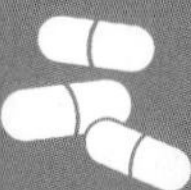

SUPPLEMENTS

Alpha CRS®+, PB Assist®+, **DigestZen® Softgels (pg. 212)**, xEO Mega, **TerraZyme® (pg. 219)**, TerraGreens®, Phytoestrogen Complex, **MicroPlex VMz (pg. 214)**

Related Ailments: Anorexia Nervosa (AN) [Weight], Avoidant/Restrictive Food Intake Disorder (ARFID), Binge Eating Disorder (BED), Bulimia Nervosa (BN) [Weight], Night Eating Syndrome (NES) [Sleep, Weight], Pica, Purging Disorder, Rumination Disorder

USAGE TIPS: Best methods of use for eating disorders

- **Aromatic:** Smell oils of choice, whether diffused, inhaled directly from bottle, swiped under nose, worn as a perfume/cologne, or placed on clothing, bedding, jewelry. Place oils in hands, rub together, cup over nose, inhale. Have on hand for immediate use.
- **Internal:**
  - › Drink oils to satisfy cravings or compulsions by placing a few drops in water.
  - › Plan ahead for typical cravings by taking supportive oils in a capsule prior to when urges hit.
  - › For more instant effects, licking a drop off back of hand to help pacify craving.
  - › Apply oils to roof of mouth (place oil on pad of thumb and then place pad on roof of mouth).
- **Topical:** Apply under nose, behind ears, to base of skull (especially in suboccipital triangles) and forehead, on roof of mouth (closest location to the amygdala; place on pad of thumb, then suck on thumb); for daily grounding, apply to bottoms of feet.

Conditions

Abdominal pain - ginger, lavender; see *Digestive & Intestinal*
Abuse, history of, healing from - frankincense, melissa, Roman chamomile; see *Mood & Behavior*
Anger - basil, bergamot, black spruce, cedarwood, frankincense, helichrysum, magnolia, Roman chamomile, rose, Balance®, InTune®, Serenity®; see *Mood & Behavior*
Anorexia* - bergamot, black pepper, cardamom, cinnamon, coriander, frankincense, ginger, grapefruit, melissa, patchouli, Roman chamomile, rose, vetiver, Citrus Bliss®, Elevation™, Peace®, Serenity®, Slim & Sassy®
Anxiety - bergamot, black spruce, cedarwood, clary sage, frankincense, green mandarin, lavender, magnolia, pink pepper, tangerine, turmeric, vetiver, wild orange, yarrow, Adaptiv®, Balance®, InTune®, Peace®, Serenity® ; see *Mood & Behavior*
Apathetic/emotionally flat/lack of emotion - lime, ylang ylang; see *Mood & Behavior*
Appetite, lack of/refusal to eat - blue tansy, cardamom, fennel, grapefruit, Slim & Sassy®, red mandarin; see *Digestive & Intestinal*
Appetite, loss of control - ginger, kumquat, peppermint, Slim & Sassy®; see *Digestive & Intestinal, Weight*
Binging/overeating until "stuffed"* - basil, cedarwood, cinnamon, ginger, grapefruit, kumquat, peppermint, thyme, Elevation™, Slim & Sassy®
Bulimia* - arborvitae, bergamot, cinnamon, ginger, grapefruit, melissa, patchouli, Balance®, DigestZen®, Forgive®, Passion®, Slim & Sassy®
Cold, frequently being - cassia, cinnamon, ginger, oregano, patchouli; see *Cardiovascular*
Constipation - cardamom, cilantro, fennel, ginger, green mandarin, lavender, lemongrass, marjoram, DigestZen®, Tamer™, Zendrocrine®; see *Digestive & Intestinal*
Control, feeling out of, of behavior - black spruce, Adaptiv®; See *Mood & Behavior*
Dehydration - cypress, juniper berry; see *Urinary*
Denial of hunger - cardamom, fennel, Slim & Sassy®
Depression - bergamot, grapefruit, magnolia, wild orange, ylang ylang, Adaptiv®, Cheer®, Elevation™; see *Mood & Behavior*
Digestive issues - cardamom, fennel, ginger, green mandarin, peppermint, lavender, DigestZen®, Tamer™; see *Digestive & Intestinal*
Dry skin - cedarwood, geranium, myrrh, patchouli, sandalwood, Immortelle; see *Integumentary*
Emotionality/overly emotional - cypress, geranium, Adaptiv®
Excessive exercising - cypress, patchouli, vetiver, Balance®, Purify
Expressing/managing emotions/feelings, difficulty - Balance®, InTune®; see *Mood & Behavior*
Family patterns/runs in family - lemon, white fir
Fear of eating in public - cardamom, wild orange, Serenity®, Slim & Sassy®
Guilt - bergamot, coriander, geranium, lemon, white fir, Breathe®, HD Clear®, Purify, TerraShield®
Gum damage - clove, myrrh, Immortelle; see *Oral Health*
Helpless - cedarwood, clove, ginger, tangerine, white fir, Citrus Bliss®, DigestZen®, On Guard®, PastTense®
Hormone imbalance - See *Men's* or *Women's Health*
Impatient - basil, Breathe®, ClaryCalm®, Elevation™, PastTense®
Intense fear of gaining weight - cypress, juniper berry, melissa
Irregular heartbeat (arrhythmia) - basil, lavender, ylang ylang; see *Cardiovascular*
Irritability - coriander, jasmine, Roman chamomile, rose, tangerine; see *Mood & Behavior*
Loneliness - black spruce, cedarwood, frankincense, marjoram, myrrh, Roman chamomile, Citrus Bliss®, Immortelle, Purify,
Low blood pressure - basil, cardamom, helichrysum, lavender, lime, rosemary, DDR Prime®, Purify; see *Cardiovascular*
Low self-esteem/self-worth - bergamot, cassia, grapefruit, jasmine, lemon, patchouli, rose, spearmint, tangerine, Slim & Sassy®; see *Mood & Behavior*
Menstrual irregularities or loss of menstruation (amenorrhea) - basil, clary sage, fennel, geranium, juniper berry, rosemary, ylang ylang, ClaryCalm®; see *Women's Health*
Obsessive/compulsive - oregano, Adaptiv®, Balance®, Serenity®; see *Mood & Behavior*
Out of sync with natural urges of body - thyme, Forgive®
People-pleasing - black pepper, cinnamon, lavender, lime, peppermint, Purify
Perfectionistic - cypress, melissa, tangerine, Balance®, TerraShield®

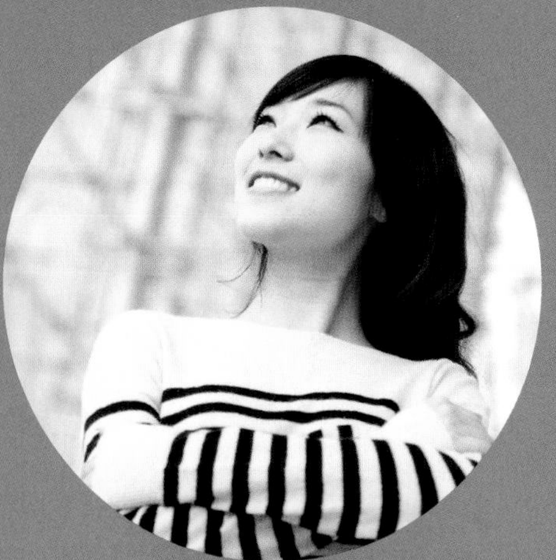

Preoccupation with food - cypress, grapefruit, lavender, vetiver, Elevation™
Purging urge - Douglas fir, lime, patchouli, rose, tangerine, wintergreen, Slim & Sassy®, Zendrocrine®
Self image, distorted/negative - bergamot, grapefruit, spearmint, Slim & Sassy®
Shame - bergamot, cypress, Douglas fir, frankincense, thyme, On Guard®
Shame, body - grapefruit, patchouli, Slim & Sassy®
Social withdrawal - cassia, cinnamon, cedarwood, frankincense, ginger, myrrh, spearmint
Sores, throat and mouth - frankincense, lemon, melaleuca, melissa, myrrh, thyme, Breathe®, DDR Prime®; see *Oral Health*
Sores, scars, calluses on knuckles or hands - see *Integumentary*
Stress - black spruce, frankincense, lavender, lime, ylang ylang, wild orange, Adaptiv®, Citrus Bliss®, Elevation™, Serenity®; see *Stress*
Swollen salivary glands in cheeks - marjoram, vetiver, Citrus Bliss®, Elevation™, PastTense®, Purify
Teeth damage - birch, clove, helichrysum, wintergreen, On Guard®; see *Oral Health*
Trouble sleeping - lavender, vetiver, Serenity®; see *Sleep*
Vomiting, addiction to forcing - Douglas fir, fennel, ginger, grapefruit, lavender, DigestZen®, Slim & Sassy®

EATING DISORDERS

** See remedy on pg. 283*

Remedies

ANOREXIC ASSIST
2 drops vetiver
4 drops bergamot
Combine and diffuse around meal times or during emotional vulnerability.

BULIMIA OR ANOREXIA: Place one drop of bergamot, grapefruit oils and DigestZen® under tongue each morning. Inhale oils of choice (choose what aroma is most impactful) throughout day. Can be inhaled from bottle, diffused or worn. Additionally, take a few drops during the day internally in water or in a capsule. Choose from bergamot, cinnamon, grapefruit, melissa, patchouli, thyme, DigestZen®, and Slim & Sassy®. Combine or use individually. Suggestions:
- Drink 2 drops cinnamon + 3 drops grapefruit in glass of water
- Wear 3 drops patchouli + 2 drops bergamot as a perfume on wrists, neck, etc.
- Combine 2 drops cinnamon, 3 drops melissa, 2 drops thyme, 3 Slim & Sassy® in a capsule and consume.

OVEREATING CONTROL
2 drops black pepper
2 drops ginger
2 drops grapefruit
2 drops lemon
2 drops peppermint
Apply to bottoms of feet or take in a capsule before eating. Additionally, diffuse any of the oils.

KILL SUGAR CRAVINGS
Choose one or more as needed:
- Use 1-3 drops of basil (smell)
- Cinnamon (lick, drink)
- Grapefruit (drink, smell)
- Thyme (capsule) and/or
- Slim & Sassy® (drink, capsule)

For more ideas, download the app at app.essentiallife.com

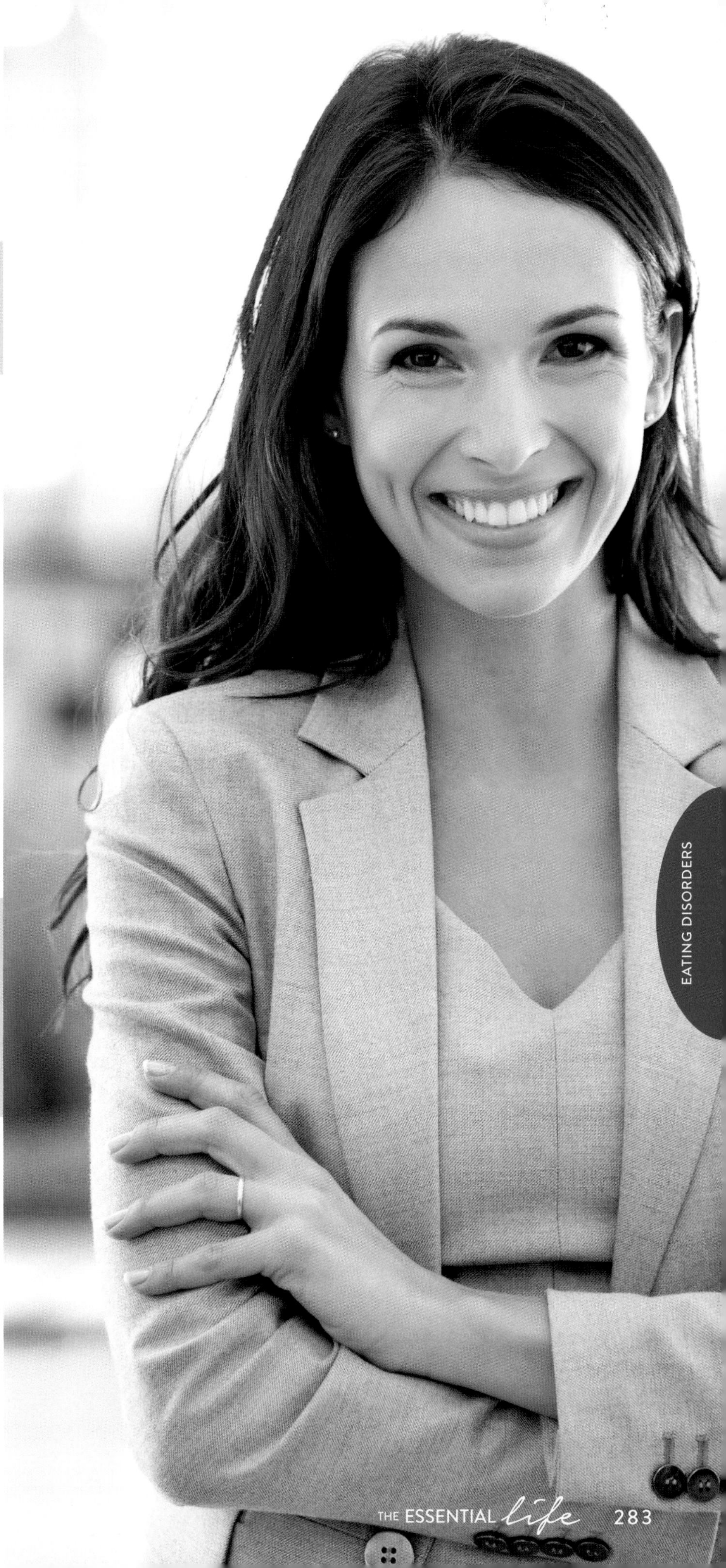

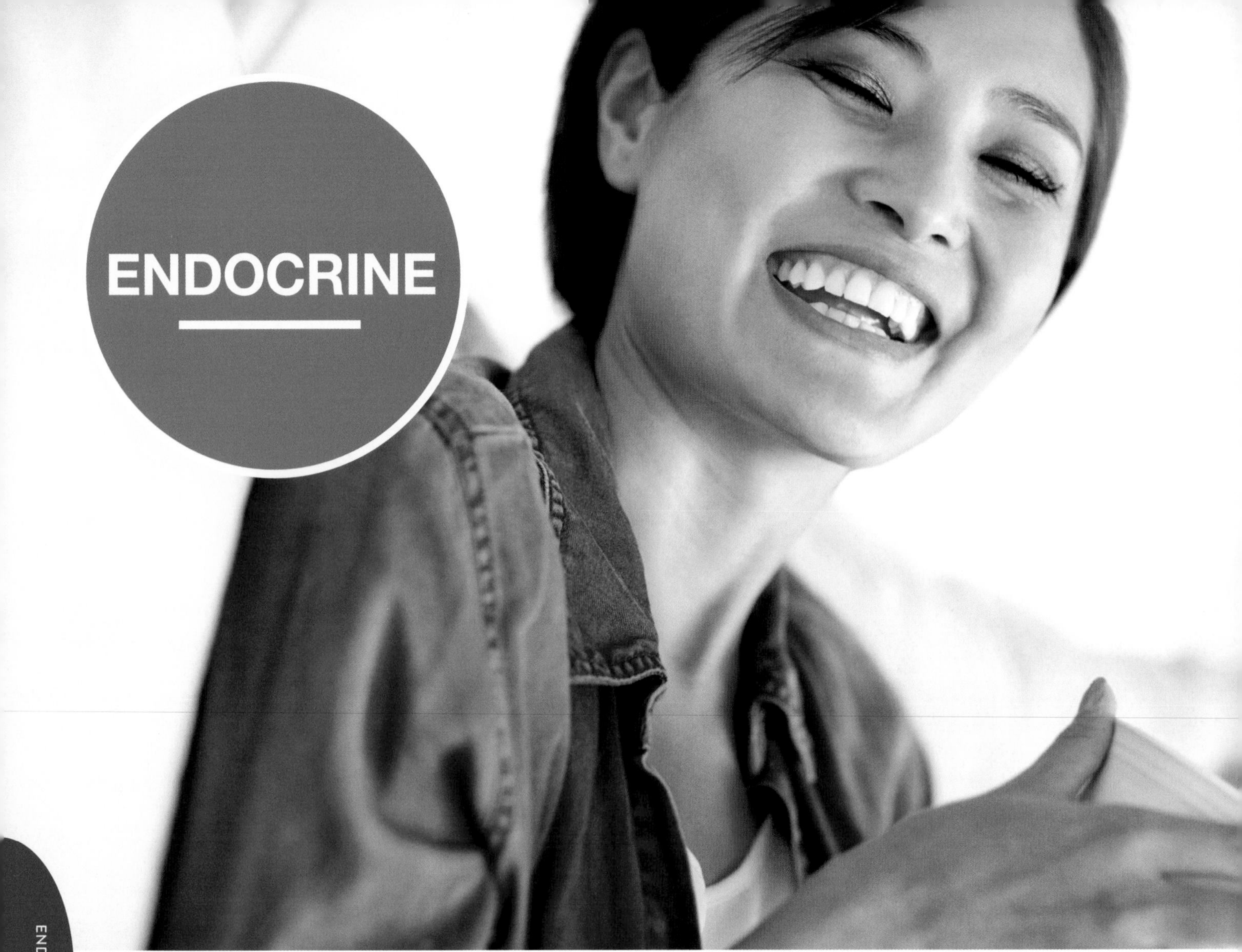

ENDOCRINE

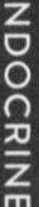

THE ENDOCRINE SYSTEM consists of glands in the body that produce and secrete hormones directly into the circulatory system. The hormones are carried to targeted organs and tissues where they bind only to cells with necessary specific receptor sites. The endocrine system is responsible for bodily functions and processes such as cell growth, tissue function, sleep, sexual and reproductive functions, metabolism, blood sugar management, how the body responds to injuries and stress, energy, water and electrolyte balance, and more. It basically tells the cells in the body exactly what to do.

The glands of the endocrine system include the pituitary gland (the master gland which helps regulate the other glands within the endocrine system), pineal gland, thyroid and parathyroid glands, adrenal glands, hypothalamus, thalamus, pancreas, gastrointestinal tract and reproductive glands (ovaries/testicles). Many organs that are part of other body systems (such as the liver, kidneys and heart) also secrete hormones, and this is recognized as a secondary endocrine function. The exocrine system also secretes hormones, but uses glands with ducts -- such as sweat glands or salivary glands -- to deliver these secretions.

Endocrine disorders are common, and include such conditions as obesity, thyroid malfunction, and diabetes. Endocrine disorders typically occur when hormone levels are too high or too low, a condition that can be caused by unregulated hormone release, cellular messaging problems (lack of response to signaling), when endocrine glands are not operating at full capacity, or when important organs/tissues become enlarged or malfunctioned. Stress, electrolyte or fluid imbalances in the blood, infection, tumors, and medication can also affect endocrine function. Hypofunction of endocrine glands means there isn't enough endocrine activity, whereas hyperfunction refers to too much activity; both types of imbalance can cause serious problems.

Because of the unique delivery system of the endocrine system (sending hormones to targeted organs & tissues via the circulatory system), essential oils can be especially beneficial since they use the same delivery system! Essential oils are able to profoundly benefit cells they encounter throughout the body as they circulate. There are also specific oils that have been shown to be incredibly supportive with certain gland/organ functions. Individuals can work together with their medical providers, when necessary, to consider the benefits of natural solutions as well as modern medical treatment options.

TOP SOLUTIONS

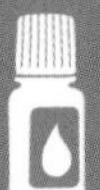

SINGLE OILS

Frankincense and sandalwood - for pineal, pituitary, and hypothalamus support (pg. 110)
Geranium and ylang ylang - hormone/glandular and adrenal support (pgs. 112 & 165)
Blue tansy, clove and lemongrass - for thyroid support (pgs. 86, 97 & 126)
Rosemary - stimulates glands and brain function; adrenal support (pg. 149)

By Related Properties

For more, See Oil Properties on pages 477 - 481

Anti-inflammatory - arborvitae, basil, blue tansy, cassia, cinnamon, clary sage, clove, copaiba, eucalyptus, fennel, helichrysum, jasmine, lemongrass, litsea, manuka, myrrh, neroli, patchouli, peppermint, pink pepper, rosemary, Siberian fir, spikenard, tangerine, turmeric, yarrow
Calming - basil, black pepper, blue tansy, cassia, copaiba, frankincense, green mandarin, juniper berry, litsea, magnolia, melissa, oregano, Roman chamomile, tangerine, yarrow
Detoxifier - arborvitae, cilantro, citronella, geranium, green mandarin, lime, litsea, tangerine, turmeric, yarrow
Regenerative - clove, coriander, helichrysum, manuka, neroli, sandalwood, wild orange, yarrow
Relaxing - blue tansy, cedarwood, clary sage, geranium, litsea, manuka, marjoram, myrrh, neroli, white fir
Sedative - basil, bergamot, blue tansy, coriander, geranium, lavender, magnolia, melissa, neroli, patchouli, rose, spikenard, tangerine, ylang ylang, yarrow
Stimulant - basil, blue tansy, cardamom, cinnamon, coriander, dill, ginger, grapefruit, myrrh, Siberian fir, spearmint, tangerine
Uplifting - bergamot, clary sage, lemon, litsea, tangerine
Vasodilator - lemongrass, marjoram, rosemary, Siberian fir, thyme

Related Ailments:

- **Adrenal:**
  Addison's Disease [located in Autoimmune], Adrenal Fatigue/Exhaustion, Cortisol Imbalance, Cushing's Syndrome
- **Pancreas:**
  Pancreas, Pancreatitis; for all other pancreas ailments related to blood sugar management, see the following section, Blood Sugar
- **Thyroid:**
  Goiter, Night sweats [Immune & Lymphatic, Women's Health], Grave's Disease [located in Autoimmune], Hashimoto's Disease [located in Autoimmune], Hyperthyroidism, Hypothyroidism, Silent Thyroiditis, Thyroid
- **Additional Endocrine Ailments:**
  Acromegaly, Endocrine System, Glands, Growth Problems, Melatonin Imbalances/Insufficiencies, Parathyroid, Pineal, Pituitary, Precocious Puberty, Schmidt's Syndrome (adrenals, thyroid) [located in Autoimmune], Thymus, Turner Syndrome

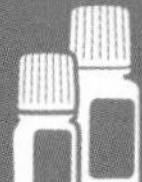

BLENDS

DDR Prime® - nerve repair; glandular support (pg. 184)
Zendrocrine® - adrenal and glandular support (pg. 206)
Whisper® - glandular support and mood stabilizer (pg. 205)

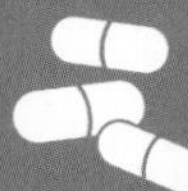

SUPPLEMENTS

Alpha CRS®+, a2z Chewable™, **Mito2Max® (pg. 214)**, DDR Prime® Softgels, **xEO Mega (pg. 222)**, IQ Mega®, MicroPlex VMz

General Gland Support

Adrenal - basil, geranium, rosemary, ylang ylang, Citrus Bliss®, Zendrocrine®
Glandular sluggishness - black spruce, citronella, clove, DDR Prime®
Hypothalamus - cardamom, cedarwood, clove, frankincense, jasmine, sandalwood, Siberian fir, Balance®, DDR Prime®, InTune®
Pancreas - basil, cassia, cinnamon, coriander, dill, eucalyptus, fennel, geranium, ginger, grapefruit, helichrysum, jasmine, lavender, lemon, lemongrass, oregano, rosemary, wild orange, ylang ylang, Cheer®, On Guard®, Serenity®, Slim & Sassy®
Parathyroid - basil, clary sage, clove, geranium, ginger, melissa, Roman chamomile, Balance®, ClaryCalm®
Pineal - arborvitae, basil, cedarwood, frankincense, helichrysum, lavender, sandalwood, Balance®, Immortelle
Pituitary - basil, black spruce, cedarwood, frankincense, geranium, ginger, patchouli, sandalwood, ylang ylang, Citrus Bliss®, DDR Prime®, On Guard®, Purify
Thalamus - clary sage, frankincense, jasmine, melissa, Siberian fir, vetiver, Purify
Thymus - blue tansy, clary sage, lemongrass, Breathe®, On Guard®; see *Immune & Lymphatic*
Thyroid - blue tansy, clove, geranium, lemongrass, myrrh, DDR Prime®, On Guard®, Purify

USAGE TIPS: For endocrine support, a variety of methods can be successful. Suggestions:
- **Internal:** Consume selected oils in capsule, under tongue, or place in water to drink.
- **Topical:** Apply selected oils directly over location of gland or the bottoms of feet on reflex points (see *Reflexology*) twice daily. Use a carrier oil to prevent sensitivity.
- **Aromatic:** Diffuse 5-10 drops of oils of choice, or inhale from product bottle or self-made blend, apply a few drops to clothing, or other inhalation methods.

Conditions

ADRENAL:

Adrenal cortex, sluggish - basil, cinnamon, frankincense, geranium, rosemary, DDR Prime®, On Guard®
Adrenal fatigue/exhaustion* - basil, black pepper, black spruce, geranium, ginger, rosemary, wild orange, ylang ylang, Citrus Bliss®, Console®, Motivate®, Passion®, Zendrocrine®; see *Energy & Vitality*
Constantly feeling sick - bergamot, lemon, DDR Prime®, On Guard®, Zendrocrine®; see *Immune & Lymphatic*
DHEA levels - clary sage, frankincense, geranium, lavender, Roman chamomile, ylang ylang, Whisper®
Difficulty concentrating - cedarwood, vetiver, InTune®; see *Focus & Concentration*
Mild depression - basil, bergamot, geranium, jasmine, magnolia, lavender, wild orange, Cheer®, Citrus Bliss®, Elevation™; see *Mood & Behavior*
Trouble sleeping - lavender; see *Sleep*
Weight gain - ginger, grapefruit, lemon, Slim & Sassy®; see "Thyroid" below, *Weight*

PANCREAS:

Balance cortisol levels - basil, bergamot, black spruce, clove, lavender, magnolia, rosemary, wild orange, ylang ylang, Adaptiv®
Blood sugar issues (too high/too low) - See *Blood Sugar*
Eyesight, poor/vision - coriander, frankincense, geranium, helichrysum, lemongrass, sandalwood, DDR Prime®, Immortelle
Hunger pains - fennel, peppermint; see *Digestive & Intestinal*
Low sex drive - basil, clary sage, wild orange, ylang ylang, Whisper®; see *Intimacy*
Obesity - cinnamon, fennel, ginger, grapefruit, lemon, peppermint, Slim & Sassy®; see *Weight*
Pancreatic duct, congested/blocked - cardamom, clary sage, helichrysum, rosemary
Pancreas, congested - grapefruit, Zendrocrine®; see *Detoxification*
Pancreas sluggish/under-active* - black pepper, helichrysum, lime, Passion®
Pancreas support* - cinnamon, dill, fennel, frankincense, geranium, ginger, Cheer®, Passion®
Pancreatitis - basil, cinnamon, coriander, geranium, lemon, marjoram, rosemary, thyme, DDR Prime®, On Guard®, Slim & Sassy®, Zendrocrine®; see *Immune & Lymphatic*
Urinary issues associated with pancreatic/blood sugar imbalances - See *Blood Sugar, Urinary*

THYROID:

Body temp, cold - black pepper, cinnamon, clove, eucalyptus, ginger, rosemary, On Guard®, Slim & Sassy®; see *Cardiovascular* "Warming" property
Cold intolerance - black pepper, cinnamon, eucalyptus; see *Cardiovascular* "Warming" property
Compromise - basil
Constipation - cardamom, ginger, DigestZen®; see *Digestive & Intestinal*
Cortisol, low - basil, birch, thyme, wintergreen
Cortisol, high - black spruce, cedarwood, clary sage, geranium, lavender, magnolia, marjoram, neroli, ylang ylang, Adaptiv®
Grave's disease - clove, frankincense, ginger, lemongrass, rosemary, On Guard®, Slim & Sassy®; see *Autoimmune*
Hashimoto's - blue tansy, frankincense, ginger, lemongrass, myrrh, patchouli, rosemary, DDR Prime®, On Guard®, Zendrocrine®; see *Autoimmune*
Hair falling out - arborvitae, cedarwood, clary sage, Douglas fir, eucalyptus, frankincense, geranium, juniper berry, Roman chamomile, rosemary, sandalwood, wintergreen, yarrow, ylang ylang, DDR Prime®, Whisper®; see *Integumentary*
Heat intolerance - eucalyptus, peppermint, spearmint, PastTense®
Hyperthyroid* - black spruce, cedarwood, clary sage, clove, frankincense, geranium, ginger, jasmine, juniper berry, lavender, lemon, lemongrass, myrrh, neroli, peppermint, rosemary, sandalwood, ylang ylang, DDR Prime®
Hypothyroid* - bergamot, black pepper, blue tansy, cedarwood, clove, frankincense, geranium, ginger, lemongrass, myrrh, peppermint, spearmint, DDR Prime®, Zendrocrine®
Overheated/night sweats/hot flashes - cedarwood, clary sage, eucalyptus, ginger, lemon, lime, peppermint, AromaTouch®, ClaryCalm®, PastTense®, Whisper®; see "Hypothyroid" above, *Blood Sugar*, *Women's Health*
Thyroid hormones, false - lemongrass, myrrh, neroli; see *Candida*

** See remedy on pg. 287*

ENDOCRINE

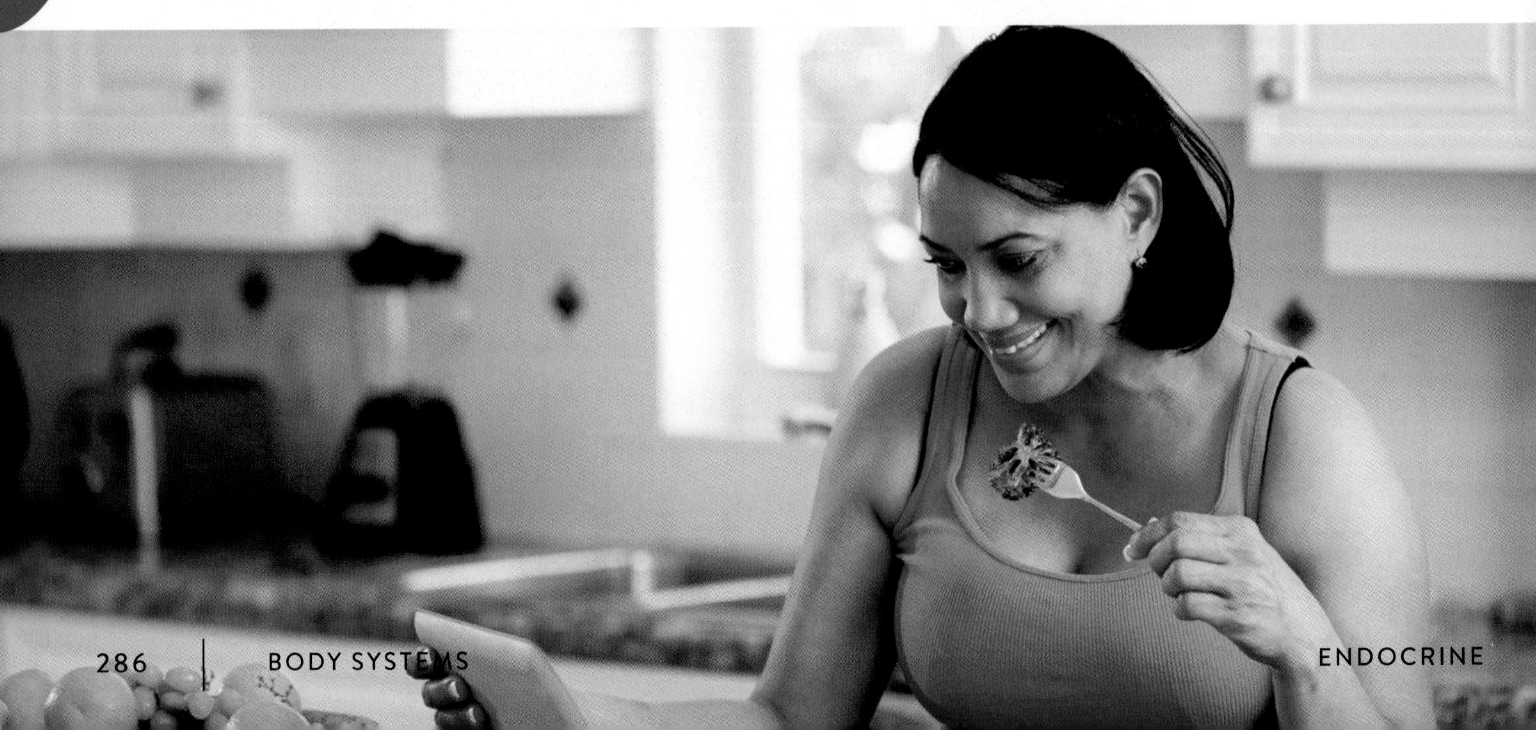

Remedies

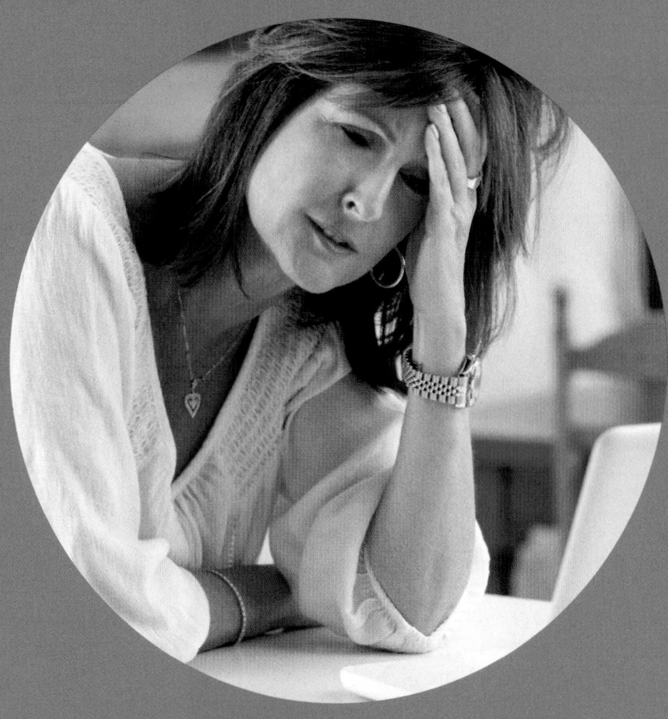

GLANDULAR HEALTH BASIC PROGRAM

- Supplement daily with:
  MicroPlex VMz
  xEO Mega
  Mito2Max®
- Choose from the following for additional support:
  DDR Prime® Softgels and/or DDR Prime®
  Slim & Sassy®
- Consider candida program - see *Candida*

ADRENAL ENERGY PUMP UP - use Mito2Max® 2 capsules twice per day.

ADRENAL AID

3 drops clove
4 drops lemon
3 drops frankincense
7 drops rosemary
Combine in a 5ml bottle/roller bottle, fill remainder with carrier oil. Apply over kidneys (on both sides of back just below rib cage), follow with a warm, damp washcloth as a compress.

SIMPLE ADRENAL SUPPORT

2 drops basil internally in water one to two times per day or massage in 1 drop on back of neck.

PANCREATIC PROMOTER

30 drops basil
25 drops vetiver
25 drops cypress
Combine in 10ml roller bottle, fill remainder with carrier oil. Apply over pancreas (on abdomen just below sternum) morning and evening for pancreatic support.

THYROID BOOST

20 drops clove
20 drops myrrh
25 drops frankincense
15 drops lemongrass
Combine in a 10ml roller bottle, fill remainder with carrier oil. Apply at least once daily over thyroid (on both sides of neck just below Adam's apple).

INTERNAL THYROID ASSIST

- Take DDR Prime® Softgels, morning and evening (may be combined with the thyroid boost treatment).
- Take 2 drops each frankincense, clove, peppermint, 1 drop each myrrh, lemongrass oils in a capsule three times per day.

THYROID CALMER

1 drop myrrh
1 drop lemongrass
Layer a base of carrier oil on thyroid area (on both sides of neck just below Adam's apple) and then massage oils on top. Apply to bottoms of feet focusing on base of big toe.

THYROID REMEDIES

- Use one of following recipes in 10ml roller bottle. Initially, apply directly to thyroid area and/or bottoms of feet two to four times per day to boost activity. As progress is made, apply once or twice per day.
  - Recipe #1: 10 drops myrrh, 10 drops lemongrass, 2-3 drops clove, 2-3 drops peppermint; add carrier oil to fill.
  - Recipe #2: 25 drops each lemongrass, clove, peppermint; fill remainder with carrier oil.
- Other variations:
  - Apply 1 drop of any single oil alone or combine with one or two others to thyroid area twice per day. Use with carrier oil. Choose from:
    - Clove, frankincense, lemongrass, myrrh, Immortelle
    - OR trade off weekly - first week lemongrass and myrrh; second week geranium and Balance®; repeat.

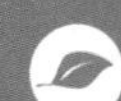

For more ideas, download the app at app.essentiallife.com

ENDOCRINE

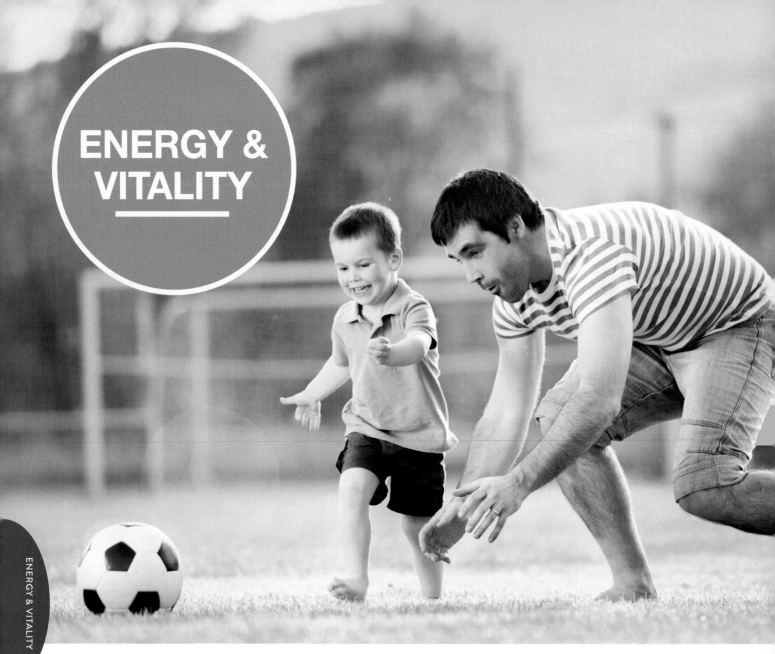

LACK OF ENERGY or diminished vitality can be described as tiredness, weariness, lethargy or fatigue and can contribute to symptoms like depression, decreased motivation, or apathy. Lack of energy can be a normal response to inadequate sleep, overexertion, overworking, stress, lack of exercise, or even boredom. When lack of energy is part of a normal response, it's often resolved with adequate rest and sleep, stress management, and good nutrition.

Persistent lack of energy that does not resolve with routine self-care may be an indication of an underlying physical or psychological disorder. Common causes may include allergies and asthma, anemia, cancer and its treatments, chronic pain, heart disease, infection, depression, eating disorders, grief, sleeping disorders, thyroid problems, medication side effects, alcohol use, or drug use.

Observing patterns and symptoms of lack of energy may be helpful in discovering its cause. Persistent fatigue with no clear diagnosis may result from chronic fatigue syndrome, which can start with a flu-like illness and may not be relieved with rest. Other symptoms, such as cognitive difficulties, long-term exhaustion and illness after activity, muscle or joint pain, sore throat, headache, and tender lymph nodes, are common. Lack of energy by itself is rarely an emergency and can be addressed successfully with effective supplementation and natural solutions. However, if it develops suddenly or is accompanied by other serious symptoms, it may require immediate evaluation to avoid serious complications.

Resolving issues of lack of energy and fatigue can be simple. First considerations include a focus on rest, proper diet, nutrition and supplementation, and balanced blood sugar. Certain essential oils are very effective partners to creating and supporting energy. Basil oil, for example, is superb for overall energy and vitality (if used in higher amounts has the opposite effect - calming). Lemongrass has an overall whole-body stimulating effect. Lavender helps balance body systems where energy might be squandered unnecessarily in one area. Any citrus oil and blend is considered refreshing, uplifting, and rejuvenating. And one of the most popular choices for an immediate, invigorating effect is peppermint oil.

TOP SOLUTIONS

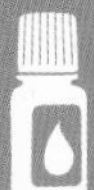

SINGLE OILS

Basil - stimulating and reviving (pg. 80)
Peppermint - invigorating and energizing (pg. 140)
Wild orange - uplifting and rejuvenating (pg. 162)
Lemon - cleansing and refreshing (pg. 123)
Lime - energizing and enlivening (pg. 127)

By Related Properties

For more, See Oil Properties on pages 477 - 481

Antidepressant - basil, bergamot, clary sage, coriander, dill, frankincense, geranium, jasmine, lemongrass, magnolia, neroli, oregano, pink pepper, sandalwood, tangerine, wild orange, ylang ylang
Energizing - basil, clove, cypress, grapefruit, lemongrass, rosemary, Siberian fir, wild orange, yarrow
Immunostimulant - cassia, cinnamon, clove, copaiba, eucalyptus, frankincense, ginger, lemon, lime, melaleuca, melissa, rosemary, Siberian fir, spearmint, vetiver, white fir, wild orange, yarrow
Invigorating - grapefruit, lemon, litsea, peppermint, Siberian fir, spearmint, wild orange, wintergreen
Refreshing - cypress, geranium, grapefruit, green mandarin, lemon, lime, melaleuca, peppermint, pink pepper, Siberian fir, wild orange, wintergreen
Restorative - basil, black spruce, frankincense, lime, neroli, patchouli, rosemary, sandalwood, spearmint, tangerine
Stimulant - arborvitae, basil, black spruce, bergamot, birch, black pepper, blue tansy, cardamom, cedarwood, cinnamon, clove, coriander, cypress, dill, eucalyptus, fennel, ginger, grapefruit, juniper berry, lime, melaleuca, myrrh, patchouli, rosemary, Siberian fir, spearmint, tangerine, thyme, vetiver, white fir, wintergreen, ylang ylang

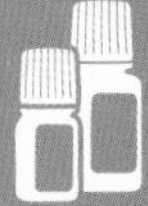

BLENDS

Citrus Bliss® - rejuvenating and energizing (pg. 181)
Breathe® - invigorating and reviving (pg. 172)
Motivate® - stimulating, renewing, and strengthening (pg. 193)
Passion® - promotes excitement, passion and joy (pg. 195)
Elevation™ - uplifting and energizing (pg. 187)
Purify - refreshing and cleansing (pg. 198)

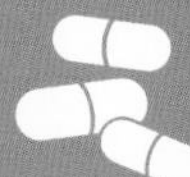

SUPPLEMENTS

Alpha CRS®+ (pg. 209), a2z Chewable™, DDR Prime® Softgels, xEO Mega, **Mito2Max® (pg. 214)**, **MicroPlex VMz (pg. 214)**

Related Ailments: Chronic Fatigue, Exhaustion, Fatigue, Nervous Fatigue, Poor Endurance, Scurvy

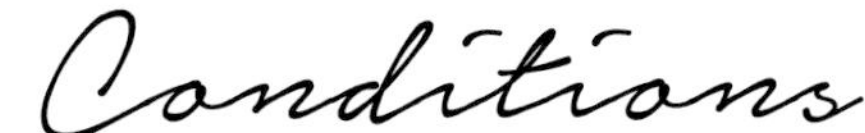

Conditions

Adrenal exhaustion/fatigue - basil, black spruce, geranium, rosemary, ylang ylang, Citrus Bliss®; see *Endocrine (Adrenals)*
Alertness, decreased/drowsiness – basil, frankincense, ginger, lemon, lemongrass, lime, peppermint, rosemary, ylang ylang, white fir, Adaptiv®, Breathe®, Citrus Bliss®, InTune®, Motivate®; see *Focus & Concentration*
Debility - cinnamon, Douglas fir, ginger, helichrysum, lavender, lemon, lime, neroli, On Guard®, Purify, Zendrocrine®
Energy, lack of* - basil, black pepper, cardamom, cinnamon, coriander, cypress, eucalyptus, ginger, grapefruit, jasmine, juniper berry, lemon, lime, melissa, patchouli, peppermint, rosemary, thyme, sandalwood, Siberian fir, tangerine, white fir, wild orange, Breathe®, Citrus Bliss®, Forgive®, Motivate®, On Guard®, Purify
Exhaustion/fatigue* - arborvitae, basil, black spruce, cinnamon, Douglas fir, eucalyptus, geranium, green mandarin, jasmine, lemon, lime, patchouli, peppermint, pink pepper, rosemary, sandalwood, wild orange, wintergreen, ylang ylang, AromaTouch®, Breathe®, Citrus Bliss®, DDR Prime®, Motivate®, Passion®, Purify, Slim & Sassy®, Zendrocrine®
Hyperactivity/restlessness/wound up - cedarwood, coriander, frankincense, lavender, patchouli, Roman chamomile, vetiver, wild orange, Adaptiv®, Balance®, InTune®, Serenity®; see *Focus & Concentration*
Jet lag - geranium, grapefruit, patchouli, peppermint, DDR Prime®, Motivate®; see *Sleep*
Lethargy/lack of motivation - Douglas fir, grapefruit, helichrysum, jasmine, lemon, lime, lemongrass, spearmint, yarrow, Adaptiv®, Breathe®, Citrus Bliss®, Purify, Motivate®
Nervous exhaustion - arborvitae, basil, black spruce, cedarwood, cinnamon, coriander, ginger, grapefruit, helichrysum, lemongrass, patchouli, rosemary, Breathe®, Motivate®, PastTense®
Oxygen, lack of - frankincense, peppermint, Siberian fir, Breathe®; see *Respiratory*
Weakness, physical after illness - basil, Douglas fir, frankincense, thyme, On Guard®, Purify, Zendrocrine®

USAGE TIPS: For best success in support optimal energy and vitality

- **Internal:** Consume energy-producing oils, products (e.g. energy & vitality complex); for oils, place a few drops of selected oils (e.g. citrus oils) in a capsule for systemic or on-going support. Also, drinking oils in water or dropping under the tongue is effective.
- **Topical** & **Aromatic:** Rubbing selected and energy-producing oils on tired/sore shoulders, neck, back, legs and feet is invigorating, improves circulation, blood flow and oxygen levels in the body both by aroma and topical sensation.

* See remedy on pg. 290

Remedies

DAILY ROUTINE FOR SUPPORTING HEALTHY ENERGY LEVELS

- Rub 1-2 drops of Balance® on bottoms of feet morning and night.
- Consume 3-5 drops of frankincense under tongue morning and night.
- Use a daily supplement routine to create long-term results with the following: Alpha CRS®+, xEO Mega, Mito2Max®, MicroPlex VMz, PB Assist®+, DDR Prime® Softgels.
- Add a favorite citrus oil to drinking water; consume throughout day.
- Use any of the blends below to create and support increase in energy and vitality.
- Rub 2-3 drops of DDR Prime®, followed by lavender oil, on bottoms of feet at night prior to sleep.

BRING THE ZING

Use grapefruit oil alone or in combination with frankincense oil, geranium oil, and/or bergamot oil. Diffuse, inhale, apply to bottoms of feet, back of neck. Dilute as desired.

ENERGY BOOST

6 drops Slim & Sassy®
3 drops peppermint
3 drops wild orange
Take oils in capsule as needed or desired.

INVIGORATING BLAST

1 drops frankincense
1 drops peppermint
2 drops wild orange
Inhale from cupped hands, massage on the back of neck.

MID AFTERNOON SLUMP BUSTER

15 drops peppermint
20 drops wild orange oil
Combine in 15ml roller bottle; fill remainder with carrier oil; apply to the back of neck, rub up into base of the skull, swipe across forehead near hairline, inhale.

ENERGY BOOSTING DIFFUSER BLEND:

Use 3-4 drops each Tangerine, Spearmint, and Lemongrass.

For more ideas, download the app at app.essentiallife.com

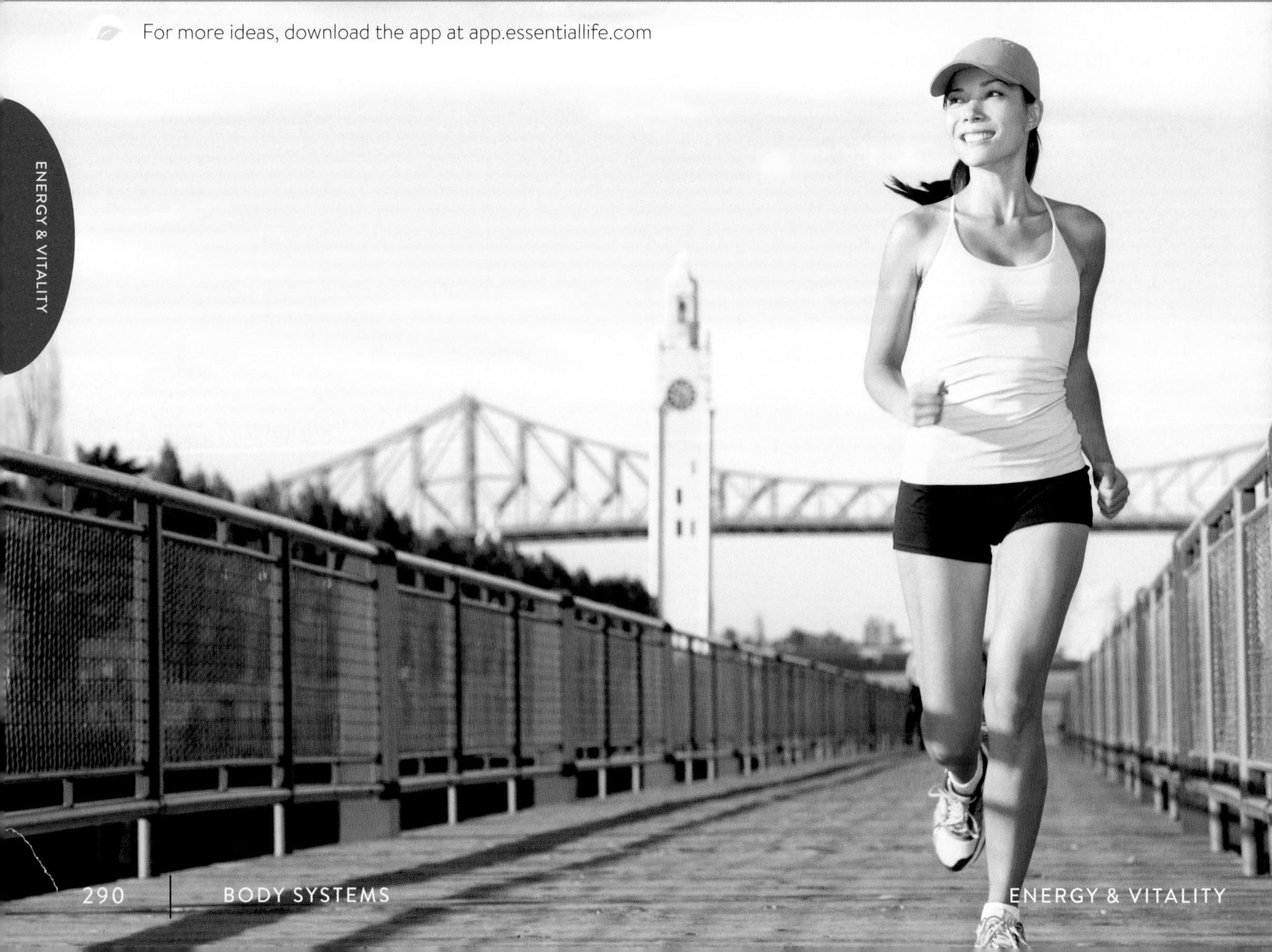

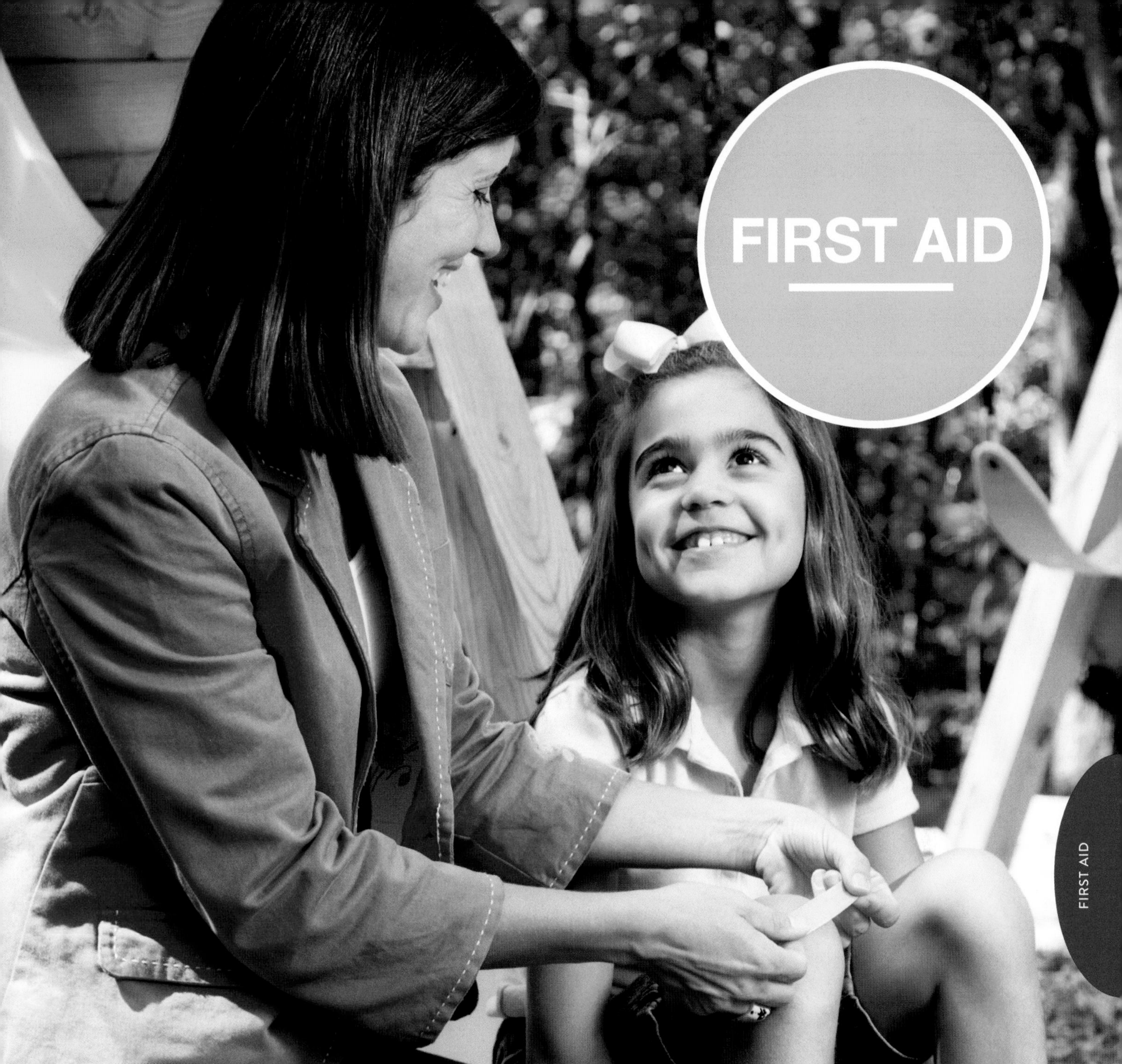

FIRST AID RESPONSE is required whenever there is an injury, illness, or an emergency situation that must be immediately addressed. Situations requiring first aid can include insect bites and stings, snake bites, scratches and cuts, bleeding and hemorrhaging, burns, bruises, shock, sudden vertigo, heart issues, breathing issues, fever, food poisoning, sprained muscles, broken and dislocated bones, heat exhaustion and sunstroke, hypothermia, and more.

In these situations it is important to have basic equipment readily available, such as antibiotic ointments, adhesive bandages, splints, etc., and to know how to respond in the event emergency personnel are required.

Essential oils and natural remedies make a great addition to complete any first aid kit. Particular oils have powerful antibiotic properties, help lower or raise body temperature, assist the respiratory system, help to settle nausea and other digestive problems, address burns, help to slow or stop bleeding, and more. Best of all, if the lids are secure and the first aid kit is kept in temperatures under 120° F, the oils typically last much longer than over-the-counter medications.

When assembling a first aid kit, it is important to consider lifestyle and risk factors for specific activities (e.g. hiking, camping, boating, traveling, etc.), and to use common sense to anticipate future needs. See below for lists of ideas for both single and blend essential oil and supplemental suggestions.

TOP SOLUTIONS

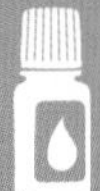

SINGLE OILS

Clove - powerful analgesic for numbing wounds (pg. 97)
Frankincense - universal healing properties, wound antiseptic/analgesic/healing, anti-scarring (pg. 110)
Helichrysum, yarrow - stop bleeding; wound repair/healing, powerful pain reliever (pgs. 117 & 164)
Lavender, blue tansy - antihistamine activity; wound, burn care, shock treatment; bite/sting recovery (pgs. 122 & 86)
Lemon - sanitize, neutralize acid; universal for immune, skin, respiratory needs (pg. 123)
Lemongrass - connective tissue repair, sore muscle/cramp relief (pg. 126)
Marjoram - muscle repair, digestive/eliminative support, sore muscle/cramp relief (pg. 131)
Melaleuca - gentle/powerful wound antiseptic, antimicrobial activity (pg. 132)
Oregano - anti-inflammatory, powerful antibacterial/antiviral (pg. 138)
Peppermint - cooling, burn care, pain reliever; relieve nausea, vomiting (pg. 140)

By Related Properties

For more, See Oil Properties on pages 477 - 481

Analgesic - arborvitae, basil, bergamot, birch, black pepper, blue tansy, cassia, cinnamon, clary sage, clove, copaiba, cypress, eucalyptus, fennel, frankincense, ginger, helichrysum, juniper berry, lavender, lemongrass, litsea, marjoram, melaleuca, oregano, peppermint, ravensara, rosemary, Siberian fir, turmeric, white fir, wild orange, wintergreen, yarrow
Anti-allergenic - blue tansy, geranium, helichrysum, manuka
Anticonvulsant - clary sage, fennel, geranium, lavender, neroli, tangerine
Antihemorrhagic - geranium, helichrysum, myrrh, yarrow
Anti-infectious - arborvitae, basil, cardamom, cedarwood, cinnamon, clove, copaiba, cypress, eucalyptus, frankincense, geranium, lavender, litsea, marjoram, melaleuca, myrrh, patchouli, Roman chamomile, rosemary, turmeric
Anti-inflammatory - bergamot, black pepper, blue tansy, cassia, cinnamon, clove, copaiba, cypress, eucalyptus, fennel, frankincense, ginger, jasmine, lemongrass, litsea, manuka, melaleuca, myrrh, neroli, oregano, patchouli, peppermint, pink pepper, rosemary, sandalwood, Siberian fir, spikenard, tangerine, turmeric, wintergreen, yarrow
Antiseptic - arborvitae, bergamot, black pepper, cedarwood, cinnamon, clove, copaiba, frankincense, ginger, grapefruit, helichrysum, juniper berry, lemon, marjoram, melaleuca, neroli, oregano, rosemary, Siberian fir, tangerine, thyme, vetiver, wild orange, ylang ylang
Antispasmodic - basil, blue tansy, cardamom, cassia, cinnamon, clove, eucalyptus, fennel, helichrysum, lavender, lemon, litsea, marjoram, neroli, peppermint, rosemary, sandalwood, Siberian fir, spearmint, tangerine, thyme, vetiver, wintergreen, yarrow, ylang ylang
Calming - bergamot, black pepper, blue tansy, clary sage, copaiba, coriander, frankincense, geranium, green mandarin, juniper berry, lavender, litsea, patchouli, Roman chamomile, tangerine, vetiver, yarrow
Hypotensive - blue tansy, clary sage, copaiba, lavender, lemon, litsea, manuka, neroli, yarrow, ylang ylang
Insect repellent - arborvitae, birch, blue tansy, cedarwood, celery seed, cinnamon, citronella, eucalyptus, geranium, lemon eucalyptus, lemongrass, litsea, patchouli, pink pepper, thyme, turmeric, vetiver, ylang ylang
Vasoconstrictor - helichrysum, peppermint, Siberian fir
Warming - birch, black pepper, cassia, cinnamon, clary sage, clove, eucalyptus, ginger, lemongrass, marjoram, neroli, oregano, peppermint, pink pepper, thyme, wintergreen

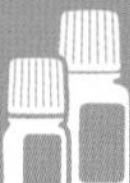

BLENDS

DDR Prime® - antitrauma, cellular, cognitive support (pg. 184)
Purify - antiseptic properties; sanitize, bug bite/sting recovery (pg. 198)
Zendrocrine® - anti-allergenic, blood cleansing, anti-infectious support (pg. 206)
DigestZen® - excellent to resolve nausea, vomiting (pg. 186)
AromaTouch® - for injured tissue recovery; sore muscle/cramp relief (pg. 169)
On Guard® - immune protection, analgesic (pg. 194)
TerraShield® - bug repellent (pg. 201)
Serenity® - for shock, trauma recovery (pg. 199)
HD Clear® - antiseptic, wound care (pg. 189)
Deep Blue® - bone/pain relief support; sore muscle/cramp relief (pg. 185)

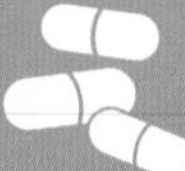

SUPPLEMENTS

Bone Nutrient Lifetime Complex, **Mito2Max® (pg. 214), Deep Blue Polyphenol Complex (pg. 212)**

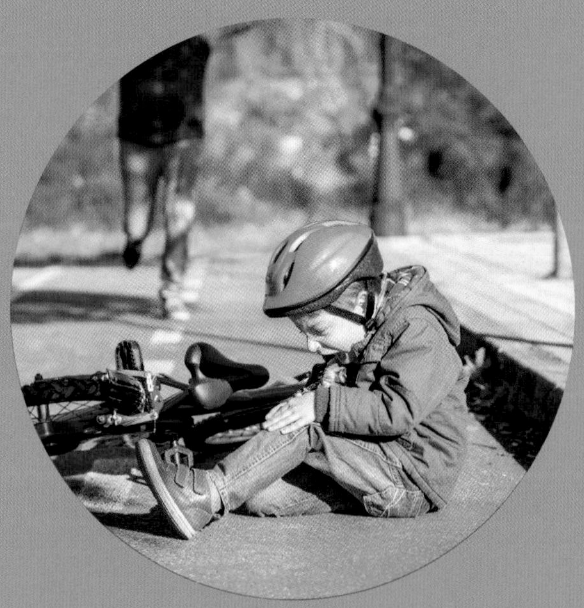

Related Ailments: Bee Sting, Chiggers, Fainting, Heat Exhaustion, Heat Illness/Dehydration, Heat Stroke, Hypothermia, Injury, Insect Bite, Insect Repellent, Mosquito Bites, Shock, Snake Bites, Tick Bites, Wasp Sting, Wounds

Conditions

Allergies to insect bite or sting - basil, blue tansy, lavender, lemon, melaleuca, melissa, peppermint, Roman chamomile, rosemary, thyme, Breathe®, Purify, TerraShield®, Zendrocrine®; see *Allergies*

Bed Bugs - arborvitae, blue tansy, cedarwood, eucalyptus, lavender, melaleuca, peppermint

Bites, insect - arborvitae, basil, blue tansy, cinnamon, copaiba, coriander, eucalyptus, frankincense, lavender, lemon, lemongrass, melaleuca, melissa, patchouli, Roman chamomile, thyme, ylang ylang, Passion®, Peace®, Purify

Bleeding/hemorrhaging - frankincense, geranium, helichrysum, lavender, myrrh, wild orange, yarrow, Console®; see *Cardiovascular*

Blood vessels, broken - cypress, frankincense, geranium, helichrysum, lemon, lime, yarrow, Purify, Zendrocrine®; see *Cardiovascular*

Breathing, shortness of breath - eucalyptus, peppermint, Breathe®; see "Allergies to insect bite" above, *Respiratory*

Bruising - arborvitae, blue tansy, clove, copaiba, cypress, fennel, geranium, grapefruit, helichrysum, lavender, neroli, oregano, Roman chamomile, white fir, ylang ylang, AromaTouch®, Citrus Bliss®, DDR Prime®, Deep Blue® or rub, Passion®, Purify, Peace®, Zendrocrine®

Burns - copaiba, eucalyptus, frankincense, geranium, helichrysum, lavender, lemon eucalyptus, myrrh, peppermint, sandalwood, Siberian fir, spearmint, tangerine, Immortelle, InTune®

Cellulitis - lime, oregano (internally), On Guard®; see *Immune & Lymphatic, Integumentary*

Chills (shock) - basil, ginger, grapefruit, lemon, melaleuca, melissa, myrrh, peppermint, Roman chamomile, rosemary, wild orange, ylang ylang, Balance®, Citrus Bliss®, Motivate®, On Guard®, Slim & Sassy®

Cuts/wounds, cleaning* - black spruce, blue tansy, cassia, cedarwood, copaiba, cypress, frankincense, juniper berry, lavender, lemon, lemongrass, melaleuca (superb disinfectant), magnolia, myrrh, HD Clear®, On Guard®, Peace®

Cuts/wounds, healing* - basil, black spruce, copaiba, cypress, eucalyptus, frankincense, geranium, helichrysum (apply to cleaned wound), lavender, lemon eucalyptus, lime, magnolia, melaleuca, myrrh, peppermint, petitgrain, sandalwood, Siberian fir, vetiver, yarrow, HD Clear®, Immortelle, Purify,

Cuts/wounds, pain (numbing)* - cassia, clove, copaiba, eucalyptus, frankincense, helichrysum, melaleuca, neroli, Siberian fir, yarrow, On Guard®

Dehydration - cypress, juniper berry, lemon, petitgrain, wild orange, Slim & Sassy®, Zendrocrine®

Dizziness/lightheaded - geranium, ginger, peppermint, Balance®, DDR Prime®, Deep Blue®, PastTense®, Whisper®, Zendrocrine®

Drop in blood pressure (allergic reaction) - cypress, helichrysum, lavender, peppermint, rosemary, thyme, white fir, ylang ylang; see *Allergies*, "Allergies to insect bite or sting" above

Fainting - basil, peppermint, rosemary, Balance®, Citrus Bliss®, Motivate®

Fleas - arborvitae, cedarwood, citronella, eucalyptus, lavender, lemon, lemon eucalyptus, lemongrass, peppermint, Purify, TerraShield®

Food poisoning - black pepper, cinnamon, clove, ginger, juniper berry, lemon, melaleuca, oregano, thyme, DigestZen®, On Guard®, Purify, Zendrocrine®

Heat exhaustion* - basil, bergamot, eucalyptus, lemon, lemon eucalyptus, lime, peppermint, spearmint, Deep Blue®, PastTense®

Hypothermia - birch, cassia, cinnamon, clove, cypress, eucalyptus, ginger, lemongrass, marjoram, oregano, patchouli, peppermint, thyme, wild orange, wintergreen, AromaTouch®, DDR Prime®, On Guard®

Infections - juniper berry, melaleuca, oregano, On Guard®, Purify; see *Immune & Lymphatic*

Insect repellent - arborvitae, basil, bergamot, birch, blue tansy, cedarwood, celery seed, cinnamon, citronella, cypress, Douglas fir, eucalyptus, geranium (mosquito), lavender (flies, gnat, midge, mosquito), lemon eucalyptus, lemongrass, lime, patchouli, pink pepper, rosemary, thyme, turmeric, vetiver, ylang ylang, Forgive®, Passion®, Purify, TerraShield®

Itching, excessive - blue tansy, cilantro, lavender, lemon, melaleuca, melissa, patchouli, peppermint, Roman chamomile, vetiver, wild orange, Immortelle, Slim & Sassy®, Zendrocrine®; see *Integumentary*

Lice - citronella, geranium, melaleuca, rosemary, thyme, TerraShield®; see *Parasites*

Mites (e.g. chiggers, scabies) - See *Parasites*

Mosquito bites - arborvitae, juniper berry, lavender, melaleuca, Roman chamomile, Purify; see "Bites, insect" above

Motion sickness - bergamot, ginger, peppermint, Cheer®, DigestZen®; see *Digestive & Intestinal*

Nausea/vomiting - basil, bergamot, cardamom, cassia, clove, coriander, fennel, ginger, lavender, melissa, pink pepper, DigestZen®; see *Digestive & Intestinal*

Nosebleeds - cypress, helichrysum, geranium, lavender, lemon, lime, yarrow; see *Cardiovascular*

Poison - black pepper, juniper berry, lemongrass, Passion®

Poison ivy - frankincense, geranium, lavender, lemon, melaleuca, Roman chamomile, Immortelle, Purify

Poison oak - clove, lavender, rose, vetiver, Immortelle

Shivering/low body temp - see "Hypothermia" above

Shock - bergamot, coriander, Douglas fir, frankincense, geranium, helichrysum, lavender, magnolia, marjoram, melaleuca, melissa, neroli, peppermint, Roman chamomile, tangerine, vetiver, wild orange, ylang ylang, Console®, DDR Prime®, InTune®, Motivate®, PastTense®, Peace®, Serenity®

Snake bite - basil, clove, coriander, helichrysum, frankincense, geranium, melaleuca, patchouli, sandalwood, Purify

Spider bite* - basil, juniper berry, lavender, melaleuca, melissa, Roman chamomile, thyme, On Guard®, Purify

Stinging nettle - clove, lemon (neutralizes acid), Citrus Bliss®, Purify

Stings - basil, cinnamon, clove, lavender, lemon, lime, melaleuca, Roman chamomile, thyme, Purify

Sunburn - arborvitae, blue tansy, eucalyptus, frankincense, helichrysum, lavender, peppermint, sandalwood, spearmint, Immortelle

Sunstroke/heatstroke - Douglas fir, eucalyptus, lavender, lemon, peppermint, rosemary, spearmint, PastTense®, Zendrocrine®

Tick bites - lavender, melaleuca; see *Parasites*

Tick prevention - lemon eucalyptus

Trauma - cypress, frankincense, geranium, juniper berry, myrrh, Balance®, DDR Prime®, Immortelle, Motivate®, Purify, Serenity®, TerraShield®; see "Shock" above

** See remedy on pg. 294*

Remedies

SPIDER BITE RECOVERY: Combine basil, Purify, rosemary, and lemon to take "sting" away and reduce inflammation. When helichrysum is added at end of treatment, the bite location is encouraged to heal faster and leave little to no scar.

OWIE SPRAY
5 drops lemon
10 drops melaleuca
10 drops lavender
5 drops helichrysum
Add to 4-ounce glass spray bottle and fill with purified water.

NATURAL FIRST AID SPRAY
5 drops lavender
3 drops melaleuca
2 drops cypress
Place oils in a spray bottle with 1/ 2 teaspoon salt and 8 ounces of distilled water. Spray on before applying bandages. Repeat several times a day for three days.

HEAT EXHAUSTION RECOVERY:
Place 2-4 drops of lemon oil in drinking water and sip to rehydrate.
Place 1 drop of peppermint oil in drinking water and sip to cool down.
Combine the two as desired.

USAGE TIPS: For first aid success

- **Topical:**
  - Apply oils directly to area(s) of concern such as on cuts, bruises, bites, stings, injury sites and burns whenever possible. Otherwise, get as close as possible to site or use bottoms of feet as alternative location.
  - For acute situations, apply frequently, even every couple minutes as needed for pain relief, to stop bleeding, etc. Clean site (e.g. with melaleuca) prior to stopping bleeding and sealing up a cut site with helichrysum.
  - To cool or raise body temperature, place cooling or warming oils on back of neck, down spine, bottoms of feet, or spray on an oil/water (cooling only) mixture (shake first). For sunburn, apply to site.
- **Aromatic:** Use for emotional support for times like shock or trauma by offering immediate inhalation from a bottle or drops placed on hands. Create continue inhalation with a diffuser or by topical application that allows for ongoing exposure.
- **Internal:** for any allergic response, place a drop of anti-histamine oil (e.g. lavender) under tongue for older children/adults or bottoms of feet for any age (dilute for infants/toddlers); inhale as well. For nausea/ vomiting place oil(s) on abdomen, lick off back of hand, drop in mouth, and/or bottoms of feet.

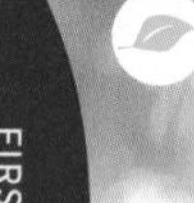

For more First Aid ideas, download the app at app.essentiallife.com

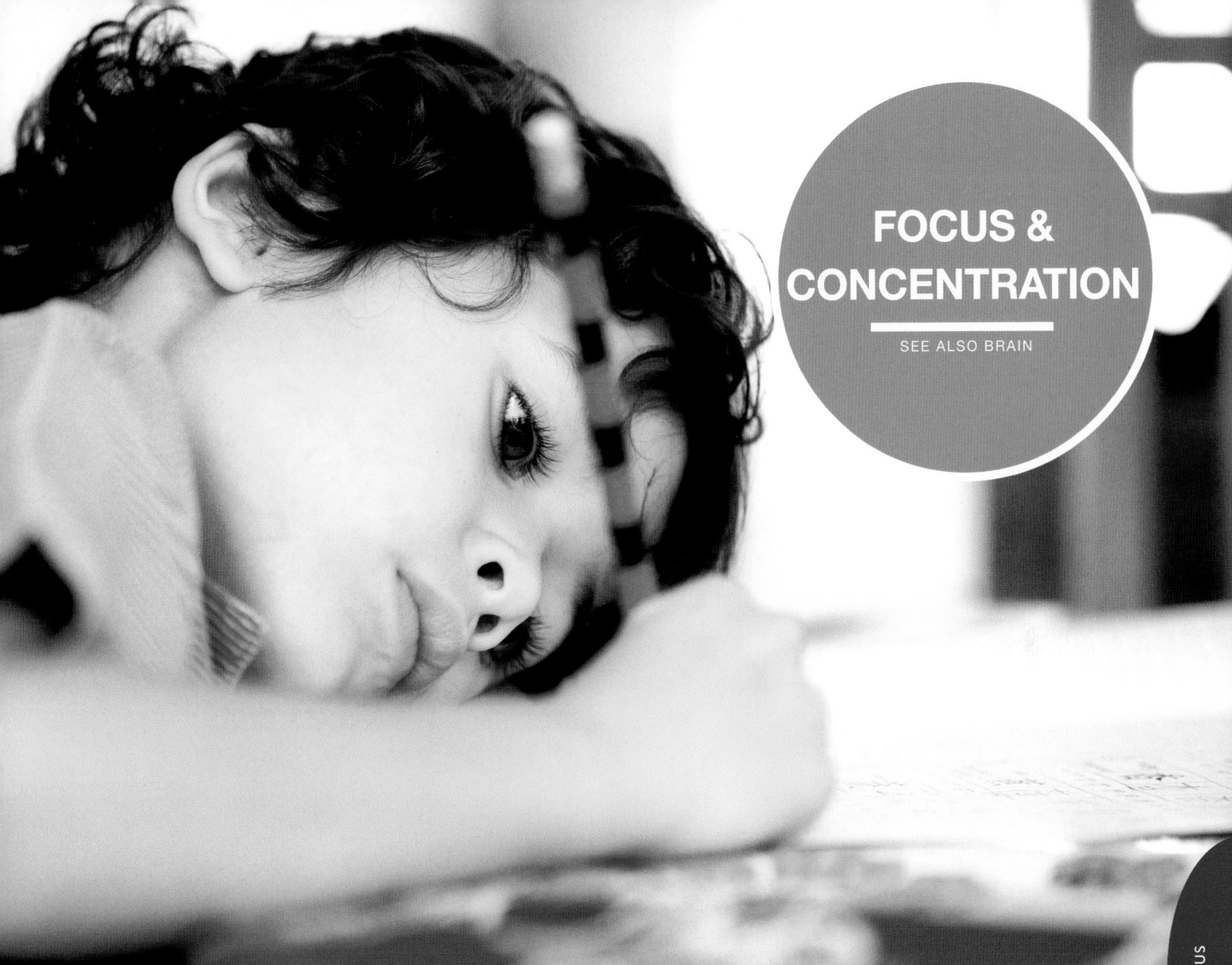

FOCUS & CONCENTRATION

SEE ALSO BRAIN

THE ABILITY TO FOCUS requires adequate neural connections in the brain to process incoming sensory data (sights, sounds, smells, etc.). When the brain is unable to assimilate this data, the stimuli becomes overwhelming or "noisy," and symptoms such as frustration, irritation, and even fatigue can occur. An increasing number of individuals of any age are experiencing a decreasing ability to focus and concentrate. It is important to consider factors that contribute to the decline of optimal focus and concentration in order to reverse or prevent this trend.

Given the innate complexity of the human brain, it is not surprising that issues of focus and concentration and contributing factors are vast. Tiredness or lack of sleep, stress, hormonal changes (such as during pregnancy or puberty), medication side effects, alcohol, drugs, chronic illness, infection, brain injury, anxiety, depression, bipolar disorder, and emotional trauma are just a few that impact neural connections necessary to make sense of the vast sensory stimuli the brain receives moment to moment. For example, individuals with ADHD consistently struggle to "think over the noise" in their brains as stimuli come in without the necessary processing ability to make sense of it all.

The very nature of the brain's structure allows for improvements in function and ability. To summarize this complex process in a simple way, the more neurons available to make connections with other neurons, the easier and more efficient focus and learning will be. While traditional medicine and neurological specialists contribute great expertise to the science of improving brain activity, there are a myriad of natural remedies that can greatly impact and benefit brain activity, specifically in the area of focus and concentration.

When an individual inhales an essential oil (or other aroma) the olfactory bulb is activated and directly links to brain processes that stimulate and encourage neural connections. The simple act of diffusing an essential oil like lavender in the classroom, or inhaling peppermint from a bottle, can have immediate and effective impact on the learner. Simple yet powerful suggestions through both single oils or blends and remedies have demonstrated that essential oils and nutritional support are powerful tools for improving focus, concentration, and much more!

TOP SOLUTIONS

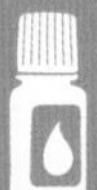

SINGLE OILS

Roman chamomile - reduces anxiety, promotes confidence (pg. 147)
Vetiver - promotes focus, concentration, mental performance (pg. 160)
Lavender - supports mental adaptability, performance (pg. 122)
Clary sage - supports a calm, clear, focused mind (pg. 96)
Cedarwood - calms mind, supports improved mental performance (pg. 89)

By Related Properties

For more, See Oil Properties on pages 477 - 481

Antidepressant - bergamot, frankincense, green mandarin, lemon, melissa, neroli, ravensara, Roman chamomile, tangerine, wild orange
Antifungal - arborvitae, bergamot, blue tansy, cedarwood, cinnamon, clary sage, copaiba, coriander, litsea, manuka, melaleuca, myrrh, oregano, sandalwood, Siberian fir, tangerine, thyme, turmeric
Antioxidant - bergamot, clove, copaiba, helichrysum, grapefruit, juniper berry, lemon, lemongrass, melaleuca, neroli, rosemary, patchouli, tangerine, thyme, turmeric, yarrow
Calming - black spruce, blue tansy, cedarwood, clary sage, copaiba, coriander, fennel, jasmine, lavender, litsea, magnolia, patchouli, Roman chamomile, sandalwood, tangerine, vetiver, yarrow
Energizing - basil, bergamot, cinnamon, cypress, ginger, rosemary, Siberian fir, tangerine, wild orange, yarrow
Grounding - black spruce, blue tansy, cedarwood, frankincense, magnolia, Siberian fir, vetiver, ylang ylang
Invigorating - lemon, lime, lemongrass, litsea, peppermint, pink pepper, Siberian fir, wild orange
Neuroprotective - frankincense, magnolia, myrrh, Roman chamomile, sandalwood, turmeric
Refreshing - any citrus oil, melaleuca, Siberian fir
Relaxing - blue tansy, cypress, geranium, green mandarin, litsea, magnolia, neroli, Roman chamomile
Sedative - bergamot, blue tansy, cedarwood, clary sage, frankincense, lavender, magnolia, melissa, neroli, patchouli, Roman chamomile, tangerine, vetiver, yarrow
Stimulant - arborvitae, basil, bergamot, black pepper, black spruce, blue tansy, cardamom, cedarwood, cinnamon, coriander, cypress, dill, eucalyptus, ginger, grapefruit, juniper berry, lime, pink pepper, melaleuca, rosemary, Siberian fir, spearmint, tangerine, vetiver, wintergreen
Uplifting - bergamot, grapefruit, green mandarin, lime, litsea, melissa, tangerine, wild orange

Related Ailments: Absentmindedness, ADD or ADHD [Brain], Concentration, Confusion, Focus, Hyperactivity [Mood & Behavior], Mental strength/clarity, Poor Concentration, Poor Memory [Brain]

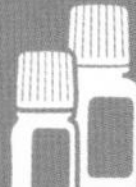

BLENDS

Serenity® - relaxes the mind (pg. 199)
InTune® - calms and stimulates the mind (pg. 192)
Motivate® - promotes motivation, mental stimulation and movement (pg. 193)
Balance® - promotes a grounded state of mind (pg. 170)
Thinker™ -calms and stimulates the mind (pg. 180)

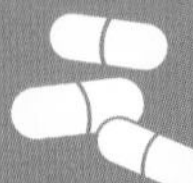

SUPPLEMENTS

Bone Nutrient Lifetime Complex, Alpha CRS®+, PB Assist®+, Zendocrine® Softgels, Zendocrine® Complex, Mito2Max®, DDR Prime® Softgels, **xEO Mega (pg. 222)**, TerraZyme®, MicroPlex VMz, **IQ Mega® (pg. 213)**

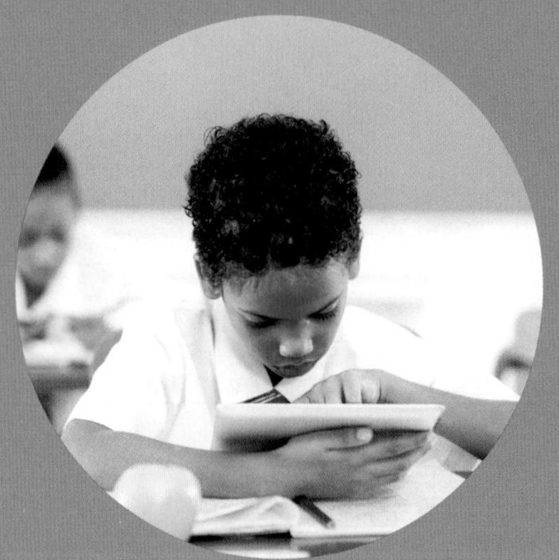

USAGE TIPS: For best methods of use for focus and concentration consider:

- **Aromatic:** Choose to diffuse 5-10 drops of oils of choice, inhale from product bottle or self-made blend, apply a few drops to clothing, bedding, or any other method that supports inhalation for oils to enter brain via nose and olfactory system.
- **Topical:** Apply on forehead, under nose, back of neck (especially in suboccipital triangles), roof of mouth (place oil on pad of thumb, place on roof, "suck").

FOCUS

Conditions

EMOTIONAL STATES:

(See *Mood & Behavior* for additional emotional support)

Afraid/unadventurous - black pepper, patchouli, ravensara, Brave™

Agitated* - arborvitae, bergamot, black spruce, patchouli, Balance®, Deep Blue®, InTune®, Serenity®, Thinker™

Angry* - bergamot, cardamom, cedarwood, frankincense, geranium, helichrysum, Roman chamomile, Balance®, InTune®, Serenity®

Antisocial - bergamot, black pepper, cedarwood, oregano, patchouli

Anxious - basil, cedarwood, frankincense, juniper berry, patchouli, vetiver, Adaptiv®, Balance®, InTune®, Serenity®

Apathetic/lacking of motivation* - birch, black pepper, cardamom, frankincense, jasmine, juniper berry, melissa, patchouli, rose, vetiver, wild orange, ylang ylang, Adaptiv®, Balance®, Breathe®, Elevation™, InTune®, Motivate®, Passion®

Defensive - ginger, lemon, melaleuca, patchouli, wintergreen, ClaryCalm®, Deep Blue®, On Guard®, PastTense®, TerraShield®

Depressed - bergamot, green mandarin, jasmine, patchouli, Roman chamomile, vetiver, wild orange, ylang ylang, Citrus Bliss®, Elevation™, Passion®

Easily bugged/bothered - black spruce, lemongrass, rose, white fir, TerraShield®

Fearful - frankincense, juniper berry, wild orange, ylang ylang, Balance®, Brave™, Breathe®, On Guard®, Serenity®, Zendrocrine®

Frustrated* - black spruce, cardamom, ylang ylang, Calmer™, InTune®, Serenity®

Hypersensitive - lavender, melissa, Roman chamomile, rosemary, vetiver

Obsessed/preoccupied - cedarwood, frankincense, jasmine, oregano, sandalwood, vetiver, Adaptiv®, InTune®, Serenity®

Performance stress/stage fright - bergamot, patchouli, ravensara, rose, wild orange, ylang ylang, Adaptiv®, Breathe®

Shy/timid/unsure - bergamot, cassia, clove, ginger, jasmine, juniper berry, melissa, patchouli, ravensara, spearmint, yarrow, ylang ylang, Brave™, Breathe®, InTune®, Motivate®, Passion®

Stubborn/willful - birch, ginger, lemongrass, melaleuca, oregano, wintergreen

Unsafe/vulnerable, feeling* - bergamot, cardamom, cilantro, cinnamon, ginger, jasmine, oregano, ravensara, Roman chamomile, ylang ylang, AromaTouch®, Breathe®, On Guard®, Serenity®, TerraShield®, Whisper®

MENTAL STATES:

Attention deficit - lavender, vetiver, Adaptiv®, InTune®, Motivate®, Peace®, Serenity®, Thinker™

Autistic - basil, bergamot, clary sage, frankincense, geranium, lemon, peppermint, rosemary, vetiver, Balance®, DDR Prime®, Deep Blue®, Immortelle, InTune®, Serenity®

Brain fogged* - arborvitae, bergamot, Douglas fir, eucalyptus, frankincense, juniper berry, lemon, lime, peppermint, Siberian fir, Motivate®, InTune®, Thinker™

Brain oxygen, lack of - cedarwood, cypress, eucalyptus, frankincense, ginger, lemon, patchouli, peppermint, sandalwood, vetiver, Passion®; see "Antioxidant" property

Chemically imbalanced - See *Brain*

Concentration/focus, lack of* - arborvitae, cedarwood, Douglas fir, eucalyptus, frankincense, lavender, lemon, lime, patchouli, peppermint, rosemary, vetiver, Adaptiv®, Calmer™, InTune®, Motivate®, Thinker™

Confusion/disorganized - arborvitae, frankincense, peppermint, rosemary, vetiver, white fir, Balance®, Elevation™, InTune®, Motivate®

Coping skills, lack of - bergamot, black spruce, clove, eucalyptus, ginger, juniper berry, lavender, oregano, rosemary, wintergreen, Adaptiv®, Balance®, Calmer™, Citrus Bliss®, Deep Blue®, Elevation™, InTune®, PastTense®, Serenity®

Daydreamer - cedarwood, frankincense, peppermint, ravensara, rosemary, vetiver, ylang ylang, AromaTouch®, Breathe®, Motivate®, Thinker™

Dendrite and neuron support - vetiver

Distracted/bored easily - frankincense, peppermint, Roman chamomile, vetiver, wild orange, Motivate®

Environmental tension - lemon, wintergreen, yarrow, Steady™

Equilibrium/balance, lack of - arborvitae, frankincense, lavender, rosemary, spearmint, ylang ylang, Balance®, Citrus Bliss®, InTune®, Steady™, Zendrocrine®

Fatigued - basil, black spruce, cassia, cinnamon, coriander, ginger, lemon, pink pepper, thyme, DDR Prime®, Motivate®, Slim & Sassy®, Zendrocrine®; see *Energy & Vitality*

Fixated - black pepper, lemongrass, tangerine, ylang ylang

Hyperactive/restlessness/wound up* - coriander, frankincense, lavender, lemon, ravensara, Roman chamomile, vetiver, Adaptiv®, Balance®, Breathe®, Calmer™, Peace®, Serenity®, Thinker™

Impulsive/acting without thinking - white fir, Balance®

Learning difficulties - cedarwood, patchouli, peppermint, vetiver, Balance®, InTune®, Motivate®, Passion®, Thinker™

Left brain, lack of activity - lemon

Mentally fatigued - basil, bergamot, black spruce, cardamom, Douglas fir, frankincense, lavender, lemon, lemongrass, peppermint, rose, rosemary, sandalwood, spearmint, white fir, ylang ylang, Breathe®, Citrus Bliss®, Console®, Motivate®, Passion®

Mentally sluggish - basil, eucalyptus, peppermint, pink pepper, rosemary, Siberian fir, Motivate®

Mentally strained/stressed - bergamot, cedarwood, grapefruit, lavender, Roman chamomile, spearmint, Adaptiv®, Calmer™, Immortelle, Thinker™

Memory, lack of/unreliable/poor sense of time - bergamot, Douglas fir, lemon, lemongrass, lime, juniper berry, melissa, peppermint, thyme, Elevation™, InTune®, Passion®

Memory, poor* - black spruce, frankincense, ginger, peppermint, rosemary, sandalwood, thyme, Adaptiv®, InTune®, Motivate®, Passion®

Memory, loss of short term - basil, black spruce, cedarwood, peppermint, rosemary, ylang ylang, Adaptiv®, Balance®, Forgive®, InTune®, Peace®

Neurotransmitter production capacity, compromised - fennel, ginger

Oxygen deprived (brain) - cedarwood, cypress, eucalyptus, frankincense, ginger, lemon, melaleuca, patchouli, peppermint, sandalwood, vetiver, On Guard®; see "Antioxidant" above

Restless/fidgety/squirming* - lavender and vetiver, ravensara, wild orange, Adaptiv®, Balance®, Breathe®, Citrus Bliss®, Serenity®, Steady™

Right brain, lack of activity - Douglas fir, Roman chamomile, wild orange

Sensory systems, closed/blocked - birch, wintergreen, Motivate®

FOCUS

* *See remedy on pg. 298*

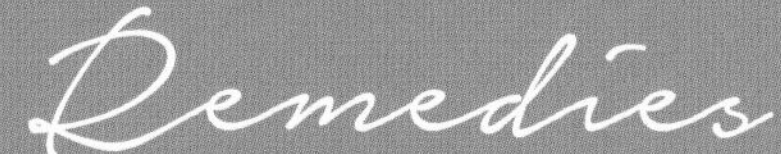

CONCENTRATION: Apply vetiver on feet or base of neck; for school children that need help during the school day, place a drop of oil on collarbone area so body heat will "diffuse" during day; apply oil to top of hand or on a necklace with a pendant made to diffuse oils for easy access to smell all day. If aroma is offensive, add an oil such as wild orange over top of vetiver to "deodorize" as desired.

FOCUS SUPPORT: Blend 2-4 drops frankincense or grapefruit with a few drops of carrier oil and massage temples.

FOCUS, MEMORY, RECALL

- Option #1: Combine frankincense with wild orange or peppermint; inhale or sniff.
- Options #2: In a 1/3 ounce roller bottle combine 20 drops each of wild orange, peppermint; fill the rest of the bottle with fractionated coconut oil and apply
- Option #3: Combine 1-2 drops each cedarwood, lavender, and vetiver and apply. Recipe can also be used in a 10ml roller bottle with a carrier oil. Place 7-13 drops of each oil depending on user's preference of aromas.

FRUSTRATION/ANGER: Use oils and blends that calm - helichrysum, lavender, magnolia, ylang ylang, Balance®, Serenity®; apply to feet, back of neck, behind ears, behind knees; diffuse.

HEALTHY TOUCH: Allow individual to choose their favorite oils (up to three) by smelling for preference or make a personal blend; massage feet prior to bedtime then cover them with warm, weighted blankets.

HYPERACTIVITY: Apply Balance® to the feet and Serenity® and/or lavender to the base of the neck, or on and behind the ears; healthy touch can be a welcomed calming support for an individual, and the action of applying oils can create a calming effect.

PEACE AND CALM: Combine 10 drops of lavender, 20 drops of vetiver, and 10 drops of Serenity® in a 10 ml roller bottle; top off with fractionated coconut oil; apply to feet, back of neck or head; diffuse or inhale; use at least two times per day.

"CHILL PILL"
10 drops clary sage
15 drops bergamot
20 drops grapefruit
25 drops wild orange
15 drops frankincense
10 drops lemon
Diffuse or apply topically at the base of the skull, back of the neck, along the spine, behind the ears, over the heart, and on the wrist.

MOTIVATION POWER
3 drops basil
3 drops grapefruit
2 drops bergamot
2 drops sandalwood
1 drop rosemary
1 drop ylang ylang
Combine oils and diffuse.

CALM AND CONFIDENT
8 drops vetiver
4 drops ylang ylang
2 drops frankincense
2 drops Roman chamomile
2 drops clary sage
2 drops marjoram
1 drops ginger
Combine oils in a 10 ml roller bottle. Fill remainder of bottle with fractionated coconut oil. Rub behind ears, on occipital triangle area, bottoms of feet, and/or down the spine before bedtime and as needed.

MELLOW OUT
10 drops Roman chamomile
10 drops lavender
10 drops wild orange
2 drops marjoram
2 drops frankincense
Combine oils in a 10 ml roller bottle. Fill remainder of bottle with fractionated coconut oil. Rub behind ears, on suboccipital triangle area, bottoms of feet, and/or down the spine before bedtime and as needed.

FIDGET FIXER
3 drops cedarwood
6 drops Balance®
2 drops frankincense
2 drops lavender
Combine oils in a 10 ml roller bottle. Fill remainder of bottle with fractionated coconut oil. Apply to ears, forehead, back of neck, down spine, bottoms of feet; massage into tissue to enhance absorption. If desired, drops can be multiplied by two or three to increase intensity of blend. Consider age, size, need, and tolerance of the intended user to determine strength desired.

IMPROVED CONCENTRATION
2 drops cedarwood
2 drops lavender
1 drop Roman chamomile
1 drop sandalwood
1 drop vetiver
Combine and apply to feet.

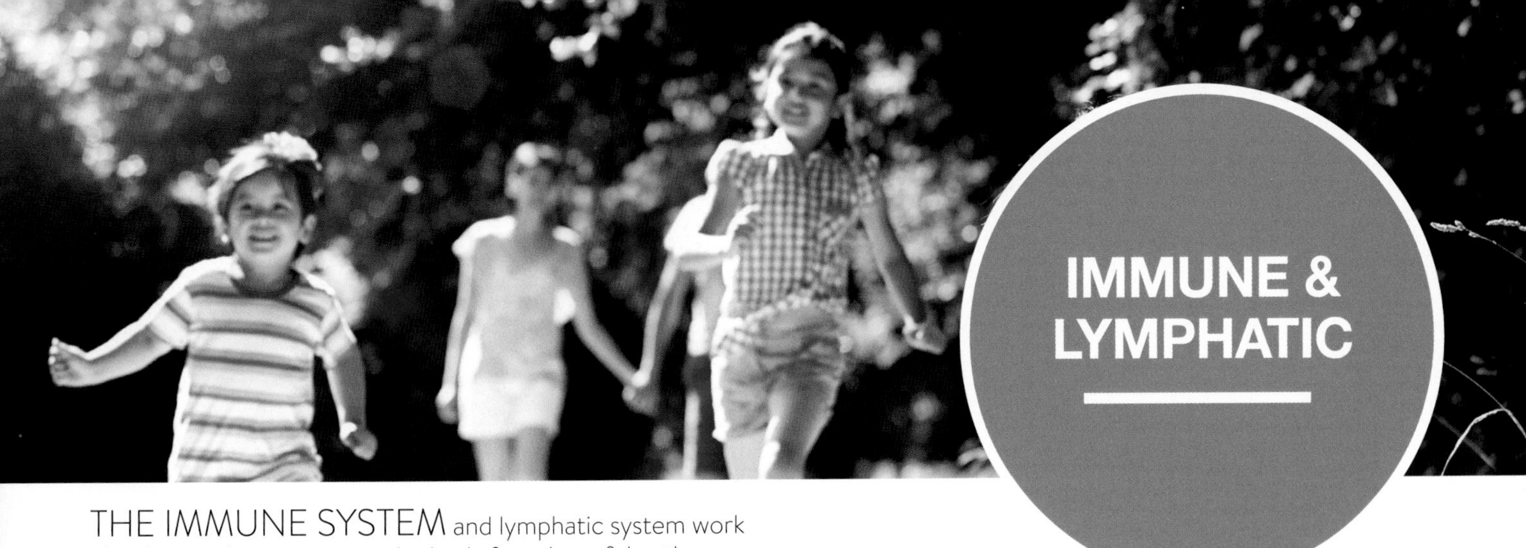

THE IMMUNE SYSTEM and lymphatic system work closely together to protect the body from harmful pathogens and disease. These systems include white blood cells, bone marrow, the spleen, tonsils, adenoids, appendix, thymus, lymph, and lymph nodes. A healthy immune response consists of the body's ability to properly identify a pathogen and engage in a series of responses designed to prevent pathogens from entering targeted cells/tissues.

The immune system consists of:

- The innate immune system--prevents pathogens from entering the body; it also provides a generalized response that destroys any pathogens that bypass the barriers.
- The adaptive immune system--analyzes the pathogen so the body can respond with an army of protective cells created specifically to destroy that particular pathogen. This system also supports the immune system by delivering nutrients to the cells and removing toxins and waste products.

The lymphatic system includes:

- Bone marrow--creates T-cells and creates and grows B-cells to maturation. B-cells travel via the blood system to destroy any lurking pathogens. T-cells, which attack pathogens and any toxic molecules, travel to the thymus, where they mature and later join the B-cells. These T-cells and B-cells are lymphocytes that travel in lymph.
- Lymph--a watery fluid, yellowish in color, that carries white blood cells. It circulates through tissues and picks up unwanted fats, bacteria, and other substances and filters it through the lymphatic system.

The first line of defense is the innate immune system, which includes physical barriers, such as skin, fingernails, mucous membranes, tears, and earwax that help prevent invaders from entering the body, and chemical barriers, such as fatty acids, stomach acid, proteins, and secretions that naturally help destroy pathogens.

When pathogens are undeterred by the innate immune response, the adaptive immune system, which is more complex than the innate, processes the pathogen in a way that allows it to design specific immune cells to combat it effectively. Then it produces huge numbers of those cells to attack the pathogen and any toxic molecules it creates. The cells that carry out this specific immune response are called lymphocytes and are created and delivered by the lymph system.

As part of the adaptive immune system response, humans have sophisticated defense mechanisms that include the ability to adapt over time to recognize specific pathogens more efficiently. This is accomplished by creating immunological memory after the initial response is rendered, leading to an enhanced response to subsequent encounters with that same pathogen.

Certain lifestyle choices can either provide great strength or can seriously weaken immune response. Nutrition is a key factor in a healthy immune system; if cells don't have the energy they need to provide critical safeguards for the body, pathogens can more easily penetrate and multiply. Detoxification is another critical activity that helps promote the body's natural defenses; many times when an individual gets sick it is simply the body's way to naturally eliminate toxins.

Natural essential oils, which have a chemical footprint compatible with the human body, have the unique ability to help the immune system bring itself to balance because they are lipophilic (soluble in fat) and thus are able to penetrate the cell membrane. Viruses are also lipophilic. Most pure essential oils are naturally drawn to the inside of the cell to help the body eradicate threats within the cell.

Interestingly, when essential oils are adulterated because the oil is synthetic (created in a laboratory), the signal molecule approaching the cell is the mirror-image of what it should be and thus is limited in the support it can give the body.

Note that for threats that exist outside the cell, namely, bacterial infections, essential oils can assist in warding off such risks. Oregano essential oil, for example, also has hydrophilic properties that allow it to effectively target threats that exist in the extracellular fluid (outside the cell). Knowledge of these powerful properties can help individuals provide effective reinforcements for the immune system.

Additional consideration for immune support:
When threats to the body from various pathogens are combined with a weakened immune system, illness can occur. Ideally, one would target pathogens within the body while simultaneously strengthening the immune system. The Oil Touch technique discussed in the introduction to this book accomplishes both objectives. The Oil Touch technique is a systematic application of eight different essential oils that serves to strengthen the immune system, eliminate pathogens, reduce stress, and bring the body into homeostasis, enabling the body to function more optimally. See *Oil Touch technique*, page 19.

TOP SOLUTIONS

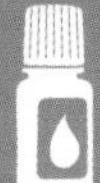

SINGLE OILS

Melaleuca - fights bacteria and viruses (pg. 132)
Cinnamon - fights bacteria and viruses (pg. 93)
Copaiba - fights bacteria and viruses (pg. 99)
Black or Pink pepper - supports digestion and boosts immunity (pg. 83), (pg. 144)
Thyme - fights bacteria and viruses (pg. 157)

By Related Properties

For more, See Oil Properties on pages 477 - 481

Antibacterial - arborvitae, basil, black pepper, blue tansy, cassia, cedarwood, cilantro, cinnamon, clove, copaiba, coriander, dill, eucalyptus, frankincense, geranium, ginger, lemongrass, lime, litsea, manuka, marjoram, melaleuca, melissa, myrrh, oregano, peppermint, ravensara, rosemary, Siberian fir, tangerine, thyme, turmeric, ylang ylang
Antifungal - arborvitae, blue tansy, cassia, cedarwood, cinnamon, copaiba, coriander, cypress, eucalyptus, fennel, ginger, lemon, lemon eucalyptus, lemongrass, litsea, manuka, melaleuca, myrrh, oregano, rosemary, Siberian fir, tangerine, turmeric, wild orange
Anti-infectious - bergamot, cardamom, cinnamon, copaiba, cypress, eucalyptus, frankincense, geranium, litsea, melaleuca, myrrh, Roman chamomile, rose, rosemary
Anti-inflammatory - arborvitae, bergamot, black pepper, cardamom, blue tansy, cinnamon, clary sage, clove, copaiba, coriander, fennel, frankincense, helichrysum, lavender, litsea, manuka, melissa, neroli, oregano, peppermint, pink pepper, Roman chamomile, Siberian fir, spikenard, tangerine, turmeric, wintergreen, yarrow
Antimicrobial - arborvitae, basil, blue tansy, cassia, cilantro, copaiba, cypress, fennel, frankincense, helichrysum, lavender, lemongrass, litsea, manuka, melissa, neroli, patchouli, ravensara, Siberian fir, thyme
Antioxidant - black pepper, cassia, cinnamon, clove, copaiba, frankincense, grapefruit, helichrysum, lemon, lime, melaleuca, neroli, oregano, tangerine, turmeric, vetiver, wild orange, yarrow
Antiseptic - basil, bergamot, cardamom, cedarwood, clary sage, copaiba, cypress, geranium, ginger, helichrysum, jasmine, lavender, lemon, lime, marjoram, melissa, myrrh, neroli, manuka, peppermint, ravensara, rosemary, Siberian fir, spearmint, tangerine, thyme, vetiver, wild orange, wintergreen
Antiviral - basil, black pepper, blue tansy, cassia, cinnamon, clove, copaiba, eucalyptus, ginger, helichrysum, lemon eucalyptus, litsea, manuka, melaleuca, melissa, myrrh, peppermint, rose, Siberian fir, thyme, turmeric, yarrow
Immunostimulant - arborvitae, cassia, cinnamon, clove, copaiba, eucalyptus, fennel, frankincense, ginger, lemon, lime, melaleuca, melissa, oregano, ravensara, rosemary, Siberian fir, spearmint, thyme, vetiver, white fir, wild orange, yarrow
Stimulant - arborvitae, basil, blue tansy, cardamom, cedarwood, clove, cypress, dill, eucalyptus, fennel, grapefruit, melaleuca, myrrh, pink pepper, Siberian fir, spearmint, tangerine, vetiver, wintergreen, ylang ylang
Warming - birch, black pepper, cassia, cinnamon, clary sage, clove, eucalyptus, ginger, lemongrass, marjoram, neroli, oregano, peppermint, pink pepper, thyme, wintergreen

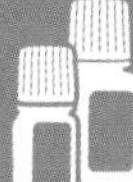

BLENDS

On Guard® - stimulates immune system and fights bacteria/viruses (pg. 194)
Zendrocrine® - supports proper detoxification (pg. 206)
DDR Prime® - manages abnormal cell activity and stimulates immune system (pg. 184)
Purify - disinfects and sanitizes (pg. 198)

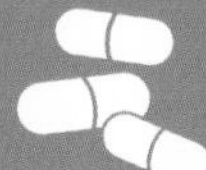

SUPPLEMENTS

Bone **Nutrient** Lifetime Complex, Alpha CRS®+, a2z Chewable™, **PB Assist®+ (pg. 216)**, Zendocrine® Complex, DDR Prime® Softgels, xEO Mega, TerraZyme®, **GX Assist® (pg. 213), On Guard Softgels (pg. 215)**, On Guard Throat Drops, TriEase Softgels, MicroPlex VMz

Related Ailments: Adenitis, AIDS or HIV, Anthrax, Antiseptic, Bacteria, Body Temperature Issues, Chemical Sensitivity Reaction [Allergies], Chest Infections, Chicken Pox, Cholera, Common Cold, Conjunctivitis (Pink Eye), Cystitis, Cytomegalovirus Infection, Dengue Fever, E. Coli, Ebola, Epstein-Barr, Ehrlichiosis, Fever, Flu, H.Pylori, Hand Foot & Mouth Disease, Hepatitis, Herpes Simplex, Infection, Legionnaires' Disease, Listeria Infection, Lockjaw (Tetanus), Lyme Disease, Measles, Meningitis, Mesenteric Lymphadenitis, Mold, Mononucleosis, MRSA, Mumps, Plague, Polio [Nervous], Q Fever, Radiation Damage [Cellular Health], Rubella [Integumentary], Reiter's Arthritis, Scurvy, Sepsis, Shigella Infection, Shingles, Staph Infection, Strep Throat [Oral Health], Tularemia, Typhoid, Virus

USAGE TIPS: For most effective use of essential oils for immune and lymphatic benefits:

- **Topical:** Apply oils topically on bottoms of feet, especially on back side of toes, rub oils down the spine and/or on any specific area of concern. Use Oil Touch technique.
- **Internal:** Take oils in capsule, place a drop(s) under or on tongue near back of throat or sip from a glass of water.
- **Aromatic:** Diffuse for associated respiratory symptoms and to clear pathogens from air.
- **Surfaces:** Sanitize surfaces with essential oil(s) mixed with water and emulsifier.

Remedies

LYME DISEASE

LYME DISEASE SUPPORT

Important facts regarding chemistry of essential oils for – Lyme protocol:

- Oregano - 60-90% carvacrol, kills bacteria, interrupts communication stream (quorum sensing) between harmful bacteria
- Thyme - 55% thymol, 10% carvacrol; protective agent for neurological tissue in brain
- Clove - 85% eugenol, controls symptoms, kills bacteria Carvacrol, eugenol, thymol are the most effective compounds for destroying pathogens; more powerful when used together
- Cassia - 80-90% cinnamaldehyde; Co2 inhibitor, antibacterial
- Cinnamon - 50% cinnamaldehyde; Co2 inhibitor, antibacterial
- Melissa - 65% aldehydes, 35% sesquiterpenes; antiviral, antibacterial; disrupts microorganism communication, immunostimulant, anti-inflammatory; antidepressant On Guard® contains cinnamon, clove, wild orange, eucalyptus, rosemary
- Frankincense - analgesic, anti-inflammatory, effective for pain management
- Patchouli - 63% sesquiterpenes; antioxidant, relief from secondary neurological effects in chronic Lyme

LYME DISEASE INTENSE RESOLVE BLEND

3 drops oregano
3 drops thyme
3 drops clove
3 drops cassia or cinnamon
2 drops On Guard®
2 drops melissa
2 drops frankincense
Place oils in capsule and take once or twice daily for two weeks depending upon intensity of symptoms. Rest from the blend for one week. Repeat this pattern until symptoms are gone for at least two months.

For greater intensity or for more chronic situations, use: Topical application option (can do while taking a break from internal use or instead of): Apply 2 drops lemongrass + 1 drop oregano to the bottom of each foot before bed. Add melissa and/or On Guard®, and/or other above suggested oils as needed.

NOTE: If rash or other discomfort occurs, reduce amount of oils being used or take a break until resolved. Consider improving intestinal elimination, removing certain foods from diet (foods that encourage microorganism growth), drink more water.

LYME DISEASE BOMB RECIPE

2 drops cinnamon or clove
2 drops cassia
2 drops oregano or thyme (alternate; use oregano in ten-day cycles; take break for twenty days)
2 drops frankincense
Place in a capsule; consume two times per day. Dilute with carrier oil if necessary or desired. Add melissa, On Guard®, and/or GX Assist® as needed.

ADDITIONAL LYME SUPPORT

- Get an Oil Touch technique weekly. See page 19 in this book.
- Apply patchouli to bottoms of feet twice per day to support nervous system. Can add other oils as desired. Consider frankincense and wild orange.
- Supplementation program - consider the following - do a minimum of a four-month program :
- Basic: MicroPlex VMz, xEO Mega
- Digestive/intestinal support: TerraZyme®, Zendocrine® Complex (mild detox support as well), GX Assist®, PB Assist®+
- Anti-inflammatory/pain relief: Alpha CRS®+ or Deep Blue Polyphenol Complex
- Cell vitality: DDR Prime® Softgels
- Immune support: On Guard Softgels AM and PM
- GI cleanse: Consider a focused cleanse followed by probiotic support: GX Assist® and PB Assist®+.

See *Candida* for a superb detox program that is beneficial for Lyme Disease.

PAIN REMEDY

10 drops lavender
8 drops Balance®
8 drops Deep Blue®
8 drops rosemary
6 drops lemongrass

- Combine above oils in 10ml roller bottle; fill remainder with carrier oil. Apply topically directly to painful joints and bottoms of feet several times each day as needed.
- Apply 1-3 drops each On Guard®, melissa, frankincense, and patchouli to bottoms of feet.
- **Sleep support ideas** (see *Sleep*):
  Apply 3 drops vetiver, 3 drops juniper berry, and 3 drops lavender to the bottoms of feet.
- **Better by morning:**
  Rub one drop each basil and lemon at night behind ears to clear symptoms of physical illness by morning.
- **Muscle range of motion support** (see *Muscular, Skeletal*):
  Apply a few drops of bergamot and cypress topically.

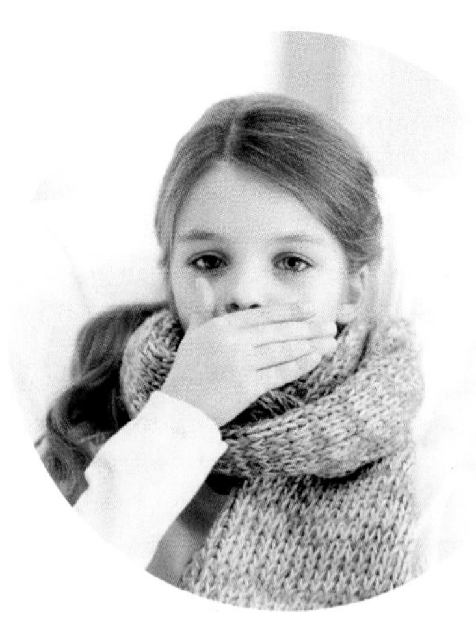

SKIN WOUND ANTISEPTIC

6 drops lavender
5 drops melaleuca
2 drops Roman chamomile
1 ounce aloe vera gel
Blend in a glass bottle or bowl. Apply using cotton swab to affected areas of skin.

COLD & FLU DRINK

2 drops lavender
2 drops lemon
2 drops peppermint
2 drops melaleuca
Mix oils in ½ cup water. Add another ½ cup water, stir, and drink.

COLD & FLU BOMB

5 drops On Guard®
5 drops melaleuca
3 drops oregano
Place in an empty capsule and swallow. Repeat every three to four hours while symptoms last.

SEASONAL WINTER-TO-SPRING BLEND

2 drops oregano
2 drops black pepper
4 drops grapefruit
Rub on the bottoms of feet five consecutive nights. Helps protect against seasonal and environmental elements.

SEASONAL SUMMER-TO-FALL BLEND

3 drops clove
2 drops Siberian fir
4 drops lemon
Rub on the bottoms of feet five consecutive nights. Helps protect against seasonal and environmental elements.

COLD SUPPORT

When a cold is coming on, blend Siberian fir, eucalyptus, and melaleuca. Place a few drops of each in a pan of steaming water. Inhale steam. Place a towel over head to make a tent to trap steam for greater potency.

HIV/AIDS SUPPORT

INITIAL CLEANSE:

- Add 2-4 drops of lemon in water daily (in glass container only).
- Take 3-4 drops each of On Guard®, oregano or melissa, and peppermint in a capsule daily for ten days followed by five days of PB Assist®+. This process can be repeated monthly as needed.
- Dietary restrictions are important. Avoid processed foods, refined sugars; increase fresh fruits and vegetables.

ONGOING SUPPORT:

- Consume 2-4 drops of lemon in water daily (in glass container only).
- Take 3-4 drops each of frankincense, On Guard®, melaleuca, rosemary in capsule daily
- Take MicroPlex VMz, Alpha CRS®+, xEO Mega daily
- Rub 2-3 drops each of Balance® and On Guard® on bottoms of feet twice a day (morning & night). Can also apply 2-4 drops of lavender for stress relief or sleep aid at night.
- Rub 1-2 drops frankincense on base of neck daily.
- Diffuse Elevation™ during day for energy and Serenity® at night for relaxation.
- Apply a hot compress for fifteen minutes after lightly massaging oils into back along the spine area for desired comfort and relief.
- For any other specific issue, refer to the respective Body System or Focus Area sections.

Perform the Oil Touch technique once a week. See *Oil Touch technique*. Benefits include:

- Strengthening the immune system
- Relieving stress and depression

ENHANCE IMMUNITY SUGAR SCRUB

2 cups brown or white sugar
1 cup fractionated coconut oil
15 drops black spruce essential oil
6 drops tea tree (melaleuca) essential oil
5 drops eucalyptus essential oil
5 drops lemon essential oil
Mix and store in glass container. Scoop out with fingers per use. For added benefits, soak in bath after scrubbing extremities.

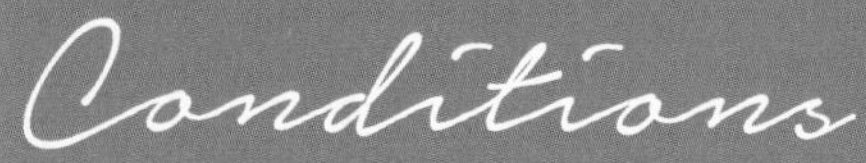

Abnormal cellular activity - frankincense, DDR Prime®; see *Cellular Health*
AIDS/HIV* - arborvitae, cassia, cinnamon, clove, helichrysum, melaleuca, melissa, myrrh, rosemary, thyme, DDR Prime®, On Guard®
Airborne germs and bacteria - arborvitae, cedarwood, eucalyptus, white fir, Breathe®, On Guard®, Purify; see "Antimicrobial" property
Allergies* - See *Allergies*
Bacteria - arborvitae, basil, black pepper, blue tansy, cassia, cedarwood, cilantro, cinnamon, citronella, clove, copaiba, coriander, eucalyptus, frankincense, geranium, kumquat, lemongrass, lime, marjoram, melaleuca, melissa, myrrh, neroli, oregano, petitgrain, red mandarin, rose, rosemary, Siberian fir, tangerine, thyme, DDR Prime®, On Guard®, Purify, Zendrocrine®
Bacteria, staph - arborvitae, celery seed, cinnamon, helichrysum, melissa, rosemary, Cheer®; see "Antibacterial" property
Boils/carbuncles - eucalyptus, frankincense, lavender, marjoram, myrrh, sandalwood, Immortelle
Body temperature issues, too cold - See "Warming" property
Body temperature issues, too hot - bergamot, black pepper, eucalyptus, lemon, peppermint
Catch colds/get sick easily - see "Weakened/suppressed immune system" below
Cellulitis - cardamom, juniper berry, lemongrass, melaleuca, oregano, sandalwood, see "Antibacterial" property
Chicken Pox - black pepper, blue tansy, eucalyptus, frankincense, melaleuca, patchouli, thyme, On Guard®
Chills - basil, black pepper, cinnamon, ginger, wintergreen, On Guard®; see "Warming" property
Cholera - black pepper, cinnamon, eucalyptus, melissa, rosemary, Zendrocrine®; see "Antibacterial" property
Cold, chronic - basil, cardamom, cypress, On Guard®, Zendrocrine®
Cold/flu - black pepper, blue tansy, cassia, celery seed, cinnamon, clove, eucalyptus, frankincense, ginger, juniper berry, lemon, lime, melaleuca, oregano, peppermint, rose, rosemary, Siberian fir, thyme, wild orange, yarrow, Breathe®, On Guard®; see "Antiviral" property, remedies this page

** See remedy this page*

† See remedy on pg. 301

Cold/flu, reduce aches/pains from† - black pepper, cypress, cedarwood, coriander, magnolia, oregano, peppermint, thyme, white fir, wild orange, AromaTouch®, Breathe®, Deep Blue®, On Guard®, PastTense®
Cold sores - arborvitae, bergamot, clove, geranium, helichrysum, lavender, lemon, lemon eucalyptus, melaleuca, melissa, myrrh, On Guard®, Zendrocrine®; see "Antiviral" property, *Oral Health*
Common Cold - see "Cold/flu" above
Conjunctivitis/pinkeye - clary sage, Douglas fir, frankincense, lavender, melaleuca, jasmine, melissa, rosemary, spikenard, corrective ointment; see "Antibacterial" property
Contagious diseases - clove, cinnamon, ginger, juniper berry, DDR Prime®, On Guard®, Purify; see "Antibacterial, Anti-infectious, Antimicrobial, Antiviral" properties
Earache - basil, cypress, ginger, helichrysum, lavender, Breathe®, Citrus Bliss®, Deep Blue®, Passion®; see *Respiratory*
Epidemics - basil, Douglas fir, ginger, juniper berry, lemon, peppermint, DDR Prime®, On Guard®
Fever - arborvitae, basil, birch, black pepper, cypress, eucalyptus, helichrysum, juniper berry, lavender, lemon, lemon eucalyptus, lemongrass, lime, patchouli, peppermint, pink pepper, Roman chamomile, rose, Siberian fir, spearmint, wild orange, yarrow, Forgive®, Passion®, PastTense®
Fever blisters - see "Cold sores" above
Flu - see "Cold/flu" above
Fungus/candida - arborvitae, basil, blue tansy, cassia, cedarwood, cilantro, cinnamon, clove, copaiba, coriander, lemongrass, marjoram, melaleuca, myrrh, oregano, patchouli, rosemary, Siberian fir, thyme, turmeric, Purify; see *Candida,*
Germs - blue tansy, grapefruit, lemon, lemon eucalytpus, lime, wild orange, Citrus Bliss®, On Guard®, Purify; see "Antimicrobial, Antiseptic" properties
Glands, swollen - cardamom, cypress, Douglas fir, frankincense, ginger, lemon, melaleuca, rosemary, sandalwood, Breathe®, On Guard®, Purify
Herpes simplex - basil, bergamot, black pepper, clove, eucalyptus, frankincense, helichrysum, lavender, melaleuca, melissa, myrrh, oregano, patchouli, peppermint, sandalwood, thyme, Console®, On Guard®; see "Antiviral" property
Illness prevention - clove, cinnamon, oregano, thyme, Adaptiv®, On Guard®
Illness recovery - cinnamon, Douglas fir, juniper berry, lemon, lemongrass, thyme, wild orange, Adaptiv®, Slim & Sassy®
Immune, weakness - cinnamon, clove, copaiba, Douglas fir, frankincense, green mandarin, melaleuca, petitgrain, sandalwood, tangerine, Citrus Bliss®, DDR Prime®, On Guard®, TerraShield®, Zendrocrine®
Infection - black pepper, cardamom, cassia, cinnamon, clove, lavender, melaleuca, melissa, oregano, thyme, wintergreen, On Guard®; see "Antibacterial, Anti-infectious, Antimicrobial, Antiviral" properties
Infectious diseases - bergamot, cassia, lemongrass, melissa, oregano, rosemary, thyme; see "Antibacterial, Anti-infectious, Antimicrobial, Antiviral" properties
Leprosy - arborvitae, cedarwood, frankincense, melissa, myrrh, peppermint, sandalwood, thyme, DDR Prime®
Lymph, congestion/stagnation - birch, cassia, cypress, Douglas fir, frankincense, geranium, grapefruit, lavender, lemon, lemongrass, lime, petitgrain, pink pepper, sandalwood, tangerine, wintergreen, Breathe®, Citrus Bliss®, Motivate®, Passion®, Purify; see *Respiratory*
Malaria - bergamot, cardamom, cinnamon, Douglas fir, eucalyptus, lemon, lemongrass, melaleuca, thyme, Breathe®, Zendrocrine®; see *Parasites*
Measles - blue tansy, clove, coriander, eucalyptus, juniper berry, lavender, melaleuca, wild orange, DDR Prime®, On Guard®; see "Antiviral" property
Microorganisms (bacterial/viral) - black pepper, cinnamon, clove, copaiba, lemongrass, melaleuca, oregano, Siberian fir, tangerine, thyme, yarrow, On Guard®
MRSA - cinnamon, clove, frankincense, geranium, juniper berry, lemon, melaleuca, melissa, oregano, peppermint, thyme, DDR Prime®, On Guard®; see "Antibacterial" property
Mumps - basil, blue tansy, cinnamon, lavender, lemon, melaleuca, rosemary, DDR Prime®, On Guard®, Zendrocrine®
Night sweats - ginger, lime, peppermint, DDR Prime®, **DigestZen®**, Zendrocrine®; see *Women's Health, Endocrine (Thyroid)*
Parasites - clove, See *Parasites*
Paralysis, facial - frankincense, helichrysum, marjoram, melissa, rosemary, thyme, DDR Prime®
Rheumatic fever - arborvitae, basil, coriander, eucalyptus, ginger, melissa, oregano, patchouli, thyme, wintergreen
Rubella - basil, black pepper, clove, frankincense, lemon, melaleuca, melissa, oregano, thyme, On Guard®, Slim & Sassy®
Ringworm - geranium, melaleuca, neroli, oregano, Roman chamomile, thyme, HD Clear®; see *Integumentary*
Scurvy - cypress, geranium, ginger, grapefruit, helichrysum, lemon, lemongrass, Zendrocrine®
Sore throat - cinnamon, copaiba, lemon, melaleuca, melissa, oregano, Siberian fir, thyme, Breathe®, On Guard®
Spleen - bergamot, cardamom, clary sage, lemon, rose, On Guard®
Spleen, congestion - cinnamon, fennel, helichrysum, lemon, sandalwood, InTune®
Spleen obstruction - basil, frankincense, ginger, marjoram, melissa
Staph - cinnamon, frankincense, geranium, lemon, melaleuca, melissa, oregano, peppermint, thyme, HD Clear®, On Guard®, Purify
Strep - cinnamon, frankincense, lemon, oregano, On Guard®
Sexually transmitted disease
· **Chlamydia** - arborvitae, basil, clove, melaleuca, thyme, On Guard®
· **Gonorrhea** - basil, copaiba, frankincense, melaleuca, rosemary, sandalwood
· **Syphilis** - black pepper, frankincense, melaleuca, melissa, myrrh, rosemary
Stomach flu (viral gastroenteritis) - arborvitae, celery seed, oregano, thyme, DDR Prime®, On Guard®, Zendrocrine®; see "Antiviral" property
Strep throat - cardamom, cinnamon, eucalyptus, lemon, melaleuca, oregano, thyme, Breathe®, On Guard®; see "Antibacterial" property
Throat, sore - cinnamon, geranium, lavender, lemon, lime, oregano, thyme, Breathe®, On Guard®, Passion®; see *Respiratory*
Tonsillitis - cinnamon, copaiba, eucalyptus, frankincense, ginger, lavender, lemon, melaleuca, myrrh, Roman chamomile, Breathe®, On Guard®; see *Oral Health*
Typhoid fever - basil, blue tansy, cinnamon, clove, eucalyptus, lemon, melaleuca, oregano, peppermint, On Guard®, Zendrocrine®
Virus - arborvitae, bergamot, black pepper, blue tansy, cassia, cinnamon, clove, copaiba, eucalyptus, frankincense, helichrysum, marjoram, melaleuca, melissa, myrrh, oregano, patchouli, peppermint, rosemary, thyme, turmeric, yarrow, Console®, On Guard®; see "Antiviral" property
Viral, hepatitis - basil, cedarwood, clove, geranium, myrrh, rosemary, Motivate®, Zendrocrine®
Virus, spinal - melaleuca, melissa, thyme, wintergreen; see "Antiviral" property
Weakened/suppressed immune system - frankincense, melaleuca, myrrh, thyme, Forgive®, On Guard®
White blood cells (leukocytes), low count/lack of formation - frankincense, lavender, lemon, lime, myrrh
Zoonosis - cedarwood, clove, eucalyptus, frankincense, melaleuca, melissa, myrrh, thyme, On Guard®

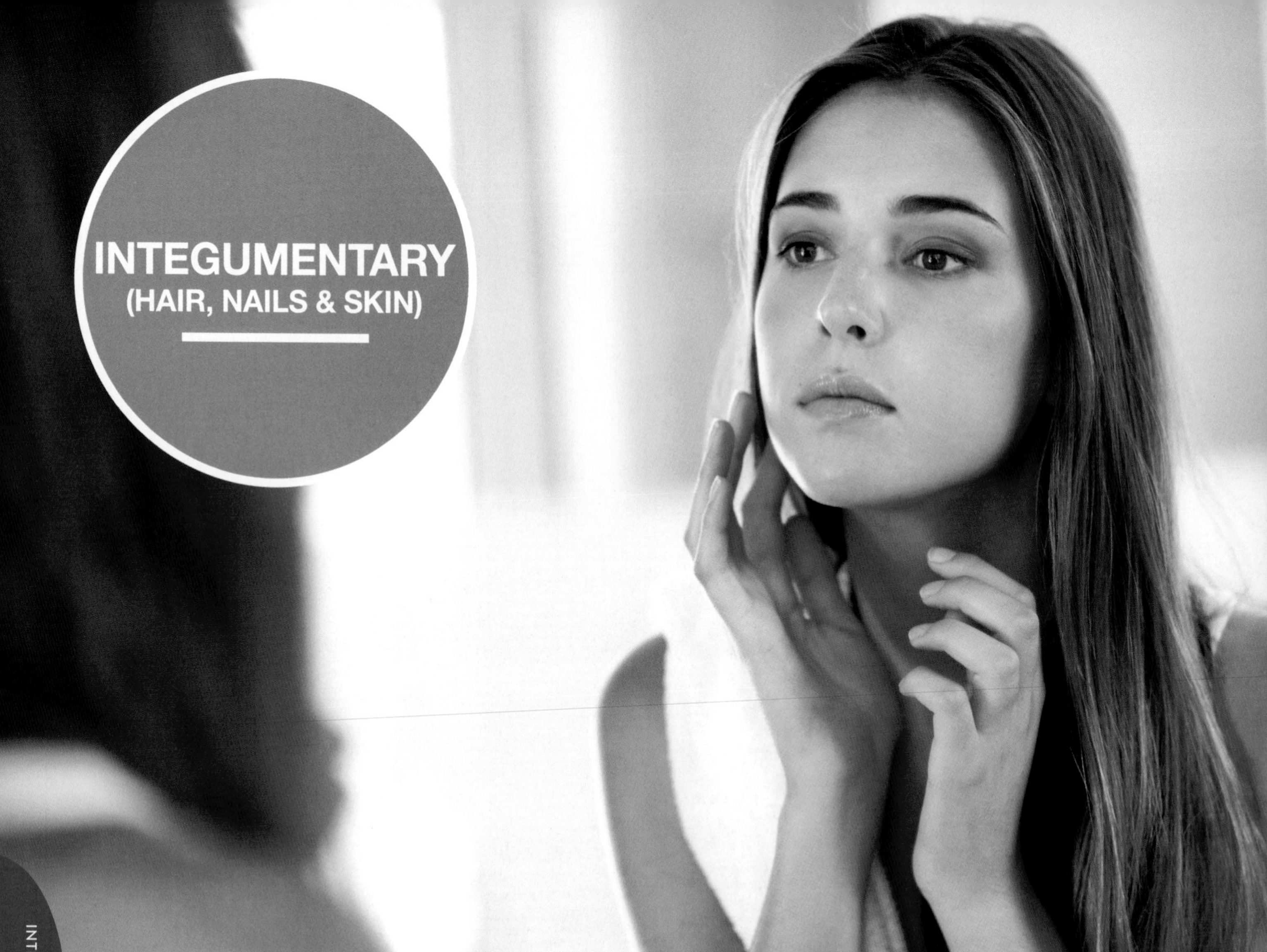

THE INTEGUMENTARY SYSTEM consists of the skin, hair, and nails. On the broadest scale, this system supports immune function and regulates homeostasis, as it constitutes the body's first line of defense against things that would disrupt its delicate balance and registers external stimuli through sensory receptors that communicate touch, pain, and pressure.

With a surface area averaging eighteen square feet, the skin is the largest organ of the body. It has two layers: the inner layer is called the dermis. The epidermis, or outer layer, consists of several strata that produce keratin, which gives strength and elasticity to the skin; melanin, which gives it its color; Merkel's cells, which facilitate touch reception; and Langerhans' cells, which produce antigens to support the immune system. And as a living organ, deep-level cells continually divide and push older cells to the surface to be worn off—millions every day— leaving behind a new epidermis every five to seven weeks.

The skin protects the internal organs, guards against infection, regulates temperature change and hydration levels through perspiration, and stores water, fat, and glucose. It excretes waste, generates vitamin D when exposed to ultraviolet light, and secretes melanin to protect against sunburn. It also has the capacity to form new cells to repair minor cuts and abrasions.

The array of dermatological conditions that may afflict people ranges from warts, eczema, acne, and moles to psoriasis, vitiligo, and a variety of skin cancers. Hair and nail conditions can be unsightly, uncomfortable, or even painful. Since many skin, hair, and nail conditions are an outward reflection of other imbalances going on inside the body, it is important to focus on detoxing, cleansing, and supplementing vital nutrition to the cells and internal organs in addition to essential oil applications that can easily target the area of concern.

Natural solutions are very effective and can be used as a first line of defense toward various integumentary conditions. If problems or conditions persist or cause concern, proper medical attention should be sought. Keep in mind that natural solutions can be used safely together with medical treatments if the latter become necessary. Many essential oils that are beneficial for integumentary support are diverse in the number of conditions they can impact. Some oils are more obvious choices, such as lavender and geranium with their marvelous healing properties. Other oils target more of the underlying factors. For example, birch oil is great used in ointments, creams, and compresses, especially for inflamed skin (eczema, boils, dermatitis, psoriasis, ulcers, etc.). There are a diverse number of oils and solutions that can be realized.

TOP SOLUTIONS

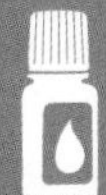

SINGLE OILS

Lavender - supports healing and maintaining healthy tissue (pg. 122)
Sandalwood - promotes regeneration and toning (pg. 150)
Geranium - regenerates tissue and tones skin (pg. 112)
Frankincense - invigorates skin, reduces inflammation (pg. 110)
Helichrysum - regenerates tissue and reduces scarring (pg. 117)

By Related Properties

For more, See Oil Properties on pages 477 - 481

Analgesic - arborvitae, basil, black pepper, blue tansy, cassia, cinnamon, copaiba, coriander, cypress, eucalyptus, fennel, frankincense, ginger, juniper berry, lavender, litsea, melaleuca, peppermint, rosemary, Siberian fir, turmeric, yarrow
Antifungal - arborvitae, blue tansy, cassia, cinnamon, clary sage, copaiba, coriander, dill, ginger, helichrysum, lemon eucalyptus, lemongrass, litsea, manuka, melaleuca, patchouli, ravensara, Siberian fir, spearmint, thyme, turmeric
Anti-infectious - cedarwood, cinnamon, clove, copaiba, cypress, frankincense, geranium, lavender, litsea, marjoram, melaleuca, Roman chamomile, rosemary
Anti-inflammatory - arborvitae, basil, birch, black pepper, blue tansy, cedarwood, cinnamon, clove, copaiba, coriander, fennel, frankincense, ginger, lavender, lime, litsea, manuka, myrrh, neroli, patchouli, Siberian fir, spearmint, spikenard, tangerine, turmeric, wintergreen, yarrow
Antimicrobial - basil, blue tansy, cardamom, cinnamon, clary sage, copaiba, cypress, dill, frankincense, helichrysum, green mandarin, lemon, lemongrass, litsea, manuka, myrrh, neroli, oregano, rosemary, Siberian fir, thyme
Antimutagenic - cinnamon, copaiba, ginger, lavender, lemongrass, neroli, tangerine, turmeric
Antiseptic - bergamot, birch, clary sage, clove, copaiba, fennel, frankincense, ginger, grapefruit, juniper berry, lavender, lemon eucalyptus, manuka, marjoram, melaleuca, myrrh, neroli, oregano, ravensara, sandalwood, Siberian fir, spearmint, tangerine, vetiver, wintergreen, yarrow, ylang ylang
Antiviral - arborvitae, basil, blue tansy, cassia, clove, copaiba, dill, eucalyptus, ginger, helichrysum, lime, litsea, manuka, melissa, myrrh, rose, turmeric, Siberian fir, yarrow
Astringent - cassia, cedarwood, clary sage, cypress, geranium, grapefruit, green mandarin, helichrysum, lemon, litsea, myrrh, sandalwood, wintergreen, yarrow
Cytophylactic - arborvitae, frankincense, geranium, lavender, manuka, neroli, rosemary, tangerine
Deodorant - bergamot, clary sage, citronella, copaiba, cypress, eucalyptus, geranium, lavender, lemon eucalyptus, lemongrass, litsea, manuka, neroli, patchouli, Siberian fir, spikenard
Insect repellent - arborvitae, birch, blue tansy, cedarwood, cinnamon, eucalyptus, geranium, lemongrass, litsea, patchouli, thyme, vetiver, ylang ylang
Regenerative - basil, cedarwood, clove, coriander, geranium, jasmine, lavender, lemongrass, manuka, melaleuca, myrrh, neroli, patchouli, sandalwood, wild orange, yarrow
Revitalizer - coriander, juniper berry, lemon, lemongrass, lime, manuka
Tonic - arborvitae, basil, birch, cardamom, clary sage, coriander, cypress, fennel, frankincense, geranium, ginger, grapefruit, green mandarin, lavender, lemon, lime, marjoram, myrrh, neroli, patchouli, pink pepper, Roman chamomile, rose, rosemary, sandalwood, Siberian fir, tangerine, thyme, wild orange, ylang ylang, yarrow

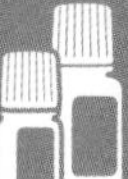

BLENDS

Immortelle - restores and tones skin (pg. 191)
HD Clear® - cleanses skin and reduces inflammation (pg. 189)

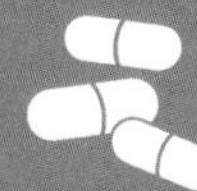

SUPPLEMENTS

Bone **Nutrient** Lifetime Complex, Alpha CRS®+, PB Assist®+, **xEO Mega (pg. 222)**, Zendocrine® Complex, TerraZyme®, GX Assist®, **IQ Mega® (pg. 213)**, MicroPlex VMz

Related Ailments: Acne, Actinic Keratosis, Age Spots, Bags Under Eyes, Baldness, Bed Sores, Blisters, Blisters from Sun, Boils, Brittle Nails, Burns, Calluses, Chapped Skin, Clogged Pores, Cold Sores, Corns, Cuts, Cyst [Cellular Health], Dandruff, Dehydrated Skin, Dry Hair, Dry Lips, Dry Skin, Eczema, Excessive Perspiration, Fragile Hair, Genital Warts, Hair Loss, Head Lice, Hernia (incisional), Ichthyosis Vulgaris, Impetigo [Immune], Infected Wounds, Ingrown Toenail, Itching [Allergies], Lichen Nitidus, Moles [Cellular Health], Oily Hair, Oily Skin, Plantar Warts, Poison Ivy [Allergies], Porphyria, Psoriasis, Rashes [Allergies], Ringworm, Rosacea, Scabies, Scarring, Sebaceous Cyst, Skin Ulcers, Stevens-Johnson Syndrome, Stretch Marks [Pregnancy], Sunburn, Swimmer's Itch [Candida], Tissue Regeneration [Cellular Health, Muscular], Ulcers – Leg and Varicose [Cardiovascular], Vitiligo, Warts, Wounds, Wrinkles

USAGE TIPS: For best support of hair, skin and nails:
- **Topical:** Apply oils directly to hair, scalp, nails, and skin. Use a carrier oil to dilute and reduce sensitivity to skin when necessary, especially with infants, elderly, and compromised skin.
- **Internal:** Consume specified oils by either capsule or under tongue. Gut health is a major component of integumentary health. See *Digestive & Intestinal, Candida*.

Conditions

HAIR:

Dandruff - cedarwood, cypress, lavender, lemon eucalyptus, melaleuca, patchouli, petitgrain, rosemary, tangerine, thyme, wintergreen, Cheer®, Elevation™, Purify
Dirty - lemon, lime, Citrus Bliss®, Purify
Dry - copaiba, geranium, lavender, patchouli, rosemary, sandalwood, spikenard, wintergreen, Breathe®, Clary-Calm®, Elevation™, Zendrocrine®
Dull - lemongrass, lime (has mild bleaching action), melaleuca, rosemary, Breathe®, TerraShield®
Fragile/brittle - clary sage, cedarwood, geranium, lavender, Roman chamomile, rosemary, sandalwood, thyme, wintergreen, Breathe®, DDR Prime®
Greasy/oily* - arborvitae, basil, cedarwood, citronella, cypress, juniper berry (scalp), lemon, melaleuca, peppermint, petitgrain, rosemary, thyme, Breathe®, Elevation™
Growth, poor - cedarwood, clary sage, geranium, ginger, grapefruit, lavender, lemon, rosemary, thyme, ylang ylang, Citrus Bliss®, Elevation™, Motivate®
Lice* - arborvitae, cedarwood, cinnamon, citronella, clove, eucalyptus, geranium, melaleuca, oregano, rosemary, thyme, TerraShield®, Zendrocrine®; see *Parasites*
Loss* - arborvitae, cedarwood, clary sage, cypress, eucalyptus, grapefruit, juniper berry, lavender, lemongrass, myrrh, Roman chamomile, rosemary, thyme, wintergreen, yarrow, ylang ylang, DDR Prime®
Scalp, itchy/flaky - cedarwood, lavender, rosemary, wintergreen, Forgive®, Zendrocrine®
Split ends - cedarwood, clary sage, lavender, rosemary, ylang ylang, Zendrocrine®

NAILS:

Brittle Nails - arborvitae, cypress, eucalyptus, frankincense, grapefruit, lavender, lemon, marjoram, myrrh, Roman chamomile, rosemary, sandalwood, wild orange, ClaryCalm®, Immortelle; see *Cardiovascular*
Fungus† - arborvitae, citronella, copaiba, eucalyptus, geranium, oregano, lemongrass, melaleuca, myrrh, thyme, DDR Prime®, HD Clear®, On Guard®, Zendrocrine®; see *Candida*
Hangnail* - basil, black pepper, cilantro, coriander, lavender, rosemary, sandalwood, ylang ylang, Breathe®
Missing (injury) - eucalyptus, frankincense, myrrh, Elevation™, On Guard®, TerraShield®
Ridges - eucalyptus, melaleuca, thyme, Zendrocrine®
Ripped/split† - eucalyptus, geranium, lemon, melaleuca, Citrus Bliss®, Elevation™, HD Clear®
Soft/weak† - eucalyptus, fennel, frankincense, grapefruit, lemon, lime, white fir, Citrus Bliss®, Purify
Swelling/red/tender - arborvitae, eucalyptus, lemongrass, melaleuca, myrrh, thyme, DDR Prime®, On Guard®, Zendrocrine®
Yellowed/infected - eucalyptus, frankincense, lemon, melaleuca, myrrh, thyme, AromaTouch®, Elevation™, On Guard®, Zendrocrine®

** See remedy on pg. 308*
† See remedy on pg. 309

SKIN:

NOTE: See *First Aid* for Bites & Stings; *Allergies* for Hives, Rashes, etc. for additional suggestions.
Acne - arborvitae, bergamot, black spruce, blue tansy, citronella, copaiba, cedarwood (astringent), clary sage, coriander, cypress, frankincense, geranium, grapefruit, green mandarin, helichrysum, juniper berry, lavender, lemon, magnolia, melaleuca, myrrh, neroli, patchouli, petitgrain, rosemary, sandalwood, spearmint, thyme, white fir, wintergreen, yarrow, ylang ylang, DDR Prime®, Forgive®, HD Clear®, Immortelle, Purify
Aging/age spots - basil, copaiba, coriander, fennel, frankincense, geranium, helichrysum, lavender, lemon, lime, myrrh, neroli, petitgrain, Roman chamomile, rose, sandalwood, spikenard, tangerine, vetiver, yarrow, DDR Prime®, Immortelle, Whisper®
Athlete's foot - arborvitae, cinnamon, citronella, clove, coriander, lemon eucalyptus, lemongrass, melaleuca, myrrh, oregano, patchouli, thyme, DDR Prime®, Purify; see *Candida*
Appearance, poor/dull - basil, cedarwood, Douglas fir, fennel, frankincense, geranium, lemon, lemongrass, lime, myrrh, sandalwood, wild orange, HD Clear®, Immortelle
Bags under eyes - cedarwood, frankincense, helichrysum, juniper berry, lavender, lemon, lime, Roman chamomile, sandalwood, Immortelle, Serenity®, Zendrocrine®
Blister, friction/heat/liquid-filled - copaiba, eucalyptus, frankincense, lavender, myrrh, patchouli, sandalwood, Immortelle
Body odor - arborvitae, cilantro, citronella, copaiba, coriander, Douglas fir, eucalyptus, lemon eucalyptus, lemongrass, melaleuca, neroli, patchouli, Siberian fir, tangerine, Elevation™, Whisper®, Zendrocrine®
Boils/carbuncles - bergamot, frankincense, helichrysum, lavender, marjoram, myrrh, neroli, Roman chamomile, sandalwood, Immortelle
Bruises - arborvitae, blue tansy, copaiba, clove, cypress, fennel, geranium, helichrysum, lavender, Roman chamomile, white fir, ylang ylang, AromaTouch®, DDR Prime®, Deep Blue®, Zendrocrine®
Bumps - clary sage, frankincense, patchouli, wild orange, Slim & Sassy®, Zendrocrine®
Burns - copabia, eucalyptus, frankincense, geranium, helichrysum, lavender, lemon eucalyptus, myrrh, peppermint, Roman chamomile, Siberian fir, spearmint, tangerine, Immortelle; see *First Aid*
Calluses - cypress, Douglas fir, lavender, oregano, Roman chamomile, white fir, HD Clear®
Capillaries, broken - geranium, lemon; see *Cardiovascular*
Cell renewal - arborvitae, basil, cedarwood, lavender, frankincense, helichrysum, jasmine, lemongrass, lime, melaleuca, myrrh, patchouli, rosemary, sandalwood, spearmint, thyme, wild orange, DDR Prime®, Immortelle
Cellulitis - see *Immune & Lymphatic*
Chapped/cracked/dry/peeling - copaiba, frankincense, green mandarin, jasmine, magnolia, myrrh, neroli, patchouli, petitgrain, sandalwood, spearmint, tangerine, turmeric, Purify, corrective ointment, Immortelle
Circulation, poor - geranium, lemongrass, marjoram, rose
Collagen, lack of - helichrysum, lemongrass, sandalwood
Corns - arborvitae, clove, grapefruit, lemon, peppermint, ylang ylang, Citrus Bliss®, DDR Prime®, TerraShield®
Cuts/wounds* - basil, cardamom, dill, frankincense, geranium, green mandarin, magnolia, helichrysum, juniper berry, lavender, lemongrass, marjoram, melaleuca, myrrh, rose, sandalwood, On Guard®
Damaged - arborvitae, basil, cedarwood, cilantro, cypress, frankincense, geranium, helichrysum, lemongrass, lime, neroli, sandalwood, wild orange, DDR Prime®, Immortelle
Dermatitis* - black spruce, blue tansy, geranium, helichrysum, patchouli, Siberian fir, thyme, Elevation™, HD Clear®
Diseased - birch, cedarwood, geranium, lavender, oregano, thyme, wintergreen, Zendrocrine®

Eczema/psoriasis* - arborvitae, bergamot, birch, black spruce, blue tansy, cedarwood, copaiba, Douglas fir, geranium, helichrysum, juniper berry, lavender, melissa, myrrh, neroli, oregano, patchouli, peppermint, Roman chamomile, rosemary, Siberian fir, spearmint, thyme, turmeric, wintergreen, yarrow, ylang ylang, Adaptiv®, Forgive®, HD Clear®; see *Candida*
Facial, thread veins - rose, Immortelle
Fine lines or cracks - lavender, sandalwood, vetiver, DDR Prime®, Immortelle
Flushed - wild orange, Breathe®, Purify
Fungus - arborvitae, cedarwood, clove, frankincense, lavender, lemon eucalyptus, melaleuca, myrrh, patchouli, Roman chamomile, thyme, turmeric, Zendrocrine®, HD Clear®; see *Candida*
Growth, small/fleshy/rough/grainy - fennel, grapefruit, thyme, HD Clear®, Elevation™, Slim & Sassy®, Zendrocrine®
Heels, cracked - myrrh, sandalwood, vetiver, corrective ointment
Hemorrhoids - cypress, geranium, helichrysum, myrrh, patchouli, Roman chamomile, sandalwood, yarrow, AromaTouch®, DigestZen®, Zendrocrine®
Hernia, incision - arborvitae, basil, geranium, helichrysum, lemongrass, melissa, On Guard®, Zendrocrine®
Impetigo - geranium, lavender, oregano, vetiver, Purify, Whisper®, Zendrocrine®
Infection - arborvitae, cassia, cinnamon, clove, copaiba, Douglas fir, eucalyptus, frankincense, juniper berry, lavender, melaleuca, melissa, myrrh, oregano, patchouli, peppermint, rose, sandalwood, thyme, On Guard®, Purify
Inflammation/redness - cedarwood, geranium, jasmine, juniper berry, lavender, helichrysum, magnolia, peppermint, Roman chamomile, rose, sandalwood, wild orange, ylang ylang, DDR Prime®, Immortelle, On Guard®, Serenity®
Itching - blue tansy, cilantro, lavender, melaleuca, patchouli, peppermint, Roman chamomile, sandalwood, vetiver, wild orange, Immortelle, Slim & Sassy®, Zendrocrine®
Lips, chapped/cracked/dry/peeling - cedarwood, jasmine, lavender, myrrh, sandalwood, Whisper®, corrective ointment
Moles - frankincense, geranium, juniper berry, lavender, oregano, sandalwood, wild orange, DDR Prime®, Elevation™, HD Clear®, TerraShield®, Zendrocrine®
Oily - bergamot, cedarwood, coriander, frankincense, geranium, grapefruit, green mandarin, jasmine, petitgrain, sandalwood, wild orange, ylang ylang, Breathe®, Forgive®, HD Clear®
Pores, clogged - cedarwood, lemon, melaleuca, juniper berry, petitgrain, sandalwood, DDR Prime®, HD Clear®, Immortelle, Purify
Pores, enlarged - lemongrass, sandalwood, DDR Prime®, HD Clear®, Immortelle
Perspiration, excessive - cilantro, coriander, cypress, Douglas fir, geranium, lemon, lemongrass, peppermint, petitgrain, Zendrocrine®
Perspiration, lack of - arborvitae, basil, black pepper, citronella, cypress, ginger, melaleuca, Siberian fir, wild orange, yarrow, Zendrocrine®
Pigmentation, excess - basil, cedarwood, frankincense, lavender, lemon, Roman chamomile, sandalwood, spearmint, ylang ylang, Citrus Bliss®, Immortelle, Whisper®
Pigmentation, lack of - bergamot, cedarwood, Douglas fir, sandalwood, vetiver, DDR Prime®, Immortelle
Radiation wounds - arborvitae, basil, cedarwood, clove, frankincense, geranium, helichrysum, jasmine, lavender, melaleuca, myrrh, patchouli, rosemary, sandalwood, thyme, wild orange, DDR Prime®, Immortelle
Rashes - arborvitae, frankincense, lavender, lemon, melaleuca, Roman chamomile, sandalwood, vetiver, ClaryCalm®, Immortelle, Purify, Serenity®, Slim & Sassy®, Zendrocrine®; see *Candida*
Ringworm - cardamom, clove, geranium, lemongrass, melaleuca, neroli, oregano, petitgrain, Roman chamomile, thyme, HD Clear®
Rough, dry, scaly cracked - black spruce, cedarwood, jasmine, lavender, myrrh, Roman chamomile, sandalwood, Whisper®, corrective ointment
Sagging - basil, coriander, frankincense, geranium, grapefruit, helichrysum, jasmine, juniper berry, lime, melaleuca, myrrh, sandalwood, Citrus Bliss®, DDR Prime®, Immortelle
Scabs - arborvitae, basil, birch, coriander, eucalyptus, frankincense, geranium, helichrysum, juniper berry, lavender, lemon, lemongrass, lime, spearmint, Citrus Bliss®, Elevation™, Immortelle
Scarring - cypress, frankincense, geranium, helichrysum, lavender, magnolia, neroli, rose, sandalwood, yarrow, vetiver, Immortelle
Sensitive/tender - arborvitae, frankincense, ginger, helichrysum, jasmine, lavender, marjoram, melaleuca, rosemary, wild orange, DDR Prime®, Elevation™, TerraShield®, Whisper®
Skin disorders - arborvitae, black pepper, cilantro, coriander, frankincense, geranium, helichrysum, oregano, rosemary, tangerine, wild orange, Immortelle
Skin tags - cedarwood, coriander, frankincense, geranium, lavender, oregano, sandalwood
Sores - lavender, myrrh, patchouli, sandalwood, spearmint, On Guard®, Purify
Stretch marks - arborvitae, cypress, Douglas fir, frankincense, geranium, lavender, myrrh, neroli, sandalwood, tangerine, AromaTouch®, ClaryCalm®, Immortelle
Sunburns* - arborvitae, blue tansy, eucalyptus, frankincense, helichrysum, lavender, myrrh, peppermint, sandalwood, spearmint, Immortelle
Sunburns, prevent (sunscreen) - arborvitae, helichrysum, lavender, myrrh
Tightened/hardened - frankincense, patchouli, DDR Prime®, Purify, Zendrocrine®
Tone, lack of/imbalanced* - arborvitae, basil, cypress, Douglas fir, frankincense, lemon, lemongrass, rose, sandalwood, ylang ylang, Citrus Bliss®, Immortelle
Ulcers (open crater, red, tender edges) - cedarwood, coriander, frankincense, geranium, helichrysum, lavender, lemongrass, melaleuca, myrrh, sandalwood, wild orange, Immortelle
UV radiation - clove, coriander, helichrysum, lavender, myrrh, sandalwood, DDR Prime®
Varicose ulcer - cedarwood, coriander, frankincense, geranium, yarrow, AromaTouch®, DDR Prime®
Varicose veins - bergamot, cardamom, cypress, geranium, helichrysum, lemon, lemongrass, rosemary, yarrow, AromaTouch®, DDR Prime®, DigestZen®
Vitiligo - bergamot, sandalwood, vetiver, Immortelle, DDR Prime®, Whisper®, Zendrocrine®
Warts* - arborvitae, cedarwood, cinnamon, clove, frankincense, lemon, lemongrass, lime, melaleuca, melissa, oregano, thyme, DDR Prime®, AromaTouch®, Forgive®, On Guard®
White patches on skin, inside mouth - bergamot, black pepper, frankincense, melaleuca, myrrh, sandalwood
Wounds, weeping (yellow/green pus)* - bergamot, clary sage, copaiba, frankincense, helichrysum, melaleuca, wild orange, yarrow
Wrinkles - arborvitae, Douglas fir, fennel, geranium, grapefruit, green mandarin, frankincense, helichrysum, jasmine, lavender, myrrh, neroli, petitgrain, Roman chamomile, rose, sandalwood, spikenard, white fir, wild orange, Forgive®, Immortelle

** See remedy on pg. 309*

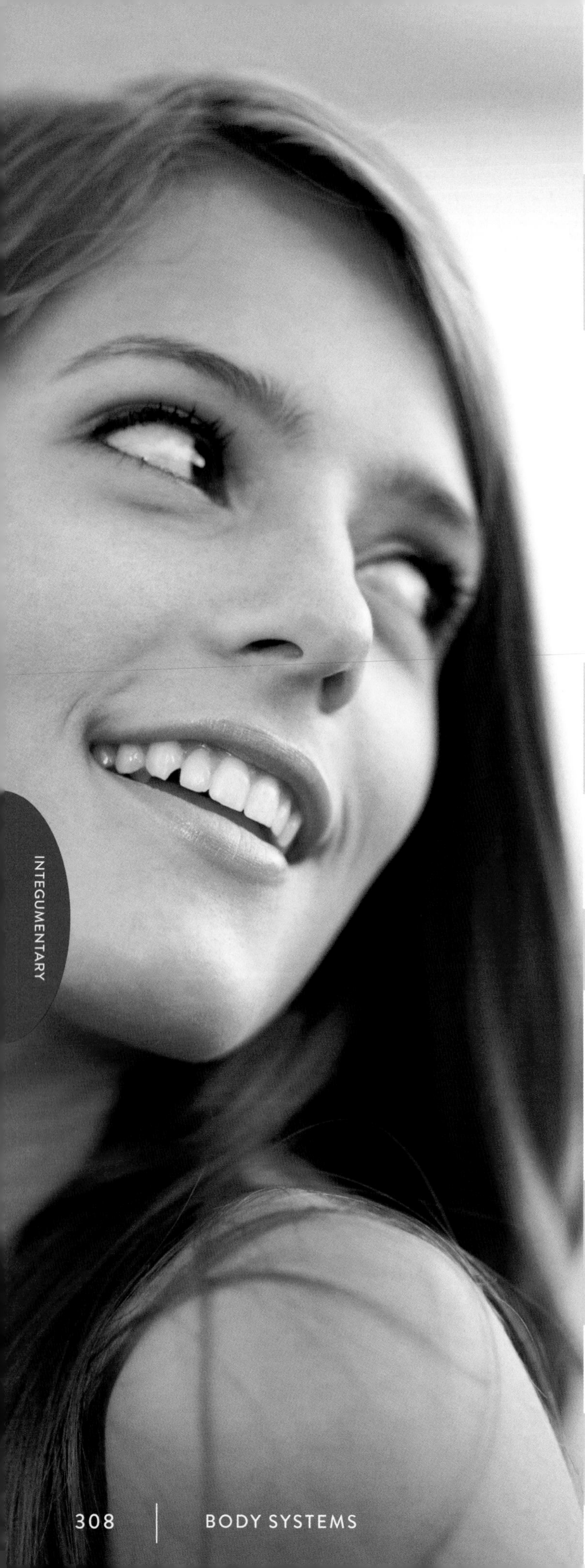

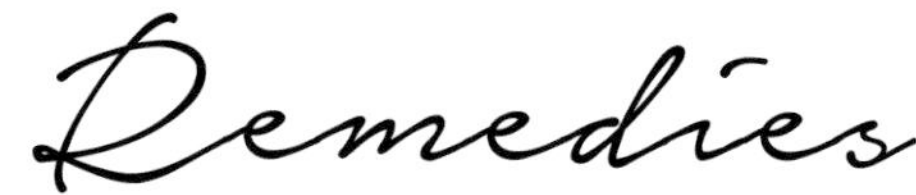

SKIN:

DERMATITIS/ECZEMA BLEND

10 drops frankincense
10 drops lavender
10 drops melaleuca
10 drops helichrysum
3 drops lemongrass
4 drops juniper berry
5 drops geranium
45 drops fractionated coconut oil
Add ingredients to spray bottle and apply as needed.

GRAPEFRUIT EXFOLIATING SCRUB - to boost circulation and tone skin (Do not use this scrub on sensitive or inflamed skin)

30ml fractionated coconut oil
3 ounces fine sea salt
10 drops of grapefruit essential oil

- Pour carrier oil into a glass bowl for blending, add grapefruit oil, mix slightly; then add sea salt in stages, stirring until a thick paste is formed. Add more carrier oil if a looser consistency is desired.
- Once prepared, mixture keeps for six months; place contents in dark jar to preserve qualities of grapefruit oil. Make note of date it was made.
- Application: massage scrub in circular motion directly onto skin. Rinse with warm water.

NATURAL ACNE BLEND

Add in the following order:
4 drops copaiba
4 drops frankincense
2 ounces witch hazel
3 drops green mandarin
3 drops lavender
Combine into glass sprayer bottle and spray to affected area.

REFRESHING SUGAR SCRUB:

Scrub: Mix 2 c. brown sugar, ¼ c. coconut oil, and 10 drops each tangerine and spearmint essential oils. Store in an airtight glass container.

SKIN REJUVENATION

Apply magnolia and neroli topically, followed by 1 drop each lavender and Roman chamomile.

SKIN TONE AND TEXTURE HEALTH

Add in the following order:
10 drops helichrysum
6 drops lavender
8 drops lemongrass
4 drops patchouli
5 drops myrrh
Add to roller bottle, top with 1 ounce carrier oil; gently shake to mix before each use. Apply to desired areas of skin three to four times daily.

SUNBURN REMEDY

25 drops lavender
25 drops helichrysum
25 drops peppermint
Add to 10ml roller or spray bottle; fill with carrier oil and apply gently to sunburn.

WART

Use 1 drop or less oregano oil (depending on size of area) twice daily for two weeks.

WOUND CARE - heal and prevent infection

Apply 1 drop melaleuca to affected area to clean wound; apply corrective ointment.

NAILS:

ANTIFUNGAL NAIL BLEND

5 drops melaleuca
1 drop cinnamon
2 drops lavender
½ ounce carrier oil
Mix and apply around and under affected nails two to three times per day until gone. Avoid contact with eyes.

HANGNAIL: Apply 1 drop arborvitae to area of concern, massage.

NAIL GROWTH: combine 1 drop of grapefruit essential oil with 10ml of carrier oil. AromaTouch® into nail bed, then with upward strokes towards nail tip

NAIL SOAK AND CUTICLE CURE - to stimulate circulation and promote healthy shine
4 drops lavender
2 drops bay leaf
3 drops sandalwood
½ ounce carrier
Soak in formula for ten minutes, buff, moisturize.

NAIL STRENGTHENER TREATMENT

2 drops lemon
2 drops frankincense
2 drops myrrh
2 drops fractionated carrier
Combine in glass bowl. Dip fingernails in blend; massage. Use twice per week.

NOURISH YOUR NAILS

15 drops lavender
10 drops lemon
4 drops myrrh
2 tablespoons fractionated coconut oil or choice of carrier oil
Mix in 2-ounce glass bottle with a dropper lid; fill remainder of bottle with carrier oil. Shake vigorously for two minutes. Warm to body temp. Let sit 24 hours. Apply 1 drop of mixture per nail; massage in each nail for one minute. Follow with a moisturizer.

SPLIT OR DAMAGED NAIL REPAIR

4 drops sandalwood
2 drops ClaryCalm®
1 drops wild orange
1 tablespoon carrier oil
Soak nail in formula each night; massage in thoroughly to promote absorption; wipe off excess with tissue; follow with moisturizer. Add 1 drop myrrh oil to formula three times per week.

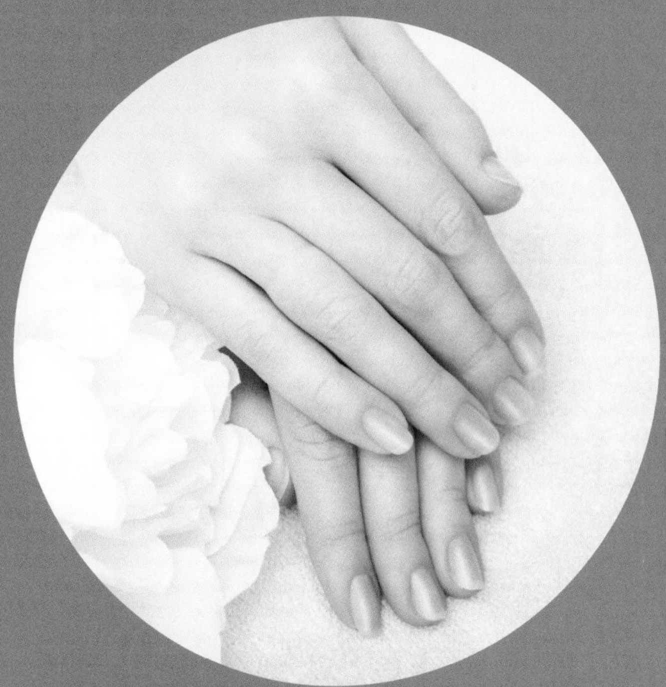

HAIR:

GREASY HAIR RESOLVE: Grapefruit oil rids scalp of impurities and residual styling products without drying out hair. It also promotes hair growth and helps rejuvenate hair.
1 teaspoon natural shampoo
1 drop of grapefruit essential oil
Combine shampoo and grapefruit oil; massage gently into scalp with fingertips. Rinse.

HAIR GROWTH: Add 2 drops of grapefruit essential oil to 8ml (just under one tablespoon) of jojoba and stir the blend. Massage the liquid into your scalp, using a circular motion with your fingertips. Leave on for thirty minutes and then wash your hair with a gentle shampoo.

HAIR LOSS REMEDY OPTIONS: Use 5 drops each of cedarwood, cypress, lavender, rosemary oils; add to 2 ounces of a natural shampoo and use when shampooing.
Blend with 2 drops of each oil listed above with 2 tablespoons of fractionated coconut oil. Massage into scalp, cover with a shower cap, and let sit for a few hours or overnight; shampoo and condition.

More intense blend: Combine 8 drops rosemary + 10 drops lavender + 10 drops sandalwood + 10 drops cedarwood + 10 drops melaleuca oils with 3 ounces of natural shampoo; work oils into scalp several times a week and let sit for twenty minutes prior to shampooing.

NATURAL BEARD OIL with copaiba, fractionated coconut oil, and Peppermint.

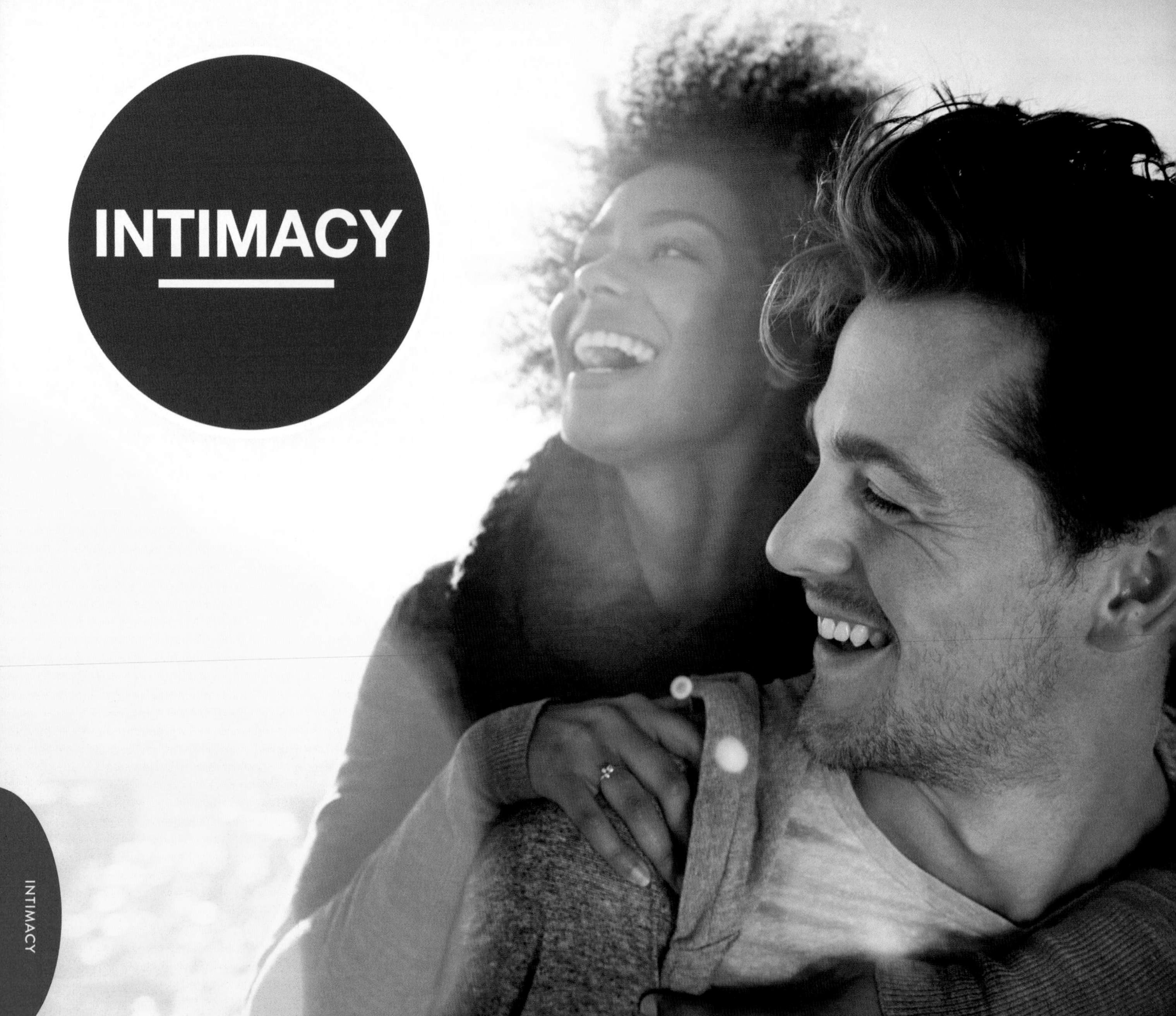

ALL HUMANS have a basic need to love and feel loved; intimate relationships that include a sexual component help to fulfill this need. If a couple desires to improve their emotional intimacy, they can attend seminars, read books, or go to marriage counseling to get some ideas. Because of past experiences and current health concerns, physical intimacy can have inherent challenges including low sex drive, exhaustion/fatigue, aches and pains, chronic illness, hemorrhoids, yeast infections, endometriosis, vaginal dryness, impotence, lack of nitric oxide, oxytocin production, and more.

At times, individuals may be interested in an aphrodisiac, which is a substance that enhances or stimulates passion and sexual arousal. An aphrodisiac can also help reduce physical, psychological, or emotional conditions that interfere with passion and sexual arousal. Certain essential oils have long been praised for their aphrodisiac qualities. One of the reasons why they are so effective is that their natural chemical composition works quickly on the circulatory, endocrine, and reproductive systems when applied to the skin (usually diluted).

Additionally, essential oils are an effective aphrodisiac because their aromatic qualities affect mood, thought, and feelings via olfaction; once inhaled, the odor molecules register a response in the limbic portion of the brain, which is also responsible for sexual behavior and memory and can influence the body's sexual response.

Essential oils can produce desired effects for oneself and/or one's partner. Most aphrodisiac essential oils work by raising the body temperature through their warm and rich aromas. Once the body has reached an ideal temperature, the sensual and euphoric properties of essential oils are most effective.

Essential oils can also help balance hormones, reduce fatigue and exhaustion, help support the body's physical health, and promote emotional wellness, which in turn promotes emotional and physical intimacy. Additionally, certain essential oil applications can help individuals relax and "get in the mood."

TOP SOLUTIONS

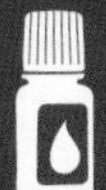

SINGLE OILS

Jasmine, Neroli , and Magnolia - enhances mood and libido, euphoric (pgs. 118, 136 , & 129)
Ylang ylang - supports a healthy libido and endocrine function (pg. 165)
Patchouli - improves circulation, raises body temperature, enhances mood (pg. 139)
Clary sage - supports the endocrine system, enhances libido (pg. 96)
Bergamot and Pink pepper - balances hormones, enhances libido (pg. 81), (pg. 144)

By Related Properties

For more, See Oil Properties on pages 477 - 481

Anaphrodisiac - arborvitae, marjoram (avoid if interested in libido enhancement)
Antidepressant - bergamot, cinnamon, coriander, dill, frankincense, geranium, grapefruit, jasmine, lavender, lemon, lemongrass, magnolia, neroli, patchouli, ravensara, sandalwood, tangerine, wild orange, ylang ylang
Aphrodisiac - black pepper, cardamom, cinnamon, clary sage, clove, coriander, jasmine, juniper berry, magnolia, neroli, patchouli, peppermint, pink pepper, ravensara, rose, rosemary, sandalwood, spearmint, thyme, turmeric, vetiver, wild orange, ylang ylang
Calming - basil, bergamot, black pepper, blue tansy, cassia, clary sage, copaiba, coriander, frankincense, geranium, jasmine, juniper berry, lavender, litsea, oregano, patchouli, sandalwood, tangerine, vetiver, yarrow
Energizing - basil, clove cypress, grapefruit, lemongrass, rosemary, Siberian fir, tangerine, wild orange
Grounding - basil, black spruce, blue tansy, cedarwood, clary sage, cypress, melaleuca, Siberian fir, vetiver, ylang ylang
Invigorating - grapefruit, lemon, litsea, peppermint, spearmint, Siberian fir, wild orange, wintergreen
Relaxing - basil, blue tansy, cassia, cedarwood, clary sage, cypress, fennel, geranium, lavender, litsea, manuka, marjoram, myrrh, neroli, ravensara, Roman chamomile, turmeric, white fir, ylang ylang
Rubefacient - bergamot, birch, juniper berry, lavender, lemon, magnolia, rosemary, Siberian fir, vetiver
Sedative - bergamot, blue tansy, cedarwood, coriander, frankincense, geranium, juniper berry, lavender, magnolia, melissa, neroli, Roman chamomile, rose, sandalwood, spikenard, tangerine, vetiver, ylang ylang, yarrow
Stimulant - basil, bergamot, birch, black pepper, black spruce, blue tansy, cinnamon, clove, cypress, dill, eucalyptus, fennel, ginger, grapefruit, juniper berry, lime, myrrh, patchouli, pink pepper, rosemary, Siberian fir, spearmint, tangerine, vetiver, white fir, ylang ylang
Uplifting - bergamot, cedarwood, clary sage, cypress, green mandarin, lemon, lime, litsea, melissa, sandalwood, tangerine, wild orange
Vasodilator - blue tansy, copaiba, lemongrass, litsea, manuka, marjoram, neroli, rosemary, thyme
Warming - birch, cassia, cinnamon, clary sage, ginger, neroli, pink pepper, turmeric, wintergreen

BLENDS

Whisper® - support healthy libido (pg. 205)
Passion® - promotes passion, excitement and joy (pg. 195)
Elevation™ - uplifts mood, energizes (pg. 187)
AromaTouch® - supports circulation, relieves tension (pg. 169)

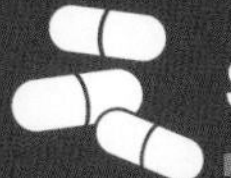

SUPPLEMENTS

Alpha CRS®+, Zendocrine® Softgels, Zendocrine® Complex, **Mito2Max® (pg. 214)**, DDR Prime® Softgels, xEO Mega, GX Assist®, **Deep Blue Polyphenol Complex (pg. 212)**, MicroPlex VMz

USAGE TIPS: For best results to support optimal intimacy

- **Aromatic:** Set the mood by diffusing oils of choice that are calming, warming and arousing to both parties.
- **Topical:** Enjoy using specified oils to obtain desired results. When in sensitive areas be sure to use a carrier oil.

Remedies

ACTIVATE HER APHRODITE
4 drops ylang ylang
2 drops clary sage
2 drops geranium
2 drops patchouli
2 drops sandalwood
1 drop bergamot
Combine and store in a glass bottle. Apply to pressure points, or diffuse.

APHRODISIAC AROMA AROUSER: Combine 12 drops sandalwood, 5 drops ylang ylang, 1 drop cinnamon, 1 drop jasmine. Apply on back of neck and behind ears. Dilute with a carrier oil if desired or necessary for sensitive skin.

BODY WARMER
2 drops rose or geranium
3 drops sandalwood
2 drops ylang ylang
3 drops clary sage
In a 2-ounce glass bottle, combine oils, swirl, fill with carrier oil. Use as a massage oil to warm the body temperature and create arousal.

DREAMMAKER BLEND: Combine 25 drops frankincense, 20 drops bergamot, and 15 drops Roman chamomile in a 10ml roller bottle; fill remainder with carrier oil. Apply topically.

ECSTASY EXTENDER AROMATOUCH® Combine 1-2 drops each geranium, cinnamon, ginger, pink pepper, and peppermint in a 2-ounce glass bottle with a orifice reducer; fill remainder with fractionated coconut oil. Blend supports reaching and prolonging climax. Use 10-15 drops at a time and massage lightly on genitals.

KISS AND MAKE UP: Combine 6 drops clove, 2 drops lemon, and 2 drops frankincense. Use blend to "diffuse" an argument or calm a partner. Diffuse or apply topically with a carrier oil.

INTIMACY RELAXATION BATH: Add 1-2 cup pink Himalayan Salt to warm bath and swish until dissolved. Layer rose, jasmine, and neroli with 2 drops green mandarin on body and step into a blissful bath. Add ½ cup of milk or cream for a soothing skin treatment.

LET'S GET IT ON - a men's formula
6 drops sandalwood
4 drops ylang ylang
2 drops clary sage
2 drops wild orange
Combine and apply to pressure points, or diffuse.

MOOD MAKER: Combine 1 drop each cinnamon, patchouli, rosemary, sandalwood, white fir, and ylang ylang oil. Diffuse to set the mood.

WARM-IT-UP!: In a 15 mL glass bottle, combine: 2 drops neroli, 2 drops wild orange, or pink pepper, 8 drops ginger, 2 drops black pepper. Shake and then fill with fractionated coconut oil. Apply to erogenous zones to support sexual arousal.

EDIBLE MASSAGE AND LUBRICATING BLEND: Melt ½ cup organic coconut oil and 2 teaspoons raw honey in a jar or bowl placed over hot water. Add oils and stir. Use warm if preferred. Can be stored for up to 6 months in airtight container. Rewarm as desired.

For more ideas, download the app at app.essentiallife.com

INTIMACY

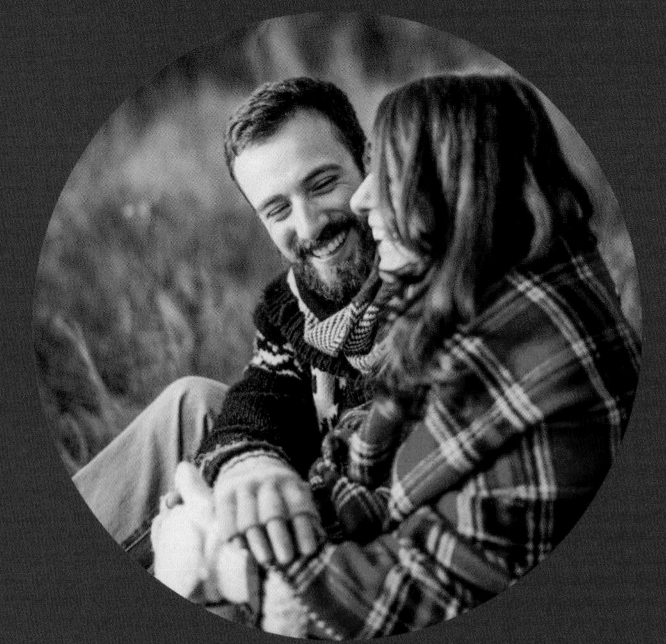

Conditions

Depressed - bergamot, rose, wild orange, ylang ylang, ClaryCalm®, Elevation™, Motivate® ; see *Mood & Behavior*
Emotional issues, female sexuality* - clary sage, jasmine, magnolia, Roman chamomile, rose, ylang ylang, Motivate®, Whisper®; see *Mood & Behavior*
Endometriosis - basil, clary sage, cypress, frankincense, ginger, lemon, rosemary, sandalwood, thyme, ylang ylang; see *Women's Health*
Exhaustion/fatigue - arborvitae, bergamot, black spruce, cinnamon, cypress, grapefruit, pink pepper, peppermint, wild orange, DDR Prime®, Motivate®, Passion®, Zendocrine®; see *Energy & Vitality*
Frigidity* - cinnamon, jasmine, neroli, patchouli, rose, sandalwood, ylang ylang, Passion®, Peace®; see *Mood & Behavior*
Headache - cinnamon, frankincense, geranium, lavender, peppermint, rose, wintergreen, PastTense®; see *Pain & Inflammation*
Hemorrhoids - cypress, helichrysum, myrrh, Roman chamomile, sandalwood, DigestZen®, Zendocrine®; see *Cardiovascular*
Impotence* - cinnamon, clary sage, cypress, geranium, ginger, neroli, rose, sandalwood, thyme, turmeric, ylang ylang, Forgive®, Passion®, Purify, Whisper®; see *Men's Health*
Lack of confidence - bergamot, blue tansy, cedarwood, jasmine, lime, melissa, rose, Citrus Bliss®, InTune®; see *Mood & Behavior*
Lack of nitric oxide - cinnamon, Oil Touch technique
Oxytocin production - clary sage, fennel, geranium, myrrh, ylang ylang
Sex drive, excessive - arborvitae, marjoram
Sex drive, low (low libido)* - black pepper, cardamom, cassia, cinnamon, clary sage, clove, coriander, geranium, ginger, jasmine, juniper berry, magnolia, neroli, patchouli, peppermint, pink pepper, Roman chamomile, rose, rosemary, sandalwood, spearmint, tangerine, vetiver, wild orange, ylang ylang, Cheer®, Console®, Forgive®, Passion®, Peace®, Whisper®; see *Men's Health* and *Women's Health*
Tension - black spruce, geranium, ginger, jasmine, lavender, lemongrass, peppermint, rose, wild orange, wintergreen, ylang ylang, Adaptiv®, PastTense®, Serenity®; see *Muscular*
Vaginal dryness - clary sage, Balance®
Warming, localized - bergamot, birch, cassia, cinnamon, clary sage, juniper berry, lavender, lemon, neroli, pink pepper, rosemary, vetiver, white fir, wintergreen; see *Cardiovascular*
Yeast infection - basil, clary sage, coriander, frankincense, lemon, melaleuca; see *Candida*

** See remedy this page*

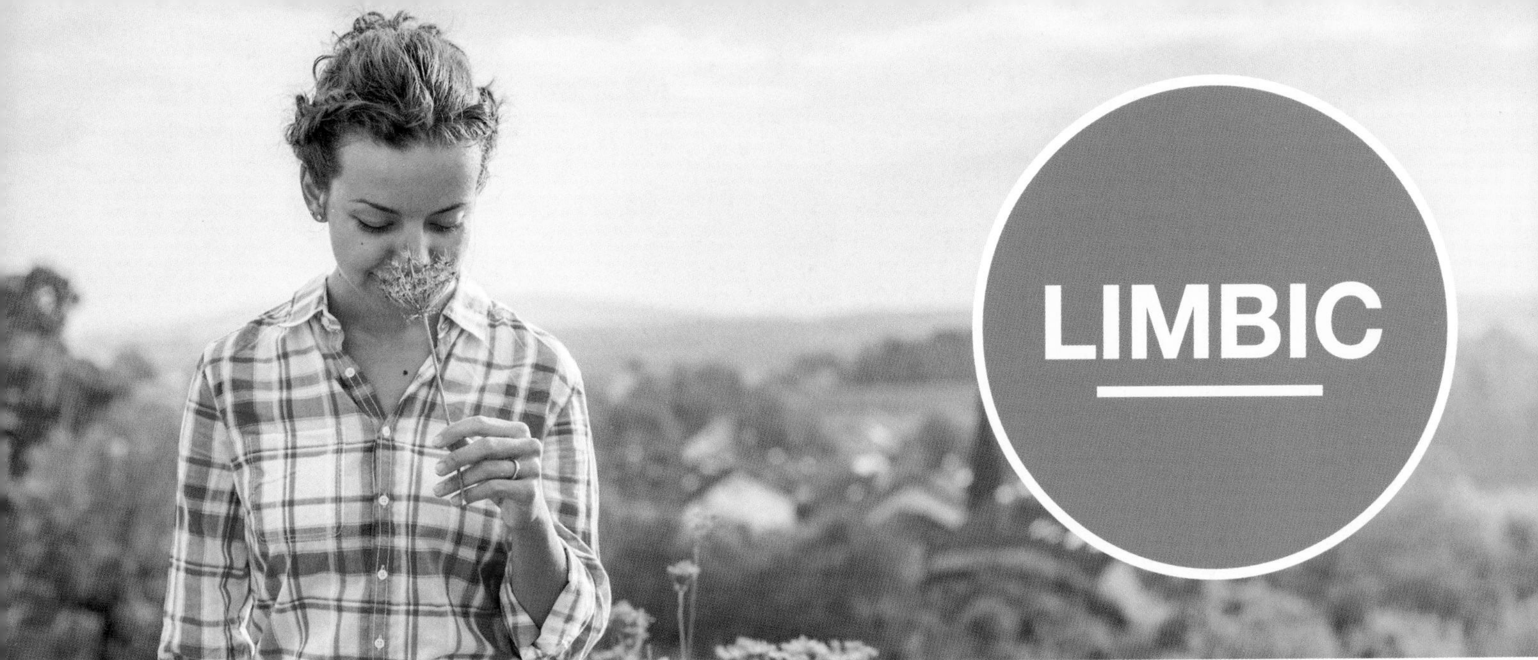

LOCATED IN THE CENTER of both hemispheres of the brain just under the cerebrum, the limbic system includes the amygdala, hippocampus, hypothalamus, olfactory cortex, and thalamus. The limbic system is a busy part of the brain, responsible for regulating both our emotional lives and higher mental functions such as learning, motivation, formulating and storing memories, controlling adrenaline and autonomic response, and regulating hormones and sexual response, sensory perception (optical and olfactory), and motor function.

Since the limbic system is involved in so many of the body's activities, and because it works so closely with several other systems, the actual anatomical parts of the limbic system are somewhat controversial. It is the reason there is pleasure in activities such as eating and sexual intimacy, and why stress manifests in the physical body and directly impacts health.

The limbic system is directly responsible for the processes of intercellular communication that affect how an individual responds to situations and all sensory stimuli and forms and stores memories about those situations and the resulting emotions. The limbic system works closely with the endocrine system to help with hormone regulation. It partners with the autonomic nervous system, the part of the body responsible for the "fight-or-flight" response, that helps the body recuperate during periods of rest, that regulates heart rate and body temperature, and that controls gastrointestinal functions. It also works with the nucleus accumbens, the pleasure center of the brain which is involved with sexual arousal and euphoric response to recreational drugs.

Deep in the core of the limbic system lies the amygdala, which is involved in many of the limbic activities listed above. It serves as the "watchtower," evaluating situations to help the brain recognize potential threats and prepare for fight-or-flight reactions. One of the ways it performs its duties is through the sense of smell. Aromas, via the olfactory system, have a quick, unfiltered route to the amygdala where emotions and memories are stored. Why? Because the sense of smell is necessary for survival.

The sense of smell is one of the more complex and discerning senses and is ten thousand times more powerful than our sense of taste. Aromas have a direct and profound effect on the deepest levels of the body systems, emotions, and psyche. Interestingly, we have only three types of receptors for sight, but an amazing one hundred distinct classes of smell receptors. We can distinguish an infinite number of smells even at very low concentrations. It is the ONLY sense linked directly to the limbic brain. The response is instant and so are the effects on the brain's mental and emotional responses and our body chemistry.

Herein lies the power and beauty of using essential oils for limbic health. Their aromas are one hundred to ten thousand times more concentrated and more potent than the solid form of a plant. Due to their unique ability to bypass the blood-brain barrier and their concentrated aromatic compounds, pure essential oils can provide significant benefits to individuals who desire to improve limbic system function.

When inhaled, essential oils enter the olfactory system and directly affect the amygdala and therefore impact mood and emotional response; thus they can be beneficial in reprogramming the significance that individuals have attached to past experiences and can initiate rapid responses both physically and emotionally in the brain and the rest of the body. Inhalation of essential oils with the resulting aromatic exposure is the most effective method of impacting the brain.

It is important to know that many apparently physical and seemingly unrelated symptoms are associated with limbic system imbalance because activities of the limbic system are so deeply integrated with other body systems. For any other related condition not listed in this section, see the corresponding body system in which the symptom tends to occur. For example, chronic fatigue - see *Energy & Vitality*; anxiety, depression, or irritability - see *Mood & Behavior*.

Specific sections in this book are complementary to the topic of limbic health. See *Addictions*, *Eating Disorders*, and *Mood & Behavior* following this section and *Emotional Usage* later in the book.

TOP SOLUTIONS

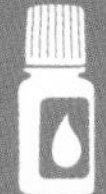

SINGLE OILS

Melissa - reduces depression and supports trauma recovery (pg. 134)
Juniper berry - helps release fears, trauma, and nightmares (pg. 119)
Frankincense - balances brain activity; supports a sense of protection, safety and releases traumatic memories (pg. 110)
Patchouli - sedates, grounds, stabilizes; supports central nervous system (pg. 139)
Turmeric - antioxidant and anti-inflammatory (pg. 158)

By Related Properties

For more, See Oil Properties on pages 477 - 481

Antidepressant - frankincense, green mandarin, lavender, magnolia, melissa, neroli, tangerine, vetiver
Calming - black spruce, blue tansy, copaiba, frankincense, litsea, melissa, patchouli, sandalwood, tangerine, vetiver, yarrow
Grounding - black spruce, blue tansy, cedarwood, clary sage, cypress, magnolia, Siberian fir, vetiver, ylang ylang
Relaxing - blue tansy, cedarwood, clary sage, cypress, lavender, litsea, manuka, myrrh, neroli, ravensara, Roman chamomile, white fir, ylang ylang
Sedative - bergamot, blue tansy, cedarwood, clary sage, frankincense, magnolia, lavender, melissa, neroli, patchouli, rose, sandalwood, tangerine, vetiver, ylang ylang, yarrow

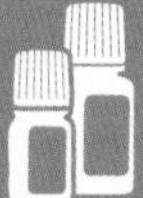

BLENDS

Serenity® - calms feelings of fear, anger, jealousy, and rage (pg. 199)
Cheer® - brings feelings of cheerfulness, optimism and positivity (pg. 173)
Motivate® - stimulates self-belief, courage and confidence (pg. 193)
Elevation™ - stabilizes mood and promotes courage and cheerfulness (pg. 187)
Balance® - calms an overactive mind; promotes sense of connectivity (pg. 170)

Related Ailments: Electrical Hypersensitivity Syndrome, Focal Brain Dysfunction (brain injury), Gulf War Syndrome, Hallucinations, Hypersexuality (excessive sex drive), Obsessive Compulsive Disorder, Post Traumatic Stress Disorder (PTSD)

Examples of other ailments that are associated with limbic imbalance:
Chronic Fatigue Syndrome - see *Energy & Vitality*
Fibromyalgia - see *Muscular*
Food Sensitivity - see *Allergies*
Chronic Pain - see *Pain & Inflammation*

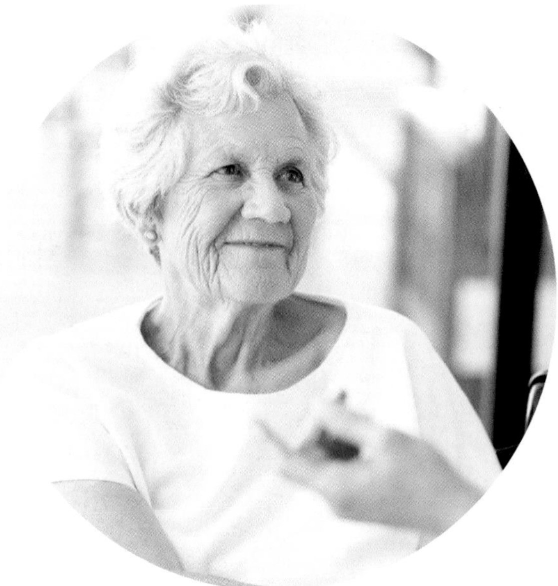

Conditions

Bipolar disorder* - bergamot, cedarwood, frankincense, lavender, melissa, vetiver, Balance®, Citrus Bliss®, Elevation™, Peace®, Serenity®; see *Mood & Behavior*
Delusions (false belief) - black pepper, clary sage, frankincense, green mandarin, helichrysum, juniper berry, kumquat, patchouli, pink pepper, vetiver, Balance®, Deep Blue®, Elevation™, Motivate®, Passion®
Environmental sensitivity - lemongrass, ylang ylang, Balance®, DDR Prime®, Serenity®
Excessive sex drive - arborvitae, marjoram
Hallucinations - cedarwood, cilantro (small amounts), clove, coriander (small amounts), frankincense, juniper berry, melissa, myrrh, sandalwood, thyme, vetiver, Balance®, DDR Prime®, InTune®
Nightmares* - cinnamon, clary sage, cypress, dill, eucalyptus, geranium, grapefruit, juniper berry, lavender, melissa, Roman chamomile, white fir, wild orange, vetiver, ylang ylang, Balance®, Elevation™, Serenity®; see *Sleep*
Obsessive/compulsive thoughts/behaviors* - bergamot, black pepper, cedarwood, cypress, frankincense, geranium, lavender, patchouli, sandalwood, vetiver, ylang ylang, Adaptiv®, Balance®, Elevation™, Forgive®, InTune®, Serenity®; see *Mood & Behavior*
Overreacting - black spruce, cedarwood, clary sage, magnolia, melissa, Roman chamomile, sandalwood, vetiver, wintergreen, Balance®, On Guard®, TerraShield®
Psychiatric conditions (not a substitute for medical care) - jasmine, melissa, patchouli, sandalwood, Balance®, Elevation™, InTune®, Serenity®
PTSD/Stress, traumatic (past, present)* - blue tansy, cedarwood, frankincense, helichrysum, jasmine, lavender, magnolia, melissa, neroli, patchouli, Roman chamomile, sandalwood, vetiver, wild orange, ylang ylang, Adaptiv®, Balance®, Citrus Bliss®, Deep Blue®, Elevation™, Forgive®, Motivate®, Peace®, Serenity®; see *Stress*

** See remedy on pg. 315*

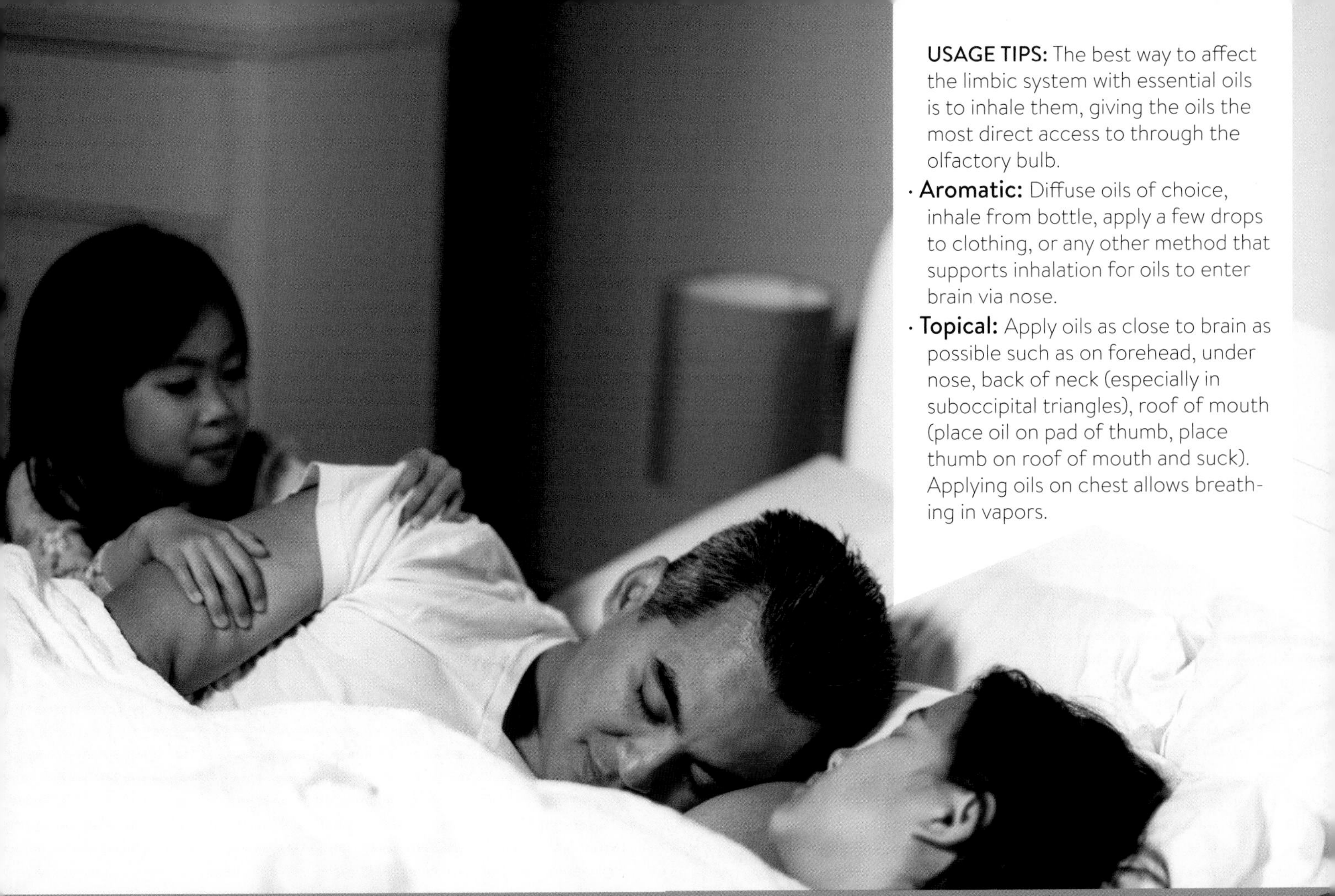

USAGE TIPS: The best way to affect the limbic system with essential oils is to inhale them, giving the oils the most direct access to through the olfactory bulb.

- **Aromatic:** Diffuse oils of choice, inhale from bottle, apply a few drops to clothing, or any other method that supports inhalation for oils to enter brain via nose.
- **Topical:** Apply oils as close to brain as possible such as on forehead, under nose, back of neck (especially in suboccipital triangles), roof of mouth (place oil on pad of thumb, place thumb on roof of mouth and suck). Applying oils on chest allows breathing in vapors.

Remedies

BIPOLAR BLENDS: Best used aromatically (inhale, diffuse); topically on back of neck, on wrists.

- Recipe #1: 3 drops bergamot and 2 drops clary sage
- Recipe #2: 1 drop lavender oil, 1 drop ylang ylang oil and 3 drops grapefruit
- Recipe #3: 2 drops frankincense, 1 drop lemon and 2 drops jasmine

POST TRAUMATIC STRESS BLEND: Combine 2 drops each cedarwood, frankincense, sandalwood, lavender, vetiver oils with a small amount of carrier oil and apply to back of neck, forehead, and bottoms of feet.

RELEASING OBSESSIONS & COMPULSIONS: In a 5 ml roller bottle, place 20 drops patchouli + 30 drops Balance® (or other oils as desired) and apply behind ears, on wrists, bottoms of feet two or three times daily. If aroma is inviting, drop 2-3 drops of each individual oil on palms of hands, cup over nose, and inhale deeply.

NIGHTMARES BE GONE

- Dilute 1 drop juniper berry with 1 teaspoon fractionated coconut oil for children. Apply to back of neck, forehead, behind ears, bottoms of feet
- Diffuse juniper berry in bedroom at bedtime.

CLEAR MINDED

3 drops frankincense
3 drops ylang ylang
2 drops cedarwood
2 drops melissa
5 drops wild orange
Combine oils in a 10ml roller bottle and fill remainder of bottle with fractionated coconut oil. Roll onto forehead, back of neck, and inside of wrists.

RESET ENTHUSIASM : Combine 1 drop ylang ylang and 3 drops wild orange and diffuse to reset, uplift and boost energy.

OH HAPPY DAY! Diffuse Elevation™ throughout the day to promote a sense of joy and well-being.

OBSESS NO MORE: Apply InTune® to back of neck and forehead to support mind in letting go of obsessive thoughts and focusing instead on what really matters.

PEACEFUL PERFUME

3 drops ylang ylang
2 drops geranium
1 drop patchouli
1 drop juniper berry
Combine oils in a 10ml roller bottle; fill remainder with fractionated coconut oil. Roll onto forehead, back of neck, and inside of wrists.

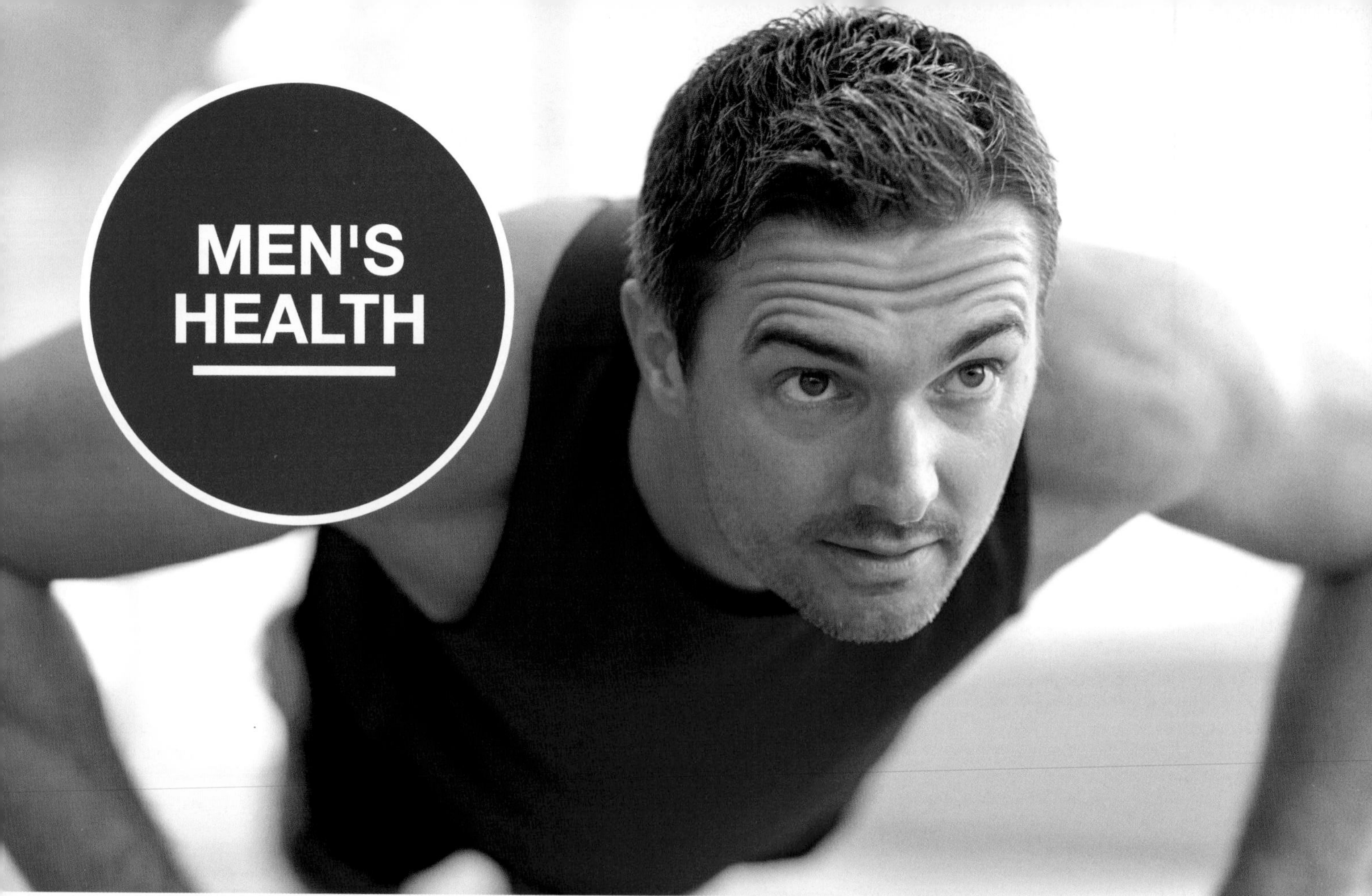

MEN'S HEALTH encompasses issues that are unique to men as well as those that are particularly common and challenging for the male gender.

The primary sex organs in the male reproductive system have dual functions. The testes produce sperm and the hormone testosterone. The penis allows sperm access to the female reproductive system during intercourse and also serves an excretory function for urine. Testosterone is primarily secreted by the testicles in men, and small amounts are also secreted by the adrenal glands. It is the principal male sex hormone and an anabolic steroid. It is responsible for the development of the testes and prostate as well as secondary sex characteristics, including increased muscle and bone mass, body hair, and a deeper voice. Testosterone levels gradually decrease over a man's lifetime.

The prostate is located beneath the bladder and connects the bladder and seminal vesicles to the penis. It produces part of the seminal fluid that is alkaline, which helps lengthen the life of sperm as they enter the vagina. It also has involuntary muscles that contract to expel the sperm during ejaculation. Normally it is a little larger than a walnut in size, but the cells that make up the prostate continue to multiply throughout a man's life. The enlarged organ can become a problem (benign prostatic hyperplasia) if it pinches off the urethra that runs through it, causing difficulty in emptying the bladder. Symptoms include urgency to urinate, hesitancy, frequency, incontinence, and an inability to completely empty the bladder. This can also lead to infection, stones, damaged bladder and kidneys, and erectile dysfunction. As men age they are at greater risk for prostate cancer as well. Next to skin cancer, prostate cancer is the most common cancer in men.

Sexual health is important for a healthy lifestyle. The ability for a man to participate in intercourse depends on hormones, the brain, nerves, and blood vessels that supply the penis. For an erection to occur all these mechanisms need to be in place. Erectile dysfunction or impotence can be caused by a complication in any of these areas and may be attributed to diabetes, peripheral vascular disease, smoking, medications, prostate cancer, and more.

As far as general health goes, compared to women, men make more risky or unhealthy choices, smoke and drink more, and put off making health decisions. Some of the most common health issues men deal with are heart disease, high blood pressure, liver disease, influenza and pneumococcal infection, skin cancer, and diabetes (which can contribute to impotence and low testosterone levels, which can in turn contribute to depression and anxiety). Regardless of the cause, many men suffer from depression that goes untreated. This can be a byproduct of a decline in physical health. Self-confidence is often at stake when a man does not feel healthy. It is common for men to hide negative emotions as they continue to function on a daily basis.

Since men are independent by nature, empowering themselves with knowledge and practical application of natural remedies can help them reduce health risks while managing mood and helping the body maintain better overall health.

TOP SOLUTIONS

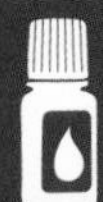

SINGLE OILS

Frankincense - promotes longevity, supports brain and prostate health (pg. 110)
Melaleuca - fights bacteria and fungus with antiseptic action (pg. 132)
Juniper berry - supports urinary and prostate health, wound healing (pg. 119)
Cardamom - supports digestive, muscular, and respiratory health (pg. 87)
Lemon - detoxifies and has an alkalizing effect (pg. 123)

By Related Properties

For more, See Oil Properties on pages 477 - 481

Anti-inflammatory - arborvitae, basil, bergamot, birch, black pepper, blue tansy, cardamom, cassia, cedarwood, cinnamon, copaiba, coriander, cypress, dill, eucalyptus, frankincense, geranium, ginger, helichrysum, jasmine, lavender, lemongrass, lime, litsea, manuka, melaleuca, melissa, myrrh, neroli, oregano, patchouli, peppermint, Roman chamomile, sandalwood, Siberian fir, spearmint, spikenard, tangerine, turmeric, wild orange, wintergreen, yarrow
Cardiotonic - cassia, copaiba, cypress, ginger, lavender, litsea, manuka, marjoram, pink pepper
Restorative - basil, frankincense, lime, neroli, patchouli, rosemary, sandalwood, spearmint, tangerine
Steroidal - basil, bergamot, birch, cedarwood, clove, fennel, patchouli, rosemary, thyme

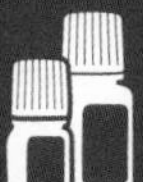

BLENDS

Balance® - makes great cologne, aftershave; brain support (pg. 170)
On Guard® - supports cardiovascular and immune health (pg. 194)
Zendocrine® - supports urinary, prostate; prevents hair loss (pg. 206)
DDR Prime® - assists with cellular repair and longevity (pg. 184)

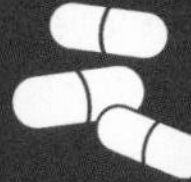

SUPPLEMENTS

Alpha CRS®+ (pg. 209), Mito2Max® (pg. 214), DDR Prime® Softgels (pg. 211), xEO Mega (pg. 222), Deep Blue Polyphenol Complex (pg. 212), MicroPlex VMz (pg. 214)

Related Ailments: Abnormal Sperm Morphology, Erectile Dysfunction, Men's Hormonal Imbalance, Impotence, Infertility, Libido (low) for Men, Prostate, Prostate Problems, Prostatitis, Testes, Testosterone (low)

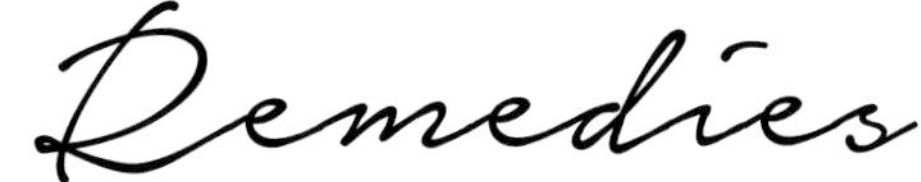

GIDDY UP (for erectile dysfunction): Restore: Apply Immortelle to genital area two to three times daily.

- Encourage and stimulate hormonal balance: 1 drop sandalwood, 2 drops clary sage, and 1 drop ylang ylang. Apply topically on lower abdomen; diffuse; take internally in a gel capsule.
- Circulation support: Apply 1-2 drops cypress, pink pepper, or AromaTouch® to inner thighs and lower abdomen.
- Anxiety and stress relief: Diffuse 1-2 drops of basil, lavender, magnolia, or ylang ylang. Inhale in cupped hand, put a few drops on pillow.
- Support healthy nutrition: Take xEO Mega, MicroPlex VMz.

PROSTATE RELIEF

- Apply 2-3 drops Balance® to bottoms of feet morning and evening before sleep.
- Consume 1-2 DDR Prime® softgels two to three times daily at mealtimes.
- Apply 2-3 drops DDR Prime® topically on feet (focusing on heel area), lower abdomen, and inner thigh. Add 2-3 drops juniper berry on abdomen area. Dilute with carrier oil for sensitive skin. Apply morning and night.
- Consume 3-5 drops frankincense under tongue morning and evening.

HAIR STAY THERE

24 drops rosemary
18 drops cedarwood
14 drops geranium
12 drops peppermint
8 drops lavender
40 drops carrier oil
Combine in 5ml bottle. Apply daily before bed or just after shower. Put 4-7 drops in palm of hand, dip fingertips, gently massage throughout scalp, paying special attention to thinning or balding spots.

EARTHY SPICE COLOGNE

18 drops bergamot
13 drops Siberian or Douglas fir
10 drops clove
8 drops lemon
Combine into 10ml roller bottle, top off with carrier oil, apply to pulse points.

LIME DELIGHT COLOGNE

2 drops lime
1 drop vetiver
Rub vetiver over heart, layer lime over top, dilute with carrier oil for sensitive skin.

AFTERSHAVE: Use Immortelle in a roller bottle and add 1-2 drops frankincense and lavender for sensitive skin relief. Rub together in palms, then apply gently to the neck and face in an upward motion.

For more ideas on Men's Health, download the app at app.essentiallife.com

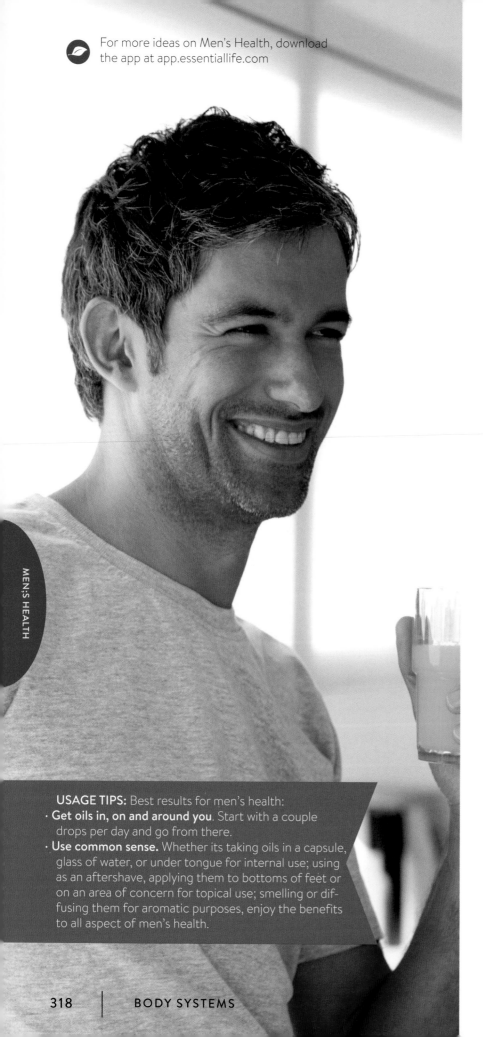

USAGE TIPS: Best results for men's health:

- **Get oils in, on and around you**. Start with a couple drops per day and go from there.
- **Use common sense.** Whether its taking oils in a capsule, glass of water, or under tongue for internal use; using as an aftershave, applying them to bottoms of feet or on an area of concern for topical use; smelling or diffusing them for aromatic purposes, enjoy the benefits to all aspect of men's health.

Conditions

Baldness* - cedarwood, cypress, geranium, lavender, rosemary, thyme, ylang ylang, Console®, Zendocrine®

Dihydrotestosterone, levels too high (male pattern baldness, enlarged prostate) - see "Testosterone (DHT), high" below

Estrogen dominance - basil, clove, geranium, thyme, Purify

Genital warts - arborvitae, frankincense, geranium, melaleuca, melissa, lemongrass, thyme

Hormones, imbalanced - citronella, frankincense, geranium, rosemary, ylang ylang, Cheer®, Console®, DDR Prime®, Whisper®, Zendocrine®

Impatience - Balance®; see *Mood & Behavior*

Impotence, erectile dysfunction* - cassia, cinnamon, clary sage, clove, cypress, dill, Douglas fir, ginger, jasmine, neroli, pink pepper, sandalwood, ylang ylang, AromaTouch®, DDR Prime®, Passion®, Whisper®, Zendocrine®

Infertility - basil, cinnamon, clary sage, geranium, jasmine, melissa, rosemary, sandalwood, spikenard, thyme, ylang ylang, DDR Prime®, Passion®, Zendocrine®

Jock itch - cypress, lavender, lemon eucalyptus, melaleuca, myrrh, patchouli, petitgrain; see *Candida*

Prostate issues* - basil, cinnamon, fennel, frankincense, helichrysum, jasmine, juniper berry, magnolia, myrrh, rose, rosemary, Cheer®, DDR Prime®, Passion®

Prostate, congested - cinnamon, cypress, juniper berry, lemon, lemongrass, peppermint, rosemary, DDR Prime®, Passion®, Zendocrine®

Prostate infection - citronella, neroli, oregano, thyme; see *Immune & Lymphatic*

Prostate, enlarged - fennel; see *Detoxification*

Prostate, inflamed* - basil, cypress, Douglas fir, eucalyptus, juniper berry, lavender, Roman chamomile, rosemary, sandalwood, Siberian fir, thyme, AromaTouch®, DDR Prime®, On Guard®

Semen production, low - celery seed, frankincense, rose, DDR Prime®, Purify, Whisper®, Zendocrine®

Sperm count, low - basil, cedarwood, celery seed, clary sage, geranium, ginger, juniper berry

Testosterone, low - black spruce, cassia, celery seed, clary sage, fennel, ginger, myrrh, rose, rosemary, sandalwood, ylang ylang, Passion®, Whisper®

Testosterone (DHT), high - celery seed, juniper berry, rosemary, DDR Prime®, Zendocrine®

* *See remedy on pg. 317*

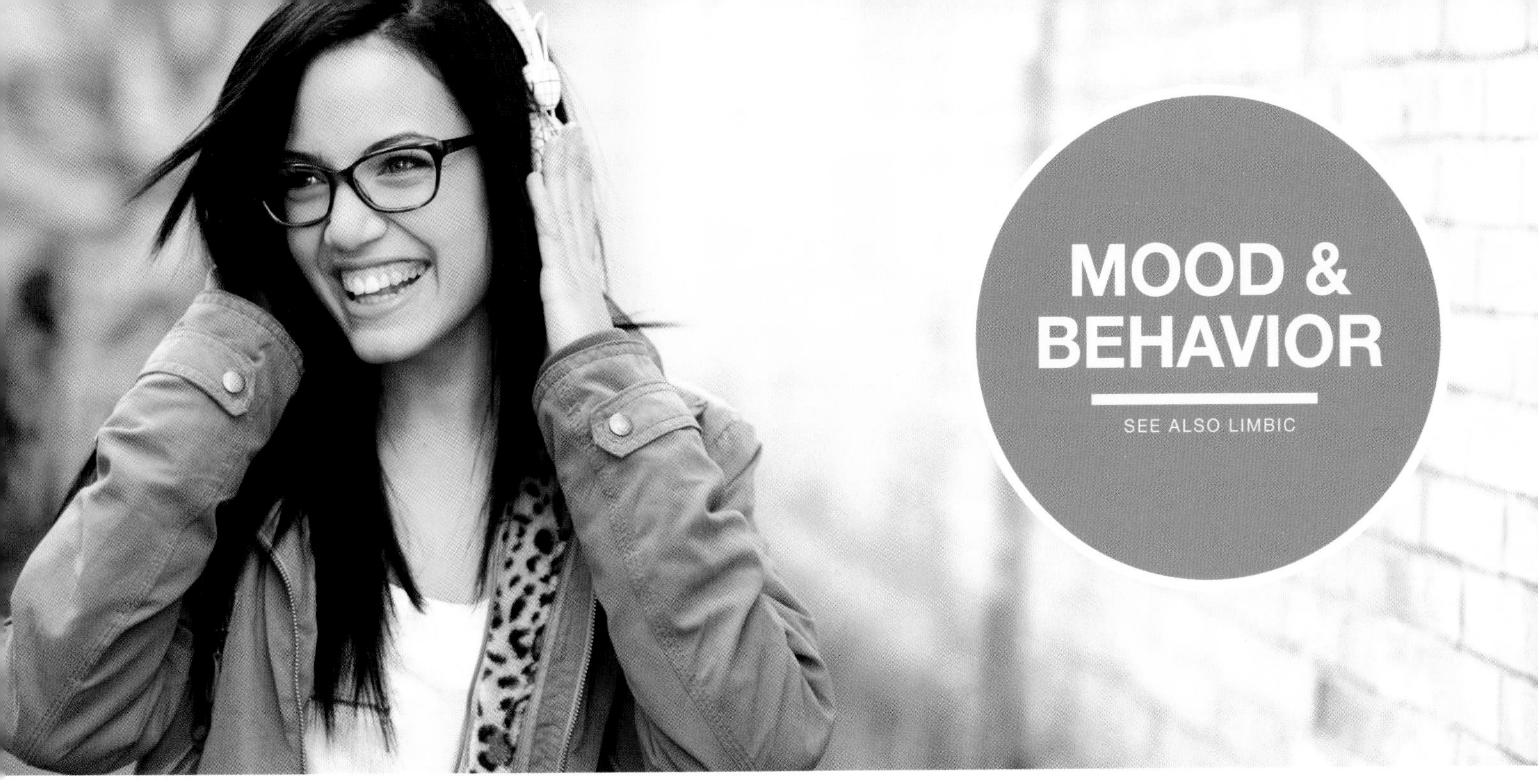

MOOD CHALLENGES and disorders are becoming more prevalent, especially in industrialized nations where computers, technology, and other conveniences have become a way of life. People are increasingly disconnected in their personal relationships, but they may have upward of half a million "friends" on social media sites, and it isn't uncommon to see teenagers texting each other, rather than conversing, while standing right next to each other!

Digestive issues and disorders are rampant, in part because of the refined and processed foods that many individuals eat. In recent years, scientists have discovered that there are more neurotransmitters in the gut than there are in the brain, and, among other things, healthy mood management depends on how well these neurotransmitters relay messages to each other. How can an individual hope to experience healthy moods if their cells are depleted of nutrition, their emotional needs for social connection are unmet, and if their neurotransmitters reside in an area with blockages and inflammation? The list of contributors to mood challenges is extensive.

The limbic system in the brain has glands that help relay and respond to emotions. It includes the amygdala, hippocampus, hypothalamus, and thalamus. The hippocampus, specifically, is involved in storing memories and producing emotions. It works effectively at full capacity when it is producing new neurons and solid nerve connections to assist with these key activities. When an individual experiences stress, the blood flow around the hippocampus changes -- and individuals in their later years can often experience up to 20% loss in the nerve connections of the hippocampus, which can drastically affect mood and memory.

One of the challenges with balancing brain functions is that the brain is well-protected by a layer of high density cells called the blood-brain barrier that restricts passage of all but a small, select group of substances. This is actually a good thing; this layer of cells helps keep neurotoxins, viruses, and other invaders out of the control center of the body. Among the few substances that can bypass this barrier are natural fat-soluble substances such as sesquiterpenes, a compound found in many essential oils.

Since the brain is the origin and relayer of messages that produce emotions, and the brain functions on a chemical level, it stands to reason that natural remedies with strong chemical messages (signal or messenger molecules) can help balance and cleanse the very processes that need assistance. Essential oils can assist with cleansing and balancing the GI tract (see *Digestive & Intestinal*, *Detoxification* sections for further information), benefit brain functions, specifically those involving focus, concentration (see *Focus & Concentration*), mood, and memory with both aromatic and topical application.

When inhaled, natural aromatic compounds enter the olfactory system and pass the olfactory bulb, which leads directly to the limbic center of the brain. Oils can be inhaled by smelling directly from the bottle, rubbing a drop of essential oil in the palms of the hands and cupping over the nose, or by utilizing a diffuser (a device that disperses essential oils into the air.) Inhalation is the fastest way to get an essential oil into the body and has significant benefits on mood as it alters the chemical messages being relayed within the limbic system.

When applying essential oils topically to assist mood, it is important to get the oils as close to the limbic system as possible and apply them where they can best bypass the blood-brain barrier. Directly below the base of the skull, on both sides of the neck, there is an "indentation" that can be felt with the fingers. This area is called the suboccipital triangle, and when pure essential oils are applied here, they are able to enter the circulatory system of the brain prior to entering the circulatory system of the body. Oils may also be topically applied on the mastoid bones behind the ears, across the front of the forehead, directly under the nose, and may even be applied to the roof of the mouth (place oil on pad of thumb and then place on roof of mouth) for more direct access to the limbic system.

TOP SOLUTIONS

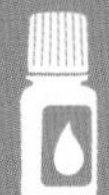

SINGLE OILS

Lavender - calms and relaxes, increases the ability to express feelings (pg. 122)
Wild orange and tangerine - melts away anxiousness and energizes (pgs. 162 & 156)
Cedarwood - grounds, promotes a sense of belonging and being connected socially (pg. 89)
Bergamot - helps increase self-confidence (pg. 81)
Neroli or Magnolia - calms and sedates (pg. 136), (pg. 129)

By Related Properties

For more, See Oil Properties on pages 477 - 481

Antidepressant - arborvitae, basil, bergamot, cinnamon, clary sage, coriander, dill, frankincense, geranium, grapefruit, jasmine, lavender, lemon, lemongrass, melissa, neroli, oregano, patchouli, ravensara, rose, sandalwood, tangerine, wild orange, ylang ylang
Calming - bergamot, birch, black pepper, black spruce, blue tansy, cassia, clary sage, copaiba, coriander, fennel, frankincense, geranium, jasmine, juniper berry, lavender, litsea, melissa, oregano, patchouli, Roman chamomile, sandalwood, tangerine, vetiver, yarrow
Energizing - basil, clove, cypress, grapefruit, pink pepper, lemongrass, rosemary, Siberian fir, spearmint, tangerine, white fir, wild orange, yarrow
Grounding - arborvitae, basil, birch, black spruce, blue tansy, cedarwood, clary sage, cypress, magnolia, melaleuca, patchouli, Siberian fir, vetiver, ylang ylang
Invigorating - grapefruit, lemon, litsea, peppermint, spearmint, Siberian fir, wild orange, wintergreen
Relaxing - basil, cassia, blue tansy, cedarwood, clary sage, cypress, fennel, geranium, jasmine, lavender, litsea, manuka, marjoram, myrrh, neroli, ravensara, Roman chamomile, white fir, ylang ylang
Sedative - basil, bergamot, blue tansy, cedarwood, clary sage, coriander, frankincense, geranium, jasmine, juniper berry, lavender, lemongrass, marjoram, melissa, neroli, patchouli, Roman chamomile, rose, sandalwood, spikenard, tangerine, vetiver, ylang ylang, yarrow
Stimulant - arborvitae, basil, bergamot, birch, black pepper, blue tansy, cardamom, cedarwood, cinnamon, clove, coriander, cypress, dill, eucalyptus, fennel, ginger, grapefruit, juniper berry, lime, melaleuca, myrrh, patchouli, rosemary, Siberian fir, spearmint, tangerine, thyme, vetiver, white fir, wintergreen, ylang ylang
Uplifting - bergamot, cardamom, cedarwood, clary sage, cypress, grapefruit, lemon, lime, litsea, melissa, sandalwood, tangerine, wild orange, ylang ylang

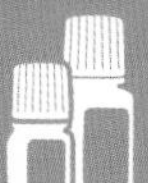

BLENDS

Citrus Bliss® - stimulates the mind and mood; encourages creativity (pg. 181)
Elevation™ - energizes, balances hormones; restores a sense of buoyancy (pg. 187)
Cheer® - promotes a cheerful, positive attitude (pg. 173)
Serenity® - encourages a restful state for mind and body (pg. 199)
Motivate® - stimulates belief, courage and confidence (pg. 193)
Balance® - promotes a state of balance and calm (pg. 170)

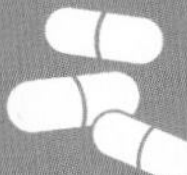

SUPPLEMENTS

Mito2Max® (pg. 214), DDR Prime® Softgels, **xEO Mega (pg. 222)**, TerraZyme®, **IQ Mega® (pg. 213)**, **Phytoestrogen Multiplex (pg. 217)**, MicroPlex VMz

Related Ailments: Abuse Trauma, Agitation, Agoraphobia, Anger, Anxiety, Apathy, Attachment Disorder (RAD), Depression, Emotional Trauma, Fear, Fear of Flying, Grief, Hysteria, Lack of Confidence, Mood Swings, Nervousness, Oppositional Defiant Disorder, Overwhelm, Panic Attacks, Seasonal Affective Disorder, Social Anxiety Disorder

USAGE TIPS: For best effect for mood and behavior

- **Aromatic:** Diffuse oils of choice, inhale from bottle, apply a few drops to clothing, or any other method that supports inhalation for oils to enter brain via nose.
- **Topical:** Apply oils as close to brain as possible such as on forehead, under nose, back of neck (especially in suboccipital triangles), roof of mouth (place oil on pad of thumb, place thumb on roof of mouth and suck). Applying oils on chest allows breathing in vapors.
- **Internal:** Place one to five drops of chosen oil in water to drink or take in a capsule, drop under tongue, lick a drop off back of hand, apply to roof of mouth (place oil on pad of thumb and then place pad on roof of mouth).

Conditions

Abandoned - birch, cilantro, clary sage, dill, frankincense, myrrh, Forgive®, InTune®
Abuse, healing from - frankincense, geranium, juniper berry, melissa, Roman chamomile, spikenard, ylang ylang, white fir, Console®, Motivate®, Serenity®
Angry - bergamot, blue tansy, cardamom, cedarwood, copaiba, frankincense, helichrysum, magnolia, melissa, neroli, Roman chamomile, rose, spearmint, tangerine, thyme, wild orange, ylang ylang, Balance®, Console®, InTune®, On Guard®, PastTense®, Serenity®
Antisocial - black pepper, clove, lemongrass, marjoram, oregano, patchouli, rosemary, spearmint, yarrow, Purify
Anxious or worried - arborvitae, basil, bergamot, blue tansy, cedarwood, cilantro, clary sage, copaiba, cypress, Douglas fir, frankincense, geranium, grapefruit, green mandarin, jasmine, juniper berry, kumquat, lavender, lemon, lime, magnolia, marjoram, melissa, neroli, patchouli, petitgrain, pink pepper, Roman chamomile, rose, sandalwood, Siberian fir, spikenard, tangerine, turmeric, vetiver, wild orange, wintergreen, yarrow, ylang ylang, Adaptiv®, Balance®, InTune®, PastTense®, Peace®, Motivate®, Serenity®, Whisper®
Apathetic/indifferent - basil, cardamom, cassia, coriander, eucalyptus, fennel, ginger, jasmine, lemon, lime, rosemary, peppermint, wild orange, ylang ylang, Breathe®, Cheer®, Citrus Bliss®, Elevation™, InTune®, Motivate®, Passion®, Zendocrine®
Betrayed/deceived - cardamom, cinnamon, green mandarin, juniper berry, lemon, marjoram, melissa, peppermint, rose, Console®, Motivate®, Whisper®
Blaming/bitter* - black spruce, cardamom, cinnamon, geranium, helichrysum, lemon, oregano, pink pepper, rosemary, thyme, wintergreen, Forgive®, Passion®, Purify, Zendocrine®
Confidence, lack of/timid/self-rejection - bergamot, black spruce, blue tansy, Douglas fir, grapefruit, jasmine, juniper berry, melissa, patchouli, Roman chamomile, rosemary, Siberian fir, spearmint, vetiver, yarrow, Adaptiv®, Balance®, Breathe®, Cheer®, Console®, DigestZen®, HD Clear®, InTune®, Motivate®, Passion®
Conflicted - clary sage, frankincense, geranium, juniper berry, patchouli, pink pepper, Roman chamomile, rosemary, sandalwood, Adaptiv®, Console®, Immortelle, Whisper®, Zendocrine®
Confused - basil, cedarwood, cinnamon, clary sage, cypress, frankincense, ginger, jasmine, juniper berry, lemon, neroli, peppermint, patchouli, wild orange, Adaptiv®, Citrus Bliss®, InTune®, Motivate®, Peace®
Crying - cypress, frankincense, geranium, lavender, neroli, Roman chamomile, rose, wild orange, white fir, ylang ylang, Balance®, Cheer®, Console®, Elevation™, Serenity®
Denial/dishonest - birch, black pepper, cinnamon, coriander, grapefruit, juniper berry, marjoram, peppermint, thyme, Purify, Zendocrine®
Depressed/sad* - basil, bergamot, black spruce, Douglas fir, frankincense, geranium, grapefruit, green mandarin, helichrysum, jasmine, lavender, lemon, lime, melissa, neroli, patchouli, peppermint, Roman chamomile, rose, sandalwood, spearmint, rose, thyme, tangerine, wild orange, ylang ylang, Adaptiv®, Cheer®, Citrus Bliss®, ClaryCalm®, Elevation™, Motivate®, Passion®
Discernment, lack of/double-minded - arborvitae, basil, cinnamon, clary sage, frankincense, juniper berry, lavender, melissa, pink pepper, Roman chamomile, rosemary, sandalwood, Siberian fir
Disconnected - cedarwood, cinnamon, coriander, frankincense, green mandarin, marjoram, myrrh, neroli, Roman chamomile, rose, white fir, wintergreen, vetiver, Balance®, Elevation™, Motivate®, Whisper®
Distrusting/suspicious - black pepper, cedarwood, cilantro, eucalyptus, frankincense, lavender, marjoram, melaleuca, rose, spearmint, spikenard, white fir, Adaptiv®, Breathe®, Citrus Bliss®, Motivate®, Peace®
Expression, lack of - birch, fennel, lavender, ravensara, Roman chamomile, wild orange, Passion®, Whisper®
Fearful/lack of courage/nervousness - basil, bergamot, birch, black pepper, black spruce, copaiba, coriander, Douglas fir, frankincense, green mandarin, jasmine, juniper berry, patchouli, tangerine, turmeric, wild orange, yarrow, ylang ylang, Balance®, Console®, Motivate®, Passion®, On Guard®, Peace®, Serenity®, TerraShield®
Frustrated - black spruce, cardamom, lemongrass, rosemary, wintergreen, ylang ylang, Adaptiv®, InTune®, Serenity®, Whisper®
Grieving - bergamot, cedarwood, frankincense, geranium, helichrysum, magnolia, marjoram, melissa, neroli, rose, sandalwood, tangerine, Balance®, Console®, Deep Blue®, Elevation™, Forgive®, Peace®, Serenity®
Heartbroken - geranium, lime, magnolia, rose, spikenard, wild orange, ylang ylang, Elevation™, Serenity®, Whisper®
Hopeless - jasmine, lime, patchouli, rose, vetiver, wild orange, ylang ylang, Elevation™
Humiliated - bergamot, birch, cassia, fennel, grapefruit, myrrh, patchouli, ylang ylang, On Guard®
Impatient - arborvitae, cardamom, cilantro, frankincense, grapefruit, lavender, lemongrass, marjoram, ravensara, Roman chamomile, Siberian fir, wintergreen, Adaptiv®, PastTense®, Serenity®
Indecisive - cassia, cinnamon, ginger, lemon, magnolia, marjoram, melaleuca, rosemary, Adaptiv®, On Guard®, Zendocrine®
Insecure/feeling unsafe or vulnerable - bergamot, black spruce, clary sage, copaiba, grapefruit, melaleuca, myrrh, ravensara, Roman chamomile, Siberian fir, yarrow, ylang ylang, AromaTouch®, Breathe®, On Guard®
Irritable/agitated - arborvitae, bergamot, black spruce, coriander, geranium, green mandarin, lavender, lemon, magnolia, neroli, Roman chamomile, rose, tangerine, wild orange, Adaptiv®, Console®, Forgive®, Serenity®, TerraShield®
Jealous - cinnamon, grapefruit, myrrh, patchouli, Roman chamomile, rose, ylang ylang, white fir, Serenity®
Melancholy - basil, bergamot, ginger, grapefruit, jasmine, lemon, lime, melissa, spearmint, tangerine, wild orange, yarrow, Citrus Bliss®, Elevation™
Night terrors/nightmares - clove, juniper berry, melissa, neroli, pink pepper, Roman chamomile, sandalwood, vetiver, Adaptiv®, On Guard®, Peace®, TerraShield®
Obsessive/compulsive - arborvitae, bergamot, black pepper, clary sage, cedarwood, cypress, frankincense, grapefruit, lavender, neroli, oregano, patchouli, Roman chamomile, sandalwood, vetiver, ylang ylang, Adaptiv®, Balance®, Elevation™, Forgive®, InTune®, Serenity®
Overwhelmed/burdened - basil, black spruce, blue tansy, clary sage, Douglas fir, lemon, lemongrass, neroli, pink pepper, rosemary, tangerine, wild orange, ylang ylang, Balance®, Console®, Citrus Bliss®, Elevation™, InTune®, Motivate®, PastTense®, Peace®, Serenity®
Over sensitive or reactive/defensive - black spruce, clove, geranium, ginger, lavender, lemon, melaleuca, melissa, patchouli, Roman chamomile, rosemary, spikenard, vetiver, white fir, wintergreen, Adaptiv®, Deep Blue®, On Guard®, PastTense®, Serenity®, TerraShield®
Powerless, feeling - bergamot, black spruce, cedarwood, cinnamon, coriander, dill, fennel, frankincense, ginger, grapefruit, jasmine, lime, melaleuca, rose, Siberian fir, vetiver, white fir, wild orange, Adaptiv®, On Guard®, Whisper®
Rejected - bergamot, fennel, frankincense, geranium, grapefruit, lime, patchouli, Citrus Bliss®, Elevation™, Whisper®
Resentful - cardamom, frankincense, geranium, lemon, lemongrass, oregano, Roman chamomile, thyme, Purify
Restless - dill, lavender, lemon, neroli, patchouli, vetiver, white fir, yarrow, Adaptiv®, Balance®, InTune®, Peace®, Serenity®, Whisper®; see "Anxious" above

* See remedy on pg. 322

Selfish - arborvitae, cardamom, cedarwood, oregano, thyme, wintergreen
Sexual Frustration - see *Intimacy*
Shame, feel - bergamot, fennel, grapefruit, helichrysum, jasmine, lavender, oregano, vetiver, ylang ylang
Shocked - bergamot, frankincense, geranium, helichrysum, magnolia, neroli, Roman chamomile, InTune®; see *First Aid*
Sluggish/stuck - black spruce, cypress, ginger, juniper berry, lemongrass, peppermint, rosemary, Adaptiv®, AromaTouch®, DigestZen®, DDR Prime®
Spiritual connection, lack of - cinnamon, frankincense, juniper berry, melissa, Roman chamomile, sandalwood, Siberian fir, spikenard, yarrow, Elevation™, Forgive®
Stiffnecked/arrogant - birch, cedarwood, cypress, Douglas fir, lemongrass, oregano, thyme, white fir, wintergreen, AromaTouch®, PastTense®
Stubborn/willful/defiant/controlling - black spruce, cardamom, coriander, lemongrass, oregano, thyme, wintergreen, Balance®, Forgive®, PastTense®, Peace®
Tense/uptight - basil, blue tansy, juniper berry, lavender, magnolia, melissa, neroli, patchouli, turmeric, vetiver, ylang ylang, Adaptiv®, Serenity®
Terror/panicked/hysterical - clary sage, jasmine, lavender, magnolia, melissa, neroli, patchouli, Roman chamomile, spikenard, wild orange, ylang ylang, Balance®, Peace®, Serenity®
Traumatized - basil, frankincense, helichrysum, melissa, rose, spikenard, tangerine, Balance®, Console®, Deep Blue®, Motivate®, Peace®, Serenity®
Weary/faint - black spruce, cassia, cinnamon, lime, peppermint, rosemary, spearmint, wild orange, Citrus Bliss®, Elevation™
Wounded, deep emotionally* - birch, copaiba, eucalyptus, frankincense, geranium, helichrysum, lime, myrrh, neroli, Roman chamomile, rose, Siberian fir, spikenard, white fir, yarrow, Deep Blue®, Cheer®, Immortelle, Motivate®
Worthless - bergamot, black pepper, black spruce, blue tansy, clove, frankincense, geranium, grapefruit, myrrh, patchouli, rose, wild orange, ylang ylang, Elevation™, On Guard®, Whisper®

* *See remedy this page*

Remedies

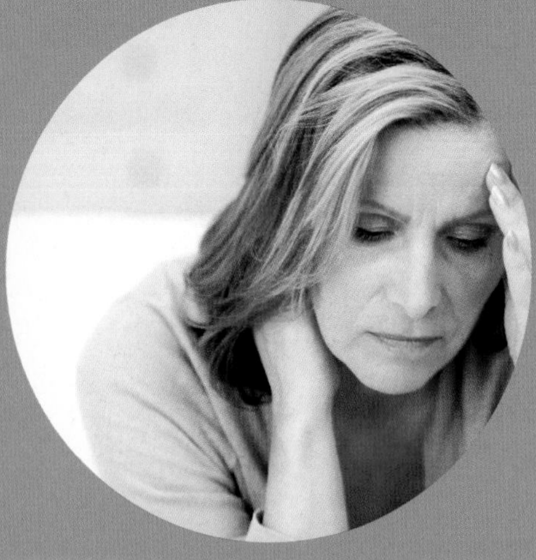

DIFFUSER BLENDS: Diffuse several times a day to manage issues and as needed for emotional support.
NOTE: Diffuser recipes can be made into topical blends. Place the oils for a particular blend into a roller bottle, multiplying the number of drops by approximately four; fill remainder with carrier oil and used on "perfume" points.

ORANGE YOU HAPPY
3 drops basil
3 drops wild orange

HEART'S DESIRES
3 drops jasmine, rose or magnolia
3 drops sandalwood
1 drop rose or geranium
1 drop sandalwood
1 drop wild orange or bergamot
1 drop ylang ylang

BRIGHTEN
3 drops bergamot
1 drop grapefruit
1 drop ylang ylang

REFRESH
2 drops bergamot
2 drops clary sage
1 drop frankincense

LIFT
3 drops bergamot or wild orange
2 drops clary sage
2 drops frankincense
1 drop jasmine or ylang ylang
1 drop lemon

UNCONDITIONAL LOVE
7 drop wild orange
4 drops frankincense
2 drops bergamot
1 drop ylang ylang
1 drop geranium
Combine in 10ml roller bottle; fill remainder with carrier oil; apply to pulse points, rub on neck, center of back, then cup hands together and inhale. For more potency, double the amount of oils in a 15ml bottle, fill remainder with carrier oil. Premix without carrier oil for use in a diffuser.

BETTER THAN BITTER AND BROODING
1 drop bergamot
1 drop helichrysum
1 drop Roman chamomile
Put oil into palms, rub hands together vigorously, cup your hands together, and slowly inhale.

AGGRESSION-LESS
(to reduce aggression)
4 drops bergamot
3 drops sandalwood
3 drops ylang ylang
2 drops lemon
2 drops Siberian fir
Combine in 15ml bottle/roller bottle; fill with carrier oil. Put 4-5 drops in palms and rub on bottoms of feet and at base of rib cage over top of liver, cup hands together and slowly inhale.

NOT SO SAD: (reduce/eliminate effects of Seasonal Affective Disorder)
3 drops grapefruit
2 drops bergamot
Combine in hands, rub hands together and then rub on pulse points, back of neck into hairline and then slowly inhale. For a 5ml roller bottle blend and less intensity, follow same ratio, multiply by 4 for 12 and 8 drops respectively; fill with carrier oil; use throughout day.

CLEAR-THE-AIR DIFFUSER BLEND
4 drops blue tansy
4 drops wild orange
2 drops melaleuca
2 drops lemon
Combine all ingredients and diffuse. Enjoy this pure, vibrant, energizing aroma.

For more ideas, download the app at app.essentiallife.com

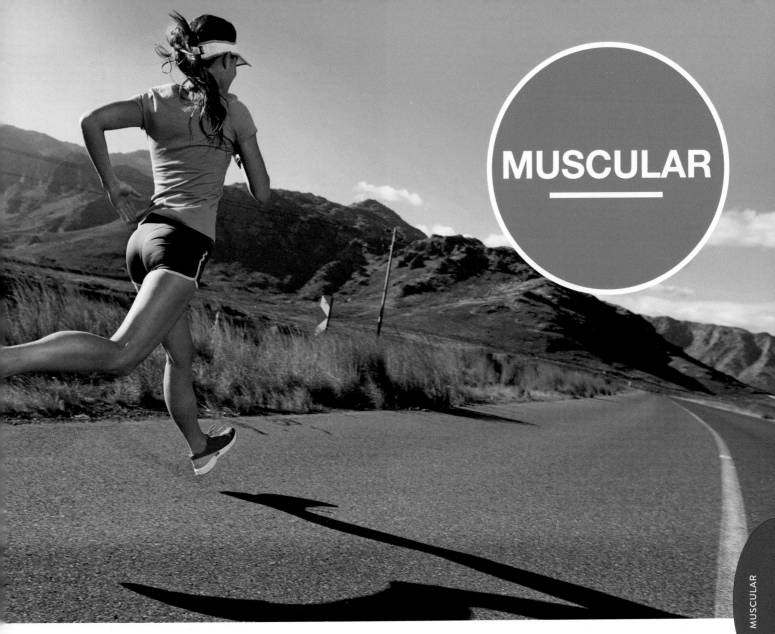

THE MUSCULAR SYSTEM consists of 650 muscles in three main categories: skeletal, smooth, and cardiac muscles. It is controlled by the nervous system via two pathways: somatic and autonomic. Only skeletal muscles fall into the somatic category, meaning that they are under voluntary control; these are the muscles attached to the skeleton. They are striated in appearance and provide strength, balance, posture, movement, and heat for the body.

Tendons are bands of fibrous tissue attached to the skeletal muscles that allow movement in the body. When a skeletal muscle contracts, it pulls on the tendon to which it is attached, causing the tendon to pull on the bone and resulting in movement. Ligaments, on the other hand, are the fibrous material that connects bone to bone and holds the skeletal structure together. Once injured, both require long healing times and are prone to weakness or re-injury. Rest is required, as scar tissue usually takes at least ninety days to form; once formed, the fibers can take up to another seven to nine months to reach maximum strength again.

Autonomic muscles contract and relax involuntarily and include both smooth and cardiac muscles. Smooth muscles are non-striated and are typically found in layers, one behind the other. They can be found in the walls of internal organs (excluding the heart), such as blood vessels, intestines, bladder, digestive system, and stomach. They are constantly at work, performing their functions throughout the body.

Cardiac muscles are specific to the heart and are also known as myocardium. These involuntary muscles contract to pump blood through the heart, then relax to allow blood to return after it has carried vital oxygen and nutrients to the body.

The muscular system is constantly in motion and supporting vital body functions. Essential oils have a unique ability to affect muscles and connective tissue and to support muscle function on a cellular level. Once oils are applied, users often experience near-instant relief. Minor issues and injuries are easily managed with either topical and internal application. For more serious muscle and tendon issues, professional medical care is appropriate. Traditional treatment methods can be enhanced and supported with essential oil and nutritional supplement solutions.

TOP SOLUTIONS

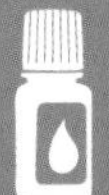

SINGLE OILS

Lemongrass - soothes muscle aches, supports connective tissue repair (pg. 126)
Cypress - promotes blood flow to muscle and connective tissue, reduces pain and spasms (pg. 103)
Marjoram - relaxes muscles and decreases spasms (pg. 131)
Ginger and Turmeric - reduces spasms and muscle aches and pain (pg. 113), (pg. 158)

By Related Properties

For more, See Oil Properties on pages 477 - 481

Analgesic - basil, bergamot, birch, black pepper, blue tansy, cinnamon, clove, copaiba, coriander, eucalyptus, fennel, frankincense, helichrysum, juniper berry, lavender, lemongrass, litsea, marjoram, melaleuca, oregano, peppermint, pink pepper, rosemary, Siberian fir, turmeric, white fir, wintergreen, yarrow
Anticonvulsant - clary sage, fennel, geranium, lavender, neroli, tangerine
Anti-inflammatory - arborvitae, basil, birch, black pepper, blue tansy, cardamom, cassia, cedarwood, cinnamon, copaiba, coriander, cypress, dill, eucalyptus, fennel, frankincense, geranium, ginger, helichrysum, jasmine, lavender, lemongrass, lime, litsea, manuka, melaleuca, melissa, myrrh, neroli, oregano, patchouli, peppermint, pink pepper, Roman chamomile, rosemary, Siberian fir, sandalwood, spearmint, spikenard, tangerine, turmeric, wild orange, wintergreen, yarrow
Antispasmodic - basil, bergamot, birch, black pepper, blue tansy, cardamom, cassia, cinnamon, clary sage, clove, coriander, cypress, dill, eucalyptus, fennel, ginger, helichrysum, jasmine, juniper berry, lavender, lemon, lime, litsea, marjoram, melissa, neroli, patchouli, peppermint, ravensara, Roman chamomile, rosemary, sandalwood, Siberian fir, spearmint, tangerine, thyme, vetiver, wild orange, wintergreen, yarrow, ylang ylang
Energizing - clove, cypress, grapefruit, lemongrass, pink pepper, rosemary, Siberian fir, tangerine, white fir, wild orange, yarrow
Regenerative - basil, cedarwood, clove, coriander, frankincense, geranium, helichrysum, jasmine, lavender, lemongrass, manuka, melaleuca, myrrh, neroli, patchouli, sandalwood, wild orange, yarrow
Relaxing - basil, blue tansy, cassia, cedarwood, clary sage, cypress, fennel, geranium, jasmine, lavender, litsea, manuka, marjoram, myrrh, magnolia, neroli, ravensara, Roman chamomile, white fir, ylang ylang
Steroidal - basil, bergamot, birch, cedarwood, clove, fennel, patchouli, rosemary, thyme, wintergreen
Tonic - arborvitae, basil, bergamot, birch, cardamom, cedarwood, clary sage, coriander, cypress, eucalyptus, fennel, frankincense, geranium, ginger, grapefruit, juniper berry, lavender, lemon, lemongrass, lime, marjoram, melissa, myrrh, neroli, patchouli, Roman chamomile, rose, rosemary, sandalwood, Siberian fir, tangerine, thyme, vetiver, white fir, wild orange, yarrow, ylang ylang
Warming - birch, black pepper, cassia, cinnamon, clary sage, ginger, marjoram, neroli, peppermint, wintergreen

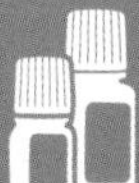

BLENDS

AromaTouch® - promotes circulation and relieves pain (pg. 169)
Deep Blue® - soothes muscle and joint pain and inflammation (pg. 185)
PastTense® - soothes sore muscles and tissue; releases tension (pg. 196)
DDR Prime® - helps with connective tissue repair and soothes pain (pg. 184)

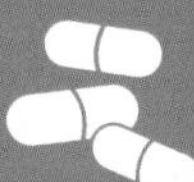

SUPPLEMENTS

Bone Nutrient Lifetime Complex (pg. 210), Alpha CRS®+, Zendocrine® Complex, Zendocrine® Softgels, **Mito2Max® (pg. 214)**, DDR Prime® Softgels, **xEO Mega (pg. 222)**, **Deep Blue Polyphenol Complex (pg. 212)**, MicroPlex VMz

Related Ailments: Aches, Back Muscle Fatigue, Back Pain, Back Stiffness, Body Myositis, Bruised Muscles, Connective Tissue Injury, Convulsions, Cramps/Charley Horse, Do Quervain's Tenosynovitis, Fibromyalgia, Frozen Shoulder, Growing Pains, Headache, Inflammatory Myopathies, Leg Cramps, Lumbago, Metabolic Muscle Disorders, Migraine, Muscle Pain, Muscle Spasms, Muscle Stiffness, Muscle Strains, Muscle Weakness, Muscular Dystrophy, Myasthenia Gravis, Myotonic Dystrophy, Neck Pain, Neuromuscular Disorders (drooping eyelids, double vision, slurred speech, difficulty swallowing, difficulty breathing), Over-exercised, Polymyositis, Rheumatism, Sore Feet, Sore Muscles, Sprains, Tendonitis, Tension, Tension Headache, Tissue Pain, Tissue Regeneration, TMJ, Whiplash

Conditions

Bruising - birch, black pepper, blue tansy, copaiba, fennel, geranium, helichrysum, lavender, neroli, Roman chamomile, white fir, AromaTouch®, Deep Blue®

Circulation (increase) - basil, black spruce, cypress, eucalyptus, green mandarin, lavender, marjoram, pink pepper, turmeric, AromaTouch®, Deep Blue®, HD Clear®, Motivate®; see *Cardiovascular*

Collagen, lack of - helichrysum, lemongrass, sandalwood

Connective tissue/fascia (tendons) - basil, birch, clove, cypress, geranium, ginger, helichrysum, lavender, lemongrass, marjoram, oregano, peppermint, Roman chamomile, rosemary, thyme, vetiver, white fir, wintergreen, AromaTouch®, Deep Blue®, PastTense®

Cramping/charley horse* - arborvitae, basil, birch, black pepper, blue tansy, cardamom, cedarwood, celery seed, cilantro, cinnamon, clary sage, clove, copaiba, cypress, dill, Douglas fir, grapefruit, jasmine, lavender, lemongrass, marjoram, peppermint, Roman chamomile, rosemary, vetiver, white fir, wintergreen, AromaTouch®, Cheer®, Deep Blue®, PastTense®, Peace®, Zendocrine®

Fatigued/overused - basil, black pepper, cinnamon, cypress, Douglas fir, eucalyptus, grapefruit, marjoram, peppermint, rosemary, Siberian fir, tangerine, thyme, white fir, Adaptiv®, AromaTouch®, DDR Prime®, Motivate®, Zendocrine®

Fibromyalgia - basil, birch, blue tansy, clove, copaiba, frankincense, marjoram, oregano, peppermint, ginger, helichrysum, lavender, Roman chamomile, rosemary, thyme, white fir, wintergreen, AromaTouch®, DDR Prime®, Deep Blue®, Zendocrine®

Headaches - frankincense, lavender, peppermint, wintergreen, Cheer®, Deep Blue®, PastTense®; see *Pain & Inflammation*

Headaches, migraine - basil, helichrysum, Roman chamomile; see *Pain & Inflammation*

Heart - cassia, cinnamon, copaiba, Douglas fir, frankincense, geranium, marjoram, lavender, peppermint, rosemary, sandalwood, ylang ylang, AromaTouch®

Hernia, inguinal - fennel, frankincense, ginger, helichrysum, lavender, vetiver

Inflammation, acute (with swelling, redness or pain)* - basil, blue tansy, clary sage, clove, coriander, eucalyptus, frankincense, ginger, helichrysum, marjoram, peppermint, rosemary, sandalwood, Siberian fir, white fir, wintergreen, AromaTouch®, Cheer®, Deep Blue®, PastTense®; see *Pain & Inflammation*

Inflammation, chronic - basil, birch, copaiba, cypress, eucalyptus, frankincense, marjoram, oregano, peppermint, patchouli, rosemary, sandalwood, Siberian fir, vetiver, white fir, wintergreen, AromaTouch®, Deep Blue®; see *Pain & Inflammation*

Injuries - birch, black spruce, frankincense, helichrysum, lavender, lemongrass, myrrh, sandalwood, white fir, wintergreen, yarrow, AromaTouch®, Deep Blue®

Muscle development - basil, birch, Douglas fir, lemongrass, marjoram, rosemary, wintergreen, AromaTouch®, Deep Blue®

Muscle, neuralgia - basil, Douglas fir, eucalyptus, frankincense, lemongrass, marjoram, neroli, peppermint, rosemary, wintergreen, AromaTouch®, Deep Blue®, PastTense®; see *Pain & Inflammation*

Numbness - arborvitae, basil, cypress, frankincense, ginger, lemongrass, patchouli, wintergreen, AromaTouch®

Pain, burning/intense - black pepper, eucalyptus, frankincense, juniper berry, lavender, petitgrain, peppermint, spearmint, turmeric, DDR Prime®, Deep Blue®, PastTense®; see *Pain & Inflammation*

Pain, dull/chronic/achy* - birch, black pepper, blue tansy, celery seed, copaiba, eucalyptus, ginger, helichrysum, lemongrass, marjoram, pink pepper, rosemary, Siberian fir, wintergreen, AromaTouch®, Deep Blue®, Immortelle; see *Pain & Inflammation*

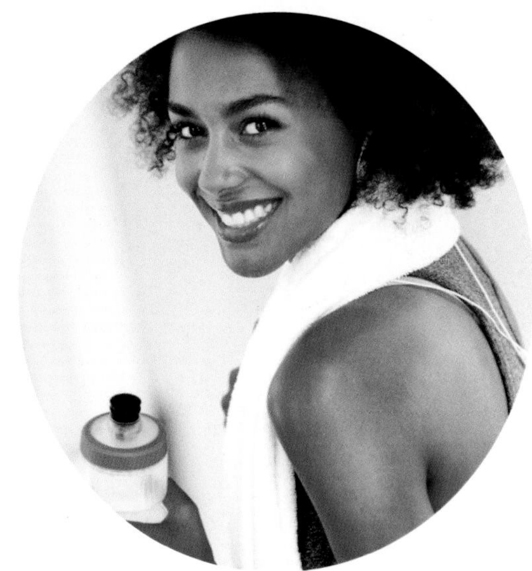

Pain, sharp/acute - basil, birch, black pepper, black spruce, blue tansy, copaiba, frankincense, ginger, helichrysum, lemongrass, peppermint, rosemary, Siberian fir, turmeric, wintergreen, yarrow, AromaTouch®, Deep Blue®, PastTense®; see *Pain & Inflammation*

Paralysis - basil, Douglas fir, frankincense, ginger, lavender, lime, melissa, patchouli, peppermint, rosemary, sandalwood, AromaTouch®, Balance®, DDR Prime®, Motivate®, PastTense®

Parkinson's disease - See *Brain, Addictions "Conditions Associated with Addictions"* - dopamine

Spasms* - basil, bergamot, black pepper, celery seed, cypress, marjoram, melissa, neroli, peppermint, rosemary, thyme, yarrow, AromaTouch®, Motivate®, Passion®, PastTense®

Sprain/strain - birch, black pepper, black spruce, clove, copaiba, eucalyptus, frankincense, ginger, helichrysum, jasmine, lavender, lemongrass, marjoram, Roman chamomile, rosemary, thyme, vetiver, white fir, wintergreen, AromaTouch®, Deep Blue®, PastTense®, Peace®

Tender tissues, swollen, red - frankincense, helichrysum, lemongrass, myrrh, wintergreen, Deep Blue®, PastTense®, Zendocrine®

Tendons/tendonitis - copaiba, lemongrass, white fir; see "Connective Tissue" above

Tension/stiffness, nervous - basil, bergamot, black spruce, cedarwood, celery seed, copaiba, coriander, cypress, Douglas fir, frankincense, ginger, grapefruit, helichrysum, lavender, lemongrass, marjoram, melissa, patchouli, peppermint, petitgrain, Roman chamomile, rose, rosemary, sandalwood, Siberian fir, turmeric, vetiver, white fir, wild orange, wintergreen, ylang ylang, AromaTouch®, Deep Blue®, Motivate®, Passion®, PastTense®, Peace®

Tingling - cedarwood, frankincense, ginger, white fir, AromaTouch®, DDR Prime®, Deep Blue®, PastTense®

Walking on toes - basil, rosemary, white fir, Balance®, DDR Prime®, Zendocrine®

Weakness/loss of mass or tone/degeneration - basil, bergamot, birch, black pepper, clove, coriander, cypress, lavender, marjoram, melissa, rosemary, wintergreen, Adaptiv®, DDR Prime®, Deep Blue®, PastTense®, Whisper®

Whiplash - birch, coriander, frankincense, helichrysum, lemongrass, peppermint, white fir, Deep Blue®, PastTense®

* *See remedy on pg. 326*

Remedies

FOOT LOVE
1 drop frankincense
2 drops of spearmint or peppermint
4 drops of rosemary
Stir oils into ¼ cup Epsom salts; mix well, add to warm water in foot bath. Soak for 20 minutes.

ACHE-Y BRAKE-Y BATH (muscle relief)
4 drops Siberian fir
4 drops frankincense
1 drop clove
Stir oils into ½ cup Epsom salts; mix well, add to hot bath water. Soak for 20 minutes.

MASSAGE IN A BOTTLE
Apply AromaTouch® and/or Deep Blue® to any unhappy muscle. Reapply every thirty minutes for acute pain and twice per day for more chronic issues.

ANTI-SPAZ (for muscle spasms)
12 drops Siberian fir
9 drops lemongrass
6 drops basil
Combine oils in 10ml roller bottle; fill remainder with carrier oil. Apply topically on or near affected area as needed.

COLD COMPRESS RELIEF RECIPES
Drop oils into small bowl of ¼ - ½ cup cold water. Dip washcloth onto to oils. Apply moistened cloth directly to muscle.
- **Muscular Pain Relief:** 3 drops Roman chamomile, 3 drops lavender
- **Muscle Inflammation Relief:** 3 drops peppermint, 3 drops yarrow
- **Pulled Muscle Relief:** 3 drops Roman chamomile, 2 drops marjoram

MUSCULAR

READY ROLLERBALL RECIPES
Combine in a 5ml roller bottle; fill remainder with carrier oil. Apply to affected area as needed.

- **Leg Muscle Cramps**
  4 drops ginger
  8 drops black pepper
  8 drops cinnamon
- **Loosen Tight Muscles**
  4 drops ginger
  8 drops lavender
  8 drops rosemary
- **Muscle Spasm Relief**
  6 drops cypress
  3 drops lemongrass
  8 drops marjoram
  4 drops ginger
- **Soothe Aching Muscles**
  2 drops of cardamom
  4 drops lemongrass
  5 drops ginger
  6 drops lavender

AROMATOUCH®
Add to a 2 oz glass bottle: 7 drops of blue tansy, 3 drops of lavender, 4 drops of frankincense, 6 drops of copaiba. Fill remainder of bottle with carrier oil. Shake well and apply as desired to sore muscles.

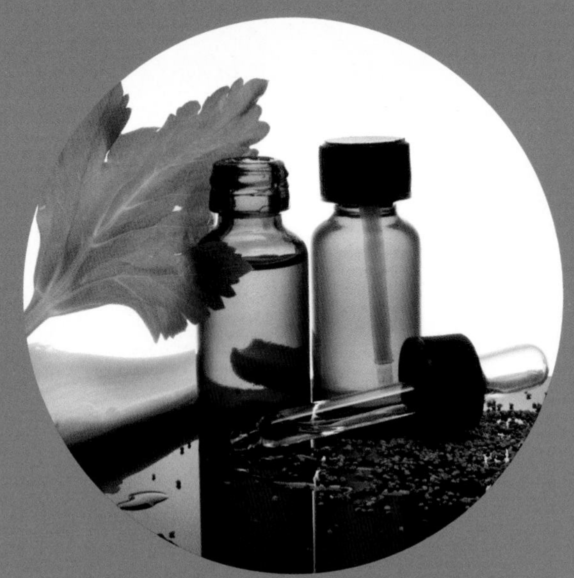

MUSCLE & PAIN RELIEF
Add 5 drops celery seed essential oil with 1-2 teaspoons fractionated coconut oil, gently massage on affected areas. Alternatively, add 3 drops to tub of warm water for a relaxing foot soak.

MUSCLE-RELAXING BLEND
Mix well and apply to tense, overexerted muscles, or for an overall relaxing massage.
4 drops black spruce essential oil
3 drops roman chamomile essential oil
3 drops cedarwood essential oil
2 drops copaiba essential oil
1 ounce carrier oil

MUSCLE RELIEF BLEND
Combine in 10 ml roller bottle; top off with carrier oil. Apply to areas of concern. Repeat as needed.
6 drops turmeric
6 drops marjoram
3 drops black pepper
3 drops rosemary
3 drops peppermint
3 drops copaiba

USAGE TIPS: For best results with muscles and connective tissue:
- **Topical:** Apply oils directly to area of concern, massage in thoroughly whenever possible. Drive oils in with heat, cold, or moisture. Use carrier oil as needed or desired. Layering multiple oils over affected area, placing them on tissue one at a time, is very effective. Any kind of cream or carrier barrier will slow absorption if placed on first and improve it if placed on last.
  - **Acute:** Apply often, every 20-30 minutes, until symptoms subside, then reduce to every two to six hours.
  - **Chronic:** Apply two to three times daily.
- **Internal:** Consume oils to support resolving inflammation in a capsule or under tongue.

For more ideas, download the app at app.essentiallife.com

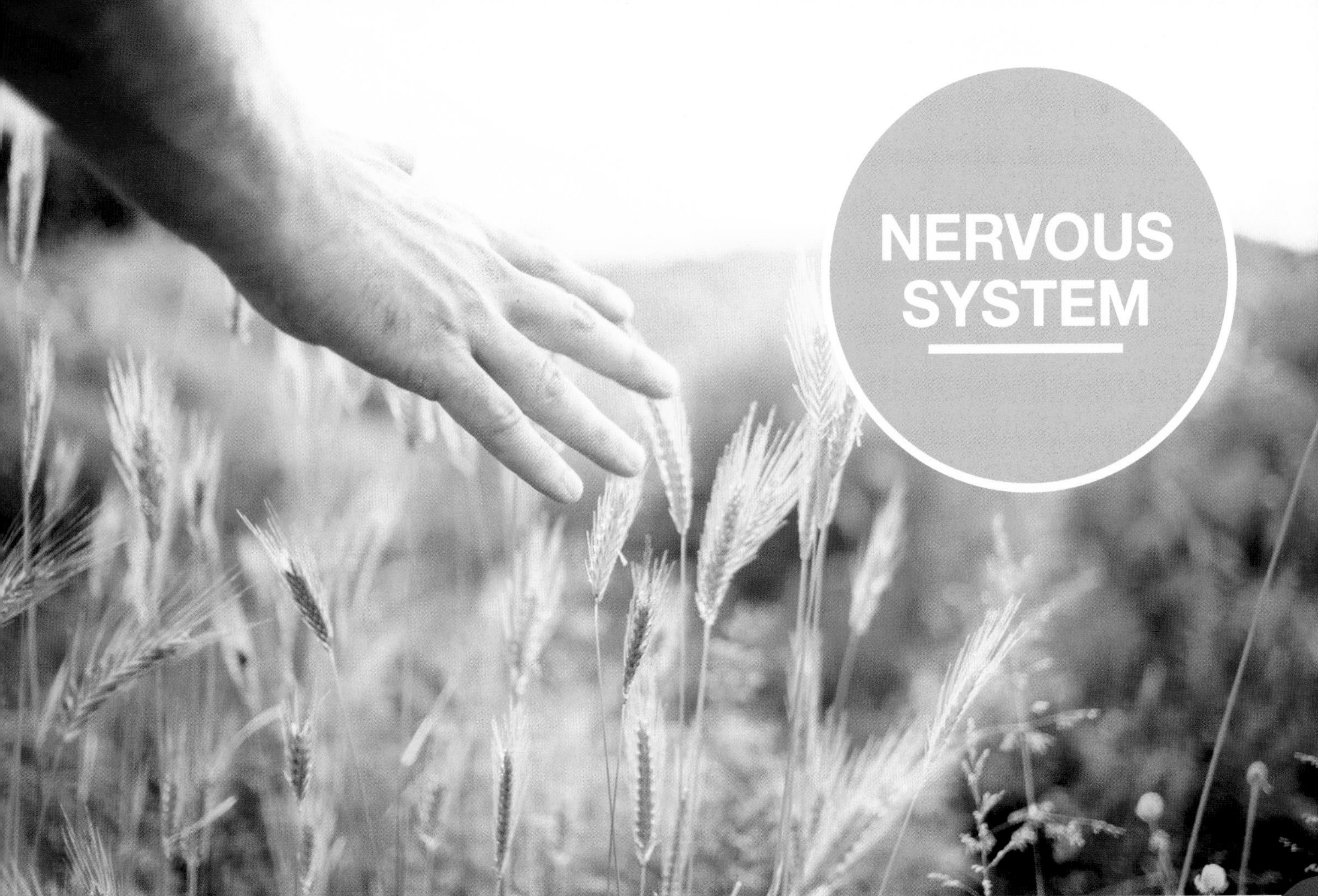

THE NERVOUS SYSTEM is a complex system of nerves and specialized cells that allows the body to transmit and receive messages. It serves as the body's primary control and communications center, responsible for transmitting and receiving messages between every other system in the body.

The sensory function involves transmitting data from sensory receptors, which register internal and external stimuli to the central nervous system (CNS), where it is processed by the brain. The CNS relies on the conscious and subconscious signals from the body's sensory receptors to make it aware of any threats. It is also charged with the higher functions of language, imagination, emotion, and personality.

When the CNS receives sensory input, a complex network of neurons in the brain and brain stem evaluates, categorizes, and files this information, making it available for decision-making and future retrieval. After the incoming sensory signals are evaluated, a signal is sent through the nerves of the peripheral nervous system (PNS) to effector cells, which release hormones or otherwise cause the body to respond to the stimulus.

The somatic nervous system (SNS), which is part of the PNS, directs the conscious, voluntary movements of the body. The autonomic nervous system (ANS), on the other hand, controls all the involuntary neurons, those that do not require conscious direction to function, such as cardiac, visceral, and glandular tissues.

The ANS is further divided into the sympathetic and parasympathetic systems. The sympathetic system is responsible for the body's fight or flight response which, when activated, increases respiration, heart rate, and adrenaline and stress hormone levels in the blood, while suppressing digestive functions. The parasympathetic system takes over when the body rests and digests. This system tries to undo what the sympathetic system does when it encounters a threat, e.g. decreasing respiration and heart rate, while increasing digestion and waste elimination.

The enteric nervous system (ENS) is yet another division of the autonomic nervous system and is in charge of regulating the digestive system. As mentioned above, it receives input from both the sympathetic and parasympathetic divisions of the ANS, instructing it what to do. The majority of the ENS's functions, however, are regulated independently, warranting the nickname "the second brain," and rightly so, for it alone boasts as many neurons as exist in the spinal cord.

Essential oils can facilitate the complex messaging that occurs throughout the nervous system. They help with homeostasis, circulation, and brain function (see Limbic System) as the brain interprets and sends out data. They even help the neurons transmitting and receiving messages to be more efficient due to their regenerative and soothing properties. They address root causes of ailments connected to the nervous system, helping improve symptoms because the body has support in helping itself.

TOP SOLUTIONS

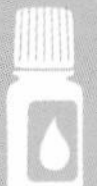

SINGLE OILS

Helichrysum - invigorates nerves and relieves pain (pg. 117)
Peppermint - stimulates nerves and supports repair (pg. 140)
Lemongrass - stimulates nerves and electrical system of body (pg. 126)
Patchouli - provides nerve protection and supports regeneration; removes toxins (pg. 139)
Basil - stimulates, energizes and restores nerves; relaxes tension (pg. 80)
Frankincense - provides nerve protection and supports regeneration (pg. 110)
Neroli or Magnolia - calms and sedates (pg. 136), (pg. 129)

By Related Properties

For more, See Oil Properties on pages 477 - 479

Analgesic - arborvitae, basil, bergamot, birch, blue tansy, cassia, cinnamon, clary sage, copaiba, coriander, eucalyptus, fennel, frankincense, ginger, jasmine, juniper berry, lavender, lemongrass, litsea, marjoram, melaleuca, oregano, peppermint, ravensara, rosemary, Siberian fir, white fir, wild orange, wintergreen, yarrow
Anti-inflammatory - arborvitae, basil, bergamot, birch, black pepper, blue tansy, cardamom, cassia, cedarwood, cinnamon, copaiba, coriander, cypress, dill, eucalyptus, fennel, frankincense, geranium, ginger, helichrysum, jasmine, lavender, lemongrass, lime, litsea, manuka, melaleuca, melissa, myrrh, oregano, neroli, patchouli, peppermint, Roman chamomile, rosemary, sandalwood, Siberian fir, spearmint, spikenard, tangerine, turmeric, wild orange, wintergreen, yarrow
Calming - bergamot, birch, black pepper, black spruce, blue tansy, cassia, clary sage, copaiba, coriander, fennel, frankincense, geranium, jasmine, juniper berry, lavender, litsea, melissa, oregano, patchouli, Roman chamomile, sandalwood, tangerine, vetiver, yarrow
Grounding - basil, black spruce, blue tansy, cedarwood, clary sage, cypress, melaleuca, vetiver, Siberian fir, ylang ylang
Nervine - basil, clary sage, clove, helichrysum, juniper berry, lavender, lemongrass, melissa, patchouli, peppermint, rose, rosemary, thyme
Neuroprotective - frankincense, lavender, magnolia, Roman chamomile, thyme, turmeric, vetiver
Neurotonic - arborvitae, basil, bergamot, black pepper, clary sage, cypress, ginger, melaleuca, neroli
Regenerative - basil, cedarwood, citronella, clove, coriander, frankincense, geranium, helichrysum, lavender, lemongrass, manuka, melaleuca, myrrh, neroli, patchouli, sandalwood, wild orange, yarrow
Relaxing - basil, blue tansy, cassia, cedarwood, cypress, fennel, geranium, jasmine, lavender, litsea, magnolia, manuka, marjoram, myrrh, neroli, ravensara, Roman chamomile, white fir, ylang ylang
Steroidal - basil, bergamot, birch, cedarwood, clove, fennel, patchouli, rosemary, thyme, wintergreen
Stimulant - arborvitae, basil, bergamot, birch, black pepper, black spruce, blue tansy, cardamom, cedarwood, cinnamon, clove, coriander, cypress, dill, eucalyptus, fennel, ginger, grapefruit, juniper berry, lime, melaleuca, myrrh, patchouli, pink pepper, rosemary, Siberian fir, spearmint, tangerine, thyme, vetiver, white fir, wintergreen, ylang ylang

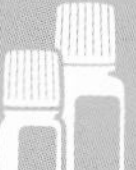

BLENDS

InTune® - helps with mental focus and reduces inflammation (pg. 192)
AromaTouch® - increases circulation (pg. 169)
Deep Blue® - invigorates and stimulates nerves (pg. 185)
DDR Prime® - regenerates and protects nerves (pg. 184)
Immortelle - regenerates nerves and increases clarity (pg. 191)

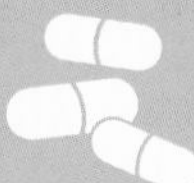

SUPPLEMENTS

Bone Nutrient Lifetime Complex, Alpha CRS®+, Mito2Max®, **DDR Prime® Softgels (pg. 211)**, **xEO Mega (pg. 222)**, TerraZyme®, **IQ Mega® (pg. 213)**, Deep Blue Polyphenol Complex, MicroPlex VMz

Targeted Nervous System Support

Autonomic nervous system - basil, bergamot, dill, fennel, lemon, Balance®, DigestZen®, Serenity®
Central nervous system - basil, black pepper (circulation to nerves), frankincense, grapefruit, lavender, patchouli, peppermint, rosemary (stimulant), DDR Prime®, Immortelle
Parasympathetic nervous system - lavender, lemongrass (regulates), marjoram, patchouli, wild orange, Balance®, Breathe®, PastTense®, Serenity®
Sympathetic nervous system - cedarwood, eucalyptus, fennel (stimulant), ginger, grapefruit (stimulant), peppermint, DDR Prime®

Related Ailments: Bell's Palsy, Blurred Vision, Carpal Tunnel Syndrome, Cataracts, Floaters, Glaucoma, Iris Inflammation, Macular Degeneration, Neuralgia, Neuritis, Neuropathy, Numbness, Multiple Sclerosis, Optic Neuritis, Ocular Rosacea, Phantom Pains, Poor Taste, Poor Vision, Porphyria, Retinitis Pigmentosa, Sciatica, Shock, Spina Bifida, Tourette Syndrome, Transverse Myelitis, Trigeminal Neuralgia, Uveitis

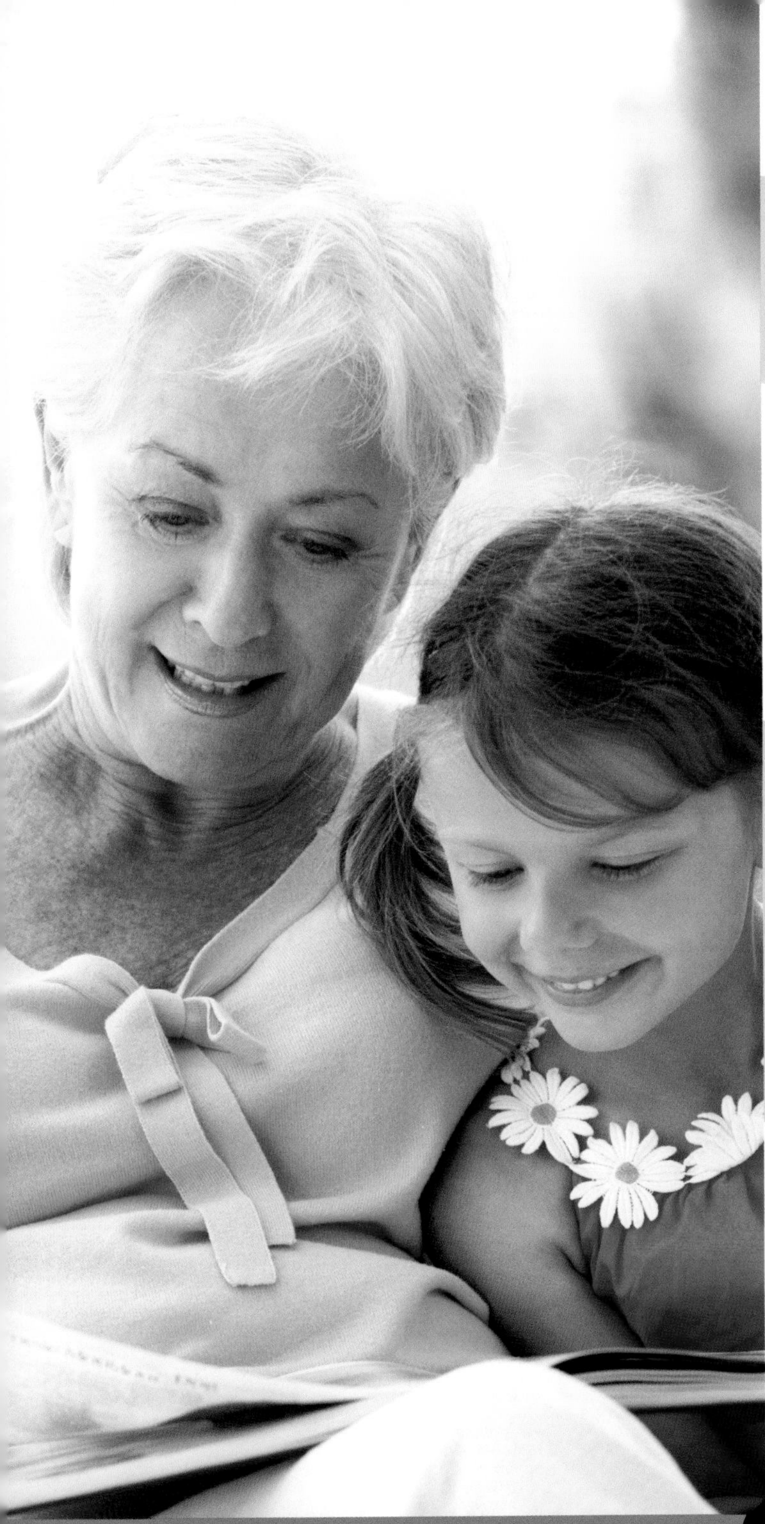

Remedies

INTERNAL NERVE BATH (nervous system cleanse: for brain and organ function):
4 drops frankincense
4 drops thyme
4 drops clove
Combine oils and take in a capsule daily.

BRAIN REVITALIZER
7 drops helichrysum
7 drops patchouli
6 drops sandalwood
5 drops Roman chamomile
3 drops cypress
2 drops pink pepper
Combine in a 5ml roller bottle; fill remainder with carrier oil. Apply to mastoid bone behind ears, back of neck into hairline, and forehead, morning and night.

BRAIN DEFOGGER DAILY ROUTINE

- Use as directed Alpha CRS®+, DDR Prime® Softgels, xEO Mega, Mito2Max®, MicroPlex VMz, PB Assist®+.
- Rub 1-2 drops of Balance® on bottoms of feet morning and night.
- Place 1-2 drops of frankincense, and/or turmeric under tongue morning and night.
- Consume water with favorite citrus oil throughout day.
- Use "Mid-Afternoon Slump Buster" blend - see *Energy & Vitality*, use as needed for focus boost.
- Layer Immortelle and InTune® up back of neck into hairline morning and evening.

NERVOUS SYSTEM

NERVE DAMAGE
14 drops frankincense
10 drops helichrysum
10 drops Roman chamomile
8 drops vetiver
6 drops peppermint
Combine into 5mil roller bottle; fill remainder with carrier oil. Massage into spine or affected area daily.

SHINGLES SPRITZER
10 drops eucalyptus
10 drops marjoram
10 drops melaleuca
10 drops Roman chamomile
10 drops On Guard®
5 drops frankincense
Combine into 2-ounce spritzer bottle; fill remainder of bottle with half fractionated coconut oil and half distilled water. Spray affected area every twenty to thirty minutes. Shake bottle before each use.

SIMPLE SHINGLES REMEDY
Combine equal parts melaleuca and frankincense in 5-10ml roller bottle. Use NEAT (directly on skin without dilution).

USAGE TIPS: For best success in support the nerves and nervous system

- **Topical:** Apply selected oil(s) directly to any area of concern remembering to use a carrier oil if necessary to prevent sensitivity.
- **Internal:** Consume oils in a capsule or under tongue to address nervous issues and bring a particular chemical message to affected areas.
- **Aromatic:** Inhaling from a preparation or diffusing selected oils can have direct impact on brain and nervous system via olfactory pathways.

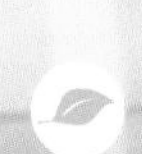

Conditions

Carpal tunnel, pain/tingling - basil, cypress, ginger, lemongrass, marjoram, oregano, peppermint, spearmint, AromaTouch®, DDR Prime®, Deep Blue®; see *Skeletal*
Decreased ability to taste - black pepper, ginger, peppermint, spearmint
Dendrites, lack of - vetiver
Dizziness - basil, bergamot, black pepper, clove, frankincense, ginger, juniper berry, peppermint, Roman chamomile, tangerine, Citrus Bliss®, DDR Prime®, Slim & Sassy®, Whisper®, Zendocrine®
Dropsy - basil, black pepper, dill, frankincense, ginger, juniper berry, marjoram, myrrh, patchouli, peppermint, vetiver, wintergreen, AromaTouch®, Breathe®, DDR Prime®, Immortelle, On Guard®, Serenity®
EYES
⚠**CAUTION** - do not put oils in eyes; place oils on skin near eyes; use very small amounts, dilute with carrier oil; use reflex point on toes for eyes - consult Reflexology chapter in this book.

- **Cataracts**- birch, black pepper, cardamom, clary sage, frankincense, lemongrass
- **Dry, itchy, red/redness, tear duct (blocked), watery** - See *Respiratory*
- **Fatigue** - cypress, lavender
- **Optical nerve** - arborvitae, frankincense, juniper berry (regeneration), patchouli, Immortelle
- **Pain** - frankincense, lavender, melaleuca
- **Sensitivity to light/glare** - arborvitae, basil, frankincense, helichrysum, patchouli, Roman chamomile, vetiver, DDR Prime®, Immortelle
- **Stinging/burning/scratching** - frankincense, helichrysum, lavender, patchouli, rosemary, DDR Prime®
- **Swollen** - cypress, frankincense
- **Vision, clouded/blurred/poor** - basil, bergamot, black pepper, cardamom, clary sage, clove, cypress, frankincense, ginger, helichrysum, juniper berry, lemongrass, melaleuca, DDR Prime®, Immortelle
- **Vision, double in one eye** - clary sage, helichrysum, lavender, lemongrass
- **Vision, fading or yellowing of colors** - basil, black pepper, clary sage, cypress, frankincense, lavender, vetiver, AromaTouch®, DDR Prime®
- **Vision, weak** - clove, frankincense, helichrysum, lemongrass, Immortelle

Headache - basil, copaiba, frankincense, lavender, neroli, patchouli, peppermint, Siberian fir, thyme, wintergreen, PastTense®
Headache, migraine - blue tansy, copaiba, frankincense, lavender, marjoram, melissa, peppermint, Roman chamomile, spearmint, PastTense®; see *Pain & Inflammation*
Huntington's disease - See *Autoimmune*
Impaired gait, posture, and balance - frankincense, marjoram, patchouli, peppermint, thyme, Balance®, Immortelle
Increased sensitivity to sound - helichrysum, Immortelle
Multiple Sclerosis - bergamot, clove, copaiba, cypress, frankincense, helichrysum, melissa, oregano, patchouli, peppermint, rosemary, sandalwood, Console®, DDR Prime®, Immortelle, InTune®; see *Autoimmune*
Myelin sheath, compromised - frankincense, patchouli, peppermint, rosemary, sandalwood, vetiver, Immortelle
Nausea - basil, bergamot, fennel, ginger, juniper berry, lavender, DigestZen®, Tamer™, Zendocrine®; see *Digestive & Intestinal*
Nerve damage* - basil, ginger, helichrysum, lemongrass, patchouli, Deep Blue®
Nerve degeneration* - basil, citronella, copaiba, frankincense, geranium, helichrysum, juniper berry, patchouli, peppermint, Deep Blue®, Immortelle, InTune®, Motivate®, Zendocrine®
Nerve inflammation - blue tansy, cedarwood, clove, copaiba, eucalyptus, frankincense, juniper berry, lavender, lemongrass, magnolia, patchouli, peppermint, Roman chamomile, turmeric, vetiver, wintergreen, Deep Blue®, InTune®
Nerve, lack of tone - black pepper, cardamom, fennel, patchouli, peppermint, sandalwood, spearmint, Forgive®
Nerve pain (neuralgia) - basil, bergamot, birch, cedarwood, cinnamon, clove, coriander, eucalyptus, frankincense, geranium, ginger, helichrysum, juniper berry, lavender, marjoram, neroli, patchouli, peppermint, Roman chamomile, rosemary, thyme, wintergreen, Deep Blue®, Immortelle, PastTense®
Nerve problems* - black pepper, cinnamon, grapefruit, lemon, lime, patchouli, peppermint, Roman chamomile, sandalwood, vetiver, Citrus Bliss®, Forgive®, Peace®
Nerve, virus - clove, frankincense, lemongrass, melissa, myrrh, turmeric, DDR Prime®, Motivate®
Nervous debility/exhaustion - coriander, ginger, grapefruit, helichrysum, patchouli, Deep Blue®
Nervous disorders - bergamot, blue tansy, cedarwood, citronella, frankincense, melissa, neroli, patchouli, Roman chamomile, spikenard, vetiver, Deep Blue®, InTune®, Peace®
Nervous tension - basil, bergamot, black spruce, Douglas fir, geranium, grapefruit, jasmine, lavender, melissa, Roman chamomile, rose, sandalwood, turmeric, vetiver, wild orange, ylang ylang, Adaptiv®, PastTense®

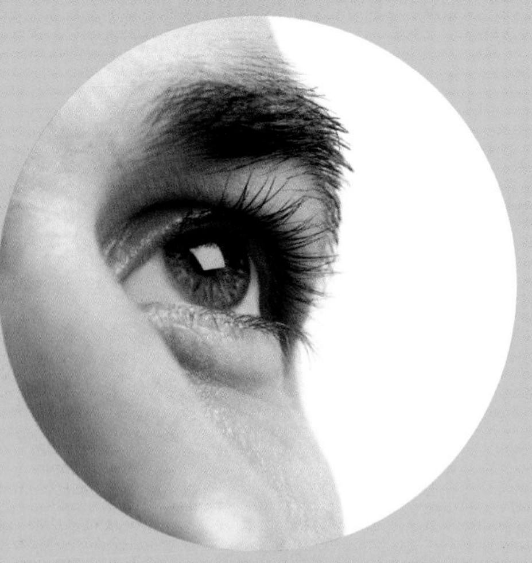

Neurons, impaired activity - Roman chamomile, vetiver, PastTense®
Neuropathy, peripheral - celery seed
Numbness/prickling - basil, cypress, helichrysum, marjoram, wintergreen, AromaTouch®, Deep Blue®, PastTense®
Paralysis - cardamom, cypress, Douglas fir, frankincense, geranium, ginger, helichrysum, juniper berry, lemongrass, melissa, peppermint, sandalwood, AromaTouch®, Balance®, DDR Prime®, Purify
Paralysis, side of face - helichrysum, marjoram, patchouli, peppermint, rose, rosemary, thyme; see "Paralysis" above
Paralysis, temporary - frankincense, rosemary, AromaTouch®
Sciatica, issues with - basil, birch, blue tansy, cardamom, copaiba, cypress, Douglas fir, frankincense, helichrysum, lavender, peppermint, sandalwood, thyme, white fir, wintergreen, Deep Blue®
Sedation, need - cedarwood, coriander, geranium, magnolia, melissa, neroli, patchouli, wild orange, ylang ylang
Shock - bergamot, frankincense, helichrysum, magnolia, neroli, peppermint, Roman chamomile, Adaptiv®, Peace®; see *First Aid*
Speech impediment - frankincense, rosemary, InTune®
Teeth grinding - frankincense, geranium, lavender, marjoram, Roman chamomile, wild orange, Serenity®; see *Parasites*

* *See remedy on pg. 329*

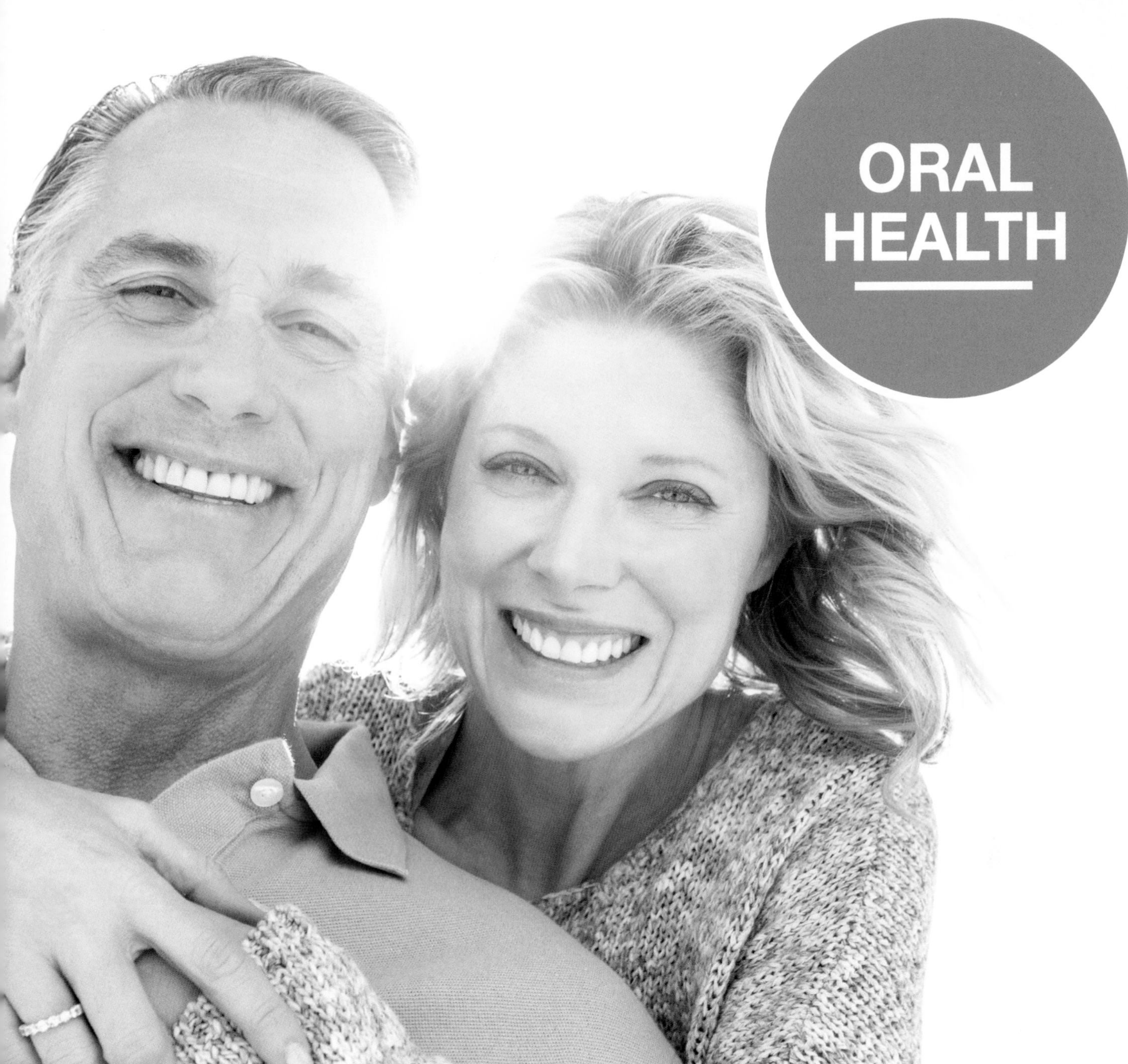

ORAL HEALTH

ALTHOUGH ORAL HEALTH is often treated separately from the body as a whole, the health of the oral cavity - the mouth and its tissues - impacts overall health. Poor oral health may be the cause of a more serious underlying disease process, or it may predispose an individual to other health conditions.

The mouth is colonized by hundreds of different bacterial species that inhabit dental plaque. These species adhere in layers to oral surfaces. They are not easily eliminated by the body's natural immune responses and must be mechanically removed. Bacteria increase tenfold when the mouth is not sufficiently cleaned.

A clean mouth contains several hundred billion bacteria, and this number increases when poor oral care exists. Using saliva and gingival fluid to supply their nutrients, bacteria inhabit all areas of the mouth, threatening oral and systemic health. Bacteria beneath the gums, or gingiva, have been reported to be involved in numerous systemic diseases. Oral health care, primarily proper cleaning and caution in the consumption of and ongoing exposure to intensely acidic and sugary foods (e.g. soda pop), contributes to a healthy lifestyle.

Essential oils are a particularly effective means of supporting oral health, partly because they are antibacterial and antifungal in nature. Clove oil helps to relieve oral pain, cinnamon and peppermint are effective against plaque and gum disease, melaleuca is soothing and helpful in eradicating canker sores, and lavender is soothing to sore muscles that result from teeth grinding. Oil pulling is also particularly beneficial to restoring and maintaining oral health. Specific essential oils can be chosen as part of that routine to target desired results. See *Detoxification* for further instruction.

TOP SOLUTIONS

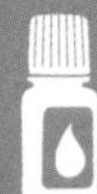

SINGLE OILS

Myrrh - fights gum disease, infections and sores; soothes gums (pg. 135)
Clove - protects nerves, soothes pain; prevents tooth decay (pg. 97)
Peppermint - freshens breath; reduces swelling, inflammation, and tenderness (pg. 140)
Wintergreen - protect nerves, soothes pain; prevents tooth decay (pg. 163)
Turmeric - relieves pain and inflammation (pg. 158)

By Related Properties

For more, See Oil Properties on pages 477 - 481

Analgesic - arborvitae, bergamot, black pepper, blue tansy, cassia, cinnamon, clove, copaiba, coriander, cypress, eucalyptus, fennel, frankincense, ginger, jasmine, juniper berry, lavender, lemongrass, litsea, marjoram, melaleuca, oregano, ravensara, Siberian fir, turmeric, wild orange, wintergreen, yarrow
Antibacterial - arborvitae, basil, bergamot, birch, black pepper, cardamom, cassia, cedarwood, cilantro, cinnamon, clary sage, clove, copaiba, coriander, cypress, dill, eucalyptus, geranium, ginger, grapefruit, helichrysum, lemongrass, lime, litsea, manuka, marjoram, melaleuca, melissa, myrrh, oregano, patchouli, peppermint, pink pepper, ravensara, rosemary, Siberian fir, sandalwood, spearmint, spikenard, tangerine, thyme, turmeric, wild orange, ylang ylang
Anti-infectious - arborvitae, bergamot, cardamom, cedarwood, cinnamon, clove, copaiba, cypress, eucalyptus, frankincense, geranium, lavender, litsea, marjoram, melaleuca, myrrh, Roman chamomile, rosemary
Anti-inflammatory - arborvitae, bergamot, birch, black pepper, blue tansy, cardamom, cassia, cedarwood, cinnamon, copaiba, coriander, dill, eucalyptus, fennel, frankincense, geranium, ginger, helichrysum, jasmine, lavender, lemongrass, lime, litsea, manuka, melaleuca, myrrh, neroli, oregano, patchouli, peppermint, Roman chamomile, rosemary, sandalwood, Siberian fir, spearmint, spikenard, tangerine, turmeric, wild orange, wintergreen, yarrow
Detoxifier - arborvitae, cassia, geranium, juniper berry, lemon, lime, litsea, rosemary, tangerine, yarrow
Immunostimulant - arborvitae, cassia, cinnamon, clove, copaiba, eucalyptus, fennel, frankincense, ginger, lemon, lime, melaleuca, melissa, oregano, ravensara, rosemary, Siberian fir, spearmint, thyme, turmeric, vetiver, wild orange, yarrow

Related Ailments: Abscess (tooth), Bleeding Gums, Canker Sores, Cavities, Dental Infection, Dysphagia [Digestive & Intestinal], Gingivitis, Gum Disease, Hoarse Voice, Halitosis, Laryngitis, Mouth Ulcers, Plaque, Pyorrhea, Sore Throat [Respiratory], Teeth Grinding, Teething Pain, Tonsillitis, Toothache

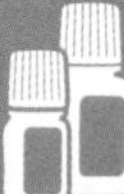

BLENDS

On Guard® - helps fight infection and bacteria; prevents tooth decay (pg. 194)
DDR Prime® - protects nerves, soothes pain; prevents tooth decay (pg. 184)
PastTense® - reduces tension, inflammation, swelling, and pain in jaw (pg. 196)

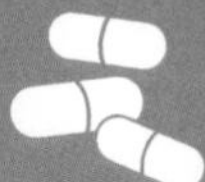

SUPPLEMENTS

Bone Nutrient Lifetime Complex (pg. 210), Alpha CRS®+, detoxification softgels, xEO Mega, food enzymes, TerraGreens®, On Guard Softgels, MicroPlex VMz

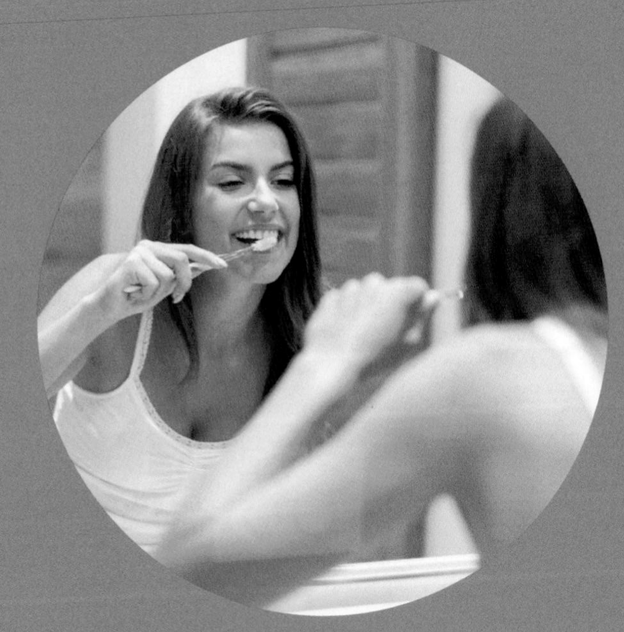

USAGE TIPS: For oral health support

- **Topical:** Apply oils directly to area of concern in mouth such as gums, teeth, tongue, sores, etc. To relieve pain, also apply pain-relieving oils to outside cheek/jaw area (can use a carrier oil as needed); apply frequently as needed for acute situations.
- **Internal:** Place oils on toothbrush and brush teeth with selected oils to affect surface of teeth. Ingest oils (e.g. lemon) to change pH (alkalize) in body/mouth which affects tooth and oral health.

Remedies

For more ideas, download the app at app.essentiallife.com

COLD SORE ROLLER BOTTLE
6 drops peppermint
6 drops melaleuca
1 drop helichrysum
2 drops clove
3 drops lavender
2 drops cinnamon
Add to a 5ml roller bottle. Fill remainder of bottle with a carrier oil and apply to the area until healed and then one day more.

CANKER SORE REMEDY
1 drop melissa
2 drops geranium
2 drops helichrysum
2 drops black pepper
1 drop clove
Combine with 2 teaspoons carrier oil and apply as needed.

BRACES PAIN: Place helichrysum or PastTense® on jaw; dilute with carrier oil if desired.

TMJ: Use Serenity® or PastTense® on neck and jaw.

MOUTHWASH
5 drops melaleuca
5 drops peppermint
3 drops clove
2 drops cinnamon
2 drops myrrh
Combine in a 4-ounce glass bottle. Fill remainder with purified water. Shake before use.

Conditions

Bleeding gums - cardamom, clove, dill, frankincense, helichrysum, lemon, lime, melaleuca, myrrh, oregano, patchouli, peppermint, rosemary, spearmint, thyme, wild orange, DDR Prime®, On Guard®, Zendocrine®
Bleeding, tooth extraction - cardamom, frankincense, helichrysum, lavender, lemon, lime, DDR Prime®, Zendocrine®
Breath, bad (halitosis) - bergamot, cardamom, cilantro, juniper berry, lavender, peppermint, spearmint, turmeric, DDR Prime®, DigestZen®, Slim & Sassy®, Zendocrine®
Canker sore* - birch, black pepper, helichrysum, melaleuca, myrrh, oregano, wild orange, DDR Prime®, On Guard®, Slim & Sassy®
Cavities - see *Tooth decay*
Cold sores* - arborvitae, basil, bergamot, clove, fennel, geranium, lavender, lemon, marjoram, melaleuca, melissa, myrrh, oregano, wild orange, DDR Prime®, On Guard®, Zendocrine®
Fever blisters - see "Cold sores" above
Gum disease - cinnamon, clove, grapefruit, melaleuca, myrrh, On Guard®
Gums, infection - basil, geranium, myrrh, DDR Prime®, On Guard®
Gums, inflammation - birch, cinnamon, clove, melaleuca, myrrh, peppermint, Console®, On Guard®
Gums, receding - clove, geranium, myrrh, DDR Prime®, On Guard®
Gums, tender - birch, cardamom, cinnamon, clove, frankincense, helichrysum, lavender, lemon, lime, melaleuca, myrrh, peppermint, rosemary, spearmint, thyme, wild orange, DDR Prime®, On Guard®
Headache, jaw-related - basil, frankincense, lavender, marjoram, peppermint, wintergreen, Balance®, DDR Prime®, PastTense®, Serenity®
Mouth, dry - frankincense, grapefruit, lemon, tangerine, wild orange
Mouth, infection - bergamot, cinnamon, clove, frankincense, helichrysum, lavender, lemon, lime, melaleuca, oregano, rosemary, thyme, turmeric, DDR Prime®, On Guard®
Mouth, injury/trauma - frankincense, helichrysum, myrrh, white fir, On Guard®
Mouth ulcers and sores - basil, bergamot, cinnamon, clove, frankincense, geranium, helichrysum, lavender, lemon, marjoram, melaleuca, melissa, myrrh, oregano, wild orange, DDR Prime®, On Guard®, Zendocrine®
Oral Health - green mandarin, turmeric
Pain with pressure of chewing/biting - helichrysum, myrrh, thyme, Zendocrine®
Plaque - clove, grapefruit, lemon, lime, myrrh, tangerine, thyme, wild orange, On Guard®, Zendocrine®
Root canal - copaiba, turmeric
Salivary glands, blocked/congested - cypress, grapefruit, lemon, lemongrass, AromaTouch®, Citrus Bliss®, On Guard®, Purify, Zendocrine®
Swallowing, difficulty/inability/gagging - peppermint, rosemary
Swollen cheek - basil, cypress, frankincense, helichrysum, peppermint, wintergreen, AromaTouch®, Deep Blue®
Tartar - black pepper, coriander, lemon, lime, ravensara, tangerine, On Guard®, Slim & Sassy®, Zendocrine®
Teeth grinding - frankincense, lavender, marjoram, Roman chamomile, Serenity®; see *Parasites*
Teeth, new spaces between - clary sage, frankincense, patchouli, DDR Prime®
Teeth, sensitivity to hot/cold - frankincense, helichrysum, lavender, myrrh, DDR Prime®, On Guard®, Zendocrine®
Tooth abscess - cinnamon, clove, frankincense, helichrysum, lavender, melaleuca, myrrh, rosemary, thyme, DDR Prime®, On Guard®
Throat, sore - cinnamon, helichrysum, lemon, melaleuca, myrrh, thyme, wild orange, Breathe®, DDR Prime®, On Guard®; see *Respiratory*
Throat, tickling/raw - frankincense, helichrysum, rosemary, wild orange, On Guard®
Tingling/burning sensation in mouth - grapefruit, lemon, Zendocrine®
Tongue, indentations - On Guard®
Tonsils, red/swollen/white patches - melaleuca, oregano
Tooth abscess - cinnamon, clove, frankincense, helichrysum, lavender, melaleuca, myrrh, rosemary, thyme, DDR Prime®, On Guard®
Toothache - bergamot, birch, black pepper, blue tansy, clove, cinnamon, frankincense, helichrysum, lavender, melaleuca, myrrh, peppermint, Roman chamomile, wintergreen, yarrow, On Guard®, Zendocrine®
Tooth decay - birch, clove, copaiba, green mandarin, helichrysum, melaleuca, wintergreen, On Guard®
Tooth enamel, worn - white fir, wintergreen
Tooth, loose - bergamot, cinnamon, clove, frankincense, green mandarin, helichrysum, lavender, myrrh, peppermint, rose, rosemary, yarrow, DDR Prime®, On Guard®
Tooth stains, black/brown/white - frankincense, lemon, lime, myrrh, peppermint, wild orange
Voice, weak, hoarse, or loss/laryngitis - basil, cardamom, cinnamon, eucalyptus, fennel, frankincense, ginger, lavender, lemon, lemongrass, lime, myrrh, peppermint, rosemary, sandalwood, thyme, vetiver, wintergreen, ylang ylang, Breathe®, On Guard®, PastTense®, Purify, Zendocrine®

** See remedy on this page*

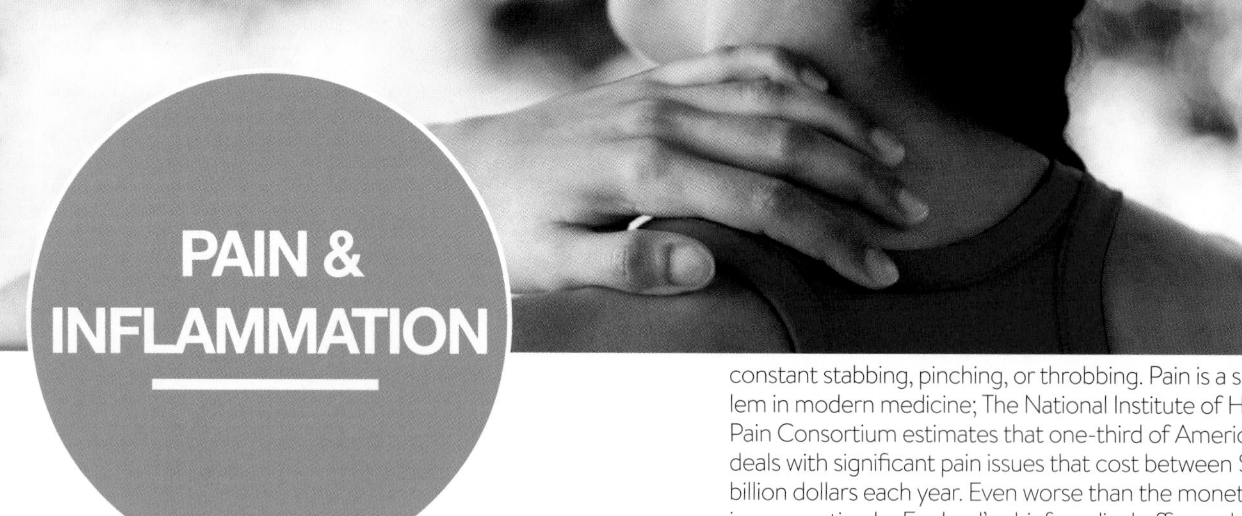

PAIN & INFLAMMATION

INFLAMMATION is the body's biological response to anything the body considers harmful, including pathogens, irritants, infection, allergens, injury, and pain. Healthy inflammation is part of the innate immune system (see Immune), which responds to pathogens with an "automatic" generalized response aiming to clear tissues and cells of harmful stimuli and initiate cellular repair. It works closely with the local vascular system to deliver the plasma and leukocytes that are the "first responders." Sometimes trying to reduce swelling too quickly can actually slow down the body's healing processes! Symptoms of inflammation can include swelling, redness, pain, heat, and at times, reduced function. Healthy inflammation is necessary for the body to prevent breakdown of body tissues due to pathogens or injury. Note that inflammation is not infection, but is part of the body's response to it.

There are two types of inflammation: acute and chronic. Acute inflammation occurs when there is a one-time trigger or event, and the body responds immediately to that trigger by moving plasma and leukocytes into the compromised tissues. Situations that can cause acute inflammation are intense physical training, cold or flu, an infected ingrown toenail, a scratch or cut, sore throat, appendicitis, etc.

Chronic inflammation is long-term inflammation and can occur because the body was unable to repair the initial cause of acute inflammation or because of an autoimmune response, in which the body mistakes healthy tissue as harmful and thus attacks healthy tissue on an ongoing basis. Conditions contributing to chronic inflammation include asthma, arthritis, any chronic condition, and any autoimmune condition.

While wounds, infections, and disease would not be able to heal without acute inflammation, chronic inflammation can cause a myriad of undesirable diseases or conditions that can include cancers, other chronic conditions, and hay fever. When chronic inflammation occurs, the type of cells at the site shift, and the result is the concurrent repair and destruction of the tissue. Inflammation must be regulated to serve as nature intended.

Cortisol, which is a hormone produced by the adrenal glands, is the most powerful anti-inflammatory substance in your body. When the adrenal glands become stressed or fatigued, insufficient amounts of cortisol are produced, resulting in increased inflammation. Therefore, proper care of the adrenal glands is a critical component to ensuring an appropriate inflammatory response.

Pain, which is very closely related to inflammation, can be slight, moderate or severe, and can manifest in a myriad of ways including constant stabbing, pinching, or throbbing. Pain is a significant problem in modern medicine; The National Institute of Health National Pain Consortium estimates that one-third of America's population deals with significant pain issues that cost between $560 and 635 billion dollars each year. Even worse than the monetary cost of pain is an assertion by England's chief medical officer who estimated that more than five million people in the UK develop chronic pain each year, but only two-thirds recover. Chronic pain, in addition to the extreme discomfort it causes, can lead to loss of ability to work or function in relationships, addiction to pain medications, and feelings of frustration and helplessness.

There are several ways to classify pain. These include:

- **Acute:** typically intense and short-lived, caused by an injury that heals in time and pain subsides
- **Chronic:** Ongoing, can be mild or intense
- Nociceptive: includes somatic and visceral pain
  - Somatic: Includes all musculo-skeletal pain, includes sore/strained muscles, cuts on skin, etc.
  - Visceral: Refers to internal organs and body cavities such as the thorax, abdomen and pelvis; includes cramping and aching sensations
- **Non-nociceptive:** Includes neuropathic and sympathetic
  - Neuropathic: Refers to nerve pain that can be caused by nerves between tissues and the spinal cord, or between the spinal cord and the brain--sometimes referred to as pinched nerves; can also be caused by degenerative disease (e.g. stroke or loss of myelin sheath) or infection, as in the case of shingles
  - Sympathetic: Refers to pain of the sympathetic nervous system (controls blood flow, etc.) which typically occurs after a fracture or soft-tissue injury. Though there are no specific pain receptors, the affected area can become extremely sensitive, causing the individual to forego use of the injured limb or area.
- **Referred pain:** When pain is felt in an area other than the original site of injury/infection, such as when the arm or back hurts in case of a heart attack

When considering how best to treat pain, medical professionals take into account the original site of pain, what other areas are affected, the type of pain, what activities lessen or worsen the pain, when pain is more aggravated, and the effect the pain has on an individual's mood and ability to function.

Responding to both inflammation and pain with natural remedies can be highly effective, since both these topics involve systematic bodily responses to injury or disease; natural remedies support the body in doing its job. When dealing with chronic injury and/or inflammation, it is important to participate in a wellness regimen that interrupts the continuation of chronic inflammation, so that the body can be liberated to properly address acute conditions that occur. Supplementation is critical so that cells and tissues have the nourishment they need to subdue more chronic conditions, and when the cells and tissues are well-nourished they respond readily to the powerful chemical influence of pure essential oils.

TOP SOLUTIONS

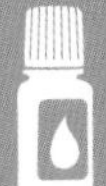

SINGLE OILS

Copaiba - relieves pain and inflammation (pg. 99)
Turmeric - relieves pain and inflammation (pg. 158)
Helichrysum - reduces pain; accelerates healing; chelates toxins (pg. 117)
Wintergreen, Birch - soothes aches and pain, warms; has a cortisone-like effect; supports bone healing (pg. 163)
Peppermint - reduces inflammation and pain, cools, invigorates, and stimulates (pg. 140)
Ginger - invigorates nerves, promotes circulation and healing to bones and muscles (pg. 113)
Black pepper - reduces inflammation, relieves pain, increases circulation (pg. 83)
Basil, Rosemary - calms nerves, improves circulation and healing; steroidal action (pg. 80)

By Related Properties

For more, See Oil Properties on pages 477 - 481

Analgesic - arborvitae, basil, bergamot, birch, black pepper, blue tansy, cassia, cinnamon, clary sage, clove, copaiba, coriander, cypress, eucalyptus, frankincense, ginger, helichrysum, jasmine, juniper berry, lavender, lemongrass, litsea, marjoram, melaleuca, oregano, peppermint, rosemary, Siberian fir, turmeric, white fir, wild orange, wintergreen, yarrow
Anti-inflammatory - arborvitae, basil, bergamot, birch, black pepper, blue tansy, cardamom, cassia, cedarwood, cinnamon, copaiba, coriander, dill, eucalyptus, fennel, frankincense, geranium, ginger, helichrysum, jasmine, lavender, lemongrass, lime, litsea, manuka, melaleuca, melissa, myrrh, neroli, oregano, patchouli, peppermint, Roman chamomile, sandalwood, Siberian fir, spearmint, spikenard, tangerine, turmeric, wild orange, wintergreen, yarrow
Calming - bergamot, birch, black pepper, blue tansy, cassia, clary sage, copaiba, coriander, fennel, frankincense, geranium, jasmine, juniper berry, lavender, litsea, melissa, oregano, patchouli, Roman chamomile, sandalwood, tangerine, vetiver, yarrow
Neurotonic - arborvitae, basil, bergamot, black pepper, clary sage, cypress, ginger, melaleuca, neroli
Purifier - arborvitae, cinnamon, eucalyptus, grapefruit, lemongrass, lime, manuka, marjoram, melaleuca, oregano, Siberian fir, tangerine, wild orange, yarrow
Relaxing - basil, blue tansy, cassia, cedarwood, clary sage, cypress, fennel, geranium, jasmine, lavender, litsea, manuka, marjoram, myrrh, neroli, ravensara, Roman chamomile, white fir, ylang ylang
Sedative - basil, bergamot, blue tansy, cedarwood, clary sage, coriander, frankincense, geranium, jasmine, juniper berry, lavender, lemongrass, magnolia, marjoram, melissa, neroli, patchouli, Roman chamomile, rose, sandalwood, spikenard, tangerine, vetiver, ylang ylang, yarrow
Steroidal - basil, bergamot, birch, black spruce, cedarwood, clove, fennel, magnolia, patchouli, rosemary, thyme, wintergreen

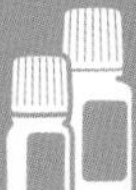

BLENDS

Deep Blue® - invigorates nerves and reduces inflammation (pg. 185)
DDR Prime® - protects cells against free-radical damage while supporting healthy cellular function and renewal (pg. 184)
PastTense® - soothes joints and tissues (pg. 196)
AromaTouch® - stimulates circulation and blood flow (pg. 169)

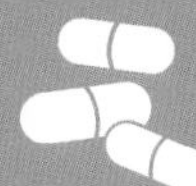

SUPPLEMENTS

Alpha CRS®+ (pg. 209), PB Assist®+, **DDR Prime® Softgels (pg. 211)**, **xEO Mega (pg. 222)**, **Deep Blue Polyphenol Complex (pg. 212)**, MicroPlex VMz

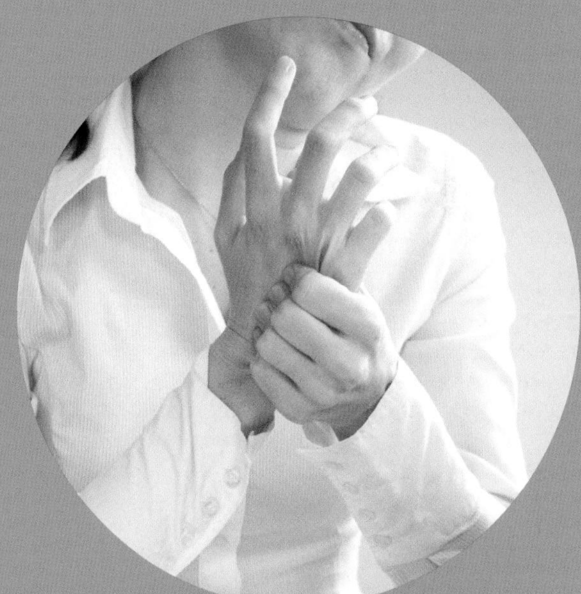

Related Ailments: Aches, Back pain, Chronic pain, Inflammation, Pain, Rheumatic fever

For other ailments of Pain & Inflammation, see the appropriate section. For example *Autoimmune, Brain, Cellular Health, Digestive & Intestinal, Endocrine, Immune & Lymphatic, Muscular, Nervous, Skeletal, Urinary*. Pain and inflammation can occur in any region or part of the body.

Conditions

GENERAL:

Emotional cause - basil, bergamot, black spruce, cardamom, frankincense, geranium, patchouli, Adaptiv®, Serenity®, Whisper®; see *Mood & Behavior*
Inflammation* - birch, bergamot, cardamom, cassia, cinnamon, clove, copaiba, coriander, cypress, frankincense, geranium, jasmine, lavender, peppermint, Roman chamomile, rosemary, turmeric, wintergreen, AromaTouch®, DDR Prime®, Deep Blue®, Elevation™, Forgive®, PastTense®, Peace®, Whisper®
Pain, acute/sharp* - black pepper, black spruce, clove, copaiba, ginger, helichrysum, lavender, peppermint, rosemary, turmeric, wintergreen, AromaTouch®, DDR Prime®, Deep Blue®, PastTense®, Serenity®
Pain, chronic* - birch, black pepper, cardamom, cilantro, cinnamon, clary sage, clove, copaiba, coriander, cypress, eucalyptus, frankincense, ginger, helichrysum, juniper berry, lavender, lemon, lemongrass, magnolia, marjoram, melaleuca, oregano, peppermint, Roman chamomile, rosemary, sandalwood, turmeric, vetiver, white fir, wintergreen, AromaTouch®, Console®, DDR Prime®, Deep Blue®, Motivate®, PastTense®, Peace®, Purify, Whisper®, Zendocrine®
Unexplained/undefined - arborvitae, frankincense, helichrysum, Adaptiv®, DDR Prime®, Deep Blue®, PastTense®, Purify, Zendocrine®; see *Cellular Health*

VISCERA (organ pain):

Abdominal, lower or side/back - bergamot, black pepper, cardamom, clary sage, cypress, ginger, lemongrass, Purify, Zendocrine®; see *Urinary*
Abdominal, upper/mid - cardamom, cinnamon, fennel, frankincense, ginger, lavender, marjoram, peppermint, petitgrain, DigestZen®; see *Digestive & Intestinal, Parasites*
Breathing issues - blue tansy, cardamom, cypress, Douglas fir, eucalyptus, frankincense, peppermint, Breathe®, Deep Blue®; see *Respiratory, Skeletal*
Chest - marjoram, ylang ylang, AromaTouch®, Immortelle; see *Cardiovascular*
Deep, glandular - basil, myrrh, Balance®, DDR Prime®, Immortelle, Zendocrine®; see *Endocrine* to address specific glandular issues
Illness/infection - cinnamon, helichrysum, melissa, peppermint, rosemary, yarrow, On Guard®; see *Immune & Lymphatic*

SOMATIC (skeletal muscular pain):

Backaches - basil, bergamot, birch, copaiba, coriander, cypress, eucalyptus, frankincense, helichrysum, lavender, lemongrass, marjoram, peppermint, turmeric, wintergreen, ylang ylang, AromaTouch®, DDR Prime®, Deep Blue® ; see *Skeletal*
Cramping/charley horse - arborvitae, basil, cypress, lemongrass, marjoram, peppermint, pink pepper, AromaTouch®, Deep Blue®; see *Muscular*
Headache* - basil, blue tansy, cardamom, cilantro, copaiba, frankincense, helichrysum, juniper berry, lavender, lemongrass, marjoram, peppermint, rose, rosemary, Siberian fir, wintergreen, Balance®, Cheer®, DDR Prime®, Deep Blue®, Forgive®, Passion®, Peace®, PastTense®, Serenity®
Headache, migraine* - basil, bergamot, clove, coriander, frankincense, helichrysum, lavender, melissa, patchouli, peppermint, marjoram, Roman chamomile, rosemary, rose, spearmint, Cheer®, Forgive®, Passion®, PastTense®, Peace®, Zendocrine®
Joints* - birch, copaiba, Siberian fir, turmeric, Deep Blue®; see *Skeletal*
Referred - frankincense, helichrysum, juniper berry, DDR Prime®, Deep Blue®, PastTense®
Spinal conditions - birch, lemongrass, white fir, DDR Prime®, Deep Blue®; see *Skeletal*
Tissue damage/injury - birch, cedarwood, clary sage, copaiba, frankincense, helichrysum, lemongrass, marjoram, myrrh, sandalwood, vetiver, Deep Blue®; see *First Aid*

NEUROPATHIC (damaged nerve fiber pain):

Facial nerve - arborvitae, basil, clary sage, clove, frankincense, neroli, patchouli, DDR Prime®, Deep Blue®, Serenity®; see *Nervous*
Nerve damage - arborvitae, black pepper, clary sage, clove, frankincense, ginger, helichrysum, lavender, lemongrass, Balance®, DDR Prime®, PastTense®; see *Nervous*
Phantom pains - arborvitae, basil, copaiba, cypress, frankincense, helichrysum, lavender, turmeric, DDR Prime®, AromaTouch®, Deep Blue®, PastTense®; see *Nervous*
Shooting/burning - arborvitae, basil, bergamot, black pepper, clary sage, clove, frankincense, helichrysum, juniper berry, lavender, patchouli, peppermint, Roman chamomile, thyme, vetiver, DDR Prime®, Deep Blue®, Passion®
Spinal cord injury - arborvitae, basil, clary sage, frankincense, helichrysum, lemongrass, thyme, DDR Prime®, Deep Blue®, Immortelle, PastTense®; see *Nervous*
Tingling/numbness - arborvitae, basil, black pepper, clary sage, clove, cypress, DDR Prime®, Immortelle, PastTense®; see *Nervous*

USAGE TIPS: Best practices for essential oil use for relief from pain and inflammation
- **Topical:** Very effective for many situations especially when it is more structural; most importantly, apply oils directly to any area of concern remembering to use a carrier oil if necessary to prevent sensitivity. Apply often, every 20-30 minutes, until symptoms subside, then reduce to every two to six hours for acute pain. For chronic pain, apply two to three times daily. Layering is also very effective for using multiple oils at the same time; apply one at a time.
- **Internal:** Highly effective for more chronic or internal pain; place oils in a capsule or drop under tongue (hold for 30 seconds; swallow).

Remedies

ARTHRITIS RUB
Mix 2 drops each of wintergreen, lemongrass, frankincense, and eucalyptus oils with a small amount of fractionated coconut oil and massage into painful areas.

JOINT & ARTHRITIS PAIN RELIEF
4 drops juniper berry
3 drops marjoram
3 drops Roman chamomile
3 drops ginger
3 drops helichrysum
Mix essential oils in roller bottle with 1 teaspoon carrier oil, shake, and use as needed OR add essential oils to 1/2 cup Epsom salt, stir; use in hot bath.

MIGRAINE INTERRUPTER: Place 1-2 drops juniper berry oil and helichrysum oil on back of neck. Dilute if desired.

HEADACHE RESOLVE (also works to reduce swelling): Layer or mix prior to application 1-2 drops each cedarwood, peppermint, frankincense oils to areas of need. Reapply every thirty minutes until headache or swelling is gone. Dilute as desired.

HEADACHE BLEND
7 drops peppermint
5 drops lavender
5 drops frankincense
Combine oils into a 5ml roller bottle. Fill bottle with fractionated coconut oil or other carrier oil. Apply as needed. Reapply every thirty minutes until relief is achieved.

PAIN AWAY (Deep Blue® for jaw, knee, foot pain): Immediately use helichrysum oil, Deep Blue®, and frankincense oil on site of pain. Reapply frequently (every twenty to sixty minutes) until relief is achieved. Continue to apply to support healing process.

SORE MUSCLE SALVE
1 tablespoon beeswax
4 tablespoons carrier oil
10-30 drops each of wintergreen, lemongrass, marjoram and/or lavender
Gently melt the beeswax with the carrier oil over very low heat, stirring frequently. Remove from heat, and allow to cool. While still soft, stir essential oils into mixture. Pour into small glass storage container. Cool completely before putting on lid. Apply to sore muscles or any aches or pains.

SORE MUSCLE SOAK
Mix 4 drops black pepper, 2 drops rosemary, 1 drop ginger into ½ cup Epsom salt. Add to a bathtub of hot water and soak for up to thirty minutes. Remember to drink lots of water while soaking and thereafter.

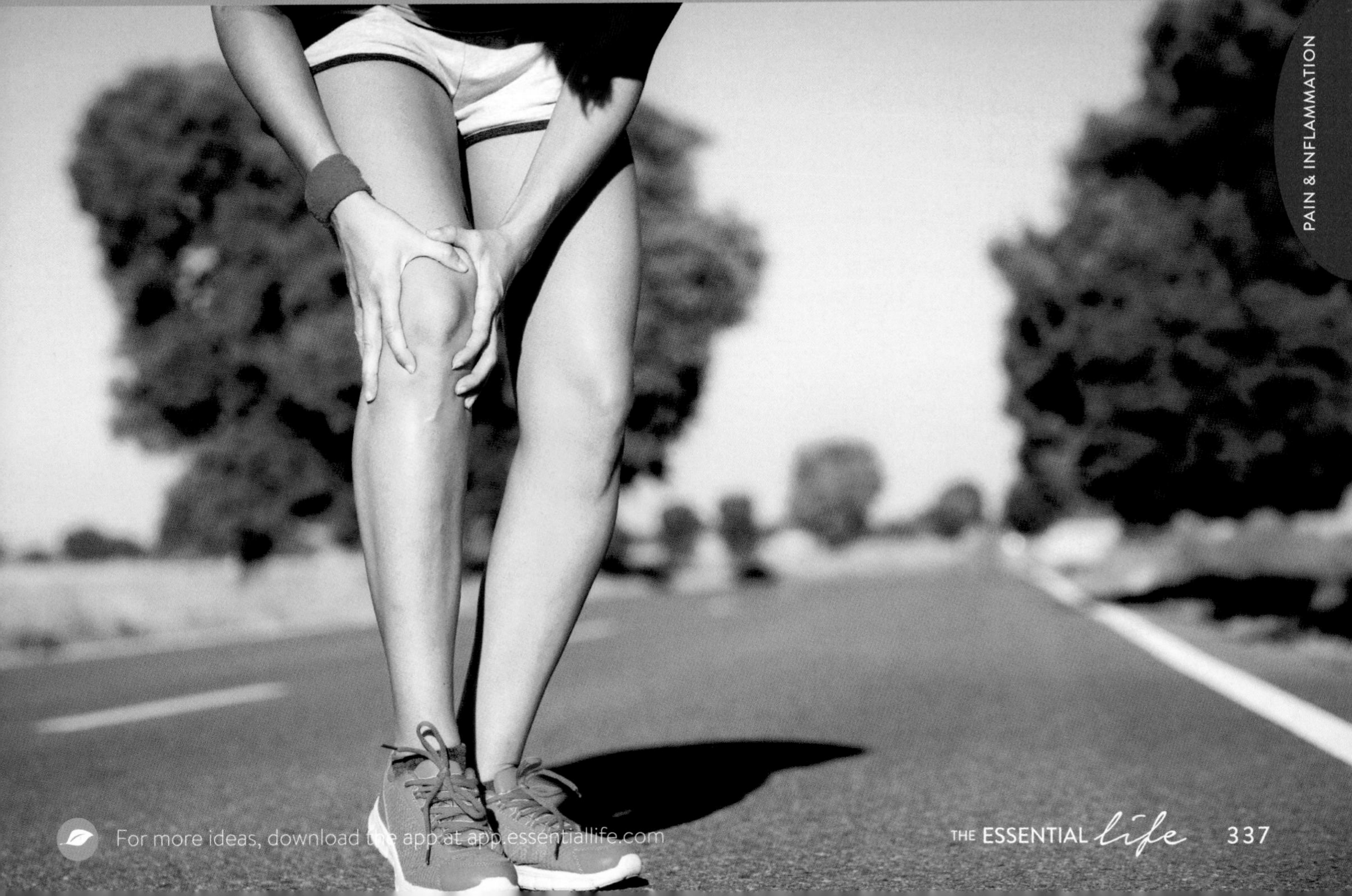

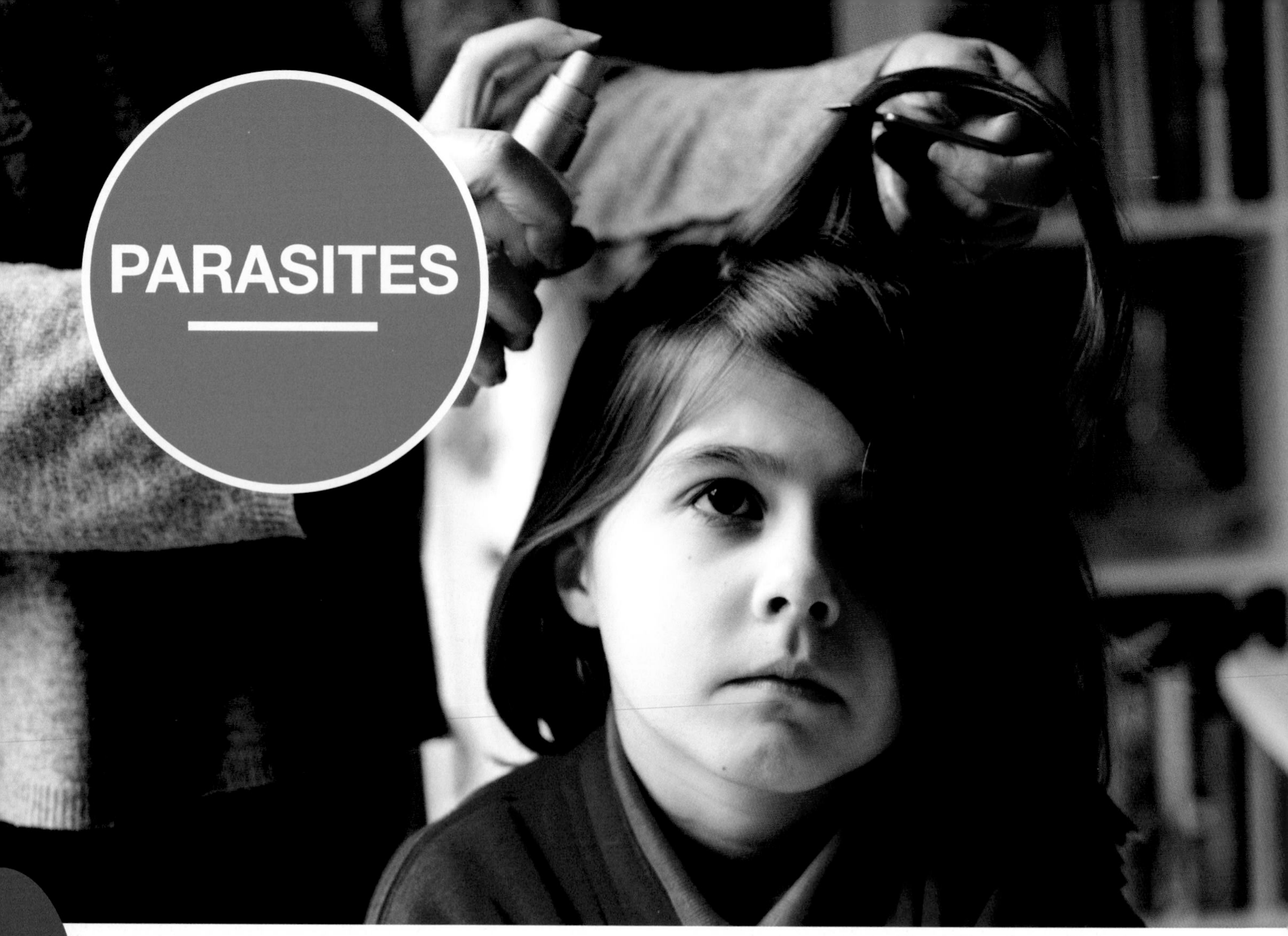

A PARASITE is an organism that lives on or in another organism, and gets food at the expense of its host. The majority of human parasites are microscopic (not visible to the naked eye), and contrary to common belief, can actually infest tissues all over the body -- not just in the intestines. Not all parasites cause sickness, but those that do can cause incredible damage to the human body. Most parasites reproduce very quickly and infest human tissues and organs. There are over a thousand types of parasites, which can be broken down into six major categories:

1--Protozoa make up about 70 percent of parasites that invade humans. They are one-celled microscopic organisms that can quickly colonize the intestinal tract and from there move on to blood and other tissues and organs. A well-known protozoa parasite is giardia lamblia.

2--Nematoda are worm-like, multicellular organisms that reproduce by laying eggs that typically grow in soil or within an intermediate host before infecting humans. Many people don't show signs of nematode infestation unless it is very heavy. Experts estimate that 75 percent of the world's population has some type of parasite infestation. Commonly known nematodes are roundworm, hookworm, and pinworm; nematodes typically infect the intestinal tract, blood, and tissues. Ascaris parasites are roundworms typically found in the intestines. Ascaris lumbricoides is probably the best known parasite in humans. Throughout their life cycle, they infect various organs/tissues of the body that can include the intestines, the lungs, and the brain. When they infiltrate sensitive tissues, they can cause serious health problems.

3--Platyhelminthes. In this group, cestodes, or tapeworms, can be seen with the naked eye. The head attaches to the intestinal wall, and they feed on partially digested particles in the intestinal tract. As long as the head is intact, new tapeworms can grow. Beef, pork, fish, and dog tapeworms are well-recognized in the cestode category. Trematodes, also called flatworms or flukes, are leaf-shaped flatworm parasites that originate from infected snails. They can penetrate human skin or infiltrate a human host after the host has eaten an infected fish, plant, or crustacean. They can infect the intestines, blood, liver, and lungs. Common trematodes include Intestinal flukes, blood flukes, and liver flukes.

5--Acanthocephala, or thorny-headed worms, in their adult form, live in the intestines. They are considered by many to be the intermediary between nematodes and cestodes. They have elongated appendages with spines they use to pierce and attach to the organ walls of their hosts. Infections by acanthocephalans in humans are relatively rare.

6--Arthropoda are part of a classification called ectoparasites. This includes every kind of arthropod that receives its nourishment from other hosts (such as mosquitoes), but more specifically refers to the arthropods that burrow into and attach to the skin and remain for a time, such as chiggers, ticks, fleas, lice, scabies, and mites. Arthropods cause disease, and are common transmitters of pathogens that cause disease.

Certain dietary and lifestyle habits encourage parasitic invasion. Poorly and improperly digested food particles, mucus-forming foods, and sick/unhealthy tissue and organs encourage the proliferation of internal parasitic populations that rely on such substances or circumstances for their food. Unsanitary conditions, contact with infected individuals, certain outdoor activities such as walking barefoot in infested sand or soil, swimming in infested water, and even improper hand washing can bring exposure.

Symptoms of parasitic infestation are: diarrhea, constipation, gas, history of food poisoning, difficulty sleeping, difficulty staying asleep, skin irritations, unexplained skin rashes, hives, rosacea, eczema, teeth grinding (during sleep), pain or aching in muscles or joints, fatigue, exhaustion, depression, feelings of apathy, feeling satiated only after meals, iron-deficiency anemia. Since many of these symptoms are commonly associated with other conditions, it is important to work with a medical professional who can properly diagnose the presence of parasites.

The use of essential oils has at times been referred to as "intelligent medicine" because these oils have a unique ability to recognize what is supposed to be present in an organism and what should be eliminated. Parasites can be especially threatening due to their mobile nature (they move from tissue to tissue, wreaking havoc in their wake) and ability to reproduce so quickly. Essential oils should be considered as part of a well-planned approach to regain systemic balance after parasitic damage is discovered.

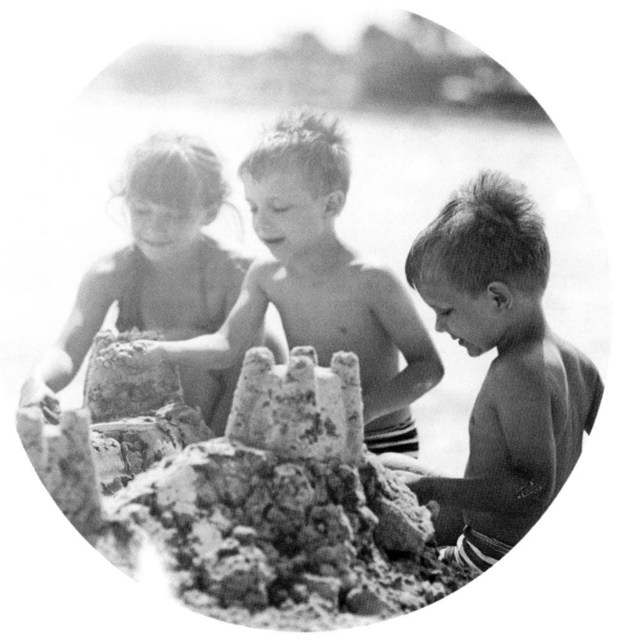

TOP SOLUTIONS

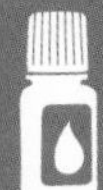

SINGLE OILS

Blue tansy (pg. 86), Cinnamon (pg. 93), clove (pg. 97), lemongrass (pg. 126), oregano (pg. 138), Roman chamomile (pg. 147), thyme (pg. 157), turmeric (pg. 158) - to establish an unfriendly environment for parasites and encourage elimination

By Related Properties

For more, See Oil Properties on pages 477 - 481

Anti-parasitic (indicated for the treatment of parasitic diseases such as nematodes, cestodes, trematodes, and infectious protozoa) - bergamot, black pepper, blue tansy, cinnamon, citronella, clove, fennel, frankincense, juniper berry, lavender, lemon eucalyptus, melaleuca, oregano, Roman chamomile, rosemary, tangerine, thyme, turmeric
Vermicide (a substance toxic to worms) - blue tansy, clove, kumquat, lavender, oregano, wintergreen
Vermifuge (an agent that destroys or expels parasitic worms) - arborvitae, basil, bergamot, black cumin oil (skin clearing), cedarwood, cinnamon, clove, eucalyptus, fennel, geranium, lavender, lemon, melaleuca, peppermint, Roman chamomile, rosemary, thyme, vetiver, wild orange, wintergreen

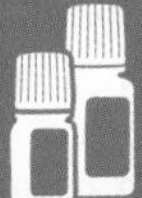

BLENDS

DDR Prime® (pg. 184), Purify (pg. 198) Zendocrine® (pg. 206), DigestZen® (pg. 186), On Guard® (pg. 194), HD Clear® (pg. 189) - to establish an unfriendly environment for parasites and encourage elimination

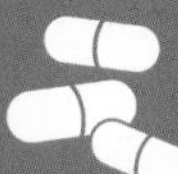

SUPPLEMENTS

DDR Prime® Softgels, PB Assist®+, **Zendocrine® Complex (pg. 223)**, DigestZen® softgels, TerraZyme®, **GX Assist®** (pg. 213) (When conducting an intestinal parasite cleanse, it is essential to keep the intestinal tract moving so toxins do not remain in the body.)

Related Ailments: Ear Mites, Head Lice, Malaria [Immune & Lymphatic], Parasites, Pinworms, Swimmer's Itch, Worms

USAGE TIPS: For parasite elimination
The goal is to get oils to location(s) where parasite(s) lives (e.g. on skin or in gut). Consume or apply topically accordingly. Use a carrier oil to prevent sensitivity wherever needed.

Remedies

PARASITE INFECTION

2 drops cinnamon
4 drops clove
2 drops rosemary
3 drops oregano
3 drops lemon
3 drops melaleuca

Put into a capsule or dilute with water in a shot glass. Take twice a day for ten to fourteen days. If you suspect parasites or worms; drink lemon water several times a day for two weeks. Additional blend suggestions:

- Tapeworms - combine: cinnamon + clove + cypress; OR lemon + oregano + sandalwood; thyme
- Thorny-headed worms - combine: arborvitae, peppermint, thyme, wintergreen

MITES BE GONE: topical formula for humans (e.g. chiggers and scabies)

- Blend 4 drops of peppermint and 4 drops lavender with a teaspoon of carrier oil (recipe can be multiplied and stored in a small glass bottle for future use) and apply generously to all affected areas of skin at least twice per day, preferably after a bath. Do a patch test first to insure there is no skin reaction.
- To make the bath more effective, add 2 drops lavender and 2 drops rosemary mixed in a teaspoon of milk to encourage elimination of mites.
- To assist skin in recovery from dry, blotchy patches, apply lavender and myrrh, 2 drops of each per 1 teaspoon of carrier oil. Apply at least twice per day.

MITE CONTROL - for household invasion

Use eucalyptus, lemon, lavender, melaleuca, and peppermint oils. Eucalyptus and melaleuca are the most important oils in this blend, so be sure you use those even if you don't have the others. Blend 35 drops each of the above oils in 24 ounces of water in a spray bottle. Add 2 ounces witch hazel (optional). Generously spray carpets, beds, curtains, pillows, furniture, etc. Clean your mattress with 1 cup of baking soda and 4 to 5 drops of the recommended oils mixed into a small mason jar. Use a screen or punch holes in the lid. This is enough for a twin mattress. Sprinkle on your mattress and let sit for one or two hours. Vacuum up the residue.

COMBAT LICE

- Prevent - add 5 drops of TerraShield® to a 30 ml spray bottle and fill with water. Spray on the scalp each day before school.
- Treat & Repel - mix 5 drops each of melaleuca and TerraShield® with shampoo in the palm. Massage thoroughly into hair and scalp and rinse well. Add 2 drops of melaleuca to conditioner. Follow a regular comb-through protocol.

BED BUGS

Repel bed bugs with lavender, eucalyptus, peppermint, and melaleuca. Use lavender and melaleuca to kill them. For a concentrated dose, add 1 drop of each recommended oil on the corners of your mattress each week. For a spray solution, add 5 drops of each oil and 16 oz of water to a spray bottle. Spray across your mattress every two weeks.

Source: Williamson, E. M., Priestley, C. M., & Burgess, I. F. (2007). An investigation and comparison of the bioactivity of selected essential oils on human lice and house dust mites. Fitoterapia, 78(7-8), 521-525.

Conditions

Fleas - arborvitae, cedarwood, eucalyptus, lavender, lemon, lemongrass, peppermint, Purify, TerraShield®
Giardia - bergamot, cardamom, clove, frankincense, ginger, lavender, melaleuca, oregano, patchouli, rosemary, thyme, Zendocrine®
Lice, head* - arborvitae, cedarwood, cinnamon, clove, eucalyptus, geranium, lavender, melaleuca, oregano, rosemary, thyme, Citrus Bliss®, TerraShield®, Zendocrine®
Lice, pubic or crab - melaleuca, rosemary
Mites, ear* - arborvitae, basil, cedarwood, clove, lavender, lemongrass, melaleuca, oregano, rosemary, thyme, InTune®, Purify, TerraShield®
Parasites, general* - cinnamon, clove, lemongrass, oregano, turmeric, On Guard®
Parasites, intestinal worms - bergamot, citronella, clove, geranium, lemon, lemon eucalyptus, peppermint, Roman chamomile, thyme, turmeric, HD Clear®, On Guard®, Zendocrine®
Scabies (caused by Sarcoptes scabiei mite) - bergamot, blue tansy, cinnamon, clove, frankincense, lavender, melaleuca, oregano, peppermint, Roman chamomile, rosemary, thyme, Cheer®, DDR Prime®, Deep Blue®, HD Clear®, On Guard®, Purify
Tick bites - eucalyptus, juniper berry, lavender, lemon, lemongrass, melaleuca, peppermint, HD Clear®, Purify; see *First Aid*
Trombiculosis (caused by chiggers mite) - arborvitae, clove, lavender, lemongrass, melaleuca, peppermint, thyme, vetiver, On Guard®, TerraShield®
Worms - black pepper, blue tansy, cinnamon, clove, fennel, lavender, lemon, lemon eucalyptus, lemongrass, oregano, Roman chamomile, thyme, turmeric, Forgive®
Flukes - clove, oregano, Purify, turmeric
Hookworms - clove, thyme, turmeric
Pinworms - bergamot, clove, lemon, lemongrass, oregano, Roman chamomile, thyme, turmeric, On Guard®
Roundworms - blue tansy, cypress, geranium, oregano, sandalwood, turmeric
Tapeworms - cinnamon, clove, cypress, lemon, oregano, sandalwood, thyme, turmeric
Thorny-headed worms - arborvitae, peppermint, thyme, wintergreen

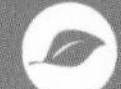
For more ideas, download the app at app.essentiallife.com

* *See remedy on this page*

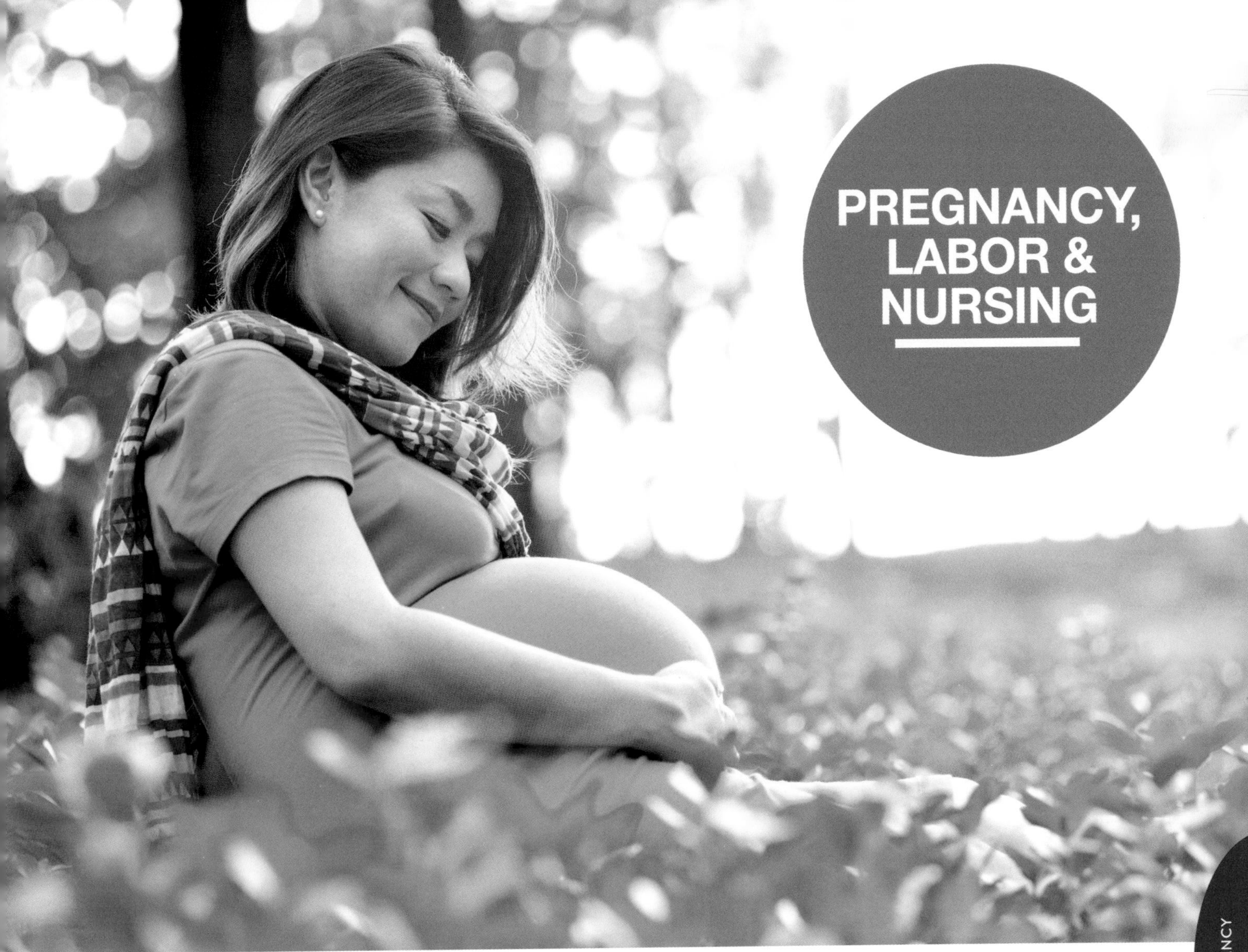

PREGNANCY, LABOR & NURSING

PREGNANCY can be a unique, exciting and joyous time in a woman's life. For a woman to become pregnant, she must release an egg from her ovary – ovulation. Next, the egg and sperm must meet and form a single cell – fertilization. Then pregnancy begins when and if the fertilized egg attaches to a woman's uterus and begins to grow – implantation.

The growing fetus depends entirely on its mother's healthy body for all needs. Pregnant women must take steps to remain as healthy and well nourished as they possibly can. After an approximate nine-month gestation period a woman's body begins the work of opening up and pushing the baby out into the world. This work is called labor.

Labor is a process by which the baby inside the womb adjusts itself to its surroundings and passes out of the uterus to be born as an infant into the world. Every labor is different. It can be long or short, very difficult or not. Each labor, however, follows a basic pattern:

- Contractions (labor pains) open the cervix
- The womb pushes the baby down through the vagina
- The baby is born, and then
- The placenta (afterbirth) is born

Once the baby is born it no longer receives nutrients from the umbilical cord. Breastfeeding is the normal way of providing young infants the nutrients they need for healthy growth and development. Typically most mothers can breastfeed, provided they have accurate information. Exclusive breastfeeding is recommended up to six months of age, with continued breastfeeding along with appropriate complementary foods as desired.

It is difficult to get all the proper vitamins and minerals needed in a normal diet, so supplementation is usually necessary both during pregnancy and while nursing. Taking whole food nutrients is key. This makes the vitamins and minerals bioavailable to the body so it is better equipped to provide adequate nutrition for both mother and baby. Many synthetic or non-food based supplements are not able to be absorbed by the body and can sometimes cause more harm than good

Essential oils can assist with some of the uncomfortable changes that take place in a woman's body during pregnancy, labor, and postpartum periods as well as during breastfeeding. The oils may be applied topically, diffused, or ingested for breast soreness, constipation, depression, fatigue, high blood pressure, nausea/ vomiting, sleep, stretch marks, swelling, and more.

TOP SOLUTIONS

pregnancy

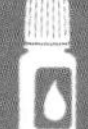

SINGLE OILS

Wild orange - energizes and lifts mood (pg. 162)
Ginger - relieves nausea and morning sickness (pg. 113)
Peppermint - relieves digestive upsets and supports memory (pg. 140)

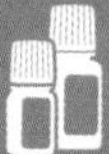

BLENDS

Deep Blue® - soothes aches and pains (pg. 185)
PastTense® - relieves tension (pg. 196)
Slim & Sassy® - balances glucose levels and metabolism (pg. 200)
DigestZen® - supports digestion and relieves morning sickness (pg. 186)
Whisper® - balances hormones (pg. 205)

labor

SINGLE OILS

Clary sage - broad-spectrum support to labor process (pg. 96)
Jasmine - assists with labor and afterbirth (pg. 118)
Geranium - supports perineum, labor performance, mood and healing (pg. 112)
Lavender and neroli - calms and soothes mood and tissues (pgs. 122 & 136)
Frankincense - lessens stress and trauma; promotes healing (pg. 110)
Basil - relieves pain; enhances labor performance (pg. 80)
Helichrysum - slows/stops bleeding and promotes healing (pg. 117)

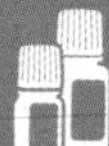

BLENDS

Balance® - improves coping capacity (pg. 170)
PastTense® - relieves tension (pg. 196)
ClaryCalm® - enhances labor performance (pg. 182)
Deep Blue® - soothes aches and pains (pg. 185)

nursing

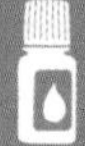

SINGLE OILS

Fennel - promotes milk production; prevents clogged ducts, infection, and thrush (pg. 108)
Ylang ylang - alleviates tender breasts and depression (pg. 165)
Clary sage - promotes milk supply and hormone balancing; boosts mood (pg. 96)
Lavender - promotes milk production; prevents/heals tender sore breasts, nipples, and clogged milk ducts (pg. 122)

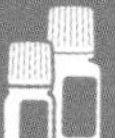

BLENDS

Whisper® - balances hormones and increases libido (pg. 205)
Elevation™ - supports mood and alleviates depression (pg. 187)

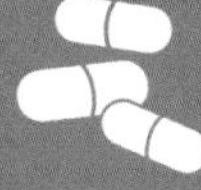

SUPPLEMENTS

Bone Nutrient Lifetime Complex (pg. 210), PB Assist®+ (pg. 216), DigestZen® softgels, DDR Prime® Softgels, **essential oil xEO Mega (pg. 222), TerraZyme® (pg. 219),** MicroPlex VMz

By Related Properties

See Oil Properties on pages 477 - 481

Analgesic - arborvitae, basil, bergamot, blue tansy, cassia, cinnamon, clary sage, copaiba, fennel, frankincense, ginger, helichrysum, litsea, peppermint, rosemary, Siberian fir, turmeric, white fir, wintergreen, yarrow
Antidepressant - bergamot, clary sage, frankincense, geranium, grapefruit, jasmine, lemon, melissa, neroli, patchouli, rose, sandalwood, tangerine, wild orange, ylang ylang
Anticoagulant - clary sage, helichrysum, lavender, tangerine
Antiemetic - basil, cardamom, cassia, clove, copaiba, coriander, fennel, ginger, lavender, patchouli, peppermint, pink pepper
Antihemorrhagic - geranium, helichrysum, lavender, myrrh, yarrow
Antispasmodic - basil, bergamot, black pepper, blue tansy, cardamom, cassia, cinnamon, clary sage, clove, cypress, eucalyptus, fennel, ginger, helichrysum, lavender, lemon, litsea, marjoram, neroli, patchouli, peppermint, pink pepper, Roman chamomile, rose, rosemary, sandalwood, Siberian fir, spearmint, tangerine, vetiver, wild orange, wintergreen, ylang ylang, yarrow
Calming - bergamot, blue tansy, clary sage, copaiba, frankincense, geranium, jasmine, lavender, litsea, patchouli, Roman chamomile, sandalwood, tangerine, vetiver, yarrow
Carminative - basil, bergamot, blue tansy, cardamom, cinnamon, clary sage, copaiba, fennel, ginger, green mandarin, lavender, lemon, litsea, myrrh, neroli, patchouli, peppermint, Roman chamomile, rosemary, sandalwood, spearmint, tangerine, turmeric, vetiver, wild orange, wintergreen, yarrow
Digestive stimulant - basil, bergamot, black pepper, cardamom, cinnamon, coriander, fennel, frankincense, grapefruit, litsea, myrrh, patchouli, spearmint, tangerine, wild orange, yarrow
Energizing - basil, cypress, grapefruit, lemongrass, rosemary, Siberian fir, white fir, wild orange, tangerine, yarrow
Galactagogue - basil, clary sage, dill, fennel, jasmine, lemongrass, wintergreen
Immunostimulant - arborvitae, cassia, cinnamon, clove, copaiba, frankincense, ginger, lemon, lime, melaleuca, melissa, oregano, rosemary, Siberian fir, spearmint, thyme, vetiver, wild orange, yarrow
Invigorating - grapefruit, lemon, litsea, peppermint, spearmint, Siberian fir, wild orange, wintergreen
Regenerative - basil, cedarwood, clove, coriander, frankincense, geranium, helichrysum, jasmine, lavender, manuka, melaleuca, myrrh, neroli, patchouli, sandalwood, wild orange, yarrow
Relaxing - basil, blue tansy, cassia, cedarwood, clary sage, cypress, fennel, geranium, jasmine, lavender, litsea, manuka, marjoram, myrrh, neroli, ravensara, Roman chamomile, white fir, ylang ylang
Sedative - basil, bergamot, blue tansy, cedarwood, clary sage, frankincense, geranium, jasmine, lavender, magnolia, marjoram, melissa, neroli, patchouli, Roman chamomile, rose, sandalwood, tangerine, vetiver, ylang ylang
Stomachic - blue tansy, cardamom, cinnamon, clary sage, coriander, fennel, ginger, marjoram, peppermint, rosemary, tangerine, turmeric, wild orange, yarrow
Uplifting - bergamot, clary sage, grapefruit, lemon, lime, litsea, melissa, sandalwood, tangerine, wild orange, ylang ylang
Warming - birch, black pepper, cassia, cinnamon, clary sage, clove, eucalyptus, ginger, lemongrass, marjoram, oregano, peppermint, pink pepper, thyme, wintergreen

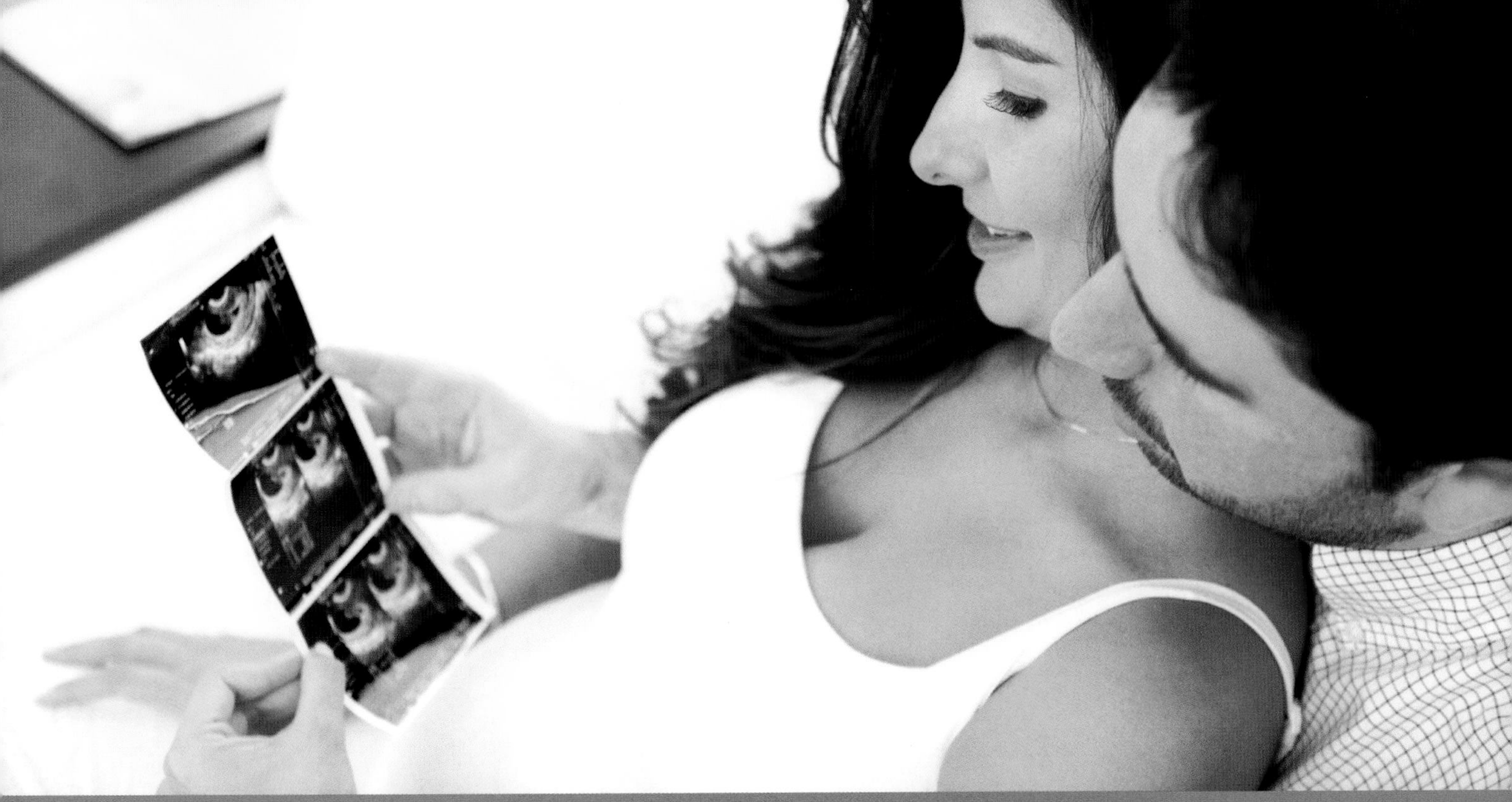

ESSENTIAL OIL USAGE FOR PREGNANT & NURSING WOMEN

There are differing opinions regarding essential use and safety during pregnancy as well as nursing. It is common to find warnings everywhere about which oils one should and should not use during pregnancy. The most commonly expressed concern is over the topical and internal use of essential oils.

When using essential oils that are laden with impurities there is a legitimate threat posed to a developing fetus. However, if the user has ensured they are using only pure, unadulterated essential oils, many of those concerns become unwarranted. It is recommended a pregnant women be under the care of a physician and/or midwife and consult with them prior to taking/using new products.

Here are a few safety guidelines to use when selecting oils for use during pregnancy:

- **Use truly therapeutic, superior grade essential oils** that are certified as pure, potent, genuine and authentic and subjected to rigorous testing to ensure no harmful ingredients are present. Many products on the market contain synthetic components/ingredients and are to be avoided altogether.
- **Be aware.** When using pure and potent oils, be aware of what they might do before using them. When using more powerful oils, use small amounts and dilute with a carrier oil.
- **Be a wise steward.** The first three months are the time baby develops rapidly. Simply be more cautious during the first trimester.
- **Pay attention to how the body responds** to dosages**.** As body weight increases, there may be a need to increase dosage accordingly. OR use less due to heightened sensitivity. Once again, pay attention to the body's responses. Consider using oils diluted (especially if particularly strong or "hot") as a habit during pregnancy versus using them NEAT (undiluted). The bottoms of the feet are an excellent conservative application location (commonly used with children). Another option is to do a patch test if concerned. Simply apply a single drop on skin and observe results prior to use.
- **Use oils aromatically** as a safe method during pregnancy. They are excellent for boosting mood and energy and creating an uplifting environment. The also support stress and tension reduction and promote a good night's sleep.
- **Consider the source.** When it comes to trying to decipher facts regarding essential oil use during pregnancy and nursing, human studies are not conducted. Rather animal studies, mainly on rats, are the source of the majority of information. During these studies inordinately high doses of essential oils are injected at levels that exceed human consumption and fail to duplicate the human experience. Frankly, no human would consume or use these quantities nor do they inject them as a form of use.
- **Err on the side of safety**. In conclusion, use prudence, dilute, and avoid anything that simply doesn't feel right. Some oils will be better diluted such as the "hot" oils listed in the usage section located earlier in this book. Consult with healthcare practitioner about usage as desired or needed.

NOTE: The use of clary sage by women who have a history of preterm labor or miscarriage or are experiencing such should be avoided. The use of peppermint oil while nursing can limit milk production for some women and therefore it is recommended for them to reduce or stop usage while breastfeeding. Some women report that minor use is acceptable but advise avoiding regular use so as to avoid a significant decrease in milk production. Fennel, clary sage, or basil can counteract effects of peppermint on lactation as they increase milk supply.

Remedies

Optimal Pregnancy and Post-pregnancy Success Suggestions

BASIC SUPPLEMENT PROGRAM

Benefits: basic nutrition, gut health, energy, stamina, emotional stability, regulate blood pressure, avoid postpartum depression, support proper digestion and absorption of nutrients, prepare for rich breast milk supply; prevent infection; ease leg/muscle/ligament cramps or spasms; support healthy connective tissue and skin, prepare cervix for birth

- Microplex VMz - delivers multivitamins and minerals
- xEO Mega - supplies essential fatty acids
- TerraZyme® - provides digestive enzyme support
- PB Assist®+ - provides and promotes prebiotics and probiotics
- Bone Nutrient Lifetime Complex - supplies needed calcium, magnesium, and more

In addition to the above basic supplementation program, choose as needed:

- **Prevent/overcome** - use as often as needed; don't wait for upset, prevent if possible
  - Morning sickness - DigestZen®, ginger, peppermint; support liver/gallbladder: apply topically - lemon, grapefruit, pink pepper, turmeric, Zendocrine®
  - Heartburn - DigestZen®
- **Stay calm, grounded** - use one or more of following at least twice daily as needed:
  - Frankincense, wild orange, Balance®, Serenity®
- **Balance metabolism, sugar cravings, appetite** - choose one; use three times daily:
  - Grapefruit or Slim & Sassy® or kumquat
- **Maintain optimal elimination and antioxidant support** - use one or more daily
  - DDR Prime®, Zendocrine®, lemon and/or other citrus oils
  - Gut cleanse - 2 drops each lemon, melaleuca, thyme at least two times a day for ten days, rest; take extra PB Assist®+
- **Prevent/overcome leg/muscle/ligament cramps or spasms** -
  - Use as needed: cypress, lavender, marjoram, AromaTouch®, Deep Blue®

PREGNANCY SWELLING RELIEF

3 drops ginger
2 drops cypress
2 drops lavender
Combine oils with 2 teaspoons carrier oil; massage onto legs and feet.

NO MORE STRETCH MARKS BLEND

10 drops cypress
10 drops lavender
10 drops wild orange
10 drops Citrus Bliss®
5 drops geranium
Place oils in a 10ml roller bottle; fill remainder with carrier oil. Use twice daily.

STRETCH MARK RELIEF

2 drops each of green mandarin, helichrysum, lavender, myrrh mixed with ½ - 1 teaspoon carrier oil (depending on surface area intended to cover) and apply to abdomen.

HEALING HEMORRHOIDS

20 drops helichrysum
20 drops geranium
20 drops arborvitae or cypress
10 drop peppermint
Make blend in 2-ounce glass bottle with an orifice-reduction seal; mix oils; fill remainder with carrier oil. Apply at least once or twice daily and/or after every bowel evacuation. For additional, more intense support if needed, 1 drop of each oil can be applied NEAT. Any burning sensation should subside within five to ten minutes, or apply carrier oil prior to oil application if desired.

THE FINAL COUNTDOWN ROLL-ON (reduces swelling and bleeding at labor)

10 drops clary sage
10 drops ginger
10 drops lavender
10 drops lemon
10 drops AromaTouch®
Combine oils in 10ml roller bottle; fill remainder with carrier oil. Twice daily apply a thin layer of carrier oil to target areas to improve distribution of oils; then apply oils. Apply blend to low back and ankles every day during the last week of pregnancy. Massage into skin thoroughly.

JUMP START CONTRACTIONS

Apply 1-2 drops each of myrrh and clary sage to wrists and abdomen as well as on uterine and cervical reflex points under inside ankle bones once labor begins, but has slowed/stalled.

INCREASE MILK SUPPLY SALVE

7 drops basil
6 drops clary sage
4 drops geranium
Combine 4 tsp carrier oil to 2 tsp beeswax (approx ⅛ stick).
Melt over low heat. Cool. While still soft, add oils to make a salve. Rub onto breasts throughout the day.

HELLO WORLD! - recovery for mom and baby; use as desired at least two times daily to support optimal recovery for mom and bonding with baby. Use any or all as desired, a drop or few at a time. Diffuse and/or use topically. A few drops of each:
- fennel, frankincense, lavender, lemon, Elevation™

POSTPARTUM DEPRESSION BLENDS: Apply topically or diffuse. These are single-use quantities; multiply as desired.
- Recipe #1: 1 drop rose, 1 drop wild orange, and 3 drops sandalwood
- Recipe #2: 1 drop lavender, 3 drops grapefruit, and 1 drop ylang ylang
- Recipe #3: 1 drop bergamot, 1 drop grapefruit, 1 drop clary sage, 1 drop wild orange, and 3 drops frankincense

PREGNANCY

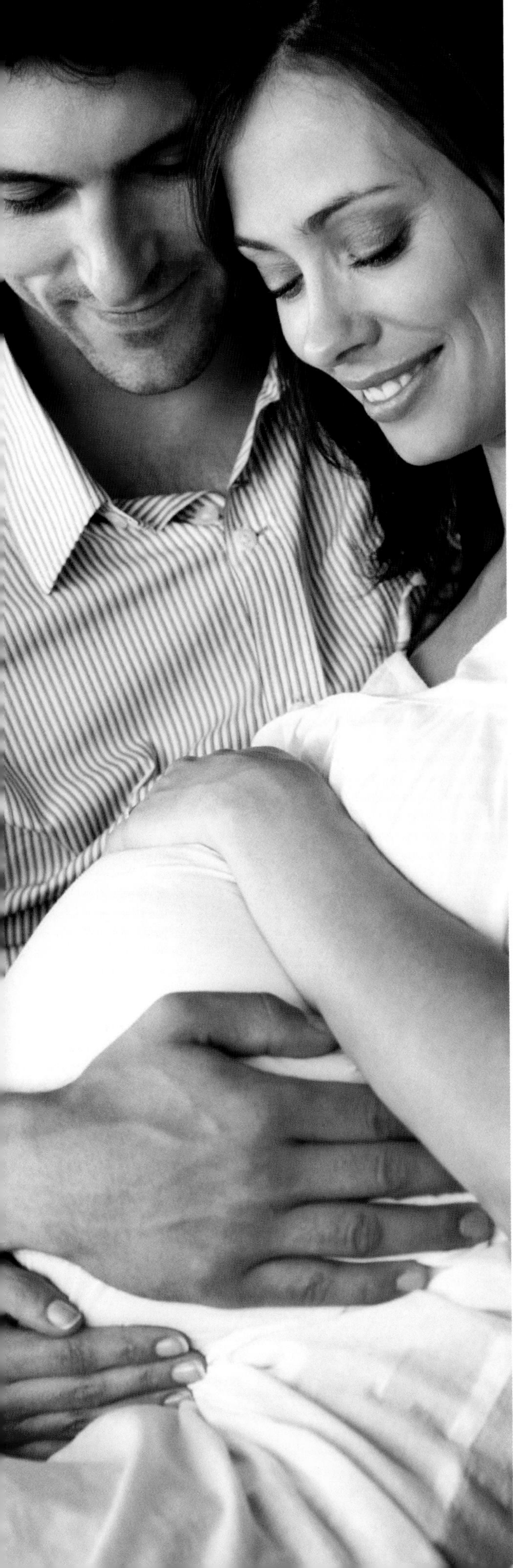

Pure essential oils are a powerful aid during pregnancy, especially since side effects from medication can be so detrimental. Essential oils support the general health of mom and baby, and go beyond to address other common discomforts.

HEMORRHOID RELIEF SPRAY

1 drop peppermint
2 drops helichrysum
2 drops geranium
2 drops cypress
Carrier oil
Mix together in a spray bottle and apply.

AFTER BIRTH TEAR RELIEF

1 bottle of witch hazel
4 drops lavender
4 drops melaleuca
Aloe vera gel
Add lavender and melaleuca to bottle of witch hazel and shake to mix. Then cut large menstrual pads into thirds. Spray the solution over the pads. Squirt aloe gel down the center and freeze them. Apply any remaining solution with peri bottle as needed.

ITCHY SKIN BELLY BUTTER

½ cup shea butter
¼ cup carrier oil
¼ cup sweet almond oil
10 drops Deep Blue®
Add oils and shea butter and place in oven-safe glass bowl. Fill a pot with a couple inches of water and place glass bowl on top. Melt butter and oils over medium heat until translucent. Remove from heat, cool slightly, then add Deep Blue® essential oil, and place in the refrigerator for about 2 hours until solid. Whip for about 2-3 minutes into buttery consistency. Spoon into jar, cover and refrigerate 1 more hour. Will store for 6 months at room temperature. Apply directly to belly or itchy spots to nourish and moisturize skin. Another solution is to add coriander essential oil to your lotion.

STRETCH MARK BLEND

5 drops lavender
5 drops myrrh
5 drops helichrysum
10 ml carrier oil
Mix oils and apply on affected area. Repeat frequently as desired to lighten stretch marks.

Conditions

PREGNANCY:

Appetite cravings/blood sugar imbalance - Slim & Sassy®
Backache - peppermint, rosemary, AromaTouch®, Deep Blue®
Bleeding - geranium, helichrysum, lavender, myrrh; see *Cardiovascular*
Blood pressure, high - eucalyptus, lavender, lemon, marjoram, ylang ylang
Breast tenderness - geranium, grapefruit, lavender, ylang ylang, ClaryCalm®
Constipation - cilantro, copaiba, fennel, ginger, green mandarin, lemon, lemongrass, marjoram, peppermint, DigestZen®, Zendocrine®; see *Digestive & Intestinal*
Cramps - arborvitae, basil, cypress, marjoram, AromaTouch®, Deep Blue®
Depression - basil, bergamot, frankincense, geranium, lavender, lemon, melissa, patchouli, ravensara, rose, sandalwood, vetiver, wild orange, ylang ylang, Adaptiv®, Balance®, Citrus Bliss®, ClaryCalm®, Elevation™; see *Mood & Behavior*
Energy, low/fatigue - black spruce, cypress, grapefruit, green mandarin, lemon, peppermint, pink pepper, wild orange, Adaptiv®, Citrus Bliss®, Elevation™; see *Energy & Vitality*
Headaches - frankincense, green mandarin, lavender, peppermint, wintergreen, Deep Blue®, PastTense®
Heartburn/gas/bloating - green mandarin, peppermint, pink pepper, wild orange, DigestZen®; see *Digestive & Intestinal*
Hemorrhoids* - See "Varicose veins" below
Infection - lemon, melaleuca, oregano, On Guard®
Labor, preterm/cramping - arborvitae, frankincense, lavender, marjoram, neroli, patchouli, Roman chamomile, wild orange + ylang ylang, ClaryCalm®, Whisper®, Zendocrine®
Leg cramps - basil, cypress, lavender, lemongrass, marjoram, wintergreen, Adaptiv®, AromaTouch®, Deep Blue®
Miscarriage, prevents - blue tansy, myrrh, patchouli, rose, thyme, Console®, DDR Prime®, Elevation™, Immortelle
Miscarriage, recovery - clary sage, frankincense, geranium, grapefruit, lavender, myrrh, patchouli, Roman chamomile, rose, ClaryCalm®, DDR Prime®, Deep Blue®, Elevation™, Immortelle, Purify, Zendocrine®

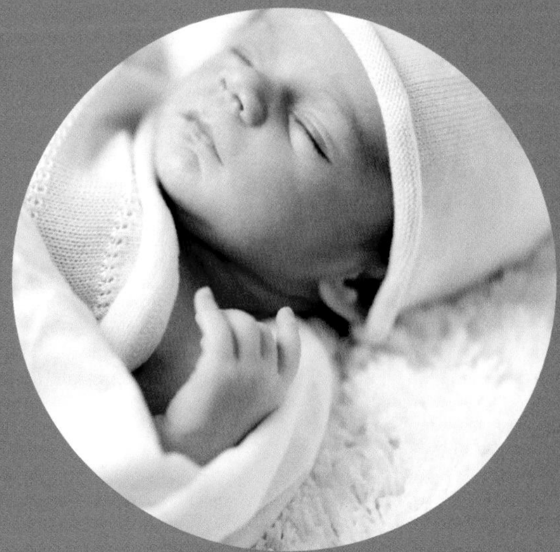

Miscarriage, process and recovery - clary sage, lavender, white fir, ClaryCalm®, Console®, DDR Prime®, Deep Blue®, Purify
Morning sickness/nausea - arborvitae, bergamot, cardamom, cinnamon, coriander, fennel, geranium, ginger, lavender, lemon, peppermint, Deep Blue®, DigestZen®, Tamer™
Muscles, sore - arborvitae, basil, birch, black pepper, clary sage, copaiba, coriander, frankincense, geranium, helichrysum, juniper berry, marjoram, peppermint, turmeric, white fir, wintergreen, Adaptiv®, AromaTouch®, Breathe®, Deep Blue®
Preeclampsia - cinnamon, cypress, frankincense, ginger, lavender, marjoram, Roman chamomile, AromaTouch®, Serenity®, Slim & Sassy®
Postbirth healing - cypress, frankincense, geranium, helichrysum, lavender, myrrh, Roman chamomile, On Guard®
Progesterone, low - geranium, grapefruit, oregano, thyme
Skin, itching/pregnancy mask - geranium, lavender, Roman chamomile, sandalwood, Immortelle
Sleep, restless/insomnia - frankincense, lavender, Roman chamomile, wild orange, Adaptiv®, Balance®, Serenity®; see *Sleep*
Stretch marks* - cypress, frankincense, geranium, green mandarin, lavender, myrrh, sandalwood, tangerine, wild orange, Citrus Bliss®, Forgive®, Immortelle,
Uterus, weak - clary sage, frankincense, ginger, jasmine, lemongrass, marjoram, DDR Prime®, Forgive®
Urinary tract infections - basil, cassia, cinnamon, cypress, lemon, lemongrass, melaleuca, oregano, thyme, On Guard®
Varicose veins - bergamot, cardamom, cypress, geranium, helichrysum, lemon, lemongrass, melaleuca, patchouli, peppermint, rosemary, Zendocrine®; see *Cardiovascular*
Water retention (edema)/blood pressure elevated - cypress, ginger, green mandarin, juniper berry, lavender, lemon, patchouli, spikenard, AromaTouch®, Citrus Bliss®; see *Cardiovascular, Urinary*

LABOR:

Afterbirth/placenta delivery - clary sage, geranium, jasmine, lavender
Bleeding - geranium, helichrysum, myrrh, ClaryCalm®, Serenity®
Calm nerves, relax mind - basil, frankincense, jasmine, lavender, magnolia, Balance®, Motivate®, Serenity®
Contractions, slow/weak/stalled labor* - cinnamon, clary sage, fennel, jasmine, lavender, myrrh, Balance®, Elevation™, Motivate®, Zendocrine®
Coping, poor/overwhelmed, low confidence/fearful mindset, mood issues - basil, clary sage, geranium, jasmine, lavender, neroli, peppermint, wild orange, Adaptiv®, AromaTouch®, Balance®, Citrus Bliss®, Deep Blue®, Elevation™, Motivate®, Serenity®
Difficult - basil, cedarwood, clary sage, fennel, geranium, lavender, myrrh, neroli, rose, spearmint, AromaTouch®, Balance®, Serenity®
Increase awareness, lift mood - basil, lavender, Citrus Bliss®, Elevation™
Labor pains, management/lower back/support circulation - arborvitae, basil, birch, black pepper, clary sage, coriander, cypress, frankincense, geranium, helichrysum, juniper berry, lavender, marjoram, neroli, white fir, wintergreen, AromaTouch®, Balance®, Deep Blue®, Peace®, Serenity®
Overall support for optimal labor - basil, clary sage, geranium, ClaryCalm®, Peace®

* See remedy on pg. 344

Overheated - birch, eucalyptus, peppermint, wintergreen
Pain - cypress, lavender, marjoram, Deep Blue®, PastTense®
Perineum, prep/avoid episiotomy - frankincense, geranium, lavender, Roman chamomile, sandalwood
Position of baby needs work - peppermint
Prep for labor - basil, clary sage, geranium, jasmine, ClaryCalm®
Tension, excess - clary sage, geranium, lavender, magnolia, neroli, ylang ylang, AromaTouch®, PastTense®
Transition - basil, Whisper®
Uterus, performance during labor - clary sage, frankincense, jasmine, myrrh, rose, ClaryCalm®, Elevation™

POST-DELIVERY & NURSING:

After pains/uterine cramping that occurs while nursing - bergamot, birch, clary sage, coriander, frankincense, helichrysum, myrrh, Whisper®
Breasts, tender - frankincense, geranium, grapefruit, lavender, ylang ylang; see *Women's Health*
Clogged milk ducts - cypress, fennel, grapefruit, lavender, patchouli, pink pepper, Purify
Constipation - cilantro, Douglas fir, fennel, ginger, lemon, lemongrass, marjoram, peppermint, DigestZen®, Tamer™, Zendocrine®; see *Digestive & Intestinal*
Depression, postpartum* - bergamot, black spruce, clary sage, frankincense, geranium, grapefruit, lemon, Roman chamomile, sandalwood, vetiver, wild orange, ylang ylang, Adaptiv®, Cheer®, Citrus Bliss®, ClaryCalm®, Console®, DDR Prime®, Elevation™, Peace®, Whisper®, Zendocrine®; see *Mood & Behavior*
Engorgement - peppermint, AromaTouch®, Deep Blue®
Episiotomy/healing from - black pepper, cypress, frankincense, helichrysum, myrrh, Immortelle
Infection (mastitis) - fennel, frankincense, lavender, melaleuca, patchouli, rosemary, wild orange, Citrus Bliss®, DDR Prime®, Purify; for internal use only - cinnamon, clove, lemongrass, melaleuca, oregano, thyme
Milk production (lactation), lack of * - basil, cardamom, clary sage, dill, fennel, geranium, jasmine, lavender, lemongrass (avoid nipple area if applying topically); *avoid peppermint or blends with peppermint as it can decrease milk supply
Milk production, to stop - peppermint
Nipple vasospasms (nipple compressed after nursing) - lime, Whisper®
Nipples dry,cracked/sore - frankincense, geranium, lavender, myrrh, neroli, Roman chamomile, sandalwood, wild orange, Immortelle, Zendocrine®; see "Thrush" below
Recovery from childbirth - clary sage, coriander, cypress, geranium, frankincense (soothe perineum or circumcision), helichrysum, jasmine (supports expulsion of placenta), lavender (supports expulsion of placenta; soothes perineum or circumcision), neroli, sandalwood, white fir, ylang ylang, Adaptiv®, Balance® (for emotional stability, recovery), Immortelle (cesarean-section recovery), Serenity® (to overcome distress, deal with newness of breastfeeding), Whisper®
Thrush - clary sage, dill, fennel, frankincense, lemon, melaleuca, Siberian fir, wild orange; see *Candida*

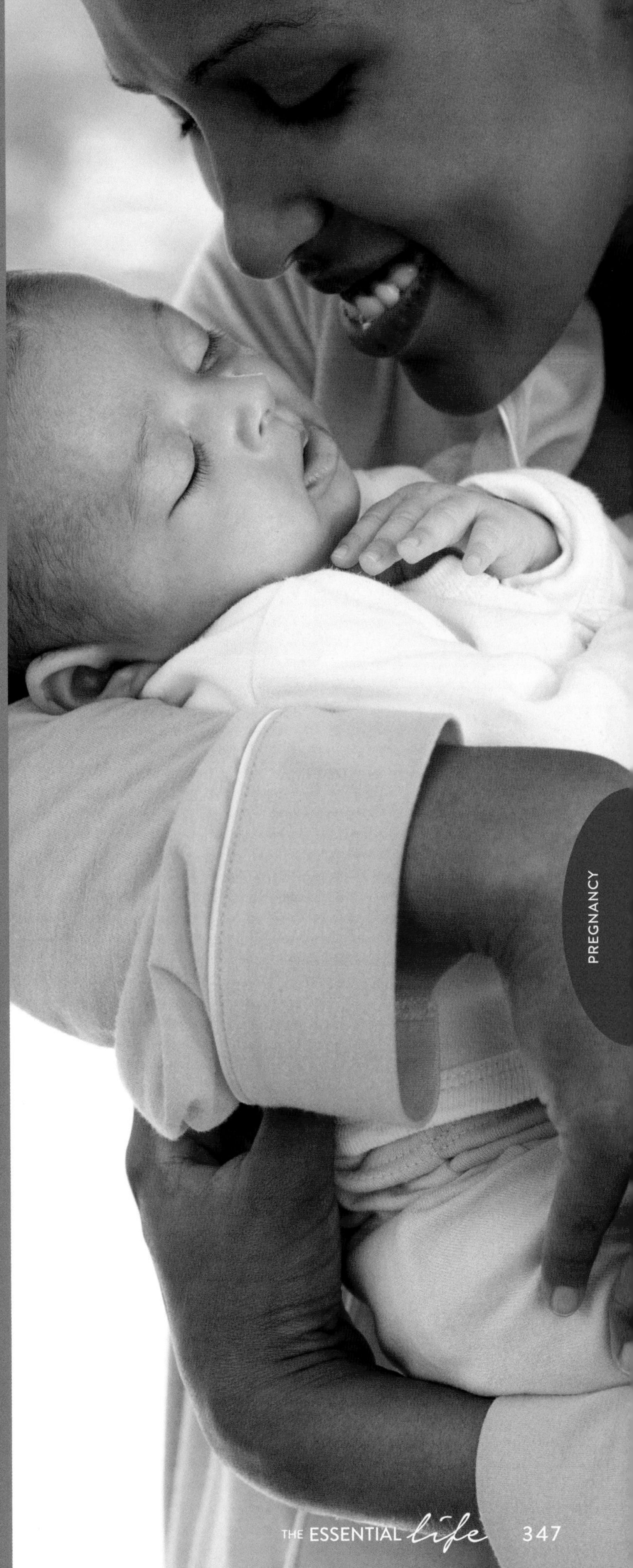

** See remedy on pg. 344*

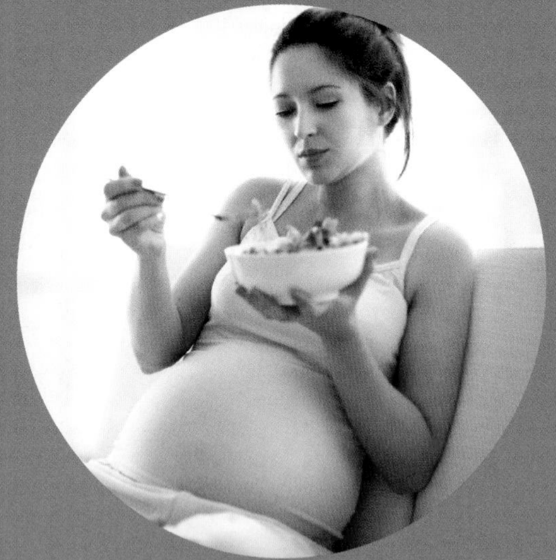

PREGNANCY

- **Allergy support** - take 2 drops each of lemon and peppermint in a capsule or in water.
- **Headache relief** - apply PastTense® or peppermint topically on forehead, temples, back of neck, and under nose.
- **Heartburn** - apply DigestZen®, peppermint, or ginger directly on breastbone.
- **Increase sex drive** - diffuse or apply wild orange or ylang ylang topically.
- **Morning sickness** - apply Zendocrine® and Zendocrine® Complex during first trimester.
- **Morning sickness** - apply under nose or put in water or in a capsule. Use peppermint, DigestZen®, fennel, or ginger.
- **Muscle cramps** - apply marjoram, AromaTouch® to muscle
- **Relaxation and deep sleep:** rub lavender or Serenity® topically, under nose, forehead, heart, and/or feet.
- **Sciatica and muscle pain** - apply Deep Blue® topically to area of concern.
- **Swelling** - apply AromaTouch®, Deep Blue®, or lemongrass to the bottoms of your feet or area of swelling. Add a few drops of lemon to your drinking water or take in a capsule.

BIRTH

- **Back pain during labor** - apply peppermint or AromaTouch® on back to help with the pain.
- **Energy during labor** - add peppermint topically or internally to drinking water or ice.
- **Increase perineum elasticity** - massage myrrh and or helichrysum on perineum prior to labor.
- **Protect the birth canal from group B strep** - add frankincense and oregano or basil to douche prior to birth.
- **Promote or induce labor** - apply ClaryCalm® to abdomen, ankles, and to pressure points when labor has stalled.
- **To support labor** - apply clary sage to ankles and other pressure points when you need contractions to increase.
- Add a small amount of neroli to baby's first bath.

tips

- When using superior grades of essential oils, use during pregnancy is expanded to most oils. For more information see the Body Systems section of this book under Pregnancy, Labor & Nursing
- Baby brain development: Take an additional 2-3 xEO Mega day during pregnancy and nursing.
- Calming emotional support: apply Balance® or frankincense to the bottoms of feet.
- Fatigue: add 2-3 drops of lemon, grapefruit, or wild orange in water, 2-3 times a day.
- Sleep support: apply lavender on feet at nap or bedtime, place a couple drops in bath water, or diffuse 30 minutes before bed. Add a few drops to a spray bottle with water and spray on sheets. Too much lavender can act as a stimulant, use wisely.
- Uplifting emotional support: apply Elevation™ topically under nose, to ears, or bottoms of feet.

POST PARTUM

- **After-birth pains** - apply Deep Blue® to abdomen.
- **Body aches and pains** - apply magnolia, Deep Blue®, AromaTouch®, or clary sage to areas of concern.
- **Bowels moving** - take 2-3 drops of DigestZen® in water or in a capsule.
- **Engorgement** - apply basil around breast.
- **Depression** - apply Elevation™, frankincense, melissa, or Citrus Bliss® under nose and on ears
- **Fatigue** - take 6 drops of Slim & Sassy® and 3 drops each of peppermint and wild orange in a capsule daily.
- **Hemorrhoid relief** - apply Balance® directly to affected area.
- **Increase milk production** - apply fennel and/or rosemary to breasts.
- **Prevent baby infection** - combine frankincense with colloidal silver and spritz or apply over baby's whole body.
- **Sore nipples** - apply helichrysum directly to nipples to bring healing and elasticity.
- **Tearing, inflammation and soreness** - apply frankincense, helichrysum, and/or lavender topically. Put drops of lavender and frankincense on frozen feminine pads.

NEWBORN

- **For swelling, baby blemishes, or skin discoloration** - apply frankincense topically to any area of concern.
- **To assist in baby's transition and release any trauma** - diffuse or apply frankincense or Balance® along baby's spine and bottom of feet.
- **To help avoid infection and release umbilical cord remains** - place several drops of myrrh on umbilical cord.

RESPIRATORY

RESPIRATION is the process of inhaling, warming, filtering, controlling the humidity of, and exhaling air. Lungs exchange oxygen for carbon dioxide, and the heart pumps oxygenated blood to the rest of the body. Additionally, the cilia in the lungs secrete mucus as they move back and forth, carrying out of the lungs; dust, germs, and other matter, where it is expelled by sneezing, coughing, spitting, and swallowing.

Breathing is controlled by the diaphragm, located at the base of the ribcage. When the diaphragm contracts it pulls down on the thoracic cavity, causing the lungs to expand and air to be inhaled. When the diaphragm relaxes, the lungs retract and air is exhaled. The breathing process, one of the most basic and important functions performed by the body, often is taken for granted...until something goes wrong. For some individuals, breathing can be challenging, especially if they suffer from some type of respiratory condition or disease.

Respiratory disease is a broad term used to refer to a series of conditions that affect the respiratory system. Therefore, any condition that affects the lungs, bronchial tubes, upper respiratory tract, trachea, pleural cavity, or even nerves and muscles used for breathing can be termed as a respiratory disease.

Infection, histamine reaction, or prolonged irritation can negatively impact the respiratory system. A variety of ailments may result, ranging from mild allergies or stuffy nose to more severe asthma or diphtheria.

In general, a respiratory illness can have a debilitating effect on one's overall health. Many people mistake respiratory illnesses for other health problems, particularly when they experience an overall feeling of fatigue and malaise. Loss of appetite, indigestion, severe weight loss, and headaches are also quite common in respiratory diseases.

Medical attention and diagnosis is absolutely essential for any respiratory ailment that is severe or persistent. However, milder conditions can be easily resolved with the support of natural and simple home remedies. The scope of home remedies is vast. They can be used alone or in combination with conventional treatments.

TOP SOLUTIONS

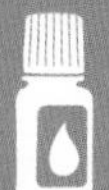

SINGLE OILS

Black pepper or Pink pepper- reduces inflammation and mucus (pg. 83), (pg. 144)
Eucalyptus - opens airways, supports proper respiratory function (pg. 108)
Peppermint - opens airways, expels mucus (pg. 140)
Rosemary - helps with many different respiratory issues (pg. 149)

By Related Properties

For more, See Oil Properties on pages 477 - 481

Anticatarrhal - basil, black pepper, cardamom, clary sage, eucalyptus, fennel, frankincense, helichrysum, neroli, oregano, rosemary, sandalwood, spearmint, white fir, wild orange
Anti-inflammatory - arborvitae, basil, bergamot, birch, black pepper, blue tansy, cardamom, cassia, cedarwood, cinnamon, copaiba, coriander, cypress, dill, eucalyptus, fennel, frankincense, geranium, ginger, helichrysum, jasmine, lavender, lemongrass, litsea, manuka, melaleuca, melissa, myrrh, neroli, oregano, patchouli, peppermint, Roman chamomile, rosemary, sandalwood, Siberian fir, spearmint, spikenard, tangerine, turmeric, wild orange, wintergreen, yarrow
Antispasmodic - blue tansy, clary sage, litsea, neroli, Roman chamomile, Siberian fir, tangerine, yarrow
Decongestant - basil, black spruce, cardamom, cassia, copaiba, cypress, eucalyptus, ginger, grapefruit, green mandarin, lemon, lemongrass, melaleuca, patchouli, Siberian fir, turmeric, yarrow
Expectorant - arborvitae, basil, black pepper, black spruce, cardamom, cedarwood, clove, dill, eucalyptus, fennel, frankincense, ginger, green mandarin, helichrysum, jasmine, marjoram, melaleuca, myrrh, lemon, lemon eucalytpus, oregano, peppermint, pink pepper, ravensara, rosemary, sandalwood, Siberian fir, thyme, turmeric, white fir
Immunostimulant - arborvitae, basil, black pepper, cassia, cinnamon, clove, copaiba, eucalyptus, fennel, frankincense, ginger, lemon, lime, magnolia, melaleuca, melissa, oregano, ravensara, rosemary, sandalwood, Siberian fir, spearmint, thyme, vetiver, wild orange, yarrow
Mucolytic - basil, cardamom, cedarwood, cinnamon, clary sage, copaiba, cypress, fennel, helichrysum, lemon, myrrh, sandalwood, tangerine, wild orange, yarrow
Steroidal - basil, birch, cedarwood, clove, fennel, patchouli, rosemary, thyme

Related Ailments: Acute Respiratory Distress Syndrome (ARDS), Anosmia, Asthma, Auditory Processing Disorder, Blocked Tear Duct, Breathing Problems, Bronchitis, Congestion, Cough, Croup, Cystic Fibrosis, Diphtheria, Dry Eyes, Dry Nose, Earache, Ear Infection (Otitis Media), Emphysema, Hearing in a Tunnel, Hearing Problems, Hiccups, Hyperpnea (increased deep and/or rapid breathing to meet demand following exercise, lack of oxygen, high altitude, as the result of anemia), Legionaire's Disease, Loss of smell, Mucus, Nasal Polyp [Cellular Health], Nosebleed, Perforated Eardrum, Pleurisy, Pneumonia (viral, bacterial), Rhinitis [allergies], Sinus Congestion, Sinus Headache, Sinusitis (sinus infection), Sleep Apnea, Snoring, Stye (Eye), Swollen Eye, Tinnitus, Tuberculosis, Whooping Cough, Xerophthalmia

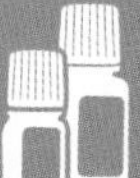

BLENDS

Purify - decongests (pg. 198)
On Guard® - fights respiratory infections, helps resolve respiratory issues (pg. 194)
Breathe® - addresses a broad spectrum of respiratory issues (pg. 172)

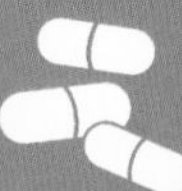

SUPPLEMENTS

DDR Prime® Softgels, xEO Mega, TerraZyme®, **On Guard Throat Drops (pg. 215), PB Assist®+ (pg. 216), Breathe Respiratory Drops (pg. 210)**, MicroPlex VMz

USAGE TIPS: Whether for preventative measures (to clear airborne pathogens and sterilize air) or to **resolve respiratory conditions**, essential oils are excellent for "clearing the air" in both the environment and the body's own respiratory system as well as addressing contributing factors such as poor digestion.

- **Aromatic:** Diffuse (using a diffuser) or inhale selected oils. For a quick treatment, drop oil(s) in hands, rub together, cup around nose and mouth area (can avoid touching face) and repeatedly, deeply inhale through mouth and nose. Additionally, use oils can be applied under the nose, on clothing or bedding, or on jewelry made for diffusing purposes or such to create long-lasting inhalation exposure.
- **Topical:** Rub oils on chest (for aromatic benefit as well), back, forehead (sinuses), and on back side of toes and ball of foot (reflex points for head and chest).
- **Internal:** Place drops of oils in a capsule or in water for systemic or chronic support.
- **Surfaces**: Make a spray mixing essential oils in water with witch hazel for surfaces such as countertops and door knobs for cleaning purposes will also support eradicating bacteria, viruses, fungi, or other harmful germs.

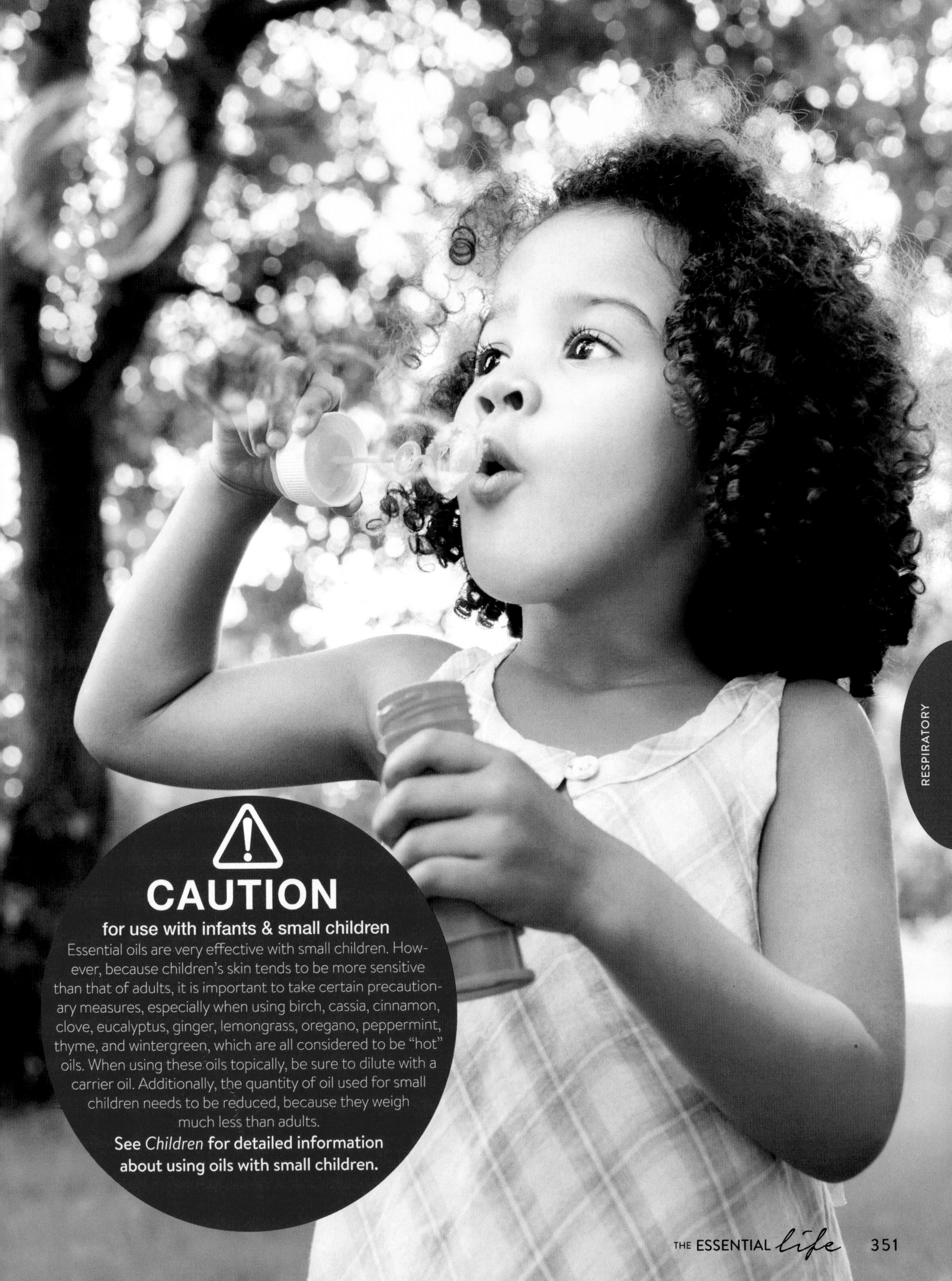

CAUTION

for use with infants & small children

Essential oils are very effective with small children. However, because children's skin tends to be more sensitive than that of adults, it is important to take certain precautionary measures, especially when using birch, cassia, cinnamon, clove, eucalyptus, ginger, lemongrass, oregano, peppermint, thyme, and wintergreen, which are all considered to be "hot" oils. When using these oils topically, be sure to dilute with a carrier oil. Additionally, the quantity of oil used for small children needs to be reduced, because they weigh much less than adults.

See *Children* for detailed information about using oils with small children.

Remedies

ALLERGY POWER TRIO
2 drops lavender
2 drops lemon
2 drops peppermint
Place drops of oil in 4-6 ounces of water. Drink. Repeat every thirty minutes as needed for relief.

GARGLE – salt, warm water, and 1-2 drops essential oil(s) of choice – at least twice per day

CLEAR THE AIR: (for snoring, respiratory or lung specific issues)
Add essential oils to a diffuser or cold-mist humidifier. Choose desired oils. Some suggested combinations:
Recipe #1: 3 drops frankincense and 3 drops Breathe®
Recipe #2: 5-10 drops Breathe®
Recipe #3: 5 drops On Guard®
Recipe #4: 1 drop white fir, 2 drops wild orange and 2 drops cinnamon
Recipe #5: 2 drops cardamom, 2 drops rosemary and 2 drops lime

ALL STEAMED UP: (using moist air to support respiratory resolve): Using a humidifier, steam from a pan or sauna, or steam from a shower, add a few drops of desired essential oils such as Breathe® or eucalyptus to hot water and inhale. If possible, drape a towel over head and source of steam, breathe for fifteen minutes three times a day.

HOT TEA: Drop a few drops of an essential oil in warm water, slowly inhale steam, then sip water when cool to relieve sore throat and breathing issues. Here are some options: cinnamon, clove, eucalyptus, lemon, oregano, rosemary, thyme.

SORE THROAT/LARYNGITIS REMEDY: Add 1 drop ginger and 3 drops lemon to a teaspoon of honey. Can be added to warm water to drink or placed on a spoon and licked.

CLEAR RESPIRATORY INFECTION: Diffuse oregano, breathe in at close range for 15-20 minutes with eyes closed.

FLU-BUSTING, LUNG-STIMULATING SMOOTHIE
1 cup orange juice
½ cup lemon juice
½ cup chopped pineapple
1 tablespoon raw honey
1 tablespoon coconut oil
1 piece of ginger (2" long up to 1" thick) or 1-2 drops of ginger
¼ tsp cayenne pepper
1-2 drops peppermint
Blend and enjoy.

PINK EYE: Mix 1 drop each lavender and melaleuca with a few drops of carrier oil. Apply small amount of mixture around eye area. Avoid the eye itself. Additionally, apply oil mixture to crooks of second and third toes.

COUGH BUSTER RUB
¾ cup virgin coconut oil
¾ cup fractionated coconut oil
4 tablespoons beeswax
Melt in glass container (double boiler or glass jar in a pot of water)
Remove from heat and add:
2 tablespoon Vitamin E
40 drops basil
40 drops frankincense
40 drops lime
40 drops marjoram
15 drops peppermint
5 drops eucalyptus
5 drops rosemary
5 drops lemon
3 drops cardamom
Mix and let cool. Rub on chest as needed.

THIN IT OUT:
2 drops fennel
2 drops green mandarin
1 drop peppermint
Mix in warm water for a tea or take internally in capsule every 2-4 hours to relieve cold and allergy symptoms with thick mucus.

HOMEMADE COUGH SYRUP
½ cup honey
8 drops peppermint
8 drops lemon
8 drops lavender
8 drops frankincense
3 drops clove
3 drops wild orange
1 drop cinnamon
Mix and take 1 teaspoon every three hours as needed.

SINGER'S OR SPEAKER'S VOICE RECOVERY SPRAY
8 drops lemon
8 drops On Guard®
4 drops peppermint
2 drops myrrh
1 drop oregano
1 drop clove
1 drop sandalwood
Add all oils to 15ml glass spray bottle. Add distilled water and shake. Spray on back of throat frequently (every 20-60 minutes) to obtain desired results.

CONGESTION RELIEF STEAM BLENDS
To a bowl of steamy water add:
Option 1: 2 drops copaiba, 1 drop lemon, 3 drops melaleuca, 4 drops eucalyptus essential oils.

Option 2: 2 drops each Siberian fir, eucalyptus, melaleuca essential oils.

Cover head with a towel to keep the steam inside. With your eyes closed, inhale through nose and breathe deeply for five minutes, or until the oils evaporate, and relief is achieved.

IMMUNE BOOSTING INHALATION
Use equal parts pink pepper, peppermint, melaleuca, and lavender in a diffuser or place 1 drop of each in palms of hands, rub together, cup over face, inhale, and then rub on chest. Dilute with carrier oil as needed.

Conditions

BRONCHIAL

Infection (e.g. bronchitis)* - cardamom, cedarwood, clary sage, clove, copaiba, eucalyptus, frankincense, green mandarin, lavender, lime, marjoram, oregano, peppermint, pink pepper, rosemary, spearmint, thyme, turmeric, Breathe®, Breathe Respiratory Drops, Console®, Forgive®, On Guard®, Peace®
Inflammation - basil, cardamom, cedarwood, clove, cypress, magnolia, rosemary, Siberian fir, spearmint, white fir, wild orange, Breathe®, Breathe Respiratory Drops

BREATHING, GENERAL NEED TO IMPROVE

General: - cinnamon, eucalyptus, patchouli, peppermint, thyme, Breathe®, Breathe Respiratory Drops, Cheer®, Motivate®, Purify
Constricted/tight airways - arborvitae, birch, black spruce, blue tansy, cardamom, cinnamon, clove, Douglas fir, eucalyptus, frankincense, helichrysum, lavender, lemon, lemongrass, marjoram, peppermint, rosemary, thyme, white fir, wild orange, wintergreen, Breathe®, Breathe Respiratory Drops, Console®, Motivate®, Passion®, Serenity®
Difficulty (hyperpnea) - cardamom, clary sage, patchouli, peppermint, Breathe®, Purify
Labored - cinnamon, ylang ylang, Purify, Serenity®
Rapid - melissa, DDR Prime®, Serenity®
Shortness of breath/breathlessness/difficulty breathing (dyspnea) - blue tansy, cinnamon, eucalyptus, frankincense, patchouli, peppermint, Breathe®, DDR Prime®, Peace®, Purify
Shortness of breath/breathlessness/discomfort while lying down (orthopnea) - melaleuca, Roman chamomile, ylang ylang, Purify
Shortness of breath/breathlessness with exertion or during exercise or activity - myrrh, oregano, wintergreen, ylang ylang, Breathe®, Peace®, Purify, Whisper®, Zendocrine®
Sleep apnea - eucalyptus, lemongrass, peppermint, rosemary, thyme, wintergreen, Balance®, Breathe®, On Guard®, Purify, Whisper®
Wheezing - birch, cinnamon, clary sage, clove, eucalyptus, fennel, frankincense, helichrysum, lavender, lemon, marjoram, myrrh, peppermint, rosemary, thyme, white fir, wintergreen, Breathe®, On Guard®, Purify, Serenity®, Whisper®

CONGESTION, GENERAL (mucus/sputum/phlegm, catarrh)

General: - blue tansy, cardamom, cassia, cypress, Douglas fir, eucalyptus, fennel, frankincense, ginger, helichrysum, lemon, lemon eucalyptus, lime, magnolia, marjoram, myrrh, peppermint, petitgrain, rosemary, Siberian fir, tangerine, white fir, Breathe®, Breathe Respiratory Drops, Console®, DigestZen®, Forgive®, Motivate®, Passion®, Slim & Sassy®, Zendocrine®
Clear mucus - black pepper, cardamom, clove, eucalyptus, ginger, lavender, lemon, melissa, peppermint, sandalwood, tangerine, Purify
Chronic discharge of mucus - basil, eucalyptus, wintergreen
Thick mucus - bergamot, birch, cardamom, cassia, cypress, eucalyptus, lemon, pink pepper, myrrh, thyme, wild orange, Breathe®, Citrus Bliss®, DDR Prime®, Forgive®, On Guard®, Passion®, Peace®, Purify, Slim & Sassy®
Yellow, green mucus - basil, cilantro, eucalyptus, ginger, lemongrass, On Guard®, Slim & Sassy®

COUGH, GENERAL*

General: arborvitae, black spruce, blue tansy, cardamom, cedarwood, copaiba, Douglas fir, eucalyptus, frankincense, ginger, green mandarin, helichrysum, juniper berry, lemon eucalyptus, magnolia, melaleuca, oregano, Siberian fir, thyme, turmeric, wild orange, Breathe®, Breathe Respiratory Drops, On Guard®
Barking (e.g. croup) - basil, bergamot, cinnamon, grapefruit, lemon, lemongrass, marjoram, oregano, patchouli, sandalwood, thyme, wild orange, Breathe®, DDR Prime®, DigestZen®, On Guard®
Chronic - cardamom, cassia, cinnamon, eucalyptus, helichrysum, lemon, melissa, oregano, rosemary, thyme, On Guard®
Coughing up blood - blue tansy, cardamom, eucalyptus, geranium, helichrysum, lavender, myrrh, oregano, rose, wild orange, wintergreen, yarrow, On Guard®, Purify, Whisper®; see "Lung - infections" below (consider radon poisoning)
Dry - eucalyptus, frankincense, lavender, white fir, ylang ylang, Breathe®, Whisper®
GERD - See *Digestive & Intestinal*
Heavy mucus - arborvitae, cinnamon, clary sage, eucalyptus, fennel, frankincense, ginger, green mandarin, lemon, melaleuca, myrrh, oregano, pink pepper, wintergreen, Citrus Bliss®, Console®, DigestZen®, Motivate®, Passion®
Moist (sputum-producing) - eucalyptus, ginger, lemon, oregano, On Guard®, Purify, Slim & Sassy®
Spastic/persistent (e.g. whooping cough) - basil, black spruce, cardamom, citronella, clary sage, cypress, frankincense, helichrysum, lavender, melissa, oregano, petitgrain, Roman chamomile, rosemary, sandalwood, thyme, yarrow, Forgive®, Peace®, Purify, Serenity®
Worsens with activity/from exposure to irritant - ginger, ylang ylang, On Guard®, Purify

EARS

Auditory processing challenges - helichrysum, Purify, Whisper®; see *Brain*
Earache/pain - basil, clary sage, cypress, fennel, ginger, helichrysum, lavender, melaleuca, peppermint, Roman chamomile, Citrus Bliss®, Deep Blue®, On Guard®, Passion®, Zendocrine®
Eardrum, perforated - arborvitae, basil, patchouli, ylang ylang, On Guard®, Purify
Ear, infection - basil, helichrysum, lavender, lemon, melaleuca, rosemary, On Guard®
Ear mites - basil, blue tansy, cedarwood, myrrh, wild orange, DigestZen®, InTune®; see *Parasites*
Hearing problems - basil, clary sage, frankincense, helichrysum, lemon, melaleuca, patchouli, Deep Blue®, PastTense®, Slim & Sassy®
Ringing/noise in the ear (tinnitus) - arborvitae, basil, cypress, frankincense, helichrysum, juniper berry, lemongrass, melaleuca, peppermint, Purify, TerraShield®, Zendocrine®

EYES

⚠ **CAUTION:** Place very small quantities of oils (highly diluted) around eyes; do not put oils in eyes; additionally or alternatively use reflex point on toes for eyes - see *Reflexology*.
Dry - lavender, myrrh, sandalwood
Itchy - lavender, oregano, patchouli, wild orange, Citrus Bliss®, DDR Prime®, Zendocrine®
Stringy mucus in or around eyes - clary sage, fennel, melaleuca, DDR Prime®
Tear duct, blocked - clary sage, eucalyptus, frankincense, lavender, lemongrass, melaleuca, myrrh, Purify
Watery/teary - arborvitae, basil, black pepper, blue tansy, frankincense, lime, patchouli, wild orange, DDR Prime®, Immortelle, On Guard®, Purify, Zendocrine®

RESPIRATORY

See remedy on pg. 352

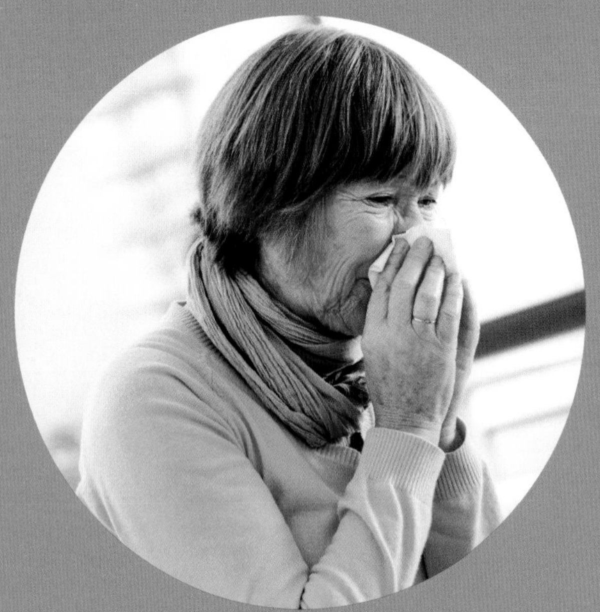

GENERAL RESPIRATORY

Infection, general respiratory* - black pepper, cardamom, cinnamon, eucalyptus, frankincense, green mandarin, lemon, magnolia, melissa, oregano, pink pepper, ravensara, rose, turmeric, Forgive®, Motivate®, On Guard®
Inflammation* - birch, black pepper, coriander, cypress, eucalyptus, ginger, marjoram, melaleuca, melissa, myrrh, rose, peppermimt, spearmint, Breathe®, On Guard®, Slim & Sassy®
Virus - cassia, cinnamon, clove, eucalyptus, melissa, oregano, ravensara, rosemary, thyme, Breathe®, On Guard®

LUNG

Infection (e.g. pneumonia) - black pepper, cedarwood, cinnamon, copaiba, Douglas fir, eucalyptus, frankincense, juniper berry, lavender, melissa, oregano, ravensara, rose, sandalwood, thyme, vetiver, white fir, Console®, On Guard®
Problems/conditions* - arborvitae, basil, bergamot, birch, cardamom, cinnamon, copaiba, Douglas fir, eucalyptus, fennel, frankincense, ginger, lemon, lemongrass, melaleuca, melissa, oregano, peppermint, rosemary, sandalwood, thyme, white fir, wild orange, wintergreen, AromaTouch®, Breathe®, Cheer®, Motivate®, Purify

NOSE

Bleeding - cypress, geranium, helichrysum, lavender, myrrh, AromaTouch®, DDR Prime®, Deep Blue®, On Guard®, Purify, Serenity®
Itchy - lavender, lemon, lemongrass, On Guard®, Purify,
Nasal polyps - frankincense, geranium, lemongrass, rosemary, sandalwood, Citrus Bliss®, melissa, myrrh, Breathe®, Deep Blue®, On Guard®, Purify, TerraShield®
Postnasal drip - cinnamon, lavender, lemon, On Guard®, Purify
Runny - lavender, lemon, peppermint, Purify, Whisper®, Zendocrine®
Smell, decreased/loss of (anosmia) - arborvitae, basil, frankincense, helichrysum, lavender, lemongrass, peppermint, Roman chamomile, rose, sandalwood, Adaptiv®, DDR Prime®, On Guard®, PastTense®
Sneezing - cilantro, coriander, lavender, lemon, peppermint, Purify, Whisper®, Zendocrine®
Stuffy - cardamom, cassia, dill, eucalyptus, fennel, frankincense, ginger, jasmine, lemon, lime, marjoram, myrrh, patchouli, peppermint, rosemary, white fir, Breathe®, DigestZen®, On Guard®, Zendocrine®

SINUS

Facial, forehead pain/pressure or tenderness, swelling and pressure around eyes, cheeks, nose, or forehead - blue tansy, cinnamon, lemongrass, peppermint, thyme, On Guard®, Purify
Infection/inflammation - basil, bergamot, cedarwood, clove, Douglas fir, eucalyptus, helichrysum, lemon, lemongrass, melissa, peppermint, rosemary, sandalwood, Siberian fir, white fir, Breathe®, DigestZen®, Forgive®
Pain in teeth - arborvitae, lavender, lemon, myrrh, DDR Prime®, On Guard®, Purify, Serenity®

THROAT

Dry - cypress, grapefruit, lemon, lime, peppermint, wild orange, Breathe®, Breathe Respiratory Drops, Purify, Zendocrine®
Sore, infection* - basil, cardamom, cinnamon, eucalyptus, lemon, lemongrass, lime, myrrh, myrrh + lemon, oregano, patchouli, rosemary, sandalwood, thyme, On Guard®, On Guard Throat Drops, Purify, Zendocrine®
Swollen, glands - lavender, lemon, peppermint, Slim & Sassy®

VOICE

Hoarse, Loss of (laryngitis) - cinnamon, eucalyptus, fennel, frankincense, ginger, jasmine, lavender, lemon, lemongrass, lime, peppermint, sandalwood, thyme, ylang ylang, Console®, On Guard®, Purify, Zendocrine®

OTHER RESPIRATORY ISSUES

Airborne germs/bacteria, fights - arborvitae, cassia, cedarwood, cinnamon, clove, eucalyptus, grapefruit, lavender, lemon, melaleuca, Siberian fir, thyme, white fir, Breathe®, On Guard®, Purify
Breath, bad - patchouli, peppermint, ylang ylang, DDR Prime®, DigestZen®, DigestZen® softgels
Chest pain - Douglas fir, consider cardiac association - see *Cardiovascular*
Hiccups - arborvitae, basil, blue tansy, lemon, peppermint, sandalwood, Zendocrine®; see *Children*
Mouth, dry - lemon, lemongrass, tangerine, vetiver, wild orange, Citrus Bliss®, On Guard®, Slim & Sassy®, Whisper®
Pleura, inflammation of - birch, cinnamon, cypress, eucalyptus, lemon, melissa, rosemary, thyme, Breathe®
Smoking, quit - See *Addictions*
Snoring* - eucalyptus, geranium, patchouli, peppermint, Breathe®, On Guard®, Purify, Zendocrine®
Taste, loss of - cinnamon, helichrysum, lemongrass, lime, melissa, peppermint, tangerine, Zendocrine®

RESPIRATORY

** See remedy on pg. 352*

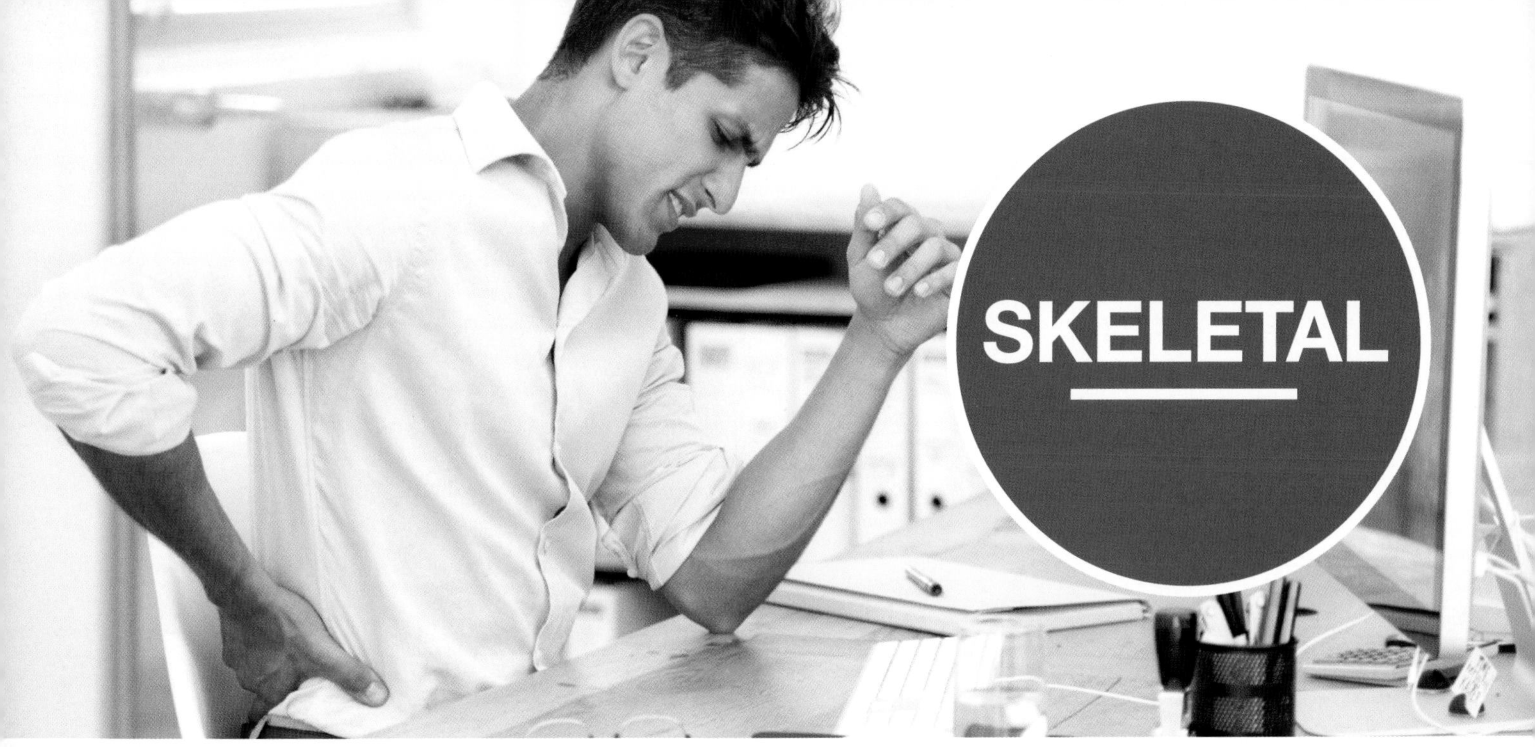

THE BODY'S SKELETAL STRUCTURE comprises the framework upon which all other organs and tissues depend for proper placement and coordination. But bones are not inert material; they are alive, and need blood and oxygen to metabolize nutrients and produce waste. They respond to external stresses by changing shape to accommodate new mechanical demands. The skeleton is often referred to in terms analogous to a tree: the trunk, or torso, supports the limbs, and so on. This system accounts for about 20 percent of the body's overall weight.

The backbone, also called the spine or vertebral column, is made up of twenty-four movable bone segments called vertebrae and is divided into three sections. The top seven are cervical vertebrae, which support the cranium, or skull. The thoracic vertebrae, twelve in all, comprise the mid-back area and support the ribs. The lower back, or lumbar spine, consists of five vertebrae that connect to the pelvis at the sacrum. Each vertebra is stacked upon another and is separated and cushioned by intervertebral discs held in place by tendons and cartilage. Through a channel formed by a hole in each of the stacked vertebrae runs the spinal cord, off of which branch root nerves. This nerve network enables the communication between the brain, the muscles,and the organs of the body system.

In addition to providing a structure to keep other body systems from lying in a heap on the floor, the skeleton protects the softer body parts. The cranium fuses around the brain, forming helmet-like protection. The vertebrae protect the spinal cord from injury. And the rib cage creates a barrier around the heart and lungs. Similarly, the majority of hematopoiesis, or the formation of blood cells, occurs in the soft, red marrow inside bones themselves.

Ligaments connect bones to each other and help to stabilize and move joints. They are composed essentially of long, elastic collagen fibers, which can be torn or injured if overworked. Gentle stretching before any strenuous activity protects the ligaments and prevents injury to joints and muscles. If ligaments are injured, healing can take ninety days and up to nine months for the fibers to regain their maximum strength.
The skeleton's dynamic functions are facilitated by a simple yet sophisticated network of levers, cables, pulleys, and winches actuated by muscles and tendons. When muscles contract, they shorten their length, thus drawing in an adjacent bone that pivots around a connecting joint, much like the boom, stick, and hydraulic lever system of a backhoe.

Since the skeletal system is in a constant state of use, it also undergoes perpetual repair and rejuvenation. It is therefore vulnerable, as is any body system, to imbalance and disease. The joints, in particular, are susceptible to damage due to constant friction, impact, and leverage. As we grow older, we may also experience challenges stemming from calcium or other mineral deficiencies—calcium being the primary material of which bones are made.

Proper pH balance in the body supports a strong skeletal structure. When pH balance is off and the body is too acidic, the blood is compelled to take minerals from the bones and organs, which can cause disease and depletion in the skeletal system. Sugar, refined and processed foods, and overconsumption of meat and dairy make the body more acidic throwing off the pH balance. Certain essential oils like dill, lemon, fennel, or lemongrass can help reduce acidity by creating a more alkaline environment. Maintaining an alkaline environment helps promote healing. Similarly, adequate nourishment with bioavailable vitamins, minerals, and trace minerals helps to maintain a proper pH balance in the blood. Adequate, high-quality supplementation will manage any chronic inflammation, and a topical use of anti-inflammatory essential oils will support joint health.

When there is a skeletal injury, the use of essential oils can accelerate the healing process and recovery time. For example, in the case of a broken bone, oils such as wintergreen and birch have been demonstrated to be useful in relieving and resolving inflammatory conditions and supporting injury recovery. Additionally, lemongrass essential oil supports the healing of any connective tissue damage.

TOP SOLUTIONS

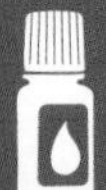

SINGLE OILS

Copaiba - relieves pain and inflammation (pg. 99)
Turmeric - relieves pains and inflammations (pg. 158)
Lemongrass - enhances connective tissue repair (pg. 126)
Wintergreen - reduces aches, pains, and inflammation; stimulates bone repair (pg. 163)
Birch - reduces inflammation and stimulates bone repair (pg. 82)
Helichrysum - relieves pain and inflammation; accelerates bone repair (pg. 117)
Siberian fir - eases bone and joint pain; reduces inflammation (pg. 152)

By Related Properties

For more, See Oil Properties on pages 477 - 481

Analgesic - arborvitae, basil, bergamot, birch, black pepper, blue tansy, cassia, cinnamon, clary sage, clove, copaiba, coriander, cypress, eucalyptus, fennel, frankincense, ginger, helichrysum, juniper berry, lavender, lemongrass, litsea, marjoram, melaleuca, oregano, peppermint, ravensara, rosemary, Siberian fir, turmeric, white fir, wild orange, wintergreen, yarrow
Antiarthritic - arborvitae, black spruce, blue tansy, cassia, copaiba, ginger, manuka, neroli, Siberian fir, yarrow
Anti-inflammatory - arborvitae, basil, bergamot, birch, black pepper, blue tansy, cardamom, cassia, cedarwood, celery seed, cinnamon, copaiba, coriander, cypress, dill, eucalyptus, fennel, frankincense, geranium, ginger, helichrysum, jasmine, lavender, lemongrass, lime, litsea, manuka, melaleuca, melissa, myrrh, neroli, oregano, patchouli, peppermint, Roman chamomile, rosemary, sandalwood, Siberian fir, spearmint, spikenard, tangerine, turmeric, wild orange, wintergreen, yarrow
Anti-rheumatic - birch, black spruce, blue tansy, cassia, clove, copaiba, coriander, cypress, eucalyptus, ginger, juniper berry, lavender, lemon, lemongrass, lime, manuka, oregano, rosemary, thyme, turmeric, white fir, wintergreen, yarrow
Regenerative - basil, cedarwood, clove, coriander, frankincense, geranium, helichrysum, jasmine, lavender, lemongrass, manuka, melaleuca, myrrh, neroli, patchouli, sandalwood, wild orange, yarrow
Steroidal - basil, bergamot, birch, black spruce, cedarwood, clove, fennel, patchouli, rosemary, thyme, wintergreen

Related Ailments: Amyotrophic Lateral Sclerosis, Ankylosing Spondylitis, Arthritis Pain [Pain & Inflammation], Bone Pain, Bone Spurs, Broken Bone, Bunions, Bursitis, Calcified Spine, Cartilage Injury, Chondromalacia Patella, Club foot, Deteriorating Spine, Frozen Shoulder, Ganglion Cyst, Gout, Herniated Disc, Joint Pain, Knee Cartilage Injury, Marfan Syndrome, Myelofibrosis, Osgood-Schlatter Disease, Osteoarthritis [Pain & Inflammation], Osteomyelitis [Immune], Osteoporosis, Paget's Disease, Plantar Fasciitis [Muscular], Rheumatism, Rheumatoid Arthritis, Scoliosis, Shin Splints, Spina Bifida [Nervous], Tennis Elbow [Muscular]

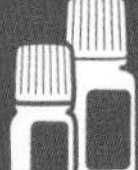

BLENDS

Deep Blue® - soothes, relaxes, and relieves aches and pains; helps with after injuries/surgery healing (pg. 185)
PastTense® - helps relieve and resolve tension, soreness, and stiffness (pg. 196)
DDR Prime® - reduces/resolves inflammation and regenerates tissue (pg. 184)

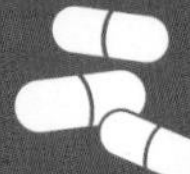

SUPPLEMENTS

Bone Nutrient Lifetime Complex (pg. 212), Alpha CRS®+, PB Assist®+, DigestZen® softgels, DDR Prime® Softgels, **xEO Mega (pg. 222)**, TerraZyme®, **Deep Blue Polyphenol Complex (pg. 212)**, MicroPlex VMz

USAGE TIPS: For best results with skeletal and connective tissue issues:

- **Topical:** Apply oils directly to area of concern for structural issues and in the case of injury, massage in thoroughly whenever possible. Drive oils in with heat, cold, or moisture. Use carrier oil as needed or desired. Layering multiple oils over affected area, placing them on tissue one at a time, is very effective. Any kind of cream or carrier oil will slow absorption if placed on first and improve it if placed on last.
  - **Acute:** Apply often, every 20-30 minutes, until symptoms subside, then reduce to every two to six hours.
  - **Chronic:** Apply two to three times daily.
- **Internal:** Consume oils (to support resolving inflammation and bone repair) in a capsule or under tongue. place oils in a capsule or drop under tongue (hold for 30 seconds; swallow).

Remedies

BROKEN BONE FIX MIX

7 drops frankincense
6 drops Siberian fir
2 drops wintergreen
11 drops helichrysum
4 drops lemongrass

Combine oils in 10ml roller bottle; fill remainder with carrier oil. Apply topically on or near affected area every two hours for two days and every four hours for the next three days. If it isn't possible to apply to area of concern, utilize sympathetic response and rub opposite arm, leg, etc.

BONE SPUR RESOLVE

5 drops frankincense
6 drops cypress
7 drops wintergreen
5 drops marjoram
4 drops helichrysum

Combine in a 10ml roller bottle, fill remainder with carrier oil. Apply topically on or near affected area morning and evening. Continue for an additional two weeks after spur is gone.

EASE-E-FLEX (for joint pain & inflammation)

15 drops frankincense
20 drops Deep Blue®
4 drops lavender

Combine in a 10ml roller bottle; fill remainder with carrier oil. Apply topically on or near affected area as needed

CONNECT REPAIR (for carpal tunnel, tendon, ligaments)

15 drops lemongrass
15 drops helichrysum
10 drops basil
10 drops ginger
10 drops copaiba
10 drops marjoram

Combine in 10ml roller bottle; fill remainder with carrier oil. Apply topically to affected area.

OH MY ACHING BACK

10 drops frankincense
10 drops helichrysum
4 drops cypress
4 drops Siberian fir
2 drops peppermint
2 drops wintergreen
10 drops turmeric

Add to 10ml roller bottle and fill remainder with carrier oil. Use along back/spine area as needed for pain. For chronic issues, apply at least morning and night.

RHEUMATIC PAIN

2 drops spikenard
2 drops lavender
4 drops ginger
4 drops turmeric

Combine in a 5ml roller bottle; fill remainder with carrier oil. Apply to affected area(s) as needed.

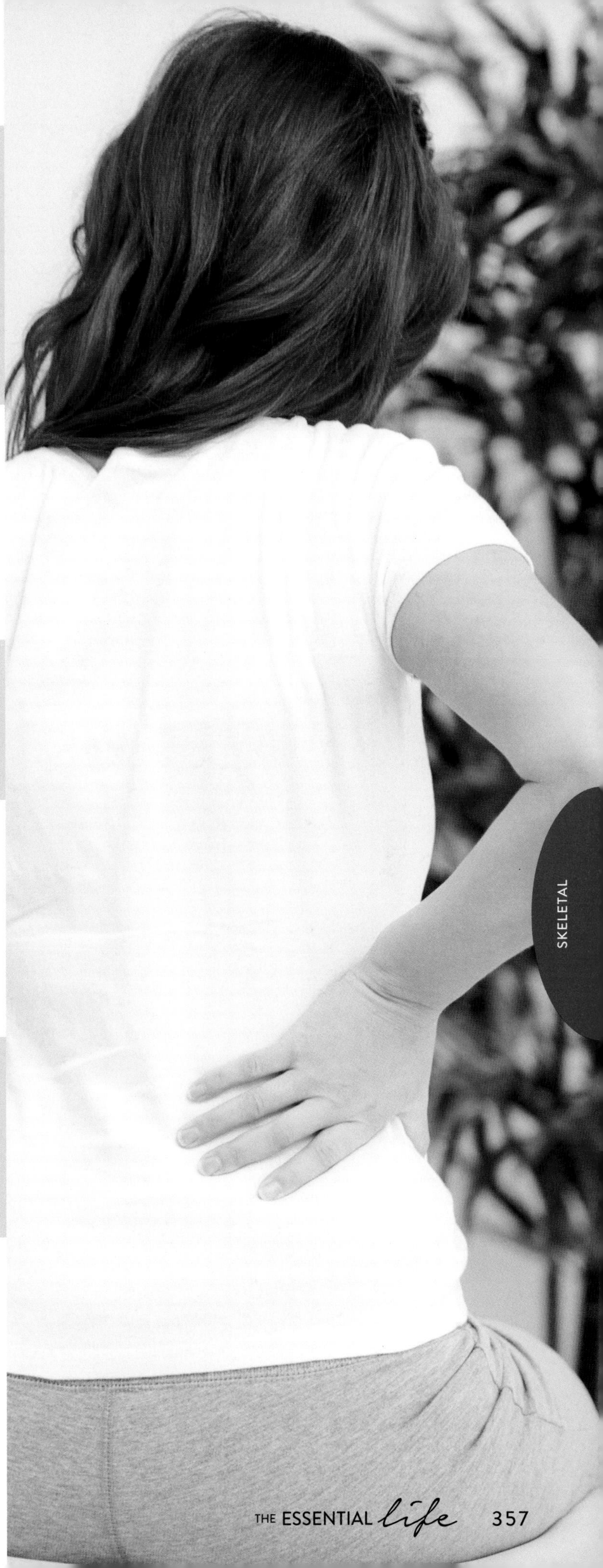

SKELETAL

For more ideas, download the app at app.essentiallife.com

Conditions

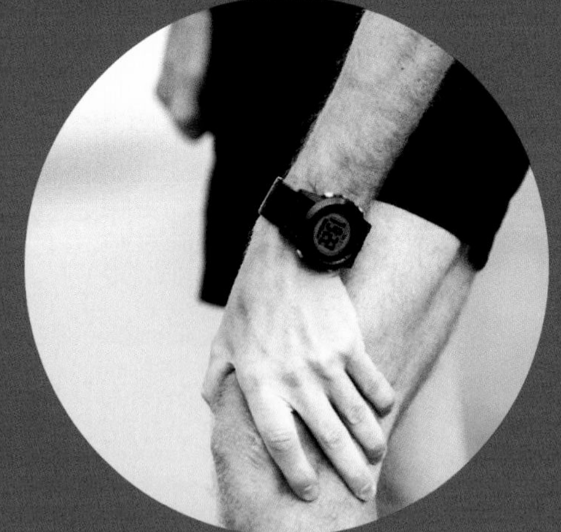

Aching pain in/around ear - arborvitae, basil, bergamot, black pepper, cedarwood, cilantro, cinnamon, clary sage, clove, cypress, eucalyptus, ginger, helichrysum, myrrh, oregano, white fir, wintergreen, AromaTouch®, DDR Prime®, Deep Blue®, Whisper®

Arthritis - basil, black pepper, black spruce, birch, blue tansy, celery seed, copaiba, cypress, Douglas fir, eucalyptus, frankincense, ginger, lavender, lemongrass, marjoram, pink pepper, rosemary, Siberian fir, turmeric, white fir, wintergreen, yarrow, AromaTouch®, DDR Prime®, Deep Blue®, Forgive®; see *Pain & Inflammation*

Back/lower back, pain* - birch, black pepper, copaiba, eucalyptus, frankincense, lemongrass, peppermint, Roman chamomile, white fir, wintergreen, AromaTouch®, Deep Blue®, PastTense®; see *Pain & Inflammation*

Bones, tender - birch, geranium, helichrysum, juniper berry, myrrh, Roman chamomile, wintergreen, DDR Prime®, Deep Blue®, On Guard®, Purify

Bones, bruised - basil, birch, clary sage, frankincense, helichrysum, wintergreen, DDR Prime®, Deep Blue®, On Guard®

Bones, breaking easily - basil, birch, clove, helichrysum, myrrh, oregano, Siberian fir, wild orange, wintergreen, DDR Prime®, Deep Blue®

Bones, broken/fractured* - birch, cypress, frankincense, ginger, helichrysum, Siberian fir, wintergreen, Deep Blue®

Bones, bumps under skin on - birch, cypress, marjoram, myrrh, oregano, rosemary, white fir, wintergreen, AromaTouch®, DDR Prime®, Deep Blue®

Bones, porous - birch, clove, cypress, geranium, helichrysum, lemongrass, peppermint, Siberian fir, wintergreen

Bones, spurs - basil, copaiba, cypress, eucalyptus, frankincense, helichrysum, ginger, peppermint, wintergreen, AromaTouch®

Bunions - basil, cypress, eucalyptus, ginger, lemongrass, thyme, wintergreen, AromaTouch®

Breathing difficulty - cardamom, cypress, Douglas fir, eucalyptus, marjoram, myrrh, oregano, peppermint, white fir, wintergreen, AromaTouch®, Breathe®, Deep Blue®, PastTense®; see *Respiratory*

Cartilage, inflamed/injured* - basil, birch, copaiba, coriander, eucalyptus, helichrysum, lemongrass, marjoram, peppermint, sandalwood, white fir, wintergreen, Deep Blue®; see *Pain & Inflammation*

Cartilage, generate - helichrysum, sandalwood, white fir

Chewing difficulty - basil, clary sage, frankincense, oregano, white fir, wintergreen, AromaTouch®, DDR Prime®, Deep Blue®, PastTense®

Club foot - arborvitae, basil, copaiba, ginger, helichrysum, lavender, lemongrass, marjoram, peppermint, Roman chamomile, rosemary, wintergreen, AromaTouch®

Connective tissue/fascia (ligaments)* - basil, birch, clary sage, copaiba, helichrysum, ginger, lemongrass, sandalwood, white fir, Deep Blue®, HD Clear®

Connective tissue (ligaments), injured/weak/aches and pains* - basil, birch, black spruce, copaiba, clove, cypress, geranium, ginger, helichrysum, lemongrass, marjoram, oregano, peppermint, Roman chamomile, rosemary, thyme, vetiver, white fir, wintergreen, AromaTouch®, Deep Blue®, PastTense®

Headaches - basil, clary sage, clove, copaiba, eucalyptus, frankincense, geranium, helichrysum, lavender, myrrh, oregano, peppermint, Roman chamomile, Siberian fir, spearmint, thyme, wintergreen, DDR Prime®, Deep Blue®, PastTense®, On Guard®

Hearing loss - basil, birch, clary sage, helichrysum, oregano, white fir, PastTense®

Inflamed/deteriorating/disc - birch, celery seed, cypress, eucalyptus, frankincense, helichrysum, peppermint, thyme, turmeric, wintergreen, AromaTouch®, DDR Prime®, Deep Blue®

Inflammation - basil, birch, clove, copaiba, eucalyptus, frankincense, ginger, peppermint, Roman chamomile, sandalwood, Siberian fir, turmeric, vetiver, wintergreen, Deep Blue®, Forgive®, PastTense®

Joint, clicking - birch, marjoram, myrrh, wintergreen, DDR Prime®, Deep Blue®, On Guard®

Joint, grinding sensation - bergamot, birch, rosemary, white fir, wintergreen, DDR Prime®, Purify

Joint, inflammation* - arborvitae, basil, bergamot, blue tansy, cardamom, cedarwood, cinnamon, clove, copaiba, coriander, cypress, Douglas fir, eucalyptus, frankincense, ginger, helichrysum, lavender, lemon, lemon eucalyptus, marjoram, peppermint, pink pepper, Roman chamomile, rosemary, thyme, turmeric, vetiver, white fir, wild orange, wintergreen, DDR Prime®, Deep Blue®, Zendocrine®

Joint, locking - basil, birch, clary sage, helichrysum, marjoram, white fir, wintergreen, AromaTouch®, DDR Prime®, Deep Blue®, On Guard®

Joint, pain/stiffness* - arborvitae, basil, birch, black pepper, cardamom, celery seed, cinnamon, copaiba, coriander, Douglas fir, eucalyptus, frankincense, geranium, lemongrass, Siberian fir, thyme, turmeric, wintergreen, AromaTouch®, Deep Blue®

Joint, swollen/warm/red/tender - citronella, eucalyptus, frankincense, lavender, Roman chamomile, AromaTouch®, Deep Blue®

Ligament strain* - copaiba, frankincense, lemongrass, marjoram, white fir, DDR Prime®, Deep Blue®

Rheumatism - basil, birch, black spruce, blue tansy, celery seed, copaiba, Douglas fir, eucalyptus, ginger, lavender, lemon eucalyptus, lemongrass, pink pepper, spikenard, Siberian fir, thyme, turmeric, white fir, AromaTouch®, Cheer®, DDR Prime®, Deep Blue®, Forgive®; see *Pain & Inflammation*

Rheumatoid arthritis* - basil, bergamot, birch, black spruce, cardamom, copaiba, cypress, Douglas fir, frankincense, ginger, lavender, lemon, marjoram, pink pepper, wintergreen, AromaTouch®, Deep Blue®, PastTense®

Sciatic issues - See *Nervous*

Shoulder, frozen - basil, birch, lemongrass, oregano, peppermint, white fir, wintergreen, DDR Prime®, Deep Blue®

Shoulder, rotator cuff - birch, white fir, wintergreen, Deep Blue®, PastTense®

Shin splints - basil, frankincense, helichrysum, lavender, lemongrass, marjoram, myrrh, patchouli, wintergreen, AromaTouch®, Deep Blue®

Stiff/limited range of motion - birch, frankincense, marjoram, white fir, wintergreen, Deep Blue® or rub, PastTense®

Vertebral misalignment - helichrysum, marjoram, rose, white fir, AromaTouch®, Deep Blue®

** See remedy on pg. 357*

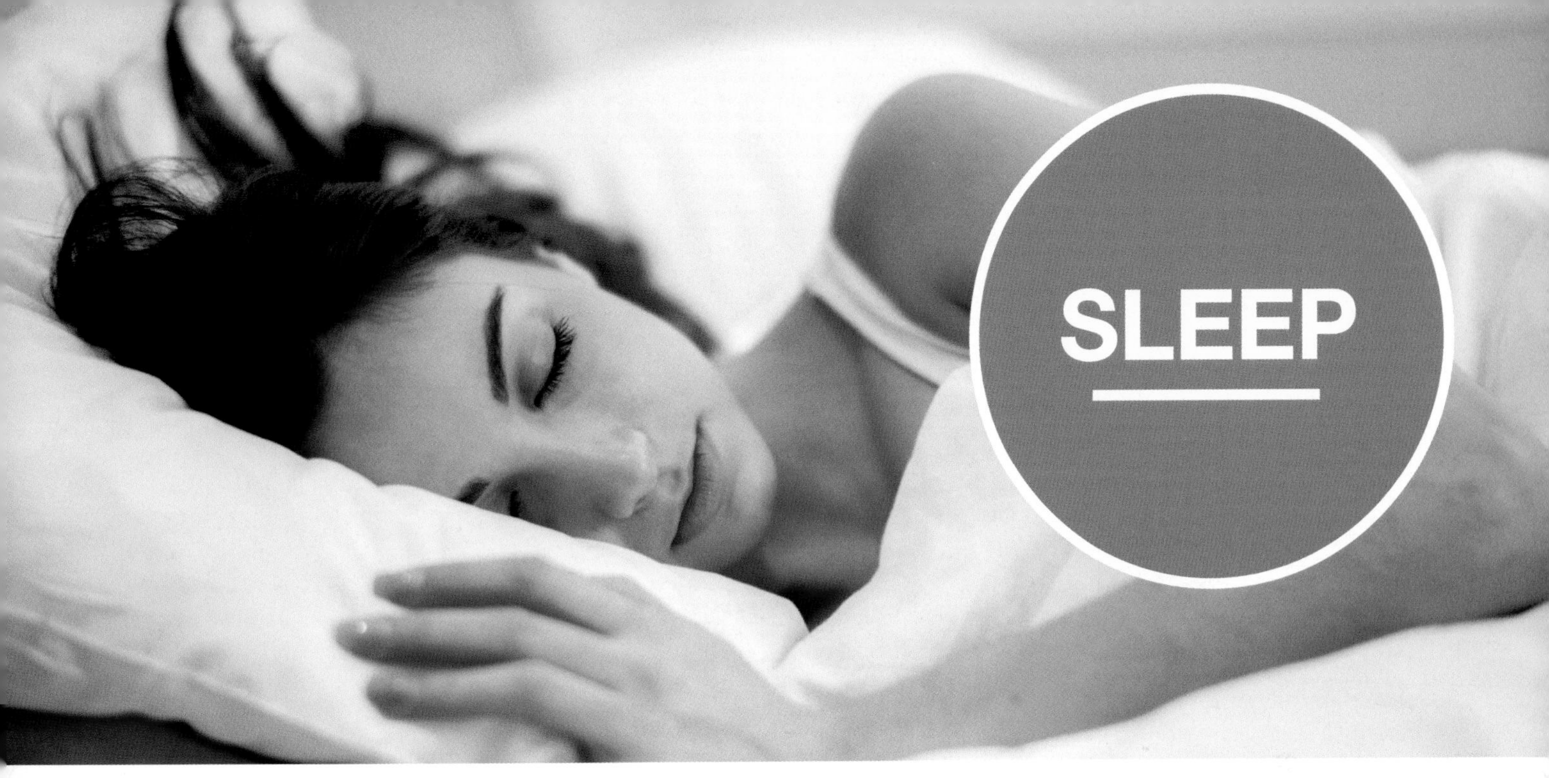

SLEEP DESCRIBES the period when the body ceases to engage in most voluntary bodily functions, thus providing an opportunity for the body to focus on restoration and repair. During this time, conscious brain activity is fully or partially suspended, a state that contributes to restoring and maintaining emotional, mental, and physical health. In recent years, doctors and organizations such as the National Sleep Foundation have encouraged the wide acceptance of sleep as one of the three pillars of health, together with nutrition and exercise.

All sleep can be divided into two states: REM and Non-REM. REM is an acronym for Rapid Eye Movement sleep, and represents a period when brain waves have fast frequency and low voltage, similar to brain activity during waking hours. However, during REM sleep all voluntary muscles cease activity except those that control eye movements. Dreams take place during REM sleep. It is the period of sleep where the body is in a deeply subconscious state, and much healing, repair, and restoration occurs.

Non-REM sleep can be further subdivided into three stages: Stage N1 sleep is the state between wakefulness and sleep; it is very light, and some people don't even recognize they are asleep during this stage. Stage N2 is a true deep sleep. Stage N3 is deep sleep or delta sleep. Interestingly, sleep typically occurs in 90-120 minute cycles, with transitions from the N-stages of sleep in the first part of the night to REM sleep in the latter.

Age plays a huge factor in normal sleeping patterns. Newborns need between sixteen to eighteen hours of sleep a day, preschoolers need ten to twelve hours, and school age children and teenagers need nine or more hours. Because deeper N3 and REM sleep states diminish as individuals age, older adults experience more difficulty getting to sleep and staying asleep. At a time when individuals tend to need more reparative and restorative sleep, they actually receive less.

Some of the most common sleep disorders include insomnia (difficulty getting to sleep and staying asleep), sleep apnea (where breathing may stop or be blocked for brief periods during sleep), sleep deprivation (not getting enough sleep), restless leg syndrome (an uncontrollable need to move legs at night, at times accompanied by tingling or other discomfort), narcolepsy (a central nervous system disease that results in daytime sleepiness and other issues, including loss of muscle tone and more), and problem sleepiness (when daytime sleepiness interferes with regular responsibilities, such as working or studying).

In addition to sleeping disorders, lack of necessary sleep can cause a myriad of other physical and emotional problems. It contributes to adrenal fatigue, poor digestion, weight gain and/or obesity, grogginess, decreased focus and concentration, memory problems, increased irritability and frustration levels and other mood challenges, heart disease, a compromised immune system, and a higher likelihood of chronic or autoimmune conditions.

When children don't get the sleep they need, both physical and emotional development can be negatively affected. The necessity for regular, healthy sleeping patterns is apparent when one considers the serious difficulties and disorders caused by lack of sleep.

Countless individuals have turned to natural remedies to promote ease in falling asleep, staying asleep, and reaching the deeper levels of sleep. There are supplements and essential oils that work together to reduce symptoms of the more serious sleeping disorders and should be considered as a viable addition or alternative to sleep treatments as advised by medical professionals. The benefits of using essential oils such as lavender to promote healthy sleep are numerous and astounding, and the results can be life-altering for the chronically sleep deprived.

TOP SOLUTIONS

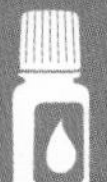

SINGLE OILS

Lavender - calms, relaxes, and sedates; supports parasympathetic system (pg. 122)
Vetiver - grounds and promotes tranquility (pg. 160)
Roman chamomile - balances hormones; sedates, calms, and relaxes (pg. 147)

By Related Properties

For more, See Oil Properties on pages 477 - 481

Analgesic - arborvitae, basil, bergamot, birch, black pepper, blue tansy, cassia, cinnamon, clary sage, clove, copaiba, coriander, cypress, eucalyptus, fennel, frankincense, ginger, helichrysum, jasmine, juniper berry, lavender, lemongrass, litsea, marjoram, melaleuca, oregano, peppermint, ravensara, rosemary, Siberian fir, wild orange, wintergreen, yarrow
Antidepressant - clary sage, coriander, frankincense, geranium, jasmine, lavender, lemongrass, magnolia, melissa, neroli, oregano, patchouli, ravensara, rose, sandalwood, tangerine, wild orange, ylang ylang
Calming - bergamot, birch, black pepper, black spruce, blue tansy, cassia, clary sage, copaiba, coriander, fennel, frankincense, geranium, jasmine, juniper berry, lavender, litsea, melissa, oregano, patchouli, Roman chamomile, sandalwood, tangerine, vetiver, yarrow
Detoxifier - arborvitae, cassia, cilantro, cypress, geranium, juniper berry, lemon, lime, litsea, patchouli, rosemary, tangerine, wild orange, yarrow
Grounding - basil, black spruce, blue tansy, cedarwood, clary sage, cypress, melaleuca, Siberian fir, vetiver, ylang ylang
Relaxing - basil, blue tansy, cassia, cedarwood, clary sage, cypress, fennel, geranium, jasmine, lavender, litsea, manuka, marjoram, myrrh, neroli, ravensara, Roman chamomile, white fir, ylang ylang
Restorative - basil, frankincense, lime, neroli, patchouli, rosemary, sandalwood, spearmint, tangerine
Sedative - basil, bergamot, blue tansy, cedarwood, clary sage, coriander, frankincense, geranium, jasmine, juniper berry, lavender, lemongrass, marjoram, melissa, neroli, patchouli, Roman chamomile, rose, sandalwood, spikenard, tangerine, vetiver, yarrow, ylang ylang

Related Ailments: Hypersomnia, Insomnia, Jet Lag, Narcolepsy, Periodic Limb Movement Disorder (PLMD), Sleep Apnea, Sleepwalking, Restless Leg Syndrome (RLS)

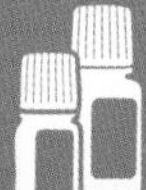

BLENDS

Serenity® - calms mind/emotions; promotes relaxation and restful sleep (pg. 199)
Balance® - promotes sense of well being and supports autonomic nervous system (pg. 170)
InTune® - balances brain activity and calms over-stimulation (pg. 192)

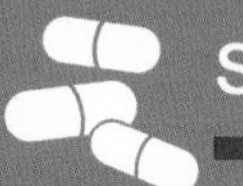

SUPPLEMENTS

Bone Nutrient Lifetime Complex (pg. 210), Alpha CRS®+, PB Assist®+, **Zendocrine® Softgels (pg. 224)**, Zendocrine® Complex, Mito2Max®, **xEO Mega (pg. 222)**, IQ Mega®, Phytoestrogen Complex, MicroPlex VMz

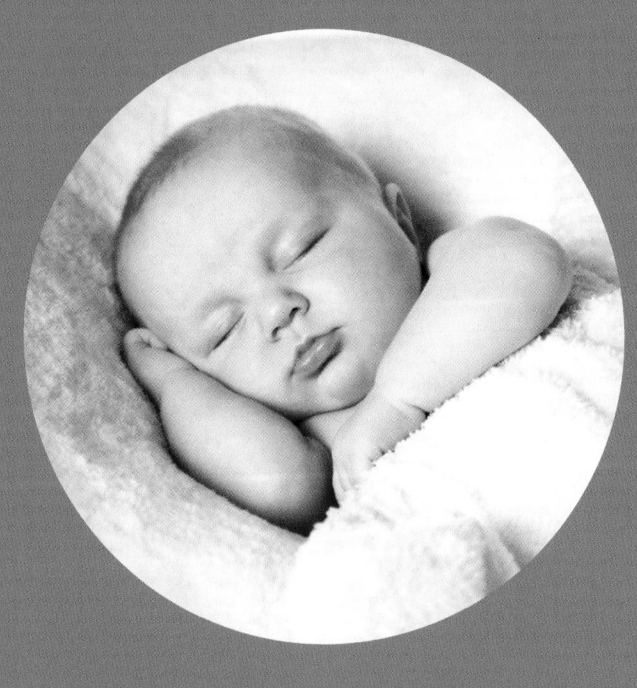

USAGE TIPS: To support optimal and restful sleep, inhalation and topical use of essential oils gives direct access to the brain through smell, relaxes tense muscles, and calms active minds.

- **Aromatic:** Diffuse selected oil(s) of choice, apply a few drops to clothing, bedding (e.g. pillow), or any other method that supports inhalation. Start exposure just before bedtime.
- **Topical:** Combine oils with soothing and relaxing massage techniques; apply oils on forehead, back, shoulders, under nose, and especially bottoms of feet from a pre-made or prepared roller bottle blend for ease. Applying oils on chest allows breathing in vapors. For chronic issues, use Oil Touch technique regularly.

Conditions

CONDITIONS (CONTRIBUTORS TO SLEEP ISSUES):

Alcohol, issues with - See *Addictions*
Anxiety* - See *Mood & Behavior*
Bedtime, chronically late - See "Night owl" below
Brain injury - See *Brain*
Breathing issues - See *Respiratory*
Caffeine (avoid consuming within four to six hours of sleep) - See *Addictions*
Chronic pain - See *Pain & Inflammation*
CPAP machine, difficulties with - See *Respiratory*
Daytime napping - See *Energy & Vitality*
Depression - See *Mood & Behavior*
Dreaming, excessive - clary sage, frankincense, geranium, juniper berry, lavender, patchouli, Roman chamomile, Balance®, PastTense®, Serenity®
Drug abuse - See *Addictions*
Drug withdrawals - See *Addictions*
Emotional discomfort - bergamot, clary sage, geranium, juniper berry, melissa, ravensara, ylang ylang; see *Mood & Behavior*
Eating, excessive, late at night - See *Eating Disorders, Weight*
Cold extremities, poor circulation - black pepper, cypress, coriander, pink pepper; see *Cardiovascular*
Fear (of sleeping, etc.) - bergamot, cardamom, coriander, patchouli, ravensara, Roman chamomile, Balance®, Deep Blue®, Serenity®; see *Mood & Behavior*
Grief - Console®; See *Mood & Behavior*
Heart symptoms (e.g. rapid heart rate) - magnolia, ylang ylang; see *Cardiovascular*
Hormone imbalances - clary sage; see *Men's Health* or *Women's Health*
Illness/chronic illness - See *Immune & Lymphatic*
Insomnia - See "Sleeplessness" below, "Sleeplessness, chronic" on next page
Insomnia, nervous tension - basil, blue tansy, lavender, magnolia, marjoram, petitgrain, Roman chamomile, rosemary, vetiver, AromaTouch®, PastTense®, Peace®, Serenity®; see *Nervous*
Interferences in normal sleep schedule - See "Jet lag" below
Jet lag, can't go to sleep - lavender, patchouli, peppermint, wild orange, Serenity®; see "Sleeplessness" next page
Jet lag, overly tired - arborvitae, basil, grapefruit, lemon, lemongrass, rosemary, tangerine, wild orange, Citrus Bliss®, InTune®, Motivate®, Slim & Sassy®
Melatonin levels low, irregular sleep cycles (REM) - black pepper, cedarwood, frankincense, ginger, lime, myrrh, rosemary (use during day), sandalwood, tangerine, ylang ylang, vetiver, InTune®, Serenity®
Mental chatter/over-thinking* - basil, black spruce, cedarwood, lavender, magnolia, neroli, rosemary, ylang ylang, Adaptiv®, Balance®, Serenity®
Muscle cramps/charley horses - See *Muscular*
Nervous tension - basil, bergamot, black spruce, Douglas fir, geranium, grapefruit, jasmine, lavender, melissa, Roman chamomile, rose, sandalwood, vetiver, wild orange, ylang ylang, AromaTouch®, Balance®, Citrus Bliss®, PastTense®, Serenity®; see *Mood & Behavior, Nervous*
Nicotine - cinnamon, clove, On Guard®; See *Addictions*
Night eating syndrome - See *Eating Disorders, Weight*
Night owl - cedarwood, lavender, vetiver, wild orange, wintergreen, Balance®, Serenity®; see "Sleeplessness," "Sleeplessness, chronic" below
Night sweats - Douglas fir, eucalyptus, ginger, lime, peppermint, AromaTouch®, ClaryCalm®, DDR Prime®, Whisper®, Zendocrine®; see *Endocrine (Thyroid), Immune & Lymphatic, Women's Health*
Nightmares - cinnamon, clary sage, cypress, eucalyptus, geranium, grapefruit, juniper berry, lavender, melissa, neroli, Roman chamomile, white fir, wild orange, vetiver, Balance®, Serenity®
Over-excited/over-stimulated - lavender, patchouli, Roman chamomile, sandalwood, wild orange; see *Mood & Behavior*
Pain or discomfort at night - copaiba, turmeric, Deep Blue®; see *Pain & Inflammation*
Periodic limb movement - marjoram, AromaTouch®; see "Twitching" below
Psychiatric disorder - See *Mood & Behavior*
Restless legs - basil, cypress, geranium, ginger, grapefruit, lavender, neroli, patchouli, peppermint, Roman chamomile, spearmint, wintergreen, AromaTouch®, Deep Blue®, PastTense®, Serenity®
Restlessness* - bergamot, black pepper, cedarwood, frankincense, lavender, neroli, patchouli, Roman chamomile, tangerine, vetiver, wild orange, yarrow, Adaptiv®, AromaTouch®, Balance®, Elevation™, PastTense®, Serenity®
Routine/schedule, poor - Balance®; see "Melatonin levels low" below
Serotonin levels low (precursor to melatonin) - bergamot, cedarwood, clary sage, grapefruit, melissa, patchouli, Roman chamomile, ylang ylang, Adaptiv®; see *Mood & Behavior*
Sleep apnea - eucalyptus, lemongrass, peppermint, rosemary, thyme, wintergreen, Balance®, Breathe®, On Guard®, Purify, Whisper®; see *Respiratory*
Sleep-walking - black pepper, geranium, lavender, vetiver, Balance®, DDR Prime®, Peace®, Serenity®
Snoring* - Douglas fir, eucalyptus, geranium, patchouli, peppermint, rosemary, Breathe®, On Guard®, Purify, Zendocrine®; see *Respiratory*
Stimulants, use of (medications, caffeine, energy drinks, supplements) - See *Addictions*
Stress - clary sage, frankincense, lavender, lime, vetiver, wild orange, Citrus Bliss®, Elevation™, Serenity®; see *Stress*
Teeth grinding - frankincense, geranium, lavender, marjoram, Roman chamomile, wild orange, Serenity®; see *Parasites*
Tranquility, lack of - cinnamon, clary sage, jasmine, melissa, neroli, Roman chamomile, Adaptiv®, PastTense®
Twitching/muscle spasms - basil, clary sage, coriander, cypress, eucalyptus, ginger, jasmine, lemongrass, marjoram, neroli, AromaTouch®, Balance®, Deep Blue®; see *Muscular*

CONDITIONS (RELATED TO, RESULT OF SLEEP ISSUES):

Adrenal fatigue - See *Endocrine (Adrenals)*
Alertness, lack of | poor daytime learning | mental fatigue; See *Energy & Vitality, Focus & Concentration*
Depression - See "Serotonin levels low" above , *Mood & Behavior*
Difficulty controlling emotions - See *Mood & Behavior*
Driving, can't stay awake (pull over!) - basil, peppermint, pink pepper, rosemary, Breathe®
Drowsiness, daytime - basil, grapefruit, lemon, rosemary, wild orange, Citrus Bliss®, InTune®; see *Energy & Vitality*
Focus, concentration compromised - See *Focus & Concentration*
Memory, poor/slow recall or response - bergamot, frankincense, rosemary; see *Focus & Concentration*
Narcolepsy - basil, frankincense, lavender + wild orange, patchouli, sandalwood, vetiver, Console®, InTune®, Motivate®, Serenity®; see *Brain*
Night eating syndrome - See *Eating Disorders, Mood & Behavior, Weight*
Physical discomfort/pain - frankincense, Deep Blue®; see *Pain & Inflammation*
Sleep, lack of/deprivation - geranium, lavender, patchouli, DDR Prime®, PastTense®, Zendocrine®; see *Energy & Vitality*
Sleep, poor - lavender, marjoram, Roman chamomile, sandalwood, vetiver, Serenity®
Sleeplessness - basil, cedarwood, clary sage, frankincense, geranium, lavender, magnolia, patchouli, petitgrain, Roman chamomile, sandalwood, vetiver, wild orange, Balance®, Console®, Forgive®, Peace®, Serenity®
Sleeplessness, chronic - bergamot, cedarwood, copaiba, cypress, jasmine, lavender, melissa, neroli, peppermint, petitgrain, Roman chamomile, sandalwood, tangerine, thyme, vetiver, wild orange, ylang ylang, Balance®, Cheer®, Console®, Forgive®, Passion®, Serenity®
Weakened immunity - See *Immune & Lymphatic*
Weight gain - See *Weight*

Remedies

Avoid using essential oils which stimulate at night, for example rosemary and peppermint. Instead opt for oils which relax, such as vetiver and Roman chamomile.

SLEEP-PROMOTING BATH RECIPES
- To help fall asleep: Add a few drops lavender to 1 cup Epsom salts; dissolve in hot bath (Epsom salts offer a good source of magnesium, which supports relaxation)
- Sleep tonight; sleep in tomorrow: Mix 5 drops patchouli oil, 2 drops wild orange oil, and 1 drop frankincense oil with Epsom salts; soak fifteen to twenty minutes.

STOP SNORING BLEND
18 drops marjoram or thyme
12 drops geranium
12 drops lavender
8 drops eucalyptus
5 drops cedarwood
Combine in spray bottle. Mist room generously, lightly spray pillow, apply to throat, inhale.

ROLLER BOTTLE REMEDIES FOR SLEEP & ANXIETY ISSUES
For all recipes use a 10ml roller bottle; after placing essential oils in bottle, fill remainder with carrier; use on feet, back of neck
- Recipe #1: 20 drops Serenity®, 10 drops vetiver, and 10 drops wild orange
- Recipe #3: 3 drops each of juniper berry, Balance®, vetiver, patchouli, ylang ylang

RESTFUL SLEEP
2 drops green mandarin, Roman chamomile, and clary sage. Diffuse at night to promote quality sleep.

SLEEPY-TIME MASSAGE RUB (Yield: ½ cup)
¼ cup cocoa butter
¼ cup coconut oil
20 drops of lavender
6 drops of Douglas fir
6 drops cedarwood
10 drops of frankincense
- Substitutions: Replace any of above oils with ylang ylang, Roman chamomile, vetiver, cedarwood, or clary sage as desired to promote relaxation and restful night's sleep.
- Instructions: Warm coconut oil and cocoa butter in a small pan until melted. Let rest on counter for ten minutes. Once cooled, add essential oils to mixture, then cool it in fridge for 1 hour. Desired texture is firm, not hard. Whip on high with electric mixer until softened and forms peaks. Apply a small, pea-sized amount and massage into feet before bed. Save remainder for additional treatments. Store in a cool place.

GOING TO & STAYING ASLEEP:
Diffuse:
1 drop each of cedarwood, patchouli, Balance®, vetiver, Roman chamomile
8 drops Serenity®
3 drops wild orange

BEDTIME "TEA" FOR RELAXATION
Steep chamomile tea and add 2 drops lavender oil (make sure you have pajamas on before finishing tea; it works great!)

QUIET THE MIND & BODY
- Stop the mind chatter: 1-3 drops each of Balance® and Serenity®, layered on bottoms of feet, back of neck, and breathe in as well.
- For more restful sleep: 3 drops DDR Prime® on bottoms feet at night

DREAMY AromaTouch®
2 drops green mandarin and 4 drops sandalwood in 1 teaspoon carrier oil. Apply with diulted rose.

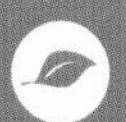

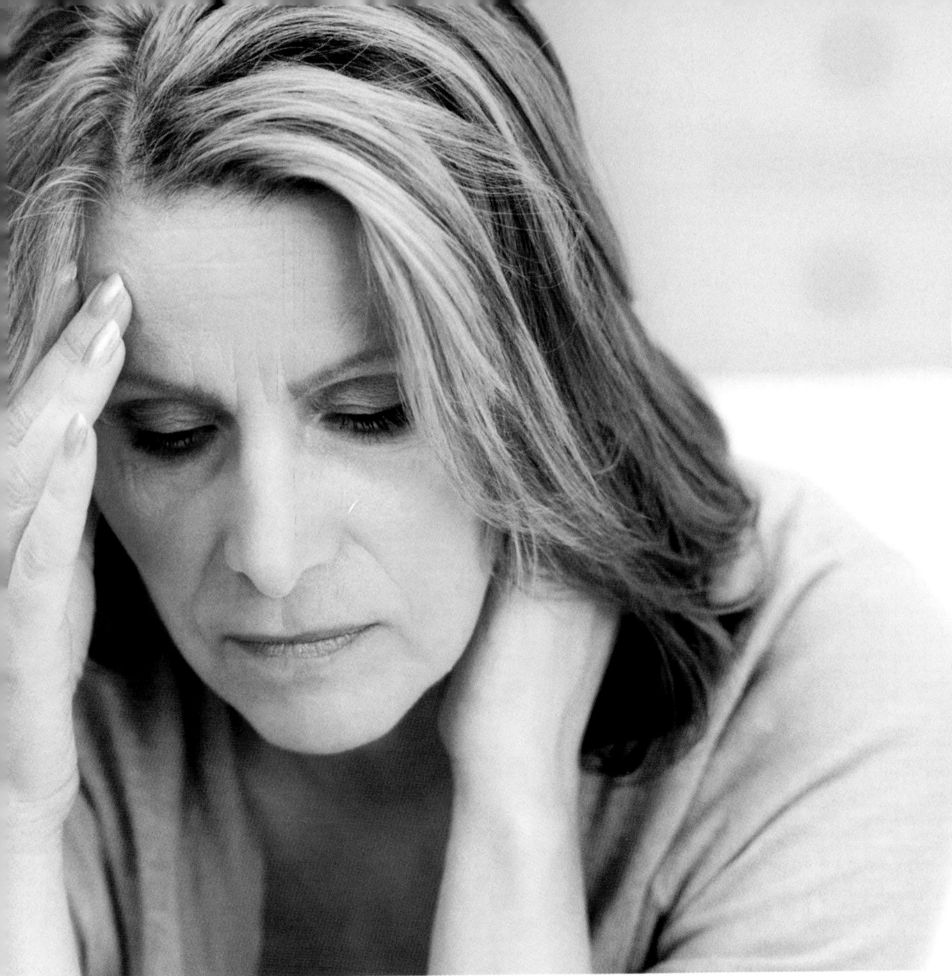

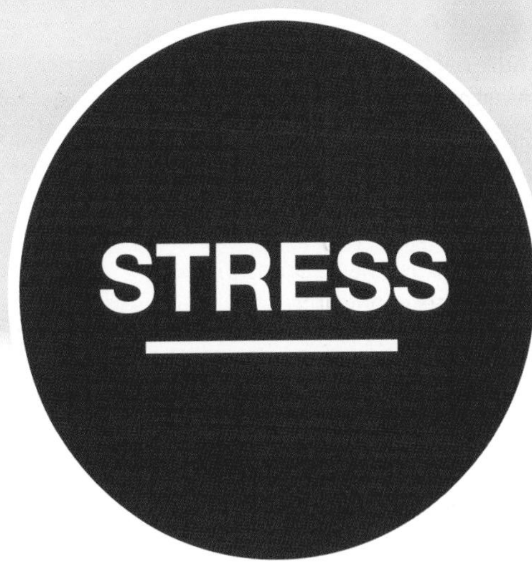

STRESS

UNDER NORMAL conditions, individuals are able to maintain homeostasis, a state where one is healthy, alert, and effective, and where body systems are operating as they should. Conversely, stress is the body's physiological response to overwhelming stimuli, a condition that directly challenges the body's ability to maintain homeostasis. When a stressful event or condition is perceived, the sympathetic nervous system is activated, which causes a fight-or-flight response in the body.

The fight-or-flight response initiates a chain reaction of activity in the body, starting with the central nervous system. Various parts of the brain, adrenal glands, peripheral nervous system (PNS), and other body systems work together to secrete hormones, such as adrenaline and cortisol, into the bloodstream. These hormones send messages instructing the immediate suspension of uncritical activities, such as those of the digestive, reproductive, and immune systems. All bodily energy and resources are directed to supporting heart and brain function.

Once the body's response to stress has been activated, a number of physical changes immediately occur. Stress reduces the blood-brain barrier's ability to block hormones and chemicals from entering the brain, thereby allowing corticosteroids to speed up the brain's ability to process information and make a decision. Cortisol deactivates the immune system, which does not cause serious problems as long as it is only a temporary, acute, response to stress.

When stress becomes chronic, however, some extremely serious situations can result. Over time, neuroplasticity of the brain is compromised, which results in the atrophy and destruction of neuron dendrites, and the brain loses the ability to form new connections or even process new sensory information (both being vital brain functions). When the immune system is repressed for an extended period of time, the body pays a significant toll. Risk of heart attack and stroke increases, anxiety and depression are more likely, and infertility can result, as well as a number of other chronic conditions including asthma, back pain, fatigue, headaches, serious digestive issues, and more.

It stands to reason that individual interpretation of relationships and other stimuli directly impact the level of stress experienced. When an individual can honestly assess a situation and choose to interpret it differently, this simple change in thinking can help reprogram an individual's stress response.

Essential oils are excellent support for effectively reprogramming the stress response on a chemical level. For example, when the cell membrane is hardened, cells suspend activity, rich nutrients and oxygen from the blood are not able to enter the cell, and toxic waste inside the cell is unable to escape. The chemical compounds in citrus oils, when inhaled, help cells to return to their normal state, thus allowing the interchange of nutrients and release of toxins to resume. On a physiological cellular level, the body's descent into fight-or-flight is interrupted, and the body is quickly able to shift towards homeostasis. There are numerous viable essential oils solutions that can interrupt unhealthy stress responses and prevent additional negative results.

TOP SOLUTIONS

SINGLE OILS

Lavender - calms and relieves stress (pg. 122)
Roman chamomile - calms reduces stress (pg. 147)
Tangerine, wild orange - energizes while reducing anxiety and depression (pgs. 156 & 162)
Frankincense - reduces depression, trauma, and tension (pg. 110)
Vetiver - improves focus and sedates (pg. 160)

By Related Properties

For more, See Oil Properties on pages 477 - 481

Calming - bergamot, birch, black pepper, black spruce, blue tansy, cassia, clary sage, copaiba, coriander, fennel, frankincense, geranium, jasmine, juniper berry, lavender, litsea, melissa, oregano, patchouli, Roman chamomile, sandalwood, tangerine, vetiver, yarrow
Energizing - basil, bergamot, clove, cypress, grapefruit, lemon, lemongrass, lime, pink pepper, rosemary, Siberian fir, tangerine, white fir, wild orange, yarrow
Grounding - basil, black spruce, blue tansy, cedarwood, clary sage, cypress, melaleuca, vetiver, Siberian fir, ylang ylang
Refreshing - cypress, geranium, grapefruit, green mandarin, lemon, lime, melaleuca, peppermint, pink pepper, Siberian fir, wild orange, wintergreen
Relaxing - basil, blue tansy, cassia, cedarwood, clary sage, cypress, fennel, geranium, jasmine, lavender, litsea, marjoram, magnolia, manuka, myrrh, neroli, ravensara, Roman chamomile, white fir, ylang ylang
Uplifting - bergamot, cardamom, cedarwood, clary sage, cypress, grapefruit, lemon, lime, litsea, melissa, sandalwood, tangerine, wild orange, ylang ylang

STRESS

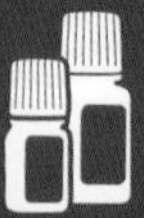

BLENDS

Citrus Bliss® - energizes while reducing anxiety and depression (pg. 181)
Balance® - balances mood while reducing stress and trauma (pg. 170)
Serenity® - reduces anxiety and stress (pg. 199)
PastTense® - relieves tension and stress (pg. 196)
Whisper® - balances hormones and calms anxiety (pg. 205)

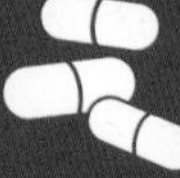

SUPPLEMENTS

Bone Nutrient Lifetime Complex (pg. 210), Alpha CRS®+, DigestZen® softgels, **Mito2Max® (pg. 214)**, **xEO Mega (pg. 222)**, IQ Mega®, Phytoestrogen Complex, **MicroPlex VMz (pg. 214)**

Conditions

For more emotions associated with stress (e.g. anxiety, depression) - see *Mood & Behavior*
Accelerated aging - frankincense, jasmine, sandalwood, ylang ylang, Immortelle, Slim & Sassy®
Anxiety* - bergamot, black spruce, cedarwood, clary sage, frankincense, kumquat, lavender, magnolia, neroli, petitgrain, pink pepper, spikenard, tangerine, turmeric, vetiver, wild orange, yarrow, Adaptiv®, Balance®, Citrus Bliss®, Forgive®, InTune®, Peace®, Serenity®; see *Mood & Behavior*
Behavioral stress - See *Addictions, Eating Disorders, Weight*
Busy-ness - juniper berry, Balance®, Serenity®
Chest pain - basil, cypress, lavender, marjoram, rosemary, sandalwood, thyme, wild orange, AromaTouch®, DDR Prime®, Deep Blue®, On Guard®; see *Cardiovascular*
Constricted breathing - bergamot, blue tansy, frankincense, lavender, Roman chamomile, Balance®, Citrus Bliss®, Passion®; see *Respiratory*
Cortisol, low or high - see *Endocrine*
Depression - bergamot, frankincense, neroli, wild orange, ylang ylang, Adaptiv®, Citrus Bliss®, ClaryCalm®, Elevation™, Serenity®; see *Mood & Behavior*
Energy, lack of stress - See *Energy & Vitality*
Endure stress and avoid illness - vetiver; see *Immune & Lymphatic*
Environmental stress - cinnamon, frankincense, geranium, juniper berry, sandalwood, wild orange, Balance®, Citrus Bliss®, Forgive®
Fainting - basil, bergamot, cinnamon, cypress, frankincense, lavender, peppermint, rosemary, sandalwood, wild orange; see *Cardiovascular*
Fatigue/exhaustion* - basil, bergamot, black spruce, cinnamon, green mandarin, lemon, lime, pink pepper, Siberian fir, Adaptiv®, Elevation™, Passion®, Motivate®, Slim & Sassy®, Zendocrine® ; see *Energy & Vitality*
Headache and migraine - copaiba, frankincense, lavender, peppermint, wintergreen, Deep Blue®, PastTense®; see *Pain & Inflammation*
Heart disease - geranium, lime, ylang ylang; see *Cardiovascular*
Illness, stress related - bergamot, copaiba, lemon, rosemary; see *Immune & Lymphatic*
Insomnia - lavender, magnolia, marjoram, neroli, Roman chamomile, vetiver, Balance®, Passion®, Serenity®; see *Sleep*
Mind/thought-related/poor memory stress - See *Brain, Focus & Concentration*
Mood-related, moodiness driven stress - See *Mood & Behavior*
Muscle tension or pain - marjoram, peppermint, wintergreen, AromaTouch®, Deep Blue®, PastTense®; see *Muscular, Skeletal, Pain & Inflammation*
Nervous tension - black spruce, Douglas fir, InTune®, Serenity®; see *Mood & Behavior, Nervous*
Obesity/overeating - bergamot, blue tansy, cinnamon, clary sage, geranium, ginger, grapefruit, jasmine, sandalwood, Siberian fir, ylang ylang, Adaptiv®, Citrus Bliss®, Slim & Sassy®, Whisper®; see *Weight, Eating Disorders*
Physical stress - geranium, lavender, Citrus Bliss®, Peace®; see *Athletes*
Sex drive, change in - neroli, ylang ylang, Passion® Whisper®; see *Intimacy*
Shock - bergamot, frankincense, geranium, helichrysum, magnolia, melaleuca, peppermint, Roman chamomile, Adaptiv®, Motivate®, Peace®; see *First Aid*
Sleep problems - lavender, wild orange, Balance®, Serenity®; see *Sleep*
Stomach, upset - peppermint, DigestZen®; see *Digestive & Intestinal*
Stress, lack of management - blue tansy, coriander, wintergreen
Teeth grinding - black spruce, frankincense, geranium, lavender, marjoram, Roman chamomile, wild orange, Serenity®; see *Parasites*
Tension - cedarwood, copaiba, ginger, lavender, lemongrass, peppermint, Siberian fir, wintergreen, PastTense®, Serenity®; see *Muscular*
Trauma stress, intense - cedarwood, frankincense, jasmine, lavender, melissa, Roman chamomile, vetiver, ylang ylang, Adaptiv®, Balance®, InTune®, Serenity®; see *Limbic, Mood & Behavior*

* *See remedy on pg. 365*

Remedies

ROLLER BOTTLE REMEDIES

LIFT AND CALM BLEND
10 drops frankincense
12 drops Citrus Bliss®
8 drops lavender
4 drops peppermint
Combine oils into a roller bottle and fill remainder with carrier oil. Apply to pulse points and behind the ears.

ANXIETY BLEND
10 drops bergamot
10 drops lemon
10 drops Citrus Bliss®
10 drops lime
10 drops lavender
5 drops Balance®
5 drops Serenity®
Combine oils into a roller bottle and fill remainder with carrier oil. Apply to pulse points and behind the ears to help reduce feelings of anxiety.

EXHAUSTION BLEND
10 drops eucalyptus
8 drops rosemary
7 drops bergamot
7 drops grapefruit
Combine oils into a roller bottle and fill remainder of bottle with carrier oil. Apply to pulse points and behind the ears to help when feeling exhausted.

MOTIVATION BLEND
10 drops lime
10 drops wild orange
5 drops frankincense
5 drops black pepper
Combine oils into a roller bottle and fill remainder with carrier oil. Apply to pulse points and behind the ears.

RELAX DIFFUSER BLEND
Add 5 drops each blue tansy, wild orange, ylang ylang to diffuser for 30-60 minutes and enjoy.

MENTAL CLARITY BLEND
12 drops lemon
8 drops rosemary
4 drops cypress
2 drops peppermint
Combine oils into a roller bottle and fill remainder with carrier oil. Apply to pulse points and behind the ears to help increase mental clarity.

CHILL PILL BLEND
10 drops clary sage
15 drops bergamot
20 drops grapefruit
25 drops wild orange
15 drops frankincense
10 drops lemon
Combine oils into a roller bottle and fill remainder with carrier oil. Apply to pulse points and behind the ears.

FROM STESSED TO CAREFREE
7 drops green mandarin
2 drops clove
Diffuse to replace discontented, agitated, nervous, or anxious feelings.

BATH REMEDIES

The Basic De-Stress Bath
1 cup Epsom salts or sea salt
1/ 2 cup baking soda
10 drops lavender
Drop oil onto dry mixture of salt and baking soda, stir. Soak in tub as desired. Repeat throughout the week as necessary. This is a basic recipe. To individualize and cater to each unique stressful situation, select appropriate oils from list below. Then simply add 10-15 drops to bath. Combining a few oils or using an existing blend is an excellent way to enjoy the benefits of multiple oils at once.

Here are some favorites to choose from:

Bliss Bath - 7 drops Serenity® and 7 drops Roman chamomile
Calming Bath - 10 drops Serenity®
De-Stress & Focus Bath - 5 drops Serenity® and 5 drops frankincense
Energizing & Calming Bath - 7 drops wild orange and 8 drops lavender or Serenity®
Get-My-Heart-Back-in-the-Project - 2 ylang ylang and 6 wild orange
Grounding Bath - 10 drops Balance®
Life-is-Good Blend - Combine 2 drops green mandarin, 1 drop spearmint, and neroli.
Quiet-the-Mind Bath - 9 drops sandalwood , 5 drops lavender and 1 drop cedarwood
Reviving & Relaxing Bath - 10 drops Citrus Bliss®
Soothing Bath - 10 drops Deep Blue®

Take Out Tantrums Bath - 4 drops

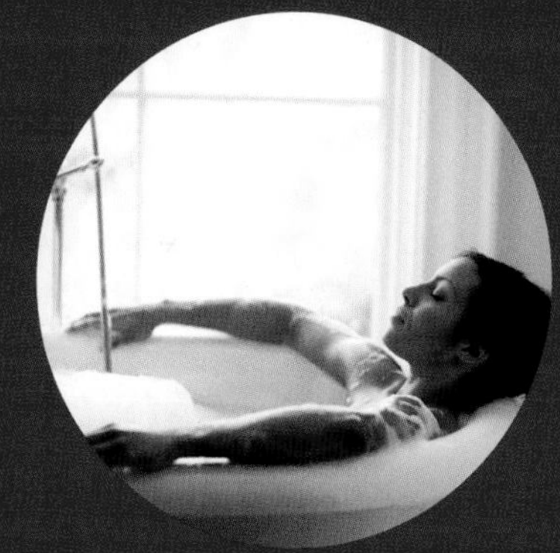

Serenity®, 3 drops lavender and 2 drops PastTense®
Tension Tamer Bath - 4 drops Serenity® and 4 drops PastTense®
Warm, Relax, Revive the Weary and Painful Bath - 4 drops ginger, 6 drops wild orange, 6 drops clove and 2 drops lavender

STRESS

USAGE TIPS: Managing and eliminating stress. Essential oils are extremely effective for stress reduction. Any method of application can be successful. Here are some primary methods:

- **Aromatic:** Get/create exposure to an aroma as a first step to success for an immediate invitation to relax, calm down, get focused or whatever is needed at the time. Diffuse favorite oils, inhale from bottle or hands, apply a few drops to clothing, or apply under nose.
- **Topical:** Apply to tense or tired muscles on back, shoulders, neck, legs, or anywhere the stress is affecting the body. This topical use also allows for an aromatic experience. Consider use on the chest, gland locations, base of skull (especially in suboccipital triangles), behind ears, or across forehead, and perfume points.
- **Internal:** Stress often affects internal activity such as digestion; choose and use oils according to needs.

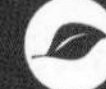

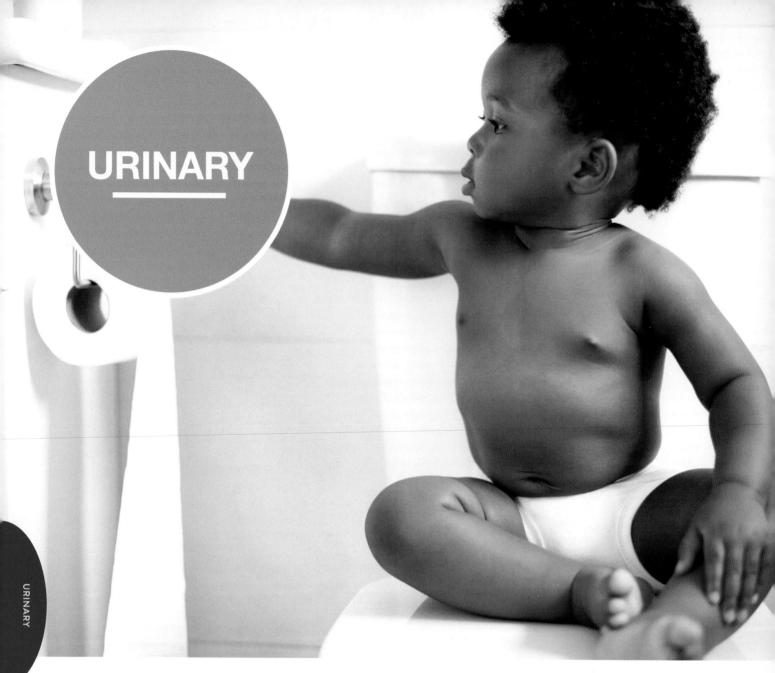

URINARY

THE URINARY TRACT consists of the kidneys, ureters, bladder, and urethra. The principal function of the urinary system is to maintain the volume and composition of body fluids within normal limits. One aspect of this function is to rid the body of waste products that accumulate as a result of cellular metabolism and, because of this, it is sometimes referred to as the excretory system. While it plays a major role in excretion, however, it relies on other organs to support this function.

The urinary system maintains appropriate fluid volumes, pH and chemical balances, and electrolyte levels through complex processes in the kidneys and by regulating the amount of water that is excreted in the urine. Urine is formed in the kidneys through a blood filtration process and carries waste products and excess fluid to the ureters, tubes made of smooth muscle fibers that propel urine toward the urinary bladder, where it is stored until it is expelled from the body.

The moving of urine from the bladder through the urethra and out of the body is called urination, or voiding.

The kidneys are also responsible for regulating sodium and potassium levels. No less important is the kidneys' ability to remove drugs from the body, release hormones that regulate blood pressure, produce an active form of vitamin D, which promotes strong, healthy bones, and control the production of red blood cells.

Most individuals operate in a constant state of dehydration, which takes its toll on overall health, but particularly impacts kidney health. In addition to adequate water intake, there are some essential oils that are extremely effective in supporting kidney health and helping the body to quickly rid itself of UTI discomfort and infections and even stones. While it is of utmost importance to utilize the services of medical professionals in the case of a prolonged or serious condition, essential oils can serve as a powerful first line of defense.

TOP SOLUTIONS

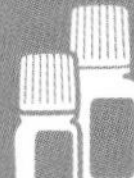

SINGLE OILS

Lemon - helps dissolve stones and acts as diuretic (pg. 123)
Juniper berry - acts as diuretic; tonifies bladder and supports urinary system (pg. 119)
Lemongrass - decongests urinary tract and fights urinary infections (pg. 126)
Cypress - resolves incontinence and excessive water/fluid retention (pg. 103)
Thyme - supports healthy prostate and circulation; fights urinary infections (pg. 157)
Eucalyptus - relieves infection, stones (pg. 107)
Celery seed - acts as diuretic, stress

By Related Properties

For more, See Oil Properties on pages 477 - 481

Anti-infectious - arborvitae, basil, bergamot, cardamom, cedarwood, cinnamon, citronella, clove, copaiba, cypress, eucalyptus, frankincense, geranium, lavender, litsea, marjoram, melaleuca, patchouli, Roman chamomile, rose, rosemary, turmeric
Anti-inflammatory - arborvitae, basil, bergamot, birch, black pepper, blue tansy, cardamom, cassia, cedarwood, cinnamon, copaiba, cypress, dill, eucalyptus, fennel, frankincense, geranium, ginger, helichrysum, lavender, lemongrass, lime, litsea, manuka, melaleuca, melissa, myrrh, neroli, oregano, patchouli, peppermint, rosemary, sandalwood, Siberian fir, spearmint, spikenard, tangerine, wild orange, wintergreen, yarrow
Cleanser - arborvitae, cilantro, eucalyptus, grapefruit, juniper berry, lemon, thyme, wild orange
Detoxifier - arborvitae, cassia, cilantro, citronella, cypress, geranium, juniper berry, lemon, lime, litsea, patchouli, rosemary, tangerine, wild orange, yarrow
Diuretic - arborvitae, basil, bergamot, birch, cardamom, cedarwood, celery seed, copaiba, cypress, eucalyptus, fennel, frankincense, geranium, grapefruit, helichrysum, juniper berry, lavender, lemon, lime, marjoram, patchouli, ravensara, rosemary, sandalwood, tangerine, thyme, white fir, wild orange, wintergreen
Purifier - arborvitae, cinnamon, eucalyptus, grapefruit, lemon, lemongrass, lime, manuka, marjoram, melaleuca, oregano, Siberian fir, tangerine, wild orange, yarrow

Related Ailments: Bed-Wetting, Berger's Disease, Incontinence, Kidney Infection, Kidney Stones, Overactive Bladder, Poor Urine Flow, Ureter Infection, Urinary Tract Infection (UTI), Urination (Painful/Frequent)

BLENDS

DDR Prime® - antioxidant; cleanses and disinfects urinary tract (pg. 184)
Zendocrine® - supports proper liver and kidney function (pg. 206)
Slim & Sassy® - acts as diuretic and detoxifies (pg. 200)
On Guard® - promotes blood flow and elimination of waste (pg. 194)

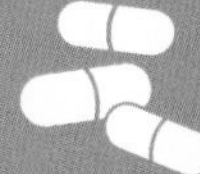

SUPPLEMENTS

Alpha CRS®+, **Zendocrine® Softgels (pg. 224), Zendocrine® Complex (pg. 223), DDR Prime® Softgels (pg. 211)**, Slim & Sassy® Softgels, **On Guard Softgels (pg. 215)**, MicroPlex VMz

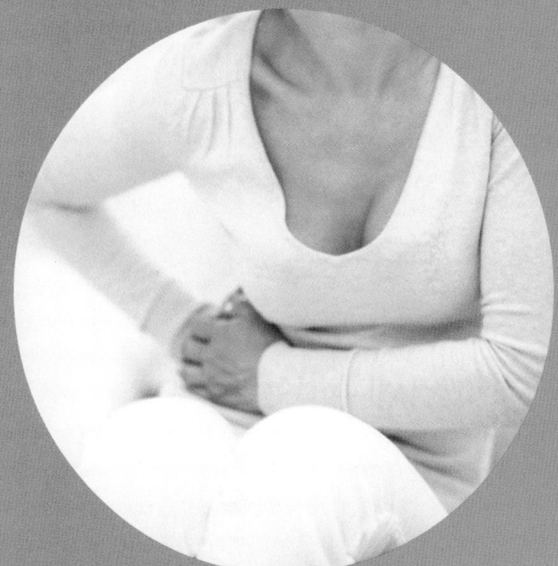

USAGE TIPS: For best success in supporting urinary conditions

- **Internal:** Use softgels or place drops of oil(s) in a capsule and consume every few hours for acute situations; or under tongue or in water.
- **Topical:** Place over urinary areas of bladder/kidneys. Use carrier oil as needed to prevent sensitivity; spine, bottoms of feet also excellent locations.
- **Aromatic:** Diffuse oils through night for nighttime concerns such as bed-wetting.

Conditions

Abdominal pain - coriander, grapefruit, ginger, lavender, oregano, rosemary, Purify; see *Digestive & Intestinal*
Bed-wetting* - black pepper, cinnamon, copaiba, cypress, frankincense, juniper berry, spearmint, rosemary, Peace®, Zendocrine®
Bladder Stones - celery seed
Disorders - basil, bergamot, birch, cypress, juniper berry, lavender, lemongrass, lime, rosemary, sandalwood, thyme, wintergreen, DDR Prime®, DigestZen®
Dribbling/minor leaks - cypress, marjoram, thyme, DDR Prime®
Edema - See "Water Retention" below
Excrete uric acid/toxins - cardamom, cypress, frankincense, juniper berry, lemon, petitgrain, rosemary, Balance®, Purify, Zendocrine®
Hesitancy, urine flow - basil, celery seed, cypress, ginger, thyme, Slim & Sassy®
Incontinence* - basil, copaiba, coriander, cypress, rosemary, spearmint, AromaTouch®, Forgive®
Incontinence, emotional (repression of emotions) - black pepper, cypress, ginger, juniper berry, lavender, thyme, vetiver, AromaTouch®, Zendocrine®; see *Mood & Behavior*
Infections, bladder - arborvitae, birch, bergamot, cedarwood, cinnamon, clove, copaiba, eucalyptus, fennel, juniper berry, lemon, lemongrass, rosemary, sandalwood, spearmint, thyme, white fir, wintergreen, Console®, On Guard®, Purify
Infections, kidney - bergamot, cardamom, cinnamon, coriander, fennel, juniper berry, lemon, lemongrass, neroli, rosemary, sandalwood, spearmint, thyme, DDR Prime®, On Guard®, Passion®, Purify
Infections, urinary - bergamot, blue tansy, cedarwood, cinnamon, citronella, copaiba, fennel, lemon, lemongrass, geranium, juniper berry, neroli, rosemary, sandalwood, Siberian fir, thyme, yarrow, DDR Prime®, On Guard®, Passion®, Purify
Ketones in urine - coriander, fennel, juniper berry, rosemary, thyme
Kidney stones* - birch, cinnamon, celery seed, clary sage, eucalyptus, fennel, geranium, juniper berry, lemon, sandalwood, spearmint, wild orange, wintergreen, Forgive®
Kidney, circulation - basil, coriander, juniper berry
Kidney, toxic - bergamot, cardamom, coriander, grapefruit, juniper berry, lemon, lemongrass, turmeric, Purify, Slim & Sassy®, Zendocrine®
Kidney, weak - geranium, helichrysum, juniper berry, lemongrass, rosemary
Low-force/volume urine stream - bergamot, cardamom, cinnamon, lemon, juniper berry, marjoram, thyme, AromaTouch®, Console®, Slim & Sassy®, Zendocrine®
Nausea/vomiting - bergamot, clove, fennel, ginger, lemon; see *Digestive & Intestinal*
Pelvic pressure - basil, cypress, clary sage, ginger, lavender, peppermint, Slim & Sassy®
Perspiration, lack of - cardamom, cilantro, ginger, juniper berry, lemongrass, oregano, Purify
Pus or blood in urine - basil, cardamom, frankincense, lemon, melaleuca, oregano, sandalwood, Citrus Bliss®, DDR Prime®, On Guard®, Purify, Zendocrine®; see *Immune & Lymphatic*
Sharp/spastic pains in kidneys or bladder when urinating - basil, cardamom, cilantro, clary sage, cypress, grapefruit, juniper berry, lavender, lemon, marjoram, Roman chamomile, thyme, white fir, PastTense®
Swollen ankles, toes, fingers - basil, cypress, frankincense, grapefruit, lemon, marjoram, patchouli, AromaTouch®
Urination, painful/burning/frequent* - basil, birch, cinnamon, juniper berry, lemongrass, sandalwood, AromaTouch®, On Guard®, Zendocrine®
Urgency of urination - cypress, frankincense, oregano, Balance®, DigestZen®
Water retention (edema) - blue tansy, cardamom, cedarwood, celery seed, cinnamon, cypress, Douglas fir, eucalyptus, fennel, frankincense, geranium, ginger, grapefruit, green mandarin, juniper berry, lemon, lemongrass, rosemary, Siberian fir, spikenard, tangerine, thyme, white fir, wild orange, wintergreen, AromaTouch®, Forgive®, Slim & Sassy®, Zendocrine®

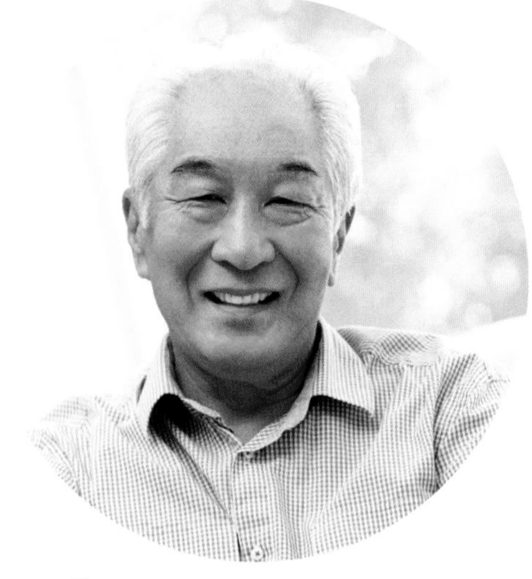

Remedies

ROCKIN' RELIEF (for kidney stones)
4 drops helichrysum
4 drops juniper berry
5 drops grapefruit
5 drops lemon
Combine in a 15ml bottle, fill remainder with carrier oil. Apply over lower back every twenty minutes and cover with hot, moist compress. Note: avoid alcohol, sugars, refined foods, and drink ample amounts of water.

FIRE EXTINGUISHER (supports resolving urinary burning/infection)
2 drops sandalwood
6 drops Purify
4 drops juniper berry
5 drops lemongrass
Combine in a 5ml roller bottle, fill remainder with carrier oil. Apply topically on lower abdomen over bladder and on lower back over kidneys every twenty minutes during daytime hours until pain no longer reoccurs. 1 drop On Guard® in a glass of water internally morning and evening. Continue bladder blend three times daily. Take On Guard® in water for three days after pain subsides.
Note: avoid alcohol, sugars, refined foods, drink ample amounts of water.

IN CONTROL (bladder control - for incontinence/bed-wetting)
1 drop juniper berry
1 drop cypress
Combine in palm and apply topically across lower abdomen, use for occasional inconvenient urges, or three-plus times a day for chronic control issues.

* See remedy on this page

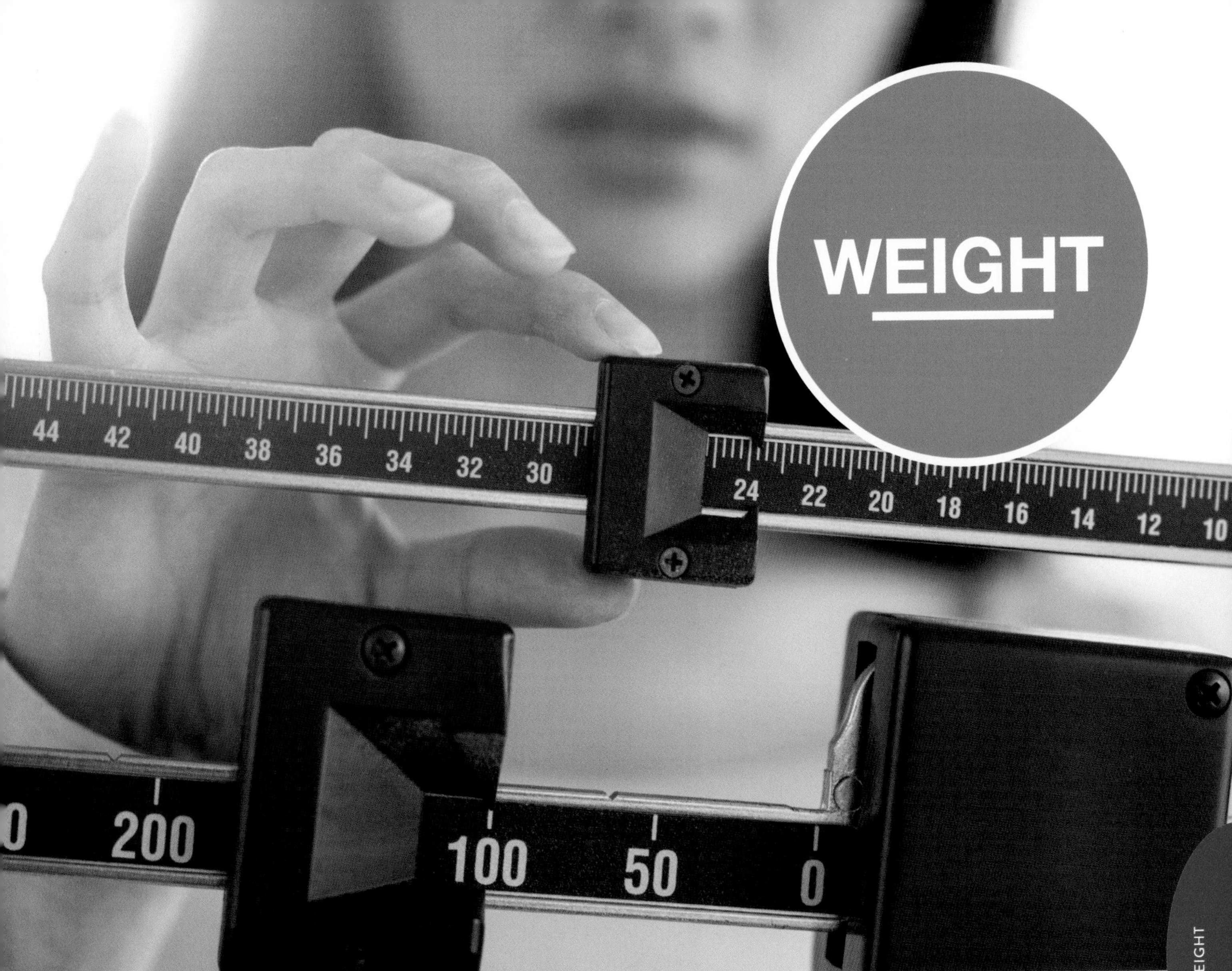

WEIGHT GAIN can result from an increase in muscle mass, fat deposits, or excess fluids such as water. The most common causes of weight gain are from excessive eating and poor nutrition. Food is made up of calories, or units of energy. Physical activity and normal body metabolism burn calories. When a person takes in more calories than the body uses, the extra calories are stored as fat subsequently enlarging or decreasing the "size" of fat cells depending on the balance of energy in the body. When fat cells build up or accumulate, it causes increased fat or obesity.

Other factors that may cause weight gain include medication, lack of lean muscle mass, inactivity, hypothyroidism, menopause, pregnancy, or slow metabolism. Sometimes toxicity levels within the body can encourage the body to hold onto fat; when there are too many toxins for the body to handle, the fats are diverted into fat cells -- the only place in the body where natural insulation provides protection for vital body organs. Later, when individuals try to lose weight, despite effort it seems to prove to be next to impossible. These protective

fat cells are programmed to guard the vital organs at all costs; therefore they cannot let go of their cargo.

Being overweight can bring about undesirable emotional effects such as depression, anxiety, and mood swings. Excess weight or obesity can cause exhaustion or fatigue and challenge individuals participating in various activities, a scenario especially difficult for overweight parents with active children. It causes undue stress on joints, bones, and muscles. Carrying excess fat can also dramatically increase the risk of developing deadly and debilitating diseases.

Essential oils and whole-food supplementation can be powerful allies in the process of maintaining a healthy weight and losing excess weight. Essential oils have the ability to coax toxic fat cells into releasing their contents, help break down the toxins, and, with proper hydration, flush them out of the body. Oils can also support the body's insulin response, reduce cravings, and provide a feeling of satiety. Supplements can give the cells the energy they need to carry out proper body function, including extra fuel for working out. Digestive enzymes help the body break down and utilize nutrients for maximum support.

TOP SOLUTIONS

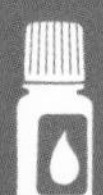

SINGLE OILS

Grapefruit - curbs cravings, reduces appetite, and induces fat burning (pg. 114)
Cinnamon - inhibits formation of new fat cells; balances blood sugar (pg. 93)
Peppermint - enhances sense of fullness; reduces cravings and appetite (pg. 140)
Ginger - encourages fat burning and promotes satiation (pg. 113)

By Related Properties

For more, See Oil Properties on pages 477 - 481

Analgesic - arborvitae, bergamot, black pepper, blue tansy, cassia, cinnamon, clary sage, clove, copaiba, coriander, cypress, eucalyptus, frankincense, helichrysum, jasmine, juniper berry, lavender, lemongrass, litsea, marjoram, oregano, peppermint, ravensara, rosemary, Siberian fir, wild orange, wintergreen, yarrow
Antidepressant - basil, bergamot, clary sage, coriander, dill, frankincense, geranium, grapefruit, jasmine, lavender, lemon, lemongrass, melissa, neroli, oregano, patchouli, ravensara, rose, tangerine, wild orange
Calming - bergamot, birch, black pepper, blue tansy, cassia, clary sage, copaiba, coriander, fennel, frankincense, geranium, jasmine, juniper berry, lavender, litsea, magnolia, oregano, patchouli, Roman chamomile, sandalwood, tangerine, yarrow
Detoxifier - arborvitae, cassia, cilantro, cypress, geranium, juniper berry, lemon, lime, litsea, patchouli, rosemary, tangerine, wild orange, yarrow
Energizing - basil, clove, cypress, grapefruit, lemongrass, pink pepper, rosemary, Siberian fir, tangerine, wild orange, yarrow
Steroidal - basil, birch, cedarwood, clove, fennel, patchouli, rosemary, thyme
Stimulant - arborvitae, basil, bergamot, birch, black pepper, blue tansy, cardamom, cedarwood, cinnamon, clove, coriander, cypress, dill, eucalyptus, fennel, ginger, grapefruit, juniper berry, lime, melaleuca, myrrh, patchouli, rosemary, Siberian fir, spearmint, tangerine, thyme, vetiver, white fir, wintergreen, ylang ylang
Stomachic - basil, blue tansy, cardamom, cinnamon, clary sage, coriander, fennel, ginger, juniper berry, marjoram, melissa, peppermint, pink pepper, rose, rosemary, tangerine, turmeric, wild orange, yarrow
Uplifting - bergamot, cardamom, cedarwood, clary sage, cypress, grapefruit, lemon, lime, litsea, melissa, sandalwood, tangerine, wild orange, ylang ylang

Related Ailments: Excessive Appetite, Autointoxication, Cellulite, Loss of Appetite, Obesity, Overeating

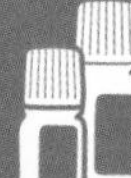

BLENDS

Slim & Sassy® - balances metabolism, eliminates cravings, and lifts mood; acts as diuretic (pg. 200)
Zendocrine® - support body's ability to remove toxins and waste effectively (pg. 224)
DDR Prime® - improves function of the endocrine system and thyroid (pg. 184)

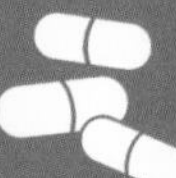

SUPPLEMENTS

Alpha CRS®+, PB Assist®+, **Zendocrine® Complex (pg. 223)**, DigestZen® softgels, xEO Mega, TerraGreens®, **TrimShake® (pg. 220)**, **Slim & Sassy® Softgels (pg. 218)**, Phytoestrogen Complex, MicroPlex VMz

USAGE TIPS: For weight management, the focus is primarily on what and how much food is consumed (appetite) and how well it is utilized as fuel by the body (metabolism). Additionally, balancing other processes such as elimination, blood sugar, and hormones is often necessary for long-lasting results. See suggested programs in "Remedies" below. With that in mind:

- **Internal:** Ingesting oils for support with appetite, cravings and metabolism, including the ability to burn fat and release it along with toxins is very effective. Place drops of oils in a capsule for systemic or on-going support. Drink oils in water; drop on tongue. Be generous with usage for this purpose.
- **Topical:** Use to assist the body to detox and target specific zones. Consider applying blends of oils to areas like the abdomen, thighs, and arms as a treatment. Use a carrier oil if necessary to prevent sensitivity especially with oils like cinnamon.
- **Aromatic:** Excellent for supporting appetite control. Inhale as needed.

Conditions

Anorexia - See *Eating Disorders*
Appetite, excess* - bergamot, cassia, cinnamon, citronella, fennel, ginger, grapefruit, juniper berry, lemon, peppermint, Peace®, Slim & Sassy®; if due to nutritional deficiencies see *Weight* - "Supplements"
Appetite, imbalanced - grapefruit, tangerine, wild orange, Slim & Sassy®
Appetite, loss of - bergamot, black pepper, cardamom, coriander, fennel, ginger, grapefruit, lemon, patchouli, spearmint, tangerine, thyme, Console®, DigestZen®, Passion®, PastTense®, Peace®, Purify, Slim & Sassy®
Blood sugar imbalance - cassia, cinnamon, coriander, fennel, green mandarin, pink pepper, rosemary, Cheer®, On Guard®, Slim & Sassy®; see *Blood Sugar*
Cellulite* - birch, cypress, Douglas fir, eucalyptus, geranium, ginger, grapefruit, lemongrass, lemon, lime, pink pepper (obesity), rosemary, Siberian fir, spikenard, tangerine, Siberian fir, wild orange, wintergreen, Slim & Sassy®; see *Detoxification*
Cravings* - ginger, grapefruit, peppermint, Slim & Sassy®
Cravings, sugar - cassia, cinnamon, clove, grapefruit, Slim & Sassy®
Eating, over/binging/compulsive - bergamot, black pepper, cedarwood, cinnamon, ginger, grapefruit, juniper berry, lemon, oregano, patchouli, peppermint, Elevation™, Slim & Sassy®
Edema/swelling/water retention - basil, cypress, ginger, green mandarin, juniper berry, lemon, lemongrass, patchouli, rosemary, tangerine, Slim & Sassy®; see *Urinary*
Emotional/stress-induced eating - bergamot, grapefruit, Slim & Sassy®; see *Eating Disorders, Mood & Behavior*
Energy, low/fatigue/exhaustion - basil, green mandarin, lime, peppermint, pink pepper, rosemary, jasmine; see *Energy & Vitality*
Excessive weight/obese - birch, cinnamon, fennel, ginger, grapefruit, juniper berry, lemon, oregano, tangerine, wild orange, wintergreen, Slim & Sassy®
Fat, breakdown/dissolve - grapefruit, lemon, neroli, spearmint, tangerine, Slim & Sassy®
Food addiction - basil, black pepper, cardamom, ginger, grapefruit, Slim & Sassy®; see *Addictions*
Hunger pains - fennel, myrrh, oregano, peppermint, InTune®; see *Digestion & Intestinal*
Inability to lose weight - cinnamon, coriander, spearmint, Slim & Sassy®, Zendocrine®; see *Candida, Detoxification*
Metabolism, slow* - cassia, clove, ginger, lemongrass, pink pepper, spearmint, tangerine, Slim & Sassy®
Metabolism, too fast - ginger, Slim & Sassy®, myrrh, Breathe® drops
Overindulgence of food* - grapefruit, juniper berry, peppermint, Slim & Sassy®
Pancreas, inflamed - dill, fennel; see *Endocrine (Pancreas)*
Satiety/satiation, lack of - bergamot, dill, fennel, ginger, grapefruit, peppermint
Sagging skin - helichrysum, grapefruit, AromaTouch®, Immortelle; see *Integumentary*
Sense of self, poor/self worth, lack of* - bergamot, grapefruit, jasmine, Elevation™; see *Mood & Behavior*
Stretch marks - frankincense, geranium, lavender, sandalwood, tangerine, Immortelle; see *Integumentary*
Thyroid imbalances - coriander, clove, frankincense, ginger, rosemary, Immortelle; see *Endocrine (Thyroid, Adrenal)*
Toxicity* - lemon, grapefruit, rosemary, Slim & Sassy®, Zendocrine®; see *Detoxification*

** See remedy on pg. 373*

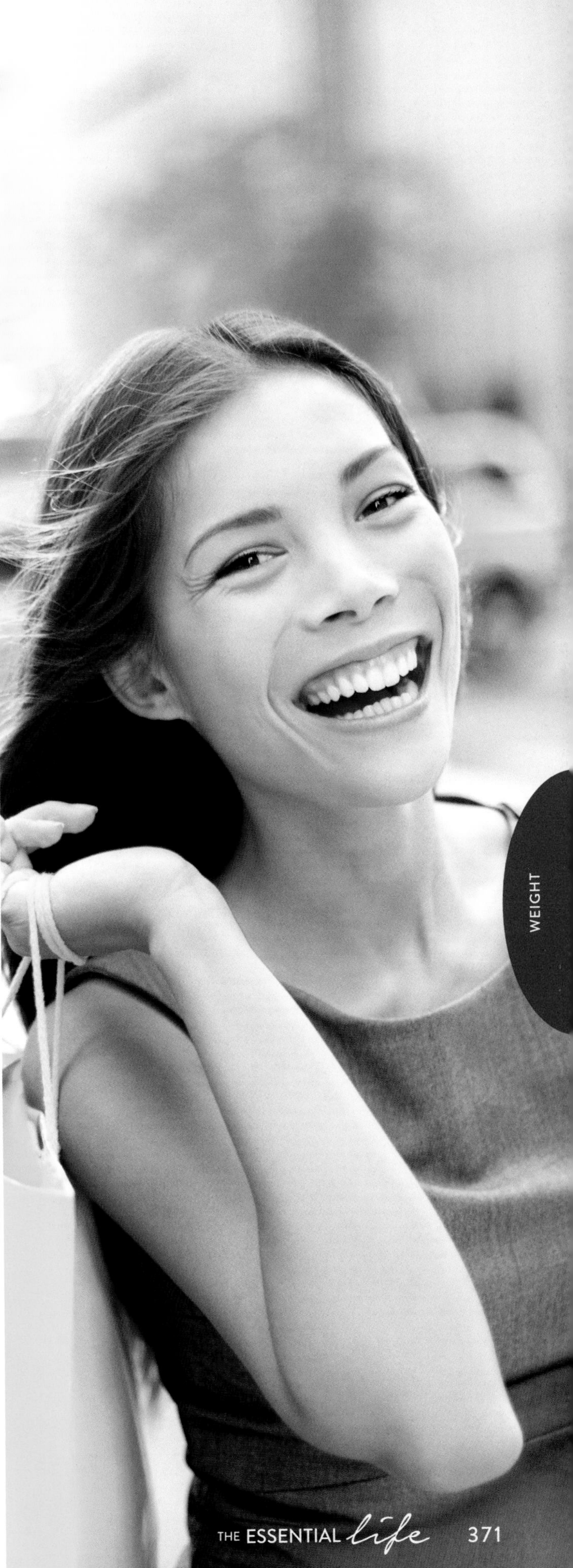

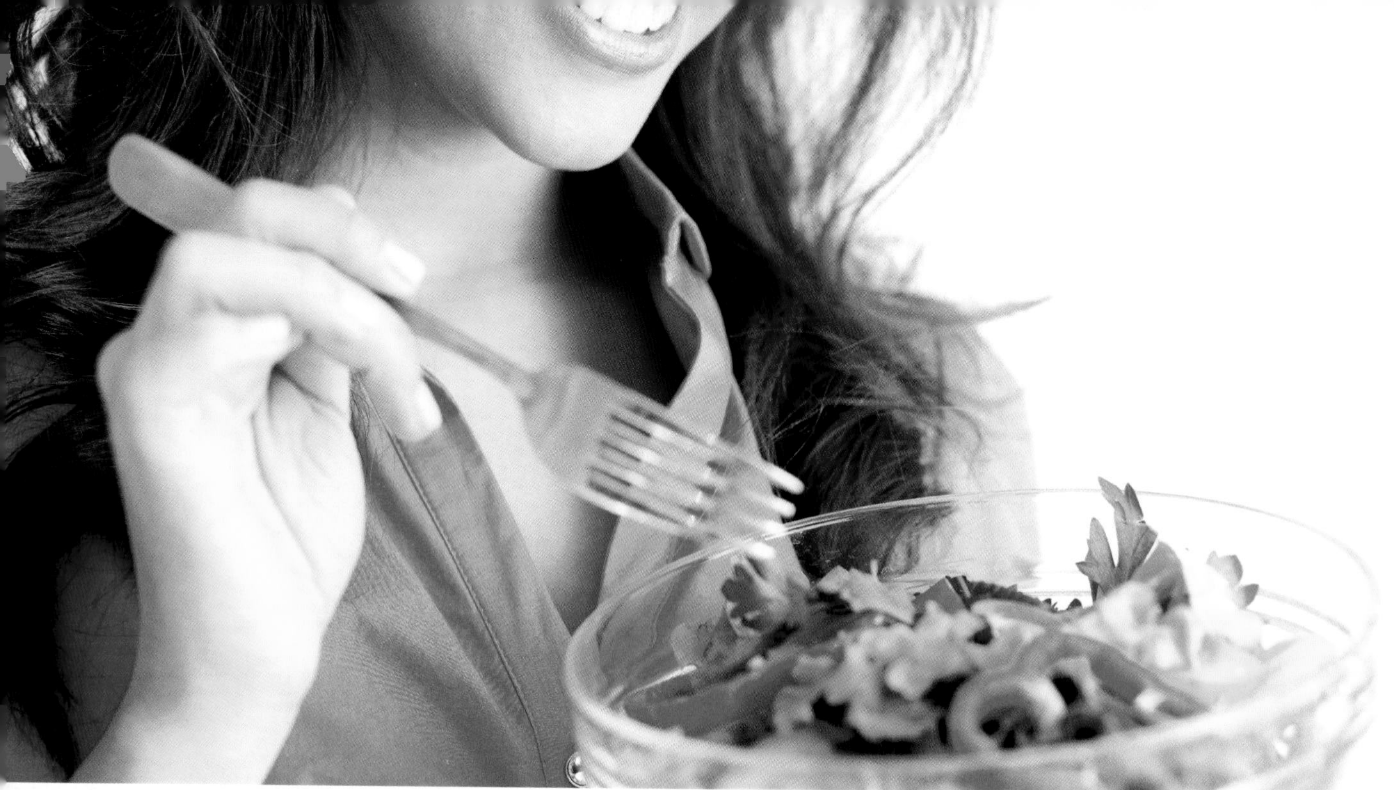

Weight Loss Program

	10-30 days (Pre-Cleanse)	10 days (Cleanse)	20 days (Restore)	30 days (Maintain)
UPON RISING	Slim & Sassy® in or with water			
MORNING MEAL	- TrimShake® - MicroPlex VMz - xEO Mega - Zendocrine® Complex - TerraZyme® ***	- TrimShake® - MicroPlex VMz - xEO Mega - GX Assist® * - Zendocrine®	- TrimShake® - MicroPlex VMz - xEO Mega - TerraZyme® *** - PB Assist®+ **	- TrimShake® - MicroPlex VMz - xEO Mega [optional: TerraZyme® ***]
BETWEEN MEALS	Slim & Sassy® in or with water			
NOON MEAL	- TrimShake® - TerraZyme® ***	- TrimShake® - GX Assist® *	- Healthy Meal or TrimShake® - TerraZyme® ***	- Healthy Meal or TrimShake® [optional: TerraZyme® ***]
BETWEEN MEALS	Slim & Sassy® in or with water			
EVENING MEAL	- Healthy Meal - MicroPlex VMz - xEO Mega - Zendocrine® Complex - TerraZyme® ***	- Healthy Meal - MicroPlex VMz - xEO Mega - TerraZyme® *** - GX Assist® * - Zendocrine®	- Healthy Meal - MicroPlex VMz - xEO Mega - TerraZyme® *** - PB Assist®+ **	- Healthy Meal - MicroPlex VMz - xEO Mega [optional: TerraZyme® ***]
BETWEEN MEALS	Slim & Sassy® in or with water			
EXERCISE	Aerobic (20+ minutes 3X per week) Resistance (10+ minutes 3X per week) Flexibility (5-20 minutes daily)			

* GX Assist® - start with 1 softgel a day, increasing to 3 a day as comfortable.
**PB Assist®+ will last for 15 days (2 capsules per day for 15 days in a 30-count bottle)
*** TerraZyme® - take 1-2 per meal

NOTE: Slim & Sassy® should be taken 5 drops 5X daily (only mentioned 4X above) fit the 5th in during the day (there are 5 drops per softgel)
CAUTION: Always follow common sense, and the advice of your health care professional***

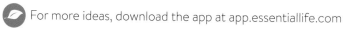

Remedies

WEIGHT LOSS DETOX AND METABOLISM BOOST

- Take 5 drops Slim & Sassy® in capsule or water two to five times per day.
- Take 3 drops Zendocrine® in capsule two times a day. Can combine oils.
- Take 1-2 capsules of TerraZyme® with every meal.
- Apply grapefruit topically to troubled areas. Dilute as needed or desired.
- Address thyroid - see Endocrine (Thyroid).
- Rub 1-2 drops of Balance® on bottoms of feet morning and evening.
- As a morning meal, use TrimShake®. Add cinnamon, cassia, or citrus oil to enhance flavor and benefits.

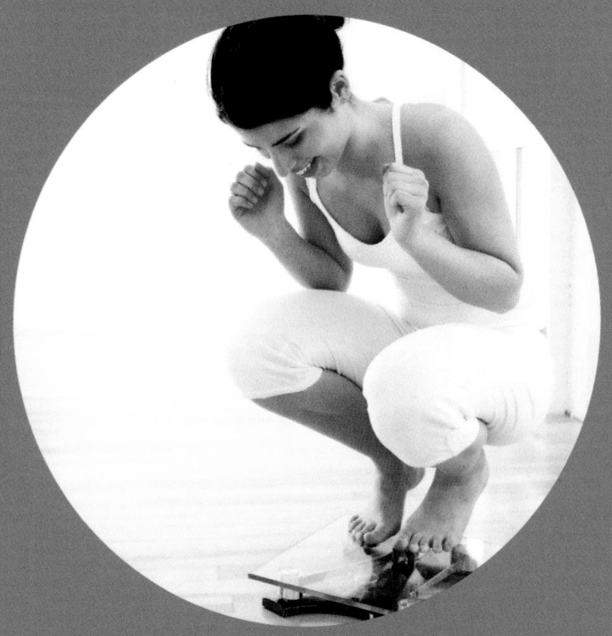

BODY SLIMMING WRAP

30 drops Slim & Sassy®
15 drops eucalyptus
15 drops peppermint
10 drops grapefruit
10 drops lavender
10 drops ClaryCalm®
5 drops wintergreen

Use a 4 ounce glass bottle with a sprayer top for ease of use. Mix oils in bottle. Swirl. Fill remainder with fractionated coconut oil. Optional: add oils to approximately 4 ounces of non-scented natural lotion as an alternative.

Instructions for use:

- Step 1: Measure the areas to be addressed prior to use.
- Step 2: Spray or apply mixture to areas of concern.
- Step 3: Place and wrap around body cotton fabric (e.g. muslin) or paper towel as a barrier between skin and plastic wrap so as not to absorb toxins from plastic (oils breakdown some plastics).
- Step 4: Using plastic wrap, wrap around about 3-4 layers
- Step 5: Leave on for anywhere from a few hours to overnight as desired and then remove.
- Step 6: Measure treated areas again and record difference.

NOTE: Drink plenty of water with lemon oil (4 drops per 16 ounces) before and after treatment. It is an excellent diuretic and helps release toxins from fat.

WEIGHT LOSS TUMMY RUB

8 drops fennel
5 drops grapefruit
4 drops patchouli
2 ounces fractionated coconut oil

Blend and store in glass bottle. Recipe can be doubled as desired. Apply to tummy. Enhance the effects by adding Slim & Sassy® to your water all day long.

CELLULITE/WEIGHT LOSS/DETOX BATH

2 cups Epsom salt
1 cups baking soda
10 drops Slim & Sassy®

Mix ingredients and use desired quantity in the bath. Soak twenty minutes or longer two to three times a week. Drink lots of water during and/or after. Add 5 drops Slim & Sassy® per 16 ounces drinking water for enhanced results and as a daily habit.

APPETITE CONTROL INHALER BLENDS

Pick a blend below and place into inhaler. Breathe in scent of blend with three long deep breaths through nostrils. Use inhaler prior to eating and when appetite is triggered.

- **Sexy Citrus**
  30 drops grapefruit
  4 drops lemon
  1 drop ylang ylang

- **Marvelous Mint**
  20 drops peppermint
  10 drops bergamot
  4 drops spearmint
  1 drop ylang ylang

- **Herbal Mix**
  15 drops basil
  15 drops marjoram
  1 drop oregano
  1 drop thyme

CRAVE AWAY

Place 1-3 drops of grapefruit or kumquat into palms, rub hands together vigorously; cup hands together and slowly inhale. May augment with a drop of patchouli.

"TONE" UP YOUR MUSCLES

Combine 4 drops basil, 3 drops cypress, 3 drops rosemary, 3 drops lavender with 1 teaspoon of carrier oil. Rub into muscles before workout. Enhances muscle tone, prevents sore muscles.

LOVE YOURSELF

Apply 1-2 drops grapefruit topically to chest or diffuse to encourage positive relationships with physical self.

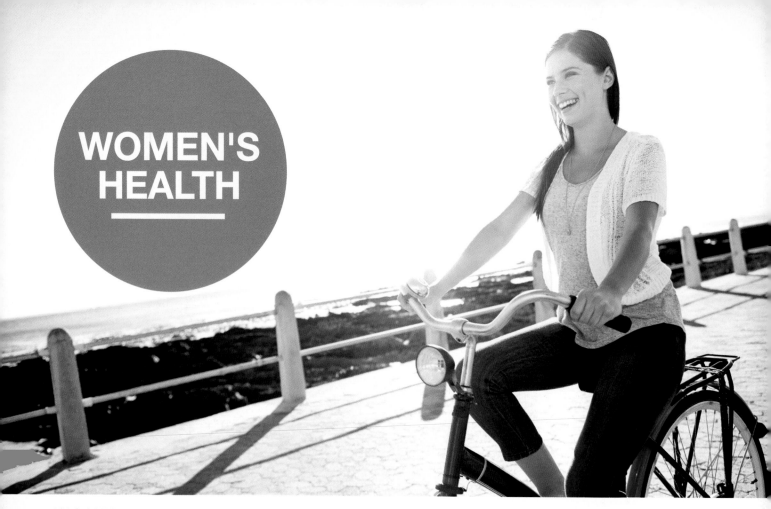

WOMEN face health challenges specific to their gender including, but not limited to, the reproductive system, brain, heart, skeleton, and hormone issues. Many women suffer from high cortisol levels, which lead to fatigue, weight changes, depression, anxiety, and digestive problems. At all stages of life, most women do their best to maintain homeostasis while multitasking. Physical and emotional stress can be a cause and symptom of many women's issues.

The female reproductive system works closely with other systems, specifically the endocrine system. The female reproductive system includes the ovaries, fallopian tubes, uterus, cervix, external genitalia, and breasts. The ovaries are responsible for producing egg cells as well as secreting the hormones estrogen and progesterone. These hormones are vital to reproductive health and fertility, but they also play a role in the balance of a woman's emotional and physical health. They influence other body tissue and even bone mass. Hydration and nutrition can directly impact the production of these hormones. Women with lower body fat sometimes do not produce enough of the sex hormones and can encounter amenorrhea (an abnormal absence of menstruation) and decreased bone density.

For approximately forty years of their lives women experience the menstruation cycle. This monthly cycle (26-35 days) involves egg development and release from the ovaries, the uterus preparing to receive a fertilized egg, and the shedding of the uterine lining if an egg is not fertilized. Many women experience difficulty during the second half of this cycle in the form of premenstrual syndrome and menstrual cramps. Irritability, anxiousness, bloating, headaches, and even migraines can be common at this time. The cycle is maintained through the secretion of the sex hormones. An imbalance of sex hormones can lead to a lack of period as well as irregular and/or extended bleeding. This can be linked to polycystic ovary syndrome or endometriosis.

As a woman ages, the sex hormones begin to diminish. Menopause refers to the time when menstruation no longer occurs due to diminished sex hormones, specifically after a lack of twelve periods. This change leads to periodic instability of functions in the body, and side effects such as hot flashes, mood swings, vaginal dryness, fluctuations in sexual desire, fatigue, forgetfulness, and urinary incontinence can occur.

Nutrition and hydration are important keys to a woman's health. Daily supplements that include a whole food nutrient supplement, essential oil xEO Mega, bone supplement complex, and phytoestrogen complex will help a woman's body be able to regulate hormones properly. The phytoestrogen complex is a natural form of estrogen-like therapy, assisting to balance not only a deficiency, but also any excess of the wrong kind and harmful estrogen metabolites. Whisper® can be applied to the wrists, ankles, and directly over the abdomen when symptoms of PMS and menopause are occurring. Grapefruit and thyme oils support healthy progesterone levels, the counterbalance hormone to estrogen. Also, mood-enhancing oils, including Elevation™, Serenity®, Citrus Bliss®, and Balance®, can help with depression and other emotions that may be prevalent for women.

TOP SOLUTIONS

SINGLE OILS

Rose - helps overcome frigidity and infertility; promotes healthy menstruation (pg. 148)
Geranium - supports hormone, emotional balance, and fertility (pg. 112)
Neroli and Ylang ylang - promotes healthy libido; relaxes (pgs. 136 & 165)
Clary sage - enhances endocrine system function and balances hormones (pg. 96)
Grapefruit - supports healthy progesterone levels and breast health (pg. 114)
Jasmine - promotes a healthy uterus, libido (pg. 118)
Ginger - promotes healthy menstruation and libido; relieves cramps (pg. 113)
Fennel - supports healthy estrogen levels and supports healthy ovaries (pg. 108)
Thyme and oregano - supports healthy progesterone levels (pg. 157) (pg. 138)

By Related Properties

For more, See Oil Properties on pages 477 - 481

Analgesic - arborvitae, basil, bergamot, birch, black pepper, blue tansy, cassia, cinnamon, clary sage, clove, copaiba, coriander, cypress, fennel, frankincense, ginger, helichrysum, jasmine, juniper berry, lavender, lemongrass, litsea, marjoram, melaleuca, oregano, peppermint, rosemary, Siberian fir, turmeric, wild orange, wintergreen, yarrow
Antidepressant - basil, bergamot, cinnamon, clary sage, coriander, dill, frankincense, geranium, grapefruit, jasmine, lemon, lemongrass, magnolia, melissa, neroli, oregano, patchouli, ravensara, rose, sandalwood, tangerine, wild orange, ylang ylang
Antihemorrhagic - geranium, helichrysum, yarrow
Aphrodisiac - black pepper, cardamom, cinnamon, clary sage, clove, coriander, ginger, jasmine, juniper berry, magnolia, neroli, patchouli, peppermint, pink pepper, ravensara, rose, rosemary, sandalwood, spearmint, thyme, vetiver, wild orange, ylang ylang
Detoxifier - arborvitae, cassia, celery seed, cilantro, cypress, geranium, juniper berry, lemon, lime, litsea, patchouli, rosemary, tangerine, turmeric, wild orange, yarrow
Emmenagogue - arborvitae, basil, cassia, cedarwood, cinnamon, clary sage, dill, fennel, ginger, jasmine, juniper berry, lavender, marjoram, myrrh, oregano, peppermint, Roman chamomile, rose, rosemary, spearmint, thyme, wintergreen, yarrow
Galactagogue - basil, clary sage, dill, fennel, jasmine, lemongrass, wintergreen

Related Ailments: Amenorrhea, Dysmenorrhea, Endometriosis, Estrogen Imbalance [Detoxification], Excessive Menstrual Bleeding, Female Hormonal Imbalance [Detoxification], Fibrocystic Breasts [Endocrine], Fibroids [Cellular Health], Hot Flashes, Infertility, Irregular Menstrual Cycle, Lack Of Ovulation, Libido (low) for Women, Menopause, Menorrhagia, Menstrual Pain, Ovarian Cyst, Pelvic Pain Syndrome, Perimenopause, PMS, Polycystic Ovary Syndrome (PCOS), Scanty Menstruation, Vaginal Yeast Infections [Candida], Vaginitis, Xenoestrogen

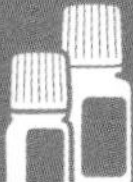

BLENDS

Whisper® - stabilizes mood and supports proper endocrine function (pg. 205)
ClaryCalm® - supports monthly cycle (pg. 182)
Motivate® - supports healthy reproductive function (pg. 193)

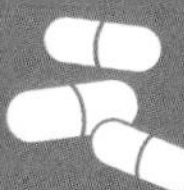

SUPPLEMENTS

Bone Nutrient Lifetime Complex (pg. 210), Alpha CRS®+, DDR Prime® Softgels, **xEO Mega (pg. 222)**, IQ Mega®, **phytoestrogen complex (pg. 217)**, **MicroPlex VMz (pg. 214)**

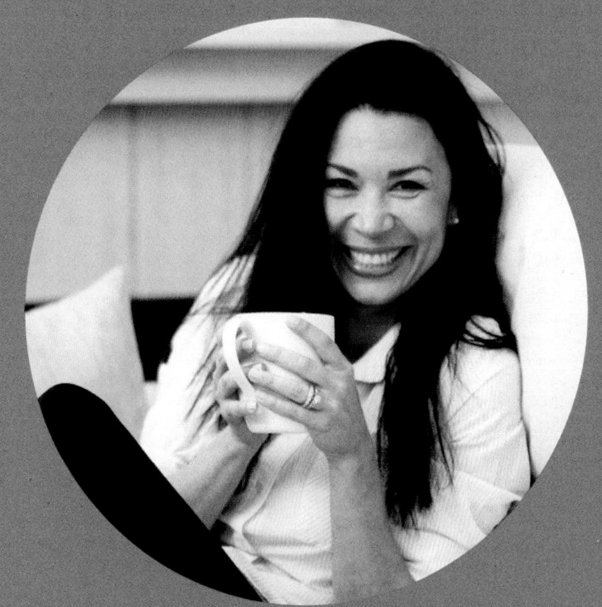

USAGE TIPS: For best results for women's health

- **Aromatic:** Women are very sensitive and emotionally responsive to aromas. Consider regular use for promoting emotional stability. Diffuse selected oils that derive desired results. Additionally, use favorite oils to wear as perfume; apply to wrists and neck. Smell wrists throughout the day. Reapply as needed.
- **Topical:** Apply selected oils to back of neck and shoulders or other areas of need (e.g. back, for menstrual cramps) to reduce tension, soothe sore muscles, reduce spasms.

Remedies

COOL YOUR HOT MESS (for PMS)

12 drops wild orange
9 drops clary sage
6 drops geranium
6 drops Roman chamomile
Combine in a 5ml bottle/roller bottle, fill remainder with carrier oil. Apply to pulse points, cup hands together over nose and mouth and inhale.

HE'LL NEVER KNOW (for symptoms of PMS/menopause)

12 drops geranium
6 drops ylang ylang
4 drops clary sage
Combine in a 5ml bottle/roller bottle, fill remainder with carrier oil. Apply over lower abdomen and lower back (female organs are in between), use on wrists for emotional support, cup hands together over nose and mouth and inhale. Or apply ClaryCalm® in same manner.

MENORRHAGIA (HEAVY FLOW)

6 drops Roman chamomile
4 drops geranium
3 drops lemon
2 drops cypress
Combine in 15 ml bottle/roller bottle, fill remainder with carrier oil. Massage onto abdomen and pelvic area (above uterus) several times daily, starting the week before menstruation.

FIXUS (PILARIS KERATOSIS)

15 drops lavender
15 drops geranium
15 drops melaleuca
15 drops myrrh
15 drops oregano
Combine in 2-ounce spray bottle, fill remainder with carrier oil. Apply three to five times a day to affected area, shaking lightly before each use.

BREAST ENHANCER

Apply 1 drop of vetiver across top of breasts two times per day until desired results are achieved (generally a couple months). Can add complimentary oils to change aroma. NOTE: This suggestion is suited for women who have lost or never had breast mass due to intense exercise levels [e.g. runners] or breastfeeding, etc. Vetiver will not have a negative impact on women with larger breasts so it is unnecessary to avoid usage for other purposes.

BREAST DETOX

- Apply 4 drops frankincense to each breast twice daily for thirty days. Do detox two to four times per year. Use a carrier oil for easier distribution.
- Eucalyptus, grapefruit, and pink pepper are also excellent for breast health, applied topically with a carrier oil. Apply for discomfort or concern.
- Apply 4 drops Frankincense to each breast twice daily for 30 days with a carrier oil (for ease of distribution and to reduce sensitivity) to relieve discomfort and concern. Consider repeating detox to two to four times per year as needed. Consider combining with: eucalyptus, grapefruit, pink pepper, and Siberian fir.

FERTILITY BLEND

12 drops clary sage
10 drops fennel
7 drops geranium
8 drops spikenard
8 drops bergamot
Bonus: add 3 drops rose if available
Combine oils in 10ml roller bottle; fill remainder with carrier oil. Apply to lower abdomen twice daily, targeting ovary and uterus areas.

FERTILITY PROTOCOL

- **Diet:** See *Candida*
- **Supplementation:** (See *Candida* for a more in-depth program):
  - Alpha CRS®+, MicroPlex VMz, essential oil xEO Mega - take as directed
  - PB Assist®+ - take 1 capsule three times on days 11-15 of monthly cycle; then take one per day on day 16 until end of monthly cycle (onset of menstruation). Repeat monthly until desired results are achieved.
  - GX Assist® - take first ten days of monthly cycle, 1-3 capsules three times a day
  - Phytoestrogen complex - take 1 capsule every day to eliminate harmful estrogen metabolites and maintain healthy estrogen levels.
- **Essential oil use:**
  - Geranium - apply two times a day over liver, adrenal glands, kidney areas to support healthy production of progesterone.
  - Grapefruit - take 16 drops under tongue or in a capsule every morning to support healthy progesterone levels.
  - Spikenard & ClaryCalm® - apply to sides of feet under ankle bones, abdomen, and wrists for hormone and mood balancing

Follow program until becoming pregnant. Then discontinue GX Assist®, phytoestrogen complex, ClaryCalm®. Continue everything else throughout pregnancy. Reduce PB Assist®+ consumption to 1-2 per day to maintain healthy terrain.

MOOD LIFTING PERFUME

In a 10 ml roller bottle, combine 3 drops ylang ylang, 3 drops bergamot, 9 drops clary sage, 9 drops lavender, and 12 drops tangerine essential oils. Top with carrier oil. Apply to pulse points throughout the day. Also consider jasmine, magnolia, neroli, rose.

CRAMP-LESS

Apply magnolia topically, followed by 2-3 drops each copaiba and marjoram to lower abdomen. Dilute as needed with carrier oil or lotion. Add geranium as desired.

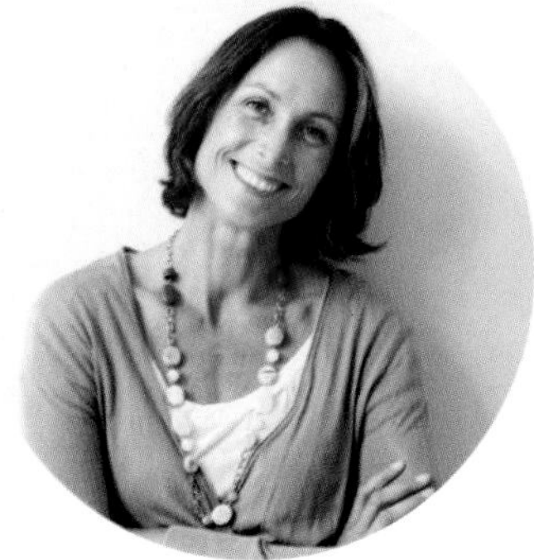

Conditions

Breast, cellular health - clary sage, eucalyptus, frankincense, geranium, grapefruit, magnolia, pink pepper, DDR Prime®
Breast size, too small (want to enlarge) - black pepper, clary sage, fennel, geranium, myrrh, vetiver, yarrow, ClaryCalm®, DDR Prime®, Peace®, Whisper® (oils will not cause already larger breasts to enlarge further)
Breasts, tender* - clary sage, fennel, geranium, helichrysum, lavender, lemon, myrrh, Roman chamomile, yarrow, Citrus Bliss®, ClaryCalm®, DDR Prime®, Whisper®, Zendocrine®
Candida - See *Candida*
Cysts, ovarian - basil, clary sage, cypress, fennel, frankincense, geranium, grapefruit, lemon, rosemary, thyme, ClaryCalm®, DDR Prime®, Purify, Slim & Sassy®, Whisper®, Zendocrine®; see *Blood Sugar*
Endometriosis - basil, bergamot, black pepper, clary sage, copaiba, cypress, eucalyptus, frankincense, geranium, ginger, lemongrass, neroli, oregano, rosemary, sandalwood, thyme, ylang ylang, yarrow, ClaryCalm®, DDR Prime®, Elevation™, On Guard®, Peace®, Whisper®, Zendocrine®
Estrogen dominance - basil, clove, lemongrass, thyme, Forgive®, Purify, Zendocrine®
Estrogen, false/xenoestrogens - clary sage, ginger, grapefruit, lemon, oregano, thyme, ClaryCalm®, DDR Prime®, Zendocrine®; see *Candida, Detoxification*
Estrogen, imbalanced/low - basil, clary sage, coriander, cypress, lavender, neroli
Fibroids - basil, clary sage, eucalyptus, frankincense, helichrysum, lemon, lemongrass, melaleuca, sandalwood, thyme, DDR Prime®, Peace®
Frigidity - jasmine, neroli, rose, ylang ylang, Adaptiv®, AromaTouch®, Passion®, Peace®, Whisper®; see "Aphrodisiacs" property, *Intimacy*
Genital warts - arborvitae, frankincense, geranium, lemongrass, melissa, thyme, Zendocrine®
Headache, migraine/cyclical - basil, clary sage, fennel, geranium, lavender, melissa, peppermint, rosemary, Roman chamomile, ClaryCalm®, DDR Prime®, PastTense®, Whisper®
Hemorrhoids - cypress, helichrysum, myrrh, Roman chamomile, sandalwood, AromaTouch®, DigestZen®, Zendocrine®; see *Cardiovascular*
Hormones, imbalanced (general) - jasmine, geranium, magnolia, ylang ylang, ClaryCalm®, Forgive®, Motivate®, Whisper®
Hot flashes - clary sage, eucalyptus, lemon, peppermint, ClaryCalm®, Whisper®; see *Endocrine (Thyroid)*
Infertility* - basil, clary sage, copaiba, cypress, fennel, frankincense, geranium, jasmine, melissa, Roman chamomile, rose, rosemary, spikenard, thyme, ylang ylang, ClaryCalm®, DDR Prime®, Passion®, Purify, Whisper®, Zendocrine®; see *Candida, Blood Sugar*, "Progesterone, low" below
Low libido - black pepper, cardamom, cinnamon, clary sage, clove, ginger, jasmine, juniper berry, magnolia, neroli, patchouli, rose, rosemary, sandalwood, spearmint, thyme, vetiver, wild orange, ylang ylang, Passion®, Whisper®; see "Aphrodisiacs" property, *Intimacy*
Mammary gland support - clary sage, geranium, grapefruit, Citrus Bliss®, DDR Prime®, Whisper®; see "Breast Detox" recipe below
Menopause problems* - basil, clary sage, cypress, fennel, geranium, lavender, neroli, Roman chamomile, rosemary, thyme, wild orange, yarrow, ClaryCalm®, Peace®, Whisper®, Zendocrine®
Menstruation (menses) cycle, irregular - cypress, fennel, jasmine, juniper berry, lavender, melissa, peppermint, rose, rosemary, thyme, yarrow, Cheer®, ClaryCalm®, DDR Prime®, Deep Blue®, Forgive®, PastTense®, Whisper®
Menstruation (menses), heavy (menorrhagia)* - clary sage, cypress, fennel, frankincense, geranium, helichrysum, thyme, yarrow, ClaryCalm®, DDR Prime®, Forgive®, Purify, Whisper®, Zendocrine®
Menstruation (menses), lack of/absence (amenorrhea) - basil, cedarwood, clary sage, dill, geranium, juniper berry, Roman chamomile, rosemary, yarrow, ClaryCalm®, DDR Prime®, Forgive®, Passion®, Whisper®, Zendocrine®
Menstruation (menses), overly light - basil, cinnamon, ginger, rosemary, ylang ylang, Citrus Bliss®, ClaryCalm®, DDR Prime®, Purify, Passion®, Whisper®, Zendocrine®
Menstruation (menses), painful (dysmenorrhea), uterine cramping - basil, black pepper, blue tansy, cardamom, celery seed, cinnamon, citronella, clary sage, copaiba, coriander, cypress, frankincense, ginger, lemongrass, jasmine, juniper berry, magnolia, neroli, peppermint, petitgrain, pink pepper, spikenard, Cheer®, ClaryCalm®, DDR Prime®, Purify, Whisper®, Zendocrine®
Menstruation (menses), prolonged - copaiba, frankincense, geranium, ClaryCalm®, DDR Prime®, Whisper®
Miscarriages (multiple) - blue tansy, clary sage, frankincense, grapefruit, lemon, oregano, thyme, Citrus Bliss®, ClaryCalm®, DDR Prime®, Purify, Whisper®, Zendocrine®
Night sweats - clary sage, eucalyptus, ginger, lime, peppermint, spearmint, AromaTouch®, ClaryCalm®, DDR Prime®, PastTense®, Whisper®, Zendocrine®; see *Endocrine (Thyroid), Immune & Lymphatic*
Ovaries - basil, clary sage, frankincense, geranium, rosemary, thyme, ClaryCalm®, DDR Prime®, Zendocrine®
Ovulation, irregular - basil, clary sage, copaiba, jasmine, melissa, rose, ylang ylang, Zendocrine®
Pelvic pain - coriander, cypress, Douglas fir, geranium, ginger, rosemary, thyme, ClaryCalm®, PastTense®
Perimenopause - cardamom, clary sage, cypress, fennel, lavender, Roman chamomile, rosemary, yarrow, ClaryCalm®, DDR Prime®, Peace®, Whisper®, Zendocrine®
PMS* - bergamot, clary sage, copaiba, cypress, fennel, geranium, grapefruit, jasmine, lavender, magnolia, neroli, pink pepper, Roman chamomile, spikenard, Adaptiv®, Cheer®, ClaryCalm®, Peace®
Postpartum depression - See *Pregnancy, Labor & Nursing*
Progesterone, low - clove, geranium, grapefruit, oregano, thyme, ClaryCalm®, Whisper®, Zendocrine®
Uterus, cleansing and purifying - clary sage, geranium, jasmine, lemon, melaleuca, rose, Citrus Bliss®, ClaryCalm®, Purify, Whisper®, Zendocrine®
Uterus, damaged/degenerated - frankincense, geranium, lemongrass, sandalwood, DDR Prime®, Whisper®
Uterus lining, unhealthy - celery seed, frankincense, geranium, grapefruit, jasmine, DDR Prime®, Whisper®
Uterus, prolapsed/lack of tone - fennel, frankincense, juniper berry (stimulates uterine muscles), melissa, rose, wild orange, ClaryCalm®, Whisper®
Vaginal, candida/thrush - melaleuca, myrrh, oregano, thyme, On Guard®, Purify, Slim & Sassy®, Zendocrine®; see *Candida*
Vaginal discharge - clary sage, frankincense, lavender (thick, yellow), DDR Prime®, On Guard®, Purify, Whisper®, Zendocrine®; see *Candida*
Vaginal dryness - clary sage, Balance®; see *Integumentary*
Vaginal infection/inflammation - clary sage, eucalyptus, frankincense, magnolia, rosemary, spearmint, DDR Prime®, On Guard®, Peace®, Whisper®, Zendocrine®

WOMEN'S HEALTH

** See remedy on pg. 376*

Emotional Well-Being

There is a significant connection between emotional and physical health. The body releases various chemicals in response to emotions. For example, the body's release of serotonin, dopamine, or oxytocin results in an uplifting emotion and positive sensation in the body. An experience of stress causes the brain to instruct the release of cortisol, and the body's response will be one of urgency and perhaps even fear.

Emotional stress, whether acute or chronic, can have profound effects on the body. A range of illnesses, from headaches to digestive issues, lack of sleep, and heart disease, can be the result of emotions such as grief, anxiety, and depression taking a toll on the immune system and other cells, tissues, and organs of the entire body.

Examining activity at a cellular level can assist in the understanding of how emotions can affect body functions. Embedded in the surface of the cell membrane are protein molecules known as receptors. These receptors face outward and continuously scan for, communicate with, and solicit needed chemicals that exist outside the cell.

These solicited chemicals attach to receptors, distribute information, and produce biochemical responses within the cell to adapt to environment and stimuli. In this way the receptors play a unique and important role in cellular communication. The binding chemical, called a ligand, is classified as a "messenger molecule," because it sends information to cells that will influence the cell's development and function. A ligand can be a neurotransmitter, hormone, pharmaceutical drug, toxin, parts of a virus, or a neuropeptide used by neurons to communicate with each other.

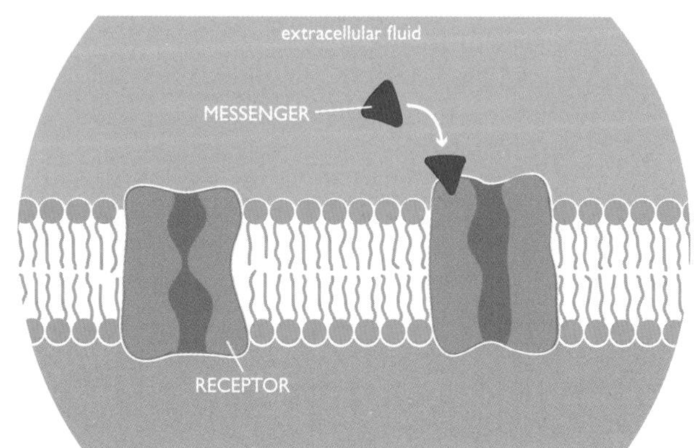

While numerous receptors are found in most cells, each receptor will only bind with ligands of a particular structure, much like how a lock will only accept a specifically shaped key. When a ligand binds to its corresponding receptor, it activates or inhibits the receptor's associated biochemical pathway.

There are two types of ligands: endogenous and exogenous. Endogenous ligands, such as serotonin, are produced in the body and can have an impact on emotions. Exogenous ligands are substances that are introduced into the body and have a similar effect. They, too, are messenger molecules and can come from a variety of sources such as medications or essential oils.

The Messages of Emotions

The hypothalamus – the "control and command center" of the brain – converts mental thoughts and emotions into hundreds of different types of ligands, specifically neuropeptides. The emotions triggered by a perceived threat, for example, are powerful and initiate the release of specific messenger molecule chemicals which, as indicated above, attach to certain receptor sites of cells and affect cell function. What the hypothalamus "believes to be true" determines what the "factory" produces, and chemical production ensues. Neuropeptides affect our chemistry, and our chemistry affects our biology. Bottom line: emotions trigger cell activity!

The Scent Alarm

The sense of smell is our most primal, and it exerts a powerful influence over our thoughts, emotions, moods, memories, and behaviors. A healthy human nose can distinguish over one trillion different aromas through hundreds of distinct classes of smell receptors. By way of comparison, we only have three types of photoreceptors used to recognize visual stimuli. Olfaction is far more complex than sight, and we are ten thousand times more capable of smelling than tasting.

It's accurate to say we "smell" danger. Our sense of smell is inextricably connected to our survival, and it plays a major role in remembering what is and isn't safe and what is pleasurable. Why remember danger, stress, trauma, and pleasure? To learn from experience so we can protect ourselves, survive, and procreate. If it wasn't safe this time, we can avoid it the next time; or if it was pleasurable (e.g. food, physical intimacy), we want to participate again. People, environments, food: smelling them is part of everyday life.

OLFACTORY SYSTEM

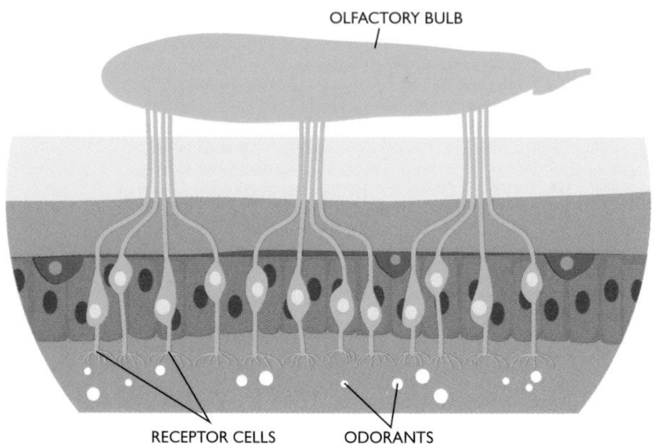

Aromas serve as exogenous ligands. They are received via olfactory receptors, which are highly concentrated in the limbic system, the primitive part of the brain and seat of emotion. In the center lies the amygdala, which instantly receives the incoming scent information before other higher brain centers. By the time the information reaches our "thinking" and decision-making cortex and we actually figure out what we smelled, the scent has already triggered emotional and body chemistry responses.

The amygdala is the storehouse of traumas and contains the densest concentration of neuropeptides, affecting cellular memory. Smell is the primary sense that unconsciously activates and affects traumatic memories stored there. Acting as the watchdog, the amygdala is constantly on the lookout for danger or threats. As it belongs to the more primitive part of our brain it doesn't have the intelligence to discern between real threats versus perceived threats (e.g. a saber-toothed tiger versus a missed bus stop or being late to work and an angry boss). It passes on its concerns and notifies the hypothalamus when safety and security are at risk, which then in turn notifies the pituitary, which alerts the adrenal glands, which sets off the alarm for fight-or-flight stress response and releases cortisol and adrenaline. Bottom line: The emotional stress triggered the release of the stress hormones.

Many researchers agree that physical illnesses are often the result of an emotional inflammatory response to trauma or negative experiences. What can begin as "emotional inflammation" can later become physical issues and disease. Although medical technology is not advanced enough to see them, memories, trauma, and painful emotions are stored in the body and eventually manifest as physical inflammation when the body's tissues follow suit.

FOOD & MOOD

What you put in your mouth has a direct impact on emotions. Nutritional deficiencies, food sensitivities, blood sugar imbalances, substance abuse, and stimulants (like caffeine) affect biochemistry and contribute to mood fluctuations and compromised emotional states.

Additives in processed foods generate adverse chemical reactions within the body and drastically affect mood and behavior in many children and adults. Some of these synthetic substances are labeled "excitotoxins" by nutritionists and wellness experts. These include additives such as high fructose corn syrup, trans-fats, artificial flavors, artificial colors, artificial sweeteners, MSG, and other preservatives. These chemicals deliver messages to the brain and cells of the body just like any exogenous ligand. More than one specific ligand can "fit" into a receptor. As heroin fits in the same opiate site as endorphins, so can these toxic food chemicals unlock receptor sites in our brain and transmit influences that, if we knew, we would never let in.

So once again, we have a choice on what chemical soup we want to ingest. The old adage, "we are what we eat," could not ring more true. Or perhaps it gets rewritten here: We emote or express emotionally what we eat.

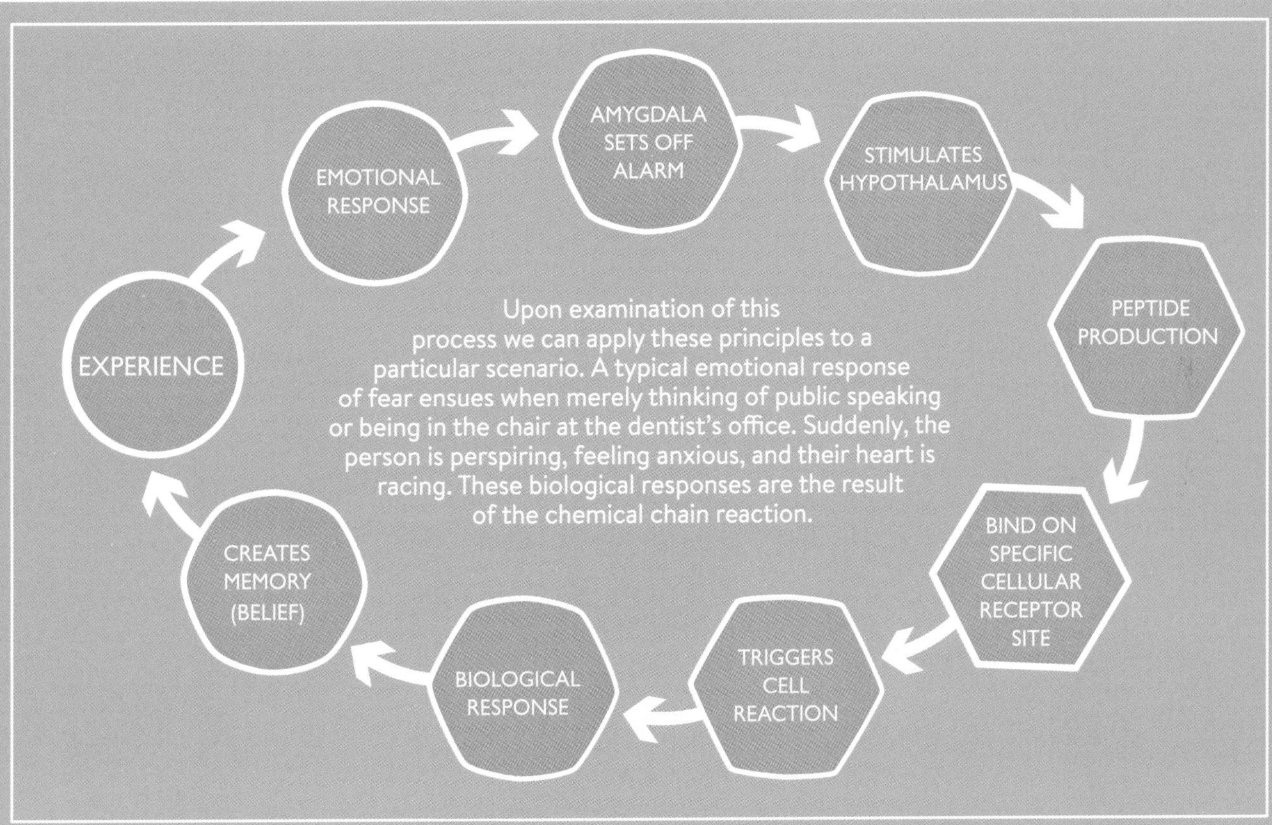
EXPERIENCE
EMOTIONAL RESPONSE
AMYGDALA SETS OFF ALARM
STIMULATES HYPOTHALAMUS
PEPTIDE PRODUCTION
BIND ON SPECIFIC CELLULAR RECEPTOR SITE
TRIGGERS CELL REACTION
BIOLOGICAL RESPONSE
CREATES MEMORY (BELIEF)
Upon examination of this process we can apply these principles to a particular scenario. A typical emotional response of fear ensues when merely thinking of public speaking or being in the chair at the dentist's office. Suddenly, the person is perspiring, feeling anxious, and their heart is racing. These biological responses are the result of the chemical chain reaction.

The Importance of the Sense of Smell

Smell can be used beneficially in healing efforts as well. Scents are experienced long before words. Whether for relieving stress, stabilizing mood, improving sleep, eliminating pain, relieving nausea, or improving memory and energy levels, scents can actually change nervous system biochemistry.

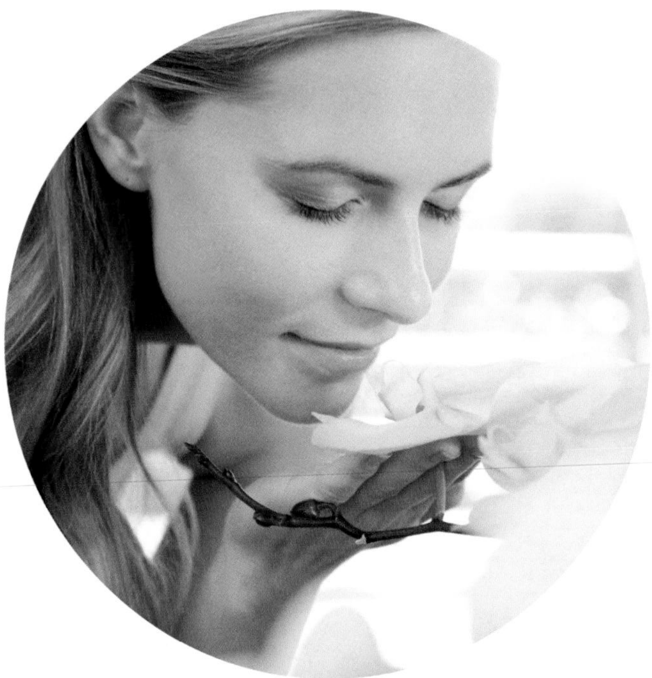

Essential oils can facilitate a rapid emotional response in the brain and the body to facilitate such a release. Essential oils are powerful biochemical agents for emotional balance, wellness, and toxic release, which can be paired or partnered with any holistic or medically-derived program to create a successful approach to mental and emotional wellness.

The Power of Essential Oils Choose Your Mood

Moods are often perceived as having chosen us, as if they are happening *to* us. Rather, the chemical impact of our emotions and other exogenous ligands is the real chooser of moods. That's why we reach for certain foods, sugar, caffeine, or a drug of choice (see "Food & Mood" for more information), interact with certain people, do certain things, and act out certain behaviors because of how it makes us feel and to get a "chemical" hit.

What if we could use this knowledge to choose the mood we want to feel and then actually feel it - without harmful substances or recreational drugs? What if we could think of a desired mood and then choose to use a healthful exogenous ligand that is capable of creating it? With essential oils, we have the ability to direct our own emotional traffic!

OUR SECOND BRAIN

Digestive issues and disorders are growing rampant, in part because of the refined and processed foods that are prevalent in today's diets. The gut is considered the body's "second brain" because of its impact on mood states. In recent years, scientists have discovered that there are more neurotransmitters (a type of ligand) in the gut than there are in the brain, and, among other things, healthy mood management depends on how well these neurotransmitters relay messages to each other.

Serotonin is a chemical responsible for maintaining mood balance, social behavior, appetite and digestion, sleep, memory, and sexual desire and function. The majority of the body's serotonin, between 80-90 percent, can be found in the gastrointestinal tract. Gut health, then, promotes emotional health and mood stabilization. How can an individual hope to experience healthy moods if their cells are depleted of nutrition and if their neurotransmitters reside in an area with blockages and inflammation? How can the over one hundred million neurons embedded in the gut influence healthy emotions when inflammation, blockages, candida, and other harmful bacteria are overpopulated and system imbalances are standard?

Detoxifying the body can improve emotional health. Toxicity symptoms in the body can directly mirror many depressive symptoms and may include insomnia, foggy thinking, low energy, digestive issues, dampened immune function, and allergies. New studies even suggest that depression may be a type of "allergic reaction" to inflammation.

Chemical compounds found in essential oils stimulate a range of gentle to more intense detoxification effects (depending on use) and promote a natural cleanse for the digestive, endocrine, immune, and lymphatic and other detoxification systems and channels of the body. This, in turn, boosts mood and restores mental and physical energy.

Blood sugar imbalances can also trigger depressive symptoms. Certain essential oils, like cinnamon, coriander, and fennel, support metabolic function and assist in moderating blood sugar levels. Omega 3-fatty acids, TerraZyme®, chelated minerals and B and D vitamins found in a MicroPlex VMz, antioxidants, and polyphenol supplements also help to regulate blood sugar levels, as well as reduce inflammation, boost energy, and support the gut with the right combination of good fats and other nourishing components.

Rather than feeling victimized by our emotional states, what if we had our own apothecary of essential oils in the home? Such a collection offers a cornucopia of emotional states for ready access. Like an eager child opening a box of candy, relishing the array of colors and designs and imagining the flavors waiting to tantalize her tongue and brighten her spirit, we, too, can delight in selecting and generating moods with the use of essential oils.

As natural exogenous ligands, essential oils can powerfully influence our emotions, much like mood-altering drugs like morphine, but with healthful results. Unlike synthetic medications or drugs that are designed to alter behavior, their complex molecular structure allows them to intelligently bind to the receptor sites of cells in our body and support a desired effect to restore balance and healthy function.

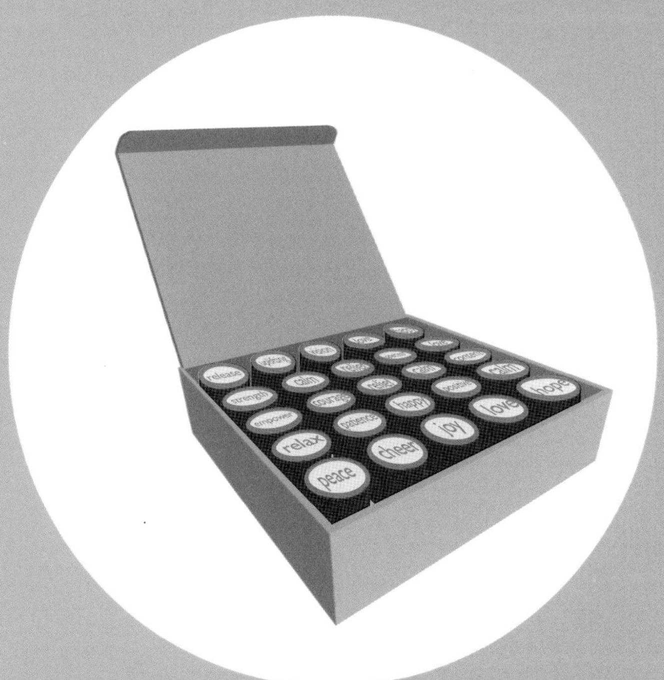

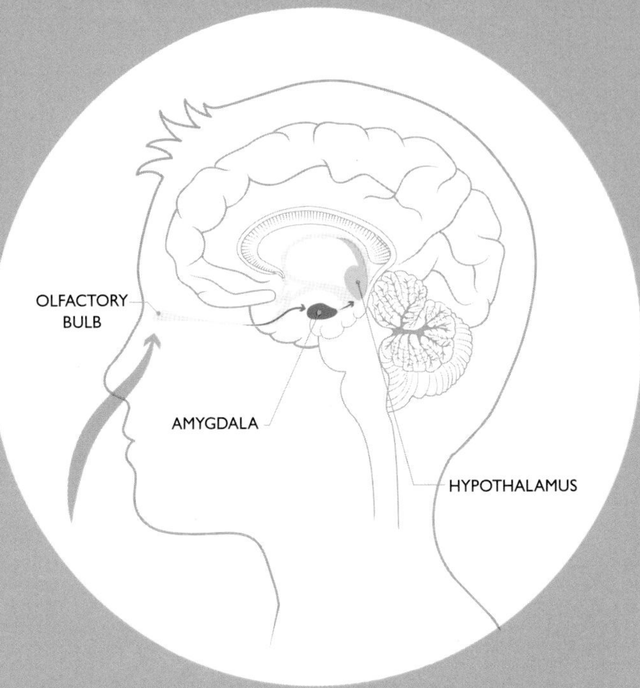

Taking It to the Next Level

Emotional healing and rebalancing of moods is accomplished when a new stimulus is introduced to the same chain of command in the brain. As we've already discussed, an aroma (stimulus) enters the olfactory system, and in turn the limbic system and amygdala, hypothalamus, and other parts of the brain and body. Depending on what aroma is introduced and the information it conveys determines the brain's response. Traumatic memories stored in the amygdala can be released by utilizing the sense of smell and essential oils. If the significance an individual attaches to a past experience can be shifted, the amygdala can release the trauma of the memory. This is what makes aromatherapy a wonderful means for emotional healing and rebalancing moods. Here is an example:

If an individual is deficient in serotonin for an extended period of time, their habitual response to life's situations might be more anxious or angry, more hopeless, more sad, more phobic, more thoughts of "what-if?". If he begins using wild orange, for example, a known antidepressant oil due to its capacity to uplift, detoxify, and calm, he would find himself irresistibly more happy and with a plausible capacity to be more hopeful, trusting, less reactive, and more calm. He also, therefore, has a potential to react to experiences and respond to memories differently.

Here's another example. A young child experiences a high level of trauma, such as a parent suffering with cancer who subsequently passes away. The child's body experiences tremendous chemical expenditures to support the experiences of stress, trauma, and grief. And then, if more trauma occurs, say the deceased parent is replaced and the surviving parent remarries, additional chemicals are released to cope with a new stepparent and step-siblings.

If, during, or after traumatic seasons of this child's life, her chemical reserves are not replenished, her coping capacity is literally chemically diminished. She might find herself crying more, experiencing meltdowns more easily, perhaps being teased for being a crybaby, or simply coping less effectively with everyday life. A missed homework deadline, low grade, or athletic performance failure may seem a crushing blow. The same exact events could happen to another person with full reserves who moves through it gracefully. What's the difference?

One of the most important chemicals we have to work in these kinds of situations is endorphins. The name itself reveals it to be an endogenous ligand: "endo-morphine," self-made morphine or *endorphin*. When endorphins are lacking, coping challenges arise. Endorphins serve us not only in our ability to experience pleasure, but also to appropriately buffer us from pain, both physical and emotional. The craving for its benefits will drive any number of behaviors when levels are low.

Typically two types of addictions may arise. One is generally met by abnormally intense levels of thrill or pleasure, as intensity is required in order to get the chemical "hit." The endogenous ligand, endorphins, is the body's "drug" of choice, received on an opiate receptor site. Activities of greater and greater intensity may be pursued to increase the production of endorphins. Bungee jumping, pornography use, playing intense video games, exaggerated sexual activity, gambling, overconsumption of comfort foods, or other behaviors known to generate endorphins become appealing in an attempt to fill a need.

The second addiction is usually focused on exogenous ligands in the form of pain-numbing opiate drugs, including opium, heroin, vicodin, oxycodone, and other prescription pain medications. Opiate drugs are received on the same opiate receptor sites. Either type of addiction is powerful as chemical needs remain unmet.

Returning to the story of the child who lost her parent, one of the main chemicals likely low, based on circumstances described, is endorphins. If those diminished reserves of endorphins were never replenished, she would potentially grow into an adult continually experiencing the inability to cope with life or fully experience pleasure, never fully recovering from the trauma, ever searching for ways to numb the pain and meet her emotional needs. Her body is simply lacking the chemical capacity to fully heal. The body needs to increase its reserves and ability to manufacture the chemicals needed.

Now to explore a potential solution, the essential oil of helichrysum. Helichrysum has powerful analgesic and pain-relieving therapeutic benefits. It is high in many chemical constituents, one known as ketones; a compound with powerful, regenerative benefits. As the child-turned-adult uses this oil and her body experiences this chemistry, she is exposed to generous amounts of healthy pain-killing/numbing chemicals. What science has yet to identify is what happens in the body from here.

Whether a chemical need is met or a pathway of reception is opened up is not known. What is happening potentially for the woman, however, is she finally feels relief from "pain." Her coping capacity is increased. She handles life better. With natural, healing chemicals on board in rich supply she finally experiences healing.

The diverse and concentrated chemical constituents in essential oils work to cleanse, ground, lift, balance, and calm the central nervous system and the emotional body. Some essential oils – like frankincense, patchouli and sandalwood – have high concentrations of sesquiterpene molecules that have been clinically demonstrated to cross the blood-brain barrier. These molecules have significant oxygen supporting effects on the brain and, when combined with aromatic stimulation, can assist the amygdala in releasing the effects of stored memories.

Here are some additional demonstrated mental and emotional benefits:

- Cleanse negative memories
- Reduce stress, anxiety, and tension
- Offset mental fatigue
- Uplift mood
- Calm the central nervous system
- Relax muscular tension
- Induce restful sleep
- Invigorate the senses
- Increase feelings of courage and determination
- Promote a cathartic effect (facilitating the release of stuck emotions)
- Support DNA correction and expression

In conclusion, aromatherapy offers many practical healing advantages, but perhaps one of the most fascinating is the relationship it has with emotional well being. Inhalation of essential oils with the resulting aromatic exposure is the most effective method of impacting the brain for emotional wellness. Some studies demonstrate that essential oils have the highest bio-frequency of any consumable natural substance.

Essential oils offer a fresh, effective support tool to aid in the emotional healing process and to shift out of old habits and ineffective coping patterns. Aromatherapy allows the individual to harness the olfactory power of plants for healing, or simply to enhance a state of well being using scents to create a powerful influence over how one thinks, feels, and behaves.

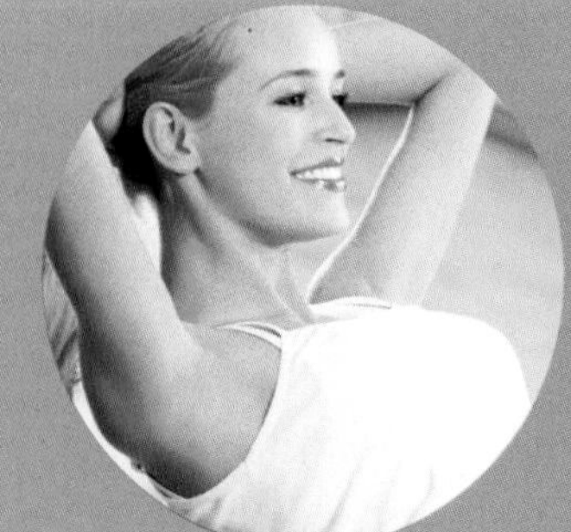

MOVE IT, MOVE IT

Studies indicate that moderate exercise of thirty minutes a day for three days a week has an antidepressant effect on a large percentage of depressed subjects. But many who are anxious or depressed lack the energy or sensory motivation to begin an exercise regime. Essential oils like peppermint, cypress, and wintergreen support the flow of blood and oxygen and the sensory "oomph" to engage in physical activity. Other oils aid in relieving muscle tension and assisting with muscle recovery. Helichrysum, for example, contains natural chemical components that have a regenerative effect both physically and emotionally.

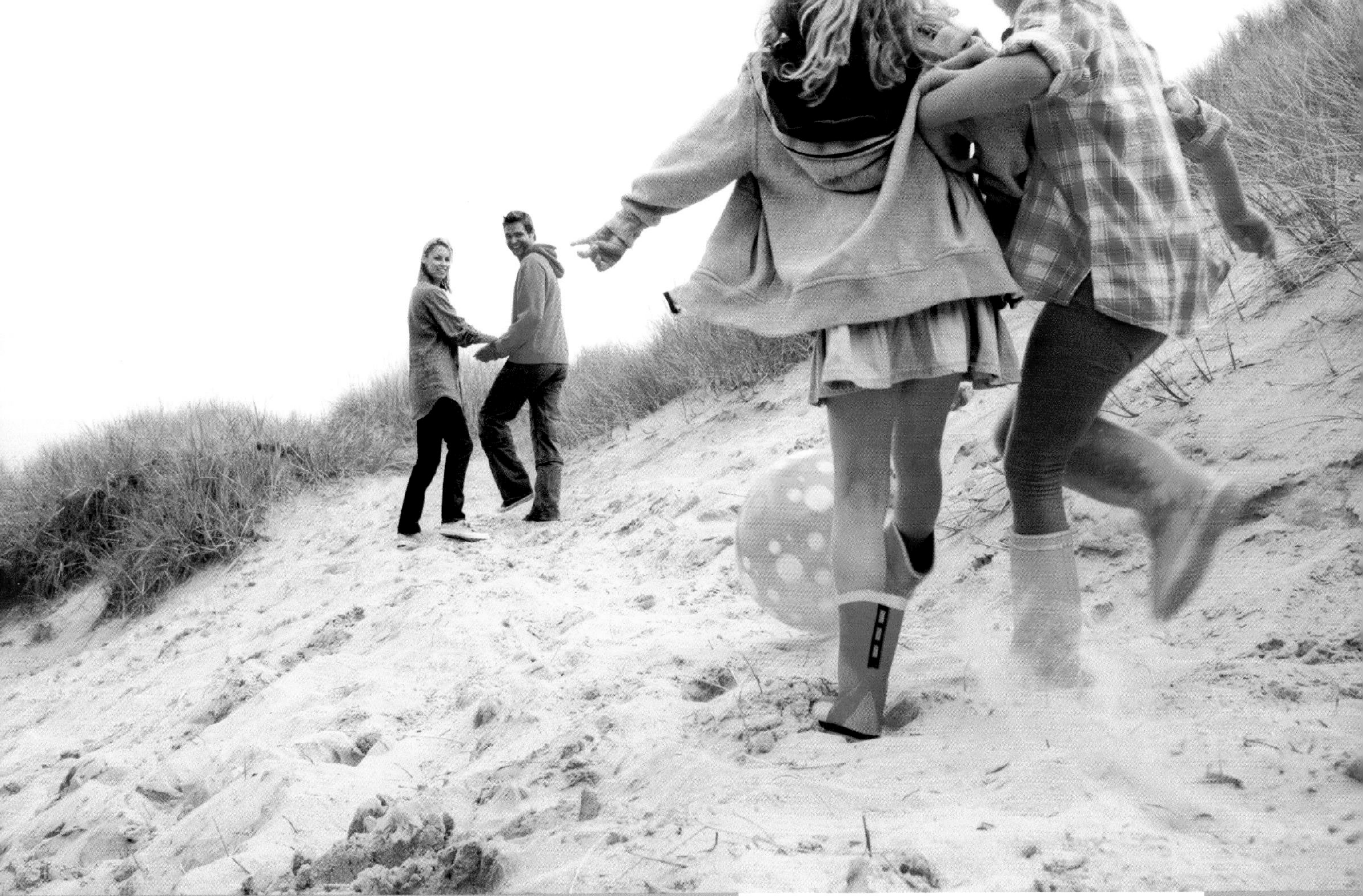

Practical Application

As essential oils are used topically, aromatically, and internally, the body's vibration is raised and its emotional frequencies are impacted, as is the capacity for emotional well being. Each individual oil with its diverse chemistry has the ability to be a tremendous multi-tasker and work in multiple areas of interest simultaneously. Additional benefits to essential oil use comes from combining oils to create synergistic blends. See Application Methods in this book to learn more.

Application methods also impact the body's response to aromatherapy in emotional health and healing:

- Aromatic use is the fastest way to access the mood center of the brain and invite the release of negative stored emotions. It is also helpful to use the oils aromatically when resetting new, healthy belief patterns.
- Topical use assists the body in moving from a stress response to a repair or restore response necessary to create an environment where emotional healing can take place.
- Internal use of essential oils supports healthy chemical reactions in the body, nourishment of cells, and release of toxins. This internal support fosters a healthy and balanced emotional environment. Cleansing the internal environment allows emotions to be recognized and processed more readily.

SWEET DREAMS

Adequate sleep is crucial to mental health and brain function. Insomnia and restless sleep are a problem for many who experience depressed or anxious mood states. Pairing a resin or tree essential oil like vetiver, cedarwood, sandalwood, or frankincense with a citrus oil like wild orange, lime, lemon, or bergamot has been found to stabilize mood fluctuations, ground the body, and promote a relaxation response in preparation for sleep. Flower oils like lavender, Roman chamomile, clary sage, geranium, and ylang ylang aid in quieting mental chatter and calming the nervous system.

Similarly, many studies have been conducted on the powerful mental, physical, and emotional benefits of meditation. Meditation is a practice that seeks to achieve a focused state of relaxation. The essential oils listed above can help to still the mind, open air pathways, and calm the mind and heart.

Emotions Index

Essential oils are some of nature's most powerful remedies for emotional health. Below are lists designed to introduce the concept of associating an oil to an emotion or vice versa as well as serve as an ongoing resource. Select specific targeted emotional states to address and then identify corresponding oils. **If you want to research specific mood conditions, refer to *Focus & Attention (pg. 295)* and *Mood & Behavior (pg. 319)* sections of this book.**

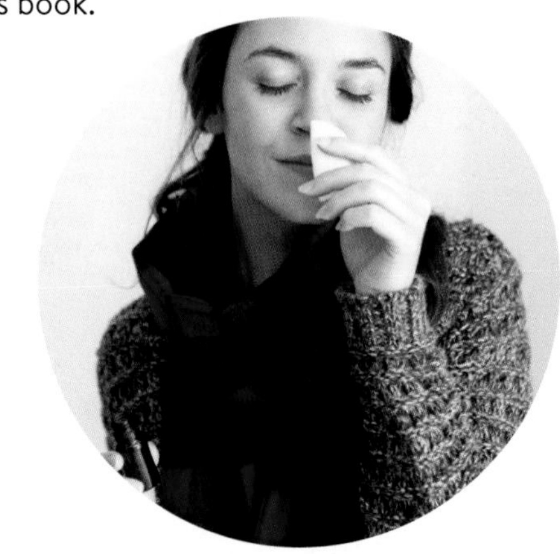

ESSENTIAL OIL	UN-BALANCED EMOTION	BALANCED EMOTION
Arborvitae	Overzealous	Composed
Basil	Inundated	Relieved
Bergamot	Inadequate	Worthy
Birch	Cowardly	Courageous
Black pepper	Repressed	Honest
Black spruce	Halted	Acclaimed
Blue tansy	Overwhelmed	Encouraged
Cardamom	Self-centered	Charitable
Cassia	Uncertain	Bold
Cedarwood	Alone	Connected
Celery seed	Aggravated	Reconciled
Cilantro	Obsessed	Easygoing
Cinnamon bark	Denied	Receptive
Citronella	Punished	Averting
Clary sage	Limited	Enlightened
Clove	Dominated	Supported
Copaiba	Plagued	Directed
Coriander	Apprehensive	Participating
Cypress	Stalled	Progressing
Dill	Avoiding	Intentional
Douglas fir	Upset	Renewed
Eucalyptus	Congested	Stimulated
Fennel	Unproductive	Flourishing
Frankincense	Separated	Unified
Geranium	Neglected	Mended
Ginger	Apathetic	Activated
Grapefruit	Rejected	Validated
Green Mandarin	Distressed	Carefree
Helichrysum	Wounded	Reassured
Jasmine	Hampered	Liberated
Juniper berry	Denying	Insightful
Kumquat	Divided	Integrous
Lavender	Unheard	Expressed
Lemon	Mindless	Energized
Lemon eucalyptus	Concealed	Revealing
Lemongrass	Obstructed	Flowing
Lime	Faint	Enlivened
Litsea	Encumbered	Purified
Magnolia	Disturbed	Confident
Manuka	Bothered	Revived
Marjoram	Doubtful	Trusting
Melaleuca	Unsure	Collected
Melissa	Depressed	Light-filled
Myrrh	Disconnected	Nurtured
Neroli	Afflicted	Released
Oregano	Obstinate	Unattached
Patchouli	Degraded	Enhanced
Pink Pepper	Impeded	Aroused
Peppermint	Hindered	Invigorated
Petitgrain	Conflicted	Harmonized
Ravensara	Uncommitted	Resolute
Red Mandarin	Troubled	Resilient
Roman chamomile	Frustrated	Purposeful
Rose	Isolated	Loved
Rosemary	Confused	Open-minded
Sandalwood	Uninspired	Devoted
Siberian fir	Excluded	Empowered
Spearmint	Weary	Refreshed
Spikenard	Agitated	Tranquil
Tangerine	Oppressed	Restored
Thyme	Unyielding	Yielding
Turmeric	Compromised	Assured
Vetiver	Ungrounded	Rooted
White fir	Blocked	Receiving
Wild orange	Drained	Productive
Wintergreen	Stubborn	Accepting
Yarrow	Invaded	Shielded
Ylang ylang	Burdened	Exuberant

If you want to feel the positive emotion listed, use the associated oil.

Accepting	wintergreen
Acclaimed	black spruce
Activated	ginger
Aroused	pink pepper
Assured	turmeric
Averting	citronella
Bold	cassia
Carefree	green mandarin
Charitable	cardamom
Collected	melaleuca
Composed	arborvitae
Confident	magnolia
Connected	cedarwood
Courageous	birch
Devoted	sandalwood
Directed	copaiba
Easygoing	cilantro
Empowered	Siberian fir
Encouraged	blue tansy
Energized	lemon
Enhanced	patchouli
Enlightened	clary sage
Enlivened	lime
Expressed	lavender
Exuberant	ylang ylang
Flourishing	fennel
Flowing	lemongrass
Guided	red mandarin
Harmonized	petitgrain
Honest	black pepper
Insightful	juniper berry
Integrous	kumquat
Intentional	dill
Invigorated	peppermint
Liberated	jasmine
Light-filled	melissa
Loved	rose
Mended	geranium
Nurtured	myrrh
Open-minded	rosemary
Participating	coriander
Productive	wild orange
Progressing	cypress
Purified	litsea
Purposeful	Roman chamomile
Reassured	helichrysum
Receiving	white fir
Receptive	cinnamon bark
Reconciled	celery seed
Refreshed	spearmint
Released	neroli
Relieved	basil
Renewed	Douglas fir
Resolute	ravensara
Restored	tangerine
Revealing	lemon eucalyptus
Revived	manuka
Rooted	vetiver
Shielded	yarrow
Stimulated	eucalyptus
Supported	clove
Tranquil	spikenard
Trusting	marjoram
Unattached	oregano
Unified	frankincense
Validated	grapefruit
Worthy	bergamot
Yielding	thyme

If you are feeling the negative emotion listed, use the associated oil.

Afflicted	neroli
Agitated	spikenard
Aggravated	celery seed
Alone	cedarwood
Apathetic	ginger
Apprehensive	coriander
Avoiding	dill
Blocked	white fir
Bothered	manuka
Burdened	ylang ylang
Compromised	turmeric
Concealed	lemon eucalyptus
Conflicted	petitgrain
Confused	rosemary
Congested	eucalyptus
Cowardly	birch
Degraded	patchouli
Denied	cinnamon bark
Denying	juniper berry
Depressed	melissa
Disconnected	myrrh
Distressed	green mandarin
Disturbed	magnolia
Divided	kumquat
Dominated	clove
Doubtful	marjoram
Drained	wild orange
Encumbered	litsea
Excluded	Siberian fir
Faint	lime
Frustrated	Roman chamomile
Halted	black spruce
Hampered	jasmine
Hindered	peppermint
Impeded	pink pepper
Inadequate	bergamot
Inundated	basil
Invaded	yarrow
Isolated	rose
Limited	clary sage
Mindless	lemon
Neglected	geranium
Obsessed	cilantro
Obstinate	oregano
Obstructed	lemongrass
Oppressed	tangerine
Overwhelmed	blue tansy
Overzealous	arborvitae
Plagued	copaiba
Punished	citronella
Rejected	cilantro
Repressed	black pepper
Self-centered	cardamom
Separated	frankincense
Stalled	cypress
Stubborn	wintergreen
Troubled	red mandarin
Uncertain	cassia
Uncommitted	ravensara
Ungrounded	vetiver
Unheard	lavender
Uninspired	sandalwood
Unproductive	fennel
Unsure	melaleuca
Unyielding	thyme
Upset	Douglas fir
Weary	spearmint
Wounded	helichrysum

SECTION 5

ESSENTIAL LIFESTYLE

Essential Lifestyle Recipes section takes living the ESSENTIAL LIFE to the next level. The recipes and tips here show how essential oils can enhance every area of life. They are the tool of choice because they contribute to most every part of a great lifestyle.

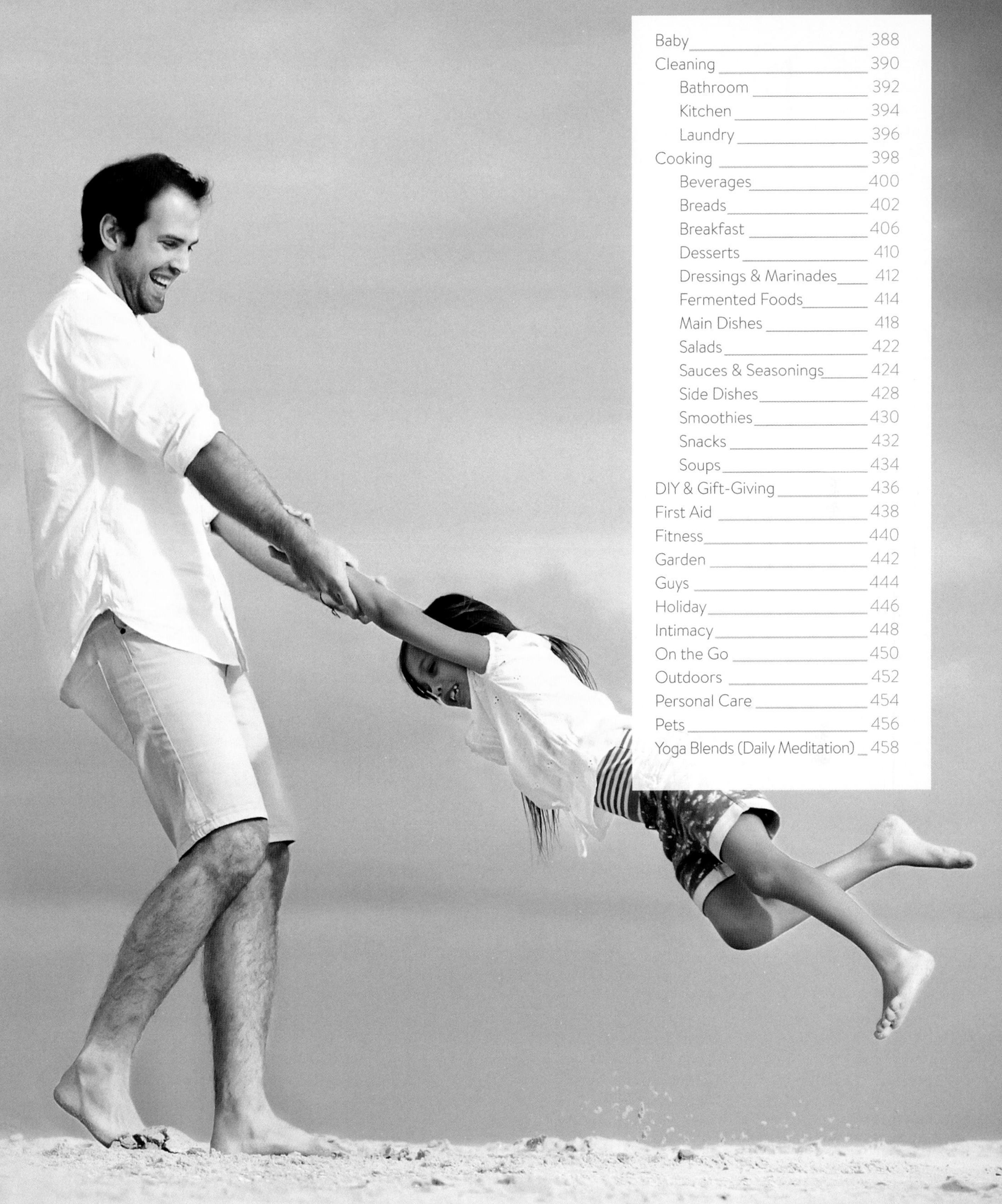

Baby

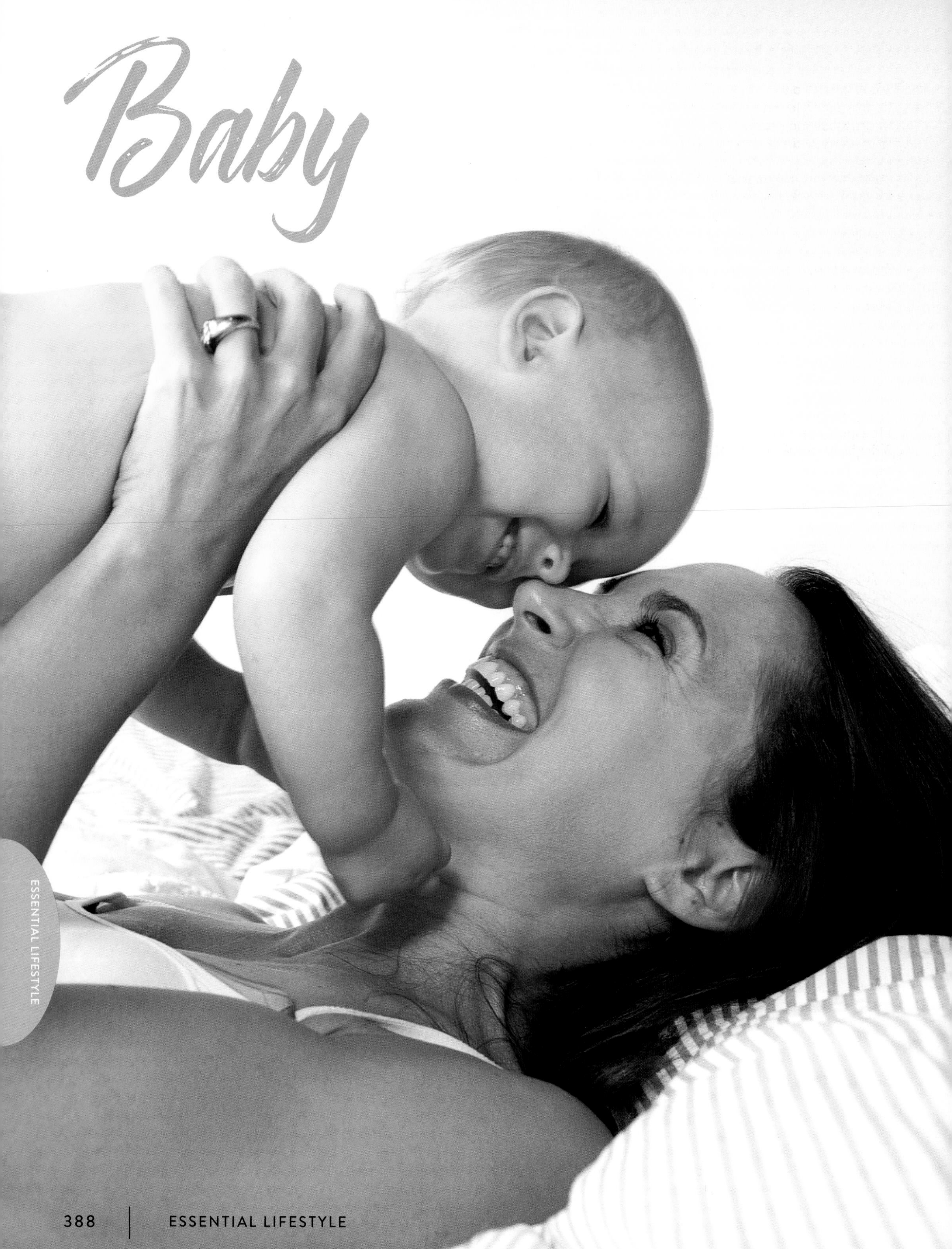

Diaper Rash Relief

½ cup carrier oil
15 drops melaleuca essential oil
15 drops lavender essential oil
15 drops frankincense essential oil

In a small glass spray bottle mix oils together. Spray a thin layer directly onto rash area and reapply as needed.

Calming Colic Blend

3 drops DigestZen® essential oil
2 drops ginger essential oil
1 teaspoon carrier oil

Mix together and massage ointment over baby's tummy and lower back. Repeat 3 to 5 times daily.

Cradle Cap Moisturizer

1 teaspoon carrier oil
3 drops lavender essential oil

Mix together in palms and rub on the baby's scalp. Add cocoa butter if additional softening as needed.

Winter Cheeks Balm

¼ cup carrier oil
¼ cup olive oil
2 tablespoon beeswax
20 drops lavender essential oil

In a small mason jar mix ingredients together, and lower the jar into a warm saucepan partially filled with water. On low heat melt beeswax, carrier oil, and olive oil together, stirring every few minutes. After wax is completely melted remove from heat and add lavender. Mix together and cool until hardened. Rub balm over reddened cheeks to ease and protect.

Baby Stain Remover Spray

8 ounces water
2 tablespoons borax
20 drops lemon essential oil

Add borax and oils to a spray bottle. Add water and shake thoroughly. Spray directly on stain and wash.

tips

- To clean baby's toys combine 2 drops lemon with 4 ounces of white vinegar in a glass spray bottle. Fill remaining with water and spray.
- To ease colic, apply 1-2 drops of DigestZen® on baby's feet.
- To calm a crying or overtired baby put 1 drop lavender or children's Serenity® under baby's nose and forehead.
- Scent children's drawers with their favorite essential oils applied to cotton balls.
- To signal safety, comfort, or time for sleep, place 2 drops of lavender, Calmer™, or Balance® near breast or nearby during feedings.
- For a soothing bath, add 2-4 drops of Roman chamomile or Serenity®.
- To soothe sore gums mix 1-2 drops of Roman chamomile, Siberian fir, or clove essential oil with carrier oil and massage into baby's gums.

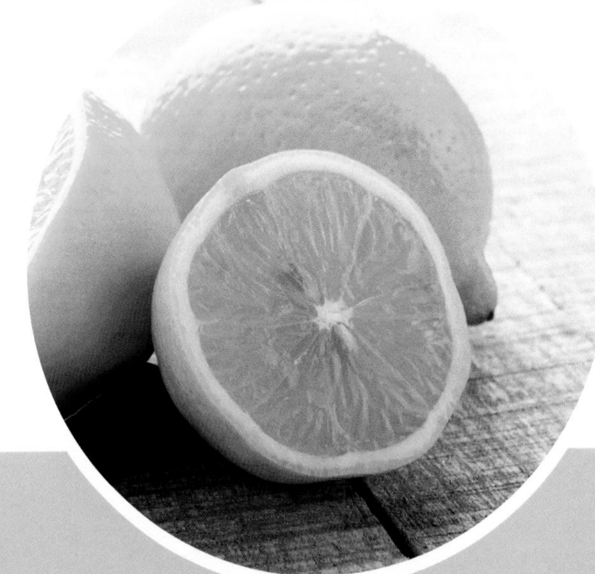

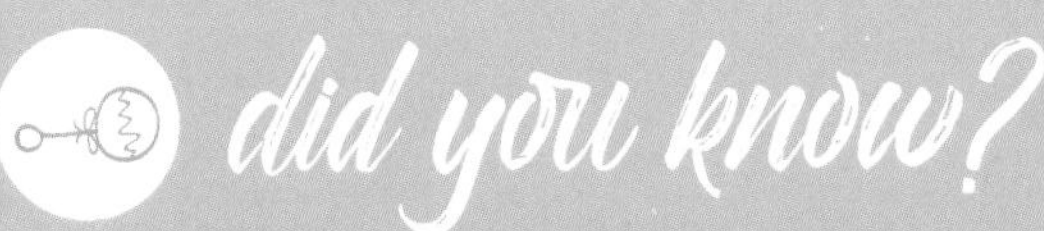

- Talc is found in most baby powders and is a known lung irritant.
- Many baby products are made with synthetic fragrances that can cause respiratory, neurological, skin, and eye damage.
- You can make natural, gentle, and safe products for your baby for a fraction of the cost of over the counter remedies.

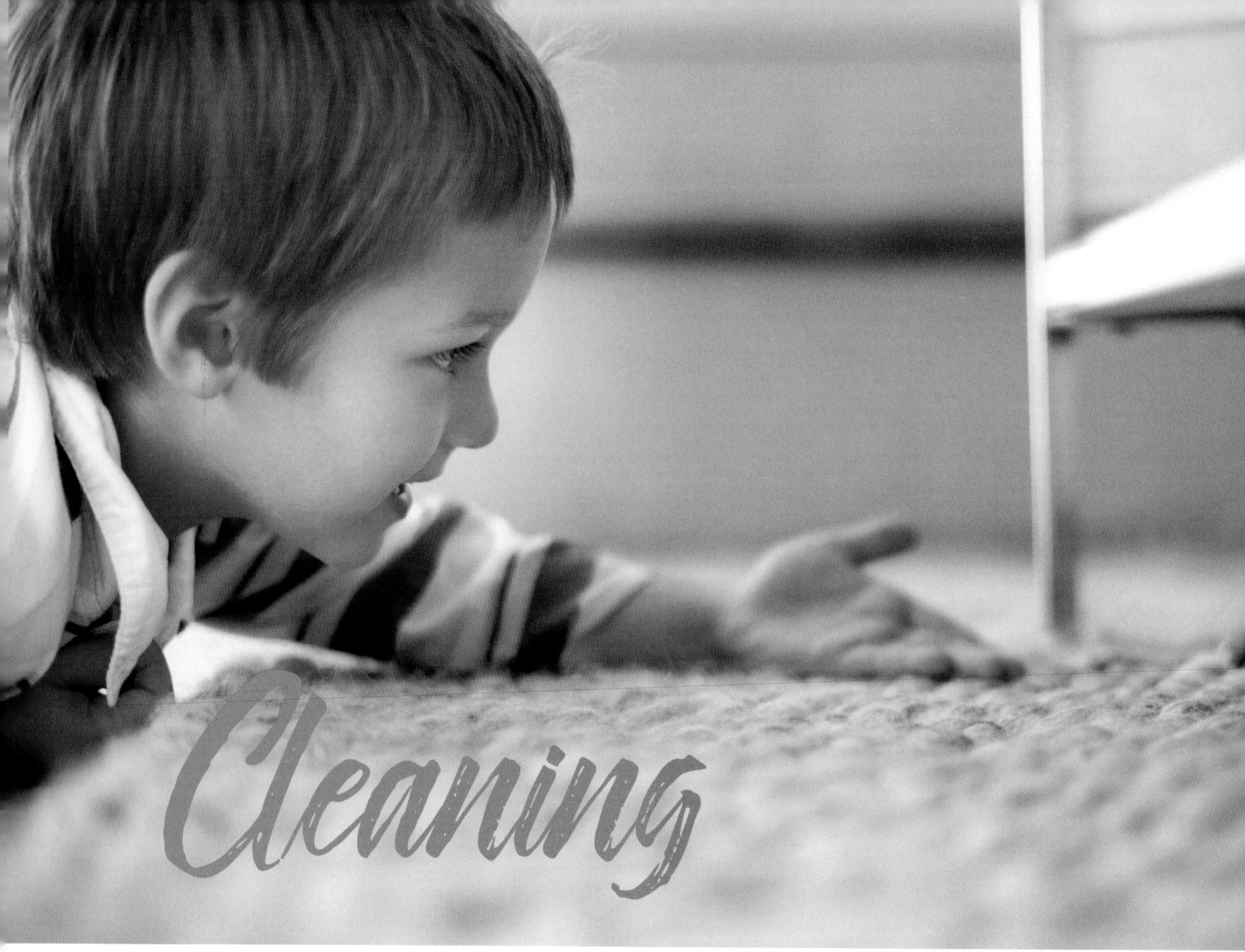

All Purpose Cleaner

1 16 oz glass spray bottle
1 mini stainless steel funnel
1 cup distilled water
1 cup white distilled vinegar
1 teaspoon natural dish soap
15 drops lemon essential oil
10 drops tea tree essential oil

Using a 16 oz. spray bottle, remove the top and secure the mini stainless steel funnel to its opening. Pour distilled water and white distilled vinegar into the bottle. Add natural dish soap, lemon essential oil, and melaleuca (tea tree) essential oils. Remove the funnel and reattach the lid; shake well. Use for any cleaning surface and reap the benefits of a natural essential oil cleaning solution!

Household Cleanser Spray

12 drops Siberian fir essential oil
12 drops lemon eucalyptus essential oil
12 drops tea tree (melaleuca) essential oil
12 drops peppermint essential oil

Combine essential oils with 8 oz water in glass spray bottle.

Wood Polish

1 16 oz glass spray bottle
1 mini stainless steel funnel
1 cup olive oil
½ cup distilled water
30 drops lemon essential oil
10 drops wild orange essential oil

Using a 16 oz. spray bottle, remove the top and secure the mini stainless steel funnel to its opening. Pour 1 cup of olive oil and distilled water into the bottle. Add lemon and orange essential oils. Remove the funnel and reattach the lid; shake well (and at every use). Spray on any wooden surface and see the shine of your essential oil wood polish!

Diy Deodorizer

2 tablespoon white distilled vinegar
30 drops citronella essential oil
Purified water
Spray bottle

Using a 16 oz. spray bottle, remove the top and secure the mini Add all ingredients to glass spray bottle. Shake well before using and store in cool, dry place.

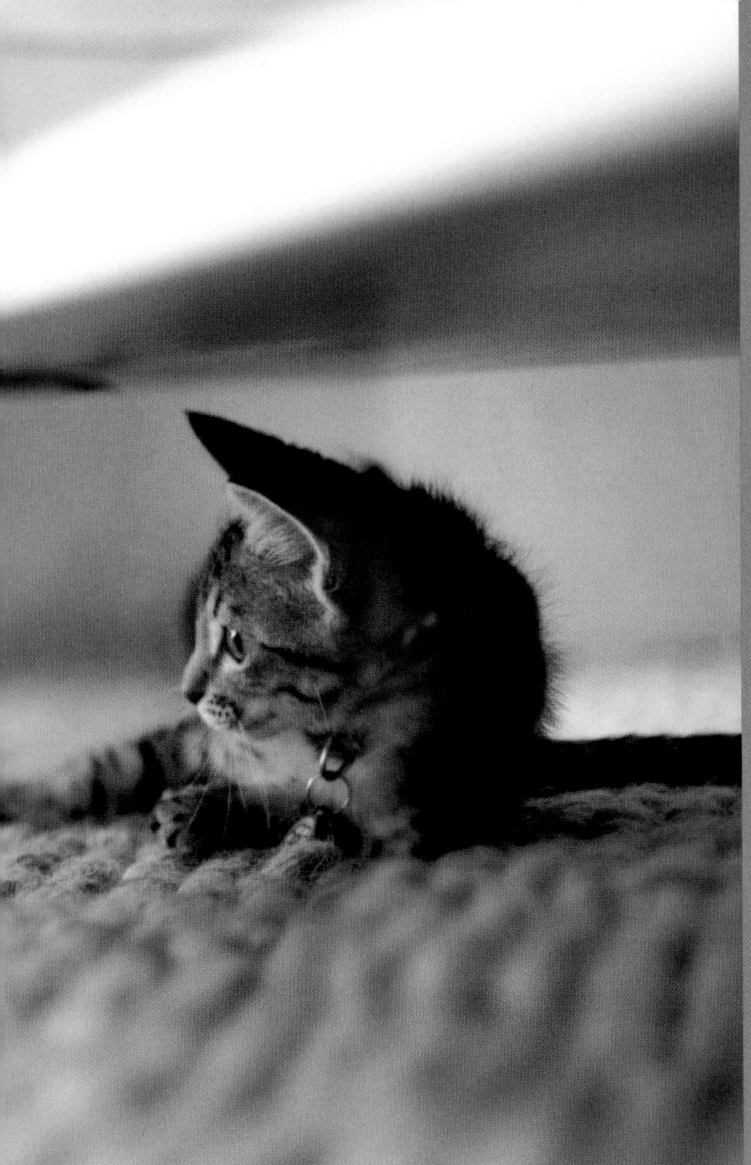

Carpet Stain Remover

4 cups warm water, divided
½ teaspoon clear castile soap or dish soap
10 drops lemon essential oil

Mix 2 cups warm water, soap, and essential oil. Soak a rag in the mixture, wring out, and gently blot the stain. Use a clean rag soaked in the remaining 2 cups warm water to remove the residue. Alternate the soap solution with the fresh water until the stain is gone. Remember to blot, not rub, to remove a carpet stain as rubbing will ruin the carpet fibers.

All-Purpose Cleaning Spray

16 oz glass spray bottle
12 ounces purified water
1 tablespoon unscented liquid castile soap
10 drops tea tree essential oil
5-10 drops citronella essential oil

Fill spray bottle with purified water, about ¾ full. Add liquid castile soap, essential oils, and remainder of bottle with additional purified water. Shake well before each use.

Stainless Steel Cleaner

16 oz glass spray bottle
2 oz liquid castile soap
5 drops lemon essential oil
5 drops On Guard® essential oil
5 drops Balance® essential oil
Distilled water

Add all ingredients to bottle. Fill the remaining space with distilled water. To use, spray on stainless steel appliances and wipe off with a rag.

Upholstered Fabric Cleaner

¼ cup warm water
2 teaspoons castile soap
3 drops lime essential oil

Mix ingredients in a container. Dip cloth in the mixture and dab onto the stain for quick spot treatments on any fabric.

Grill Cleaner

16 oz glass bottle
Baking soda
3 tablespoons castile soap
20 drops lemon essential oil
White vinegar

Combine castile soap and lemon essential oil. Fill the remainder of the spray bottle with vinegar. Sprinkle baking soda on grill and spray solution onto the grill. Let it sit on the grill for at least 30 minutes before cleaning.

Leather Cleaner

¼ cup olive oil
½ cup white vinegar
3 drops eucalyptus essential oil
8 oz spray bottle

Mix the ingredients together in your spray bottle and shake it well. Spray the leather down and wipe it clean with a cotton cloth. Please note that this recipe is perfectly safe for regular leather but is it not designed to be used on suede.

Dusting Spray

1 cup water, distilled or boiled and cooled
¼ cup vinegar
1 tablespoon olive oil
15 drops preferred essential oil (lemon, wild orange)

Combine ingredients in a spray bottle. Shake the bottle before each use. Spray on a microfiber cloth and apply to surface to clean, polish, and keep dust away.

BATHROOM Cleaning

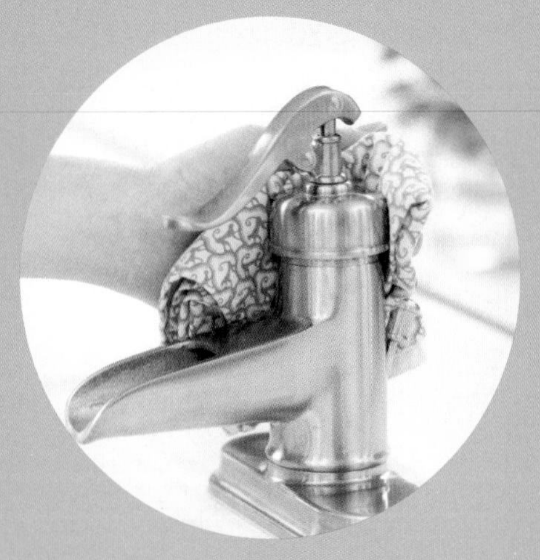

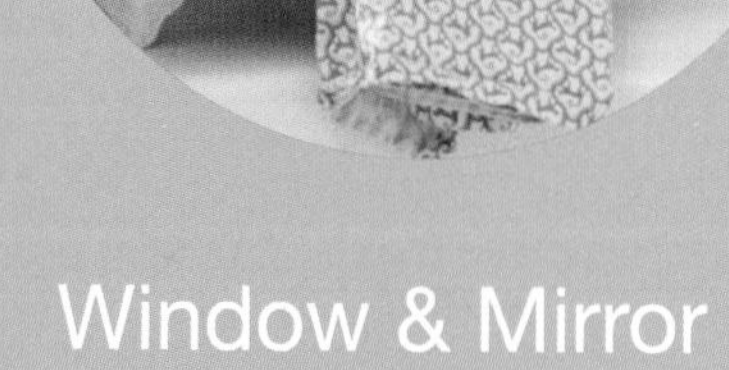

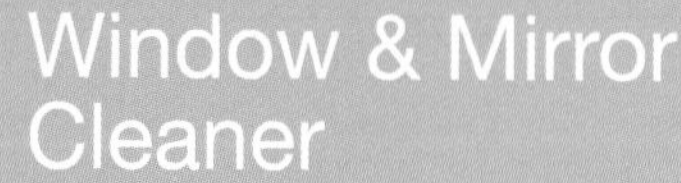

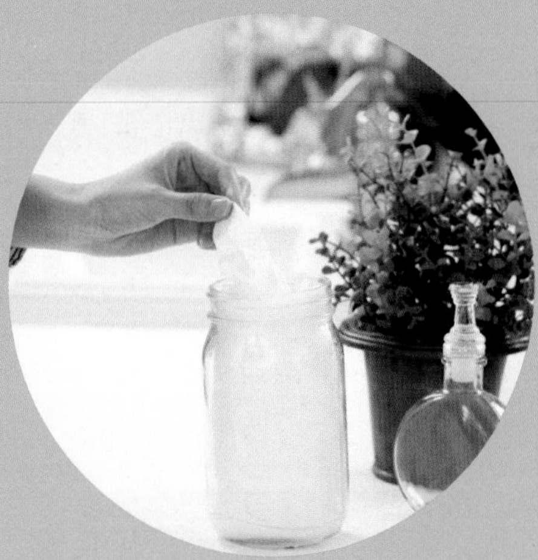

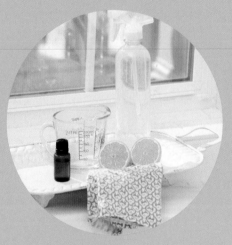

Soap Scum Remover

2 cups hot water
¼ - ½ cup borax
10 drops lemon essential oil

Add ingredients to a spray bottle and shake well. Spray surfaces and wipe dry. Store in cool place for up to two months.

Window & Mirror Cleaner

2 cups water
2 tablespoons white vinegar
2 tablespoons rubbing alcohol
5 drops peppermint essential oil

Add ingredients to a spray bottle and shake well. Spray windows or mirrors and wipe dry. Store in cool place for for up to two months.

Disinfecting Cleaning Wipes

12 thick and durable paper towels
1 cup distilled water
½ cup white vinegar
¼ cup rubbing alcohol
5 drops lavender essential oil
5 drops lemon essential oil

Cut paper towels in half and stack into a neat pile. Roll up and stuff into a quart size wide-mouth mason jar or large zip-lock bag. Mix ingredients and pour over paper towels and let absorb before using.

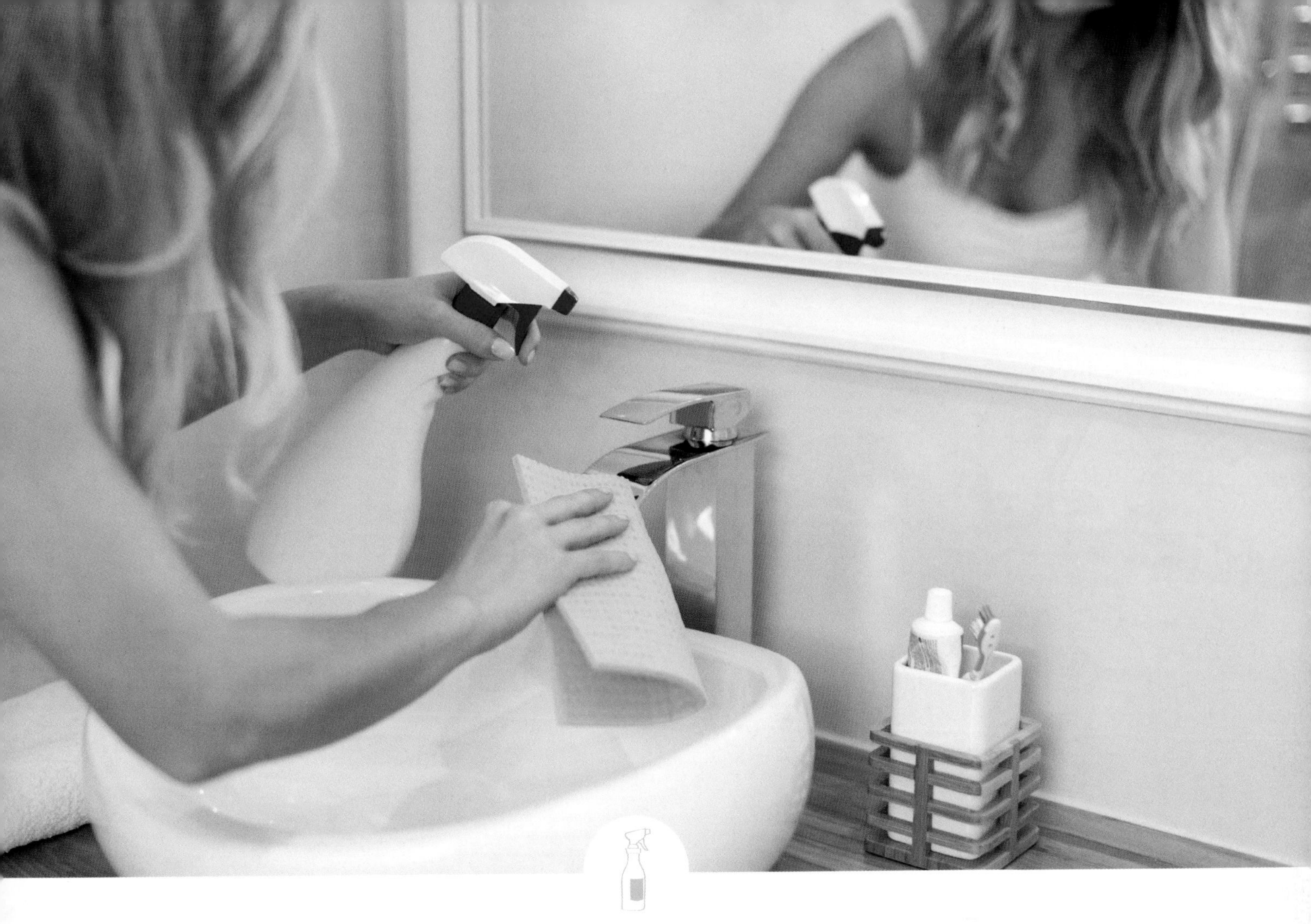

Mold & Mildew Preventer

2 cups water
30 drops tea tree essential oil
10 drops peppermint essential oil

Add ingredients to a spray bottle and shake well. Spray directly on mold or mildew. Do not rinse. Repeat daily or weekly as needed.

Disinfecting Toilet Bowl Cleaner

½ cup baking soda
¼ cup white vinegar
10 drops tea tree essential oil

Mix ingredients to dissolve baking soda. Add to toilet. Let sit for five to fifteen minutes. Scrub with a toilet brush and flush.

KITCHEN

Cleaning

Drain Cleaner

¼ cup baking soda
¼ cup distilled white vinegar
3 drops wild orange essential oil

Pour essential oil directly down drain, followed by baking soda, and then the vinegar. Allow to sit for fifteen minutes. Pour hot water down the drain, followed by cold water to unclog drains.

Sticker & Goo Remover

1 tablespoon baking soda
1 tablespoon almond or vegetable oil
2 drops lemon essential oil

Mix into a small glass bowl. Apply a small amount to the sticker or label and let sit for one to two minutes. Use a cloth or paper towel to remove. Apply again if needed.

Garbage Can Odor Tablets

2 cups baking soda
1 cup Epsom salt
¼ cup water
10 drops lemon essential oil
5 drops peppermint essential oil
Ice cube tray

Combine dry ingredients. Slowly add water, then oils, and stir. Using a spoon, transfer mixture into the ice cube tray without overfilling the tray. Allow to dry overnight or until hardened. Place one to two tablets in the bottom of your garbage can and store the rest in an airtight container. Replace tablets as needed

Grill Cleaner

¼ cup baking soda
2 tablespoons natural dish detergent
5 drops lemon essential oil
Distilled white vinegar

Combine the first three ingredients. Add vinegar until mixture has an olive-oil consistency. Brush mixture onto metal grill, and let sit for fifteen to thirty minutes. Use a damp scouring pad or grill brush to scrub surface clean. Rinse with water.

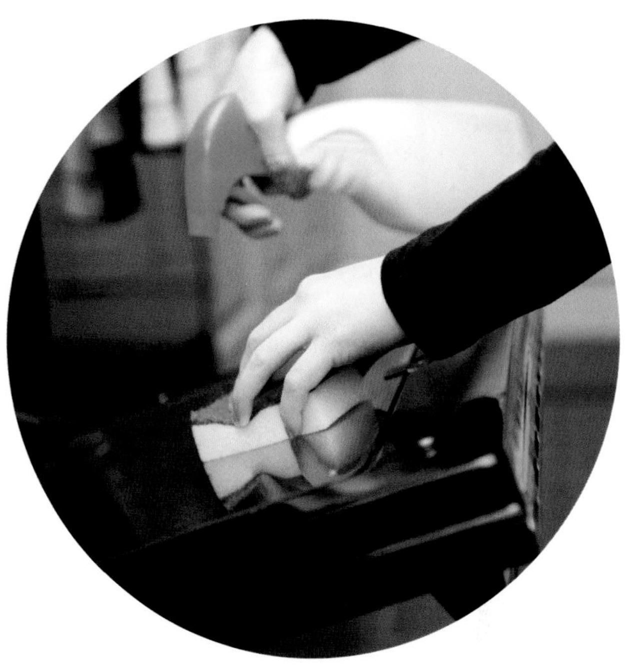

Oven Cleaner Spray

1 cup warm water
3 tablespoons baking soda
1 tablespoon castile soap
5 drops lemon essential oil
5 drops clove essential oil

Add all ingredients to a spray bottle and shake to combine. Spray liberally in the oven and let sit for fifteen minutes. Wipe clean with a sponge or cloth.

Oven Cleaner Paste

1 cup baking soda
½ cup water
1 tablespoon dish or castile soap
10 drops lemon essential oil

Combine ingredients in a bowl to form a paste. Apply with a sponge and let sit up to thirty minutes. Wipe off with clean cloth or sponge and water.

LAUNDRY Cleaning

Stain Remover

1 4 oz. glass spray bottle
½ cup white distilled vinegar
10 drops lemon essential oil
10 drops tea tree essential oil

Using a 4 oz. spray bottle, pour ½ cup of white distilled vinegar into the bottle. Add essential oils. Shake well. Spray onto any stain before washing and be amazed as this natural essential oil solution removes all unwanted marks!

Linen Spray

1 cup distilled water
1 tablespoon witch hazel
4 drops green mandarin essential oil

Combine ingredients in a glass spray bottle. Spritz pillows and linens.

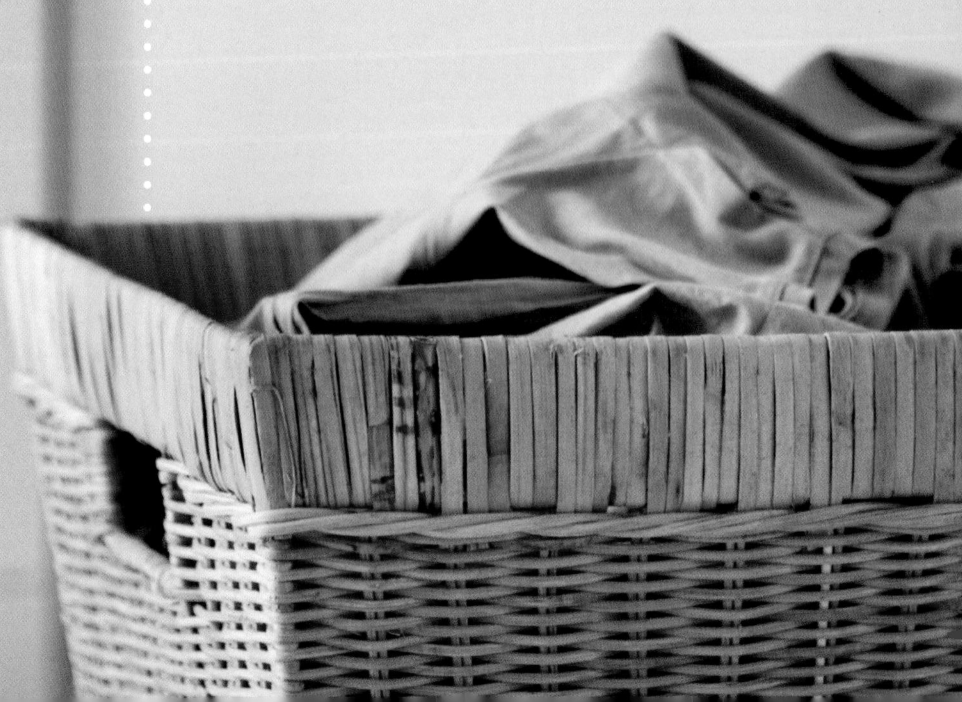

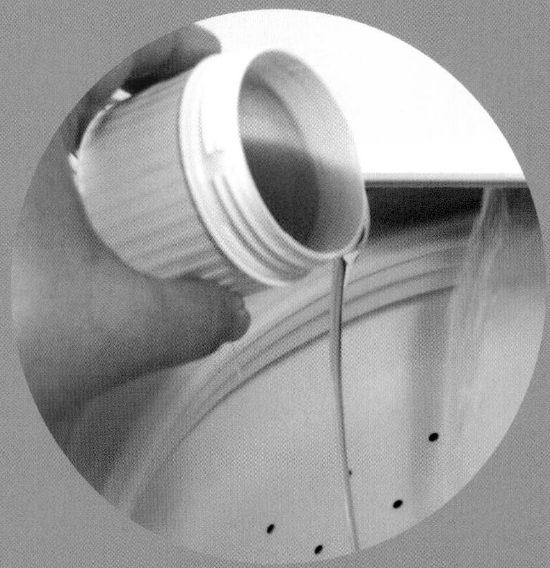

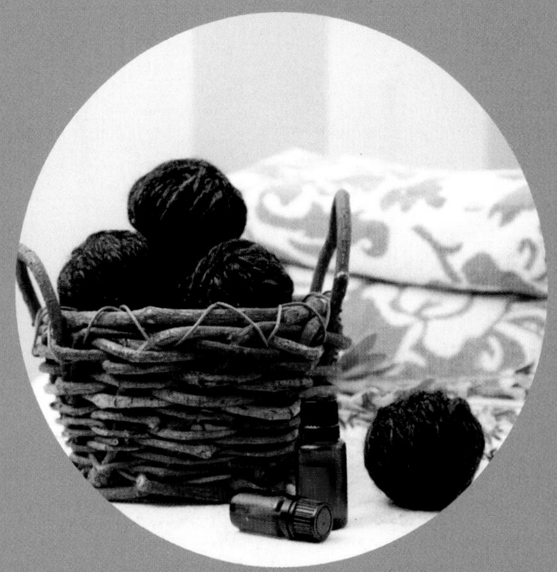

Liquid Fabric Softener

1 gallon distilled white vinegar
2 cups baking soda
20 drops clove essential oil
10 drops lemon essential oil

Combine ingredients in a large bowl or container and add ¼ to ½ cup per load. Your laundry will be softened and smell great.

Reusable Dryer Sheet

This is an easy and natural solution for a wonderfully scented dryer sheet.

1 6"x 6"piece of cotton or wool cloth (recycled T-shirts, sweaters, or socks, etc.)
2-4 drops orange or other essential oil

Place cloth in a container. Drop essential oil on fabric. Allow essential oil to dry thoroughly. Place dryer sheet on top of wet clothes in dryer and dry as usual. When sheet has lost its scent, simply add more oil.

Laundry Fragrance Booster

4 oz glass jar
Epsom salt
10-20 drops essential oil of choice

Fill jar ¾ full with Epsom salt. Add essential oils to the salt and stir well. To use, sprinkle (based on preference) into the washing machine. Start by adding a 3lb. box of kosher salt (you can substitute with Epsom salt or table salt) to a large bowl or ½ gallon mason jar. Then, add 20-25 drops of lavender essential oil. You could use lemon, lemongrass, Citrus Bliss®, or a scent of your choice.

Mix together, making sure to spread the oils throughout the salt. To use in your laundry, simply add ½ cup to your laundry and wash as usual. It is safe for high efficiency washers, and your clothes will not come out of your dryer smelling super strong, it will simply give your laundry a boost in scent.

Dryer Softener Balls

100% wool yarn or 100% animal yarn
Pantyhose (reuse pantyhose with runs in them)
4 to 6 drops essential oil of choice

Take the end of the yarn and wrap it around your middle and index finger ten times. Remove it from the fingers and then wrap two or three times around the middle. (It should look like a bow.) Keep tightly wrapping the yarn around, making a round shape the size of a tennis ball. Cut the yarn and tuck the ends into the sides of the ball. Create four or more balls. Cut one leg off pantyhose. Place one yarn ball into the bottom and tie a knot above the ball. Repeat until all the balls have been added and secured. Once secured, felt (fusing together resulting in a ball) the yarn by washing and drying on the highest heat setting. When the balls are dry, remove the pantyhose and add 4-6 drops of your favorite essential oil. Toss in dryer with clothes.

Stain Stick

This is a quick recipe for spot treatments on any fabric.

½ 5-ounce bar castile soap
3 teaspoons water
4 drops tea tree essential oil

Grate soap and place in microwave-safe bowl with water. Melt on low heat in microwave in thirty-second intervals for about a minute and a half. Once it has melted, let cool for five minutes and stir in essential oil. Pour into a stain stick container or deodorant container with a push-up bottom. Allow to cool to a solid state before using. Because melaleuca essential oil is a mild solvent, this stick will also help to remove set-in stains.

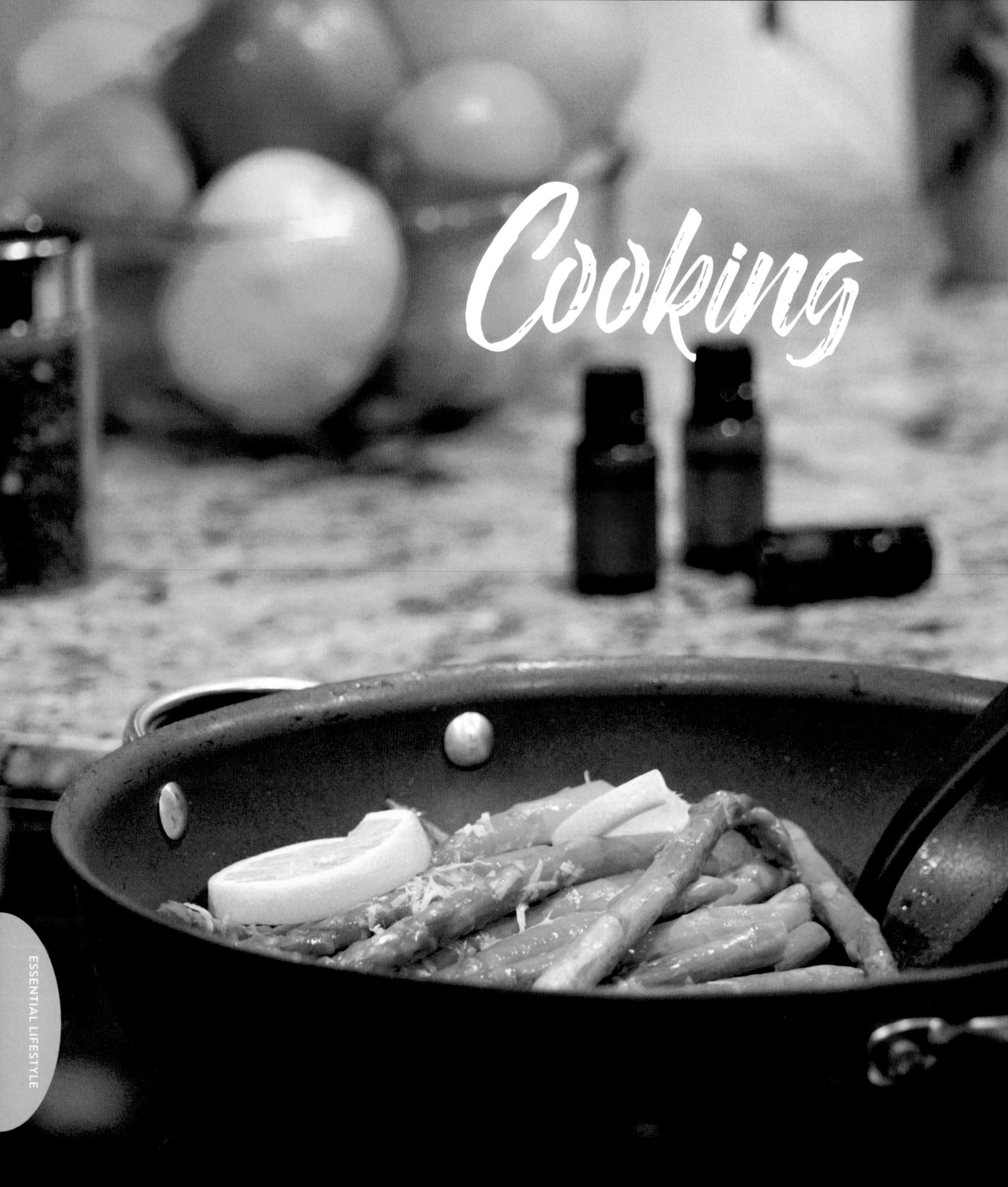

Cooking

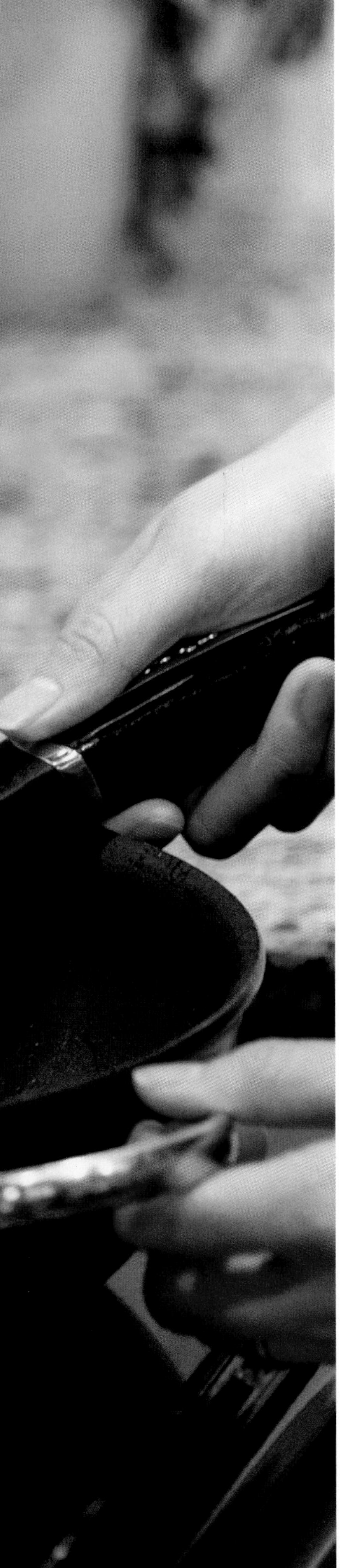

Tips for Cooking with Essential Oils

Green mandarin and pink pepper are both flavor preservatives. Use green mandarin with fruits/fruit salads to prolong flavor, use pink pepper in marinades and sauces for meats and vegetables.

Natural food preservatives: Add green mandarin (fruits) or turmeric (meats/vegetables) to naturally preserve your food.

Adding essential oils to your favorite recipes makes it easy to incorporate their healthful benefits throughout the day. There are many variables with dealing with essential oils for cooking. If you have ever used fresh herbs instead of dried, you know the flavor and the quantity used is different. The same rule applies to essential oils for cooking. The oils are super-concentrated in flavor and aroma. You may find that some essential oil brands are more potent than others—this has to do with sourcing and purity. Essential oils can add a very subtle or very strong taste to your cooked dishes, depending on how much you use. We like to enjoy and identify as many flavors in our foods as possible, so use caution and know that less is best. Start with a tiny amount, then add more as you need it. If you get too much, the flavor will dominate and can spoil your dish.

The oils all have different viscosity as well, so some are thinner and some are thicker. The type of opening in the bottle you are using will affect the size of the drop. Using a dropper or syringe can help control what you are dispersing. Another good option is to drip onto a utensil first, then pull from that amount what you want to go into your dish or beverage.

You'll notice in the following recipes there are some interesting measurements that will help you add the right amount of essential oils to your cooking recipes. The best way to control quantity is to use the toothpick method.

1 toothpick dip = dip a toothpick into the essential oil and dip it once into the recipe
1 toothpick swirl = dip a toothpick into the essential oil and swirl it around in the recipe
½ drop = Drop an essential oil into a spoon, then use the tip of a sharp knife to obtain the desired amount of oil and add it to the recipe.

Be sure to use a fresh toothpick with each use so as not to contaminate your essential oil bottles.

Hot, savory, or spicy herbs are particularly hard to judge (for example, basil oil may be much more subtle in flavor than oregano), so the general rule should be: if it isn't citrus oil, use a toothpick until you test it or have a guaranteed recipe.

It's always best to mix your essential oils with an olive or other oil or liquid when cooking to more evenly disperse the flavor in your dish.

Baking typically requires more oil flavoring than cooking does. For example, where you might use 2 or 3 toothpick swirls of oregano in spaghetti sauce, you might use 2 or 3 drops when making artisan bread.

SUBSTITUTING OILS FOR HERBS

Substitute an oil for an herb to increase the health benefits and increase the flavor of any dish.

- **½ teaspoon dried herbs = 1½ teaspoons fresh herbs = 2-3 toothpick swirls essential oil**
- **1 teaspoon dried herbs = 1 tablespoon fresh herbs = 1 drop essential oil**

SUBSTITUTING OILS FOR CITRUS

- **1 teaspoon lemon extract = ⅛ teaspoon lemon essential oil = 16 drops**
- **1 tablespoon lemon zest = 1/16 teaspoon lemon essential oil = 8 drops**

Homemade Cola

4 drops lime essential oil
4 drops orange essential oil
2 drop lemon essential oil
2 drop cardamom essential oil
⅛ teaspoon nutmeg
2 drop cinnamon essential oil
4 teaspoons vanilla extract
4 teaspoons maple syrup, honey or liquid stevia

Mix the essential oils with vanilla extract, nutmeg, and sweetener. Divide into two 8-10 oz of bubbly water. Serve chilled.

Blueberry Lavender Lemonade

Juice from 2 pounds (about 7 lemons) (should total about 1½ cups juice)
8 cups cold water
blueberry lavender simple syrup (below)
1 cup fresh blueberries
1 cup granulated sugar
2 cups water
6-8 drops lavender essential oil

Combine the lemon juice, water, and blueberry lavender simple syrup in a large jug. Serve over ice.
To Make the Blueberry Lavender Simple Syrup: Place the blueberries, sugar, and water in a small pot and bring to a simmer over medium heat. Reduce the heat to low and continue simmering for 5 minutes.
Remove from heat and allow to steep until completely cooled. Stir in the lavender essential oil.

Celery Seed Tea

2-3 drops celery seed essential oil
1 cup of hot water

Combine and drink up to three cups a day.

Sparkling Citrus Drink

12 ounces selzer water
⅛ -¼ teaspoon stevia, to taste
6 drops grapefruit essential oil
6 drops lemon essential oil

Mix ingredients together and serve chilled or over ice. Garnish with a sprig of mint or a slice of lime, if desired. For a dash of color, add a tiny bit of red food coloring to create a pink color for the pink grapefruit.

Frozen Blended Virgin Daiquiri

1 cup frozen strawberries
1 teaspoon vanilla extract
1-2 drops lime essential oil
1 cup water
Stevia to sweeten

Mix all ingredients in blender. Add more sweetener or lime to taste. Add more water for a thinner consistency. For a creamy consistency, add a little plain yogurt.

Sparkling Lavender Lemonade

1 cup water
1 cup sugar
2 drops lavender essential oil
1 cup lemon juice (about 6 lemons juiced)
3 cups cold sparkling water
1 drop purple food coloring (optional)

Create a simple syrup by combining equal parts water and sugar in a small saucepan. If using fresh or dried lavender add that to your saucepan. Bring to a simmer and cook, stirring until sugar is dissolved. Let cool to room temperature, strain and combine lemon juice, simple syrup, and water in a 1 quart pitcher. If using essential oil, add 2 drops of lavender oil. Add food coloring if desired. Serve with ice and lemon slices.

tips

- Try adding these essential oils to still or sparkling water for a delicious flavor (and zero calories!)
  - Peppermint
  - Lemon
  - Cardamom
  - On Guard®
  - Grapefruit
  - Ginger
  - Lime
  - Grapefruit & cassia
- Add essential oil to ice cube trays. To distinguish the flavor and add to the presentation, you can include a drop of food coloring, zest of fruit, or leaf (e.g. peppermint or basil; dried citrus looks appealing as well).

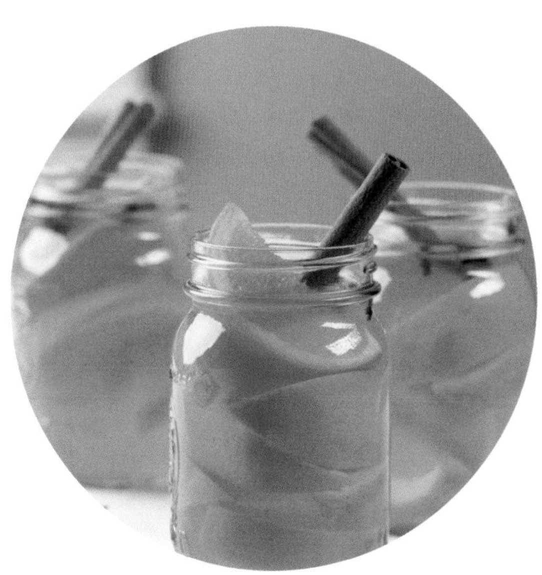

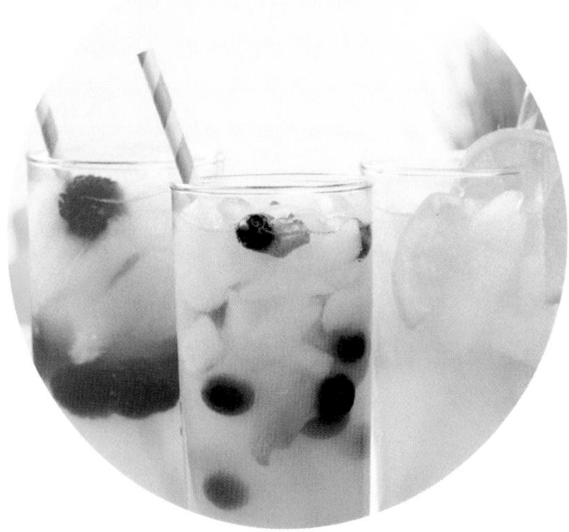

Citrus Water

16 oz. water
Glass water bottle or mason jar
1 drop lemon essential oil
1 drop orange essential oil
1 drop grapefruit essential oil
Sliced lemons, limes, berries or other fresh fruit, optional

Add 16 oz. water to a glass water bottle or mason jar. Add essential oils. Add more oils, 1 drop at a time, to taste. Optional, add fresh lemon slices, lime slices, berries or other fresh fruit. Drink and enjoy a refreshing citrus flavor in your daily water glasses.

Green Berry Protein Shake

8 ounces almond milk (or milk of your choice)
3 scoops protein shake mix
1-2 cups fresh or frozen berries
2 scoops powdered greens mix or 1 large handful of fresh, washed spinach
2 drops ginger essential oil
2 drops grapefruit essential oil

Pour ingredients in blender, blend until smooth, and serve.

Lemonade Bar

Prepared lemonade of choice (8 ounces per person).
Various fresh fruits, like raspberries, strawberries, lemons, limes.
Toothpicks for flavoring with oils.

Choose one or more of these essential oils:
- Basil essential oil, 1 toothpick dip or to taste (great with raspberry lemonade)
- Lavender essential oil, 1 toothpick swirl or to taste
- Geranium essential oil, 1 toothpick swirl or to taste
- Ginger essential oil, 1 toothpick swirl or to taste
- Grapefruit essential oil, 3-4 toothpick swirls or to taste
- Lime essential oil, 2-3 toothpick swirls or to taste

Pour prepared lemonade into glasses, allowing your guests to add fruit and their choice of essential oils with the toothpicks. This is a fun crowd-pleaser!

Lime Rickey

32 oz. Concord grape juice
16 oz. sparkling apple cider
4 drops lime essential oil
Lime slices, for garnish

Add all ingredients into a large glass pitcher, stir, and serve over ice cubes.

Breads

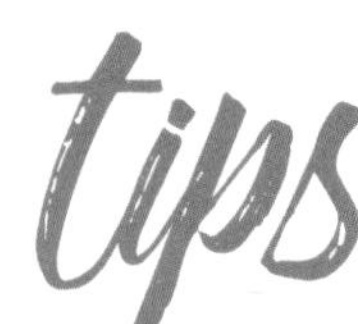

tips

Essential oils can flavor butters and oils for a savory, spicy, or sweet taste. For example, add cinnamon essential oil, stevia, and ground cinnamon to butter or oil for toast or biscuits. Add flavored butters or oil to the bread after it comes out of oven.

To your favorite bread recipes, add corresponding essential oils instead of herbs. You can also add orange essential oil-infused dried cranberries into sweet bread or muffin batters (see Snacks).

Make bread dips by flavoring olive oil with rosemary, thyme, and basil essential oils to taste. Mix balsamic vinegar with the flavored olive oil and serve with fresh bread chunks or slices.

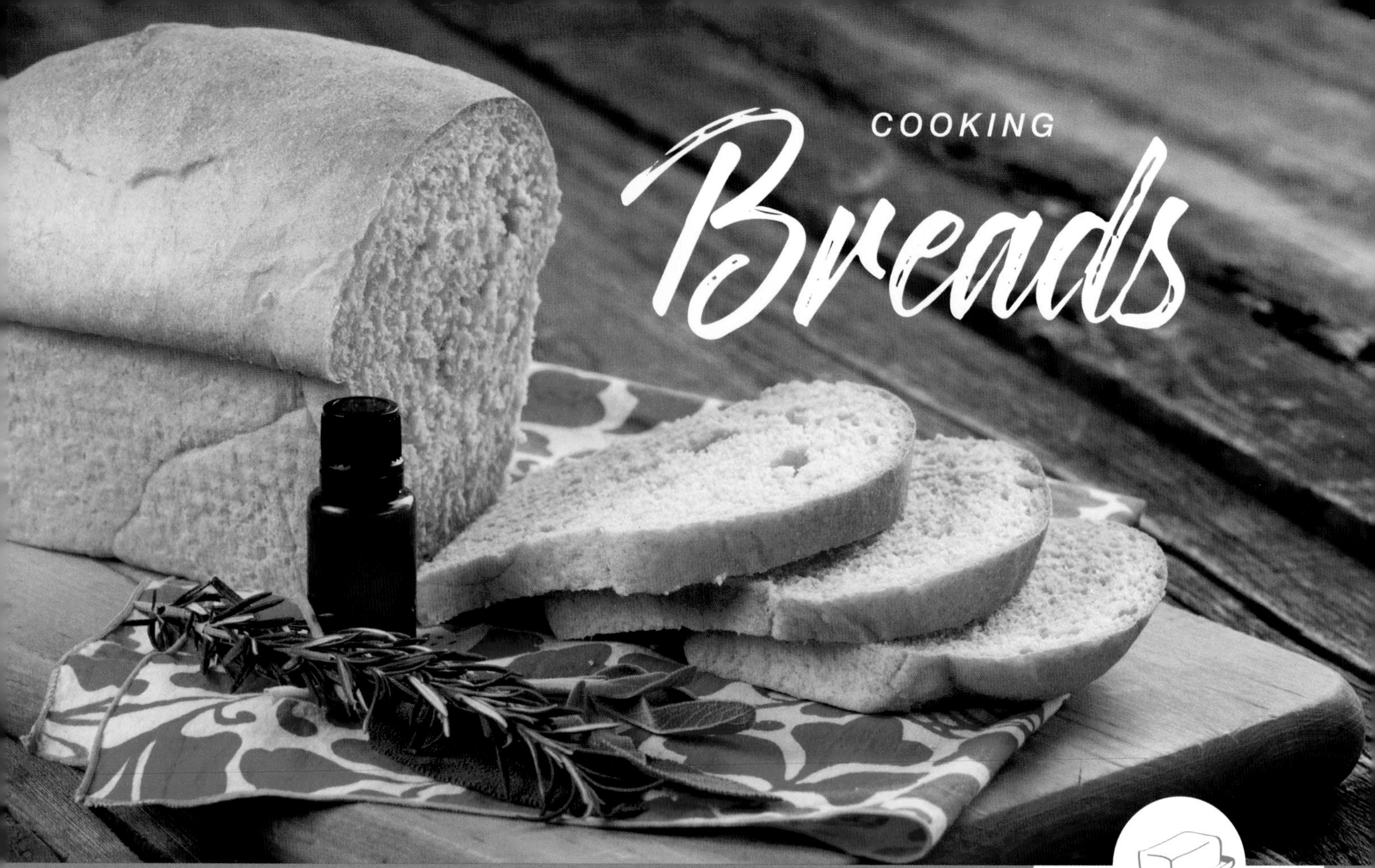

Wheat Herb Bread

2 drops thyme, sage, basil, rosemary, or oregano essential oil
1 ½ teaspoon honey (to taste)
1 ⅓ cups warm water
1 package or 2 ¼ teaspoons active dry yeast
1 ½ teaspoon sea salt
2 to 2 ¼ cups bread flour
1 ¾ cups whole wheat flour

Stir together essential oil drops and honey.

In a large bowl, combine water, yeast, and honey/essential oil mixture. Let stand for 5 minutes.

In a separate bowl, combine salt and flours. Stir flour mixture in gradually to water mixture until flour has been absorbed and the dough forms a ball.

In a mixer or by hand, knead dough until it is moderately stiff, smooth, and elastic.

Lightly spray a bowl with nonstick spray. Place dough in bowl, cover with a towel or plastic wrap (spray with nonstick spray), and let rise until doubled in size.

Remove dough from bowl, and punch down. Let rest for 10 minutes.

Spray an 8x4" bread loaf pan with nonstick spray. Shape dough to form a loaf and place in loaf pan. Let rise again until doubled in size, but not much higher than top of loaf pan. Put into a cold oven.

Bake in a 350 degrees oven for 25-30 minutes or more until golden on top and sides pull away from pan.

Tip: Great bread for dipping in your favorite olive oil (see Sauces recipes for ideas)

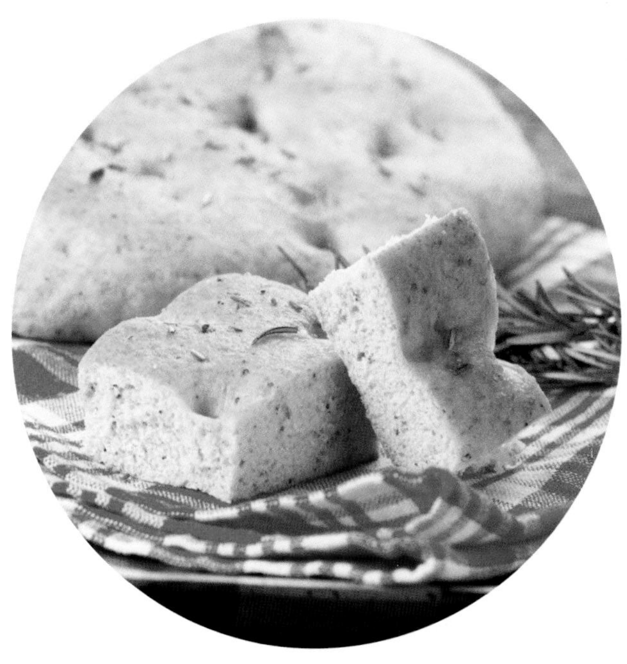

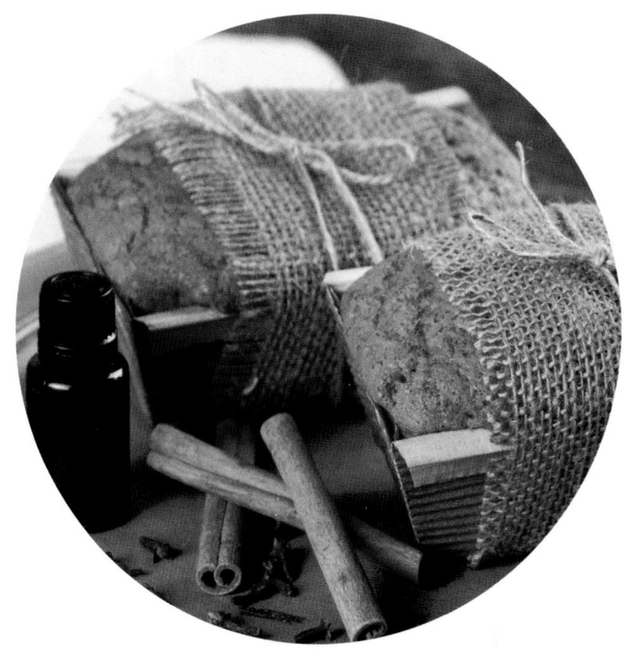

Rosemary Artisan Sourdough Bread

1 ½ cups all-purpose flour
1 ½ cups whole wheat flour
1 teaspoon salt
½ teaspoon active dry yeast (increase to 2 ¼ teaspoon if you don't want to wait all night)
1 ½ cups warm water
3–4 drops rosemary essential oil
¼ teaspoon Italian seasoning (optional)
¼ teaspoon garlic powder (optional)
¼ teaspoon black pepper (optional)
Fresh rosemary, roughly chopped, for garnish

In a large bowl, stir the flour, salt, and yeast together. Add warm water and rosemary essential oil, and stir to combine. It's fine if it looks messy or on the dry side.

Cover the bowl with plastic wrap, and set at room temperature for 8–24 hours (it is done sitting when it looks wet and bubbly and has doubled in size). Turn dough out onto a well-floured surface, and gently pull it into a squarish shape. Sprinkle on Italian seasoning, garlic powder, black pepper, and fresh rosemary. Fold the corners in like an envelope; then flip the dough over and shape it into a ball. Let it rest for 30 minutes. In the meantime, put your baking dish with high sides (we used a dutch oven) in the oven, and preheat to 450°F (230°C).

After the 30 minutes are up, flip the bread over (seam side up) or cut an "x" in the dough, sprinkle with fresh rosemary, and carefully place it in the hot dutch oven. Cover with the lid, and cook for 30 minutes. Remove the lid and continue cooking, uncovered, for 10–20 minutes, or until bread is golden brown.

Pumpkin Bread

3 ½ cups all purpose flour
1 teaspoon salt
2 teaspoons baking soda
2 ¾ cups sugar
1 teaspoon baking powder
½ cup coconut oil
½ cup unsalted butter, softened
1 (15 oz) can pumpkin puree
4 large eggs
⅓ cup water
1 cup plain yogurt
2 drops cinnamon essential oil
1 drop clove essential oil
⅛ teaspoon nutmeg
1 drop ginger essential oil
4 drops lemon essential oil

Preheat oven to 325 degrees. Spray pans with non-stick cooking spray. In a small bowl, combine flour, baking soda, baking powder, salt, and sugar and set aside. In a mixing bowl, combine the coconut oil, butter, pumpkin puree, water, yogurt, eggs, and all essential oils.

With the mixer on low, slowly add the dry ingredients to the wet, scraping the sides often to make sure all ingredients are well combined. Once they're well mixed, set the mixer to a medium speed and mx for two minutes until light and fluffy.

Divide mixture into pans and bake for 45-50 minutes or until a toothpick comes out clean from the middle of the bread.

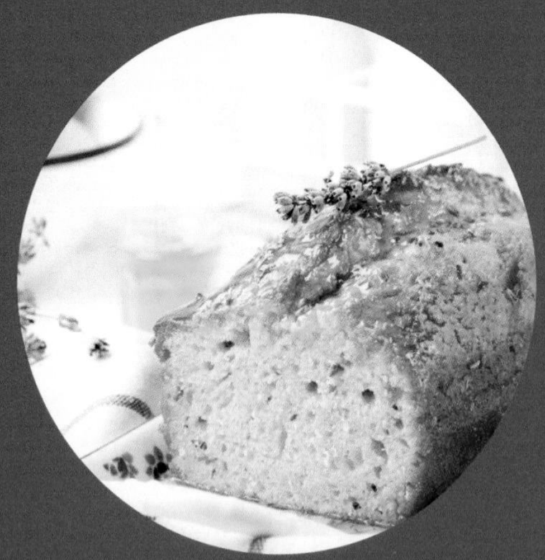

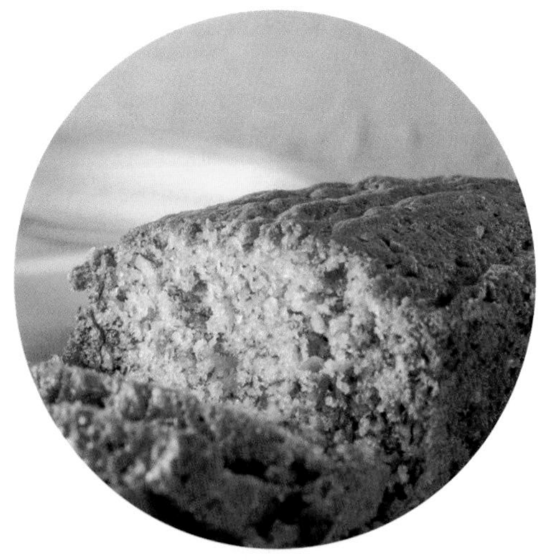

Lavender Lemon Banana Bread

2 ripe bananas, mashed
1 egg
3 drops lavender essential oil
2 drops lemon essential oil
¼ cup softened butter
1 ¾ cups superfine cake flour
½ teaspoon salt
1 teaspoon vanilla
¾ teaspoon baking powder
¼ teaspoon baking soda
⅔ cup sugar
1 tablespoon lemon zest
⅓ cup sour cream

Preheat oven to 350.

In mixing bowl, combine butter and sugar, mixing until smooth. Add in egg, sour cream, lemon zest, vanilla, lavender and lemon oils, and bananas. Mix and set aside.

In separate bowl combine flour, baking soda and powder, and salt. Whisk together until blended. In loaf pan, grease and then dust the sides with flour. Pour In batter until it fills the pan halfway. Bake for 40-45 minutes.Remove and allow to cool briefly. Serve warm or cooled.

Ginger Spice Banana Bread

4 medjool dates, washed and de-seeded
½ tablespoon maple syrup
½ cup coconut flour (almond flour)
½ teaspoon salt
¼ teaspoon baking soda
½ teaspoon nutmeg
6 eggs
½ tablespoon vanilla
¼ cup coconut oil (warmed)
½ cup very ripe bananas, mashed
½ cup walnuts, chopped
½ cup pecans, chopped
1 drops ginger essential oil
1 drop cinnamon essential oil

Preheat the oven to 350 degree. Place the dates and maple syrup in a food processor and process to combine, add the mixture to a large mixing bowl with the remaining ingredients and mix to combine.

Pour the batter into loaf pan and bake for 30-40 minutes or until golden.

Specialty Frostings/Glazes

Add 1-2 drops lemon or wild orange essential oil to glazes or frostings. If you make a lemon or citrus cake or pastry, you can try a toothpick dip of lavender essential oil with a drop of lemon essential oil in the glaze for a unique and delicious flavor combination.

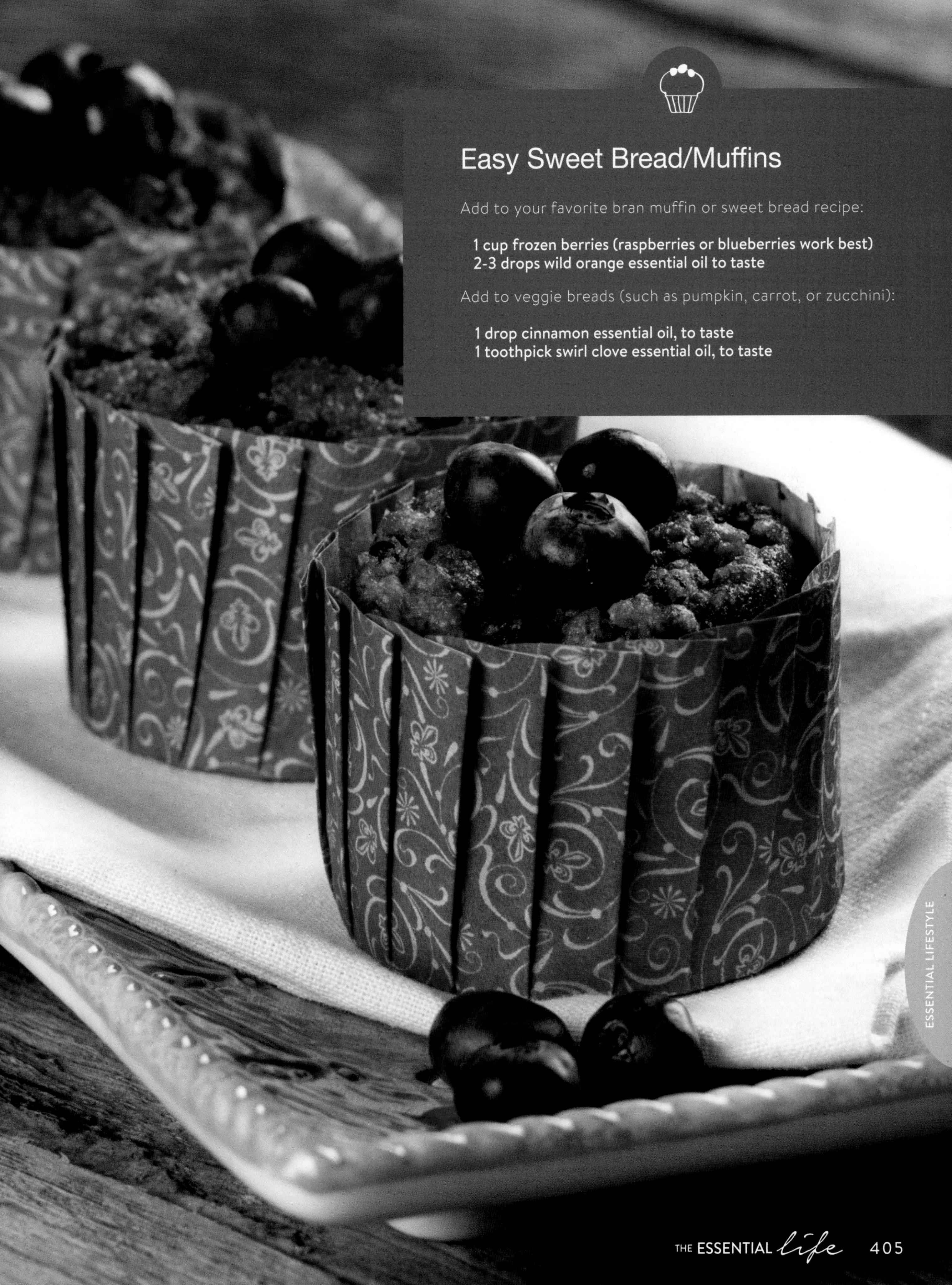

Easy Sweet Bread/Muffins

Add to your favorite bran muffin or sweet bread recipe:

1 cup frozen berries (raspberries or blueberries work best)
2-3 drops wild orange essential oil to taste

Add to veggie breads (such as pumpkin, carrot, or zucchini):

1 drop cinnamon essential oil, to taste
1 toothpick swirl clove essential oil, to taste

COOKING

Breakfast

Blueberry Cardamom Scones

3 cups all-purpose flour
⅓ cup sugar
1 tablespoon baking powder
1 teaspoon salt
12 tablespoon butter, cut into pieces
1 pint blueberries
¾ cups plus 2 tablespoon milk
2 drops cardamom essential oil
1 drops ginger essential oil
2 tablespoon turbinado sugar, for sprinkling

Preheat oven to 375 degrees. Line a rimmed baking sheet with piece of parchment paper.

In a bowl, combine flour, sugar, baking powder and salt, cut in the butter pieces until well combined, toss in the fresh blueberries, add milk and combine well. Divide dough into 2 pieces and on a floured surface, form into a round disk, about 6" in diameter, using extra flour if needed. Slice each section into 6 triangular scones. Place on lined baking sheet. Mix turbinado sugar, cardamom and ginger essential oils in small bowl, and sprinkle tops of scones. Bake in the preheated oven for 25 to 30 minutes, or until golden on top.

Grain-free Huevos Rancheros

10-12 eggs
1 medium onion, finely chopped
1 red bell pepper, finely chopped and de-seeded
2 bunches green onions or one leek, finely chopped
2 tomatoes, finely chopped
½ to 1 drop oregano essential oil to taste
¼ cup fresh cilantro, finely chopped
1 tablespoon of each of the following – cumin, coriander, oregano, and chili powder
½ tablespoon paprika
1 teaspoon Celtic Sea Salt or Himalayan Pink Salt
1 teaspoon pepper of choice – red pepper flakes or 1 drop black pepper essential oil
4 cloves minced garlic
¼ cup coconut milk or yogurt for added creaminess if desired
½ cup shredded cheese – Gruyere, Cheddar, or Colby Jack
2 drops lemon essential oil

In a large cast iron or stainless steel skillet, saute the onion until clear and slightly browned. Add the green onions/leeks until they get a little soft, but not too soft. Add the tomatoes, garlic and spices and cook for just a few minutes. Add the eggs and cook until desired consistency is reached. Top with grated cheese. Serve right out of the skillet!

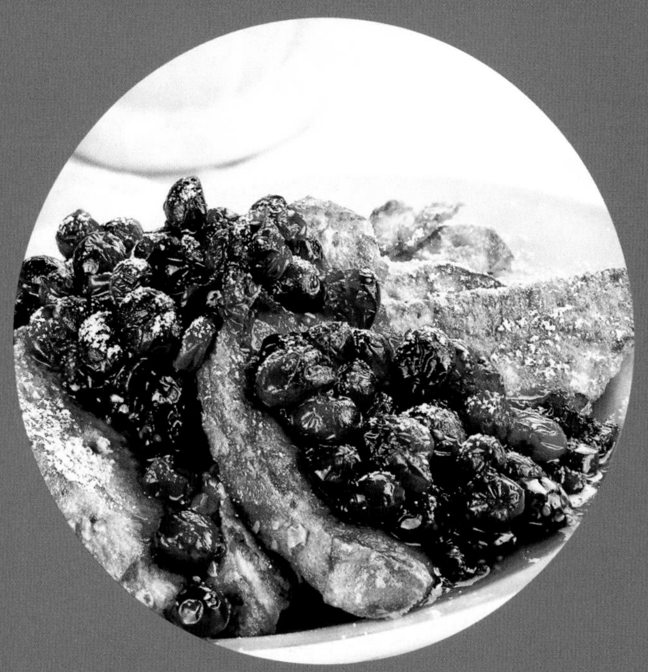

French Toast with Apple Cranberry Sauce

1 cup dried cranberries
½ cup juice (grape, apple or orange)
1 cup berry preserves
1 Granny Smith apple, chopped
4 drops orange essential oil, divided
3 drops cinnamon essential oil, divided
3 eggs
¾ cup milk
½ cup butter, melted
½ teaspoon vanilla extract
⅛ teaspoon nutmeg
1 drop clove essential oil
1 drop ginger essential oil
2 drop cinnamon bark essential oil
2 drops wild orange essential oil
8 big slices of bread or 12 regular slices

In a small stainless steel saucepan, combine the cranberries, juice, preserves, and apples. Cook over low heat until the mixture comes to a low simmer. Remove from heat and stir in orange and cinnamon essential oils and set aside.

Heat griddle to 375 degrees.

In a shallow glass or ceramic dish, combine the eggs, milk, butter, vanilla, nutmeg, clove and ginger essential oil, plus cinnamon bark and orange essential oils, stir well. Dip bread into the egg mixture and allow extra mixture drip off before cooking on the griddle, and cook on both sides until done. Spoon apple mixture over the top and serve immediately.

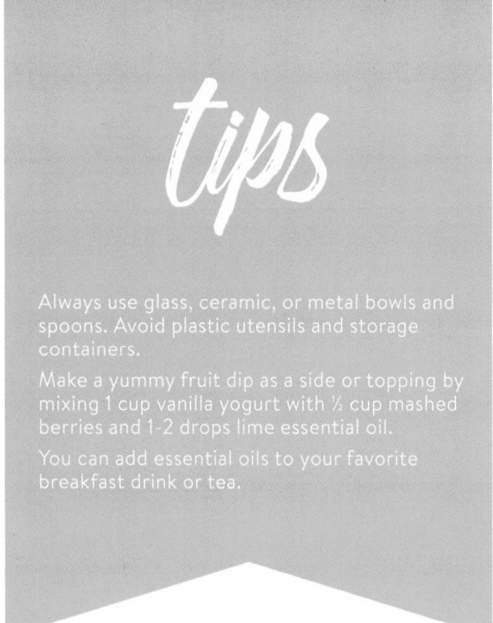

Always use glass, ceramic, or metal bowls and spoons. Avoid plastic utensils and storage containers.

Make a yummy fruit dip as a side or topping by mixing 1 cup vanilla yogurt with ½ cup mashed berries and 1-2 drops lime essential oil.

You can add essential oils to your favorite breakfast drink or tea.

Mexican Eggs

2 cups cooked black beans
½ cup salsa or more, to taste
½ teaspoon unrefined sea salt
½-1 drop lime essential oil, to taste
Bacon drippings
¼ teaspoon cumin essential oil or ground cumin to taste

Place first three ingredients in a saucepan and heat over medium until heated through and bubbling. Turn the burner off and allow beans to cool for a few minutes, and then add essential oil. Heat skillet over medium heat and add bacon drippings. Scramble eggs with a bit of salt and pepper. Combine black bean mixture and scrambled eggs in individual bowls, and add optional toppings. Enjoy!

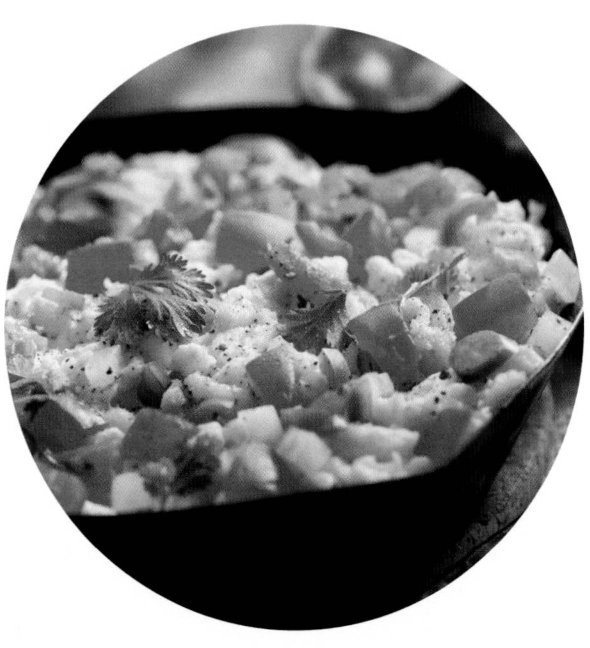

Orange Cinnamon Biscuits

2 ½ cups all-purpose flour
½ cup cornstarch (plus more for rolling)
4 ½ teaspoons baking powder
½ teaspoon salt
½ cup salted butter (cold)
1 cup whole fat plain yogurt
2 teaspoons vanilla extract + ½ teaspoon, divided
1 egg
6 drops tangerine essential oil
6 drops lemon essential oil
2 tablespoons butter, softened
¼ cups sugar
2 teaspoons ground cinnamon
2 tablespoons whole milk
10 drops wild orange essential oil
1 cup powdered sugar

Heat oven to 450 degrees. Line a baking sheet with parchment paper. In your food processor, combine flour, cornstarch, baking powder, and salt, when combined add ½ cup cold butter. Pulse about 10 seconds until crumbly and the butter is pea sized, evenly distributed throughout the flour mixture. Add yogurt, 2 teaspoons vanilla, egg, and tangerine and lemon essential oils and pulse until dough ball forms.

Remove from bowl onto rolling surface that is lightly covered with cornstarch. Knead the dough a few times turning it over onto itself and turning about 6 – 10 times. Don't overwork the dough with your hands. This will heat the dough and cause the butter to melt. This will make for less than perfect biscuits.

Use a rolling pin to roll out to 9 X 15 rectangle. It will be about ¾ inch thick.

Spread the softened 2 tablespoons of butter over the dough rectangle, and sprinkle the sugar and cinnamon over the top. Roll the long side of the dough up with the butter mixture on the inside. Slice into 15 sections (about 1 inch each).

Bake on middle rack at 450 degrees for 10 minutes until biscuits are lightly browned.

While the biscuits cool mix together the milk, ½ teaspoon vanilla extract, wild orange essential oil, and the powdered sugar in a small bowl. Stir until no lumps remain. Dip the biscuits into the glaze and allow them to sit for 5 minutes before serving.

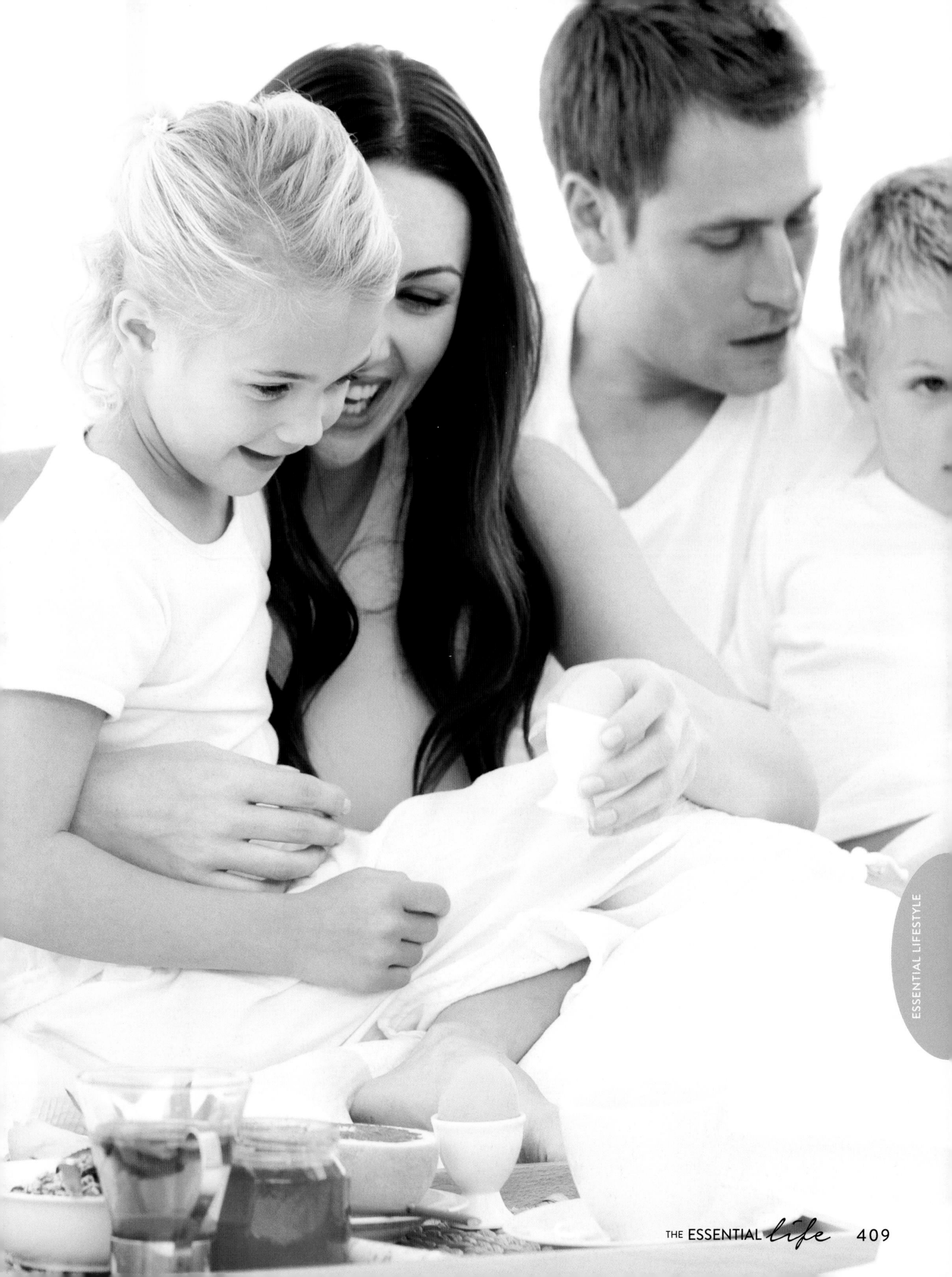

ESSENTIAL LIFESTYLE

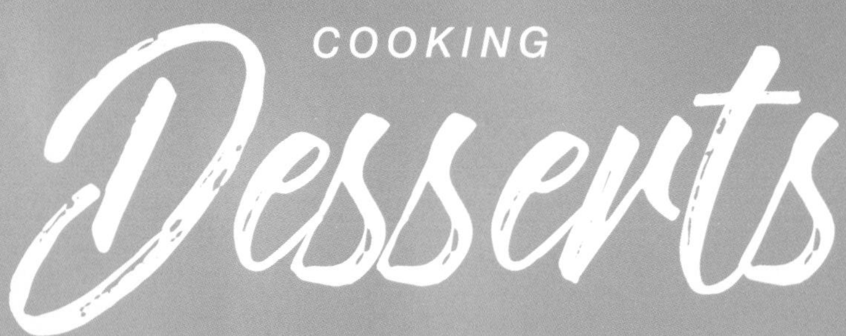

Lemon Or Lime Bars

CRUST:
1 cup butter, softened (not melted)
2 cups flour
½ cup powdered sugar
¼ teaspoon sea salt

FILLING:
4 eggs
2 cups sugar
3 tablespoon lemon or lime juice
1 tablespoon water
¼ cup cornstarch
6 drops lemon or lime essential oil (or more to taste)

TOPPING (after baking):
⅓ - ½ cup powdered sugar
1 drop lemon or lime essential oil

Mix butter, flour, ½ cup powdered sugar, and salt with pastry blender. Press into the bottom of 9x13" pan. (For nicer presentation, line pan with parchment paper so you can lift bars out of pan). Bake at 350 degrees for 15 minutes. While baking, mix eggs and sugar till light and fluffy. Add the lemon or lime juice, essential oil, water and cornstarch. Pour mixture over semi-cooked crust and bake an additional 25-30 minutes. Mix powdered sugar and citrus oil in baggie and shake it up. When lemon bars are done, sprinkle with citrus-infused powdered sugar on top by putting into metal strainer and shaking onto warm bars (let them cool a bit, but not completely).

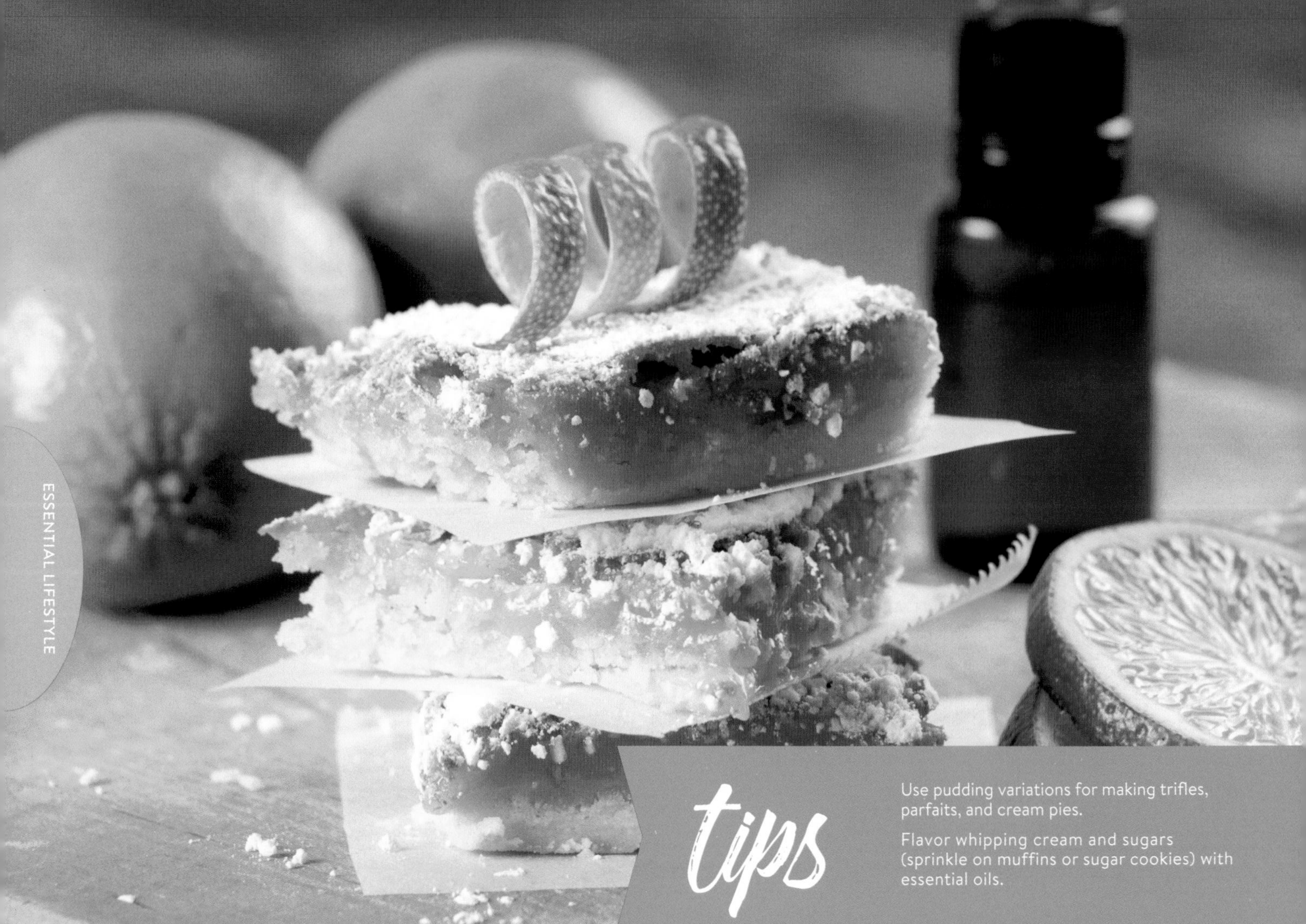

tips

Use pudding variations for making trifles, parfaits, and cream pies.

Flavor whipping cream and sugars (sprinkle on muffins or sugar cookies) with essential oils.

Strawberries Romanoff

Wash and rinse 1 quart strawberries and lay on paper towel to dry. Into sour cream or plain Greek yogurt, add 2 toothpick swirls lemon essential oil. Put brown sugar in a dish. Holding strawberry by the stem, dip into yogurt or sour cream essential oil mixture, then dab into brown sugar.

Ice Cream Log

Prepare desired cake recipe as directed. Instead of using a 9" x 13" pan, prepare a jelly roll pan with nonstick spray. Place parchment paper 2" larger than pan on all sides, and spray nonstick spray on parchment paper. Spread cake batter thinly onto the paper.

Bake on a higher oven rack for 10-12 minutes at 350 degrees. Remove pan. Lift cake out of pan by holding all corners of parchment paper, let cool.

While cake is cooling, make ice cream mixture. Into 1 quart vanilla ice cream softened to the consistency of a thick milkshake, add your desired flavoring (e.g. peppermint, orange, lime, lemon, cinnamon, cardamom essential oils, chocolate chip pieces or sprinkles) to taste. Spread ice cream evenly on top of cooled cake mixture. Roll cake and ice cream using parchment paper, removing paper as you roll. Place roll onto a parchment-paper lined pan and freeze. Once frozen, you can wrap with plastic wrap to store in freezer. Slice and serve.

Pudding Variations

Use your favorite pudding recipe.

Citrus: Add 1 drop lemon, lime, grapefruit, mandarin,tangerine or wild orange essential oils to warm pudding, after pudding has thickened slightly. If you want to add more, add in "toothpick dip" increments.

Chocolate: In a microwavable dish, melt 1 cup chocolate chips and stir into warm pudding after pudding has thickened slightly. Add 3 toothpick swirls peppermint essential oil to taste; 1 drop wild orange; 2 toothpick swirls cinnamon, cassia, or cardamom essential oils to taste.

Butterscotch: In a microwavable dish, melt 1 cup butterscotch chips and stir into warm pudding after pudding has thickened slightly. Add 1 toothpick dip ginger essential oil to taste.

Banana: Chop a banana into small pieces; add to warm pudding. Add 1 toothpick swirl of Citrus Bliss® essential oil or 1 swirl ginger essential oil.

Coconut: Add roasted coconut flakes to prepared pudding, add a dollop of whipped cream, and sprinkle shredded coconut on top.

Coconut lime: Add roasted coconut flakes to prepared pudding together with 2-3 toothpick swirls lime essential oil. Add a dollop of whipped cream and sprinkle shredded coconut on top.

Lemon Essential Oil Cookies

1 ice cream scoop
2 cups all-purpose flour
2 teaspoons baking powder
½ teaspoon salt
10 tablespoons softened butter
1 cup and 2 tablespoons organic sugar
1 large egg yolk
1 large egg
8-12 drops lemon essential oil (amount dependent on taste preference)
2 tablespoons whole milk

Preheat oven to 350 degrees. In a medium size bowl, combine flour, baking powder, salt, softened butter, organic sugar, egg yolk, and 1 whole egg. Add 8-12 drops of lemon essential oil (amount dependent on taste preference) to contents. Pour whole milk into bowl and mix well with the spatula until a dough is formed. Line a baking pan, and with the ice cream scoop, place cookie dough balls into even sections on the pan. Bake at 350 degrees for ten minutes. Let the cookies cool for 5-10 minutes, and then hoard a few lemon essential oil cookies before they are all gone!

Peppermint Brownies

12 oz. semi-sweet chocolate chips
¾ cup salted butter
1 ¼ cup organic sugar
1 tablespoon pure vanilla extract
4 large eggs
3 drops peppermint essential oil
1 teaspoon salt
1 cup of all purpose flour
1 cup of chocolate chips (optional; for richer, extra taste)

Preheat oven to 350 degrees. In a small microwaveable bowl, melt the butter and semi-sweet chocolate chips together. Stir contents with spatula to ensure the chocolate and butter are both melted and incorporated. Pour mixture into the medium size bowl. Add organic sugar, pure vanilla extract, eggs and peppermint essential oil, and mix well with the spatula. Add 1 teaspoon of salt, and stir again. Slowly, fold in flour. As an extra chocolate incentive, add additional chocolate chips and mix. Lightly dust your 13x9 baking pan with flour, and pour batter evenly into pan. Bake at 350 degrees for 30 minutes. Let cool for ten minutes, and then dig in to this masterpiece!

COOKING

Dressings & Marinades

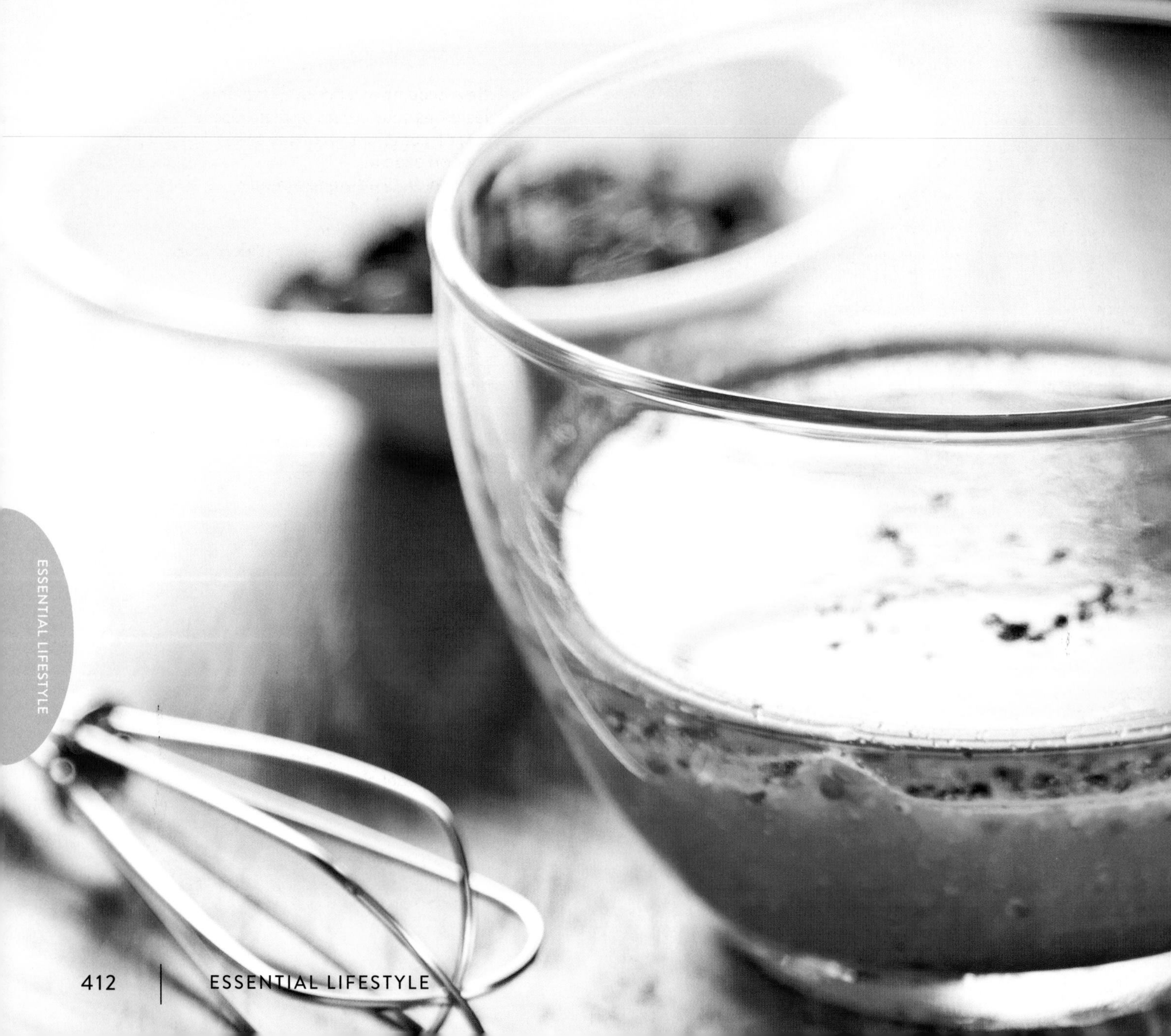

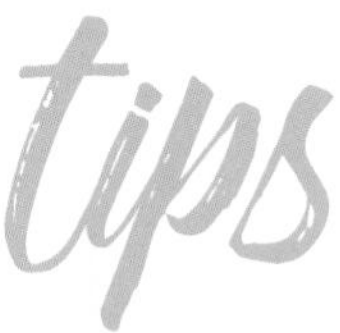

- Essential oils absorb well into meats and make great marinades.
- When making vinegar dressings, pair ingredients. Balsamic or red wine vinegar (dark vinegars) pairs with raspberry or strawberry salads, beef, and lamb. White wine vinegar, rice, or champagne vinegars (light vinegars) go well with chicken, fish, pears, chunks of grapefruit, mango, or orange.
- Candied nuts and feta cheese go well with both dressings.

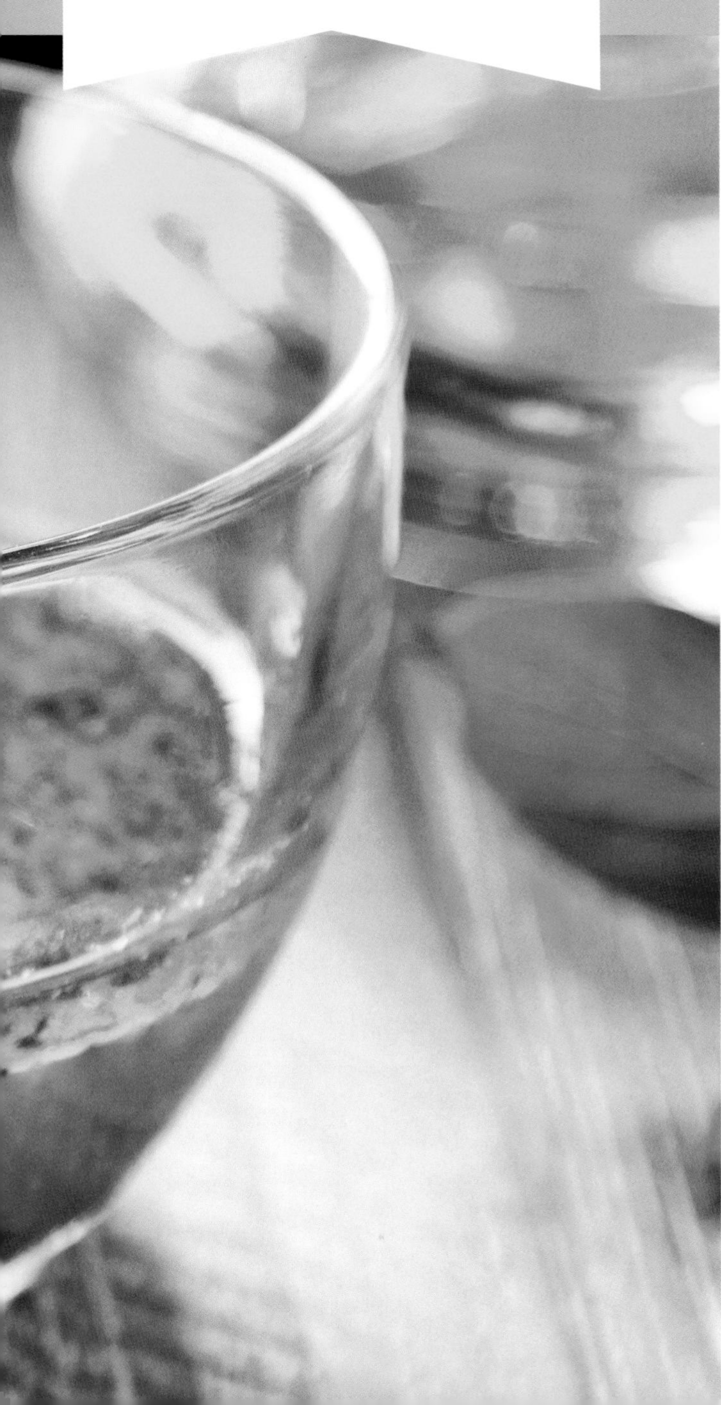

Wild Orange Vinaigrette

1 cup extra virgin olive oil
1 teaspoon Dijon mustard
½-⅓ cup balsamic vinegar
1-2 drops wild orange essential oil
2 tablespoon mayonnaise
½ cup brown sugar
Sea salt & black pepper to taste (can use black or pink pepper essential oil)

Combine ingredients in a food processor or blender until smooth. This dressing is good on all salads. Try Romaine lettuce, sliced apples, dried cranberries, & toasted sliced almonds. Stored in a glass jar, it will keep, in the fridge, for several months.

Creamy Cucumber Dill Dressing

1 seedless cucumber, chopped into chunks
4 tablespoons sour cream or plain Greek yogurt (or a combination of the two)
1 tablespoon olive oil
1 tablespoon distilled white vinegar
1 drop dill essential oil
¼ teaspoon garlic powder
Black pepper to taste (black or pink pepper essential oil)
Salt to taste

Put everything in a blender and blend until smooth. Add spices to taste and blend for a few more seconds. Chill or serve immediately. Store in the refrigerator for up to a week.

NOTE: Add more sour cream/yogurt if you like a thicker dressing.

Cinnamon Spice Salad Dressing

¼ cup olive oil
2 tablespoons raw apple cider vinegar
2 drop cinnamon essential oil
1 drop clove essential oil
⅛ teaspoon fresh ground nutmeg
1 small garlic clove, finely minced
¼ teaspoon gray salt or sea salt
⅛ teaspoon fresh ground pepper (black or pink pepper essential oil)

Mix all ingredients and place in a jar, shake well.

*Great on a bed of baby spinach, toss with thinly sliced apples, and top with toasted pine nuts and crumbled goat cheese.

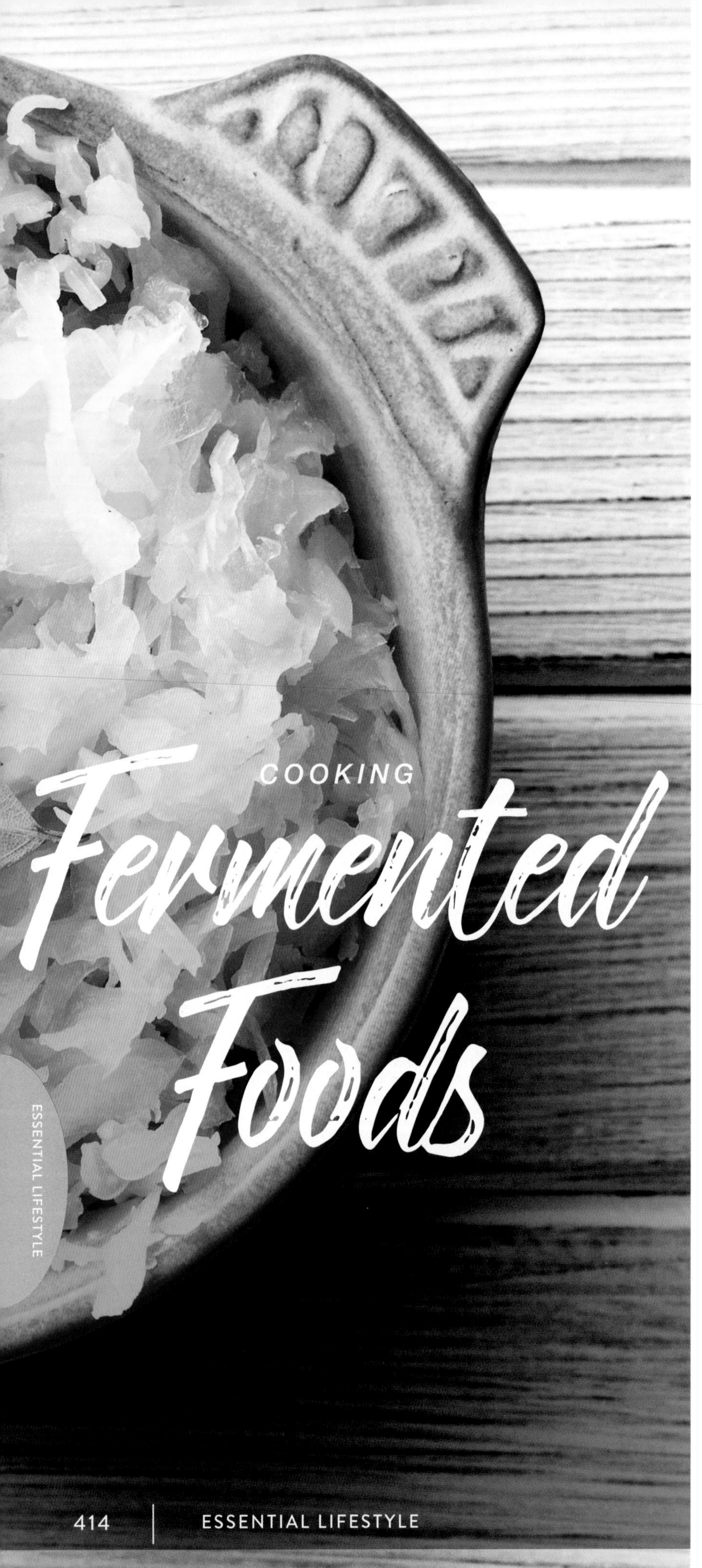

How To Make Wild Fermented Sauerkraut

Raw, unpasteurized sauerkraut delivers healthful probiotics to the digestive tract, increases body alkalinity, and increases nutrition absorption.

To make sauerkraut you will need a knife, cutting board, large mixing bowl, non-porous crock or Mason jar, and weighted jar.

Chop the cabbage into chunks of uniform size or shred into a bowl. Two heads of cabbage fill a ½ gallon jar nicely. Add any desired spices. Add coarse sea salt and mix throughout, using your hands to massage the mixture. The cabbage will begin to produce liquid (brine).

Using your fist or a wooden tamper, create an anaerobic environment by removing the air bubbles as you pack the vegetable mixture tightly into a crock or jar. Push until the brine starts to rise to the top of the veggies. Place a saucer or plate on top of the vegetables, covering them as closely to the edges as possible. Alternatively, use outer cabbage leaves to make a seal. Place a weight on top of the packed vegetables. A jar of water works well. Cover completely with a cloth and secure with a rubber band to keep bugs away.

During the first week, tamp the mixture down daily to help keep the veggies under the brine. Sometimes it takes a day or two to get the brine to stay above the veggies. This will help prevent mold from forming. Taste it after a week and see if you like it. You can let it ferment as long as you want, but most people prefer two to four weeks of fermentation in small batches. When it is too young, it will leave a carbonated feeling on your tongue, which disappears after about a week of fermentation.

The best temperature to ferment sauerkraut is 55-65 degrees. Put it in a pantry, root cellar, cupboard, or on your kitchen counter. A variation in this temperature is fine, but the best flavors develop within this range. When fermentation is complete, remove the weight, plate, or cabbage seal, scrape off the top layer, and enjoy the fresh healthy goodness below. Add essential oils after the sauerkraut is fermented.

Note: If mold forms, all is not lost. This is a test of your senses. Scrape off the mold and compost it. If the sauerkraut underneath smells okay, taste it. If it tastes "off," spit it out, and discard the batch!

Basic Sauerkraut

1 to 1 ½ heads cabbage
1 tablespoon sea salt per pound of cabbage
1 onion
2 drops dill essential oil
2-3 tablespoons caraway seeds
2 drops lemon essential oil to a pint size container of sauerkraut (after fermentation)

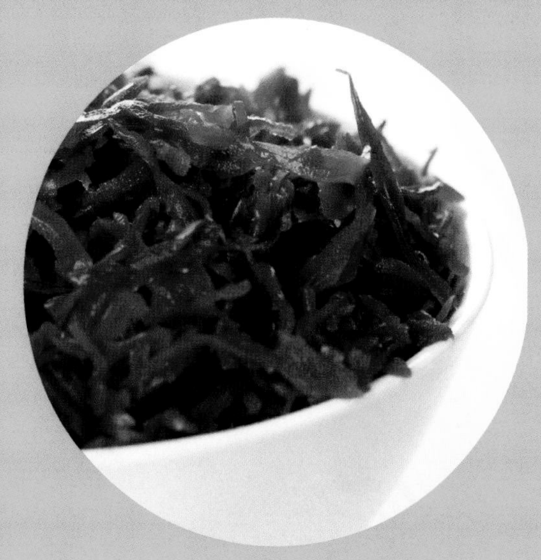

Cortido (Sauerkraut Variation)

1 head/about 1000 g Napa cabbage, cored and outer leaves removed, shredded
2 tablespoons fine Celtic sea salt
1 cup (140g) chopped carrots
1 green apple, peeled, thinly sliced
1 onion, peeled, thinly sliced
1 fresh jalapeño pepper, thinly sliced (deseed for less heat)
1 drop oregano essential oil
5 drops lime essential oil
Juice of half of a lime
1 sterilized quart size canning jar with 2 part lid

In a large non-metal bowl, mix the cabbage with the sea salt. Use clean hands to really work the salt into the cabbage, and then allow it to rest for 1-2 hours. The cabbage will wilt and brine (salty liquid) will develop.

Add the carrots, apple, onion, jalapeño, and lime juice to the cabbage and mix well.

*Follow How to Recipe.

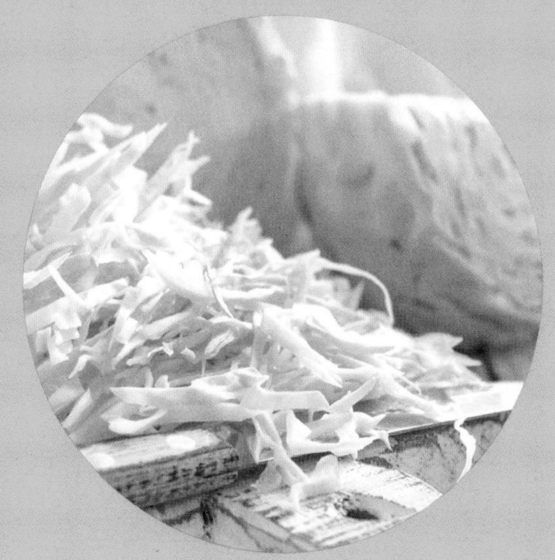

Red Cabbage & Apple Sauerkraut

1 to 1 ½ heads of red cabbage, finely shredded
2 Granny Smith apples, cored and shredded
¼ cup very thinly sliced red onion
1 tablespoon salt per pound of cabbage
5 whole peppercorns or 2 drops black pepper essential oil
2 drops clove essential oil
1 drop cardamom essential oil
¼ teaspoon coriander seeds
⅛ teaspoon cinnamon

Combine cabbage, apple, and red onion. Sprinkle with salt and massage. Place the remaining ingredients in a small bowl. Crush with the back of a spoon or mortar and pestle. Add to cabbage mixture and follow basic recipe instructions.

Juniper Berry Sauerkraut

1 ½ to 2 heads red or green cabbage, shredded
1 to 1 ½ apples, peeled, cored, and coarsely chopped
1 tablespoon caraway seeds
1 drop juniper berry essential oil
1 tablespoon salt per pound of cabbage

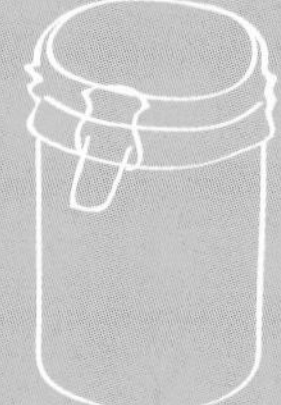

tip

You can use essential oils to flavor fermented foods after the fermenting process is completed. Simply add a toothpick-dip of your oil of choice to taste.

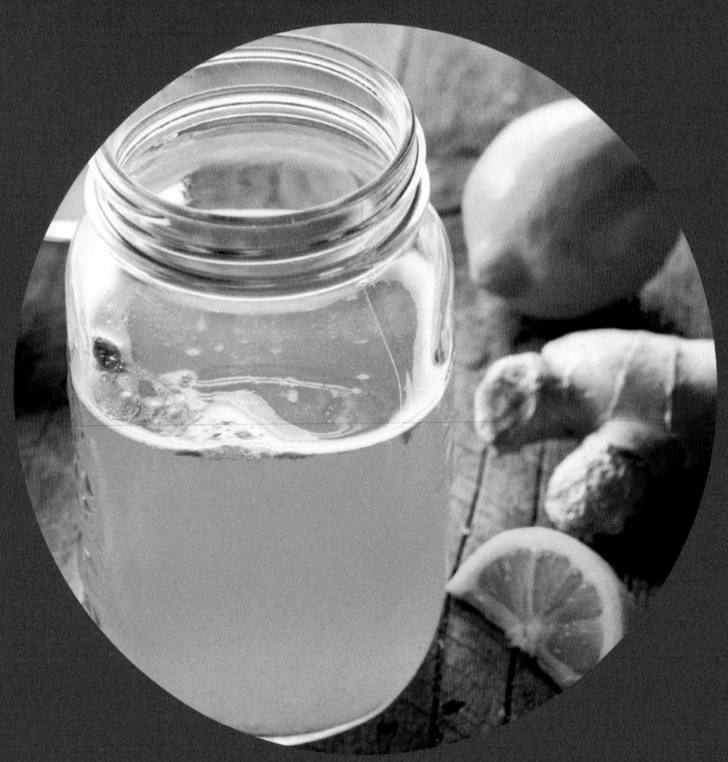

Vanilla Orange Kombucha

½ cup sugar
750ml kombucha (homemade or store bought)
Wild orange essential oil
Vanilla bean
750ml glass bottle (swing top ones work best)

Pour your homemade kombucha into your glass jar leaving a 2cm gap between the kombucha and the lid. Add 1–2 drops of wild orange and a small piece of the vanilla bean. Secure the lid and leave in a dark place to ferment for 2 days then transfer to the fridge and enjoy.
Variation: Grapefruit oil instead of orange and with a piece of a cinnamon stick instead of the vanilla bean.

Lemon and Ginger Kombucha

750ml kombucha (homemade or store bought)
Lemon essential oil
1 lemon wedge
1 drop ginger essential oil
750ml glass bottle (swing top ones work best)

Pour your homemade kombucha into your glass jar leaving a 2cm gap between the kombucha and the lid. Add 1 drop of lemon oil, the lemon wedge and the ginger essential oil. Secure the lid and leave in a dark place to ferment for 2 days then transfer to the fridge and enjoy.

Kefir

Kefir is high in enzymes and probiotics and is alkalizing to the body. It stimulates mucosal immune response to protect from microbiological invasion of mucous membranes throughout the body. Kefir contains peptides that may restore normal immune function. Kefir is also good for lactose-intolerant people. The lactose found in milk is converted to lactic acid during the fermentation process.

1 tablespoon milk kefir grains
8-16 ounces goat or cow milk (raw, unpasteurized is the best choice)

Add 1 tablespoon kefir grains to 8-16 ounces of raw milk, place in a jar with a lid. Let it sit on the counter at room temperature for 24 to 72 hours, depending on how sour you like it and how warm your house is. Shake gently a couple times a day to redistribute the grains. When fermentation is complete, strain the milk and save the kefir grains to make a new batch. Put the strained kefir in a jar with a tight lid. Let it sit at room temperature for a few hours to increase fizziness. Then store in refrigerator.

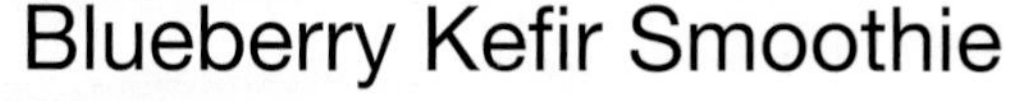

Blueberry Kefir Smoothie

Blend together:
1 cup blueberries
1 cup kefir
2 large handfuls of greens
1 apple
1 drop lemo essential oil

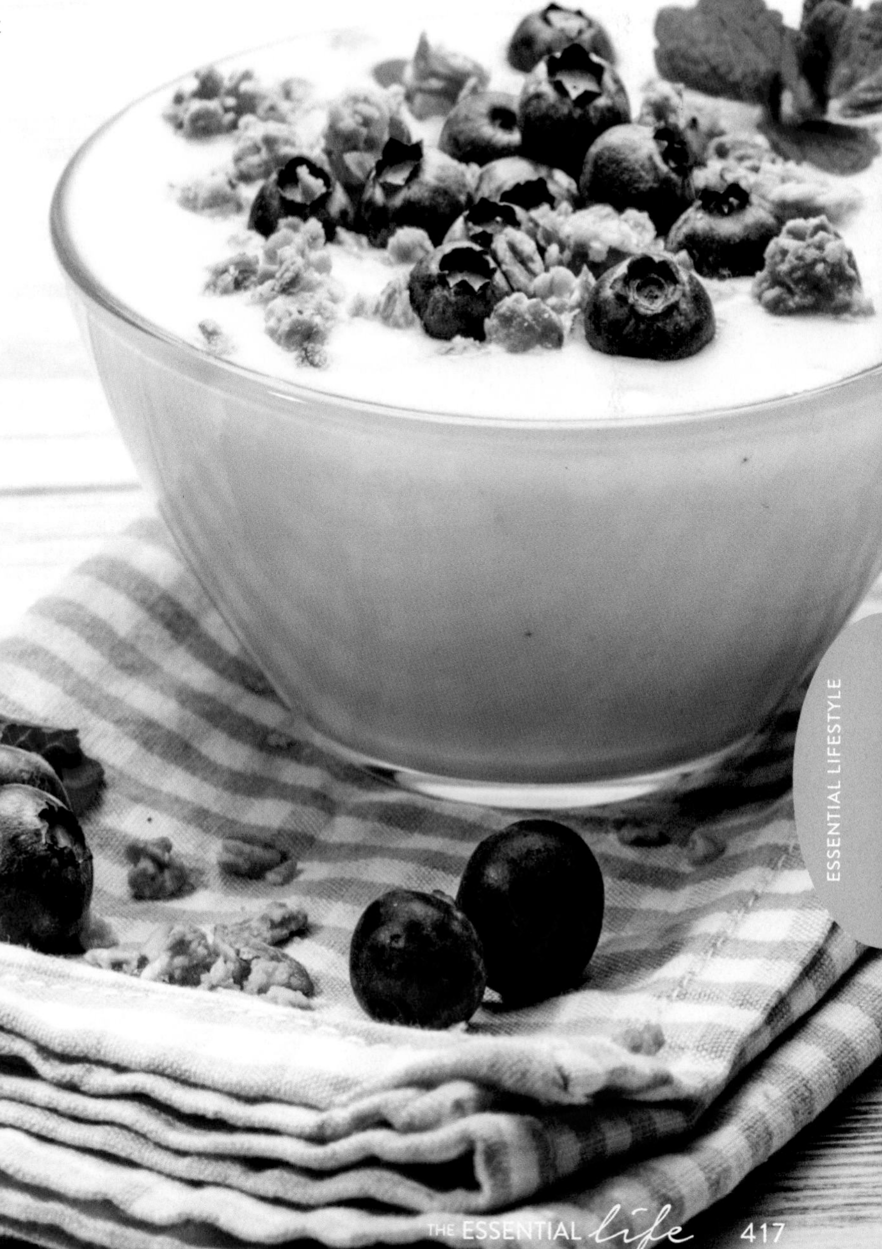

COOKING

Main Dishes

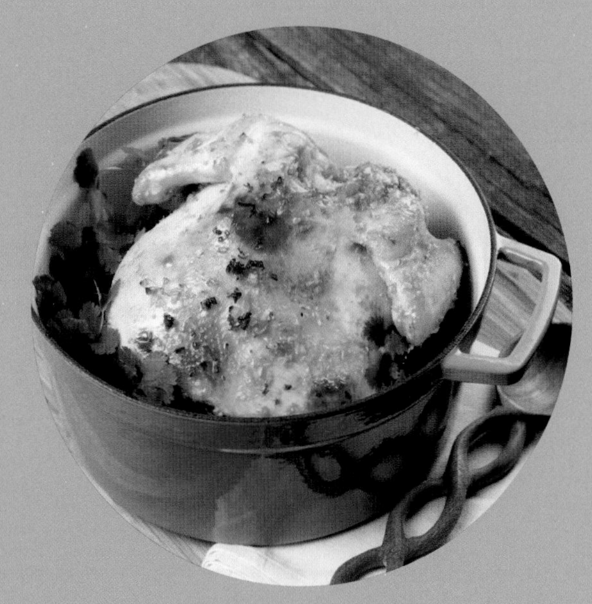

remember

Certain essential oils go best with certain dishes.

- **Chicken:** basil, bergamot, black pepper, cassia, cilantro, cinnamon, ginger, grapefruit, lemon, lemongrass, lime, rosemary, tangerine sage, thyme, and wild orange.
- **Red meats**: basil, black pepper, cassia, cilantro, cinnamon, clove, coriander, fennel, ginger, grapefruit, lemongrass, lime, marjoram, oregano, wild orange, rosemary, tangerine, and thyme.
- **Vegetables:** basil, black pepper, cardamom, cilantro, fennel, ginger, grapefruit, lemon, lemongrass, and lime.

Roast Chicken with Lemon and Thyme Essential Oil

Whole chicken
4 tablespoon olive oil
4 drops lemon essential oil
4 drops thyme essential oil
Salt and pepper to taste
Sprinkle of dried oregano
1 lemon, sliced
1 onion, sliced

Preheat oven to 350 degrees. Mix the oils and salt and pepper together in a small bowl. Set aside. Place lemon and onion slices in the bottom of the roasting pan and in the cavity of the chicken. Place whole chicken in roasting pan, breast side up, and remove giblets from cavity. Add a little water, just enough to barely cover the bottom of the pan. Add chicken to roasting pan, and using silicone basting brush, cover the entire outside of the chicken with your oil mixture. If there's some leftover, pour some in the cavity of the chicken. Sprinkle the chicken with a little dried oregano.

Cook in oven until the internal temperature reaches 180 degrees (about 1 hour 45 minutes, give or take depending on the size).Take it out and let chicken rest 10 minutes before slicing. Enjoy!

Perfect Peppered Burger

1 pound ground beef
Salt to taste
Pink or black pepper essential oil
Preheat outdoor grill to high heat and lightly oil grate.
Form ground burger into 4 patties, approximately ¾" thick and salt to liking

Place patties on the prepared grill. When meat juices appear on the top of the burgers, add a drop of black pepper essential oil per patty and spread. Cover and cook 6 to 8 minutes or to desired doneness.

Sesame Orange Chicken

1½ to 2 pounds chicken breast, cut into bite-size pieces
4 tablespoons coconut oil, divided
⅔ cup soy sauce
2 inches fresh ginger, chopped
4 cloves garlic, minced
3 tablespoons tomato paste
¼ cup honey (agave or a liquid sugar of your choice)
½ teaspoon ground black pepper
Pinch of red pepper flakes
½ cup water + 10-20 drops wild orange essential oil
1 tablespoon sesame seeds

Heat 2 tablespoons coconut oil in a cast iron skillet. Add the chicken and sauté until chicken begins to brown on the outside and is no longer pink on the inside. Set aside. In a medium saucepan, combine other 2 tablespoons coconut oil and next 7 ingredients, whisk together over low-medium heat and simmer 5 minutes. Remove from the heat and use an immersion blender and blend in the ginger and garlic. A stand-up blender will also work (careful the liquid is HOT). Transfer the sauce back to the pan and add the orange oil mix and whisk to combine. Taste the sauce, adjust as needed. Add chicken and stir to coat the chicken, add the sesame seeds, serve immediately over spaghetti squash or cauli-rice.

Lasagne Flavoring Ideas

To flavor your favorite lasagna recipes try:
- Oregano essential oil (to taste)
- Basil essential oil (to taste)
- Rosemary essential oil (to taste)

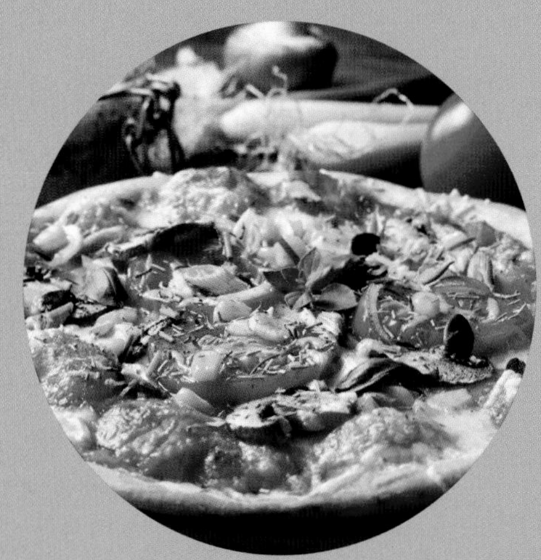

Veggie Pita Pizzas

A treat for the eyes and the palette! These pizzas are enough to create lunch-envy!

2 whole grain pita rounds
3-4 tablespoon Neufchatel cheese
1 drop basil essential oil
½ cup fresh baby spinach
⅓ red pepper, thinly slices
1-2 mushrooms, thinly sliced
¼ cup frozen sweet corn
½ cup mozzarella cheese
⅛ teaspoon garlic power

Preheat oven or toaster oven to 450°F. In a small cup or bowl, stir basil essential oil into Neufchatel cheese. Spread mixture on entire face of both pitas. Layer on spinach, red pepper, muchrooms, and corn. Top with mozzarella cheese and a sprinkling of garlic powder. Bake on cookie sheet or directly on oven rack for about 2 minutes or until cheese is melted. Slice if desired and enjoy!

Chicken Alfredo Stuffed Shells

2 lbs chicken fajita meat, pre cooked, shredded
12 oz jumbo shells
2 jars alfredo sauce
Oregano essential oil 2 drops
Salt to taste
Shredded parmesan

Preheat oven to 350. Shred chicken, add alfredo, oregano oil, salt and pepper into a skillet. Spread about ¼ of the sauce onto the bottom of a foil lined 9x13 baking dish. Fill each shell with the sauce and line in the baking dish. Sprinkle cheese over the shells

Bake for 20 minutes and serve!

Essential Broccoli Beef

½ cup soy sauce
3 tablespoons water
2 tablespoons brown sugar
2 tablespoons cornstarch
1–2 drops ginger essential oil
1 ½ pounds thin sliced steak
2 cups small broccoli florets

Combine the first 5 ingredients in a small bowl. Pour the mixture over the sliced steak. Let marinate for at least 10 minutes. Preheat your pan, and stir fry the broccoli, to desired doneness, remove from pan, and set aside. Allow pan to get hot again, and add the meat in batches. Cook about five minutes, stirring occasionally, to brown all sides. Once all the meat is cooked, add the remaining marinade and broccoli to the pan, and stir it in with your meat. Cook until the mixture thickens. Serve over your choice of rice.

Acapulco Chicken

Marinate for boneless skinless chicken (breasts and/or thighs)

1 – 6oz can pineapple juice
Juice of 1 large orange & zest the rind (plus ½ drop of wild orange essential oil)
1 good pinch of saffron (rubbed between fingers)
Garlic (finely minced about 4 large cloves)
Ginger (finely zest about an inch fresh ginger)
1 drop cardamom essential oil

Mix in a glass bowl, and let rest at least a ½ hour, turning often. Grill chicken until done. Add remaining marinade to pan on stove, and bring to a boiling, to serve with chicken, if desired. (This had raw chicken in it, so you must boil it for a minute or two; I personally boiled it, and then let it reduce until the chicken was done).

Serve with fresh cut pineapple pieces, and sliced green onions (if desired)

NOTE: served with long grain rice with 1-2 drops of wild orange and the zest of an orange added or try cardamom essential oil rice.

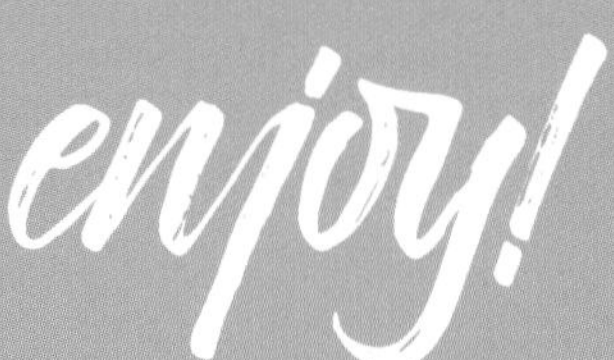

French Dip Pot Roast

Delish for dipping! Perfect for dinner! This is a recipe you'll add to your weekly menu!

3 pounds roast
½ cup soy sauce
1 drop thyme essential oil
1 drop rosemary essential oil
1 teaspoon garlic powder
1 bay leaf
2 cups water
2 drops black pepper essential oil
4-8 large romaine lettuce leaves, rinsed (may also use a healthy whole grain roll, whole wheat roll, or French roll)

Place roast in a crock-pot or baking pot. Add drops thyme and rosemary essential oils to roast and then pour soy sauce over the top of roast. Add garlic powder, bay leaf, water, and black pepper essential oil to pot, and cook for 5-6 hours until meat is tender. When roast is cooked thoroughly, pour juice into small dishes for au jus dip. Cut the meat into thin slices. Pile meat onto lettuce leaf, and roll up meal/lettuce burrito style, or place meat on a French roll. Serve with au jus for dipping and your favorite side of veggies. Delish!

Makes 6-8 servings

Pork Chops with Orange Sauce

6 loin pork chops ¾ inch thick
1 tablespoon butter
1 medium onion diced
1 tablespoon flour
2 cubes bullion
1 cup hot water
½ teaspoon minced parsley
1 tablespoon dry mustard
1 teaspoon salt
1 drop black pepper essential oil
1 drop peppermint essential oil
1 drop lemon essential oil
3 drops wild orange essential oil (or more to taste, one drop at a time only)
½ cup water or orange juice

Over medium, brown both sides of pork chops and set aside. Add butter to pan, melt and add onions sauté for approx. 5 minutes or until clear. Dissolve bullion into hot water and set aside. Stir flour into onions then slowly add water bullion mix stirring constantly as you go. Cook 5 minutes then add parsley, salt, pepper, oils and ½ cup water or orange juice. Place chops in liquid, cover and cook over low for 25-35 minutes or until meat is tender.

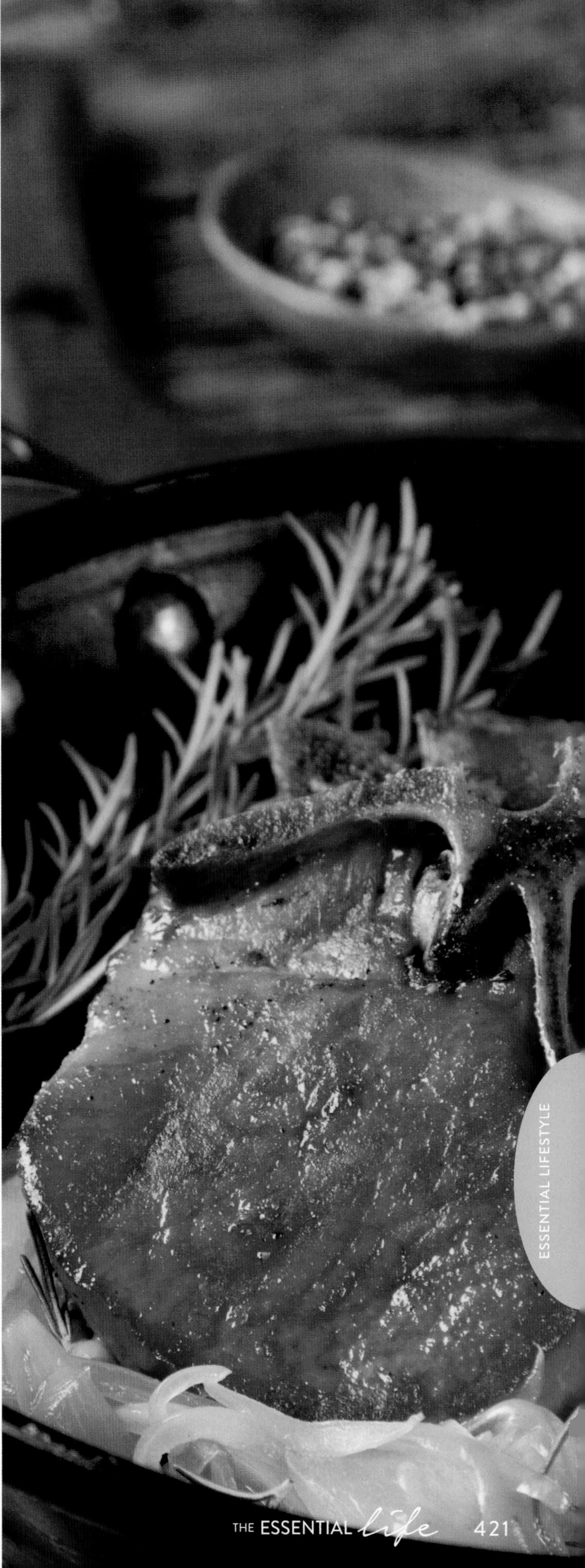

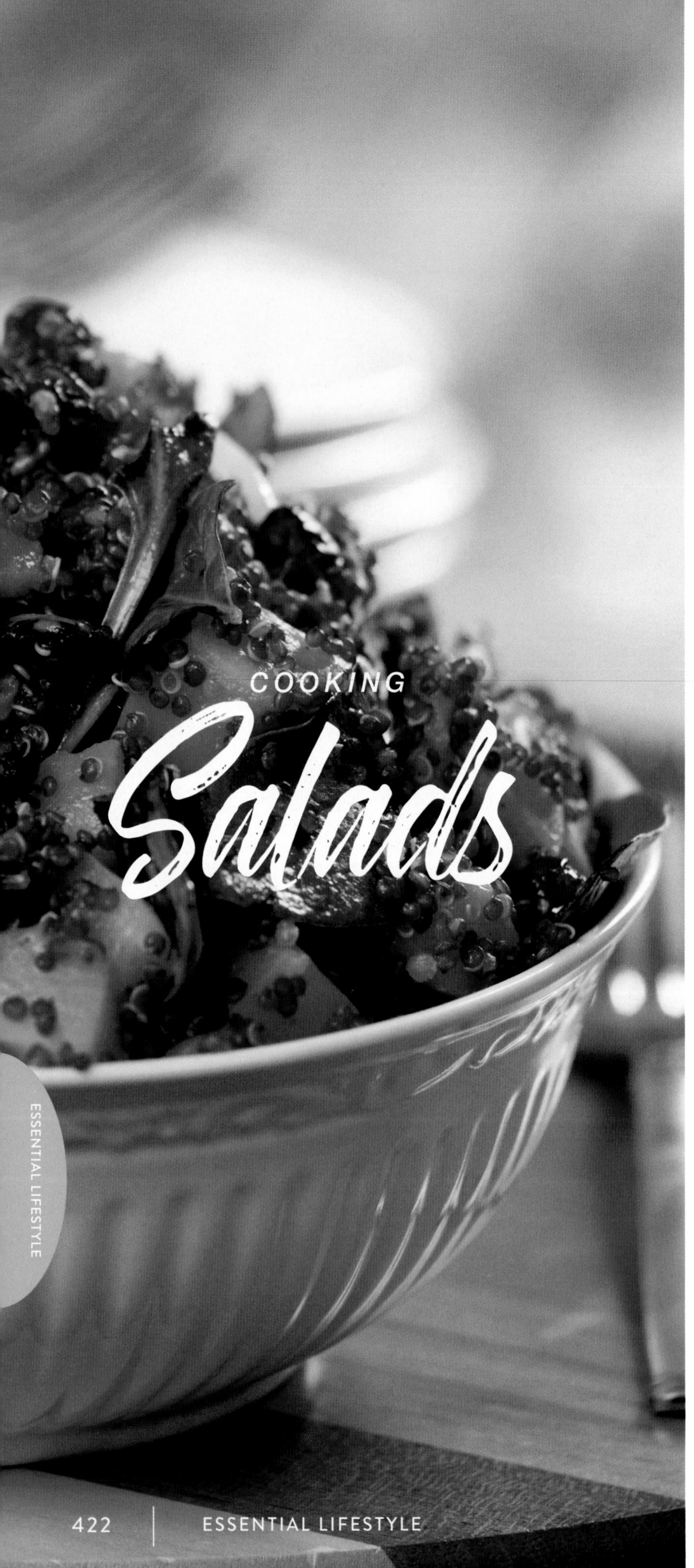

Warm Roasted Butternut Squash & Quinoa Salad

¾ cup dried cranberries
¾ cups baby spinach leaves
1 tablespoon fresh lemon juice
1 tablespoon raw honey
1 tablespoon olive oil
Large pinch of salt
1 toothpick black pepper essential oil
1 butternut squash, peeled and cut into a medium dice
½ teaspoon coarse salt
½ large sweet onion, thinly sliced
4 cups red quinoa, cooked and kept warm
1 ½ cup wheat berries, cooked kept warm

Place the spinach and dried cranberries in a large bowl. Cover and set aside.

Combine the lemon juice, honey, 1 tablespoon olive oil, pinch of salt, and black pepper essential oil in a small bowl and whisk until combined. Set aside.

Preheat the oven to 425 degrees. Line a baking pan with tin foil.

Toss the diced butternut squash with 1 tablespoon olive oil and ½ teaspoon salt. Spread the squash out evenly on the tin foil lined baking sheet.

Roast the squash on the top rack of the oven for 15-20 minutes, or until squash is tender and turning golden brown on top. Remove from oven.

While the squash is roasting, place the ½ tablespoon olive oil in a small saute pan and heat to medium/high. Add the sweet onion and saute for 2 minutes. Reduce the heat to medium and continue to saute for another 5-6 minutes until the onion is lightly caramelized.

Add the hot butternut squash, hot onions, warm quinoa and wheat berries to the bowl of spinach and cranberries. Toss together to slightly wilt the spinach. Add the dressing and toss until well coated. Serve warm.

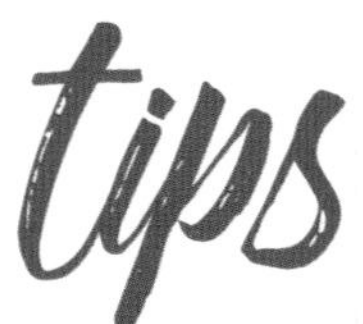

- Use essential oils to infuse into olive oil and make seasoned croutons.
- See Spiced Almond recipe in Snacks to add crunch to your salads.
- See Dressings recipes as a companion to salad recipes.
- Essential oils are a fantastic addition to pasta salads.

Peach Jerk Sausage Salad with Citrus Dressing

2 tablespoons freshly squeezed orange juice
2 tablespoons freshly squeezed lemon or lime juice
½ teaspoon kosher salt
¼ teaspoon ground cumin
1 drop black pepper essential oil
¼ cup extra-virgin olive oil
1 drop wild orange essential oil
1 (11-ounce) package peach jerk sausage (or flavored sausage of your choosing)
5 ounces baby arugula
2 oranges or 4 clementines, peeled and sliced
1 cup sugar snap peas, trimmed and thinly sliced
1 small jicama, peeled, cut into matchstick sized pieces
½ small red onion, thinly sliced

Make citrus dressing by combining the first 5 ingredients in a small bowl, whisking in the olive oil until well combined. Set aside. Cook the sausages according to the package instructions, remove from heat, drain, and slice sausage. Combine the arugula, oranges, snap peas, jicama, and onion in a large salad bowl, top with sausage. Drizzle the salad dressing over everything and toss to coat. Serve at once.

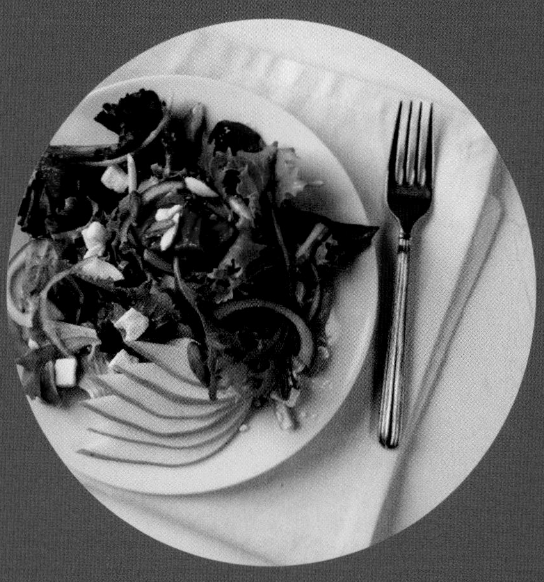

Died and Gone To Heaven Salad

1 head romaine
½ head red-leaf lettuce
½ cup red onion, chopped
2 medium artichokes, chopped
½ cup sun-dried tomatoes, chopped
½ cup olives (green, black, Kalamata, your choice!)

Dressing:

1 lemon, zested and juiced
¼ cup white wine vinegar
3-4 drops lemon essential oil
⅓ cup extra virgin olive oil
Salt & Pepper (black or pink pepper essential oil)

Top salad with some Parmesan Reggiano. Oh so yummy!

Waldorf Salad

5 apples, medium diced (soaked in On Guard® to prevent from browning)
5 ounce celery small diced
4 ounces walnuts course chopped
⅔ cup mayo or plain Greek yogurt cup
7 drops lemon essential oil

Combine all above ingredients; serve.

Celery Seed Salad Dressing

½ cup extra virgin olive oil
2 tablespoons balsamic vinegar
1 teaspoon apple cider vinegar
½ small onion, peeled and quartered
1 tablespoon raw honey
¼ teaspoon celery seed essential oil
A dash of garlic powder
Himalayan salt, to taste
Ground black pepper, to taste (black or pink pepper essential oil)

Combine ingredients in blender until smooth. Add salt and pepper to taste. Refrigerate and shake before use.

COOKING

Sauces & Seasonings

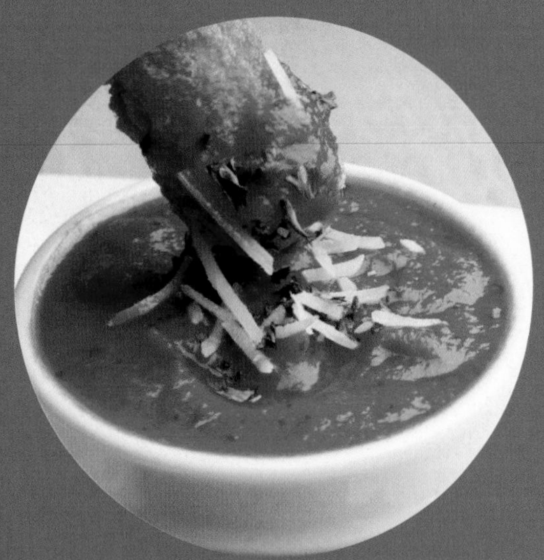

Marinara Sauce

2 pounds Roma tomatoes, halved
1 onion, sliced
4 garlic cloves
Olive oil
Sea salt
Pepper
1 drop basil essential oil
1 toothpick oregano essential oil

Preheat oven to 350° F.

Place sliced tomatoes, onions, and garlic on baking sheet. Add a generous amount of sea salt, pepper, and olive oil to top of tomatoes and onion. Cook for one to two hours or until tomatoes and onions begin to darken around the edges. Remove from oven and transfer to food processor or blender. Pulse until sauce reaches your desired consistency. Add basil and oregano oil and stir.

Barbecue Sauce

15 oz. tomato sauce
¼ cup apple cider vinegar
1 ½ tablespoon mustard
1 tablespoon lemon juice
1 tablespoon hickory liquid smoke
½ tablespoon sea salt
1 teaspoon garlic powder
1 teaspoon onion powder
1 teaspoon molasses
¼ cup brown sugar
2–3 drops black pepper essential oil
1 drop lemon essential oil

Put all the ingredients in a blender. If you have a high-speed blender, use the soup setting, and it will heat and blend your sauce at the same time. If you have a regular blender, blend on high for a minute; then transfer contents to a saucepan, and heat thoroughly. Serve in your favorite dishes calling for barbecue sauce.

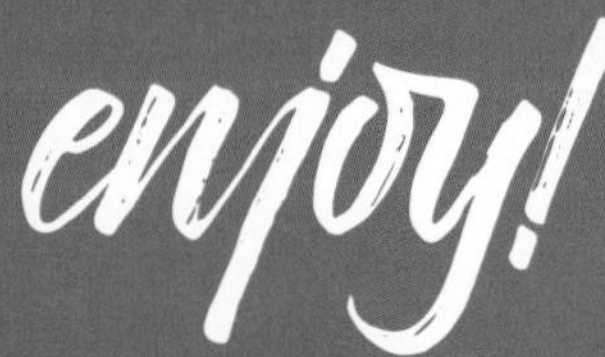

Southwest Beef Marinade

¼ cup fresh cilantro, chopped
¼ cup olive oil
¼ cup lemon or lime juice
2 teaspoons salt
1 teaspoon cumin
1 teaspoon fresh garlic, minced
5 drops black pepper essential oil
7 drops lemon essential oil

Mix all ingredients together. Marinate tenderized beef for at least an hour in the refrigerator before grilling to proper temperature (145 degrees + 3 minute rest). Delicious when served with a side of homemade guacamole.

Wild Orange Strawberry Jam

⅔ cup granulated sugar
2 tablespoons instant pectin
1 ⅔ cup prepared strawberries
2-4 drops wild orange essential oil

To prepare strawberries, wash in lemon essential oil, hull and cut into small pieces. Mash with potato masher 1 layer at a time. Combine sugar and pectin by stirring, then add the prepared fruit, drop in the essential oils and stir fro 3 minutes. Store in a clean glass jar and refrigerate to keep fresh.

Pizza Sauce

1 -6 oz can organic tomato paste
½ chopped red onion
1 chopped shallot
2 cloves garlic minced
2 drops basil essential oil
½ - 1 drop oregano essential oil
1 teaspoon sea salt
2 tablespoons raw honey

Combine all the ingredients in your blender and blend well. Add sauce to a pot, bring to a boil and then simmer for 30-40 minutes. Top your pizza.

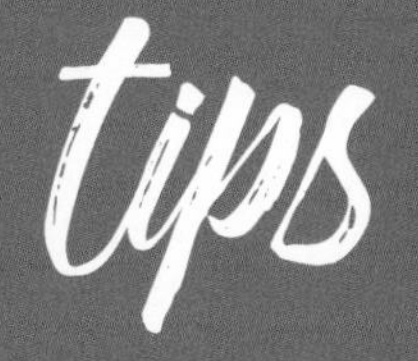

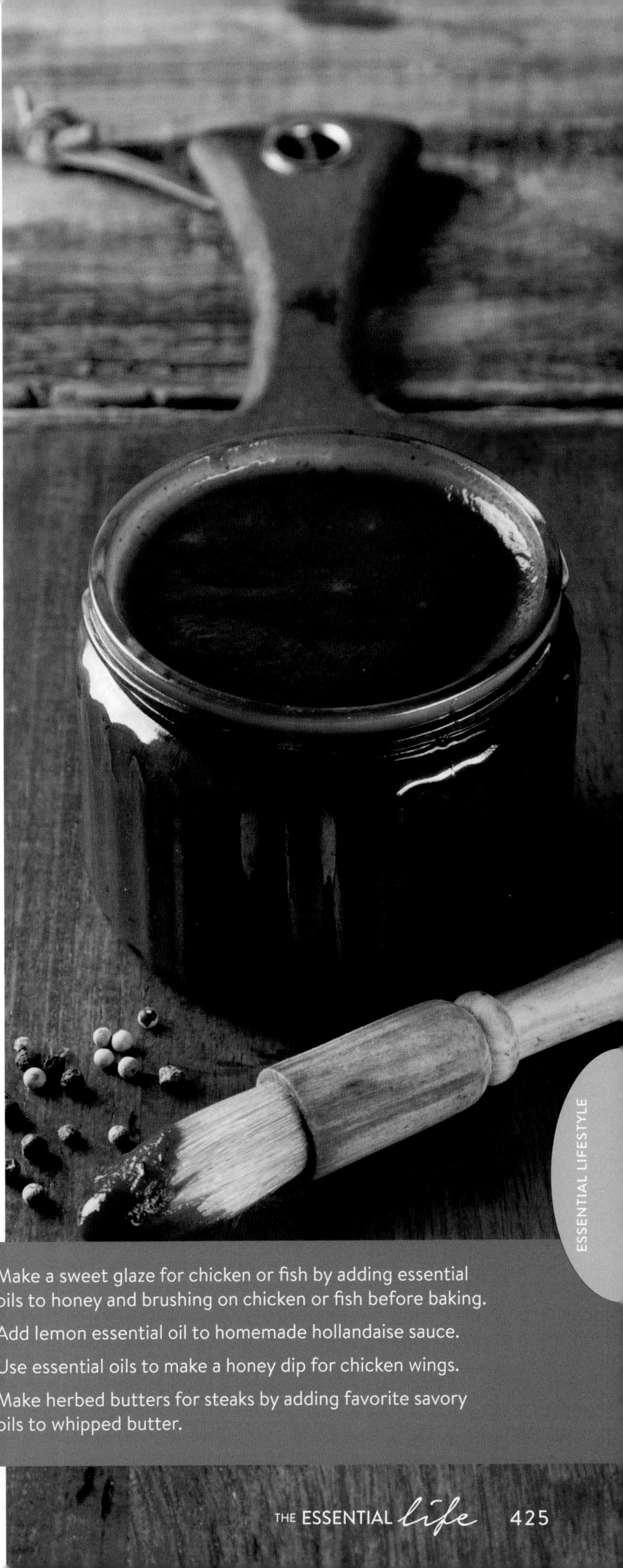

- Make a sweet glaze for chicken or fish by adding essential oils to honey and brushing on chicken or fish before baking.
- Add lemon essential oil to homemade hollandaise sauce.
- Use essential oils to make a honey dip for chicken wings.
- Make herbed butters for steaks by adding favorite savory oils to whipped butter.

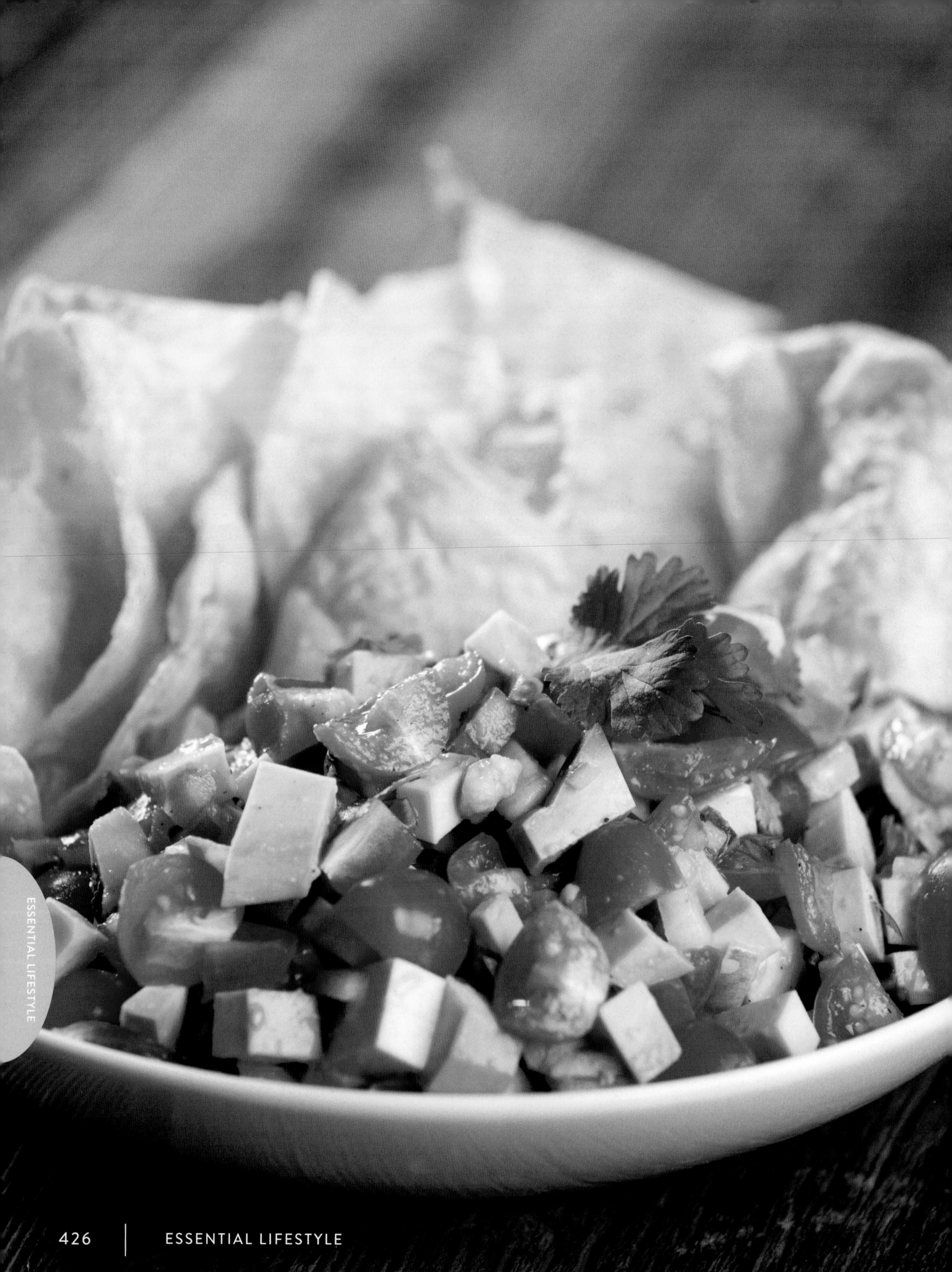

Avocado Salsa

6 medium roma tomatoes (20 ounces), seeded and diced
1 cup chopped red onion, chopped
1 large or 2 small jalapeños, seeded and chopped (¼ cup. Leave seeds if you like heat)
3 medium avocados, semi-firm but ripe, peeled cored and diced
3 ½ tablespoons olive oil
3 tablespoons fresh lime juice
1 clove garlic, finely minced
½ teaspoon salt (more or less to taste as desired)
¼ teaspoon freshly ground black pepper
½ cup loosely packed cilantro leaves, chopped

Place red onion in a strainer or sieve and rinse under cool water to remove harsh bite. Drain well. Add to a mixing bowl along with tomatoes, jalapeños and avocados.

In a separate small mixing bowl whisk together olive oil, lime juice, garlic, salt and pepper until mixture is well blended. Pour mixture over avocado mixture, add cilantro then gently toss mixture to evenly coat. Serve with tortilla chips or over Mexican entrees.

Italian Seasoning Salt

2 tablespoons sea salt
1 drop each: rosemary, basil, oregano, and thyme essential oils

Blend and reserve in airtight container.

5 Spice Sugar Seasoning Salt

2 tablespoons coarse cane sugar
1 drop cinnamon essential oil
1 drop cardamom essential oil
1 drop black pepper essential oil
1 drop wild orange essential oil
1 drop clove essential oil

Blend and reserve in airtight container.

Asian Blend Seasoning Salt

2 tablespoons sea salt
2 drops ginger essential oil
2 drops lemongrass essential oil
1 drop basil essential oil

Blend and reserve in airtight container.

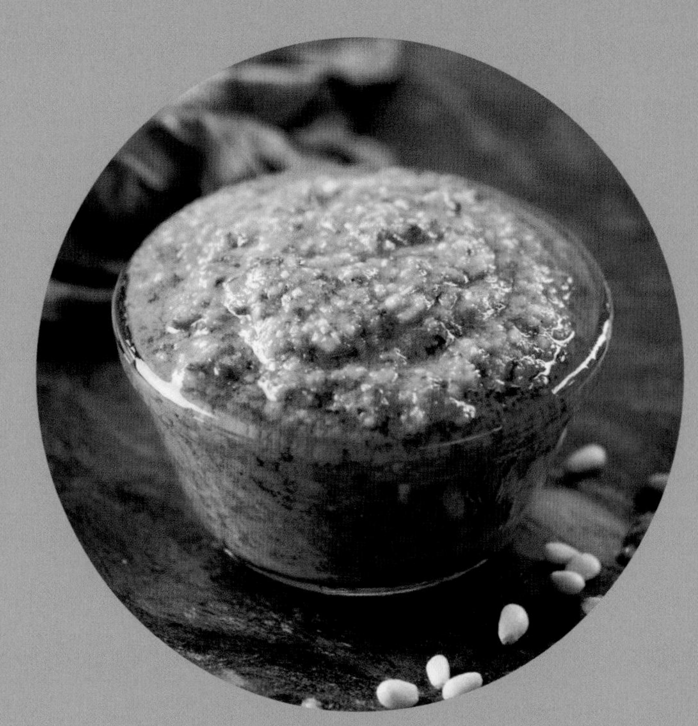

Pesto

3 cups basil leaves, loosely packed
3 small or 2 large garlic cloves
¼ cup pine nuts
⅔ - ¾ cup olive oil
1 toothpick dip black pepper essential oil
1 toothpick dip basil essential oil
1 toothpick dip lemon essential oil
½ cup freshly grated Parmesan cheese

Combine all ingredients in blender or food processor. If in blender, blend ½ the ingredients well, then add the rest and pulse-blend till pesto has reached desired consistency. Add more olive oil if too dry. If making in a food processor, add all ingredients and chop till well blended and has reached desired consistency. Store in refrigerator in air-tight container. Excellent on pasta, fish, chicken, add to fresh salsa.

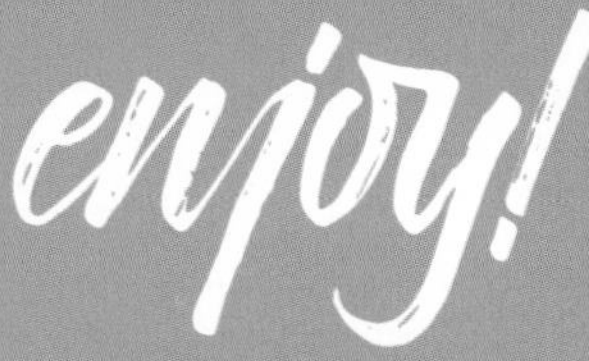

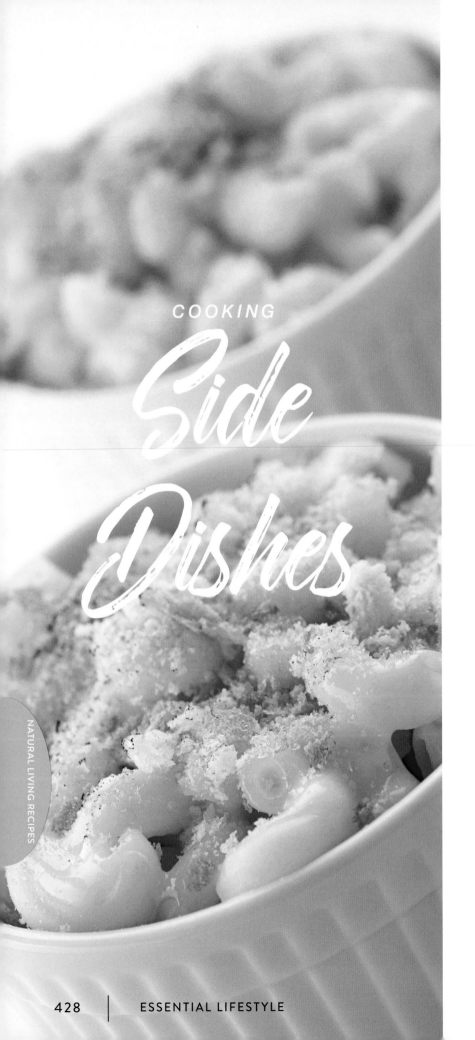

Italian Bread Dip with Essential Oils

¼ cup olive oil
1-3 tablespoons balsamic vinegar to taste
½ teaspoon Italian seasoning
1 tablespoon Parmesan cheese
1-3 drops oregano essential oil

Gently mix together all ingredients in a bowl large enough to dip into. Dip any Italian style bread in and enjoy!

Clean Eating Mac and Cheese

½ cup canned pumpkin puree
½ cup plain Greek yogurt
1 8 oz. package gluten-free pasta (or pasta of your choice)
2-4 drops black pepper essential oil
⅛ teaspoon garlic powder
⅛ teaspoon paprika
¼ teaspoon salt
½ cup shredded sharp cheddar cheese
2 teaspoon breadcrumb brand

Preheat oven to 350 degrees. Boil pasta according to package directions. In a separate bowl, combine all other ingredients, add cooked pasta and stir until thoroughly mixed. Spoon mixture into a lined muffin tins. Top with breadcrumbs and bake for 10 minutes until barely crispy brown on top.

Guacamole

2-3 ripe avocados
¼ cup diced red onion
¼ cup chopped cilantro
¼ cup chopped tomato
Garlic powder to taste
Sea salt to taste
4-6 drops lime essential oil

Mash avocados and mix all ingredients together. Enjoy with your favorite tortilla chips or as a topping on your favorite foods!

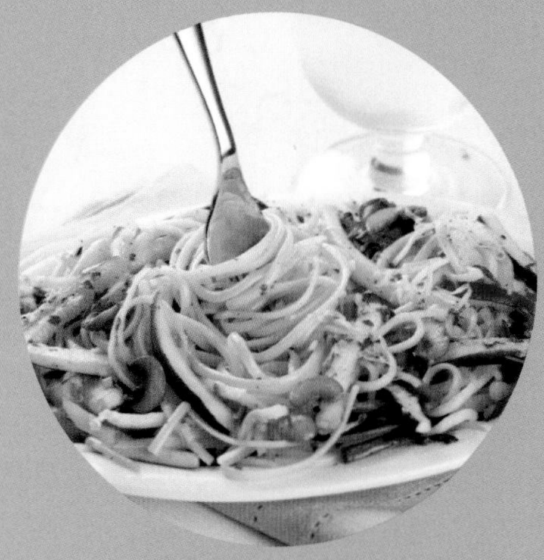

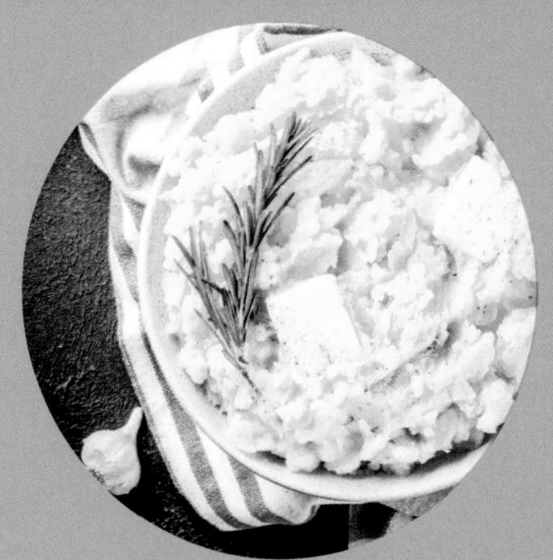

Zucchini Mushroom Pasta

1 pound medium zucchini, julienned
1 pound medium mushrooms, sliced thin
3 tablespoons olive oil
1 cup green onions, sliced thinly
2 cloves minced garlic
1-2 toothpick dips basil essential oil, to taste
1 toothpick dip black pepper essential oil
½ teaspoon sea salt
3 tablespoon butter, softened
¼ teaspoon sea salt and pepper (to taste)
2 teaspoon parsley
1 ½ cups grated Parmesan cheese, divided
1 pound noodles of your choice

Start cooking pasta in a sauce pan. In a large skillet over medium heat, sauté onions until just tender. Add garlic and cook another minute. Add zucchini and cook until fork can be inserted, but still a little firm. Sprinkle salt and pepper, then add mushrooms, and sauté until tender. Remove from heat. When pasta is done, drain and put in serving bowl. Add essential oil to butter; toss butter in with warm pasta along with parsley, green onion, and ¾ cup grated Parmesan cheese. Top with remaining freshly grated Parmesan cheese.

Fresh Caprese Skewers

½ cup cherry tomato halves
¼ cup mozzarella cheese ball halves
2–3 tablespoon olive oil
2 tablespoon balsamic vinegar
1–2 drop basil essential oil
Mini wooden skewers
Fresh basil leaves for garnish

Thread tomatoes and cheese onto mini wooden skewers and drizzle with balsamic vinegar and olive oil mixture, top with fresh basil.

Rosemary Garlic Mash Potatoes

5 pounds Yukon gold potatoes, peeled and diced
1 ½ teaspoon salt
1 teaspoon garlic powder
¾ heavy cream
6 tablespoon butter
3 tablespoon milk
1-2 drops rosemary essential oil, to taste
1 drop black pepper essential oil

Peel, dice and boil the potatoes for 20-25 minutes or until soft. Drain potatoes and place in a bowl with butter. Allow butter to melt then add cream. Mash potatoes thoroughly until desired consistency, adding milk as needed. Stir in essential oils, garlic, and salt to taste. Place in serving bowl and keep warm.

Sweet & Spicy Yogurt Topping

⅔ cup plain yogurt
1 teaspoon honey
½ to 1 drop cinnamon essential oil
¼ cup granola or chopped nuts
Sea salt to taste

Mix together and serve over yogurt.

Additional oil suggestions: Lime, lemon, grapefruit, protecting blend, or get creative and try something new.

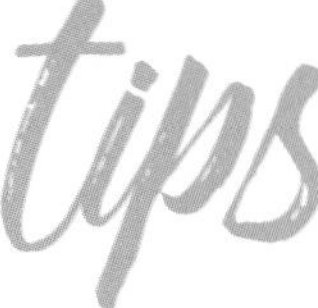

- Use a produce rinse for healthier and fresher tasting fruit, berries, and vegetables, including greens. Fill a clean glass or metal bowl with water. Add 1 tablespoon white vinegar and 2-3 drops lemon essential oil. Rinse produce, and place on clean paper towels or cotton cloth to dry.
- For oven-roasted veggies, add your favorite essential oils to taste to olive oil. Add salt and pepper until you like the flavor. Pour oil mixture over veggies and toss to cover. Spread out on cookie sheet and roast just until tender. Serve.

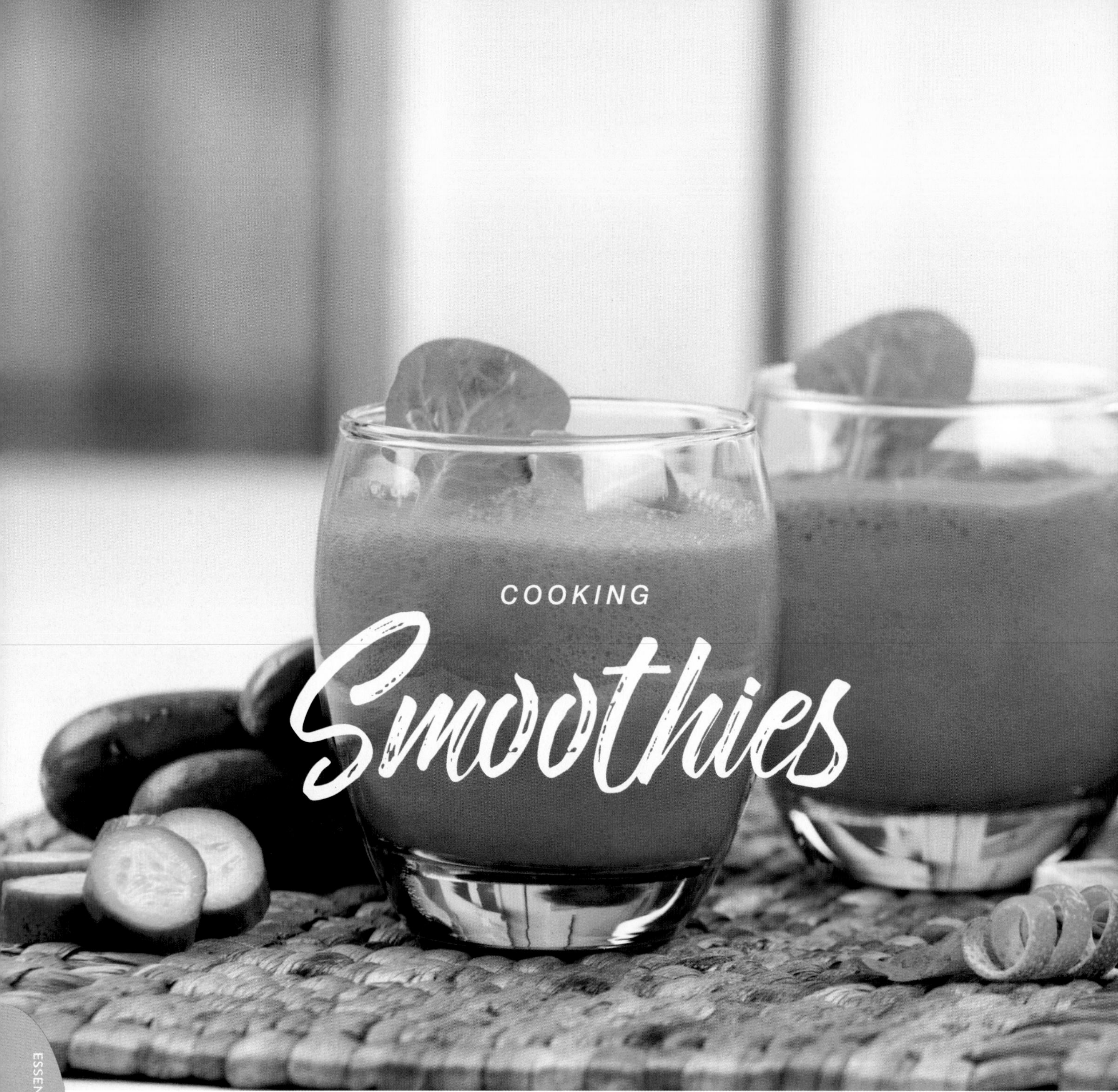

Wild Orange Smoothie

Blend together:
¾ cup vanilla yogurt
¾ cup skim milk (or coconut milk almond milk, etc.)
3-4 mandarin oranges or 1 large orange
1-2 drops wild orange essential oil
½ teaspoon vanilla extract
12-15 ice cubes

Place all ingredients in the blender and blend until smooth. Blend longer to break up extra pulp from the oranges. Recipe makes enough for 2-3 servings.

Healthy Shamrock Shake

Blend together:
1 banana, peeled
1 avocado, peeled and cut up
2 cups light coconut milk
4 drops (or more) peppermint essential oil
4 drops of organic liquid Stevia
1 cup of ice

Place all ingredients in a blender. Blend on high for 2 minutes until smooth. Top with coconut whipped cream, dark chocolate shavings and strawberries. Serve right away and enjoy!

tips

- You can use a glass regular-mouth jar (e.g. canning jar) in lieu of a regular blender container. Simply unscrew the base and blade from the blender container, put the blade over the mouth of the jar, then screw on the base. This is perfect for small portions, nuts, pestos, etc. It's a time saver too!
- Add extra nutrition to your smoothie by adding any of the following:
  - Ground flaxseed
  - Coconut oil
  - Chia seeds
  - Protein powder
- When blending, put liquid in first followed by greens and chunks of fruit and ice.

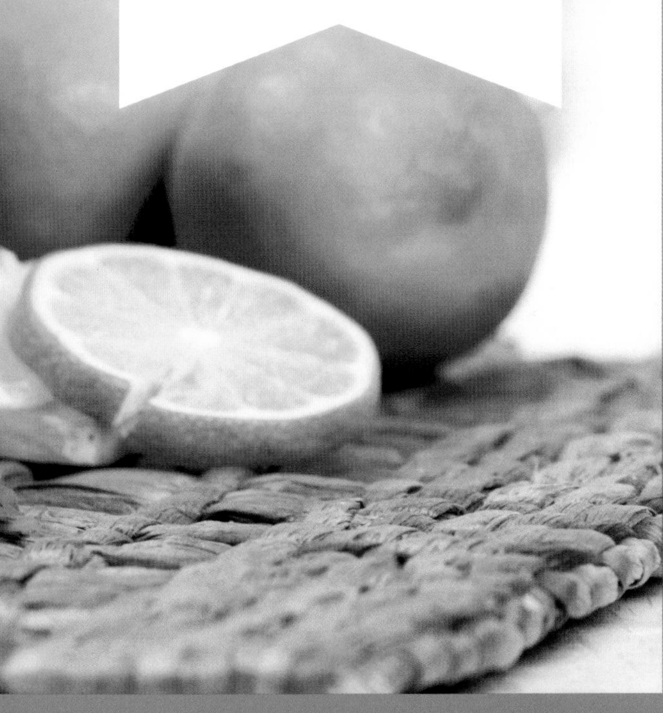

Basic formula:

2 cups liquid base
2 cups leafy greens
3 cups ripe or frozen fruit
Essential oils to taste

Berry Citrus Smoothie

1 banana
2 cup frozen mixed berries
1 cup frozen mango
1 medium avocado
3 tablespoon raw hemp seeds
2 tablespoon chia seeds
1 scoop green powder
4 cup water
2 drops wild orange essential oil
2 drops lime essential oil

Blend until smooth. Use all organic fruits for optimal taste and health benefits. Serves 2 – 4, Enjoy!

Lavender Blueberry Raspberry Smoothie

6 ice cubes
2 cups almond milk
1 cup frozen blueberries
1 cup frozen raspberries
½-1 drop lavender essential oil
2 teaspoons chia seeds

Blend all ingredients in a blender, adding more milk if desired.

Paradise in a Glass Smoothie

Blend together:
½ cup coconut milk
1 toothpick dip lime essential oil
1 cup kale
1 cup spinach
1 cup chopped pineapple
½ cup frozen mango
4 frozen strawberries
1 banana
Water as needed for consistency

Simple Veggie Smoothie

Blend together:
2 cups kale
1 cup chopped tomato or grape tomatoes
¾ cup chopped cucumber
1 toothpick dip black pepper essential oil
1-2 cups water, as desired for consistency
1 cup ice
Dash salt

COOKING

Snacks

Lavender Lemon Cookies

1 box lemon cake mix
½ cup unsalted butter, melted
1 egg
8 drops lemon essential oil
½ cup lavender colored candy melts (could also use white)
1-2 drops lavender essential oil

Preheat oven to 350°

Have an ungreased cookie sheet ready to go. In a large mixing bowl, combine the cake mix, melted butter, egg and lemon oil (or extract) and mix until combined. Using your hands, roll out golf ball sized rounds of the cake batter mixture. Place the balls 1" apart on the cookie sheet, sprinkle all with a little sugar. Bake for 9 minutes. While baking, place the candy melts in a microwave safe bowl and microwave for 45 seconds. Stir until completely melted and smooth (microwave again for 10 second increments if needed). Add one drop of lavender essential oil and test for taste, adding another drop if needed (while it may taste strong, remember the lemon cookie will also balance this out). Set the lavender infused candy melts aside to cool slightly.

Remove the cookies from the oven and allow to continue baking on the cookie sheet for another 5-6 minutes. Using your thumb or forefinger, gently press an indent or well into the center of each cookie. Using a small spoon, carefully place a teaspoon of the melted lavender infused candy into the center "well" of each cookie. Using the back of the spoon smooth out the melted candy to create a little round. Allow to cool completely until the lavender center has hardened.

Orange Creamsicle Cheesecake Fruit Dip

16 ounces cream cheese OR neufchatel cheese (2 blocks), softened to room temperature
⅔ cup vanilla greek yogurt
6 tablespoons granulated sugar
2 teaspoons vanilla extract
4-6 drops wild orange essential oil
¼ teaspoon salt

In a large mixing bowl, using an electric hand mixer, beat the cream cheese on Medium/High speed for about 2 minutes, until very smooth and fluffy. Stop the mixer and scrape down the sides of the bowl as needed during this and any of the following steps.

Add yogurt, and continue to beat for another 1-2 minutes, until very creamy.

Add sugar, vanilla, wild orange essential oil, and salt, and beat for another 1-2 minutes, until very smooth and creamy.

Makes about 3 cups. Serve with assorted fruits, cookies, or pretzels as desired.

Lemon Fruit Dip

1 package cream cheese, softened
1 cup sour cream
⅓ cup sugar
2 teaspoon vanilla extract
1-2 drops lemon essential oil

Mix together cream cheese, sour cream, sugar, vanilla, and lemon essential oil with an electric hand mixer until smooth. Serve with your choice of fresh fruits. Store leftover dip in a tightly sealed container, in the refrigerator, up to 2-3 days.

White Chocolate Lemon Cashew Bites

1 ¾ cup cashew flour or almond flour
1 tablespoon lemon juice
1 tablespoon lemon zest (1 large lemon)
3 drops lemon essential oil
Pinch of vanilla powder or teaspoon vanilla
1 tablespoon coconut oil, melted
1 tablespoon coconut nectar (or liquid sweetener of choice)
Pinch of salt
White chocolate
4 tablespoon melted cacao butter*
3 tablespoons raw coconut butter
1 tablespoon coconut nectar + 5 drops stevia (or an extra 1 tablespoon coconut nectar)
Pinch of vanilla powder or teaspoon vanilla

For the Lemon-Cashew Bites: Add all ingredients for the lemon-cashew bites to a food processor and pulse until combined. You should have a thick dough-like consistency but it shouldn't be too sticky or wet.

Roll the mixture into small balls and place on a plate covered in parchment paper in the freezer to firm up.

*For the White Chocolate Coating: Gently melt the cacao and coconut butter together over a double boiler, remove from heat and add the vanilla powder, coconut nectar or sweetener.

Set aside to thicken up slightly for 5-10 minutes at room temperature, stirring occasionally.

Dip each bite in the chocolate coating until it is completely covered. Scoop out carefully with a fork, and tap the fork handle on the edge of the bowl so that excess coating drips back into the bowl. Place back on the parchment lined plate and return to the freezer until coating is solid (about 5 minutes); then repeat the coating process once more.

COOKING

Soups

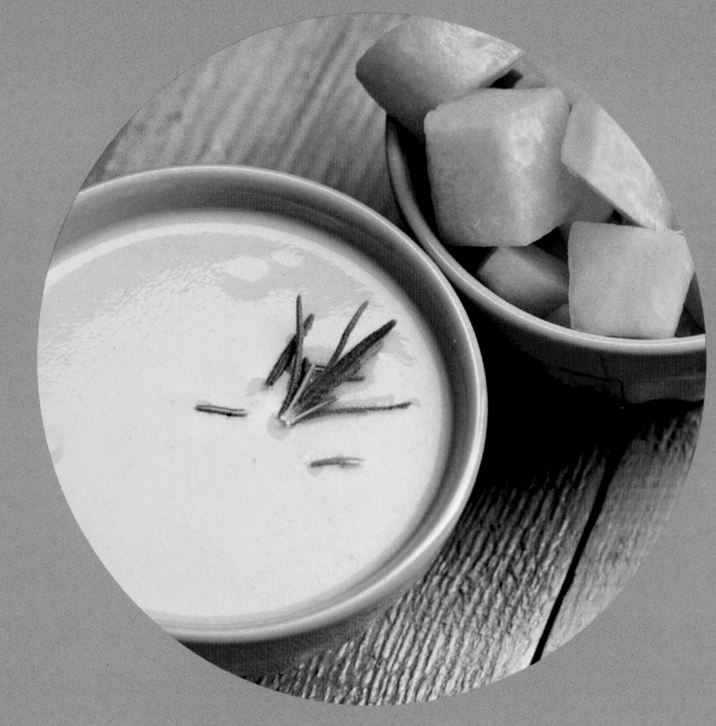

Nourishing Soup

2 pounds bone in chicken; chopped into 1 inch cubes or leave whole to shred after cooking
1 ½ gallon filtered water
1 pound carrots, sliced
2 cups winter squash, scooped or in chunks; favorite vegetables, shredded cabbage, sliced mushrooms, frozen peas etc.
1 bunch chives, finely chopped
1 tablespoon + 1 teaspoon sea salt
2-3 drops lemongrass or basil essential oil, or a combination of both
½-1 drop ginger essential oil, to taste
1 clove garlic, chopped

Place chicken, water and sea salt into pot. cook for 45 minutes on medium, strain out all bones.

Pull out chicken and let cool slightly, then shred vegetables to pot. Simmer until vegetables are tender, about 30 minutes, stirring occasionally. Add chicken back to the pot when vegetables are soft.

Add essential oils and garlic. Stir to combine. Taste, add sea salt if desired. Serve, garnished with lots of green onions or chives.

Roasted Butternut Squash Soup

¼ cup medium diced onion
¼ cup medium diced celery
¼ cup small diced carrot
3 cups medium diced butternut squash
2–3 cups vegetable stock
½ cup almond milk
1 teaspoon salt
½ teaspoon black pepper
2 drops cardamom essential oil
2 drops cinnamon essential oil

Roast first 4 ingredients in 350 degree Fahrenheit oven; when nicely browned put in sauce pan. Add 2 cups vegetable stock, almond milk, salt and pepper. Simmer until just boiling, place in food processor. Puree until smooth, add more stock if needed for smooth, soupy texture. Add essential oils. Add more seasoning if needed. Serve hot.

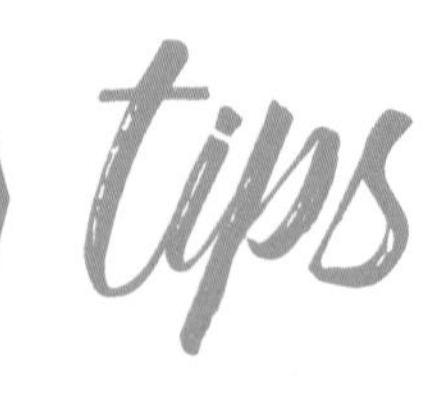

- It has been found that smelling essential oils helps curb the appetite. Every few hours, just take a sniff of a savory oil and trick the brain into feeling satiated.
- Asian soups are fantastic with a little lemongrass, lemon, and ginger essential oils.
- Remember, less is more. To retain the flavor of all of the ingredients in your dish, use the toothpick dip and add more to taste.

ESSENTIAL LIFESTYLE

Glowing Spiced Lentil Soup

2 cups diced onion
2 large garlic cloves, minced
1-2 drops turmeric essential oil
1 drop cumin essential oil
1 toothpick swirl cinnamon essential oil
1 toothpick swirl cardamom essential oil
1 15 ounce can diced tomatoes, with juice
1 15 ounce can coconut milk
¾ cup uncooked red lentils, rinsed
3 ½ cups low-sodium vegetable broth
½ teaspoon fine sea salt, or to taste
1-2 drops black pepper essential oils, to taste
Red pepper flakes or cayenne pepper, to taste
1 5 ounce package baby spinach
2 teaspoons fresh lime juice, or more to taste

In a large pot, sauté the onion, and garlic in coconut oil over medium heat for 4 to 5 minutes until the onion softens.

Add the diced tomatoes (with juice), entire can of coconut milk, red lentils, broth, salt, and plenty of black pepper essential oil. Add red pepper flakes or cayenne, if desired, to taste. Stir to combine. Increase heat to high and bring to a low boil.

Once it boils, reduce the heat to medium-high, and simmer, uncovered, for about 18 to 22 minutes, until the lentils are fluffy and tender.

Turn heat to low and stir in the spinach until wilted. Add the lime juice to taste. Stir in the turmeric essential oil, cumin essential oil , cinnamon essential oil, and cardamom essential oil until combined. Continue cooking for about 1 minute, until fragrant.

Taste and add more salt and pepper, if desired. Ladle into bowls and serve with toasted bread and lime wedges.

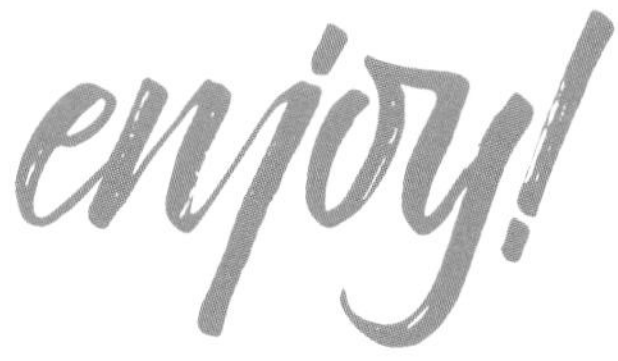

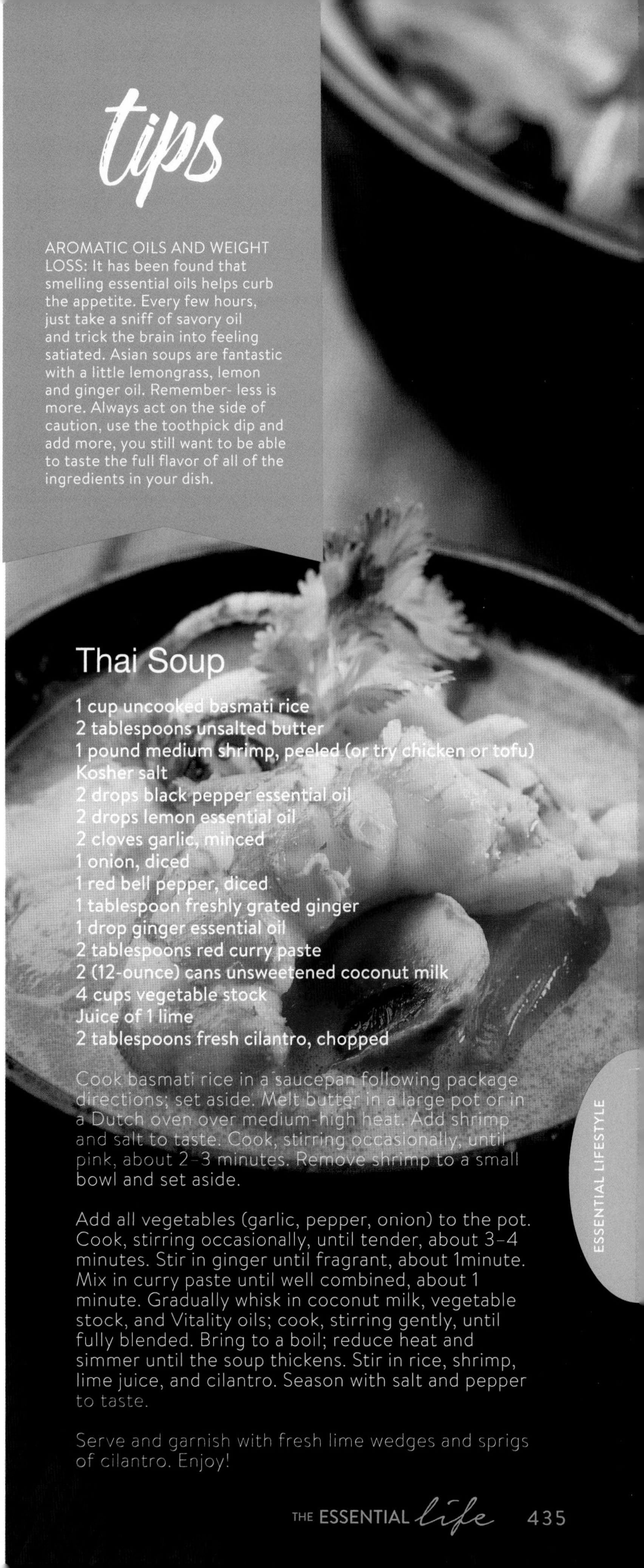

tips

AROMATIC OILS AND WEIGHT LOSS: It has been found that smelling essential oils helps curb the appetite. Every few hours, just take a sniff of savory oil and trick the brain into feeling satiated. Asian soups are fantastic with a little lemongrass, lemon and ginger oil. Remember- less is more. Always act on the side of caution, use the toothpick dip and add more, you still want to be able to taste the full flavor of all of the ingredients in your dish.

Thai Soup

1 cup uncooked basmati rice
2 tablespoons unsalted butter
1 pound medium shrimp, peeled (or try chicken or tofu)
Kosher salt
2 drops black pepper essential oil
2 drops lemon essential oil
2 cloves garlic, minced
1 onion, diced
1 red bell pepper, diced
1 tablespoon freshly grated ginger
1 drop ginger essential oil
2 tablespoons red curry paste
2 (12-ounce) cans unsweetened coconut milk
4 cups vegetable stock
Juice of 1 lime
2 tablespoons fresh cilantro, chopped

Cook basmati rice in a saucepan following package directions; set aside. Melt butter in a large pot or in a Dutch oven over medium-high heat. Add shrimp and salt to taste. Cook, stirring occasionally, until pink, about 2-3 minutes. Remove shrimp to a small bowl and set aside.

Add all vegetables (garlic, pepper, onion) to the pot. Cook, stirring occasionally, until tender, about 3-4 minutes. Stir in ginger until fragrant, about 1minute. Mix in curry paste until well combined, about 1 minute. Gradually whisk in coconut milk, vegetable stock, and Vitality oils; cook, stirring gently, until fully blended. Bring to a boil; reduce heat and simmer until the soup thickens. Stir in rice, shrimp, lime juice, and cilantro. Season with salt and pepper to taste.

Serve and garnish with fresh lime wedges and sprigs of cilantro. Enjoy!

DIY & Gift Giving

Essential Oil Bath Bomb

Molds
1 cup baking soda
⅔ cup Epsom salt
½ teaspoon mica (color dependent on your choice)
40 drops frankincense essential oil
10 drops myrrh essential oil
1 tablespoon of castor oil
½ cup citric acid
Witch hazel (in any spray bottle)

Pour 1 cup of baking soda, ⅔ cup of Epsom salt, and ½ teaspoon of mica into the blender. Add 40 drops of frankincense essential oil, 10 drops of myrrh essential oil and 1 tablespoon of castor oil. Mix ingredients in blender until incorporated; use spatula to scrape the sides. Dump contents into big bowl, and mix again with spatula. Add ½ cup of citric acid and stir again. Using the witch hazel (in any spray bottle), spray the top of the ingredients evenly, as if resembling a thin sheet, and mix; the mixture will foam a tiny bit and create clumps as you go. Once the contents can hold its shape when picked up, it's time to fit the ingredients into the molds. Compact the mixture into the molds, and let it sit for 24 hours. Gently, tap out the intact bomb from the molds, and be sure to use the essential oil bath bomb in your next soak!

Chapped Lip Balm

Lip balm tube
1 tablespoon honey
2 tablespoons beeswax
1 tablespoon shea butter
2-5 drops spearmint essential oil
Optional: lipstick color

Heat beeswax, honey, shea butter and lipstick (if desired) on medium/low heat until melted. Remove from heat, add oil, and quickly pour into balm containers.

Bubble Bath

8 oz clear plastic oval bottle
½ cup castile soap
¼ cup vegetable glycerine
15 drops lemon essential oil
5 drops lavender essential oil

Combine all ingredients and fill the remainder of the bottle with water. Shake well before use.

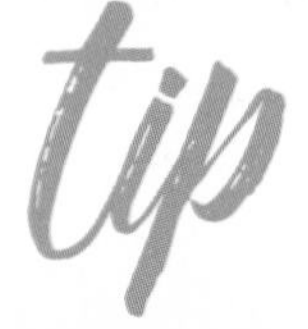

Simply mix your favorite essential oils together in a roller bottle to create your own unique aroma. Use for yourself or as a gift.

ESSENTIAL LIFESTYLE

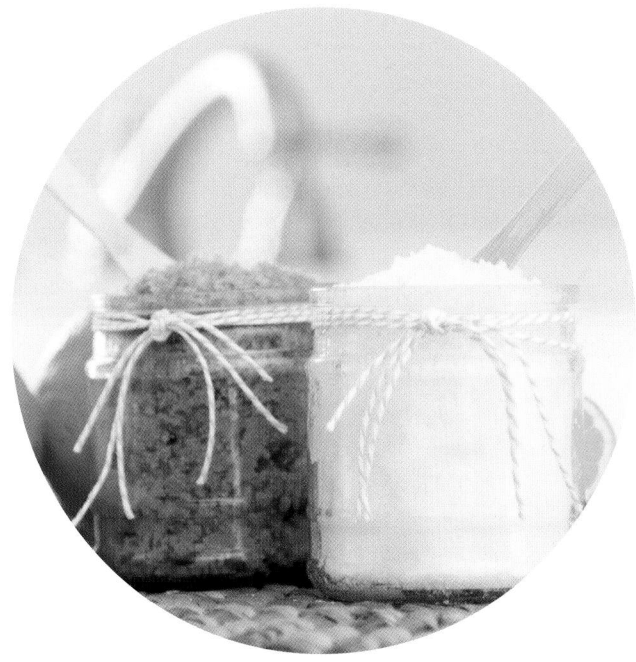

Mood-Boosting Bath Salt

8 oz jar
1 cup sea salt or Epsom salt
½ tablespoon jojoba oil (or carrier oil)
5 drops wild orange essential oil
5 drops grapefruit essential oil
5 drops tangerine essential oil

Add all ingredients to the jar and stir to mix the ingredients together well.

Lavender Essential Oil Makeup Remover

1 4 oz. glass bottle with dropper
1 mini stainless steel funnel
1 bag cotton balls/pads (for facial use)
2 tablespoons carrier oil
1 tablespoon witch hazel
4 drops lavender essential oil

Using a 4 oz. glass bottle with dropper, remove the top and secure the mini stainless steel funnel to its opening. Pour 2 tablespoons of carrier oil, and 1 tablespoon of witch hazel into the bottle. Add 4 drops of lavender essential oil. Remove the funnel and reattach the dropper lid. Shake well. Squeezing the dropper top, absorb the liquid contents and release them onto the cotton ball/pad. Dab face gently with the absorbed cotton ball/pad and feel the fresh sensation of a moisturizing essential oil makeup remover!

Essential Oil Glitter Body Spray

4 oz. glass spray bottle
1 mini stainless steel funnel
1 measuring spoon
3 teaspoons of carrier oil
2 teaspoons of gold mica
4 drops of frankincense essential oil
(or any essential oil of your choice)
Distilled water

Using a 4 oz. glass bottle, remove the top and secure the mini stainless steel funnel to its opening. Pour 3 teaspoons of carrier oil into the bottle. Add 2 teaspoons of gold mica, and 4 drops of frankincense essential oil. With the remaining space left open, fill up the bottle with distilled water. Remove the funnel and reattach the lid. Shake well (and before every use). Spray on your body, face or hair, and glow with this essential oil glitter body spray!

Light Up Your Life Candle

16 oz mason jar
13 oz of soy wax
Popsicle sticks
Wick
Candle dye (if desired)
5 drops lavender essential oil
5 drops grapefruit essential oil
5 drops Citrus Bliss® essential oil
5 drops Siberian fir essential oil

In a double boiler, melt wax slowly. Once all wax is melted, add colors if desired. Put the wick in the center and wrap the top around the popsicle stick to hold it up. Let the wax cool for about 30 minutes before pouring into the container to ensure it doesn't crack when setting. Add essential oils and pour. Let set for at least 24 hours before lighting.

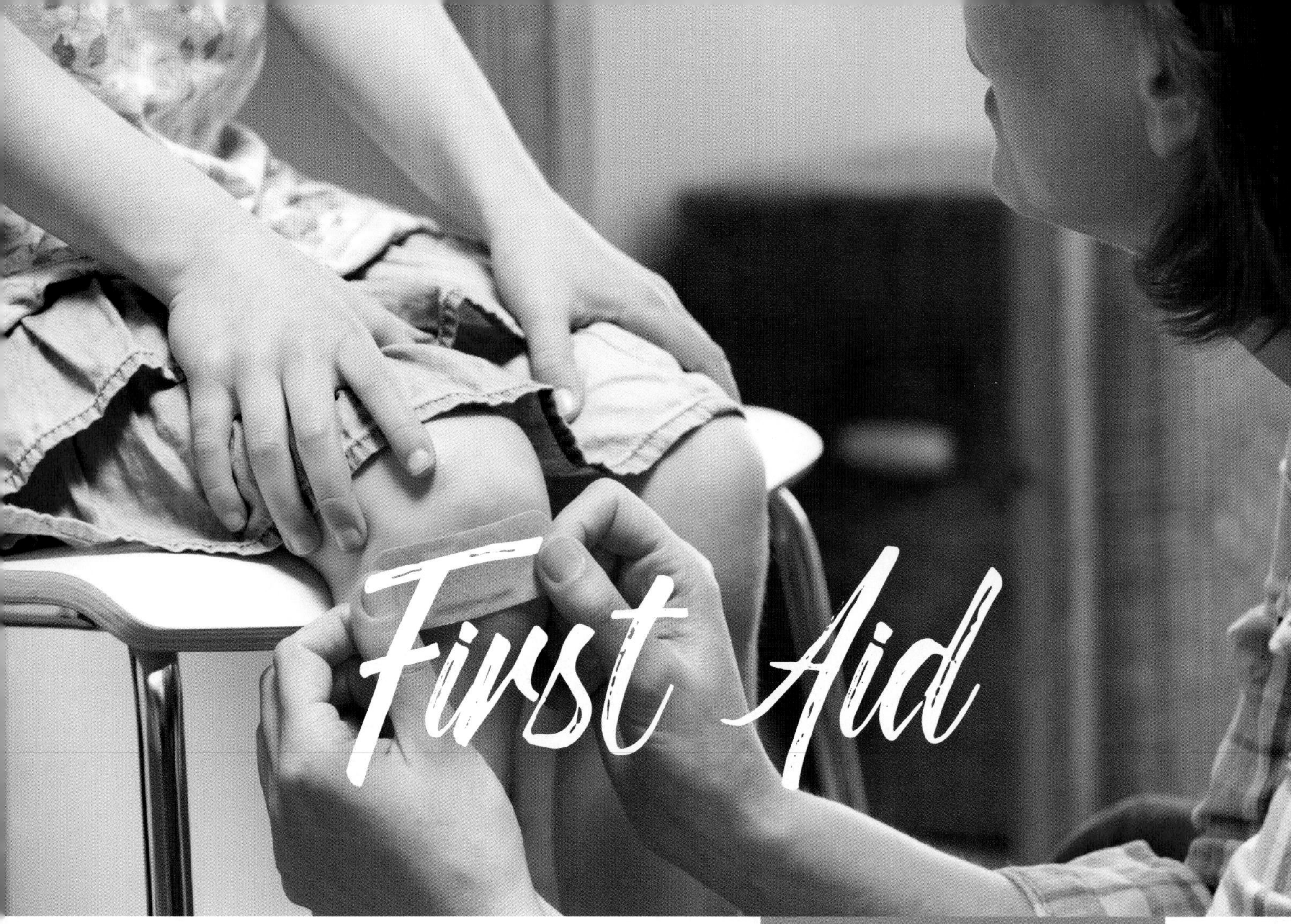

Bump & Bruise Spray

2 oz. glass spray bottle
1 mini stainless steel funnel
5 drops myrrh essential oil
5 drops frankincense essential oil
5 drops lavender essential oil
5 drops helichrysum essential oil
Distilled water (amount dependent on space left in bottle)

Using a 2 oz. glass spray bottle, remove the top and secure the mini stainless steel funnel to its opening. Add myrrh, frankincense, lavender, and helichrysum to the bottle. With the remaining space left open, fill with distilled water. Remove the funnel and reattach the lid. Shake well. Spray on any cut, bruise or scrape and kiss the tears goodbye!

Top reasons to include essential oils in your First Aid Kit

1. They're multi-faceted. You can disinfect a cut, stop bleeding, and soothe a child with a single application of a few drops of lavender essential oil.
2. They're affordable. They are pennies on the dollar for what you'd pay for most over-the-counter medications
3. They don't expire! They have an extended shelf-life that will keep you from wasting your oils.
4. They're all natural. So you'll avoid any negative side effects of synthetic medications by using nature's medicine cabinet.

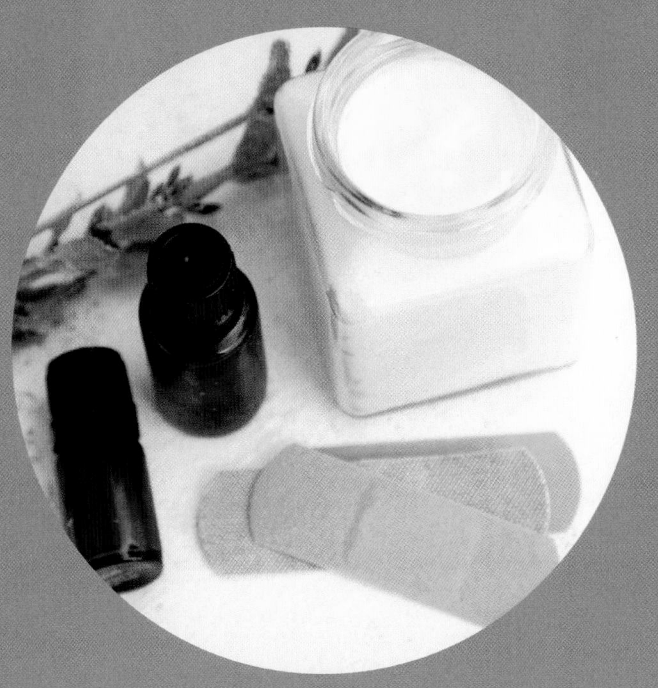

tips

- To clean a wound, apply lavender essential oil or corrective ointment to disinfect and promote healing.
- To stop bleeding quickly, apply lavender and then helichrysum essential oil.
- For splinters deep under the skin, apply clove essential oil to bring the splinter to the surface. For splinters near the surface, apply a piece of adhesive tape to the area of skin containing a splinter. Yank tape off quickly and the splinter should come out. Apply 1 drop of Deep Blue® essential oil to affected area.
- For stings, apply Purify and then lavender essential oil to soothe.
- For blister relief, apply 2 drops lavender and 2 drops tea tree essential oil. Repeat as necessary.

Cooling Salve

4 oz clear glass jar straight sided with plastic lined cap
¼ cup carrier oil
1 tablespoon shea butter
1 tablespoon aloe vera juice
1 tablespoon beeswax
2 teaspoon vitamin E oil
10 drops lavender essential oil
2 drops peppermint essential oil

Add shea butter and beeswax to glass jar and melt in hot water. Cool slightly. Add carrier oil, aloe vera, Vitamin E oil, and essential oils. Mix well. Store in cool dark place (refrigerator even) and use as needed for owies and areas that need cleaning and cooling.

Wound Spray

4 oz spray bottle
10 drops tea tree essential oil
5 drops lemon essential oil
5 drops eucalyptus essential oil
Water

Fill the bottle halfway with water, then add the oil. Fill the remainder of the bottle with water. Shake before spraying on use.

Allergy Relief

Try 1-3 TriEase Softgels for quick allergy relief.

4 drops lemon essential oil
4 drops lavender essential oil
4 drops peppermint essential oil
Carrier oil

In a small roller bottle, mix essential oils and fill remainder with carrier oil. Shake and roll on as needed.

Soothing Wipes Spray

2 oz spray bottle
Bamboo wipes
10 drops lavender essential oil
5 drops frankincense essential oil
1 teaspoon vitamin E oil
Water

Fill the bottle halfway with water, then add the oils. Fill the remainder of the bottle with water, with enough room to screw on the cap. Shake and spray on wipes. Pre-soaking is not recommended because the oils might break down the bamboo fibers.

Fitness

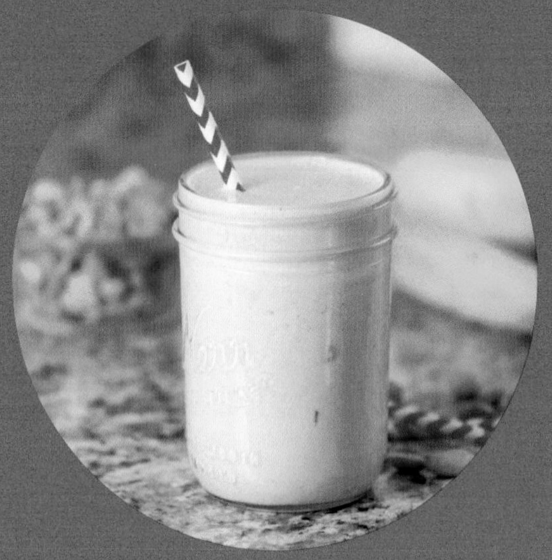

When it comes to health and fitness, isn't it nice to have cutting-edge natural products on your side?

Can you imagine the benefits of all-natural freshening and cleansing sprays for your body and workout equipment?

Can you picture overcoming cravings and keeping your metabolism active with pure, zero-calorie essential oils? Are you looking forward to more easily warming up and cooling down your muscles and effectively relieving muscle soreness?

Get ready for essential oils to maximize your efforts and help you reach your fitness goals!

Peanut Butter Heaven Protein Shake

1 scoop vanilla meal replacement powder
¾ cup vanilla almond milk (or milk)
1 tablespoon natural peanut butter
½ banana
1 cup ice

Mix in blender until smooth and creamy.

Muscle Rub

5 drops ginger essential oil
5 drops peppermint essential oil
5 drops eucalyptus essential oil
1 tablespoon argan/ carrier oil

Add oils in a bottle, shake well and massage onto sore muscles!

Muscle Soak

1 cup Epsom salt
2 drops black pepper essential oil
2 drops peppermint essential oil
3 drops juniper essential oil
3 drops lavender essential oil

In a bowl, combine Epsom salt and essential oils, run the bath slowly pouring the salt mixture into the moving water, let dissolve. Soak for 30 minutes, enjoy!

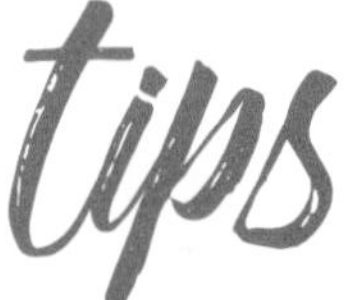

- To help flush out toxins, add 1-2 drops of lemon essential oil in your water.
- To manage appetite between meals, use 3-5 drops of Slim & Sassy® essential oil under tongue or in water.
- Open airways before, during, or after a workout by inhaling Breathe® essential oil.
- Increase your endurance by taking Mito2Max® essential oil daily.
- For sore muscles, rub or massage Deep Blue® essential oil anywhere it aches.
- To improve clarity and focus, use Balance® essential oil.
- To ease swimmers ear, rub clove essential oil behind, around, and on – but not in – the ear.
- To relieve pressure and tension, use AromaTouch® essential oil on your back and shoulders.
- For quick relief of leg cramps, apply AromaTouch® essential oil.

Leg Cramp Blend

3-4 drops Deep Blue® essential oil
3-4 drops lemongrass essential oil
1-2 drops helichrysum essential oil

Mix together and apply directly to affected area.

Post-Workout Aromatherapy

2 drops lavender essential oil
2 drops jasmine essential oil
1 drop Amavi® essential oil
Diffuser

Add essential oils to diffuser and relax after a tough workout

Sanitizing Spray

10 drops lemon essential oil
10 drops tea tree essential oil
1 oz water
Spray bottle

Pour water and essential oils into a spray bottle, mix and spray your yoga mats or gym equipment before and after use to stay sanitary!

Post-Workout Rub

1 ounce carrier oil
3 drops marjoram essential oil
2 drops thyme essential oil
4 drops Roman chamomile essential oil
4 drops cypress essential oil
3 drops lemon essential oil
2 drops peppermint essential oil

Mix together and gently massage the mixture into your muscles and joints to prevent stiffness and pain.

Cellulite Reducing Spray

4 ounces carrier oil
15 ml grapefruit essential oil (one bottle)

Mixed together in a glass spray bottle. After bathing, spray on body to reduce the appearance of cellulite.

Refreshing Body Spray

6 drops lime essential oil
2 drops lavender essential oil
2 drops lemon essential oil
1 drop peppermint essential oil

Combine essential oils in a 2-ounce spray bottle and fill with water to refresh yourself in seconds.

did you know?

- You can use cutting-edge natural products to help maximize your efforts and reach your fitness goals.
- Benefit from all-natural freshening and cleansing sprays for your body and workout equipment.
- Overcome cravings and keep your metabolism active with pure, zero-calorie essential oils.
- Easily warm up and cool down your muscles and effectively relieve muscle soreness with essential oils.

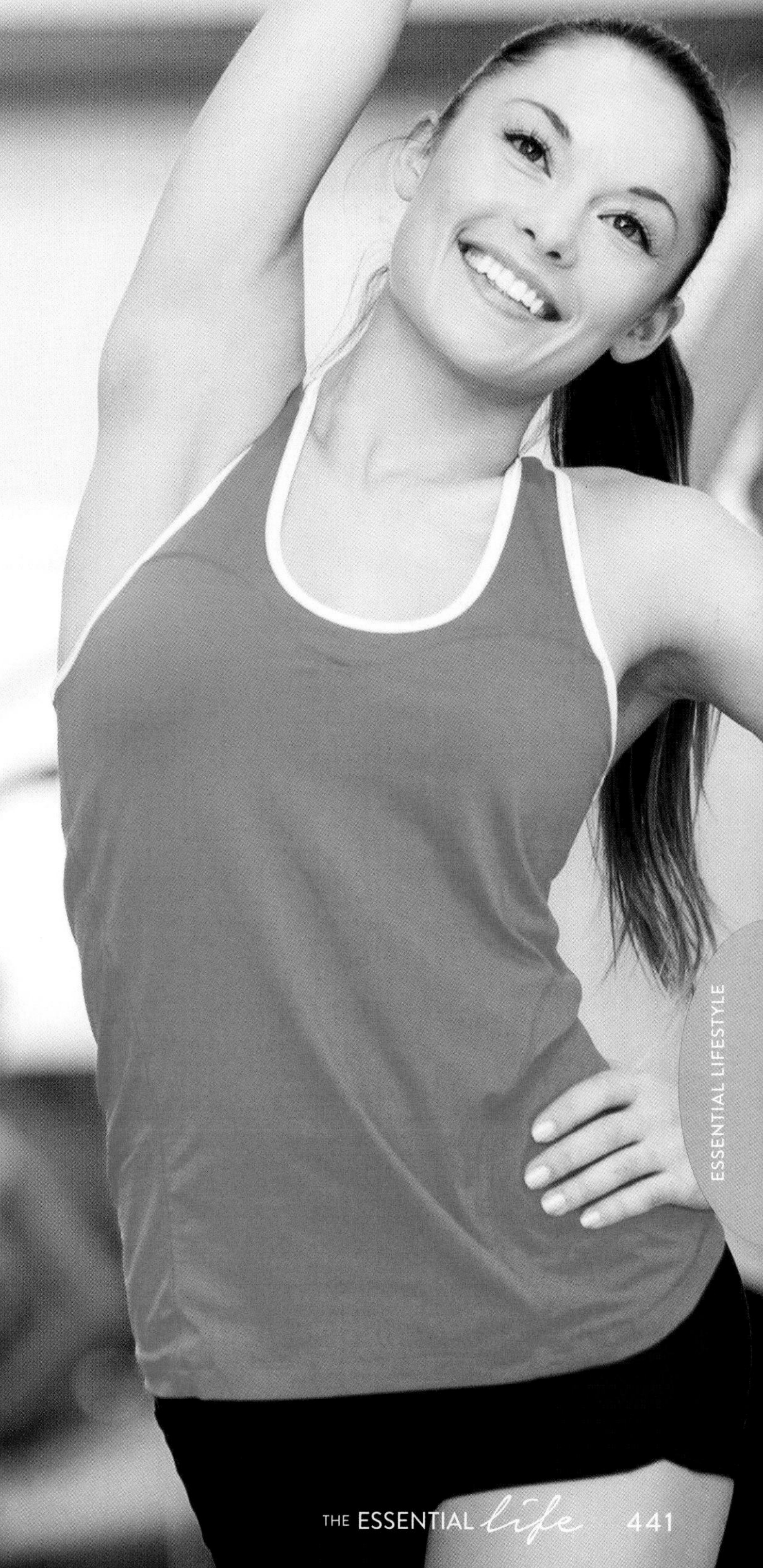

Garden

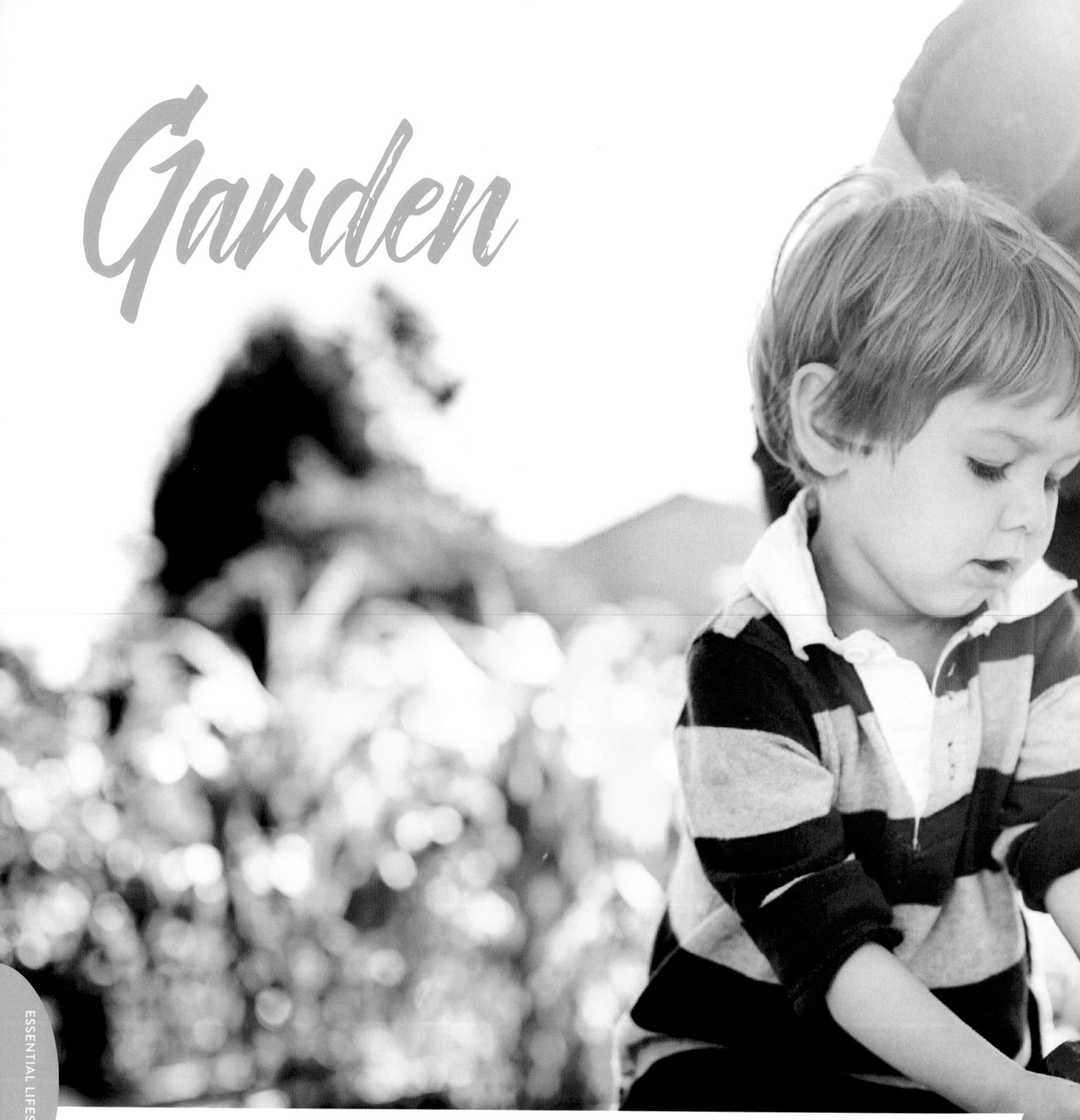

did you know?

85% of all plant disease is fungal-related. Avid gardeners love spending time outdoors, connecting with the earth and nurturing their plants in the sun. Unfortunately, there are pests and fungal diseases that can impede growth or reduce the harvest of producing plants. Rather than turning to harmful chemicals to address these challenges, try all-natural solutions and keep your garden organic.

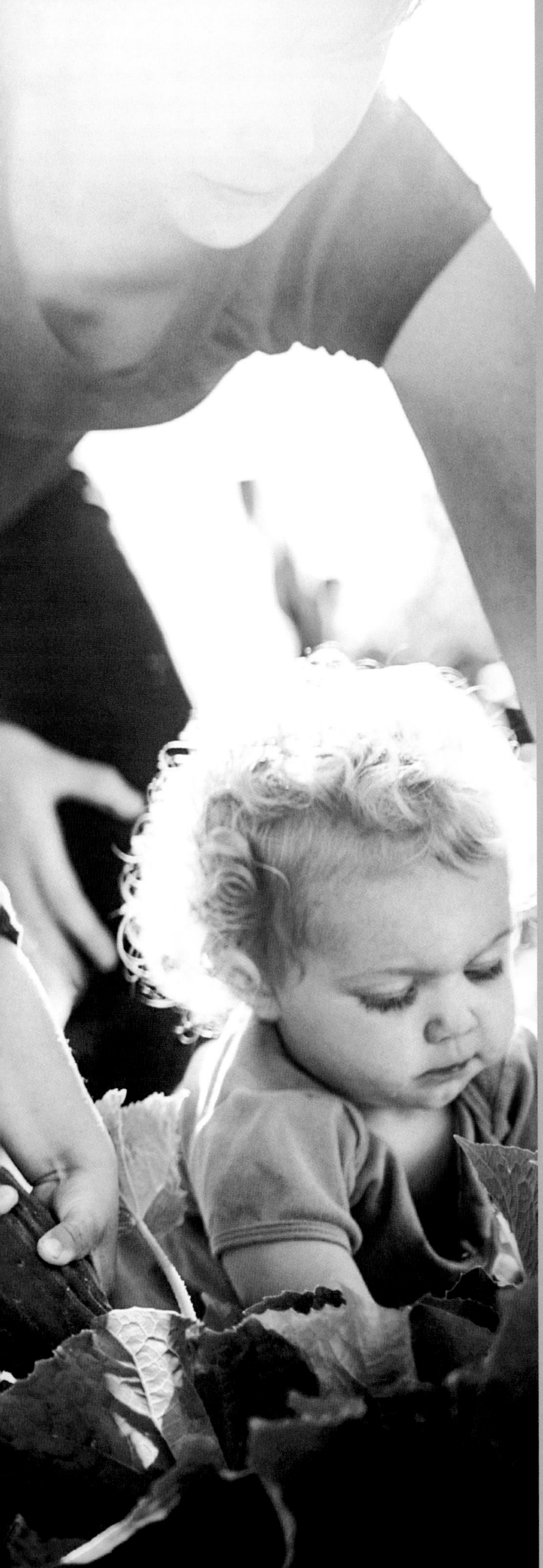

Plant Pest Control

16 oz glass bottle with sprayer
2 tablespoons castile soap
10 drops peppermint essential oil
10 drops lavender essential oil
5 drops cedarwood essential oil
5 drops lemongrass essential oil

Combine all ingredients and fill the remainder of the spray bottle with water. Spray early mornings or after the sun has set to prevent burning the leaves.

Fungus Suppressant

In a small spray bottle, combine 20 drops of tea tree essential oil and water to fill. Spray directly onto infected plants and surrounding soil, once or twice weekly.

Ant Spray

4 oz sprayer bottle
¼ cup witch hazel
10 drops peppermint essential oil

Combine all the ingredients and fill the remainder of the spray bottle with water. Spray ant trails and all areas ants have populated.

Pollinator Attractor

Add 5 to 6 drops wild orange essential oil to a spray bottle filled with 1 cup water. Spray on flowers and buds to attract bees for pollination.

Pest Repellents

Scare rodents away with 2 drops of peppermint essential oil dropped on a cotton ball. Tuck balls into mouse holes, burrows and nests to encourage them to relocate. Repel other pests with these essential oils:

- **Ants:** peppermint, spearmint
- **Aphids:** cedarwood, peppermint, spearmint
- **Beetles:** peppermint, thyme
- **Caterpillars:** spearmint, peppermint
- **Chiggers:** lavender, lemongrass, sage, thyme
- **Fleas:** peppermint, lemongrass, spearmint, lavender
- **Flies:** lavender, peppermint, rosemary, sage
- **Gnats:** patchouli, spearmint
- **Lice:** cedarwood, peppermint, spearmint
- **Mosquitoes:** lavender, lemongrass, arborvitae, TerraShield®
- **Moths:** cedarwood, lavender, peppermint, spearmint
- **Plant lice:** peppermint, spearmint
- **Slugs:** cedarwood
- **Snails:** cedarwood, patchouli
- **Spiders:** peppermint, spearmint
- **Ticks:** lavender, lemongrass, sage, thyme
- **Weevils:** cedarwood, patchouli, sandalwood

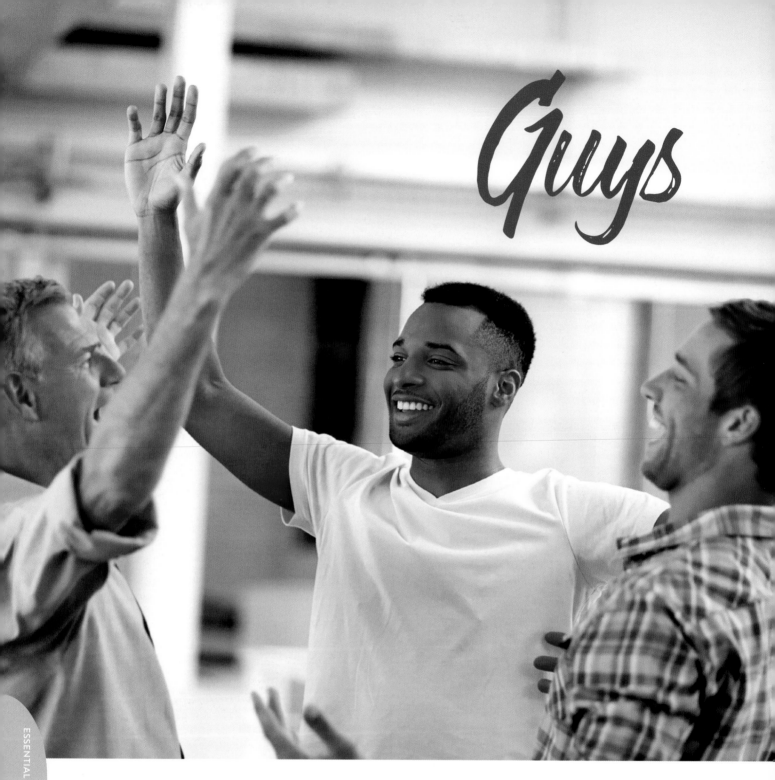

Guys

Shaving Cream

⅔ cup shea butter
⅔ cup cocoa butter
¼ cup carrier oil
5 drops sandalwood essential oil
5 drops peppermint essential oil
5 drops tea tree essential oil

Place butters in double boiler to melt and cool slightly. Mix in essential oils. Let shaving cream cool completely. Whip with hand mixer.

Earthy Aftershave

¾ cup witch hazel
1 tablespoon apple cider vinegar
10 drops sandalwood essential oil
5 drops peppermint essential oil
3 drops rosemary essential oil
2 drops tea tree essential oil

Place all ingredients in a bottle. Shake well and pat onto skin after shaving for a natural, great-smelling antiseptic and anti-inflammatory aftershave.

tips

- Remove oil, grease stains, and sticky residue with lemon essential oil.
- Clean the car battery and polish chrome wheels with tea tree and lemon essential oils diluted with water in a spray bottle.
- Most colognes and cleaners are both expensive and toxic, so use oils instead.
- To support hair growth in thinning areas, apply rosemary essential oil directly to scalp or add to shampoo.

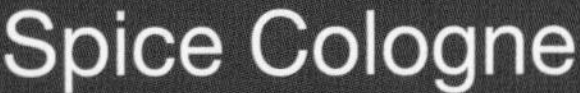

Spice Cologne

40 drops bergamot essential oil
10 drops clove essential oil
20 drops Siberian fir essential oil
5 drops lemon essential oil
3 teaspoons carrier oil

Combine essential oils with carrier oil into a glass roller bottle. Attach the roll-on cap and shake the vial until the mixture is combined. Let mixture sit for at least 24 hours before use.

Musky Deodorant

15 drops Purify essential oil
15 drops clary sage essential oil
10 drops frankincense essential oil
10 drops lime essential oil
5 drops lavender essential oil
5 drops patchouli essential oil
5 drops Balance® essential oil
5 drops cedarwood essential oil
3 drops sandalwood essential oil
Carrier oil

Combine the essential oils in an empty 2-ounce glass spray bottle. Add carrier oil to fill the bottle. Shake well before each use.

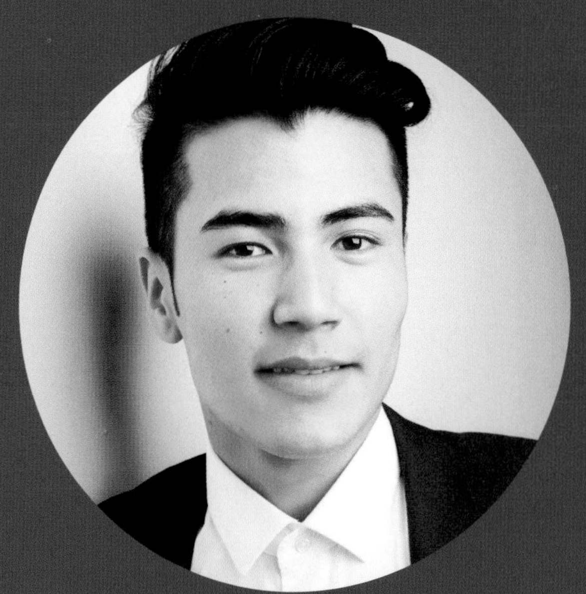

Hair & Scalp Stimulator

½ cup carrier oil
40 drops rosemary essential oil
25 drops basil essential oil
20 drops lemon essential oil
15 drops lavender essential oil
15 drops lemongrass essential oil
10 drops peppermint essential oil

Drop essential oils and carrier oil into a bottle with lid. Shake vigorously for 2 minutes. Dip fingertips into mixture and gradually massage the entire amount into your dry scalp for three to five minutes. Wrap your hair completely with plastic wrap or a shower cap and cover with a very warm, damp towel. Replace towel with another warm towel once it has cooled. Leave on thirty to forty-five minutes. Follow with shampoo and light conditioner. Use up to two times per week if hair is thinning.

Antifungal Foot Roll-On

35 drops tea tree essential oil
8 drops lavender essential oil

Combine essential oils in a glass bottle with a roller lid and apply topically to affected areas between toes and around toenails.

Shoe Deodorizer

2 drops peppermint essential oil
2 drops wild orange essential oil

Drop essential oils onto a paper towel, used dryer sheet, or cotton balls/rounds. Place in your shoes overnight.

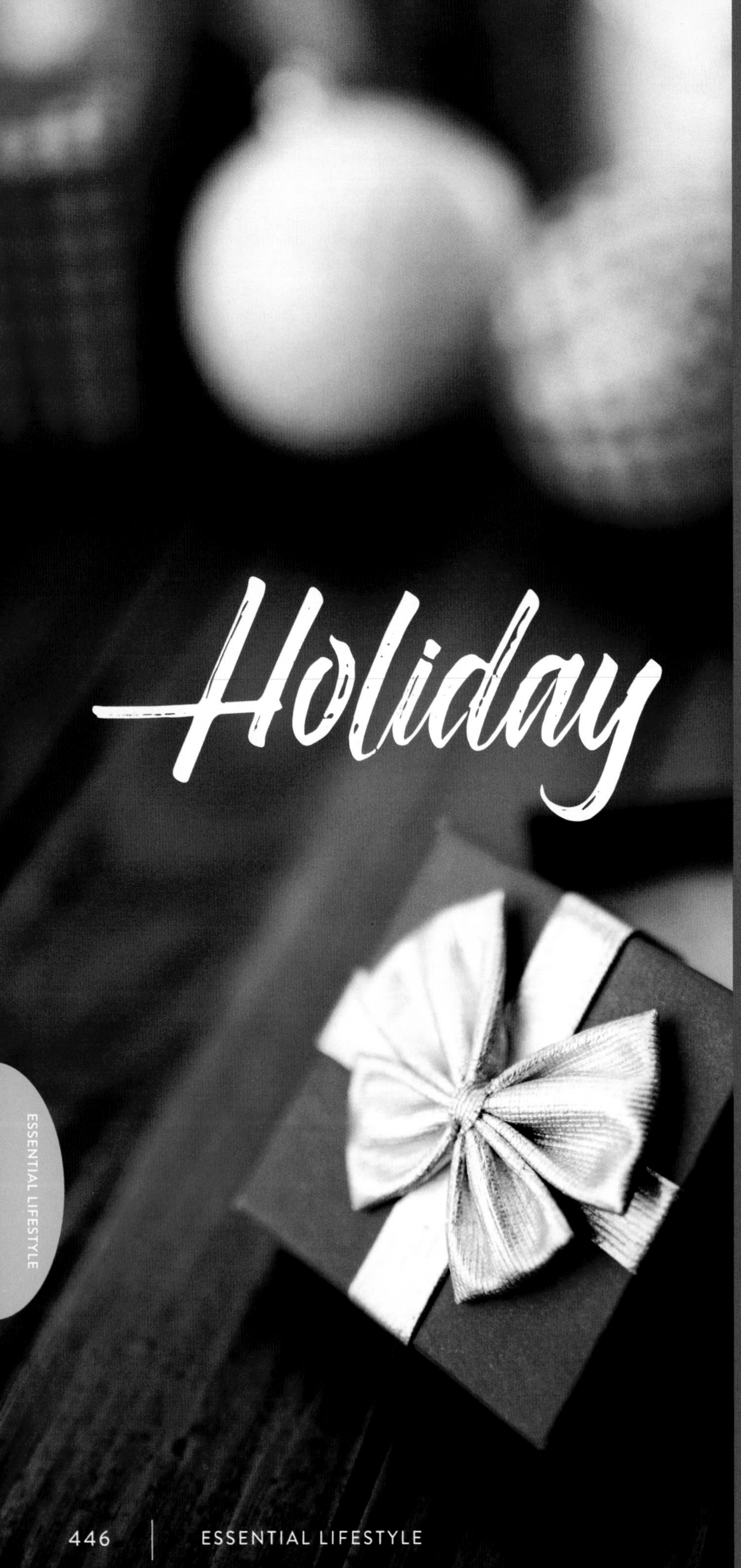

Pumpkin Bread

3 ½ cups all-purpose flour
1 teaspoon salt
2 teaspoons baking soda
2 ¾ cups sugar
½ teaspoon ground nutmeg
1 teaspoon baking powder
½ cup coconut oil
½ cup unsalted butter, softened
1 (15 oz) can pumpkin puree
4 large eggs
⅓ cup water
1 cup plain yogurt
2 drops cinnamon essential oil
1 drop clove essential oil
1 drop lemon essential oil
4 drops lemon essential oil

Preheat oven to 325 degrees. Spray pans with non-stick cooking spray. In a small bowl, combine flour, baking soda, baking powder, nutmeg, salt, and sugar and set aside. In a mixing bowl, combine the coconut oil, butter, pumpkin puree, water, yogurt, eggs, and all essential oils.

With the mixer on low, slowly add the dry ingredients to the wet, scraping the sides often to make sure all ingredients are well combined. Once they're well mixed, set the mixer to a medium speed and mx for two minutes until light and fluffy.

Divide mixture into pans and bake for 45-50 minutes or until a toothpick comes out clean from the middle of the bread. Cool slightly before serving. Nuts optional.

Scented Ornaments

1 cup baking soda
½ cup cornstarch
½ cup water
10-15 drops of cassia, Siberian fir, Holiday Joy®, wild orange, or peppermint essential oil

In a saucepan, heat together all ingredients except the oils over medium heat. Bring to a boil, stirring continuously. Once mixture has thickened into a dough-like consistency, remove from heat and mix in oils. Add glitter or food coloring, if desired. Roll cooled dough onto a cookie sheet and cut with cookie cutters. Use a large toothpick or skewer to make a hole in the top of each shape. Cool completely. String twine or ribbon through the hole to hang the ornament.

tips

- Create the scent of Christmas by diffusing Holiday Joy® essential oil.
- Create Christmas pine cones by adding 1-2 drops of cassia essential oil to a pine cone or spray a bowl of pine cones with Holiday Joy® essential oil.
- Keep your Christmas tree smelling fresh all season long by filling a small glass spray bottle with 20 drops of Douglas fir. Fill the remainder with water and spray on your Christmas tree.

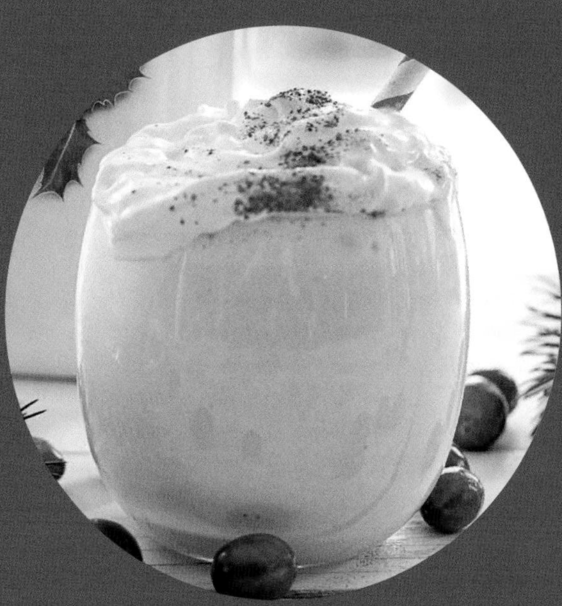

Eggnog

6 large egg yolks
½ cup sugar
1 cup heavy cream
2 cups milk
½ teaspoon nutmeg
Pinch of salt
¼ teaspoon vanilla extract
1 drop cinnamon essential oil

Whisk the egg yolks and sugar together in a medium bowl until light and creamy. In a saucepan over medium-high heat, combine the cream, milk, nutmeg, and salt. Stir often until mixture comes to a low simmer. Temper the milk into the mixture. Add a big ladle of the hot milk mixture to the egg mixture, whisking vigorously. Repeat until all combined. Once all combined, pour the mixture back into the saucepan on the stove, whisk constantly, until mixture reaches 160 degrees F. Remove from heat and stir in vanilla.

Pour eggnog into a pitcher, add cinnamon essential oil, and cover with plastic wrap. Refrigerate until chilled. Serve with whipped cream if desired.

Peppermint Bark

1 pkg white almond bark
1 pkg chocolate almond bark
1 drop peppermint essential oil
4-8 crushed candy canes or 10-15 peppermints

Cover a cookie sheet with wax or parchment paper. In a double boiler, heat chocolate bark until completely melted. Add peppermint essential oil and stir well. Carefully pour onto prepared cookie sheet and smooth out with a spatula. Transfer cookie sheet to freezer while you prepare the top layer. Wipe out the top of the double boiler and add the white bark, heating until completely melted. While heating, add the candy canes to a Ziploc bag and crush with a rolling pin. Remove the chocolate layer from the freezer and carefully smooth the white bark on to the chocolate. Top with crushed peppermints or candy canes and return cookie sheet to the freezer until set, about 10 minutes.

Cinnamon Hot Chocolate

4 cups chocolate milk
¼ cup chocolate, chopped
2 teaspoons vanilla
1 drop cinnamon essential oil
2 teaspoons chocolate, shaved
Cinnamon sticks for garnish

In a medium-sized saucepan, heat milk, chocolate and vanilla over low heat. Stir constantly until chocolate is melted. Heat to a low boil, stirring constantly. Reduce heat and simmer 5 minutes stirring frequently. Remove from heat, stir in essential oil, and garnish with a sprinkle of chocolate shavings and a cinnamon stick. Enjoy!

Intimacy

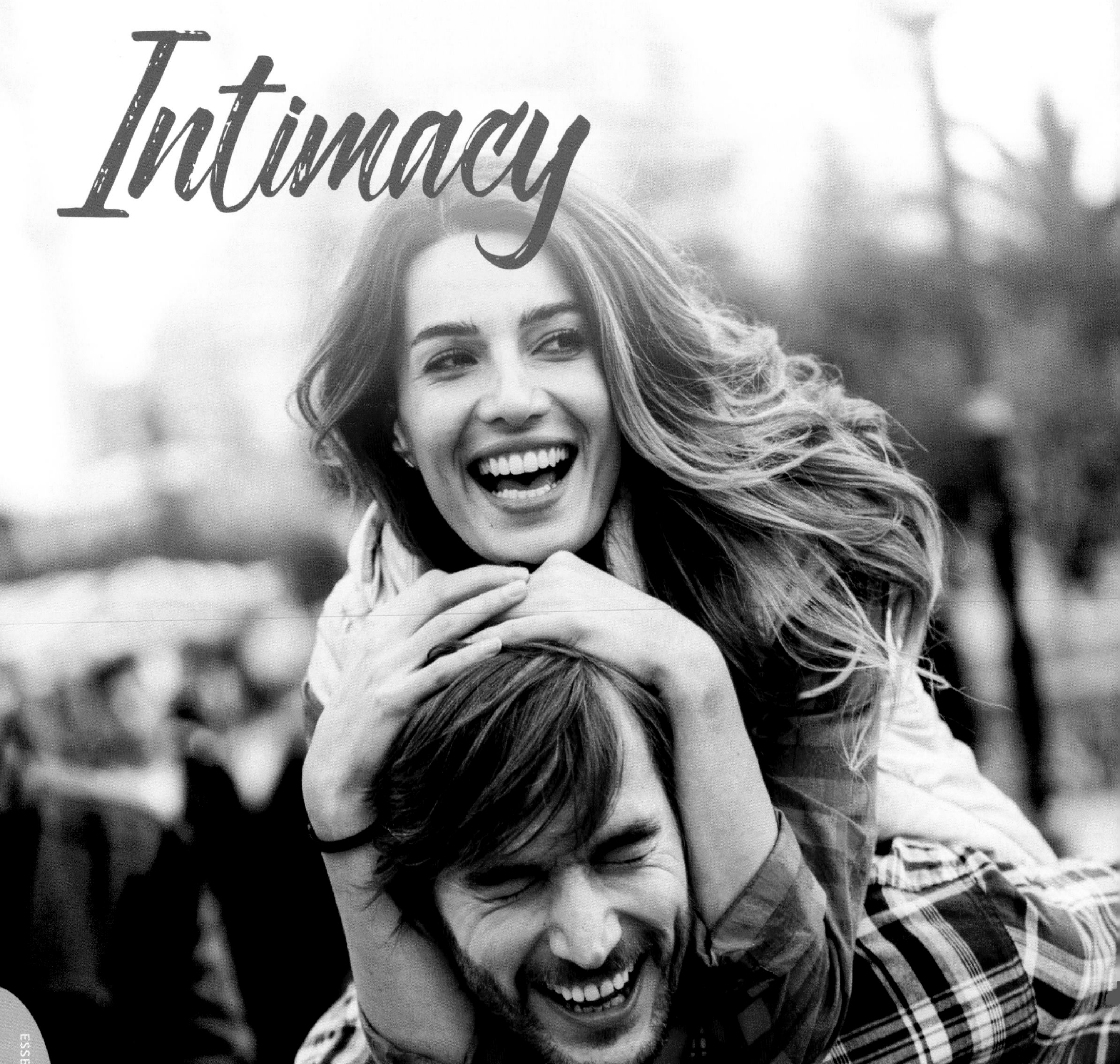

Sheet Spritzer

10 drops sandalwood essential oil
6 drops ylang ylang essential oil
14 drops bergamot essential oil
3 oz distilled water
4 oz glass spray bottle

Add essential oils to a spray bottle and fill with water. Spray lightly on sheets for a romantic evening.

Sexy AromaTouch®

2 drops ylang ylang essential oil
1 drop black pepper essential oil
1 drop ginger essential oil
1 drop wild orange essential oil

Add to 2 tablespoons lotion or massage oil. Massage onto legs, arms and body.

Aphrodisiac Blend For Diffusing

1 drop Siberian fir essential oil
1 drop cinnamon essential oil
1 drop patchouli essential oil
1 drop rosemary essential oil
1 drop sandalwood essential oil
1 drop ylang ylang essential oil

Drop these essential oils into a diffuser and fill the air with excitement.

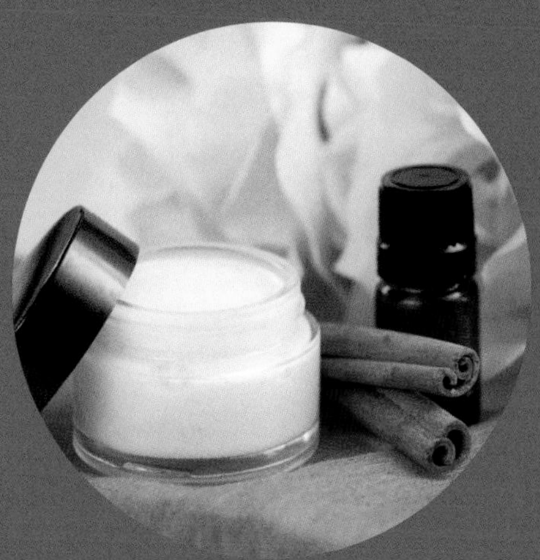

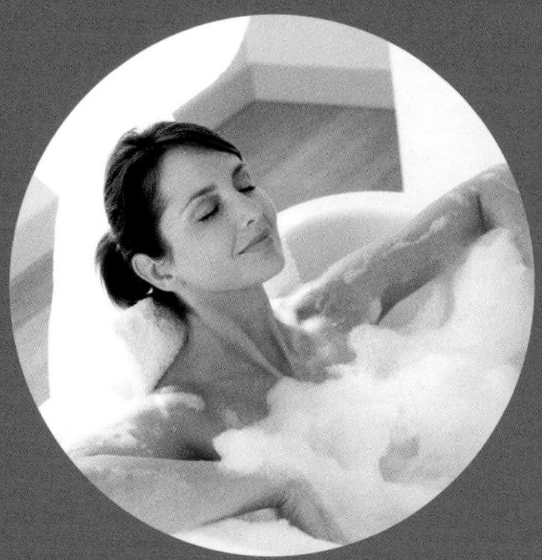

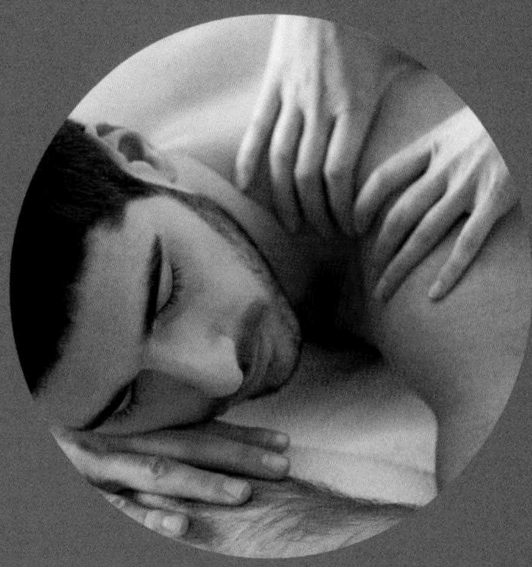

Exotic Cinnamon Love Balm

2 ½ tablespoons carrier oil
1 tablespoon cocoa butter
1 ½ teaspoons vegetable glycerin
1 teaspoons beeswax
6 drops cinnamon essential oil

Warm all ingredients, except essential oil, over low heat until the cocoa butter and beeswax are melted. Remove from heat and add the essential oil. Beat the mixture for a few minutes until it begins to thicken and becomes opaque. Pour or spoon into a storage container. Cool for fifteen minutes before capping. Let mixture sit for four hours before use as a kissing or massage balm.

Ecstasy Bubble Bath

1 ½ cups liquid castile soap
2 tablespoons vegetable glycerin
½ tablespoon white sugar
30 drops cedarwood essential oil
20 drops clary sage essential oil
10 drops ylang ylang essential oil
6 drops patchouli essential oil

Stir together ingredients in a large glass or ceramic bowl until the sugar has dissolved. Pour into bottle, shake, and let sit for 24 hours before using. To use, pour about ¼ cup of bubble bath under hot running water.

Steamy After-Bath Rub

30 drops bergamot essential oil
10 drops sandalwood essential oil
5 drops juniper berry essential oil
4 drops ginger essential oil
4 drops ylang ylang essential oil
2 drops jasmine or lavender essential oil
4 ounces coconut oil

Combine ingredients and massage on skin. Combine the deep, intoxicating effects of essential oils with sensual touch and massage to arouse intense desire.

Love Potion Diffuser Blend

4 drops jasmine
4 drops geranium

did you know?

- Essential oils have been used throughout history to increase sensuality and passion by helping provide a lovely ambience, relieve emotional exhaustion, and even increase libido.
- Essential oils, used for this purpose, are typically used topically and aromatically. Different oils appeal to different people; it's all about the journey of discovery to find out which oils work best for you and your partner.

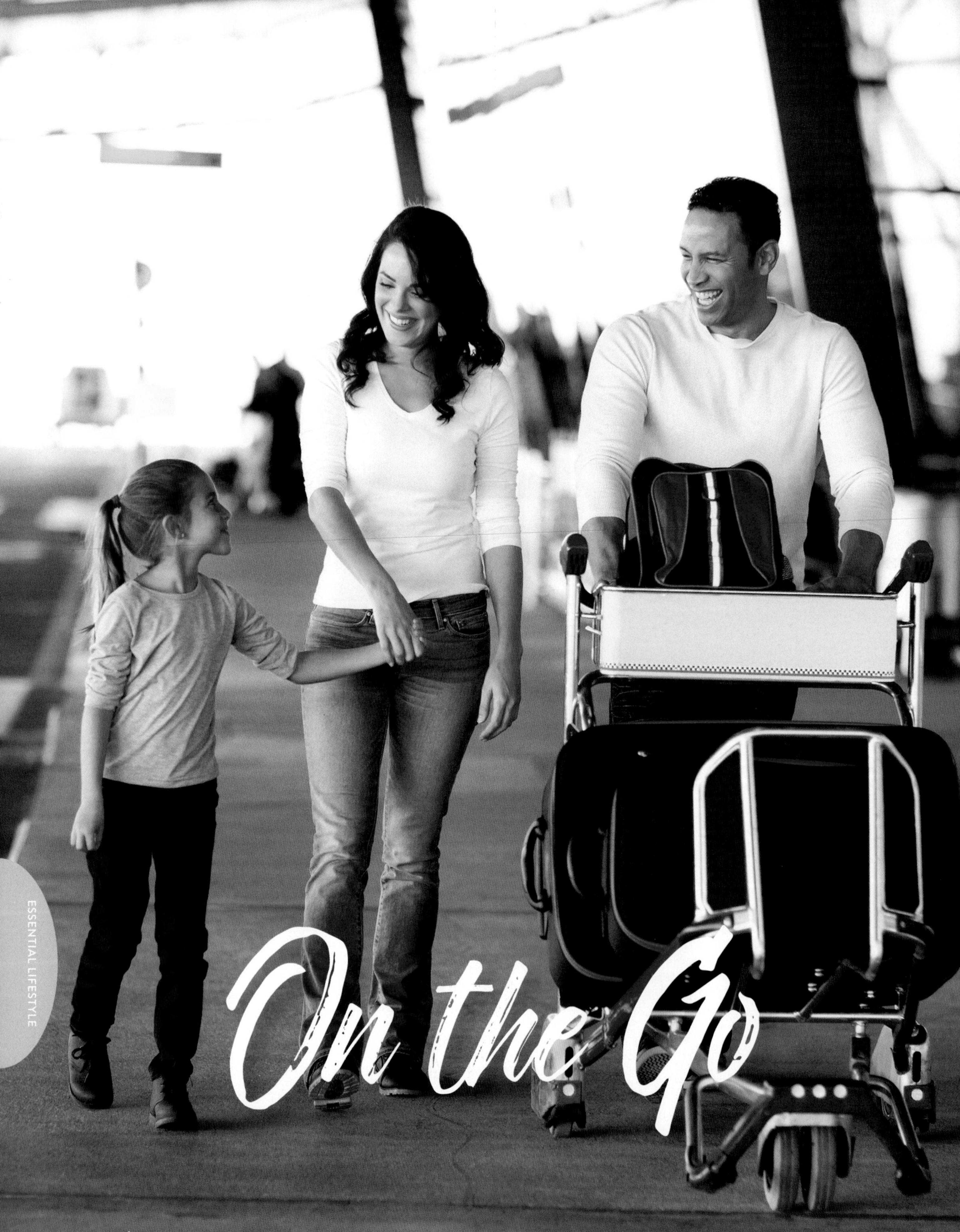

On the Go

Hand Sanitizer

5 tablespoons aloe vera gel
4 tablespoons water
½ teaspoon vitamin E oil
10 drops On Guard® essential oil
5 drops wild orange essential oil

Combine all ingredients in a squeezable container. Shake well and you are ready to clean hands anywhere without stripping off your body's natural protection barrier.

Car Air Freshener

Wool felt
Twine
10 drops of your favorite essential oils

Create non-toxic hanging car air fresheners in any shape, color, and scent you desire. Cut a simple 4" shape from wool felt and drop the oil onto the felt.
Using a small hole punch, punch a hole into the top of your shape, thread twine through it, and knot. Hang on the rear view mirror.

Bedbugs Be Gone Spray

On your travels, bring a small spray bottle filled with 10 drops of Siberian fir or peppermint essential oil mixed with water. Spray on bedding and sheets before using to deter bedbugs. Spray suitcases too, so they can't stow away home with you.

Eye Glasses Cleaner

1 cup white vinegar
¼ cup water
5 drops lemon essential oil

Mix ingredients into a small spray bottle, shake, and spray directly onto glass. Wipe with a scratch-free cloth.

Jet Lag Help

Simply add 8 drops of lavender and 8 drops of rosemary essential oils to your tub water. Bathe and enjoy. Follow with a quick cold shower to help you feel refreshed and alive in no time.

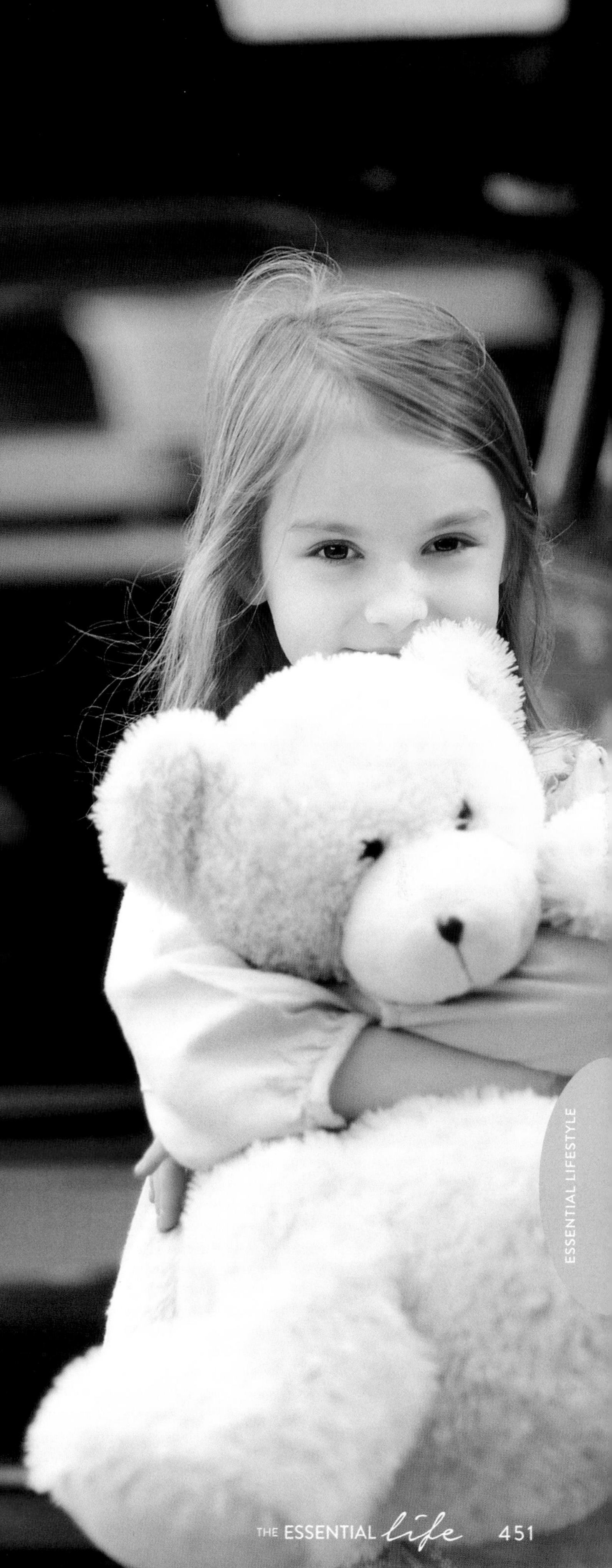

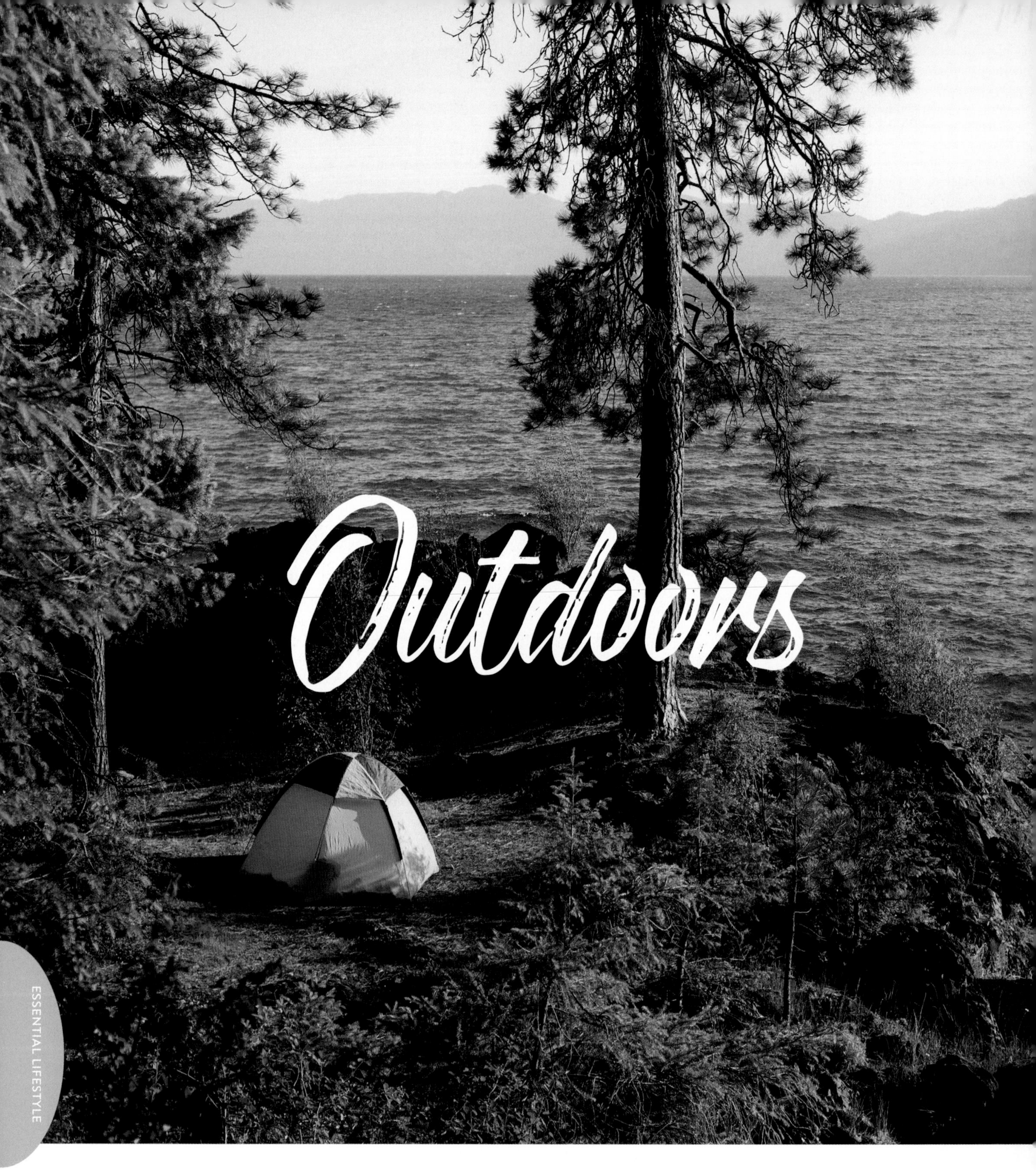

did you know?

- Out of 2,000 sunscreens reviewed, more than 75% were found to contain toxic chemicals.
- Common side effects for insect repellents include skin reactions, allergic rashes, and eye irritation.
- Many topical medicated creams for insect-bite itching and irritation have side effects causing redness, irritation, and swelling.

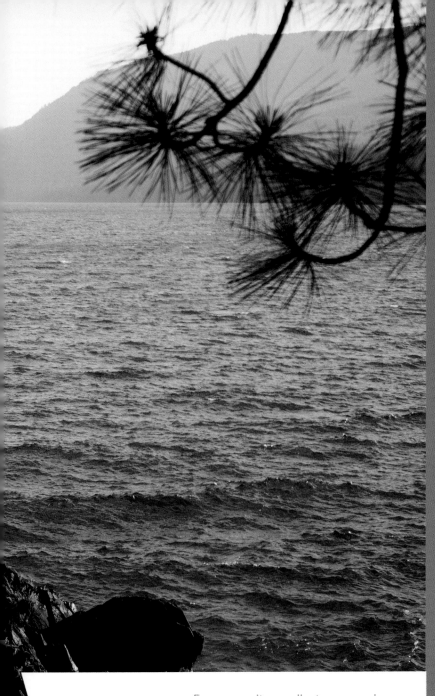

Sunburn Spray

1 cup aloe vera juice
¼ cup carrier oil
1 teaspoon vitamin E oil
8 drops lavender essential oil
8 drops tea tree essential oil
8 drops Roman chamomile essential oil

Combine ingredients in a 16-ounce glass spray bottle. Shake well and spray onto sunburned skin. Repeat as needed.

Bug Repellent

4 oz glass spray bottle
¼ cup witch hazel
10 drops peppermint essential oil
6 drops eucalyptus essential oil
6 drops melaleuca (tea tree) essential oil
5 drops cedarwood essential oil

Using a 4 oz. glass spray bottle, remove the top and secure the mini stainless steel funnel to its opening. Pour ¼ cup of witch hazel into the bottle. Add essential oils

.

Sunscreen

8 oz clear oval bottle
2 tablespoons shea butter
⅓ cup beeswax
2 tablespoons zinc oxide
½ cup olive oil
½ cup carrier oil
1 tablespoon raspberry seed oil
1 teaspoon vitamin E oil
10 drops helichrysum essential oil
5 drops myrrh essential oil
5 drops frankincense essential oil

Heat shea butter and beeswax on medium/low until melted. Mix in zinc oxide. Take off heat and add the remainder of the oils. Let cool and then pour mixture into bottle.

Cooling Spray

2 oz glass spray bottle
1 mini stainless steel funnel
1 oz water
1 oz witch hazel
4 drops peppermint essential oil
4 drops lavender essential oil

In a glass spray bottle, remove the top and secure the mini stainless steel funnel to its opening. Pour water and witch hazel into the bottle. Add peppermint and lavender essential oils. Remove the funnel and reattach the top. Shake well. Spray directly to your face to use as a cooling mist.

tips

- For a mosquito repellent, spray or drop and rub in TerraShield® essential oil.
- To relieve the discomfort of a poison ivy rash, apply lavender and Roman chamomile essential oils.
- For cooling or heat stroke apply peppermint essential oil to the back of your neck or add 10 drops of lavender essential oil to a cool washcloth. Apply to forehead or over the neck.

Bug Off

Combine 16 drops patchouli essential oil, 10 drops cedarwood essential oil, 4 drops lemon eucalyptus essential oil. Add to 2 oz witch hazel in glass spray bottle. Cover exposed areas and re-apply every 4-6 hours.

Personal Care

Texturizing Hair Spray

4 oz glass spray bottle
½ cup warm water
½ tablespoon sea salt
½-1 teaspoon carrier oil
4-5 drops lavender essential oil

Add all ingredients to bottle and shake well before each use. To use, spray all over damp hair. This will help add more texture to your dried and styled hair.

Sun-kissed Goddess Skin Bronzer

2 oz heavy wall jar
1 tablespoon cinnamon powder
1 teaspoon cocoa powder
1 teaspoon nutmeg powder
2 teaspoon arrowroot powder (or cornstarch)
15 drops lavender or rosemary essential oils
*If you prefer a loose powder, leave out the essential oils

Adjust the levels of ingredients to your shade and mix well in a small bowl, and break up any clumps until it's smooth. Place the powder in a clean, empty compact and pack it in firmly.

did you know?

- Most deodorants and antiperspirants contain ingredients linked to breast cancer and Alzheimer's disease.
- Teeth whitening products can cause sensitivity and lead to gum recession and irritation. Irritation of the oral mucous membranes, a burning feeling in the mouth, and potential to increase the risk of pharyngeal and oral cancers are common side effects from mouthwash use.
- Incorporate all-natural essential oils into your personal care regimen to bypass negative side effects and harmful chemicals.
- For easy eye and makeup remover use carrier oil.
- For a quick breath freshener, pop a peppermint essential oil beadlet.
- To pull toxins from the body and improve overall health, try oil pulling. Oil pulling has been said to help with overall oral health while pulling unwanted toxins out of the body. Apply 1-2 teaspoons carrier oil into mouth. Add desired essential oils and swish around for fifteen to twenty minutes, then spit out (in the trash, not down a drain). Rinse with warm water and brush teeth well.

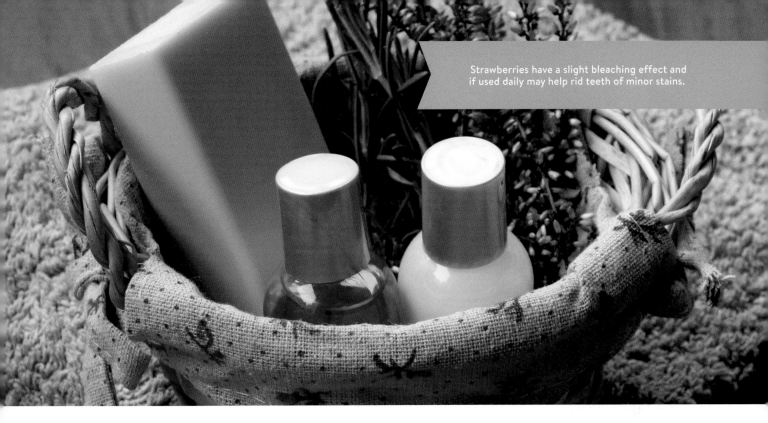

Strawberries have a slight bleaching effect and if used daily may help rid teeth of minor stains.

Floral Hair Repair

1 2 oz glass spray bottle
1 dropper
1 carrier oil
22 drops ylang ylang essential oil
13 drops rosemary essential oil
24 drops lavender essential oil

Using a 2 oz. glass spray bottle, remove the top. Pour carrier oil into the bottle until it is ¾ filled. Add ylang ylang, rosemary and lavender to the bottle. Secure the top, and shake well. Spray 2-3 times (whether on wet hair or on dry hair) before styling and love your essential oil infused soft, vibrant hair!

Dry Shampoo

8 tablespoons arrowroot
½ tablespoon cocoa powder (adjust according to hair color)
5 drops tea tree essential oil
3.5 oz plastic shaker bottle

Add powerders to bowl and mix. Add oils and mix well. Pour into shaker container. Sprinkle a light dusting of powder on your hair and comb it in through to your roots. Keep combing until you can't see the powder anymore.

Foot Soak

Combine 10 drops lemon eucalyptus essential oil, 10 drops tea tree (melaleuca) essential oil and 4 drops lavender essential oil with 2 oz of carrier oil. Stir in 2 oz pink Himalayan salt. Use spoon, scoop out 1 tablespoon in tub of warm water. Disperse well before soaking feet for 15 minutes.

Lovely Moisturizing Shampoo

8 oz clear oval bottle
½ cup liquid castile soap
¼ cup canned coconut milk
½ tablespoon aloe vera gel
½ teaspoon carrier oil
½ teaspoon magnesium gel
10 drops vitamin E oil
10 drops argan oil
10 drops lavender essential oil
10 drops tea tree essential oil
5 drops lemon essential oil

Blend ingredients together and store in 8 oz bottle.

Booty Booster Skin Firming Cream

8 oz clear oval bottle
8 oz carrier oil
15 ml copaiba essential oil
30 drops clove essential oil

Add the carrier oil to the 8 oz oval bottle. Add the entire bottle of copaiba and add clove essential oils. Make sure the mixture is mixed well and let it sit overnight. Apply twice a day to help firm your skin and help reduce cellulite.

Shampoo

Add 1 drop lemon eucalyptus essential oil + 2 drops rosemary essential oil to approximately 1 teaspoon shampoo, massage into scalp. Rinse well before conditioning.

Pets

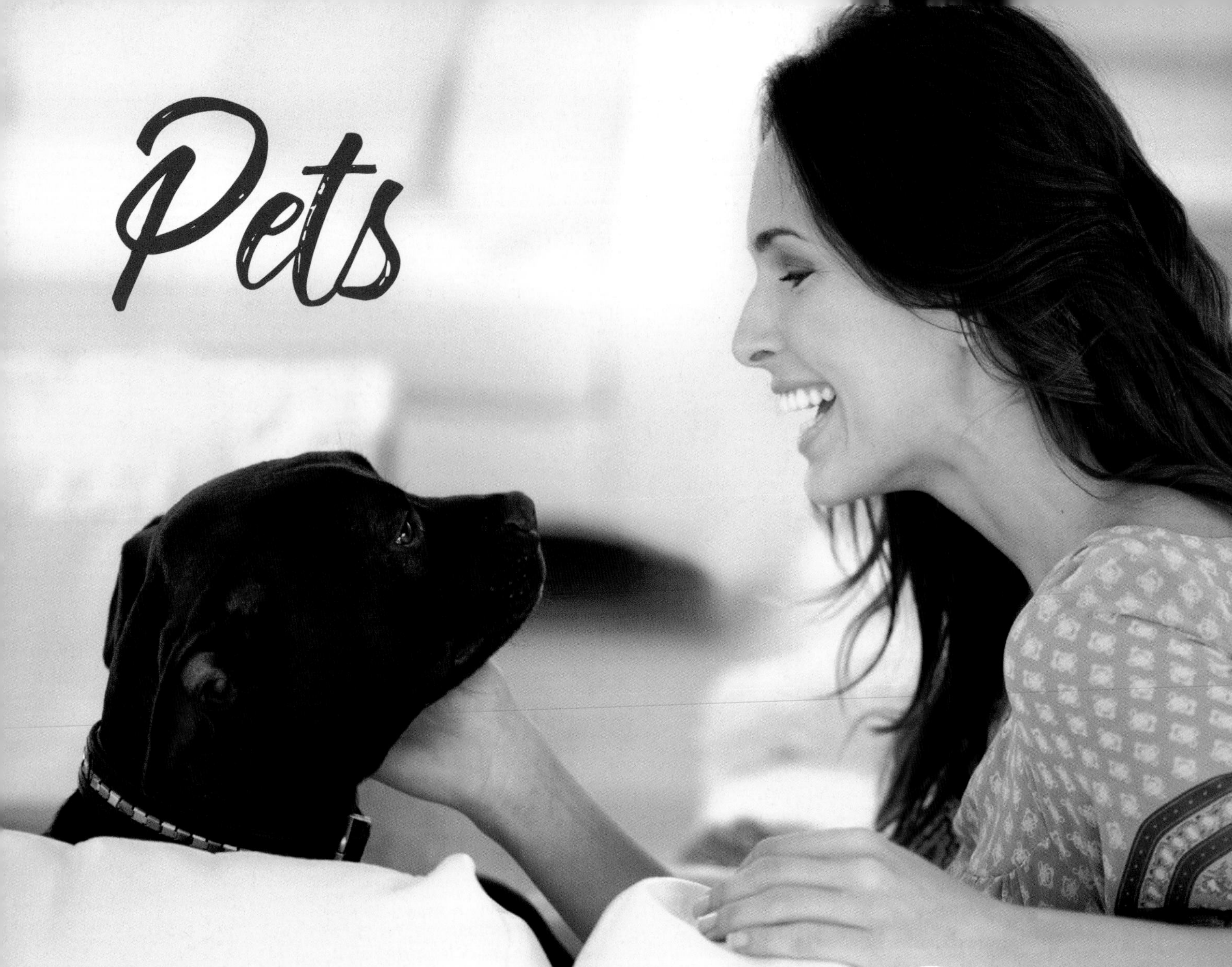

Pet Shampoo

1 cup water
1 tablespoon castile soap
¼ teaspoon vitamin E
3 drops peppermint essential oil
2 drops Roman chamomile essential oil
2 drops Purify essential oil
1 drop cedarwood essential oil

Place all ingredients in a glass jar and mix well. Apply a quarter-size amount to pet and scrub vigorously. Use more on a large pet, if needed. Shampoo will be a bit watery, but your pet will be clean and smell great for days.

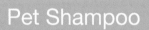

did you know?

- Common anti-flea solutions for dogs can cause adverse reactions such as skin irritation, hair loss, vomiting, diarrhea, tremors, and seizure.
- Medication commonly used to treat painful arthritis in cats and dogs often causes serious damage to the stomach, liver, and kidneys.
- Most people don't realize that pure essential oils can provide all-natural solutions for animals as well as humans.

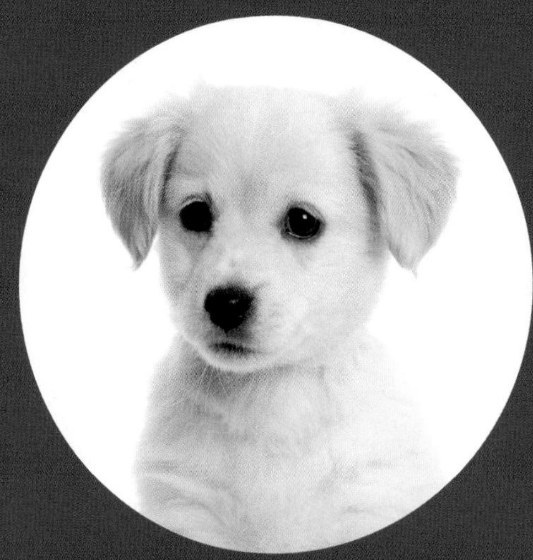

Flea Collar Repellent

¼ teaspoon rubbing alcohol
4 garlic oil capsules
1 drop cedarwood essential oil
1 drop lavender essential oil
1 drop lemon essential oil
1 drop thyme essential oil

Mix ingredients in a medium bowl. Soak a pet collar in the mixture for 25 to 30 minutes. Lay out to dry; place on animal's neck. Repeat once or twice a month.

Doggie Anxiety Spray

4 oz glass spray bottle
20 drops lavender essential oil
10 drops cedarwood essential oil
5 drops vetiver essential oil
5 drops frankincense essential oil
Distilled water

Add the essential oils to the bottle and fill the remaining space with distilled water. Shake well before each use.

Doggie Paw Balm

8 oz jar
2 tablespoons shea butter
2 tablespoons coconut oil
1 teaspoon jojoba oil
2 tablespoons of beeswax
1-2 drops lavender essential oil
1-2 drops frankincense essential oil
1-2 drops peppermint essential oil

Heat up a pot of water. Set a glass bowl in the pot and melt the shea butter, coconut oil, beeswax and jojoba together in the glass bowl. Lift the glass bowl out of the pot and let it cool enough to touch. Add essential oils to the mixture and pour into the jar.

No-Odor Kitty Litter

25 drops Purify essential oil
4 cups baking soda

Combine in a large bowl. Sprinkle 2 tablespoons onto kitty litter when cleaning box daily.

Cat Scratch Deterrent

10 drops eucalyptus essential oil
10 drops lemon essential oil
1 cup water

Fill an empty spray bottle with oils. Add water shake well, and spray on areas you do not want your cat to scratch.

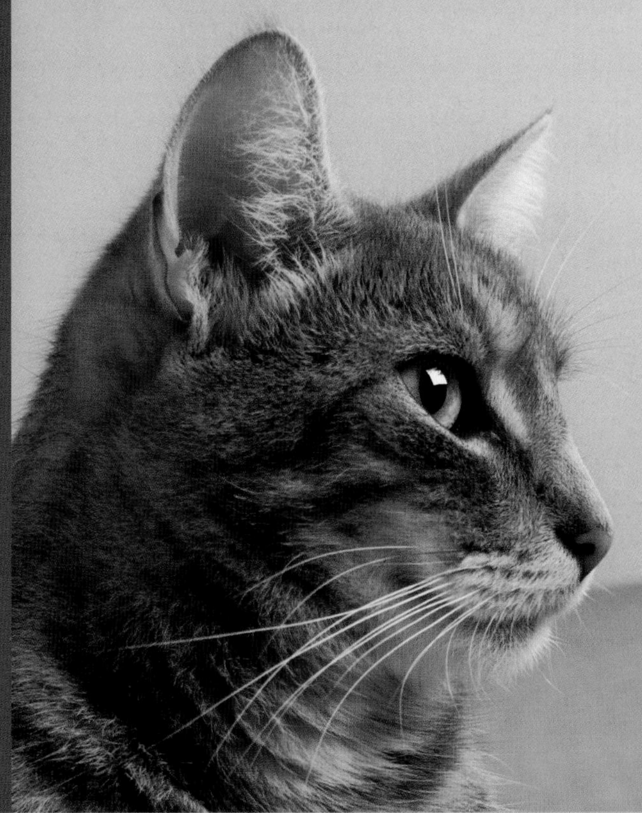

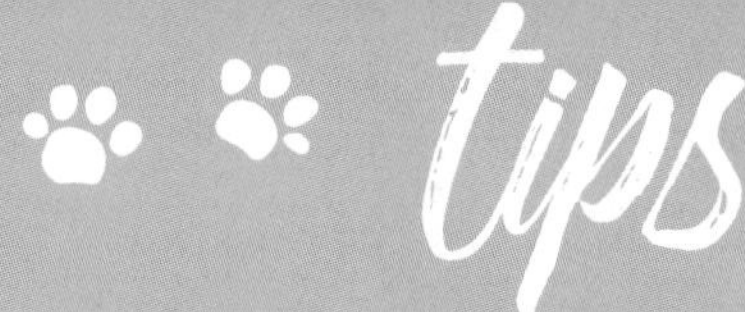

- Animals are smaller, so diluting essential oils is important.
- Avoid using melaleuca for cats.
- Animals prefer certain aromas just as humans do—you can experiment with various oils to see how your pet responds to the aroma and the benefit of the oil.
- For joint pain relief, rub frankincense and Deep Blue® essential oils directly on joints.
- To help calm and relax a stressed pet, apply 2 to 3 drops of lavender essential oil to ears and paws.

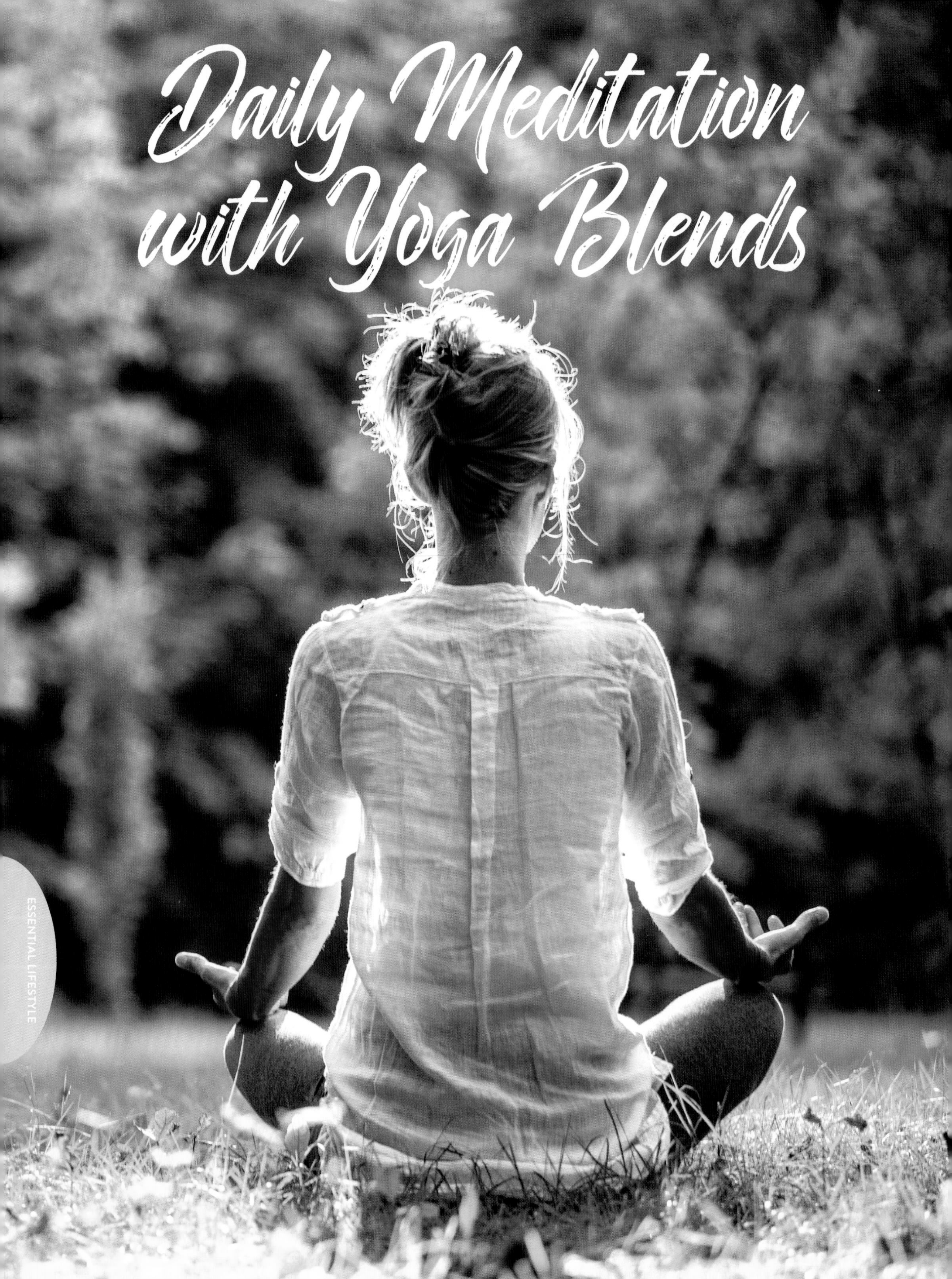
Daily Meditation
with Yoga Blends
ESSENTIAL LIFESTYLE

To be used by individuals, in a one-on-one setting, or group session to create an environment that promotes healthy emotional processing and provides a process by which to overcome emotional paralysis.

Step One: Align®

Apply Align® to the crown, base of spine, and bottoms of feet as you begin the process of bringing self into a state of focus, alignment, and singlemindedness. Visualize the intention for your meditation. Invite yourself to feel and experience what it is you envision.

Step Two: Anchor®

Once connection has been established with the intention for your meditation:

Apply the Anchor®. Get in touch with what is being felt with and within the body, identifying what may be keeping you from moving forward in life in some way. Ask yourself: *If I trust that all emotions have a higher or positive purpose and allow myself to accept and surrender to what I am feeling, then what is the higher intention for my troubled feelings? How are they alerting me to misalignment and inviting me to get out of my head and move into my heart? Continue asking until you identify the purpose of your feelings. Allow your awareness to anchor you, no longer fearful or avoiding how you feel but creating a space of safety that honors self.*

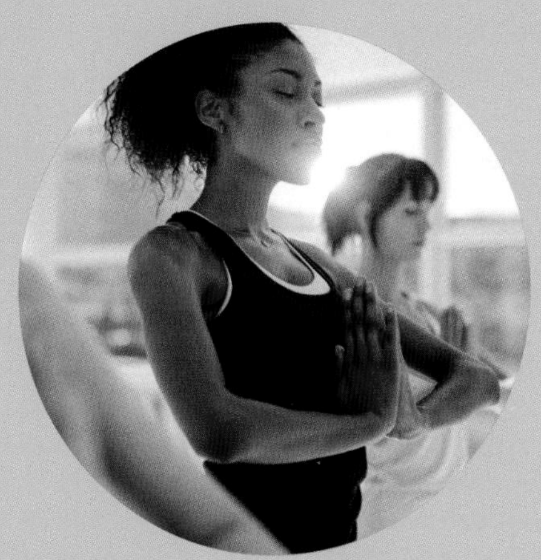

Step Three: Arise®

Once the higher intentions is identified:

Apply the Arise® to support your discoveries as you seek to understand the valuable partnership with the emotions you are feeling. Through acceptance, you are allow your emotions to be part of your life and in moving you forward. Be with your emotions and their higher intentions. Consciously find where within you your power resides so it can be accessed repeatedly.

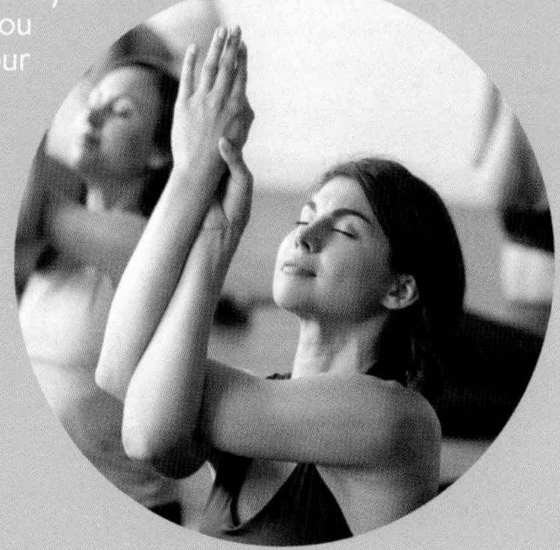

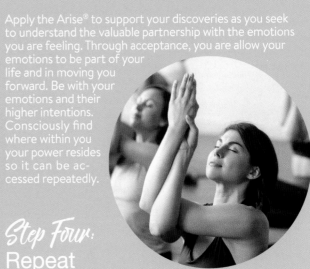

Step Four: Repeat

Once you have connected with your higher intention:

Go back to the Arise® blend multiple times throughout the day to remind you of your intention. If you find yourself slipping back into old thinking, re-align yourself with Align® or re-anchor with the Anchor®.

By choosing to accept how you feel, the very feelings most people avoid become a catalyst for moving you forward in life. With acknowledgement and focus of the higher meaning, the intention for your day is no longer cluttered, obscured, or shrouded by unnecessary confusion, overwhelm, or doublemindedness that typically arises when one is placed into a state of fight or flight when ruled by unacknowledged or addressed emotions.

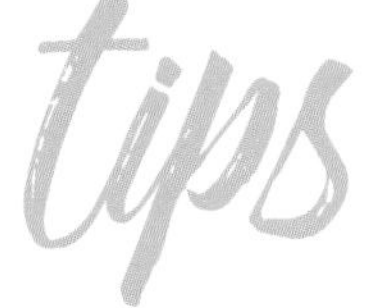

Anytime during the day when unpleasant feelings arise:

- Bring self back into alignment and apply the Align®.
- Seek to discover the purpose of your discontent and apply the Anchor®.
- Choose to move forward and apply the Arise®.

SECTION 6

SUPPLEMENTAL

Turn to these resources to explore research used, deepen understanding of ailments, and find oil properties.

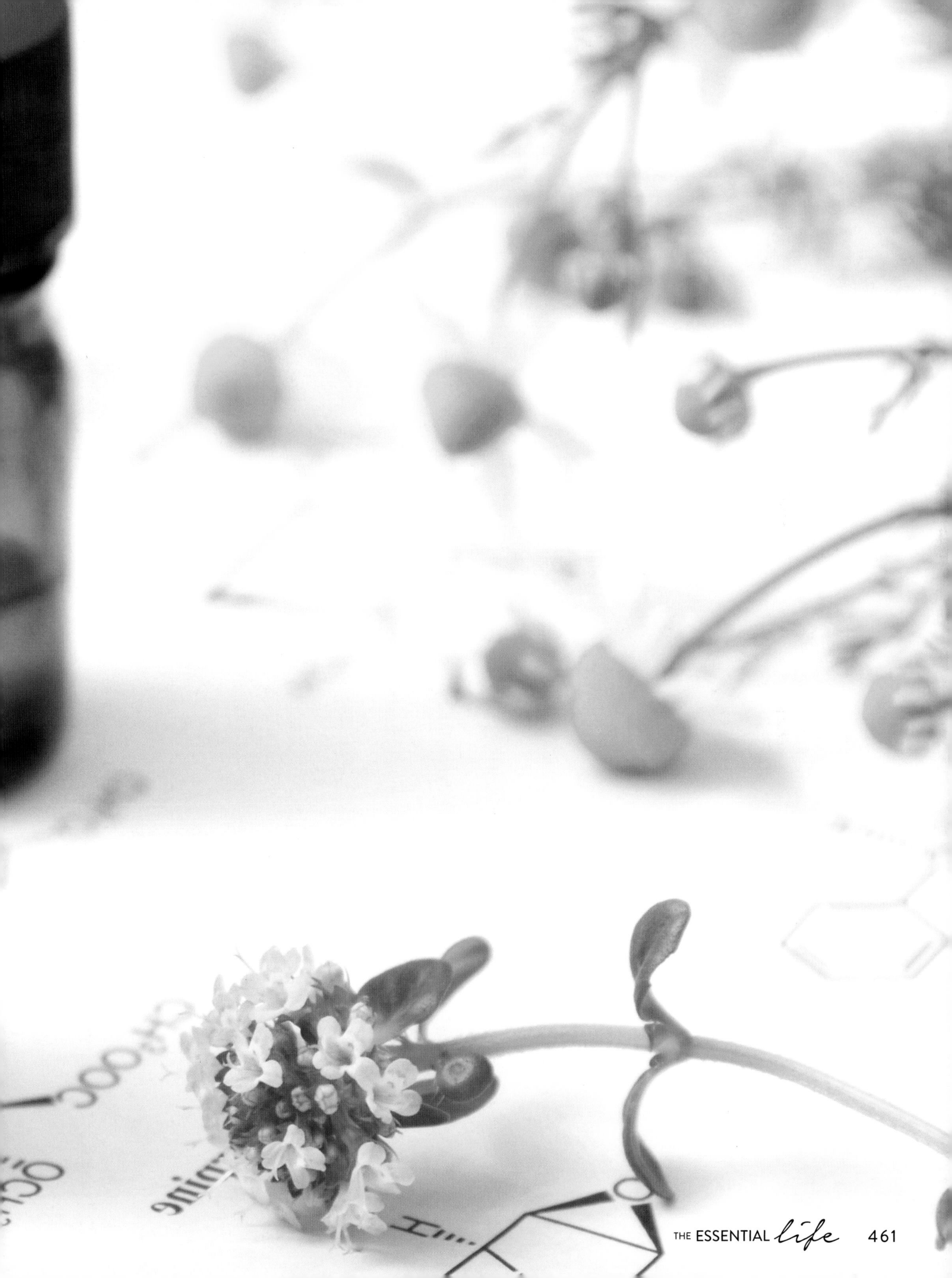

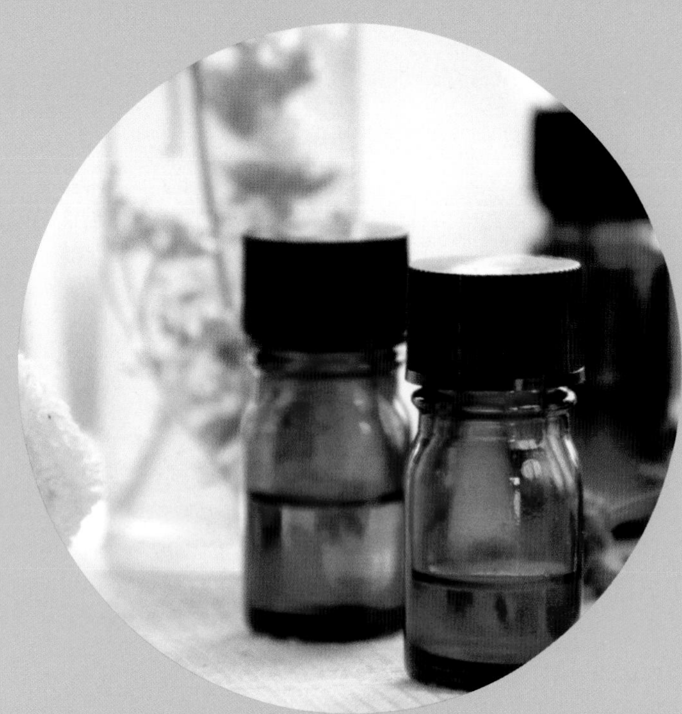

Be a Power User

The Essential Life supports you in focusing on core elements of wellness where YOU hold the power to create your personal health reality. This section teaches how to become a confident essential oil Power User with the healing tools needed to elevate your essential life.

Live an Essential Lifestyle

A first step to balanced living is considering and implementing the components that contribute to wellness, or when neglected, lack of wellness. The pages in this section are designed to assist you in successfully focusing on each of these key areas.

ESSENTIAL LIFESTYLE

BODY FUEL

What you put into your body becomes your body. If you want a high-energy, vibrant, high-functioning body, then put high-energy, vibrant, high-functioning food & fuel into your body! **Add vitality supplements and energizing oils to a great diet.**

ACTIVITY

Your body was built to move. As you enjoy some kind of active moment every day, your body systems have good reason to stay active and healthy. **Enhance activity with oils for muscle, joint, and respiratory support**

REST

Meaningful rest is necessary for every body system to reset and regenerate. Commit daily to giving yourself adequate time to recover through quality sleep and personal care. **Use oils that your body responds to for optimal relaxation and sleep.**

STRESS MANAGEMENT

Emotional and physical stressors are at the root of all illness and disease. Intentionally discover the best tools to reduce stress in your life. **Pause briefly throughout each day to support emotional balance with your oils.**

TOXIC REDUCTION

Toxicity is found in our water, air, household cleaners and chemicals, and many more things we put into our bodies. Minimize toxicity and create a clean environment inside your body. **Use oils to safely clean your home and detox your body.**

RESTORATIVE SELF-CARE

Knowing how to use safe, effective natural remedies is empowering. It allows you to restore health, prevent unwanted issues, and be prepared for the unexpected. **Discover your solutions and how to put them to work for you!**

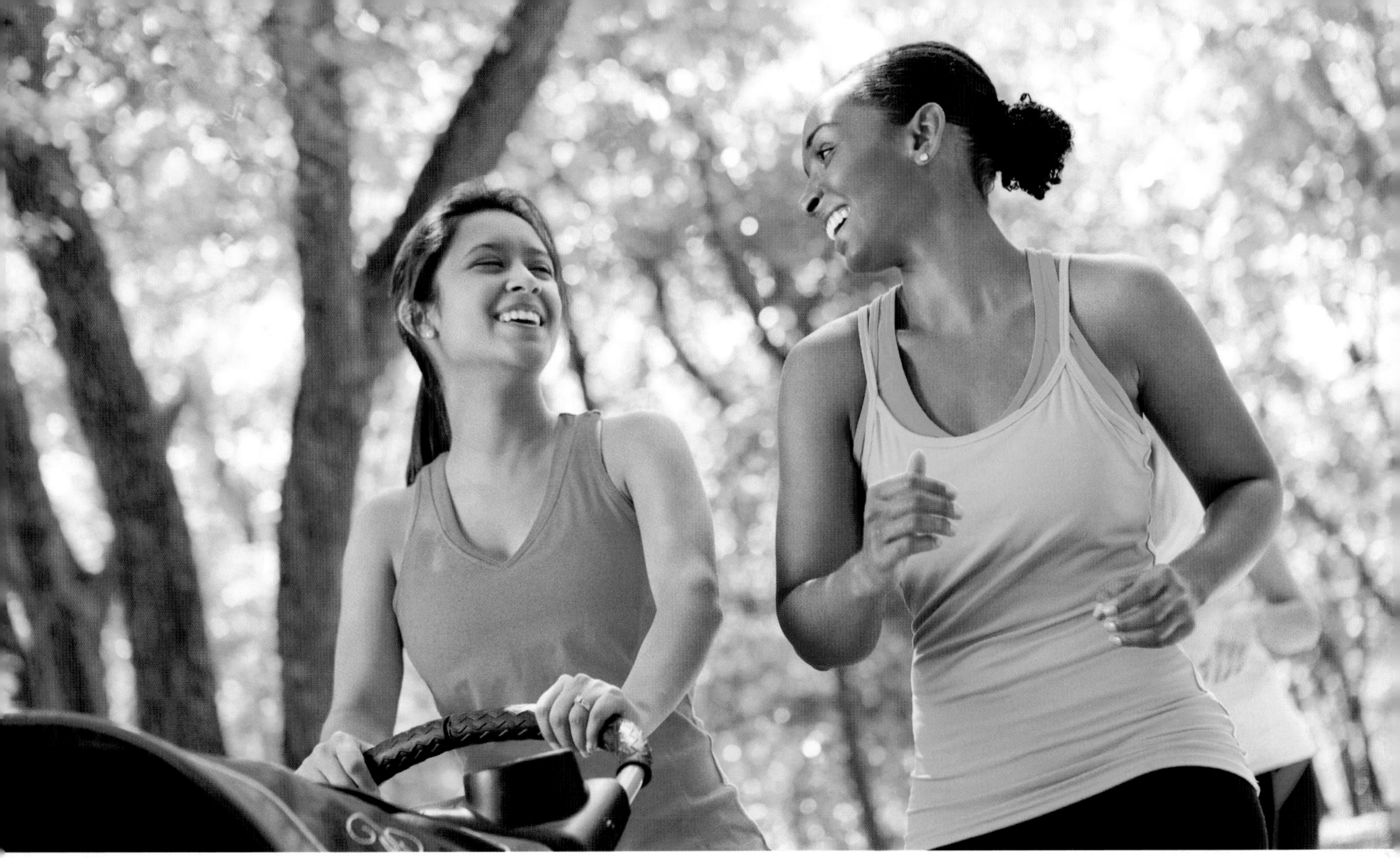

Good Health Loves Preparation

Be prepared for anything by having your essential oils and other remedies handy. Try a few of these:

- **Around the House** Keep frequently used oils handy by your bedside, in the bathroom, the kitchen, and main family living space. You'll use them more often and see better results, and your family will join in if they're easily accessible.
- **Purse or Keychain** Have a small bag of oils you need for mood support, digestive support, and immune protection when you're out and about. If you don't carry a purse or bag, get a keychain that holds small vials (5/8 dram) of your favorite oils.
- **Car** Keep oils for focus and stress management in your car to turn driving time into useful rejuvenation time.
- **Diaper Bag or Stroller** Kids love to do the unexpected, which is why you'll always be glad to have oils ready for bumps and bruises, skin irritations, and temper tantrums wherever you go.

tip Consistency makes magic. While oils are fast-acting, consistency breeds the best long-term results.

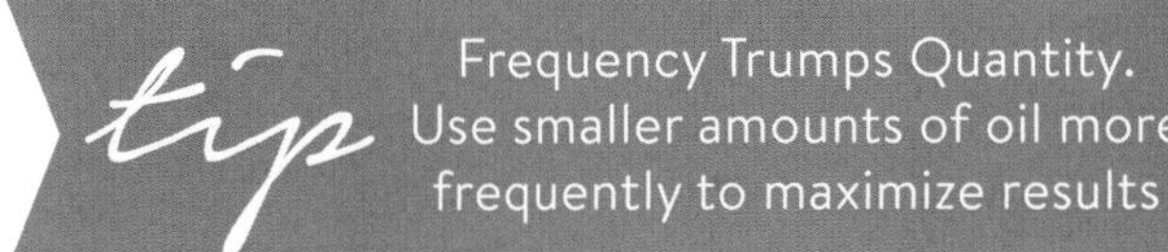

tip
Frequency Trumps Quantity.
Use smaller amounts of oil more
frequently to maximize results

Find Brilliant Answers

Learning to how to fully take ownership of your personal health and wellness can be stressful. Where do you turn to find resources, which are both trustworthy and always up-to-date?

The Essential Life team is dedicated to helping you eliminate the stress of learning to take charge of your health and wellness by providing additional resources at: www.EssentialLife.com

Go to EssentialLife.com to:

- **Buy** *The Essential Life, The Essential Basics, The Essential Quick Reference.*
- **Download** the *Essential Life* App to look up remedies on the go and stay in sync with the community as they share their remedies and insights.

Explore Different Usage Methods

- **Aromatic.** Keep a diffuser in high-traffic areas in the home and in sleeping areas. Diffusers are a great way to let everyone around enjoy the benefits of the oils.
- **Topical.** Have a carrier oil like fractionated coconut oil on hand for use on sensitive skin, and to use as a remedy if someone experiences sensitivity after an oil has been applied. Try recipes for skin creams and lotions with your oils.
- **Internal.** Keep veggie capsules near your oils for easy internal use. Try putting some in a small plastic baggie so you can have them ready on the go. Remember to only use oils internally if they are verified pure and therapeutic.

tip Layering vs. Blending: While blending oils is a valuable art, you may have success with layering. Apply one oil topically, wait several seconds, and then apply the next one, etc.

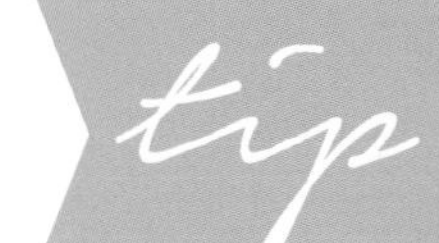

tip Focus your efforts. You'll achieve greater results as you concentrate your efforts on a few key wellness goals.

Supercharge Your Oils

While you can use oils a seemingly infinite number of ways, you'll also find methods that work best for you and your family. Try some of these tips to enhance the effectiveness of your oils:

- **Add heat** Use a hot compress to drive the oils in deeper when using topically.
- **Add frankincense** Frankincense enhances the therapeutic effects of many protocols, and brings powerful healing properties.
- **Massage** Massaging oils into the needed area stimulates tissues and increases absorption. It also provides benefit for the person giving and the person receiving the massage.
- **Combine oils that complement each other** Don't be afraid to try different oil combinations. You can find an ocean of essential oil recipes and protocols because nature complements itself in so many ways. Try different combinations, and enjoy the process of discovering what resonates with your body.

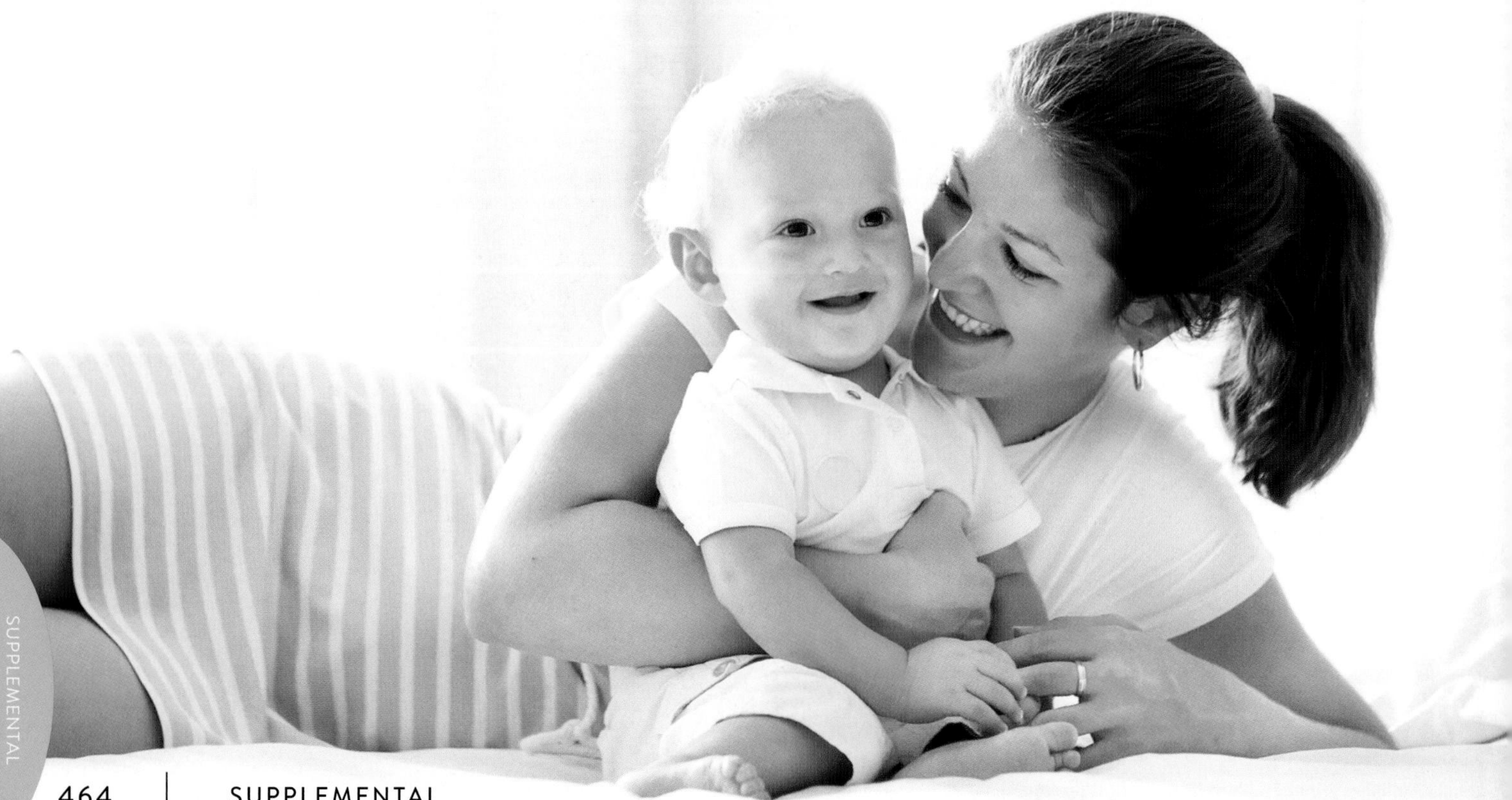

Oil Composition & Chemistry

Plants synthesize two types of oils: fixed oils and essential oils. Fixed oils consist of glycerol and fatty acids. Essential oils are a mix of volatile organic compounds that contribute to the fragrance and well being of the plant. Essential oils are made up of many compound constituents that serve several purposes for the plant:

- Protection and responses to parasites such a bacteria, viruses, fungi, and other pests
- Restoration from wounds and physical damage
- Protection from sun and other elements
- Communication through fragrance to insects or other plants of the same genus

Essential oils are volatile oils that have an intrinsic nature or essence of the plant. Essential oils are more soluble in lipophilic solvents than in water. They are complex mixtures of chemical compounds, and every biological effect displayed by an essential oil is due to the actions of one or more of its constituents.

Essential oils are secondary metabolites in plants. The oils are isolated from plants through a process called hydro-distillation: passing boiling water through the plant material and vaporizing the essential oil from the plant. As the steam rises and condenses, the water and essential oil separate and the oil product, the essential oil, is captured. The remaining water is aromatic and contains in much lower concentrations and in different ratios some of the constituents from the oil. This water is known as a hydrosol and is used and sold for its therapeutic benefits and its fragrance.

The chemical compounds in citrus essential oils come from the rind of the fruit. Most citrus essential oils are generally isolated by cold pressing rather than distillation. Citrus oils that are cold pressed also include relatively large, involatile molecules, including the phototoxic compounds. These compounds are not in distilled citrus oils.

Some fragrant oils such as rose or jasmine oil are at times extracted with organic solvents, which produces concretes, absolutes, or resinoids.

Essential oils typically contain dozens of constituents with related, but distinct, chemical structures. Each constituent has its own characteristic and has different effects when used. Even though an essential oil contains many different types of compounds, usually one or two compounds dominate their action. For example, alpha-Pinene is the main compound that is responsible for action of frankincense essential oil. Some constituents may comprise a small percentage of an oil but may play a significant role in its overall action. Because no two distillations are ever the same and because of many other variables such as elevation, harvest time, soil type, weather condition, etc., lists of compounds contained in an essential oil are usually stated as a range. For example, the compound alpha-Pinene may range from 41 percent to 80 percent of a frankincense essential oil (*Boswellia frereana*).

Because of their antimicrobial properties, essential oils are not generally subject to microbial contamination. Essential oils can be contaminated from unnatural constituents, distillation items, or adulterants. These include pesticides or herbicides, traces of solvent, and phthalates (plasticizing agents). Adulteration includes both intentional dilution and fabrication of an oil or parts of an essential oil. There are many ways and methods to test an essential oil for levels of purity. Testing by independent and properly equipped labs is critical to knowing of an oil's purity and complete profile. Adulteration could increase toxicity of an oil. Only essential oils that are tested and verified pure therapeutic grade should be used for therapeutic benefits.

It's a complex task to evaluate and unravel the chemistry of an essential oil. Many compounds in an essential oil are present in minute amounts. They may be hard to detect except through testing by laboratories with a large enough database to identify all of the constituents. Some of the modern methods and analyses that are used to determine the chemical profile of an essential oil include:

- Gas Chromatography (GC)
- Mass Spectrometry (MS)
- High Performance Liquid Chromatography (HPLC)
- Nuclear Magnetic Resonance Spectroscopy (NMR)
- Fourier Transform Infrared Spectroscopy (FTIS)
- Chiral GC Testing
- Isotope Carbon 14TPC/Microbial

The best testing involves a combination of several methods throughout the process from harvest to bottle.

Essential oils are made up of organic (carbon-based) compounds. The individual essential oil constituents contain atoms in addition to carbon(C), such as hydrogen(H) and oxygen(O). Learning the basics of essential oil chemical construction will help in understanding why different oils achieve different actions. For example, alpha-Pinene, a compound in frankincense essential oil, is written chemically as $C_{10}H_{16}$ This means the alpha-Pinene consists of ten carbon atoms and sixteen hydrogen atoms. The compound can also be shown as a diagram. The double line indicates a double bond in that part of the compound. Essential oil molecules are three-dimensional but represented in this diagram as two-dimensional.

[1] *Essential Oil Safety*, Robert Tisserand and Rodney Young, 2014, page 6.
[2] *Essential Oil Safety*, pg 7.
[3] *Essential Oil Safety*, pg 8.

Essential oil constituents are built on a framework of isoprene units. Isoprene units consist of carbon and hydrogen atoms; their chemical makeup consists of five carbon atoms and eight hydrogen atoms. Their chemical signature is C_5H_8. Most of the compounds in essential oils consist of two to four isoprene units. These units are referred to as terpenes or terpenoids. Terpenoids are terpenes that have functional groups added to them. These functional groups are made up of mostly hydrogen and oxygen and include alcohols, phenols, aldehydes, esters, and ethers. Terpenes do not have a functional group added to them; they are often referred to as hydrocarbons. The simplest and most common class of terpenes found in essential oils is the monoterpene (a double isoprene unit with ten carbon atoms). The next group of terpenes is the sesquiterpenes, and the basic structure is composed of fifteen carbon atoms or three isoprene units. They have a larger molecular size than the monoterpenes and therefore are less volatile.

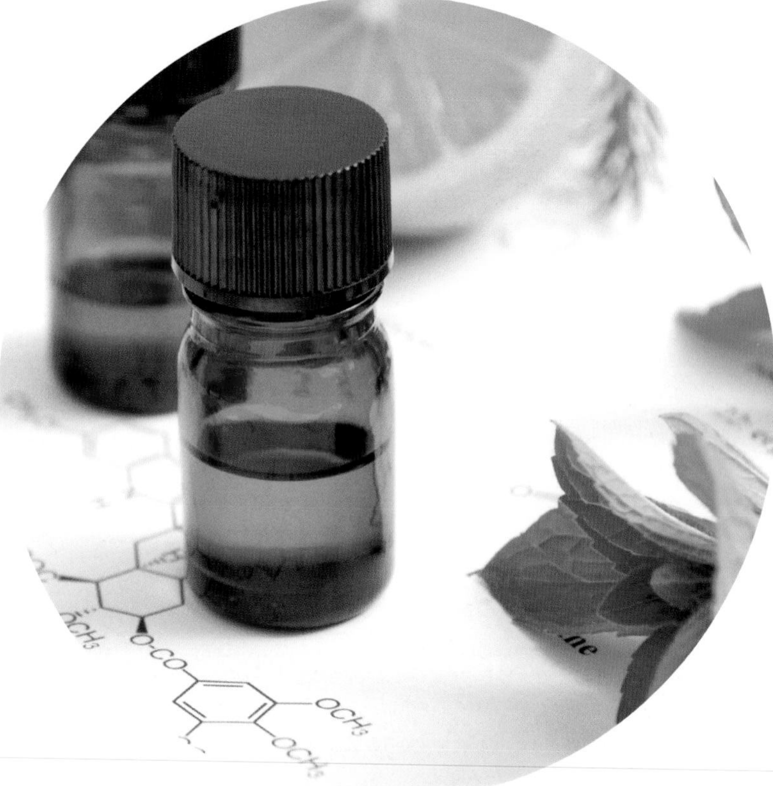

See the following table for the classes of terpenes and the number of carbon atoms in each.

Monoterpene	10 carbon atoms	Most common
Sesquiterpenes	15 carbon atoms	Larger size molecule and less volatile
Diterpenes	20 carbon atoms	Only in some essential oils
Triterpenes	30 carbon atoms	Can be present in absolutes
Tetraterpenes	40 carbon atoms	Not part of essential oils but found in cold-pressed citrus oils (beta-carotene is an example)

All of the compounds or constituents in essential oils belong to a group. These groups are defined by the number of carbon atoms they have and the type of functional group assigned to them. For example alpha-Pinene is part of the monoterpene hydrocarbon group. It has ten carbon atoms and does not have a functional group as part of its molecular makeup, which makes it a hydrocarbon. It is unique from the other compounds in the group because of the number hydrogen atoms and how the carbon and hydrogen atoms are bonded together. Another example is alpha-Santalol, a major compound in sandalwood essential oil. Alpha-Santalol chemically is $C_{15}H_{24}O$ It has an oxygen functional group and fifteen carbon atoms, so it is part of the sesquiterpene alcohol group.

The compounds and the compound groups have been researched and found to exhibit certain common therapeutic benefits. Once a compound is identified as part of an essential oil and once the group to which it belongs is identified, the possible action of the essential oil can be determined. Essential oils are made up of many compounds. Some compounds make up a larger percentage of an oil, while others may only offer a trace of the total essential oil. Though compounds that comprise larger parts of an oil definitely help guide an oil's benefit, the smaller amounts play a part in the oil's actions.

The following table lists common groups of compounds in essential oils, examples of compounds in that group, the known therapeutic benefits of that group, and some of the essential oils that contain compounds in that group.

CHEMICAL COMPOUND GROUP AND EXAMPLES	THERAPEUTIC BENEFITS	OILS CONTAINING SOME OF THE GROUP	MOLECULAR STRUCTURE
Monoterpene Hydrocarbon (alpha & beta-pinene, limonene, sabinene, phellandrene)	Inhibit the accumulation of toxins and help discharge existing toxins, anti-inflammatory, antibacterial, soothing to irritated tissues, insect repellent, cancer-preventative properties, cellular protective	basil, citrus oils, cypress, Douglas fir, frankincense, ginger, juniper berry, litsea, marjoram, melaleuca, pink pepper, rosemary, Siberian fir, thyme, yarrow	10 carbon terpenes
Sesquiterpene Hydrocarbon (chamazulene, fare-sene, zingiberene)	Anti-inflammatory, sedative, soothing, antibacterial, soothing to irritated skin and tissue, liver and glandular stimulant	black pepper, blue tansy, cedarwood, copaiba, ginger, helichrysum, myrrh, patchouli, spikenard, ylang ylang	15 carbon terpenes
Monoterpene Alcohols (borneol, geraniol, linalool)	Antimicrobial, supports immune system, restorative to skin, cleansing, antispasmodic, sedative, gentle, mild	basil, coriander, frankincense, geranium, lavender, magnolia, marjoram, melaleuca, neroli, petitgrain, rose	10 carbon terpenoids bound to a hydroxyl group, high resistance to oxidation
Sesquiterpene Alcohols	Anti-allergenic, antibacterial, an-ti-inflammatory, liver and glandular stimulant	cedarwood, patchouli, sandal-wood, vetiver, yarrow	15 carbon terpenoids bound to a hydroxyl group bound to a carbon instead of a hydrogen
Esters (geranyl acetate, linalyl acetate, methyl salicylate)	Very calming, relaxing, and bal-ancing, antifungal, antispasmodic, balancing to nervous system	arborvitae, bergamot, birch, cardamom, clary sage, heli-chrysum, jasmine, lavender, petitgrain, Roman chamomile, wintergreen, ylang ylang	Consists of a carboxyl group (carbon atom double-bonded to an oxygen atom)
Aldehydes (citral, geranial, neral)	Powerful aromas, calming to emotions, anti-infectious, anti-in-flammatory, calming to autonomic nervous system, fever-reducing, hypotensive, tonic	cassia, cilantro, cinnamon, geranium, lemongrass, lime, litsea, marjoram, melissa	Consists of a carboxyl group (car-bon atom double-bonded to an oxygen atom). Slightly fruity odor, can cause skin irritation
Ketones (camphor, jasmone)	Mucolytic, stimulate cell regener-ation, promote the formation of tissue, analgesic, sedative	fennel, helichrysum, lavender, lemongrass, manuka, myrrh, peppermint, Roman cham-omile, rosemary, spearmint, spikenard, turmeric, vetiver	Consists of a carboxyl group (carbon atom double-bonded to an oxygen atom)
Phenols (carvacrol, eugenol, thymol)	Powerful antibacterial, anti-infec-tious, antiseptic, very stimulating to the autonomic nervous system, analgesic, antifungal, cancer pre-ventative	cinnamon, clove, oregano, thyme	Consists of a benzene ring – 6 carbon atoms bound in a circle – and a hydroxyl group. May be irritating to skin, some concerns at high dosages for liver toxicity. Use for short periods of time.
Oxides (1,8 cineole)	Expectorant, mildly stimulating, respiratory support, pain relief, anti-inflammatory	basil, cardamom, clary sage, clove, cypress, eucalyptus, fennel, melaleuca, peppermint, rosemary, thyme,	An oxygen atom has become bound between two carbon atoms.
Ethers (estragole, anethole)	Balancing to autonomic nervous system, soothing, sedative	basil, fennel, marjoram, ylang ylang,	Compounds in which an oxygen atom in the molecule is bonded to two carbon atoms.
Lactones (coumarin)	Expectorant properties	In very low amounts in some essential oils	Consists of an ester group inte-grated into a carbon ring system. Has a vanilla-like odor
Coumarins (bergamottin)		bergamot	phototoxic

Blending & Layering

When using essential oils, the desired outcome may best be accomplished by using more than one essential oil at a time. To do so, the oils may be layered topically, ingested separately, or placed together in a blend. Layering is defined as applying one essential oil to the skin, waiting for it to be absorbed, and then applying another oil over the first. This may be repeated several times until all the desired oils are applied. Massage expedites and improves this absorption process. Oils are absorbed rapidly into the skin, so the wait time can be short. A carrier oil, such as fractionated coconut oil, may be applied prior to or along with an oil application. In some cases, layering is a preferred method for topical use, as it requires less skill and knowledge than blending, and allows the oil selections to be varied at every application.

Layering is particularly useful when multiple concerns must be addressed simultaneously. For example, a sprained or twisted ankle may involve tendons or ligaments (connective tissue) as well as muscle or bone. Furthermore, bruising and swelling may be present. Increasing blood flow to the injury site would also be useful for healing. Each of these concerns may be addressed through the use of layering.

Here is an example of an injured tissue layering sequence:

- 1-2 drops of lemongrass – for connective tissue; apply, massage lightly if possible, wait for absorption
- 1-2 drops of marjoram – for muscle; apply, massage lightly if possible, wait for absorption
- 1-2 drops of cypress – for circulation; apply, massage lightly if possible, wait for absorption
- 1-2 drops of helichrysum – for pain; apply, massage lightly if possible, wait for absorption
- 1-2 drops of wintergreen – for bone; apply, massage lightly if possible, wait for absorption

This layering sequence would be repeatedly applied to expedite healing. For example, application every 30-60 minutes for the first four applications may be followed by application every 4-6 hours the following few days. Finally, twice-a-day application may be used once the pain has mostly subsided and until complete healing has occurred.

In addition to layering the oils, there are times when creating an essential oil blend is a good or better way to achieve an intended result such as calming a mood, relaxing muscles, or supporting a distressed respiratory system. Blending is the process of combining multiple selected essential oils together in one bottle. The chemical profile of a blend is very different from each of the individual oils it contains. Combining essential oils together creates a synergistic effect, forming a new, unique molecular structure.

There is an art to blending, which is enhanced and improved by practice and through applying proven techniques and principles. Artistry and skill combine to creating a blend that is aromatically pleasing and that accomplishes the desired therapeutic outcome or goal. Since essential oils are potent and often expensive, care should be taken to blend appropriately so as not to waste essential oils or to create a blend that may cause an adverse reaction, such as a headache or skin sensitivity. There are many resources and educational classes on the art of blending essential oils. One excellent resource is *Aromatherapy Workbook* by Marcel Lavabre. A study of the basic chemical makeup of essential oil aids in creating therapeutically effective blends. For a foundational understanding of the main chemical constituents in essential oils refer to the "Body Systems: Oil Composition & Chemistry" section in this book.

Blending Guidelines

Some basic guidelines help in blending regardless of the method used:

1. The "Blends Well With" listings under each oil description in the "Natural Solutions: Single Oils" assist in selecting oils that blend well together.
2. Blends that have been professionally created are best used as they are.
3. Essential oils from the same botanical family usually blend well together.
4. Essential oils with similar constituents usually mix well together.
5. A blend should be aromatically pleasing.
6. It is best to use the smallest amount of oil possible when experimenting with a blend.
7. It is helpful to label your blend.
8. Be specific in defining your desired outcome.
9. Keeping a blending journal serves as a reference for making adjustments or remembering what worked.
10. As a beginner, it is best to start with blending four to six essential oils for a total of fifteen to twenty drops in the blend.

There are differing opinions and experiences as to what order oils should be added to a blend. It is has been shown in a laboratory that in small amounts, such as blends for personal use, order doesn't matter. However, if blending in large amounts (e.g. companies that create their own blends en masse to sell) the order in which oils are added may be very important.

Blending Methods

There are three suggested techniques for creating essential oil blends:

1 Blending Classifications Method.

2 Odor Types/Notes Method.

3 Combination of Techniques (Chemical Compounds and Odor Types) Method.

An in-depth description of each of these methods or techniques is beyond the scope of this book, though a summary is included here for each method. Practice and study improves the ability to create effective and aromatically pleasing blends.

Blending Classification Method

This method uses the four blending classifications: personifier, enhancer, equalizer, and modifier. Below is a description of each classification.

PLACE IN BLEND	NAME OF CLASSIFICATION	PERCENTAGE OF THE BLEND	CHARACTERISTICS	EXAMPLE OILS IN THIS CLASSIFICATION
First	Personifier	1-5%	Sharp, strong, and long-lasting aroma, dominant properties, strong therapeutic action	birch, black pepper, blue tansy, cassia, cardamom, cinnamon, clary sage, clove, copaiba, coriander, ginger, helichrysum, neroli, orange, peppermint, Roman chamomile, rose, spearmint, tangerine, vetiver, wintergreen, and ylang ylang
Second	Enhancer	50-80%	Enhances the properties of the other oils in the blend, not a sharp aroma; evaporates faster than the Personifier	arborvitae, basil, bergamot, birch, cassia, cedarwood, cinnamon, dill, eucalyptus, frankincense, geranium, grapefruit, jasmine, lavender, lemon, lemongrass, lime, litsea, manuka, marjoram, melaleuca, melissa, orange, oregano, patchouli, rose, rosemary, thyme, wintergreen, and yarrow
Third	Equalizer	10-15%	Creates balance and synergy among the oils in the blend	arborvitae, basil, bergamot, cedarwood, cilantro, cypress, fennel, white fir, frankincense, geranium, ginger, jasmine, juniper berry, lavender, lemongrass, lime, litsea, marjoram, melaleuca, melissa, myrrh, neroli, oregano, rose, sandalwood, Siberian fir, thyme, and white fir
Fourth	Modifier	5-8%	Mild; evaporates quickly, adds harmony to the blend	bergamot, black pepper, cardamom, coriander, eucalyptus, fennel, grapefruit, jasmine, lavender, lemon, melissa, myrrh, neroli, rose, sandalwood, tangerine, and ylang ylang

The table below provides an example of a blend for easing muscle strain using the Blending Classification Method. Using this recipe, mix the four oils in the order listed in a 10 ml roller bottle and fill with a carrier oil such as fractionated coconut oil for dilution.

CLASSIFICATION	AMOUNT*	ESSENTIAL OIL
Personifier	1 drop	cinnamon
Enhancer	8 drops	basil
Equalizer	2 drops	ginger
Modifier	4 drops	grapefruit

*based on a 15-drop blend

Odor Types/Notes

This second method focuses on the odor and odor intensity ascribed to each essential oil. The perfume industry has assigned perfume "notes" to essential oils. The three notes are base, middle, and top. These assignments can be used as a guide in creating a blend.

Top notes are light oils and often have fresh, sweet, citrusy, or fruity aromas. Middle notes are oils that have a floral, slight woody, or sweet aroma. Base notes are woody, heavy, earthy, rich, or deep. Some oils such as basil or fennel may be used in a blend as either a top or middle note. Clary sage and ylang ylang are examples of oils that may be used as either middle or base notes. When creating a blend, base notes are 5% to 20% of the blend, middle notes are 50% to 80%, and top notes are 5% to 20% of the blend. This blending method is more focused on aroma than therapeutic benefits.

Following is an example of a blend designed to ease muscle strain using the **Odor Types/Notes** method. Using this recipe, mix the four oils in the order listed in a 10 ml roller bottle and fill with a carrier oil such as fractionated coconut oil for dilution.

ODOR TYPE/NOTE	AMOUNT*	OIL
Base Note	3 drops	sandalwood
Middle Note	3 drops	ginger
Middle Note	4 drops	cypress
Top Note	5 drops	wild orange

*based on a 15-drop blend

Following is a table of single oils with their scent profile and assigned scent note. Knowing an oils scent note is critical in blending using the note type classification method.

OIL	SCENT PROFILE	SCENT NOTE
Arborvitae	Intense, medicinal, woody, earthy	Top to Middle
Basil	Herbaceous, spicy, anise-like, camphoraceous, lively	Top to Middle
Bergamot	Sweet, lively, citrusy, fruity	Top
Birch	Sweet, sharp, camphoraceous, fresh	Top
Black pepper	Spicy, peppery, musky, warm, with herbaceous undertones.	Middle
Blue tansy	Sweet, slightly-floral, fruity	Middle
Cardamom	Sweet, spicy, balsamic, with floral undertones	Middle
Cassia	Spicy, warm, sweet	Middle
Cedarwood	Warm, soft, woody	Middle
Cilantro	Herbaceous, citrusy, fresh	Top
Cinnamon	Spicy, earthy, sweet	Middle
Clary sage	Herbaceous, spicy, hay-like, sharp, fixative	Middle to Base
Clove	Spicy, warming, slightly bitter, woody	Middle to Base
Copaiba	Sweet, woody	Base
Coriander	Woody, spicy, sweet	Middle
Cypress	Fresh, herbaceous, slightly woody with evergreen undertones	Middle
Dill	Fresh, sweet, herbaceous, slightly earthly	Middle
Douglas fir	Clean, fresh, woody, sweet	Middle
Eucalyptus	Slightly camphorous, sweet, fruity	Middle
Fennel (sweet)	Sweet, somewhat spicy, licorice-like	Top to Middle
Frankincense	Rich, deep, warm, balsamic, sweet, with incense-like overtones	Base
Geranium	Sweet, green, citrus-rosy, fresh	Middle
Ginger	Sweet, spicy-woody, warm, tenacious, fresh, sharp	Middle
Grapefruit	Clean, fresh, bitter, citrusy	Top
Green Mandarin	Sweet, bright, citrusy, tangy	Top
Helichrysum	Rich, sweet, fruity, with tea and honey undertones	Middle
Jasmine	Powerful, sweet, tenacious, floral with fruity-herbaceous undertones	Base
Juniper berry	Sweet, balsamic, tenacious	Middle
Kumquat	Refreshing, citrus, bright, rich	Top
Lavender	Floral, sweet, herbaceous, balsamic, woody undertones	Middle
Lemon	Sweet, sharp, clear, citrusy	Top
Lemongrass	Grassy, lemony, pungent, earthy, slightly bitter	Top
Lime	Sweet, tart, intense, lively	Top
Litsea	Crisp, citrusy, fresh	Top
Magnolia	Sweet, fruity, exotic, rich, heady, radiant	Top
Manuka	Warm, rich, sweet	Middle
Marjoram	Herbaceous, green, spicy	Middle
Melaleuca	Medicinal, fresh, woody, earthy, herbaceous	Middle
Melissa	Delicate, lemony, spicy	Middle
Myrrh	Warm, earthy, woody, balsamic	Base
Neroli	Light, sweet-floral	Top or Base
Orange	Fresh, citrusy, fruity, sweet	Top
Oregano	Spicy, warm, herbaceous, sharp	Middle
Patchouli	Earthy, herbaceous, sweet, balsamic, rich, with woody undertones	Base
Peppermint	Minty, sharp, intense	Middle
Petitgrain	Fresh, floral, woody, slightly herbaceous	Top
Pink Pepper	Intense, dry, warm, sweet-spicy with a faint floral note, slightly smoky undertone	Middle
Red Mandarin	smooth, sweet-tart, citrusy, slightly floral undertone	Top
Roman chamomile	Fresh, sweet, fruity-herbaceous, apple-like, no tenacity	Middle
Rose	Floral, spicy, rich, deep, sensual, green, honey-like	Middle to Base
Rosemary	Herbaceous, strong, camphorous, with woody-balsamic and evergreen undertones	Middle
(Hawaiian) Sandalwood	Soft, woody, spicy, sweet, earthy, balsamic	Base
Siberian fir	Fresh, soft-pine	Middle to Top
Spearmint	Minty, slightly fruity, less bright than peppermint	Top
Spikenard	Earthy, woody, musty, spicy	Base
Tangerine	Fresh, sweet, citrusy	Top
Thyme	Fresh, medicinal, herbaceous	Middle
Turmeric	Woody, spicy, fresh, warm	Base
Vetiver	Earthy, heavy, woody, smoky, balsamic	Base
White fir	Fresh, woody, earthy, sweet	Middle
Wintergreen	Minty, camphorous, fresh	Top
Yarrow	Fresh, green-herbaceous, woody	Middle
Ylang ylang	Sweet, heavy, euphoric, tropical floral, with spicy-balsamic undertones	Middle to Base

Combination of Techniques (Chemistry Compounds and Scent Types)

The first two blending methods are primarily focused on creating a pleasing aroma with secondary consideration to the end therapeutic goal. The Combination of Techniques method allows for both aroma and therapeutic effectiveness to be considered. When creating a blend, first set a specific end goal. Then select specific essential oils, based on desired therapeutic benefits from their chemical compounds. By also considering scent types, both an effective and aromatically pleasing blend is created. Refer to Oil Composition & Chemistry in previous section.

The steps to create a blend by considering essential oil chemical compounds and odor types are listed below. Fine-tuning these steps necessarily includes intuitive action and experience.

1. Select the desired outcome. The more specific the outcome; the more effective the blend will be.
2. Select the essential oil chemical compound groups that will best meet the goal.
3. Select approximately eight to fifteen essential oils from these groups to draw from.
4. Note the scent profile/note for each of the selected oils.
5. Select one oil as the base note, two to three oils as the middle notes, and one oil to be the top note. (This is a guideline; use intuition and experience to alter.)
6. Decide how many drops will be used of each of the five oils selected. A fifteen-drop blend is a good ratio for a 5 ml or 10 ml bottle with a carrier oil.
7. Place the oils in the bottle and add the carrier oil. As the blend is used to meet the desired outcome, make notes in a blending journal.

The following is an example of using the steps to create a blend to ease muscle strain using Combination of Techniques Method.

For **steps 1-2**, the following table is used to identify the most helpful chemical compound groups to meet the blend goal. In this example, aldehydes, esters, sesquiterpene hydrocarbons, and ethers would be helpful.

Steps 3-4: The following is an example (see next page) of a list of oils chosen from the four selected chemical groups, which will help meet the desired outcome of easing muscle strain.

The letter next to each oil indicates the odor type assigned to that oil so as to assist with selection. (T) Top (M) Middle (B) Base

CHEMICAL COMPOUND GROUP	THERAPEUTIC BENEFITS	OILS
Monoterpene Hydrocarbon	Cellular protective, anti-inflammatory, antibacterial	basil, citrus oils, cypress, Douglas fir, frankincense, ginger, juniper berry, litsea, neroli, pink pepper, rosemary, Siberian fir, tangerine, thyme, yarrow,
Sesquiterpene Hydrocarbon	Anti-inflammatory, sedative, soothing, antibacterial	black pepper, blue tansy, cedarwood, copiaba, ginger, helichrysum, manuka, myrrh, patchouli, spikenard, white fir, ylang ylang
Monoterpene Alcohols	Antimicrobial, somewhat stimulating, tonifying and restorative to the skin, cleansing, antispasmodic, sedative, gentle, mild	basil, cilantro, coriander, frankincense, geranium, lavender, magnolia, marjoram, melaleuca, petitgrain, neroli, rose
Sesquiterpene Alcohols	Anti-allergenic, antibacterial, anti-inflammatory, liver and glandular stimulant	cedarwood, geranium, patchouli, sandalwood, vetiver, yarrow
Esters	Very calming, relaxing, balancing, antifungal, antispasmodic	arborvitae, bergamot, birch, cardamom, cassia, clary sage, clove, geranium, helichrysum, jasmine, lavender, peppermint, petitgrain, Roman chamomile, wintergreen, ylang ylang
Aldehydes	Strong aroma; calming to the emotions, anti-infectious, anti-inflammatory, calming overall, fever-reducing, hypotensive, and tonic; some are vasodilators	cassia, cinnamon, geranium, lemongrass, lime, litsea, marjoram, melissa, Roman chamomile
Ketones	Mucolytic, stimulate cell regeneration, promote the formation of tissue, analgesic, sedative	fennel, helichrysum, lavender, manuka, myrrh, peppermint, Roman chamomile, rosemary, spearmint, spikenard, turmeric, vetiver
Phenols	Powerful antibacterial, anti-infective, and antiseptic, very stimulating to the autonomic nervous system	cinnamon, clove, oregano, thyme
Oxides	Expectorant, mildly stimulating	basil, cardamom, clary sage, clove, cypress, fennel, melaleuca, peppermint, rosemary, thyme,
Ethers	Balancing to the autonomic nervous system, soothing, sedative	basil, fennel, eucalyptus, marjoram, myrrh, ylang ylang,

Aldehyde:	lemongrass (T), roman chamomile (M)
Esters:	roman chamomile (M), geranium (M), ylang ylang (M to B)
Sesquiterpene Hydrocar-bons:	cedarwood (B), white fir (M), black pep-per (M), ginger (M), ylang ylang (M to T)
Ethers:	basil (M to T), ylang ylang (M to T), marjoram (M)

Steps 5-7: Using the above list of selected oils, select five oils and the number of drops needed from each oil to create the blend that will equal a total of fifteen drops. The blend can be placed in a 5 ml or 10 ml roller bottle and topped off with a carrier oil to fill the bottle.

Base note:	cedarwood	(4 drops)
Middle note:	roman chamomile	(2 drops)
Middle note:	ginger	(2 drops)
Middle note:	black pepper	(3 drops)
Top note:	ylang ylang	(4 drops)

When using essential oils for a therapeutic goal, it is often helpful to use more than one oil. Layering these oils following the suggested steps in this section is beneficial to accomplish the desired outcome. When time permits, it may also be helpful to create a blend using oils selected based on their chemical compounds and their note type as outlined in this section. Intuition and experience improves blending skills.

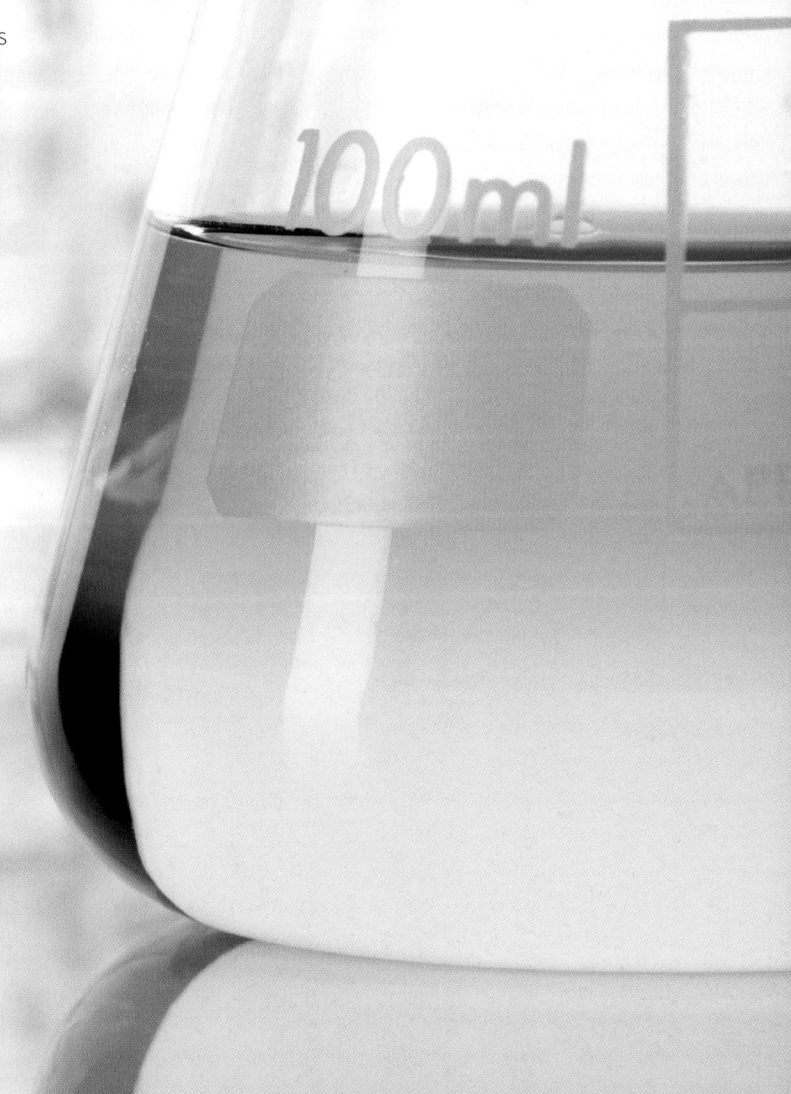

Massage with Oils

The application of essential oils topically, combined with massage, is simple to do but very powerful in the healing process. It increases the benefits of massage and the efficacy of essential oils on and within the body. Massage increases circulation and absorption, helps improve lymphatic flow, and aids in the release of toxins. It can also soothe nerve endings, relax muscles, and relieve stress and tension in the body.

Head

Apply essential oils to the fingertips and gently massage entire scalp. For headache, massage around the base of the neck and work upward to the base of the scalp.

Neck

Use circular movements, working from the base of the neck, up both sides of the vertebrae, to the base of the scalp. Work to the sides of the neck and repeat the movements, working down again.

Shoulders

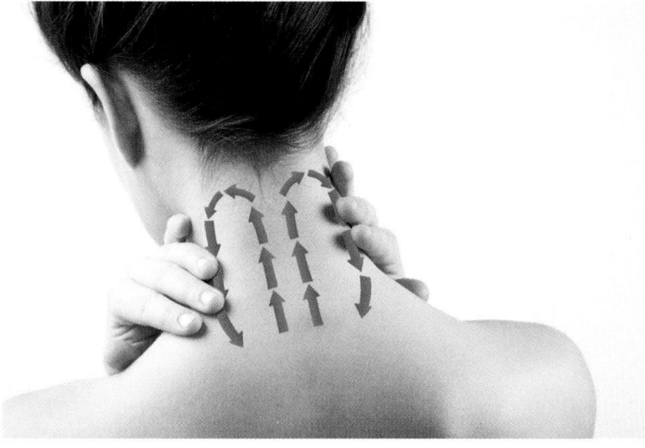

Using your thumbs and palms, make firm strokes from the shoulder to the neck and back again.

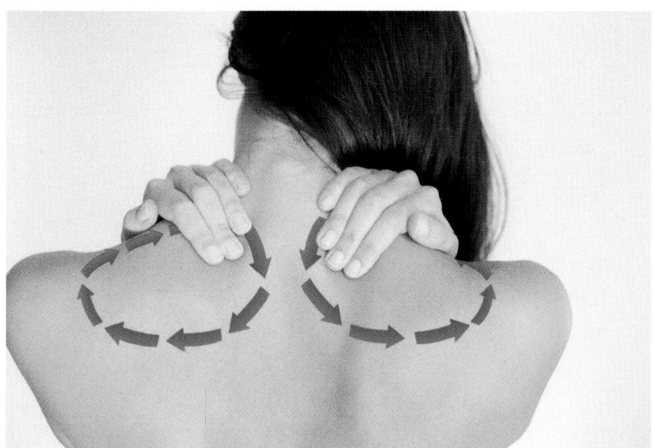

Arms

Massage up toward the armpit on the fatty or muscular areas only.

Back

Start from the lumbar region of the back, and with two hands stroke all the way up to the shoulders alongside the spine. Slide the hands over the shoulders and return down the sides of the back.

Abdomen

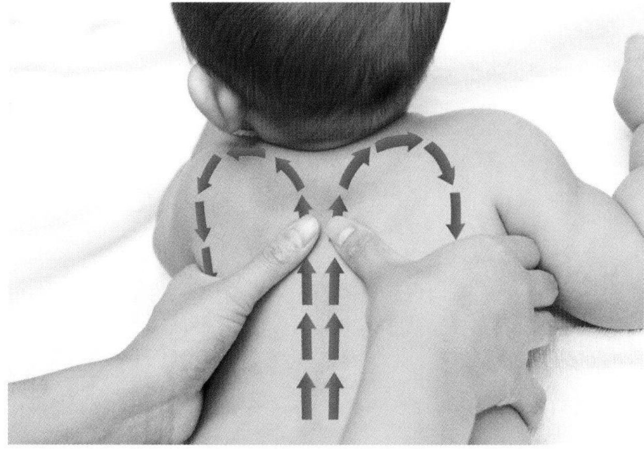

Use circular movements only, in a clockwise direction.

Legs

Always massage legs upward on the fatty or muscular areas only and avoid varicose veins.

Feet

Massage from the toes to the heel with thumbs under the foot and fingers on top.

- Massage is most effective when done with the flow of the body—and toward the heart, from hand to shoulder, foot to thigh, and so on.
- When massaging children and invalids, use gentle movements.

Reflexology

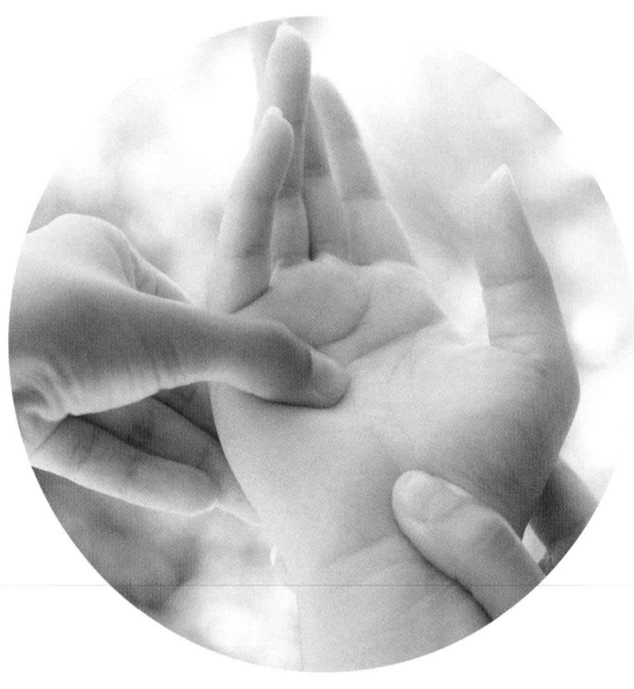

This a great technique to use personally, on family or friends, as well as with those whose hands and feet are not accessible for hand and foot reflexology. Young children are especially receptive to having their outer ears worked on, finding it calming and soothing.

Foot Reflexology is an effective method to bring the body systems into balance by applying pressure to specific places on the feet. Hand reflexology can be utilized in a similar manner. The nerves in the feet correspond with various parts of the body; thus, the entire body is mapped on the feet, telling a story of emotional and physical well being.

One way to find imbalances in the body is to massage all the areas noted on the foot reflexology chart and feel for triggers or small knots underneath the skin. When a trigger is found, apply an essential oil to the location on the foot and continue to massage the trigger until it releases. Another way to use reflexology is to address a specific ailment. For instance, if a person has a headache, locate the brain on the foot chart and the corresponding point on the foot. Apply an essential oil of choice and massage the pad of the big toe to reduce tension. If a person has a tight chest induced by stress, locate the lungs/chest on the foot chart and the corresponding point on the foot. Apply an essential oil of choice followed by medium to light circular massage on the ball of the foot.

The autonomic nervous system is then engaged, helping to alleviate symptoms and heal the body naturally.

Reflexology is the application of pressure to the feet and hands with specific thumb, finger, and hand techniques without the use of oil or lotion. It is based on a system of zones and reflex areas that reflect an image of the body on the feet and hands, with the premise that such work effects a physical change to the body.

Ear Reflexology is a simple and efficient way to relieve stress and pain by applying minimal pressure to the reflex points on the ear. Each ear contains a complete map of the body, rich with nerve endings and multiple connectors to the central nervous system. For example, if the reflex point for the bladder is tender, the body may be in the beginning stages of a bladder infection. One can take preventative measures to head off the bladder infection by applying an essential oil to the reflex point on the ear followed by minimal pressure.

To begin treatment, start at the top of the right ear and slowly work your thumb and forefinger along the outer edges. Hold each point for five seconds before continuing to the end of the earlobe. For best results, repeat this procedure at least five times. Next, work the inner crevices of the ear using the pointer finger and applying minimal pressure. Repeat procedure on left ear. If any areas in and around the crevices of the ear are sensitive, consult the ear reflexology chart to pinpoint the area of the body that may be out of balance.

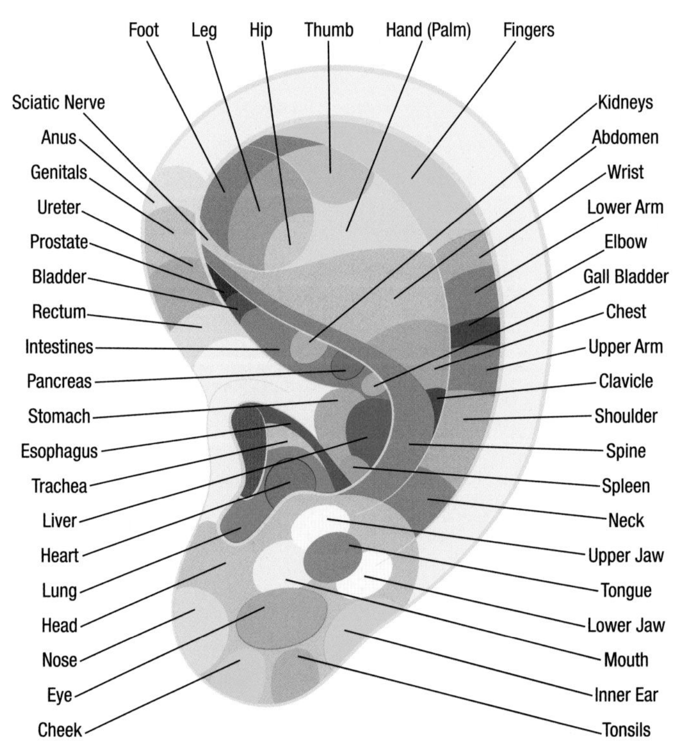

SUPPLEMENTAL

REFLEXOLOGY REFERENCE

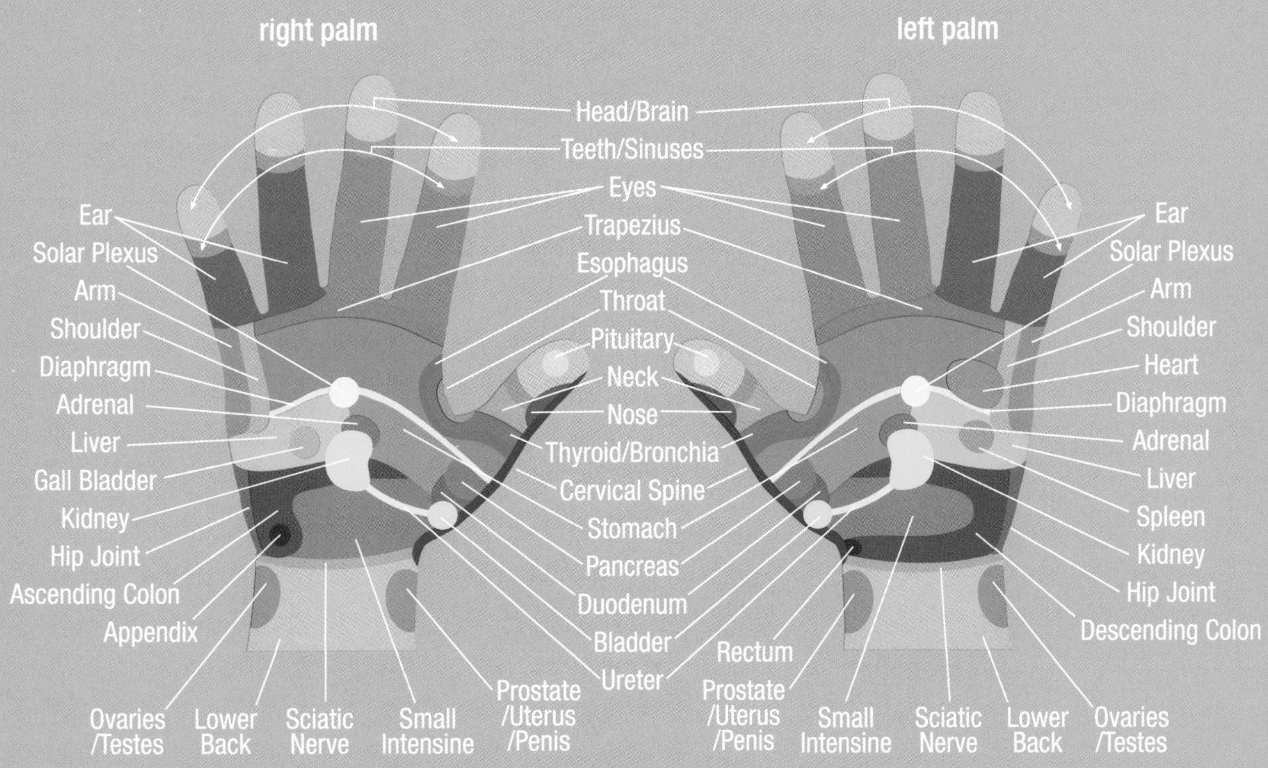

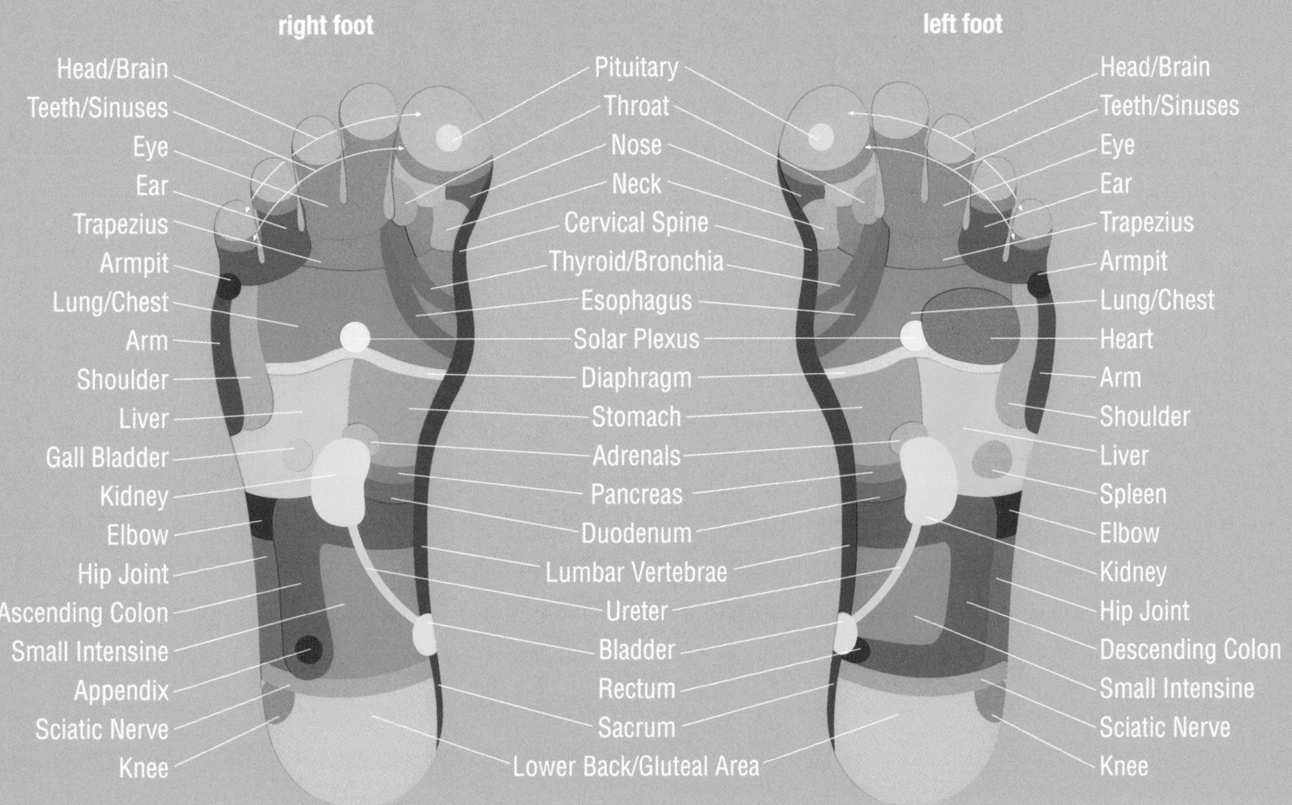

Cooking with Oils Chart

	Meat	Chicken	Fish	Eggs	Cheese	Vegetables	Rice	Pasta	Desserts	Pastries	Bread	Cakes	Sorbets	Ice Cream	Fruit	Dressings
Basil	•	•	•			•	•	•								
Bergamot		•	•						•				•	•		
Black pepper	•	•	•	•		•	•	•			•				•	•
Cardamom	•	•	•	•		•	•		•	•	•	•	•	•	•	•
Cassia			•		•	•	•	•	•	•	•	•		•	•	•
Cilantro	•	•				•		•								
Cinnamon	•	•	•	•	•	•	•	•	•	•	•	•	•	•	•	•
Clove	•	•							•	•	•	•	•	•	•	•
Coriander	•	•				•		•								
Dill	•	•	•			•	•	•		•	•				•	•
Fennel			•			•	•	•	•	•	•	•			•	•
Ginger					•	•		•	•	•	•	•	•	•	•	•
Grapefruit				•		•	•	•	•	•			•	•		•
Green Mandarin						•			•	•		•	•	•	•	•
Jasmine		•	•			•	•	•	•	•	•	•	•	•	•	
Lavender		•	•	•	•		•	•	•	•	•	•	•	•	•	
Lemon	•	•	•		•	•	•	•	•		•	•	•	•	•	•
Lemongrass		•	•	•	•	•	•	•	•	•	•	•	•	•	•	•
Lime	•	•	•			•	•	•	•	•	•	•	•	•	•	•
Marjoram	•	•	•								•					•
Melissa		•	•	•	•	•	•						•	•	•	
Oregano	•	•	•	•	•	•	•	•			•					•
Peppermint						•			•	•		•	•	•	•	
Pink Pepper	•	•	•	•		•	•	•			•				•	•
Rose		•		•	•		•		•	•	•	•	•	•	•	
Rosemary	•	•	•		•	•	•			•						•
Spearmint						•			•	•		•	•	•	•	
Tangerine	•	•	•				•	•	•	•	•	•	•	•	•	•
Thyme	•	•	•			•	•	•								•
Turmeric	•	•	•	•	•	•	•	•			•					•
Wild orange	•	•	•	•			•	•	•	•	•	•	•	•	•	•
Ylang ylang		•					•	•	•	•	•	•	•	•	•	

SUPPLEMENTAL

Oil Properties Glossary

Analgesic - relieves or allays pain
Anaphrodisiac - reduces sexual desire
Anti-allergenic - reduces allergic response
Antiarthritic - effective in treatment of arthritis
Antibacterial - kills or inhibits growth of bacteria
Anticarcinogenic - inhibits development of cancer
Anti-carcinoma - destroys or inhibits cancer cells
Anticatarrhal - removes excess mucus
Anticoagulant - prevents clotting of blood
Anticonvulsant - reduces convulsions
Antidepressant - effective in treatment against depression
Antiemetic - effective against nausea and vomiting
Antifungal - inhibits growth of fungi
Antihemorrhagic - promotes hemostasis; stops bleeding
Antihistamine - blocks histamine receptors; reduces allergic response
Anti-infectious - reduces/prevents infection
Anti-inflammatory - reduces inflammation
Antimicrobial - kills or inhibits microorganisms
Antimutagenic - reduces rate of genetic variants/mutation
Antioxidant - mitigates damage by free radicals
Anti-parasitic - destroys or inhibits growth/reproduction of parasites
Anti-rheumatic - mitigates pain and stiffness
Antiseptic - destroys microorganisms to prevent or treat infection on living tissue/skin
Antispasmodic - relieves spasms of involuntary muscles
Antitoxic - neutralizes or counteracts toxins
Anti-tumoral - inhibits growth of tumors
Antiviral - destroys viruses or suppresses replication
Aphrodisiac - heightens sexual desire
Astringent - contracts tissues, generally of the skin; reduces minor bleeding
Calming - pacifying
Cardiotonic - tones and vitalizes the heart
Carminative - reduces gas or bloating
Cleanser - cleanses body and/or household surfaces
Cytophylactic - stimulates cell growth
Decongestant - reduces respiratory congestion; opens airways
Deodorant - stops formation of odors
Detoxifier - removes toxins from the body tissues and organs
Digestive stimulant - stimulates digestion
Disinfectant - mitigates growth of microorganisms on inorganic surfaces
Diuretic - increases production and excretion of urine
Emmenagogue - regulates and induces menstruation
Energizing - generates and enhances energy
Expectorant - promotes discharge of phlegm and other fluids from the respiratory tract
Galactagogue - promotes lactation and increases milk supply
Grounding - assists one's sense of feeling centered and secure
Hypertensive - raises blood pressure
Hypotensive - lowers blood pressure
Immunostimulant - induces activation of the body's protective ability
Insect repellent - deters insects and bugs
Insecticidal - kills insects and bugs
Invigorating - revitalizes and rejuvenates
Laxative - stimulates bowel excretion
Mucolytic - loosens, thins, and breaks down mucus
Nervine - beneficial effect on nerves
Neuroprotective - protects nerves
Neurotonic - improves tone or force of nervous system
Purifier - eliminates impurities
Refreshing - renews; promotes feeling of freshness
Regenerative - promotes regeneration of body tissue
Relaxant - promotes relaxation; reduces tension
Restorative - encourages repair, recovery, restoration
Revitalizer - uplifts and energizes
Rubefacient - increases circulation; increases skin redness
Sedative - promotes calm and sleep; reduces agitation; tranquilizing
Steroidal - stimulates cortisone-like action
Stimulant - increases activity
Stomachic - assists digestion, promotes appetite
Tonic - promotes a feeling of vigor or well being
Uplifting - elevating; promotes sense of happiness and hope
Vasoconstrictor - restricts blood vessels; decreases blood flow; can increase blood pressure
Vasodilator - relaxes/dilates blood vessels; increases blood flow; can decrease blood pressure
Vermicide - kills parasitic worms
Vermifuge - stuns parasites
Warming - raises body and/or specific body tissue temperature - referred to as "localized warming"

Oil Properties Chart A-R

Oil Properties	analgesic	anaphrodisiac	anti-allergenic	antiarthritic	antibacterial	anticarcinogenic	anti-carcinoma	anticatarrhal	anticoagulant	anticonvulsant	antidepressant	antiemetic	antifungal	antihemorrhagic	antihistamine	anti-infectious	anti-inflammatory	antimicrobial	antimutagenic	antioxidant	anti-parasitic	antirheumatic	antiseptic	antispasmodic	antitoxic	anti-tumoral	antiviral	aphrodisiac	astringent	bactericidal	calming	cardiotonic	carminative	cleanser	cytophylactic	decongestant	deodorant	detoxifier
Arborvitae	•	•		•	•	•	•						•		•	•	•	•		•			•			•	•		•					•	•			•
Basil	•				•			•			•	•				•	•	•		•			•	•			•				•		•			•		
Bergamot	•				•						•		•			•	•				•		•	•	•						•		•				•	
Birch	•				•												•					•	•	•					•									
Black Pepper	•				•			•									•			•	•		•	•	•			•			•							
Black Spruce	•				•	•												•		•				•			•				•						•	
Blue Tansy	•		•	•	•								•		•		•	•			•	•		•			•				•		•					
Cardamom					•							•				•	•	•					•	•				•					•			•		
Cassia	•			•	•							•	•				•	•		•		•		•			•		•	•	•	•	•			•		•
Cedarwood					•								•			•	•						•						•									
Celery Seed	•				•												•			•											•							•
Cilantro					•								•					•		•										•			•	•				•
Cinnamon	•				•						•		•			•	•	•	•	•	•		•	•	•		•	•	•	•			•					
Citronella	•				•					•	•		•			•	•			•	•		•	•		•	•		•	•				•			•	•
Clary Sage	•				•				•	•	•		•				•	•					•	•				•	•		•		•				•	
Clove	•				•							•	•		•	•	•			•	•	•	•	•		•	•	•					•					
Copaiba	•			•	•		•					•	•			•	•	•	•	•		•	•			•	•				•	•	•			•	•	
Coriander	•				•						•	•	•				•	•		•		•		•	•			•			•		•				•	
Cypress	•				•								•			•	•	•				•	•	•					•			•	•			•	•	•
Dill					•						•		•				•	•						•			•						•					
Douglas fir	•				•															•			•						•									
Eucalyptus	•				•			•					•			•	•	•		•		•		•			•							•		•	•	
Fennel	•									•		•	•				•	•			•		•	•	•						•	•	•					
Frankincense	•					•	•	•			•					•	•	•		•	•		•			•			•		•				•			
Geranium			•		•					•	•		•	•		•	•						•	•	•				•	•	•				•		•	•
Ginger	•			•	•							•	•				•		•	•		•	•				•					•	•			•		
Grapefruit					•		•				•									•			•		•				•			•		•		•		
Green Mandarin					•	•						•					•	•		•			•	•					•		•		•	•				•
Helichrysum	•		•		•			•	•				•	•			•	•		•			•	•			•		•									
Jasmine	•										•						•						•	•				•			•	•	•					
Juniper berry	•																			•	•	•	•	•	•			•	•		•	•	•	•				•
Kumquat					•		•						•				•	•		•			•				•		•				•	•	•			
Lavender	•								•	•	•	•	•		•	•	•	•	•		•	•	•	•	•	•			•		•	•	•		•		•	
Lemon							•				•		•					•		•		•	•	•	•		•						•	•		•		•
Lemon Eucalyptus	•				•								•			•	•				•		•				•							•		•	•	
Lemongrass	•				•		•				•		•				•	•	•	•		•	•		•					•			•			•	•	
Lime					•												•			•		•	•	•			•											•
Litsea	•				•		•						•			•	•	•						•			•		•		•	•	•				•	•
Magnolia	•		•		•						•							•					•					•			•					•		•
Manuka			•	•	•								•		•		•	•				•	•				•					•			•		•	
Marjoram	•	•			•											•							•	•								•						
Melaleuca	•				•								•			•	•			•	•		•				•									•		
Melissa					•						•				•		•	•					•	•			•		•	•	•	•	•					
Myrrh					•	•	•	•					•			•	•	•					•			•	•		•			•	•					
Neroli				•	•			•		•	•						•	•	•	•			•	•				•					•		•		•	
Oregano	•				•						•		•				•	•		•	•	•	•				•				•	•	•					
Patchouli					•						•	•	•			•	•	•					•	•	•			•	•		•	•	•			•	•	•
Peppermint	•				•	•						•					•						•	•			•	•				•	•					
Petitgrain					•						•	•				•							•	•							•	•					•	•
Pink Pepper	•				•		•				•	•					•	•		•		•	•	•			•	•				•	•					
Ravensara	•				•						•		•					•					•	•			•	•										

	digestive stimulant	disinfectant	diuretic	emmenagogue	energizing	expectorant	galactagogue	grounding	hypertensive	hypotensive	immunostimulant	insect repellent	insecticidal	invigorating	laxative	mucolytic	nervine	neuroprotective	neurotonic	purifier	refreshing	regenerative	relaxant	restorative	revitalizer	rubefacient	sedative	steroidal	stimulant	stomachic	tonic	uplifting	vasoconstrictor	vasodilator	vermicide	vermifuge	warming
Arborvitae		•	•	•		•					•	•							•	•									•	•	•					•	
Basil	•	•	•	•	•	•	•	•							•	•	•		•			•	•	•			•	•	•	•	•					•	
Bergamot	•		•		•										•				•							•	•	•	•		•	•				•	
Birch		•	•									•														•		•	•		•						•
Black Pepper	•					•				•					•				•							•			•								•
Black Spruce						•		•								•	•			•				•		•		•	•	•		•					
Blue Tansy								•		•		•	•		•								•				•		•	•				•	•		
Cardamom	•		•			•																							•	•	•	•					
Cassia				•							•												•														•
Cedarwood			•	•		•		•				•	•			•						•	•				•	•	•		•	•				•	
Celery Seed	•		•						•			•								•			•				•			•							
Cilantro																																					
Cinnamon	•			•							•	•								•									•	•						•	•
Citronella			•									•	•																•	•	•	•					
Clary Sage	•			•			•	•		•						•	•		•				•				•			•	•	•			•		
Clove		•			•	•					•						•					•							•							•	•
Copaiba		•	•							•	•		•		•	•																		•			
Coriander	•												•									•			•		•		•	•	•						
Cypress			•		•			•								•			•		•		•						•		•	•	•				
Dill	•			•		•	•	•		•																			•								
Douglas fir			•		•	•									•												•		•	•							
Eucalyptus		•	•			•				•	•	•	•							•						•			•							•	•
Fennel	•		•	•		•	•	•			•				•	•							•					•	•	•	•					•	
Frankincense	•	•	•				•				•							•				•		•			•				•						
Geranium			•									•									•	•	•				•				•					•	
Ginger				•		•					•				•				•							•			•	•	•						•
Grapefruit	•	•	•		•									•						•	•								•		•	•					
Green Mandarin	•		•			•											•					•		•		•	•				•	•					
Helichrysum	•		•			•										•	•					•				•							•				
Jasmine				•		•	•	•	•													•	•				•										
Juniper berry	•		•	•													•								•	•	•		•	•	•						
Kumquat	•				•					•	•			•		•		•			•	•		•	•		•		•	•	•	•			•		
Lavender			•	•						•			•				•	•				•	•			•	•				•				•	•	
Lemon		•	•		•					•	•		•	•		•					•				•	•					•	•				•	
Lemon Eucalyptus	•	•				•					•	•				•										•				•							
Lemongrass	•				•	•	•	•					•				•			•		•			•		•				•			•			•
Lime		•	•		•						•									•	•			•	•				•		•	•					
Litsea	•	•								•		•		•									•									•		•			
Magnolia								•								•		•		•			•			•	•			•							
Manuka										•										•		•	•		•									•			
Marjoram	•			•		•				•										•			•				•			•	•			•			•
Melaleuca	•					•		•			•		•						•	•	•	•							•							•	
Melissa									•		•						•										•			•	•	•					
Myrrh	•			•		•										•						•	•						•		•						
Neroli		•								•									•			•	•	•			•				•			•			•
Oregano	•	•		•		•					•									•															•		•
Patchouli	•		•						•		•	•	•				•					•		•			•	•	•		•						
Peppermint				•	•	•								•			•				•									•			•			•	•
Petitgrain											•												•				•				•	•					
Pink Pepper	•		•		•	•						•		•	•					•	•		•			•			•	•	•	•					•
Ravensara		•	•			•					•												•								•						

Chart continues on next page ⟶

Oil Properties Chart R-Y

Oil Properties	analgesic	anaphrodisiac	anti-allergenic	antiarthritic	antibacterial	anticarcinogenic	anti-carcinoma	anticatarrhal	anticoagulant	anticonvulsant	antidepressant	antiemetic	antifungal	antihemorrhagic	antihistamine	anti-infectious
Red Mandarin					•	•						•	•			
Roman chamomile																•
Rose											•					•
Rosemary	•				•		•	•					•			•
Sandalwood					•		•	•			•		•			
Siberian fir	•				•								•			
Spearmint					•			•					•			
Spikenard					•								•			
Tangerine						•	•		•	•	•					
Thyme					•								•			
Turmeric	•		•		•	•	•			•			•			
Vetiver																
White fir	•			•				•								
Wild orange	•				•		•				•		•			
Wintergreen	•															
Yarrow	•					•	•							•	•	
Ylang ylang					•						•					

Oil Properties	anti-inflammatory	antimicrobial	antimutagenic	antioxidant	anti-parasitic	antirheumatic	antiseptic	antispasmodic	antitoxic	anti-tumoral	antiviral	aphrodisiac
Red Mandarin	•	•		•			•	•		•	•	
Roman chamomile	•				•			•				
Rose							•	•			•	•
Rosemary	•	•		•	•	•	•	•				•
Sandalwood	•						•	•		•		•
Siberian fir	•	•					•	•			•	
Spearmint	•						•	•				•
Spikenard	•											
Tangerine	•		•	•	•		•	•				
Thyme		•		•	•	•	•	•	•		•	•
Turmeric	•	•	•	•	•		•			•	•	
Vetiver				•			•	•				•
White fir						•	•				•	
Wild orange	•			•			•	•				•
Wintergreen	•					•	•	•				
Yarrow	•			•		•		•			•	
Ylang ylang							•	•				•

Oil Properties	astringent	bactericidal	calming	cardiotonic	carminative	cleanser	cytophylactic	decongestant	deodorant	detoxifier
Red Mandarin	•		•		•	•	•			•
Roman chamomile			•	•	•					
Rose		•		•	•					
Rosemary	•		•	•	•		•			•
Sandalwood	•		•	•	•					
Siberian fir								•	•	
Spearmint				•	•					
Spikenard									•	
Tangerine			•		•		•			•
Thyme				•	•	•				
Turmeric					•			•		•
Vetiver			•	•	•					
White fir	•		•					•	•	
Wild orange				•	•	•				•
Wintergreen	•		•	•	•					
Yarrow	•		•		•			•		•
Ylang ylang										

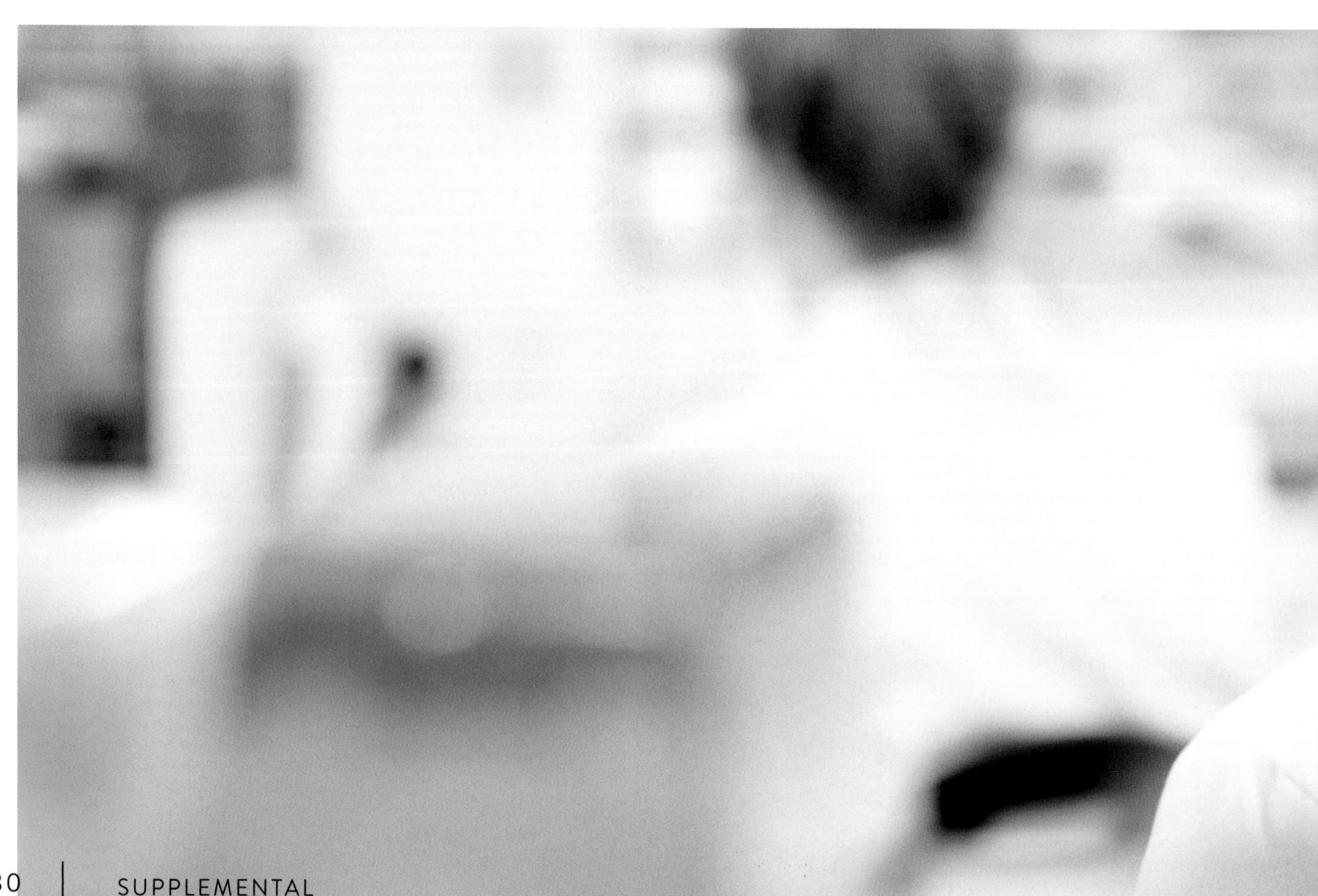

	digestive stimulant	disinfectant	diuretic	emmenagogue	energizing	expectorant	galactagogue	grounding	hypertensive	hypotensive	immunostimulant	insect repellent	insecticidal	invigorating	laxative	mucolytic	nervine	neuroprotective	neurotonic	purifier	refreshing	regenerative	relaxant	restorative	revitalizer	rubefacient	sedative	steroidal	stimulant	stomachic	tonic	uplifting	vasoconstrictor	vasodilator	vermicide	vermifuge	warming
Red Mandarin	•		•			•					•						•				•		•	•		•	•			•	•	•					
Roman chamomile				•														•					•				•				•					•	
Rose				•											•		•										•			•	•						
Rosemary			•	•	•	•			•		•						•							•		•		•	•	•	•			•		•	
Sandalwood			•			•			•				•								•	•		•			•				•	•					
Siberian fir					•	•		•	•		•			•						•	•					•			•		•		•				
Spearmint	•			•	•						•		•	•										•					•								
Spikenard															•												•										
Tangerine	•		•		•										•	•				•				•			•		•	•	•	•					
Thyme			•	•		•			•		•	•	•				•	•								•		•	•					•		•	•
Turmeric	•					•						•						•					•				•			•							•
Vetiver								•			•	•	•					•								•	•		•		•					•	
White fir			•		•	•				•	•												•			•			•		•		•				
Wild orange	•		•		•						•			•						•	•	•								•	•	•				•	
Wintergreen		•	•	•			•	•						•							•							•	•						•	•	•
Yarrow	•			•	•	•				•	•				•	•				•		•					•	•		•	•						
Ylang Ylang								•		•	•	•											•				•		•		•	•	•				

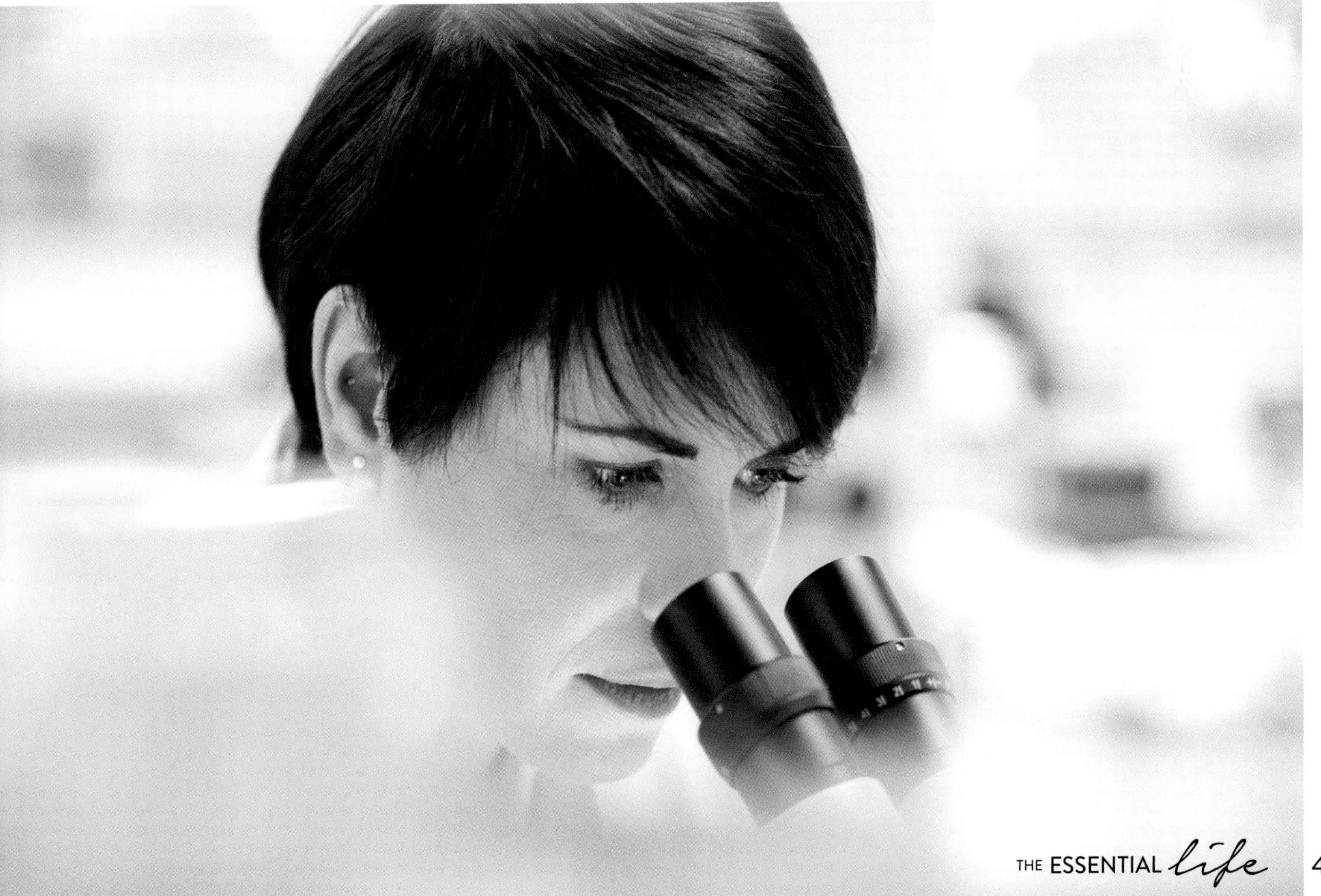

Recipe Index

Research Index

ADDICTION

The effects of aromatherapy on nicotine craving on a U.S. campus: a small comparison study, Cordell B, Buckle J, *The Journal of Alternative and Complementary Medicine*, 2013

ALERTNESS

Effects of Peppermint and Cinnamon Odor Administration on Simulated Driving Alertness, Mood and Workload, Raudenbush B, Grayhem R, Sears T, Wilson I., *North American Journal of Psychology*, 2009

The influence of essential oils on human attention. I: alertness, Ilmberger J, Heuberger E, Mahrhofer C, Dessovic H, Kowarik D, Buchbauer G, *Chemical Senses*, 2001

The influence of essential oils on human vigilance, Heuberger E, Ilmberger J, *Natural Product Communications*, 2010

Volatiles emitted from the roots of Vetiveria zizanioides suppress the decline in attention during a visual display terminal taskvi, Matsubara E, Shimizu K, Fukagawa M, Ishizi Y, Kakoi C, Hatayama T, Nagano J, Okamoto T, Ohnuki K, Kondo R, *Biomedical Research*, 2012

ALLERGIES

Cytological aspects on the effects of a nasal spray consisting of standardized extract of citrus lemon and essential oils in allergic rhinopathy, Ferrara L, Naviglio D, Armone Caruso A, *ISRN Pharm*, 2012

ALZHEIMER'S DISEASE

Effect of arborvitae seed on cognitive function and α7nAChR protein expression of hippocampus in model rats with Alzheimer's disease, Cheng XL, Xiong XB, Xiang MQ, *Cell Biochem Biophys*, 2013

Effect of aromatherapy on patients with Alzheimer's disease, Jimbo D, Kimura Y, Taniguchi M, Inoue M, Urakami K, *Psychogeriatrics*, 2009

Inhalation of coriander volatile oil increased anxiolytic-antidepressant-like behaviors and decreased oxidative status in beta-amyloid (1-42) rat model of Alzheimer's disease, Cioanca O, Hritcu L, Mihasan M, Trifan A, Hancianu M, *Physiology & Behavior*, 2014

ANTIBACTERIAL

Activity of Essential Oils Against Bacillus subtilis Spores, Lawrence HA, Palombo EA, *Journal of Microbiology and Biotechnology*, 2009

Antibacterial activity of essential oils and their major constituents against respiratory tract pathogens by gaseous contact, Inouye S, Takizawa T, Yamaguchi H, *The Journal of Antimicrobial Chemotherapy*, 2001

Antibacterial activity of Litsea cubeba (Lauraceae, May Chang) and its effects on the biological response of common carp Cyprinus carpio challenged with Aeromonas hydrophila. Nguyen HV, Caruso D, Lebrun M, Nguyen NT, Trinh TT, Meile JC, Chu-Ky S, Sarter S. J Appl Microbiol. 2016

Antibacterial activity of the essential oil from Rosmarinus officinalis and its major components against oral pathogens, Bernardes WA, Lucarini R, Tozatti MG, Flauzino LG, Soutza MG, Turatti IC, Andrade e Silva ML, Martins CH, da Silva Filho AA, Cunha WR, *Zeitschrift Fur Naturforschung C-A Journal of Biosciences*, 2010

Antibacterial and antioxidant properties of Mediterranean aromatic plants, Piccaglia R, Marotti M, Giovanelli E, Deans SG, Eaglesham E, *Industrial Crops and Products*, 1993

Antibacterial Effects of the Essential Oils of Commonly Consumed Medicinal Herbs Using an In Vitro Model, Soković M, Glamočlija J, Marin PD, Brkić D, van Griensven LJ, *Molecules*, 2010

Atomic force microscopy analysis shows surface structure changes in carvacrol-treated bacterial cells, La Storia A, Ercolini D, Marinello F, Di Pasqua R, Villani F, Mauriello G, *Research in Microbiology*, 2011

Bactericidal activities of plant essential oils and some of their isolated constituents against Campylobacter jejuni, Escherichia coli, Listeria monocytogenes, and Salmonella enterica, Friedman M, Henika PR, Mandrell RE, *Journal of Food Protection*, 2002

Bacteriostatic effect of copaiba oil (Copaifera officinalis) against Streptococcus mutans. Pieri FA et al. Braz Dent J. 2012

Chemical composition and antibacterial activity of selected essential oils and some of their main compounds, Wanner J, Schmidt E, Bail S, Jirovetz L, Buchbauer G, Gochev V, Girova T, Atanasova T, Stoyanova A, *Natural Product Communications*, 2010

Chemical composition, antibacterial activity and cytotoxicity of essential oils of Tanacetumparthenium in different developmental stages. Mohsenzadeh F, Chehregani A, Amiri H. Pharm Biol. 2011 Sep;49(9):920-6. doi: 10.3109/13880209.2011.556650. Epub, 2011

Coriander (Coriandrum sativum L.) essential oil: its antibacterial activity and mode of action evaluated by flow cytometry, Silva F, Ferreira S, Queiroz JA, Domingues FC, *Journal of Medical Microbiology*, 2011

Effects of Helichrysum italicum extract on growth and enzymatic activity of Staphylococcus aureus, Nostro A, Bisignano G, Angela Cannatelli M, Crisafi G, Paola Germanò M, Alonzo V, *International Journal of Antimicrobial Agents*, 2001

Eugenol (an essential oil of clove) acts as an antibacterial agent against Salmonella typhi by disrupting the cellular membrane, Devi KP, Nisha SA, Sakthivel R, Pandian SK, *Journal of Ethnopharmacology*, 2010

Evaluation of bacterial resistance to essential oils and antibiotics after exposure to oregano and cinnamon essential oils, Becerril R, Nerín C, Gómez-Lus R, *Foodborne Pathogens and Disease*, 2012

Growth inhibition of pathogenic bacteria and some yeasts by selected essential oils and survival o roma f L. monocytogenes and C. albicans in apple-carrot juice., Irkin R, Korukluoglu M, *Foodborne Pathogens and Disease*, 2009

Helichrysum italicum extract interferes with the production of enterotoxins by Staphylococcus aureus., Nostro A, Cannatelli MA, Musolino AD, Procopio F, Alonzo V, *Letters in Applied Microbiology*, 2002

In vitro antibacterial activity of some plant essential oils, Prabuseenivasan S, Jayakumar M, Ignacimuthu S, *BMC Complementary and Alternative Medicine*, 2006

Inhibition by the essential oils of peppermint and spearmint of the growth of pathogenic bacteria, Imai H, Osawa K, Yasuda H, Hamashima H, Arai T, Sasatsu M, *Microbios*, 2001

Investigation of antibacterial activity of rosemary essential oil against Propionibacterium acnes with atomic force microscopy, Fu Y, Zu Y, Chen L, Efferth T, Liang H, Liu Z, Liu W, *Planta Medica*, 2007

Origanum vulgare subsp. hirtum Essential Oil Prevented Biofilm Formation and Showed Antibacterial Activity against Planktonic and Sessile Bacterial Cells, Schillaci D, Napoli EM, Cusimano MG, Vitale M, Ruberto A, *Journal of Food Protection*, 2013

Potential of rosemary oil to be used in drug-resistant infections, Luqman S, Dwivedi GR, Darokar MP, Kalra A, Khanuja SP, *Alternative Therapies in Health and Medicine*, 2007

Screening of the antibacterial effects of a variety of essential oils on microorganisms responsible for respiratory infections, Fabio A, Cermelli C, Fabio G, Nicoletti P, Quaglio P, *Phytotherapy Research*, 2007

Screening of the antibacterial effects of a variety of essential oils on respiratory tract pathogens, using a modified dilution assay method, Inouye S, Yamaguchi H, Takizawa T, *Journal of Infection and Chemotherapy: Official Journal of the Japan Society of Chemotherapy*, 2001

Some evidences on the mode of action of Cinnamomum verum bark essential oil, alone and in combination with piperacillin against a multi-drug resistant Escherichia coli strain, Yap PS, Krishnan T, Chan KG, Lim SH, *Journal of Microbiology and Biotechnology*, 2014

Sub-inhibitory stress with essential oil affects enterotoxins production and essential oil susceptibility in Staphylococcus aureus. Turchi B, Mancini S, Pistelli L, Najar B, Cerri D, Fratini F. Nat Prod Res. 2017 .

Tea tree oil-induced transcriptional alterations in Staphylococcus aureus, Cuaron JA, Dulal S, Song Y, Singh AK, Montelongo CE, Yu W, Nagarajan V, Jayaswal RK, Wilkinson BJ, Gustafson JE, *Phytotherapy Research*, 2013

The anti-biofilm activity of lemongrass (Cymbopogon flexuosus) and grapefruit (Citrus paradisi) essential oils against five strains of Staphylococcus aureus, Adukwu EC, Allen SC, Phillips CA, *Journal of Applied Microbiology*, 2012

The antibacterial activity of geranium oil against Gram-negative bacteria isolated from difficult-to-heal wounds, Sienkiewicz M, Poznańska-Kurowska K, Kaszuba A, Kowalczyk E, *Burns*, 2014

The effect of lemongrass EO highlights its potential against antibiotic resistant Staph. aureus in the healthcare environment, Adukwu EC, Allen SC, Phillips CA, *Journal of Applied Microbiology*, 2012

The potential of use basil and rosemary essential oils as effective antibacterial agents, Sienkiewicz M, Łysakowska M, Pastuszka M, Bienias W, Kowalczyk E, *Molecules*, 2013

ANTIFUNGAL

Antibacterial, antifungal, and anticancer activities of volatile oils and extracts from stems, leaves, and flowers of Eucalyptus sideroxylon and Eucalyptus torquata, Ashour HM, *Cancer Biology and Therapy*, 2008

Antifungal activity of clove essential oil and its volatile vapour against dermatophytic fungi, Chee HY, Lee MH, *Mycobiology*, 2007

Antifungal mechanism of essential oil from Anethum graveolens seeds against Candida albicans, Chen Y, Zeng H, Tian J, Ban X, Ma B, Wang Y, *Journal of Medical Microbiology*, 2013

Antifungal, anti-biofilm and adhesion activity of the essential oil of Myrtus communis L. against Candida species, Cannas S, Molicotti P, Usai D, Maxia A, Zanetti S, *Natural Product Research*, 2014

Chemical composition, bio-herbicidal and antifungal activities of essential oils isolated from Tunisian common cypress (Cupressus sempervirens L.), Ismail A, Lamia H, Mohsen H, Samia G, Bassem J, *Journal of Medicinal Plants Research*, 2013

Coriandrum sativum L. (Coriander) Essential Oil: Antifungal Activity and Mode of Action on Candida spp., and Molecular Targets Affected in Human Whole-Genome Expression, Freires Ide A, Murata RM, Furletti VF, Sartoratto A, Alencar SM, Figueira GM, de Oliveira Rodrigues JA, Duarte MC, Rosalen PL, *PLoS One*, 2014

Dill (Anethum graveolens L.) seed essential oil induces Candida albicans apoptosis in a metacaspase-dependent manner, Chen Y, Zeng H, Tian J, Ban X, Ma B, Wang Y, *Fungal Biology*, 2014

In vitro antagonistic activity of monoterpenes and their mixtures against 'toe nail fungus' pathogens, Ramsewak RS, Nair MG, Stommel M, Selanders L, *Phytotherapy Research*, 2003

In-vitro and in-vivo anti-Trichophyton activity of essential oils by vapour contact, Inouye S, Uchida K, Yamaguchi H, *Mycoses*, 2001

Oil of bitter orange: new topical antifungal agent, Ramadan W, Mourad B, Ibrahim S, Sonbol F, *International Journal of Dermatology*, 1996

ANTIMICROBIAL

A novel aromatic oil compound inhibits microbial overgrowth on feet: a case study, Misner BD, *Journal of the International Society of Sports Nutrition*, 2007

Antimicrobial activities of cinnamon oil and cinnamaldehyde from the Chinese medicinal herb Cinnamomum cassia Blume, Ooi LS, Li Y, Kam SL, Wang H, Wong EY, Ooi VE, *The American Journal of Chinese Medicine*, 2006

Antimicrobial Activities of Clove and Thyme Extracts, Nzeako BC, Al-Kharousi ZS, Al-Mahrooqui Z, *Sultan Qaboos University Medical Journal*, 2006

Antimicrobial activity against bacteria with dermatological relevance and skin tolerance of the essential oil from Coriandrum sativum L. fruits, Casetti F, Bartelke S, Biehler K, Augustin M, Schempp CM, Frank U, *Phytotherapy Research*, 2012

Antimicrobial activity of clove oil and its potential in the treatment of vaginal candidiasis, Ahmad N, Alam MK, Shehbaz A, Khan A, Mannan A, Hakim SR, Bisht D, Owais M, *Journal of Drug Targeting*, 2005

Antimicrobial Activity of Copaiba (Copaifera officinalis) and Pracaxi (Pentaclethra macroloba) Oils against Staphylococcus Aureus: Importance in Compounding for Wound Care.Guimarães AL et al. Int J Pharm Compd. 2016

Antimicrobial activity of essential oils and five terpenoid compounds against Campylobacter jejuni in pure and mixed culture experiments, Kurekci C, Padmanabha J, Bishop-Hurley SL, Hassan E, Al Jassim RA, McSweeney CS, *International Journal of Food Microbiology*, 2013

Antimicrobial activity of individual and mixed fractions of dill, cilantro, coriander and eucalyptus essential oils, Delaquis PJ, Stanich K, Girard B, Mazza G, *International Journal of Food Microbiology*, 2002

Antimicrobial activity of juniper berry essential oil (Juniperus communis L., Cupressaceae), Pepeljnjak S, Kosalec I, Kalodera Z, Blažević N, *Acta Pharmaceutica*, 2005

Antimicrobial activity of the bioactive components of essential oils from Pakistani spices against Salmonella and other multi-drug resistant bacteria, Naveed R, Hussain I, Tawab A, Tariq M, Rahman M, Hameed S, Mahmood MS, Siddique AB, Iqbal M, *BMC Complementary and Alternative Medicine*, 2013

Antimicrobial Effect and Mode of Action of Terpeneless Cold Pressed Valencia Orange Essential Oil on Methicillin-Resistant Staphylococcus aureus, Muthaiyan A, Martin EM, Natesan S, Cran-

dall PG, Wilkinson BJ, Ricke SC, *Journal of Applied Microbiology*, 2012
Antimicrobial effects of essential oils in combination with chlorhexidine digluconate, Filoche SK, Soma K, Sissons CH, *Oral Microbiology and Immunology*, 2005
Antimicrobial effects of Manuka honey on in vitro biofilm formation by Clostridium difficile. Piotrowski M, Karpiński P, Pituch H, van Belkum A, Obuch-Woszczatyński P. Eur J Clin Microbiol Infect Dis. 2017
Chemical composition and in vitro antimicrobial activity of essential oil of Melissa officinalis L. from Romania, Hăncianu M, Aprotosoaie AC, Gille E, Poiată A, Tuchiluş C, Spac A, Stănescu U, *Revista Medico-Chirurgicala a Societatii de Medici si Naturalisti din Iasi*, 2008
Comparative evaluation of 11 essential oils of different origin as functional antioxidants, antiradicals and antimicrobials in foods, Sacchetti G, Maietti S, Muzzoli M, Scaglianti M, Manfredini S, Radice M, Bruni R, Food Chemistry, 2005
Comparison of essential oils from three plants for enhancement of antimicrobial activity of nitrofurantoin against enterobacteria, Rafii F, Shahverdi AR, *Chemotherapy*, 2007
Essential Oil Compositions and Antimicrobial Activities of Various Parts of Litsea cubeba from Taiwan. Su YC, Ho CL. Nat Prod Commun. 2016
Essential Oil Compositions and Antimicrobial Activities of Various Parts of Litsea cubeba from Taiwan. Su YC, Ho CL. Nat Prod Commun. 2016
Evaluation of the antimicrobial properties of different parts of Citrus aurantifolia (lime fruit) as used locally, Aibinu I, Adenipekun T, Adelowotan T, Ogunsanya T, Odugbemi T, *African Journal of Traditional, Complementary, and Alternative Medicines*, 2006
Immune-Modifying and Antimicrobial Effects of Eucalyptus Oil and Simple Inhalation Devices, Sadlon AE, Lamson DW, *Alternative Medicine Review: A Journal of Clinical Therapeutic*, 2010
Microbicide activity of clove essential oil (Eugenia caryophyllata), Nuñez L, Aquino MD, *Brazilian Journal of Microbiology*, 2012
Oregano essential oil as an antimicrobial additive to detergent for hand washing and food contact surface cleaning, Rhoades J, Gialagkolidou K, Gogou M, Mavridou O, Blatsiotis N, Ritzoulis C, Likotrafiti E, Journal of Applied Microbiology, 2013
Study of the antimicrobial action of various essential oils extracted from Malagasy plants. II: Lauraceae, Raharivelomanana PJ, Terrom GP, Bianchini JP, Coulanges P, *Arch Inst Pasteur Madagascar*, 1989
The additive and synergistic antimicrobial effects of select frankincense and myrrh oils--a combination from the pharaonic pharmacopoeia, de Rapper S, Van Vuuren SF, Kamatou GP, Viljoen AM, Dagne E, *Letters in Applied Microbiology*, 2012
The battle against multi-resistant strains: Renaissance of antimicrobial essential oils as a promising force to fight hospital-acquired infections, Warnke PH, Becker ST, Podschun R, Sivananthan S, Springer IN, Russo PA, Wiltfang J, Fickenscher H, Sherry E, *Journal of Cranio-Maxillo-Facial Surgery*, 200
Volatile composition and antimicrobial activity of twenty commercial frankincense essential oil samples, Van Vuurena SF, Kamatoub GPP, Viljoenb, AM, *South African Journal of Botany*, 2010

ANTIOXIDANT
Anti-Inflammatory and Antioxidant Actions of Copaiba Oil Are Related to Liver Cell Modifications in Arthritic Rats. Castro Ghizoni CV, Arssufi Ames AP, Lameira OA, Bersani Amado CA, Sá Nakanishi AB, Bracht L, Marçal Natali MR, Peralta RM, Bracht A, Comar JF. J Cell Biochem. 2017
Antioxidant activities and volatile constituents of various essential oils, Wei A, Shibamoto T, Journal of Agriculture and Food Chemistry, 2007
Antioxidant activity of rosemary (Rosmarinus officinalis L.) essential oil and its hepatoprotective potential, Ra Kovi A, Milanovi I, Pavlovi NA, Ebovi T, Vukmirovi SA, Mikov M, *BMC Complementary and Alternative Medicine*, 2014
Antioxidant and antimicrobial activities of essential oils obtained from oregano, Karakaya S, El SN, Karagözlü N, Sahin S, *Journal of Medicinal Food*, 2011
Antioxidant and Hepatoprotective Potential of Essential Oils of Coriander (Coriandrum sativum L.) and Caraway (Carum carvi L.) (Apiaceae), Samojlik I, Lakić N, Mimica-Dukić N, Đaković-Svajcer K, Bozin B, *Journal of Agricultural and Food Chemistry*, 2010
Antioxidant potential of the root of Vetiveria zizanioides (L.) Nash, Luqman S, Kumar R, Kaushik S, Srivastava S, Darokar MP, Khanuja SP, *Indian Journal of Biochemistry and Biophysics*, 2009
Antioxidative effects of lemon oil and its components on copper induced oxidation of low density lipoprotein, Grassmann J, Schneider D, Weiser D, Elstner EF, *Arzneimittel-Forschung*, 2001
Biological effects, antioxidant and anticancer activities of marigold and basil essential oils, Mahmoud GI, *Journal of Medicinal Plants Research*, 2013
Comparative evaluation of 11 essential oils of different origin as functional antioxidants, antiradicals and antimicrobials in foods, Sacchetti G, Maietti S, Muzzoli M, Scaglianti M, Manfredini S, Radice M, Bruni R, Food Chemistry, 2005
Evaluation of in vivo anti-hyperglycemic and antioxidant potentials of α-santalol and sandalwood oil, Misra BB, Dey S, *Phytomedicine*, 2013
In Vitro Antioxidant Activities of Essential Oils, Veerapan P, Khunkitti W, *Isan Journal of Pharmaceutical Sciences*, 2011
Minor Furanocoumarins and Coumarins in Grapefruit Peel Oil as Inhibitors of Human Cytochrome P450 3A4, César TB, Manthey JA, Myung K, *Journal of Natural Products*, 2009

ANTIVIRAL
Antiviral activities in plants endemic to madagascar, Hudson JB, Lee MK, Rasoanaivo P, *Pharm Biol.* 2000
Antiviral activity of the volatile oils of Melissa officinalis L. against Herpes simplex virus type-2, Allahverdiyev A, Duran N, Ozguven M, Koltas S, *Phytomedicine*, 2004
Antiviral efficacy and mechanisms of action of oregano essential oil and its primary component carvacrol against murine norovirus, Gilling DH, Kitajima M, Torrey JR, Bright KR, *Journal of Applied Microbiology*, 2014
Immunologic mechanism of Patchouli alcohol anti-H1N1 influenza virus may through regulation of the RLH signal pathway in vitro, Wu XL, Ju DH, Chen J, Yu B, Liu KL, He JX, Dai CQ, Wu S, Chang Z, Wang YP, Chen XY, *Current Microbiology*, 2013
Oral administration of patchouli alcohol isolated from Pogostemonis Herba augments protection against influenza viral infection in mice, Li YC, Peng SZ, Chen HM, Zhang FX, Xu PP, Xie JH, He JJ, Chen JN, Lai XP, Su ZR, International Immunopharmacology, 2012

ANXIETY
Ambient odor of orange in a dental office reduces anxiety and improves mood in female patients, Lehrner J, Eckersberger C, Walla P, Pötsch G, Deecke L, *Physiology and Behavior*, 2000
Anxiolytic-like effects of rose oil inhalation on the elevated plus-maze test in rats, de Almeida RN, Motta SC, de Brito Faturi C, Catallani B, Leite JR, *Pharmacology Biochemistry and Behavior*, 2004
Effect of sweet orange aroma on experimental anxiety in humans, Goes TC, Antunes FD, Alves PB, Teixeira-Silva F, *The Journal of Alternative and Complementary Medicine*
Essential oils and anxiolytic aromatherapy, Setzer WN, *Natural Product Communications*, 2009
The effects of prolonged rose odor inhalation in two animal models of anxiety, Bradley BF, Starkey NJ, Brown SL, Lea RW, *Physiology & Behavior*, 2007
The GABAergic system contributes to the anxiolytic-like effect of essential oil from Cymbopogon citratus (lemongrass), Costa CA, Kohn DO, de Lima VM, Gargano AC, Flório JC, Costa M, *Journal of Ethnopharmacology*, 2011

ARTHRITIS
Anti-arthritic effect of eugenol on collagen-induced arthritis experimental model, Grespan R, Paludo M, Lemos Hde P, Barbosa CP, Bersani-Amado CA, Dalalio MM, Cuman RK, *Biological and Pharmaceutical Bulletin*, 2012
The effects of aromatherapy on pain, depression, and life satisfaction of arthritis patients, Kim MJ, Nam ES, Paik SI, *Taehan Kanho Hakhoe Chi*, 2005

BEHAVIOR
Immunological and Psychological Benefits of Aromatherapy Massage, Kuriyama H, Watanabe S, Nakaya T, Shigemori I, Kita M, Yoshida N, Masaki D, Tadai T, Ozasa K, Fukui K, Imanishi J, *Evidence-based Complementary and Alternative Medicine*, 2005
The effect of gender and ethnicity on children's attitudes and preferences for essential oils: a pilot study, Fitzgerald M, Culbert T, Finkelstein M, Green M, Johnson A, Chen S, *Explore (New York, N.Y.)*, 2007

BLOOD
Black pepper essential oil to enhance intravenous catheter insertion in patients with poor vein visibility: a controlled study, Kristiniak S, Harpel J, Breckenridge DM, Buckle J, *Journal of Alternative and Complementary Medicine*, 2012
Comparative screening of plant essential oils: Phenylpropanoid moiety as basic core for antiplatelet activity, Tognolini M, Barocelli E, Ballabeni V, Bruni R, Bianchi A, Chiavarini M, Impicciatore M, *Life Sciences*, 2006
Comparison of oral aspirin versus topical applied methyl salicylate for platelet inhibition, Tanen DA, Danish DC, Reardon JM, Chisholm CB, Matteucci MJ, Riffenburgh RH, *Annals of Pharmacotherapy*, 2008
Effects of a novel formulation of essential oils on glucose-insulin metabolism in diabetic and hypertensive rats: a pilot study, Talpur N, Echard B, Ingram C, Bagchi D, Preuss H, Diabetes, *Obesity and Metabolism*, 2005
Mechanism of changes induced in plasma glycerol by scent stimulation with grapefruit and lavender essential oils, Shen J, Niijima A, Tanida M, Horii Y, Nakamura T, Nagai K, *Neuroscience Letters*, 2007
Suppression of neutrophil accumulation in mice by cutaneous application of geranium essential oil, Maruyama N, Sekimoto Y, Ishibashi H, Inouye S, Oshima H, Yamaguchi H, Abe S, *Journal of Inflammation (London, England)*, 2005

BLOOD PRESSURE
Antioxidative Properties and Inhibition of Key Enzymes Relevant to Type-2 Diabetes and Hypertension by Essential Oils from Black Pepper, Oboh G, Ademosun AO, Odubanjo OV, Akinbola IA, *Advances in Pharmacological Sciences*, 2013
Effects of Aromatherapy Massage on Blood Pressure and Lipid Profile in Korean Climacteric Women, Myung-HH , Heeyoung OH, Myeong SL, Chan K, Ae-na C, Gil-ran S, *International Journal of Neuroscience*, 2007
Effects of Ylang-Ylang aroma on blood pressure and heart rate in healthy men, Jung DJ, Cha JY, Kim SE, Ko IG, Jee YS, *Journal of Exercise Rehabilitation*, 2013
Essential oil inhalation on blood pressure and salivary cortisol levels in prehypertensive and hypertensive subjects, Kim IH, Kim C, Seong K, Hur MH, Lim HM, Lee MS, *Evidence-Based Complementary and Alternative Medicine*, 2012
Inhibitory potential of omega-3 fatty and fenugreek essential oil on key enzymes of carbohydrate-digestion and hypertension in diabetes rats, Hamden K, Keskes H, Belhaj S, Mnafgui K, Feki A, Allouche N, *Lipids in Health and Disease*, 2011
Olfactory stimulation with scent of essential oil of grapefruit affects autonomic neurotransmission and blood pressure, Tanida M, Niijima A, Shen J, Nakamura T, Nagai K, *Brian Research*, 2005
Randomized controlled trial for Salvia sclarea or Lavandula angustifolia: differential effects on blood pressure in female patients with urinary incontinence undergoing urodynamic examination, Seol GH, Lee YH, Kang P, You JH, Park M, Min SS, *The Journal of Alternative and Complementary Medicine*, 2013
The effects of the inhalation method using essential oils on blood pressure and stress responses of clients with essential hypertension, Hwang JH, *Korean Society of Nursing Science*, 2006
Neroli EO (that is extracted from flowers of Citrus aurantium) demonstrated the capacity to reduce systolic pressure in patients undergoing colonoscopy. Stea, Susanna, Alina Beraudi, and Dalila De Pasquale. "Essential Oils for Complementary Treatment of Surgical Patients: State of the Art." Evidence-based Complementary and Alternative Medicine, 2014.

BRAIN
Effects of fragrance inhalation on sympathetic activity in normal adults, Haze S, Sakai K, Gozu Y, *The Japanese Journal of Pharmacology*, 2002
Essential oil from lemon peels inhibit key enzymes linked to neurodegenerative conditions and pro-oxidant induced lipid peroxidation, Oboh G, Olasehinde TA, Ademosun AO, *Journal of Oleo Science*, 2014
Inhibition of acetylcholinesterase activity by essential oil from Citrus paradisi, Miyazawa M, Tougo H, Ishihara M, *Natural Product Letters*, 2001
Neuropharmacology of the essential oil of bergamot, Bagetta G, Morrone LA, Rombolà L, Amantea D, Russo R, Berliocchi L, Sakurada S, Sakurada T, Rotiroti D, Corasaniti MT, *Fitoterapia*, 2010
Olfactory receptor neuron profiling using sandalwood odorants., Bieri S, Monastyrskaia K, Schilling B, *Chemical Senses*, 2004
Plasma 1,8-cineole correlates with cognitive performance following exposure to rosemary essential oil aroma, Moss M, Oliver L, *Therapeutic Advances in Psychopharmacology*, 2012
The essential oil of bergamot enhances the levels of amino acid neurotransmitters in the hippocampus of rat: implication of monoterpene hydrocarbons, Morrone LA, Rombolà L, Pelle C, Corasaniti MT, Zappettini S, Paudice P, Bonanno G, Bagetta G, *Pharmacological Research*, 2007

CANCER

Alpha-santalol, a chemopreventive agent against skin cancer, causes G2/M cell cycle arrest in both p53-mutated human epidermoid carcinoma A431 cells and p53 wild-type human melanoma UACC-62 cells, Zhang X, Chen W, Guillermo R, Chandrasekher G, Kaushik RS, Young A, Fahmy H, Dwivedi C, *BMC Research Notes*, 2010

Anticancer activity of an essential oil from Cymbopogon flexuosus (lemongrass), Sharma PR, Mondhe DM, Muthiah S, Pal HC, Shahi AK, Saxena AK, Qazi GN, *Chemico-Biological Interactions*, 2009

Anticancer activity of liposomal bergamot essential oil (BEO) on human neuroblastoma cells, Celia C, Trapasso E, Locatelli M, Navarra M, Ventura CA, Wolfram J, Carafa M, Morittu VM, Britti D, Di Marzio L, Paolino D, *Colloids and Surfaces*, 2013

Antioxidant and Anticancer Activities of Citrus reticulate (Petitgrain Mandarin) and Pelargonium graveolens (Geranium) Essential Oils, Fayed SA, *Research Journal of Agriculture and Biological Sciences*, 2009

Apoptosis-mediated proliferation inhibition of human colon cancer cells by volatile principles of Citrus aurantifolia, Patil JR, Jayaprakasha GK, Chidambara Murthy KN, Tichy SE, Chetti MB, Patil BS, Food Chemistry, 2009

Biological effects, antioxidant and anticancer activities of marigold and basil essential oils, Mahmoud GI, *Journal of Medicinal Plants Research*, 2013

Composition and potential anticancer activities of essential oils obtained from myrrh and frankincense, Chen Y, Zhou C, Ge Z, Liu Y, Liu Y, Feng W, Li S, Chen G, Wei T, *Oncology Letters*, 2013

Conservative surgical management of stage IA endometrial carcinoma for fertility preservation, Mazzon I, Corrado G, Masciullo V, Morricone D, Ferrandina G, Scambia G, *Fertil Steril*, 2010

Differential effects of selective frankincense (Ru Xiang) essential oil versus non-selective sandalwood (Tan Xiang) essential oil on cultured bladder cancer cells: a microarray and bioinformatics study, Dozmorov MG, Yang Q, Wu W, Wren J, Suhail MM, Woolley CL, Young DG, Fung KM, Lin HK, *Chinese Medicine*, 2014

Effect of Vetiveria zizanioides Essential Oil on Melanogenesis in Melanoma Cells: Downregulation of Tyrosinase Expression and Suppression of Oxidative Stress, Peng HY, Lai CC, Lin CC, Chou ST, *The Scientific World Journal*, 2014

Effects of Abies sibirica terpenes on cancer- and aging-associated pathways in human cells. Kudryavtseva A, Krasnov G, Lipatova A, Alekseev B, Maganova F, Shaposhnikov M, Fedorova M, Snezhkina A, Moskalev A. Oncotarget. 2016 Medicinal plants as antiemetics in the treatment of cancer: a review, Haniadka R, Popouri S, Palatty PL, Arora R, Baliga MS, *Integrative Cancer Therapies*, 2012

In vitro effect of Knotolan, a new lignan from Abies sibirica, on the growth of hormone-dependent breast cancer cells. Zhukova OS, Fetisova LV, Trishin AV, Anisimova NY, Scherbakov AM, Yashunskii DV, Tsvetkov DE, Men'shov VM, Kiselevskii MV, Nifant'ev NE. Bull Exp Biol Med. 2010 Oct;149(4):511-4. English, Russian. Erratum in: Bull Exp Biol Med. 2011

Protective effects of lemongrass (Cymbopogon citratus STAPF) essential oil on DNA damage and carcinogenesis in female Balb/C mice, Bidinotto LT, Costa CA, Salvadori DM, Costa M, Rodrigues MA, Barbisan LF, *Journal of Applied Toxicology*, 2011

Sesquiterpenoids from myrrh inhibit androgen receptor expression and function in human prostate cancer cells, Wang XL, Kong F, Shen T, Young CY, Lou HX, Yuan HQ, *Acta Pharmacologica Sinica*, 2011

Skin cancer chemopreventive agent, {alpha}-santalol, induces apoptotic death of human epidermoid carcinoma A431 cells via caspase activation together with dissipation of mitochondrial membrane potential and cytochrome c release, Kaur M, Agarwal C, Singh RP, Guan X, Dwivedi C, Agarwal R, *Carcinogenesis*, 2005

Strawberry-Tree Honey Induces Growth Inhibition of Human Colon Cancer Cells and Increases ROS Generation: A Comparison with Manuka Honey. Afrin S, Forbes-Hernandez TY, Gasparrini M, Bompadre S, Quiles JL, Sanna G, Spano N, Giampieri F, Battino M. Int J Mol Sci. 2017

Terpinen-4-ol, the main component of Melaleuca alternifolia (tea tree) oil inhibits the in vitro growth of human melanoma cells, Calcabrini A, Stringaro A, Toccacieli L, Meschini S, Marra M, Colone M, Salvatore G, Mondello F, Arancia G, Molinari A, *Journal of Investigative Dermatology*, 2004

Topically applied Melaleuca alternifolia (tea tree) oil causes direct anti-cancer cytotoxicity in subcutaneous tumour bearing mice, Ireland DJ, Greay SJ, Hooper CM, Kissick HT, Filion P, Riley TV, Beilharz MW, *Journal of Dermatological Science*, 2012

α-Santalol, a derivative of sandalwood oil, induces apoptosis in human prostate cancer cells by causing caspase-3 activation, Bommareddy A, Rule B, VanWert AL, Santha S, Dwivedi C, *Phytomedicine*, 2012

CELLULAR REPAIR AND CELLULAR HEALTH

Carvacrol and rosemary essential oil manifest cytotoxic, DNA-protective and pro-apoptotic effect having no effect on DNA repair, Melusova M, Slamenova D, Kozics K, Jantova S, Horvathova E, *Neoplasma*, 2014

Effectiveness of aromatherapy with light thai massage for cellular immunity improvement in colorectal cancer patients receiving chemotherapy, Khiewkhern S, Promthet S, Sukprasert A, Eunhpinitpong W, Bradshaw P, *Asian Pacific Journal of Cancer Prevention*, 2013

Protective effect of basil (Ocimum basilicum L.) against oxidative DNA damage and mutagenesis, Berić T, Nikolić B, Stanojević J, Vuković-Gačić B, Knezević-Vukcević J, *Food and Chemical Toxicology*, 2008

CHEMICAL COMPOSITION AND PROPERTIES

Anethum graveolens: An Indian traditional medicinal herb and spice, Jana S, Shekhawat GS, Pharmacognosy Review, 2010

Antioxidant activities and volatile constituents of various essential oils, Wei A, Shibamoto T, *Journal of Agriculture and Food Chemistry*, 2007

Application of near-infrared spectroscopy in quality control and determination of adulteration of African essential oils, Juliani HR, Kapteyn J, Jones D, Koroch AR, Wang M, Charles D, Simon JE., Phytochem Anal. 2006 Mar-Apr

Botanical perspectives on health peppermint: more than just an after-dinner mint, Spirling LI, Daniels IR, *Journal for the Royal Society for the Promotion of Health*, 2001

Chamomile: A herbal medicine of the past with bright future, Srivastava JK, Shankar E, Gupta S, *Molecular Medicine Reports*, 2010

Chemical composition and antibacterial activity of selected essential oils and some of their main compounds, Wanner J, Schmidt E, Bail S, Jirovetz L, Buchbauer G, Gochev V, Girova T, Atanasova T, Stoyanova A, *Natural Product Communications*, 2010

Chemical composition and biological activity of the essential oil from Helichrysum microphyllum Cambess. ssp. tyrrhenicum Bacch., Brullo e Giusso growing in La Maddalena Archipelago, Sardinia., Ornano L, Venditti A, Sanna C, Ballero M, Maggi F, Lupidi G, Bramucci M, Quassinti L, Bianco A, *Journal of Oleo Science*, 2014

Chemical composition of the essential oils of variegated pink-fleshed lemon (Citrus x limon L. Burm. f.) and their anti-inflammatory and antimicrobial activities, Hamdan D, Ashour ML, Mulyaningsih S, El-Shazly A, Wink M, *Zeitschrift Fur Naturforschung C- A Journal of Biosciences*, 2013

Constituents of south Indian vetiver oils, Mallavarapu GR, Syamasundar KV, Ramesh S, Rao BR, *Natural Product Communications*, 2012

Determination of the absolute configuration of 6-alkylated alpha-pyrones from Ravensara crassifolia by LC-NMR., Queiroz EF, Wolfender JL, Raoelison G, Hostettmann K, *Phytochem Anal*. 2003

Evaluation of the chemical constituents and the antimicrobial activity of the volatile oil of Citrus reticulata fruit (Tangerine fruit peel) from South West Nigeria, Ayoola GA, Johnson OO, Adelowotan T, Aibinu IE, Adenipekun E, Adepoju AA, Coker HAB, Odugbemi TO, *African Journal of Biotechnology*, 2008

The Essential Oil of Bergamot Stimulates Reactive Oxygen Species Production in Human Polymorphonuclear Leukocytes, Cosentino M, Luini A, Bombelli R, Corasaniti MT, Bagetta G, Marino F, *Phytotherapy Research*, 2014

The essential oil of ginger, Zingiber officinale, and anaesthesia, Geiger JL, *International Journal of Aromatherapy*, 2005

Two 6-substituted 5,6-dihydro-alpha-pyrones from Ravensara anisata., Andrianaivoravelona JO, Sahpaz S, Terreaux C, Hostettmann K, Stoeckli-Evans H, Rasolondramanitra J, *Phytochemistry*. 1999

Volatile composition and biological activity of key lime Citrus aurantifolia essential oil, Spadaro F, Costa R, Circosta C, Occhiuto F, *Natural Product Communications*, 2012

Volatiles from steam-distilled leaves of some plant species from Madagascar and New Zealand and evaluation of their biological activity, Costa R, Pizzimenti F, Marotta F, Dugo P, Santi L, Mondello L, *Nat Prod Commun*, 2010

CHOLESTEROL

Hypolipidemic activity of Anethum graveolens in rats, Hajhashemi V, Abbasi N, *Phytotherapy Research*, 2008

Protective effect of lemongrass oil against dexamethasone induced hyperlipidemia in rats: possible role of decreased lecithin cholesterol acetyl transferase activity, Kumar VR, Inamdar MN, Nayeemunnisa, Viswanatha GL, *Asian Pacific Journal of Tropical Medicine*, 2011

Protective role of arzanol against lipid peroxidation in biological systems, Rosa A, Pollastro F, Atzeri A, Appendino G, Melis MP, Deiana M, Incani A, Loru D, Dessì MA, Chemical and Physics of Lipids, 2011

DECONGESTANT

Effect of inhaled menthol on citric acid induced cough in normal subjects, Morice AH, Marshall AE, Higgins KS, Grattan TJ, *Thorax*, 1994

Remedies for common family ailments: 10. Nasal decongestants, Sinclair A, *Professional Care of Mother and Child*, 1996

DEMENTIA

Aromatherapy as a safe and effective treatment for the management of agitation in severe dementia: the results of a double-blind, placebo-controlled trial with Melissa, Ballard CG, O'Brien JT, Reichelt K, Perry EK, *The Journal of Clinical Psychiatry*, 2002

DEPRESSION (INCLUDING POSTPARTUM)

Antidepressant-like effect of carvacrol (5-Isopropyl-2-methylphenol) in mice: involvement of dopaminergic system, Melo FH, Moura BA, de Sousa DP, de Vasconcelos SM, Macedo DS, Fonteles MM, Viana GS, de Sousa FC, *Fundamental and Clinical Pharmacology*, 2011

Antidepressant-like effect of Salvia sclarea is explained by modulation of dopamine activities in rats, Seol GH, Shim HS, Kim PJ, Moon HK, Lee KH, Shim I, Suh SH, Min SS, *Journal of Ethnopharmacology*, 2010

Effects of Aroma Hand Massage on Pain, State Anxiety and Depression in Hospice Patients with Terminal Cancer, Chang SY, *Journal of Korean Academy of Nursing*, 2008

Effects of lavender aromatherapy on insomnia and depression in women college students, Lee IS, Lee GJ, *Taehan Kanho Hakhoe Chi*, 2006

The effects of clinical aromatherapy for anxiety and depression in the high risk postpartum woman – a pilot study, Conrad P, Adams C, *Complimentary Therapy in Clinical Practice*, 2012

DIABETES

Ameliorative effect of the cinnamon oil from Cinnamomum zeylanicum upon early stage diabetic nephropathy, Mishra A, Bhatti R, Singh A, Singh Ishar MP, *Planta Medica*, 2010

Cinnamon bark extract improves glucose metabolism and lipid profile in the fructose-fed rat, Kannappan S, Jayaraman T, Rajasekar P, Ravichandran MK, Anuradha CV, *Singapore Medical Journal*, 2006

Comparative effects of Artemisia dracunculus, Satureja hortensis and Origanum majorana on inhibition of blood platelet adhesion, aggregation and secretion, Yazdanparast R, Shahriyary L, *Vascular Pharmacology*, 2008

Effects of a novel formulation of essential oils on glucose-insulin metabolism in diabetic and hypertensive rats: a pilot study, Talpur N, Echard B, Ingram C, Bagchi D, Preuss H, Diabetes, *Obesity and Metabolism*, 2005

From type 2 diabetes to antioxidant activity: a systematic review of the safety and efficacy of common and cassia cinnamon bark., Dugoua JJ, Seely D, Perri D, Cooley K, Forelli T, Mills E, Koren G, *Canadian Journal of Physiology and Pharmacology*, 2007

Hypoglycaemic effects of myrtle oil in normal and alloxan-diabetic rabbits, Sepici A, Gürbüz I, Cevik C, Yesilada E, *Journal of Ethnopharmacology*, 2004

Hypoglycemic and antioxidant effects of leaf essential oil of Pelargonium graveolens L'Hér. in alloxan induced diabetic rats, Boukhris M, Bouaziz M, Feki I, Jemai H, El Feki A, Sayadi S, *Lipids in Health and Disease*, 2012

Inhibitory potential of ginger extracts against enzymes linked to type 2 diabetes, inflammation and induced oxidative stress, Rani MP, Padmakumari KP, Sankarikutty B, Cherian OL, Nisha VM, Raghu KG, *International Journal of Food Sciences and Nutrition*, 2011

DIGESTION

Antigiardial activity of Ocimum basilicum essential oil, de Almeida I, Alviano DS, Vieira DP, Alves PB, Blank AF, Lopes AH, Alviano CS, Rosa Mdo S, *Parasitology Research*, 2007

Enteric-coated, pH-dependent peppermint oil capsules for the treatment of irritable bowel syn-

drome in children, Kline RM, Kline JJ, Di Palma J, Barbero GJ, *The Journal of Pediatrics*, 2001
Gastroprotective activity of essential oils from turmeric and ginger, Liju VB, Jeena K, Kuttan R, *Journal of Basic and Clinical Physiology and Pharmacology*, 2014
Gastroprotective effect of cardamom, Elettaria cardamomum Maton. fruits in rats., Jamal A, Javed K, Aslam M, Jafri MA, *Journal of Ethnopharmacology*, 2006
Olfactory stimulation using black pepper oil facilitates oral feeding in pediatric patients receiving long-term enteral nutrition, Munakata M, Kobayashi K, Niisato-Nezu J, Tanaka S, Kakisaka Y, Ebihara T, Ebihara S, Haginoya K, Tsuchiya S, Onuma A, *The Tohoku Journal of Experimental Medicine*, 2008
Peppermint oil for the treatment of irritable bowel syndrome: a systematic review and meta-analysis, Khanna R, MacDonald JK, Levesque BG, *Journal of Clinical Gastroenterology*, 2014
Randomized clinical trial of a phytotherapic compound containing Pimpinella anisum, Foeniculum vulgare, Sambucus nigra, and Cassia augustifolia for chronic constipation, Picon PD, Picon RV, Costa AF, Sander GB, Amaral KM, Aboy AL, Henriques AT, *BMC Complementary and Alternative Medicine*, 2010
Reversal of pyrogallol-induced delay in gastric emptying in rats by ginger (Zingiber officinale), Gupta YK, Sharma M, *Methods and Findings in Experimental and Clinical Pharmacology*, 2001
Systematic Review of Complementary and Alternative Medicine Treatments in Inflammatory Bowel Diseases, Langhorst J, Wulfert H, Lauche R, Klose P, Cramer H, Dobos GJ,Korzenik,J, *Journal of Crohn's & Colitis*, 2015
The cinnamon-derived dietary factor cinnamic aldehyde activates the Nrf2-dependent antioxidant response in human epithelial colon cells, Wondrak GT, Villeneuve NF, Lamore SD, Bause AS, Jiang T, Zhang DD, *Molecules*, 2010
Treatment of irritable bowel syndrome with herbal preparations: results of a double-blind, randomized, placebo-controlled, multi-centre trial, Madisch A, Holtmann G, Plein K, Hotz J, *Alimentary pharmacology and & therapeutics*, 2004

FIBROMYALGIA
Cutaneous application of menthol 10% solution as an abortive treatment of migraine without aura: a randomised, double-blind, placebo-controlled, crossed-over study, Borhani Haghighi A, Motazedian S, Rezaii R, Mohammadi F, Salarian L, Pourmokhtari M, Khodaei S, Vossoughi M, Miri R, *The International Journal of Clinical Practice*, 2010
Lavender essential oil in the treatment of migraine headache: a placebo-controlled clinical trial, Sasannejad P, Saeedi M, Shoeibi A, Gorji A, Abbasi M, Foroughipour M, *European Neurology*, 2012

HERPES
Inhibitory effect of essential oils against herpes simplex virus type 2, Koch C, Reichling J, Schneele J, Schnitzler P, *Phytomedicine*, 2008
Susceptibility of drug-resistant clinical herpes simplex virus type 1 strains to essential oils of ginger, thyme, hyssop, and sandalwood, Schnitzler P, Koch C, Reichling J, *Antimicrobial Agents and Chemotherapy*, 2007

IMMUNE SYSTEM
Chemistry and immunomodulatory activity of frankincense oil, Mikhaeil BR, Maatooq GT, Badria FA, Amer MM, *Zeitschrift fur Naturforschung C*, 2003

INFLAMMATION AND PAIN
Anti-Inflammatory and Antioxidant Actions of Copaiba Oil Are Related to Liver Cell Modifications in Arthritic Rats. Castro Ghizoni CV, Arssufi Ames AP, Lameira OA, Bersani Amado CA, Sá Nakanishi AB, Bracht L, Marçal Natali MR, Peralta RM, Bracht A, Comar JF. J Cell Biochem. 2017
Anti-inflammatory constituents from the root of Litsea cubeba in LPS-induced RAW 264.7 macrophages. Lin B, Sun LN, Xin HL, Nian H, Song HT, Jiang YP, Wei ZQ, Qin LP, Han T. Pharm Biol. 2016
Anti-Inflammatory Effects of Boldine and Reticuline Isolated from Litsea cubeba through JAK2/STAT3 and NF-kB Signaling Pathways. Yang X, Gao X, Cao Y, Guo Q, Li S, Zhu Z, Zhao Y, Tu P, Chai X. Planta Med. 2017
A review on anti-inflammatory activity of monoterpenes, de Cássia da Silveira e Sá R, Andrade LN, de Sousa DP, *Molecules*, 2013
An experimental study on the effectiveness of massage with aromatic ginger and orange essential oil for moderate-to-severe knee pain among the elderly in Hong Kong, Yip YB, Tam AC, *Complementary Therapies in Medicine*, 2008
Anti-inflammatory activity of patchouli alcohol in RAW264.7 and HT-29 cells, Jeong JB, Shin YK, Lee SH, *Food and Chemical Toxicology*, 2013
Anti-inflammatory and analgesic activity of different extracts of Commiphora myrrha, Su S, Wang T, Duan JA, Zhou W, Hua YQ, Tang YP, Yu L, Qian DW, *Journal of Ethnopharmacology*, 2011
Anti-inflammatory and anti-ulcer activities of carvacrol, a monoterpene present in the essential oil of oregano, Silva FV, Guimarães AG, Silva ER, Sousa-Neto BP, Machado FD, Quintans-Júnior LJ, Arcanjo DD, Oliveira FA, Oliveira RC, *Journal of Medicinal Food*, 2012
Anti-inflammatory and antioxidant properties of Helichrysum italicum, Sala A, Recio M, Giner RM, Máñez S, Tournier H, Schinella G, Ríos JL, *The Journal of Pharmacy and Pharmacology*, 200
Anti-inflammatory effects of Melaleuca alternifolia essential oil on human polymorphonuclear neutrophils and monocytes, Caldefie-Chézet F, Guerry M, Chalchat JC, Fusillier C, Vasson MP, Guillot J, *Free Radical Research*, 2004
Antihypernociceptive activity of anethole in experimental inflammatory pain, Ritter AM, Domiciano TP, Verri WA Jr, Zarpelon AC, da Silva LG, Barbosa CP, Natali MR, Cuman RK, Bersani-Amado CA, *Inflammopharmacology*, 2013
Antiinflammatory effects of essential oil from the leaves of Cinnamomum cassia and cinnamaldehyde on lipopolysaccharide-stimulated J774A.1 cells., Pannee C, Chandhanee I, Wacharee L, *Journal of Advanced Pharmaceutical Technology & Research*, 2014
Antiinflammatory effects of ginger and some of its components in human bronchial epithelial (BEAS-2B) cells, Podlogar JA, Verspohl EJ, *Phytotherapy Research*, 2012
Antioxidant components of naturally-occurring oils exhibit marked anti-inflammatory activity in epithelial cells of the human upper respiratory system, Gao M, Singh A, Macri K, Reynolds C, Singhal V, Biswal S, Spannhake EW, *Respiratory Research*, 2011
Antioxidant, anti-inflammatory and antinociceptive activities of essential oil from ginger, Jeena K, Liju VB, Kuttan R, *Indian Journal of Physiology and Pharmacology*, 2013
Arzanol, a prenylated heterodimeric phloroglucinyl pyrone, inhibits eicosanoid biosynthesis and exhibits anti-inflammatory efficacy in vivo, Bauer J, Koeberle A, Dehm F, Pollastro F, Appendino G, Northoff H, Rossi A, Sautebin L, Werz O, *Biochemical Pharmacology*, 2011
Arzanol, an anti-inflammatory and anti-HIV-1 phloroglucinol alpha-Pyrone from Helichrysum italicum ssp. microphyllum, Appendino G, Ottino M, Marquez N, Bianchi F, Giana A, Ballero M, Sterner O, Fiebich BL, Munoz E, *Journal of Natural Products*, 2007
Assessment of the anti-inflammatory activity and free radical scavenger activity of tiliroside., Sala A, Recio MC, Schinella GR, Máñez S, Giner RM, Cerdá-Nicolás M, Rosí JL, *European Journal of Pharmacology*, 2003
Boswellia frereana (frankincense) suppresses cytokine-induced matrix metalloproteinase expression and production of pro-inflammatory molecules in articular cartilage., Blain EJ, Ali AY, Duance VC, *Phytotherapy Research*, 2012
Chamazulene carboxylic acid and matricin: a natural profen and its natural prodrug, identified through similarity to synthetic drug substances, Ramadan M, Goeters S, Watzer B, Krause E, Lohmann K, Bauer R, Hempel B, Imming P, Journal of Natural Products, 2006
Ginger: An herbal medicinal product with broad anti-inflammatory actions, Grzanna R, Lindmark L, Frondoza CG, *Journal of Medicinal Food*, 2005
Identification of proapoptopic, anti-inflammatory, anti-proliferative, anti-invasive and anti-angiogenic targets of
essential oils in cardamom by dual reverse virtual screening and binding pose analysis, Bhattacharjee B, Chatterjee J, *Asian Pacific Journal of Cancer Prevention*, 2013
In vitro cytotoxic and anti-inflammatory effects of myrrh oil on human gingival fibroblasts and epithelial cells, Tipton DA, Lyle B, Babich H, Dabbous MKh, *Toxicology in Vitro*, 2003
In Vivo Potential Anti-Inflammatory Activity of Melissa officinalis L. Essential Oil, Bounihi A, Hajjaj G, Alnamer R, Cherrah Y, Zellou A, *Advances in Pharmacalogical Sciences*, 2013
Inhibitory effect of anethole in nonimmune acute inflammation, Domiciano TP, Dalalio MM, Silva EL, Ritter AM, Estevão-Silva CF, Ramos FS, Caparroz-Assef SM, Cuman RK, Bersani-Amado CA, *Naunyn-Schmiedeberg's Archives of Pharmacology*, 2013
Lavender essential oil inhalation suppresses allergic airway inflammation and mucous cell hyperplasia in a murine model of asthma, Ueno-Iio T, Shibakura M, Yokota K, Aoe M, Hyoda T, Shinohata R, Kanehiro A, Tanimoto M, Kataoka M, *Life Sciences*, 2014
Parthenolide inhibits proliferation of fibroblast-like synoviocytes in vitro. Parada-Turska J. Mitura A, Brzana W, Jalonkski M, Majdan M, Rzeski W. Inflammation. 2008
Results suggest that neroli possesses biologically active constituent(s) that have significant activity against acute and especially chronic inflammation, and have central and peripheral antinociceptive effects which support the ethnomedicinal claims of the use of the plant in the management of pain and inflammation. Asgarpanah, J, P Khadobakhsh, and H Shafaroodi. "Analgesic and anti-inflammatory activities of Citrus aurantium L. blossoms essential oil (neroli): involvement of the nitric oxide/cyclic-guanosine monophostphate pathway." Journal of Natural Medicines, 2015
Rose geranium essential oil as a source of new and safe anti-inflammatory drugs, Boukhatem MN, Kameli A, Ferhat MA, Saidi F, Mekarnia M, *The Libyan Journal of Medicine*, 2013
Supercritical fluid extraction of oregano (Origanum vulgare) essentials oils: anti-inflammatory properties based on cytokine response on THP-1 macrophages, Ocaña-Fuentes A, Arranz-Gutiérrez E, Señorans FJ, Reglero G, *Food and Chemical Toxicology*, 2010

INSECT REPELLENT
Bioactivity-guided investigation of geranium essential oils as natural tick repellents, Tabanca N, Wang M, Avonto C, Chittiboyina AG, Parcher JF, Carroll JF, Kramer M, Khan IA, *Journal of Agricultural and Food Chemistry*, 2013
Essential oils and their compositions as spatial repellents for pestiferous social wasps., Zhang QH, Schnidmiller RG, *Hoover DR, Pest Management Science*, 2013
Field evaluation of essential oils for reducing attraction by the Japanese beetle (Coleoptera: Scarabaeidae), Youssef NN, Oliver JB, Ranger CM, Reding ME, Moyseenko JJ, Klein MG, Pappas RS, *Journal of Economic Entomology*, 2009
Fumigant toxicity of plant essential oils against Camptomyia corticalis (Diptera: Cecidomyiidae), Kim JR, Haribalan P, Son BK, Ahn YJ, *Journal of Economic Entomology*, 2012
Insecticidal properties of volatile extracts of orange peels, Ezeonu FC, Chidume GI, Udedi SC, *Bioresource Technology*, 2001
Repellency of Essential Oils to Mosquitoes (Diptera: Culicidae), Barnard DR, Journal of Medical Entomology, 1999
Repellency to Stomoxys calcitrans (Diptera: Muscidae) of Plant Essential Oils Alone or in Combination with Calophyllum inophyllum Nut Oil, Hieu TT, Kim SI, Lee SG, Ahn YJ, *Journal of Medical Etomology*, 2010
Repelling properties of some plant materials on the tick Ixodes ricinus L, Thorsell W, Mikiver A, Tunón H, *Phytomedicine*, 2006

MENOPAUSE
Aromatherapy Massage Affects Menopausal Symptoms in Korean Climacteric Women: A Pilot-Controlled Clinical Trial, Myung-HH, Yun Seok Y, Myeong SL, *Evidence-based Complementary and Alternative Medicine*, 2008
Changes in 5-hydroxytryptamine and Cortisol Plasma Levels in Menopausal Women After Inhalation of Clary Sage Oil, Lee KB, Cho E, Kang YS, *Phytotherapy Research*, 2014
Effect of aromatherapy massage on abdominal fat and body image in post-menopausal women, Kim HJ, *Taehan Kanho Hakhoe Chi*, 2007
Inhalation of neroli oil by postmenopausal women improved their quality of life related to menopausal symptoms, increased sexual desire, and reduced blood pressure. In addition, inhalation of neroli oil may reduce stress levels and stimulate the endocrine system. Choi, Seo Yeon et al. "Effects of Inhalation of Essential Oil of Citrus AurantiumL. Var. amara on Menopausal Symptoms, Stress, and Estrogen in Postmenopausal Women: A Randomized Controlled Trial." Evidence-based Complementary and Alternative Medicine, 2014

MENSTRUAL
Effect of aromatherapy on symptoms of dysmenorrhea in college students: A randomized placebo-controlled clinical trial, Han SH, Hur MH, Buckle J, Choi J, Lee MS, *The Journal of Alternative and Complementary Medicine*, 2006
Pain relief assessment by aromatic essential oil massage on outpatients with primary dysmenorrhea: a randomized, double-blind clinical trial, Ou MC, Hsu TF, Lai AC, Lin YT, Lin CC, *The Journal of Obstetrics and Gynecology Research*, 2012

MIGRAINE
Cutaneous application of menthol 10% solution as an abortive treatment of migraine without aura: a randomised, double-blind, placebo-controlled, crossed-over study, Borhani Haghighi A, Motazedian S, Rezaii R, Mohammadi F, Salarian L, Pourmokhtari M, Khodaei S, Vossoughi M, Miri R, *The International Journal of Clinical Practice*, 2010
Lavender essential oil in the treatment of migraine headache: a placebo-controlled clinical trial, Sa-

sannejad P, Saeedi M, Shoeibi A, Gorji A, Abbasi M, Foroughipour M, *European Neurology*, 2012

MOOD

Effects of fragrance inhalation on sympathetic activity in normal adults, Haze S, Sakai K, Gozu Y, *The Japanese Journal of Pharmacology*, 2002

Evaluation of the harmonizing effect of ylang-ylang oil on humans after inhalation, Hongratanaworakit T, Buchbauer G, *Planta Medica*, 2004

Relaxing effect of rose oil on humans, Hongratanaworakit T, *Natural Product Communications*, 2009

Relaxing Effect of Ylang ylang Oil on Humans after Transdermal Absorption, Hongratanaworakit T, Buchbauer G, *Phytotherapy research*, 2006

NAUSEA

A brief review of current scientific evidence involving aromatherapy use for nausea and vomiting, Lua PL, Zakaria NS, *The Journal of Alternative and Complementary Medicine*, 2012

Aromatherapy as a Treatment for Postoperative Nausea: A randomized Trial, Hunt R, Dienemann J, Norton HJ, Hartley W, Hudgens A, Stern T, *Divine G, Anesthesia and Analgesia*, 2013

Controlled breathing with or without peppermint aromatherapy for postoperative nausea and/or vomiting symptom relief: a randomized controlled trial, Sites DS, Johnson NT, Miller JA, Torbush PH, Hardin JS, Knowles SS, Nance J, Fox TH, Tart RC, *Journal of PeriAnesthesia Nursing*, 2014

The effect of lemon inhalation aromatherapy on nausea and vomiting of pregnancy: a double-blinded, randomized, controlled clinical trial, Yavari Kia P, Safajou F, Shahnazi M, Nazemiyeh H, *Iranian Red Crescent Medical Journal*, 2014

The palliation of nausea in hospice and palliative care patients with essential oils of Pimpinella anisum (aniseed), Foeniculum vulgare var. dulce (sweet fennel), Anthemis nobilis (Roman chamomile) and Mentha x piperita (peppermint), Gilligan NP, *International Journal of Aromatherapy*, 2005

ORAL HEALTH

Efficacy of grapefruit, tangerine, lime, and lemon oils as solvents for softening gutta-percha in root canal retreatment procedures, Jantarat J, Malhotra W, Sutimuntanakul S, *Journal of Investigative and Clinical Dentistry*, 2013

Essential oil of Melaleuca alternifolia for the treatment of oral candidiasis induced in an immunosuppressed mouse model, de Campos Rasteiro VM, da Costa AC, Araújo CF, de Barros PP, Rossoni RD, Anbinder AL, Jorge AO, Junqueira JC, *BMC Complementary and Alternative Medicine*, 2014

General Toxicity and Antifungal Activity of a New Dental Gel with Essential Oil from Abies SibiricaL. Noreikaitė A, Ayupova R, Satbayeva E, Seitaliyeva A, Amirkulova M, Pichkhadze G, Datkhayev U, Stankevičius E. Med Sci Monit. 2017

Plants and other natural products used in the management of oral infections and improvement of oral health. Chinsembu KC. Acta Trop. 2016

Susceptibility to Melaleuca alternifolia (tea tree) oil of yeasts isolated from the mouths of patients with advanced cancer, Bagg J, Jackson MS, Petrina Sweeney M, Ramage G, Davies AN, *Oral Oncology*, 2006

Synergistic effect between clove oil and its major compounds and antibiotics against oral bacteria, Moon SE, Kim HY, Cha JD, *Archives of Oral Biology*, 2011

Topical lavender oil for the treatment of recurrent aphthous ulceration, Altaei DT, *American Journal of Dentistry*, 2012

PHYSICAL AGILITY

Effects of lavender (lavandula angustifolia Mill.) and peppermint (Mentha cordifolia Opiz.) aromas on subjective vitality, speed, and agility, Cruz AB, Lee SE, Pagaduan JC, Kim TH, *The Asian International Journal of Life Sciences*, 2012

The effects of peppermint on exercise performance, Meamarbashi A, Rajabi A, *Journal of International Society of Sports Nutrition*, 2013

PREGNANCY

Aromatherapy with C. aurantium blossom oil is a simple, inexpensive, noninvasive, and effective intervention to reduce anxiety during labor. Namazi, Masoumeh et al. "Aromatherapy With Citrus Aurantium Oil and Anxiety During the First Stage of Labor." Iranian Red Crescent Medical Journal , 2014

Clinical trial of aromatherapy on postpartum mother's perineal healing, Hur MH, Han SH, *Journal of Korean Academy of Nursing*, 2004

REPRODUCTIVE SYSTEM

Development and pharmacological evaluation of in vitro nanocarriers composed of lamellar silicates containing copaiba oil-resin for treatment of endometriosis. de Almeida Borges VR, da Silva JH, Barbosa SS, Nasciutti LE, Cabral LM, de Sousa VP. Mater Sci Eng C Mater Biol Appl. 2016

Effect of different terpene-containing essential oils on permeation of estradiol through hairless mouse skin, Monti D, Chetoni P, Burgalassi S, Najarro M, Saettone MF, Boldrini E, *International Journal of Pharmaceutics*, 2002

Effect of olfactory stimulation with flavor of grapefruit oil and lemon oil on the activity of sympathetic branch in the white adipose tissue of the epididymis, Niijima A, Nagai K, *Experimental Biology and Medicine*, 2003

The Effects of Herbal Essential Oils on the Oviposition-deterrent and Ovicidal Activities of Aedes aegypti (Linn.), Anopheles dirus (Peyton and Harrison) and Culex quinquefasciatus (Say), Siriporn P, Mayura S, *Tropical Biomedicine*, 2012

SEIZURES

Anticonvulsant and neuroprotective effects of Pimpinella anisum in rat brain, Fariba K, Mahmoud H, Diana M, Hassan A, Gholam RH, Mohamad B, Maryam J, Hadi K, Ali G, *BMC Complementary and Alternative Medicine*, 2012

Increased seizure latency and decreased severity of pentylenetetrazol-induced seizures in mice after essential oil administration, Koutroumanidou E, Kimbaris A, Kortsaris A, Bezirtzoglou E, Polissiou M, Charalabopoulos K, Pagonopoulou O, *Epilepsy Research and Treatment*, 2013

The results suggest that neroli possesses biologically active constituent(s) that have anticonvulsant activity which supports the ethnomedicinal claims of the use of the plant in the management of seizure. Azanchi, T, H Shafaroodi, and J Asgarpanah. "Anticonvulsant activity of Citrus aurantium blossom essential oil (neroli): involvement of the GABAergic system." Natural Products Communication, 2014.

SKIN

A comparative study of tea-tree oil versus benzoylperoxide in the treatment of acne, Bassett IB, Pannowitz DL, Barnetson RS, *Medical Journal of Australia*, 1990

Activities of Ten Essential Oils towards Propionibacterium acnes and PC-3, A-549 and MCF-7 Cancer Cells, Zu Y, Yu H, Liang L, Fu Y, Efferth T, Liu X, Wu N, *Molecules*, 2010

Cinnamomum cassia essential oil inhibits α-MSH-induced melanin production and oxidative stress in murine B16 melanoma cells, Chou ST, Chang WL, Chang CT, Hsu SL, Lin YC, Shih Y, *International Journal of Molecular Sciences*, 2013

Cooling the burn wound: evaluation of different modalites., Jandera V, Hudson DA, de Wet PM, Innes PM, Rode H, Burns: *Journal of the International Society for Burn Injuries*, 2000

Coriandrum sativum L. protects human keratinocytes from oxidative stress by regulating oxidative defense systems, Park G, Kim HG, Kim YO, Park SH, Kim SY, Oh MS, *Skin Pharmacology and Physiology*, 2012

Effects of Abies sibirica terpenes on cancer- and aging-associated pathways in human cells. Kudryavtseva A, Krasnov G, Lipatova A, Alekseev B, Maganova F, Shaposhnikov M, Fedorova M, Snezhkina A, Moskalev A. Oncotarget. 2016

Essential oil of Australian lemon myrtle (Backhousia citriodora) in the treatment of molluscum contagiosum in children, Burke BE, Baillie JE, Olson RD, *Biomedicine & Pharmacotherapy*, 2004

Randomized trial of aromatherapy: successful treatment for alopecia areata, Hay IC, Jamieson M, Ormerod AD,, *Archives of Dermatology*, 1998

Tea tree oil as a novel anti-psoriasis weapon, Pazyar N, Yaghoobi R, *Skin Pharmacology and Physiology*, 2012

Tea tree oil reduces histamine-induced skin inflammation, Koh KJ, Pearce AL, Marshman G, Finlay-Jones JJ, Hart PH, *British Journal of Dermatology*, 2002

The effect of clove and benzocaine versus placebo as topical anesthetics, Alqareer A, Alyahya A, Andersson L, *Journal of Dentistry*, 2006

Two US practitioners' experience of using essential oils for wound care, Hartman D, Coetzee JC, *Journal of Wound Care*, 2002

SLEEP

An olfactory stimulus modifies nighttime sleep in young men and women, Goel N, Kim H, Lao RP, *Chronobiology International*, 2005

Neroli oil (citrus aurantium) to have pharmacological effects on fatigue and insomnia, Essential oils used in aromatherapy, Babar Ali, Naser Ali Al-Wabel, Saiba Shams, Aftab Ahamand, Shah Alam Khan, Firoz Anwar, Asian Pacific Journal of Tropical Biomedicine, 2015.

Preliminary investigation of the effect of peppermint oil on an objective measure of daytime sleepiness, Norrish MI, Dwyer KL, *International Journal of Psychophysiology: Official Journal of the International Organization of Psychophysiology*, 2005

Sedative effects of the jasmine tea odor and (R)-(-)-linalool, one of its major odor components, on autonomic nerve activity and mood states, Kuroda K, Inoue N, Ito Y, Kubota K, Sugimoto A, Kakuda T, Fushiki T, *European Journal of Applied Physiology*, 2005

Stimulating effect of aromatherapy massage with jasmine oil, Hongratanaworakit T, *Natural Product Communications*, 2010

Stimulative and sedative effects of essential oils upon inhalation in mice, Lim WC, Seo JM, Lee CI, Pyo HB, Lee BC, *Archives of Pharmacal Research*, 2005

STRESS

Effect of "rose essential oil" inhalation on stress-induced skin-barrier disruption in rats and humans, Fukada M, Kano E, Miyoshi M, Komaki R, Watanabe T, *Chemical Senses*, 2012

Effect of flavour components in lemon essential oil on physical or psychological stress, Fukumoto S, Morishita A, Furutachi K, Terashima T, Nakayama T, Yokogoshi H, *Stress and Health*, 2008

The physical effects of aromatherapy in alleviating work-related stress on elementary school teachers in taiwan, Liu SH, Lin TH, Chang KM, *Evidence-Based Complementary and Alternative Medicine*, 2013

STROKE

Effect of lavender oil (Lavandula angustifolia) on cerebral edema and its possible mechanisms in an experimental model of stroke,Vakili A, Sharifat S, Akhavan MM, Bandegi AR, *Brain Research*, 2014

TUMORS

Chemopreventive effects of alpha-santalol on skin tumor development in CD-1 and SENCAR mice, Dwivedi C, Guan X, Harmsen WL, Voss AL, Goetz-Parten DE, Koopman EM, Johnson KM, Valluri HB, Matthees DP, Cancer Epidemiology, *Biomarkers and Prevention*, 2003

Frankincense oil derived from Boswellia carteri induces tumor cell specific cytotoxicity, Frank MB, Yang Q, Osban J, Azzarello JT, Saban MR, Saban R, Ashley RA, Welter JC, Fung KM, Lin HK, *BMC Complementary and Alternative Medicine*, 2009

Sandalwood oil prevent skin tumour development in CD1 mice, Dwivedi C, Zhang Y, *European Journal of Cancer Prevention*, 1999

WEIGHT LOSS AND WEIGHT MANAGEMENT

Effect of aromatherapy massage on abdominal fat and body image in post-menopausal women, Kim HJ, *Taehan Kanho Hakhoe Chi*, 2007

Effects of herbal essential oil mixture as a dietary supplement on egg production in quail, Çabuk M, Eratak S, Alçicek A, Bozkurt M, *The Scientific World Journal*, 2014

Essential oil from Citrus aurantifolia prevents ketotifen-induced weight-gain in mice, Asnaashari S, Delazar A, Habibi B, Vasfi R, Nahar L, Hamedeyazdan S, Sarker SD, *Phytotherapy Research*, 2010

Low level of Lemon Balm (Melissa officinalis) essential oils showed hypoglycemic effects by altering the expression of glucose metabolism genes in db/db mice, Mi Ja Chung, Sung-Yun Cho and Sung-Joon Lee, *The Journal of the Federation of American Societies for Experimental Biology*, 2008

Olfactory stimulation with scent of grapefruit oil affects autonomic nerves, lipolysis and appetite in rats, Shen J, Niijima A, Tanida M, Horii Y, Maeda K, Nagai K, *Neuroscience Letters*, 2005

Safety assessment of Ylang-Ylang (Cananga spp.) as a food ingredient., Burdock GA, Carabin IG, *Food and chemical toxicology*, 2008

The effects of inhalation of essential oils on the body weight, food efficiency rate and serum leptin of growing SD rats, Hur MH, Kim C, Kim CH, Ahn HC, Ahn HY, *Korean Society of Nursing Science*, 2006

The metabolic responses to aerial diffusion of essential oils, Wu Y, Zhang Y, Xie G, Zhao A, Pan X, Chen T, Hu Y, Liu Y, Cheng Y, Chi Y, Yao L, Jia W, *PLOS One*, 2012

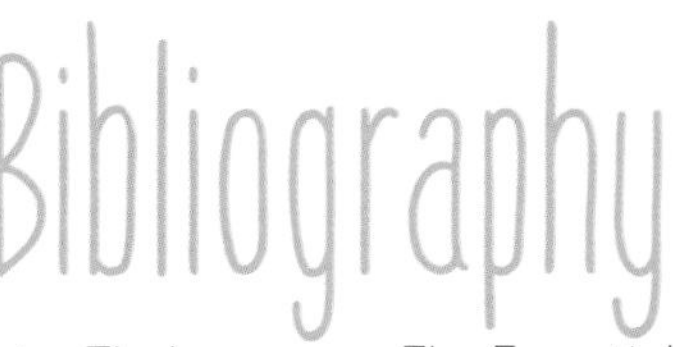

Bibliography

About Brain Tumors. Barrow Neurological Institute. Thebarrow.org, 2014.

The American Heritage Medical Dictionary. Boston: Houghton Mifflin Co., 2007.

The Aromatic Practitioners Reference. Australia: Maria Mitchell, 2011.

The Aromatherapy Encyclopedia: A Concise Guide to Over 385 Plant Oils. Basic Health Publications, Inc.: Schiller, C. and Schiller, D., 2008.

Aromatherapy Workbook. London: Price, Shirley, Thorsons, 2000.

The Art of Aromatherapy. Essex: The C W Daniel Company Ltd, Tisserand, Robert, 2009.

The Aromatherapy Encyclopedia. Laguna Beach, CA: Basic Health Publications Inc, Schiller, Carol & Schiller, David, 2008.

Aromatherapy for Health Professionals, 3rd ed. London: Churchhill Livingstone Elsevier, Price, Shirley & Price, Len, 2007.

Aromatherapy A-Z. London, England: Random House, Davis Patricia, 2005.

BabyMed.com, 2014.

Churchill Livingstone Dictionary of Sport and Exercise Science and Medicine. Philadelphia: Churchill Livingstone, 2008.

Clinical Aromatherapy Essential Oils in Healthcare, 3rd ed. St Louis, MO: Elsevier, Buckle, Jane 2015.

Collins English Dictionary. London: Collins, 2000.

The Columbia Electronic Encyclopedia. New York, NY: Columbia University Press, 2012.

The Complete Aromatherapy & Essential Oils Handbook for Everyday Wellness. Toronto: Robert Rose Inc, Purchon, Nerys & Cantele, Lora, 2014.

The Complete Guide to Aromatherapy, 2nd ed. Brisbane, QLD: The International Centre of Holistic Aromatherapy, Battaglia, Salvatore, 2003.

The Directory of Essential Oils. London: Vermillion, Sellar, Wanda, 2005.

Dorland's Medical Dictionary for Health Consumers. 2014

Emotions & Essential Oils 3rd Edition. American Fork, Utah: Enlighten Alternative Healing, 2014.

The Encyclopedia of Essential Oils. London: Thorsons, Lawless, Julia, 2002.

Essential Oil Safety, 2nd ed. London: Churchill Livingstone Elsevier, Tisserand, Robert & Young, Rodney, 2013.

Essential Oils Desk Reference, 5th ed. USA: Life Science Publishing, 2011.

The Essential Oils Handbook. London: Duncan Baird Publishers Ltd, Harding, Jennie, 2008.

Essential Oils Integrative Medical Guide. USA: Essential Science Publishing, Young, D Gary, 2006.

Essentials of the Earth, 2nd ed. Idaho USA: Essential Oils Books LLC, James, R L, 2013.

Farlex Partner Medical Dictionary. Huntingdon Valley, PA: Farlex Inc. 2014.

The Fragrant Pharmacy. Moorebank, NSW: Transworld Publishers Ltd, Wormwood, Valerie A, 1993.

Gale Encyclopedia of Medicine. Farmington Hills, MI: Gale, 1999.

The Healing Intelligence of Essential Oils. Rockester, Vermont: Healing Arts Press, Schnacbelt Kurt, 2011.

The Huffington Post; HuffingtonPost.com, 2014.

The Human Body. New York, New York: Dorling Kindersley Publishing, Inc., 2001.

Illustrated Dictionary of Podiatry and Foot Science. New York: Churchill Livingstone, 2009.

MayoClinic.org, 2014 & 2015.

McGraw-Hill Concise Dictionary of Modern Medicine. New York: McGraw-Hill, 2006.

McGraw-Hill Dictionary of Scientific & Technical Terms 6th ed., New York: McGraw-Hill, 2003.

Mind Over Medicine. Hay House, Inc.: Rankin Lissa, 2014.

Molecules of Emotion. Simon & Schuster, Pert Candance B. Ph.D., 1999.

The Mood Cure. London, England: Penguin Books, Ross Julia MA, 2003.

Mosby's Dental Dictionary, 2nd ed. C.V. Mosby Co, 2008

Mosby's Dictionary of Complementary and Alternative Medicine. St. Louis, MO: Elsevier Mosby, 2005.

Mosby's Medical Dictionary 9th ed., Philadelphia: Elsevier, 2013.

Miller-Keane Encyclopedia and Dictionary of Medicine, Nursing, and Allied Health, 7th ed. Philadelphia: Saunders, 2003.

Patient.co.uk, 2014.

Random House Kernerman Webster's College Dictionary. New York: Random House, 1997.

Saunders Comprehensive Veterinary Dictionary. Edinburgh [Scotland]: Saunders Elsevier, 2012.

Segen's Medical Dictionary. New York: McGraw-Hill, 2006.

Stedman's Medical Dictionary for the Health Professions and Nursing. Philadelphia: Lippincott Williams & Wilkins, 2005.

WebMD.com, 2014.

Index

SUPPLEMENTAL

SUPPLEMENTAL

SUPPLEMENTAL

SUPPLEMENTAL

GET AMAZING RESULTS

Anytime, Anywhere

ESSENTIAL LIFE BOOK 6.0

Comprehensive Reference Guide

The most-trusted essential oil resource! With recommendations for 600+ ailments, expansive explorations of every body system and related symptoms and conditions, and answers to top health priorities, there is no better way to become your own essential oil expert.

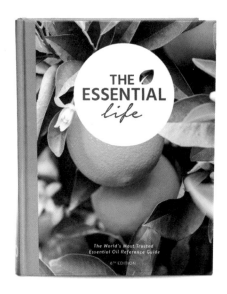

THE ESSENTIAL BASICS

On-the-Go Guide

Access essential oil solutions when out and about! This travel size guide pairs A-Z ailment solutions with much of the core information provided in the comprehensive guide and fits easily into your purse or car.

THE ESSENTIAL QUICK REFERENCE

Share the Love

This A-Z reference is the perfect way to introduce essential oil safety, storage, and quality to the new user and beyond. Include a copy with every essential oil sample you share!

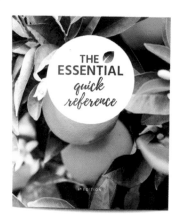